Comprehensive Textbook of Medical Physiology

Comprehensive Textbook of Medical Physiology

Vol 1

Author

Gopal Krushna Pal MBBS BNYT MD PhD DSc MD (AM) MD (Yoga) MABMS FABMS FABAP FSAB
Dean, JIPMER, Karaikal (Puducherry)
Professor of Physiology
Program Director, Advance Center for Yoga and Nodal Officer to Ministry of Health and FW
Jawaharlal Institute of Postgraduate Medical Education and Research (JIPMER)
Puducherry, India

Co-Authors

Pravati Pal MBBS MD MABMS
Professor
Department of Physiology
Jawaharlal Institute of Postgraduate Medical Education and Research (JIPMER)
Puducherry, India

Nivedita Nanda MSc PhD (Medical Biochemistry)
Assistant Professor
Department of Biochemistry
Jawaharlal Institute of Postgraduate Medical Education and Research (JIPMER)
Puducherry, India

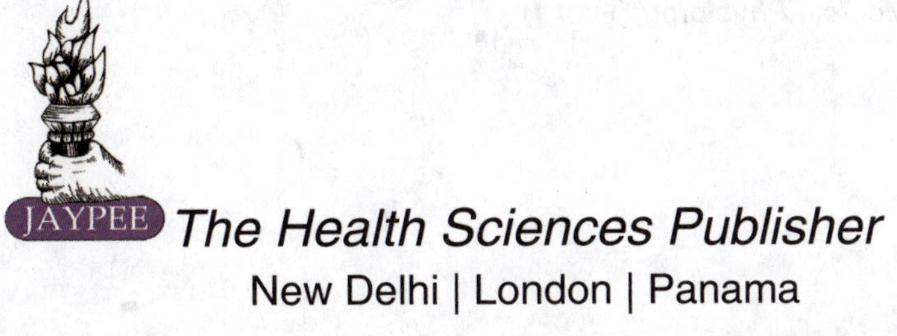

The Health Sciences Publisher
New Delhi | London | Panama

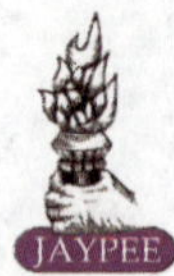

Jaypee Brothers Medical Publishers (P) Ltd

Headquarters
Jaypee Brothers Medical Publishers (P) Ltd
4838/24, Ansari Road, Daryaganj
New Delhi 110 002, India
Phone: +91-11-43574357
Fax: +91-11-43574314
Email: jaypee@jaypeebrothers.com

Overseas Offices

J.P. Medical Ltd
83 Victoria Street, London
SW1H 0HW (UK)
Phone: +44 20 3170 8910
Fax: +44 (0)20 3008 6180
Email: info@jpmedpub.com

Jaypee-Highlights Medical Publishers Inc
City of Knowledge, Bld. 235, 2nd Floor, Clayton
Panama City, Panama
Phone: +1 507-301-0496
Fax: +1 507-301-0499
Email: cservice@jphmedical.com

Jaypee Brothers Medical Publishers (P) Ltd
17/1-B Babar Road, Block-B, Shaymali
Mohammadpur, Dhaka-1207
Bangladesh
Mobile: +08801912003485
Email: jaypeedhaka@gmail.com

Jaypee Brothers Medical Publishers (P) Ltd
Bhotahity, Kathmandu
Nepal
Phone: +977-9741283608
Email: kathmandu@jaypeebrothers.com

Website: www.jaypeebrothers.com
Website: www.jaypeedigital.com

Comprehensive Textbook of Medical Physiology (Vol 1)

First Edition: 2017

Reprint: ***2017***

ISBN: 978-93-86056-97-9

Printed at Replika Press Pvt. Ltd.

Dedicated at the feet of
Sreema, the Divine Mother
and
Sri Aurobindo, the Divine Master

All Nature dumbly calls to her alone
To heal with her feet the aching throb of life
And break the seals on the dim soul of man
And kindle her fire in the closed heart of things.
All here shall be one day her sweetness' home,
All contraries prepare her harmony;
Towards her our knowledge climbs, our passion gropes;
In her miraculous rapture we shall dwell,
Her clasp shall turn to ecstasy our pain.
Our self shall be one self with all through her.
In her confirmed because transformed in her,
Our life shall find in its fulfilled response
Above, the boundless hushed beatitudes,
Below, the wonder of the embrace divine.

Sri Aurobindo (in 'SAVITRI')

Preface

Oh India, land of light and spiritual knowledge!
Wake up to your true mission in the world,
Show the way to union and harmony.

The Mother (of Sri Aurobindo Ashram, Puducherry, India)

Physiology is the key subject in medicine. Starting from the knowledge of body functions, physiology provides the concept of dysfunctions, the basis of understanding the disease processes and the insight into disease management and prevention. Physiology is the core of medical wisdom. Due to its enormous contribution to the growth of medical knowledge, the Nobel Prize in health sector has been designated as Nobel Prize in Physiology and Medicine. Physiology as a subject in medical science has changed over the years from its nonclinical to preclinical and then to the current proclinical format with the incorporation of Applied and Clinical Physiology as the essential components in its core curriculum. Physiology is the foundation of medical practice. Many clinical investigations related to neurological disorders, autonomic dysfunctions, cardiovascular and respiratory diseases, endocrinal, renal, reproductive and metabolic problems are carried out in the well-equipped laboratories of physiology departments. Further, many research investigations are conducted in physiology laboratories. Sooner, the superspecialty course in Clinical Physiology will be a reality.

In India, Physiology as a subject in medical curriculum has changed immensely over decades. With the introduction of the new Medical Council of India (MCI) guidelines in 1997, the duration of first MBBS course was reduced from its original one-and-half years to one year. With subsequent modifications by MCI, directing physiology to become a more clinically oriented subject, a need aroused in reshaping the subject, integrating it with subjects of paraclinical and clinical medicine and orienting physiology knowledge for application-based learning. Therefore, in the present textbook, we have made all our sincere efforts without diluting the core concepts of physiology that includes regulation and integration of body functions, to amalgamate the knowledge in physiology with other subjects for its application in medicine.

After the publication of our Textbook and Practical Book of Physiology, the students and teachers in Physiology across the globe have been requesting to write a comprehensive book in Physiology that can offer a holistic concept of functions, integration, dysfunctions of body systems, and physiological basis of management and prevention of diseases. With all their wishes and blessings, finally this book has been made available to them. We hope this book will fulfill the aspiration of the readers in acquiring and applying the knowledge of physiology in clinics. Nevertheless, this is a project in evolution, and needs inputs, support and encouragement from our readers for its endless progression.

Gopal Krushna Pal
Pravati Pal
Nivedita Nanda

Acknowledgments

Let us work as we pray. For indeed work is the body's best prayer to the Divine.

The Mother (of Sri Aurobindo Ashram, Puducherry, India)

With pride and privilege, we acknowledge the contribution of all our past teachers, especially the professors of VSS Medical College, Burla, Odisha for educating us acquire the principle and practice of clinical medicine. We also gratefully acknowledge our past physiology teachers at Jawaharlal Institute of Postgraduate Medical Education and Research (JIPMER), Puducherry, India for having guided us learn the essentials of physiology, and notable among them are Dr DP Thombre, Dr V Srinivasan, and Dr (Late) DB Koner.

We sincerely acknowledge the contribution of Shri Jitendar P Vij, Group Chairman, Jaypee Brothers Medical Publishers Pvt Ltd, New Delhi for personally coming to Puducherry, and motivating and inspiring us to take up this special responsibility of writing such a wonderful book. For preparing the manuscript of the present book, we are especially thankful to Ms Chetna Malhotra Vohra (Associate Director - Content Strategy) and Ms Angima Shree (Senior Development Editor) for their constant support and timely help. The contribution of Ms Angima Shree is immense and praiseworthy. We also thank the other editors and designers of the Jaypee group who helped in the preparation of this book. We acknowledge Mr Narendra Singh Shekhawat (Delhi, India), Mr Venugopal (Bengaluru, Karnataka, India), and Mr Muralidharan (Puducherry, India) of the Jaypee group for their support. We are also thankful to Jaypee Brothers Medical Publishers for providing us many of the pictures and materials of their medical publications.

We are thankful to all our colleagues and students across the globe for reading our book and providing us their inputs for its further improvement. We thank all our colleagues and residents of JIPMER for their constant inspiration and support.

Auroprajna and Auroprakash, the divine children gifted to us, have been the constant support to us in all our endeavors. We shall fail in our duty if we do not appreciate the contribution of our sister Sabita Nanda, who has been constantly taking care of all our family requirements. We always keep in high esteem our parents Dr (Late) Artatran Nanda, Smt Anupama Nanda, Sri Mrutyunjay Pal and Srimati Malatimani Pal for showering on us their love and blessings and providing us everything to come to the greater heights in our life. We take this opportunity to express our heartfelt obeisance to Ms Kumud Ben of Sri Aurobindo Ashram, who is no more physically on this earth but lives in our hearts forever.

Special Features of the Book/How to use it Best

All sincere prayers are granted, every call is answered. With my Blessings.

The Mother (of Sri Aurobindo Ashram, Puducherry, India)

This *Comprehensive Textbook of Medical Physiology* has the following special features. These tips are meant for the readers to best use the book.

Learning Objectives: The topics start with *'Learning Objectives'*. By reading the learning objectives, a student will know the gross content of the topic, and how much he should acquire from it after reading the topic. The objectives have been divided into *'Must Know'* criteria that a student should minimum acquire, and *'May Know'* criteria that a student is desirable to acquire. These *'Must Know'* and *'May Know'* criteria will help a teacher prepare the content of his lecture class and to focus more on the major criteria.

Scientists Contributed: Invariably, important topics start with the contributions of great scientists in the concerned field, especially those who have received the Nobel Prize and/or are popular for their contributions in that field. Often, examiners ask to name the scientists who have invented/discovered the concepts or profoundly contributed to the development of the subject. This will not only give the information of the history of medicine, but will also inspire students and teachers to take up research in physiology and medicine. This part the readers should not miss!

Application Box: The concepts of Physiology have lot of applications in daily life and medical practice. Therefore, a major component of physiology is *'Applied Physiology'*. These important concepts and applied aspects of the topic are depicted in the *'Application Box'* and highlighted by green-colored boxes. If a student will miss to read these boxes, he/she will miss the core concepts in physiology.

Clinical Physiology: Presently, the learning in physiology is oriented to understand the etiology of the disease, and the physiological basis of management. Therefore, the major part of physiology is devoted for **'Clinical Physiology'**. The Clinical Physiology has been depicted in this book in the following formats:

- At the end of each topic, a description has been given for the common dysfunctions and disorders or diseases. A note has been given to explain the pathophysiology of the disease process and the physiological basis of the management. This is primarily to sensitize the 1st MBBS student for learning medicine, and to highlight the importance of physiology in learning medicine.
- Constructed pictures or original photos of the common diseases have been shown at the end of the topics. This is to create interest in the mind of the 1st MBBS student for clinical medicine. It also helps to understand and memorize Clinical Physiology.
- The core concepts related to diseases and patient management have been highlighted in ***'Clinical Box'***. This provides the core concepts of understanding clinical medicine. The clinical boxes are highlighted with pink-colored bars.

The *Clinical Physiology* part is the uniqueness of this book, which is not given in any other textbook in this structured format. A student should never miss to read these clinical components in physiology.

Important Note: Some important and useful facts that are not covered in application or clinical boxes, are depicted as *'Important Note'*. These are useful information that may be asked in examinations, especially in viva voce.

Structured Presentation: Every chapter is divided into various parts by different headings and subheadings with different fonts and colors. Further, all important and complex mechanisms are structured and presented in a *point-wise description*. This structured presentation will help the student easily grasp the topic and memorize it. Further, this will ensure that a student does not miss any of the relevant points.

Flowcharts: All major concepts are simplified and summarized in *'Flowcharts'*. Not only it helps to memorize and recap the topic, but also, presenting the text along with flowcharts in examination helps the examiner easily assess the knowledge of the student. Usually, presentation with flowcharts in examination is more marks-fetching. The presentation of many flowcharts is a special feature of this book. A student must read and remember these flowcharts.

Schematic Diagrams and Graphs: All the relevant and significant mechanisms, theories and concepts are described in this book with the help of schematic diagrams and graphs. If a student is able to draw a labeled schematic diagram, it is always considered that a student has understood the topic. Especially in an examination, due to shortage of time, if a student draws a good schematic diagram and gives a brief answer with the help of flowcharts, even if he fails to give a descriptive answer, he gets good marks invariably. Therefore, the student should never miss to understand the diagrams and figures.

Tables: All important data, special concepts and lengthy information that a student needs to remember have been presented in **structured tabular format**. Reading the tables helps to revise and remember these facts quickly.

Histological Pictures: All mechanisms and manifestations of a disorder that require structural knowledge of a tissue or organ to comprehend the concept of the disease have been identified with appropriate *histological pictures*. For example, when a student sees the blood cells of an anemia in a blood smear, he understands and remembers better. A student must see these histological pictures.

Chapter Summary: All topics end with a *'Chapter Summary'* that has been divided into two parts:

1. The first part is the *'Key Concepts'*, that depicts the central theme or the major take-home message of the topic. This is not the chapter summary, rather the summary of the main concepts.
2. The second part is the *'Important to Know (Must Read)'* that provides all the probable *long questions* and *short questions* that usually come in theory examinations. Also, the questions that are usually asked in *oral (viva) examination*, are listed in this section. Students will definitely find it very useful. This will also help teachers to frame questions for the examination. A student should never miss this part.

Thus, this book is a comprehensive textbook that has incorporated all the requirements of a medical student for imparting the knowledge and skill of the subject, for acquiring all the ingredients needed to appear in the examination, and to complete the course with the best results.

Contents

Volume 1

Section–1: General Physiology 1

1. Defining the Role of Physiology in Modern Medicine 3
2. Functional Organization of Human Body 7
3. Principles of Homeostasis 9
4. Cellular Organization and Intercellular Connections 13
5. Physiology of Genetics and Apoptosis 28
6. Transport Across the Cell Membrane 40
7. Membrane Potential 58
8. Body Fluids 63

Section–2: Blood and Immunity 69

9. Composition and Functions of Blood and Plasma Proteins 71
10. Bone Marrow and Hemopoiesis 76
11. Red Blood Cells 83
12. Erythropoiesis 90
13. Destruction of Red Blood Cells 99
14. Hemoglobin and Blood Indices 103
15. Pathophysiology of Anemia and Polycythemia 109
16. Blood Groups and Physiological Basis of Blood Transfusion 116
17. White Blood Cells 127
18. Thymus, Lymphoid Tissues, and Lymph 150
19. Immunity 158
20. Platelets and Their Role in Hemostasis 183
21. Blood Coagulation 196

Section–3: Nerve and Muscle 213

Part A: Nerve

22. Structure and Functions of Neurons 215
23. Nerve Potentials 224
24. Properties, Classification and Applied Aspects of Nerve Fibers 236

Part B: Neuromuscular Junction

25. Neuromuscular Transmission 241

Part C: Muscles

26. Structure of Skeletal Muscle: Physiological Aspects 249
27. Mechanism of Skeletal Muscle Contraction 258
28. Skeletal Muscle: Properties, Fiber Types, and Applied Aspects 266
29. Smooth Muscle and Cardiac Muscle 276

Section–4: Autonomic Nervous System 285

30. Functional Organization of Autonomic Nervous System 287
31. Sympathetic System 295
32. Parasympathetic System 301
33. Control of Autonomic Functions and Applied Aspects 306
34. Autonomic Function Tests 312
35. Heart Rate Variability 317

Section–5: Gastrointestinal System 325

Part A: Introduction to GI System

36. Functional Organization of GI System and Principles of GI Regulations 327
37. Gastrointestinal Hormones 335

Part B: GI Secretions

38. Principles of GI Secretion and Secretion of Saliva 341
39. Gastric Secretion 348
40. Pancreatic Secretion 362
41. Physiology of Liver, Liver Function Tests, and Pathophysiology of Jaundice 370
42. Biliary Secretion 378
43. Intestinal Secretion 384
44. Secretion of Large Intestine 389

Part C: GI Motility

45. Introduction to GI Motility 393
46. Chewing and Deglutition 398
47. Esophageal Motility 401
48. Gastric Motility 404
49. Small Intestinal Motility 412
50. Motility of Large Intestine 416

Part D: Digestion and Absorption

51. Principles of Digestion and Absorption 421

Section–6: Endocrine Physiology 429

52. Introduction to Endocrinology 431
53. Mechanisms of Hormone Action 441
54. Hypothalamus and Hypothalamo-pituitary Axis 453
55. Pituitary Gland: The Anterior Pituitary 459
56. Posterior Pituitary 475
57. Thyroid Gland 481
58. Adrenal Gland: The Adrenal Medulla 498
59. Adrenal Cortex 506
60. Endocrine Pancreas 527
61. Calcium and Phosphate Metabolism and Physiology of Bone 547
62. Parathyroid Gland, Calcitonin and Vitamin D 556
63. Pineal Gland 566
64. Local Hormones 569

Section–7: Reproductive System 575

Part A: General Reproductive Physiology

65. Sex Differentiation and Development, Puberty and Menopause 577
66. Physiology of Puberty and Menopause 584

Part B: Male Reproductive Physiology

67. Male Reproductive System 588

Part C: Female Reproductive Physiology

68. Female Reproductive System: Functional Anatomy, Oogenesis and Follicular Development 604
69. Menstrual Cycle and Ovulation 614
70. Ovarian Hormones and Control of Ovarian Functions 623

Part D: Physiology of Conception, Pregnancy, Lactation and Contraception

71. Physiology of Copulation 630
72. Pregnancy and Parturition 634
73. Physiology of Breast Development and Lactation 649
74. Physiology of Contraception 653

Section–8: Renal System 657

75. General Introduction and Functional Anatomy of Kidney 659
76. Renal Blood Flow 671
77. Glomerular Filtration 676
78. Tubular Functions 682
79. Mechanisms of Urine Concentration and Dilution 699
80. Water Excretion, Diuresis, and Diuretics 705
81. Acidification of Urine 709
82. Kidney Function Tests and Pathophysiology of Renal Failure 715
83. Physiology of Micturition, and Bladder Dysfunctions 722

Volume 2

Section–9: Cardiovascular System 727

Part A: General Introduction

84. Functional Organization of Cardiovascular System 729

Part B: Heart

85. Functional Anatomy of Heart, Cardiac Muscle, Conducting System, and Cardiac Innervation 736
86. Properties of Cardiac Muscle 746
87. Electrophysiology of the Heart 751
88. Electrocardiogram 759
89. Cardiac Cycle 778
90. Cardiac Output 787
91. Heart Rate and Arterial Pulse 797

Part C: Circulation

92. Principles of Hemodynamics 803
93. Arterial System 809

94. Venous System 813
95. Capillary Circulation 816
96. Regulation of Blood Pressure 822
97. Integrated Regulation of Cardiovascular Functions 839
98. Regional Circulations 844
99. Fetal Circulation 859

Part D: Applied and Clinical Aspects of CVS

100. Pathophysiology of Hypertension and Hypotension 861
101. Pathophysiology of Shock 866
102. Pathophysiology of Heart Failure 871

Section–10: Respiratory System 877

103. Functional Organization of Respiratory System 879
104. Mechanics of Breathing 886
105. Alveolar Ventilation and Gas Exchange in Lungs 907
106. Pulmonary Circulation and Ventilation-Perfusion Ratio 914
107. Transport of Gases in Blood 922
108. Regulation of Respiration 931
109. Physiological Changes at High Altitude 947
110. Hypoxia and Oxygen Therapy 950
111. Hazards of Deep Sea Diving and Effects of Increased Barometric Pressure 954
112. Respiration in Abnormal Conditions and Abnormal Respirations 957
113. Artificial Ventilation and Cardiopulmonary Resuscitation 961
114. Pulmonary Function Tests 965

Section–11: Neurophysiology 973

Part A: Introduction to Neurophysiology

115. Functional Organization of Nervous System 975
116. Synaptic Transmission in Central Nervous System 981

Part B: The Sensory System

117. Introduction to Sensory System and Physiology of Receptors 995
118. Sensory Communication to Spinal Cord 1002
119. Ascending Pathways 1007
120. Physiology of Pain, Itch and Temperature 1014
121. Trigeminal System 1024
122. Thalamus 1026
123. Sensory Cortex 1033
124. Sensory Abnormalities 1037

Part C: The Motor System

125. Introduction to and Organization of Motor System 1040
126. Segmental Organization of Motor System 1044
127. Muscle Spindle and Golgi Tendon Organ 1048
128. Spinal Reflexes 1054
129. Descending Pathways 1061
130. Regulation of Posture and Movement 1070

131. Basal Ganglia 1082
132. Cerebellum 1088
133. Vestibular Apparatus 1097

Part D: Hypothalamus, EEG and Sleep; Limbic and Higher Functions; CSF

134. Functions of Hypothalamus 1104
135. Physiology of Reticular Activating System 1112
136. Electroencephalogram and Sleep 1115
137. Limbic System 1125
138. Physiology of Learning and Memory 1134
139. Physiology of Language and Speech 1143
140. Association Cortex, Cerebral Asymmetry, Lobes of the Brain, and Cortical Plasticity 1147
141. Cerebrospinal Fluid 1155

Section–12: Special Senses 1163

Part A: Vision

142. Functional Anatomy of Eye 1165
143. Image-forming Mechanism 1172
144. Photoreceptor Mechanism 1177
145. Visual Pathway and Visual Cortex 1181
146. Visual Acuity, Visual Field, Light and Dark Adaptations, and Visual Reflexes 1188
147. Color Vision 1193
148. Movements of the Eye 1198

Part B: Hearing

149. Functional Anatomy and Functions of the Ear 1202
150. Auditory Pathways 1208
151. Mechanism of Hearing 1211
152. Hearing Defects and Hearing Tests 1217

Part C: Smell and Taste

153. Physiology of Smell 1220
154. Physiology of Taste 1224

Section–13: Integrative Physiology 1231

155. Structure and Functions of the Skin 1233
156. Regulation of Body Temperature and Acclimatization to Hot and Cold Environments 1237
157. Physiology of Exercise and Sports Science 1252
158. Principles of Acid-Base Homeostasis 1266
159. Regulation of Volume, Composition and Osmolality of Body Fluid Compartments 1272
160. Physiology of Growth and Development 1278
161. Physiology of Nutrition 1282
162. Physiology of Aging and Oxidative Stress, Prevention of Aging and Physiology of Yoga 1295

Index *I-i*

SECTION–1

General Physiology

1. Defining the Role of Physiology in Modern Medicine
2. Functional Organization of Human Body
3. Principles of Homeostasis
4. Cellular Organization and Intercellular Connections
5. Physiology of Genetics and Apoptosis
6. Transport Across the Cell Membrane
7. Membrane Potential
8. Body Fluids

"All the world possibilities in man
Are waiting as the tree waits in its seed:
His past lives in him; it drives his future's pace;
His present's acts fashion his coming fate.
The unborn gods hide in his house of Life."

Sri Aurobindo (in 'SAVITRI')

CHAPTER 1

Defining the Role of Physiology in Modern Medicine

Learning Objectives

On completion of study of this chapter, the student **MUST** be able to:

1. Understand the importance of physiology in learning various aspects and branches of medicine.
2. Appreciate the role of physiology in understanding the principles of medical practice.
3. Realize the value of physiology knowledge for conducting medical research.

The student **MAY** also be able to:

1. Learn the role of physiology in health promotion and disease prevention.
2. Comprehend that physiology knowledge facilitates integral progress of human being.

Physiology is the study of body functions, their mechanisms and regulations in all living organisms. **Human physiology** is the study of functions of various cells, organs and organ systems of human body. It encompasses the integration and control of organ systems that help in smooth functioning of body systems as a single unit. **Medical physiology** is the application of knowledge of human physiology in the management of dysfunctions and diseases in human beings.

In essence, human physiology is similar to the physiology of other mammals and vertebrates. However, as human being is the highest creation in the hierarchy of nature's evolution, the physiological processes that govern human life are more refined and developed. Nevertheless, the intricacies of human mind and vital and their profound influence on body functions have made human physiology more complex. Therefore, treatment of human diseases not only requires knowledge in physiology and medicine, but also the understanding of human behavior.

PHYSIOLOGY FOR LEARNING MEDICINE

Physiology, the Mother of Medicine

Physiology provides the essential knowledge to understand the process of *homeostasis*, which is defined as the constancy of the internal environment of the body. Homeostasis is the state of internal harmony among the body systems. A disease is an expression of functional disharmony of the systems that usually occurs due to prolonged disturbances of any kind. Understanding the nature of disturbance is critical to comprehend the pathophysiology of a disease and the physiological basis of management of the disease. Therefore, to learn any branch of medicine, it is essential to acquire the basic knowledge of systemic physiology related to the specialty. The concept in physiology helps understand, diagnose and treat the disease. For example, for management of a case of acute myocardial infarction (AMI), the physician should know the physiology of coronary blood flow, electrophysiology of cardiac myocytes, homeostasis of myocardial perfusion, principle of regulation of coronary circulation, and the factors that disturb coronary hemodynamics to produce myocardial ischemia. All these physiology concepts help the physician to understand the mechanism of genesis and spread of pain of AMI, to appreciate the nature of radiation of myocardial ischemic pain to left upper arm, to interpret ECG abnormalities to diagnose AMI, and to prescribe appropriate drugs that improve coronary blood flow, re-establish myocardial perfusion and prevent progression of infarction. For many diseases, knowledge in physiology facilitates proper diagnosis and effective treatment. Therefore, the great Physiologist EH Starling had said "*Physiology of Today is the Medicine for Tomorrow*".

Scientist contributed

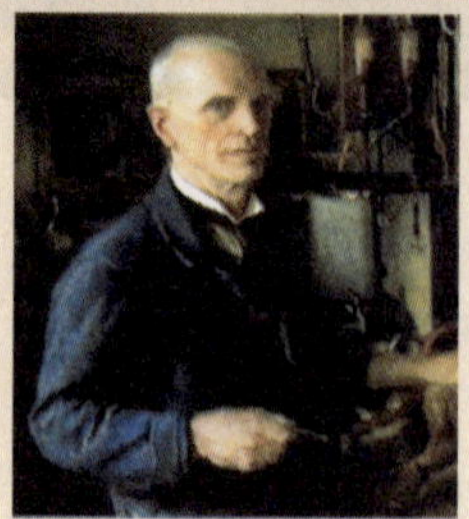
E H Starling
(1866–1927)

In this picture, Starling in the midst of an experiment upon circulation with a dog, in 1926.

Ernest Henry Starling was an English physiologist. His main collaborator was his brother-in-law, William Maddock Bayliss. His major contributions to physiology were: the Starling equation, describing fluid shifts in the body, the discovery of peristalsis (with Bayliss), the discovery of secretin, the first hormone (with Bayliss), the introduction of the concept of hormones and the discovery that the distal convoluted tubule of the kidney reabsorbs water and various electrolytes. Starling is most famous for developing the "Frank-Starling law of the heart", presented in 1915 and modified in 1919. He died in 1927 at the age of 61.

A practitioner should have basic knowledge in physiology to become a good physician. Also, a physiologist by virtue of his knowledge and experience is inherently a good physician. Therefore, I always profess *"A good physician is a physiologist, and a good physiologist is a physician"*.

For Learning Medical Subjects

A medical student with ample knowledge in physiology can easily learn pharmacology and pathology. In principle, **pharmacology is extension of physiology**. For example, while learning pharmacotherapy for bronchial asthma, the student learns the use of catecholaminergic agents, especially β-receptor agonists that cause bronchodilation and provide immediate relief. It is easy for the student to understand pharmacotherapeutics of asthma as he has studied in physiology that sympathetic stimulation causes relaxation of bronchial smooth muscle by releasing norepinephrine, acting through β-receptors. Similarly, action of all of drugs has physiological basis; and therefore, a fundamental knowledge in physiology is essential for learning pharmacology.

Physiology is **useful in learning pathology**. For example, in physiology the student learns neutrophil as the first line of defence against acute infections and monocyte as the defence for chronic infections. Therefore, in histology slide when he finds abundant neutrophils in the microscopic field, he comprehends the infection or inflammation is of acute nature, and presence of abundant monocytes or macrophages makes him realize the infection or inflammation is of chronic nature. Similarly, understanding pathological basis of diseases requires the basic knowledge in physiology. In fact, all the diseases have a pathophysiological basis.

Likewise, the student utilizes his knowledge in physiology **for learning all branches of medicine**. Etiopathogenesis, clinical manifestation, diagnosis and management of all diseases have the physiological basis. Without basic concepts in physiology, a student will not be able to understand the principle of medicine. Hence, all the chapters in medicine textbooks start with an introduction to relevant **clinical physiology**.

In surgery textbooks, there are portions for **surgical physiology**. In all branches of medicine, such as gynecology, ophthalmology, otorhinolaryngology, pediatric medicine, endocrinology, oncology, gastroenterology, pulmonology, neurology, cardiology and so on, a considerable portion is devoted to **clinical physiology** of the topic that helps reader comprehend the physiological basis of the management.

PHYSIOLOGY FOR MEDICAL PRACTICE

For Becoming a Good Physician

The knowledge in physiology guides a physician to understand the principles of medical practice and the rationality of disease management. The present-day physician often tends to provide prompt symptomatic relief by prescribing a list of medicines starting from analgesics to antibiotics. This is because the modern man is in a hurry and wants immediate relief from the sufferings. There is no time, interest and knowledge for an assisted-natural remission of the disease. The physician wants to earn his money and reputation of being a good physician by providing a quick relief. But, this type of treatment does not help the person in the long run, as often medicine suppresses immunity. Although, few diseases require prompt and aggressive treatment by modern therapeutics such as antibiotics, many diseases are cured by assisted-natural remission with minimum medicines. For example, for management of hypertension in the early stage, a good physician can advise reduction in salt intake and stress level, practice of mental relaxation, regular physical exercises and adaptation to a healthy diet and life style. Usually, these nonpharmacological practices are known to decrease blood pressure. Therefore, the physician should motivate his patient to practice natural measures, and should not prescribe a list of blood pressure reducing drugs that have known side effects. Medicines should be prescribed only when these natural means fail to show desirable results.

Physiology educates physicians that effective treatment of many diseases requires improvement of immunity of the subject as enhancement of immunity halts the spread of diseases and slowly discards the disease from the body. For, example, fever due to acute inflammation is a natural manifestation of the disease and part of the defense mechanisms of the body. Therefore, instead of immediately prescribing antibiotics, physician can reassure the patient that the body heals itself or at best he can prescribe mild antipyretic-analgesic. Administration of higher antibiotics and analgesics suppresses the immunity of the patient that exposes him to various infections. The doctor should explain to the patient that fever is a natural defence mechanism against infection, as rise in body temperature kills the organisms. Moreover, prescribing antibiotics in the early part, the course and usual manifestation of the disease is missed, and therefore the diagnosis of the disease is overlooked. Another example, a simple boil (cellulitis), which heals by itself, does not warrant prescription of antibiotics. A doctor should assure the patient about the natural course of the boil and may advise him for warm fomentation on the part that improves blood flow to the region and facilitates the process of healing. Treatment by antibiotic from the beginning may halt the healing process of the boil and in some cases may produce antibioma (tumor due to antibiotics). A doctor should know that frequent use of antibiotics suppresses immune system of the body and predisposes the body to other infections. A physician with ample knowledge in physiology helps patient in facilitating the natural remission and recovery without prescribing higher medicines. Hence, **a good physician is a physiologist.**

For Disease Prevention and Health Promotion

Pathophysiology elucidates the physiological basis of pathology. A physician with physiology knowledge understands the measures that prevent occurrence of diseases. Presently, India is the epicenter of metabolic disorders and cardiovascular risks. A physiologist knows that regular physical exercises with a good eating habit retard the process of atherosclerosis and oxidative stress that prevents occurrence of cardiovascular and cerebrovascular accidents, many metabolic diseases, and retards degeneration and decay. A physiologist not only practices healthy lifestyle himself for his personal health but also encourages others to adapt to such a life. This promotes the community health. Therefore, **a good physiologist is a physician**.

We give emphasis on preventive and promotive aspects of health, which will be more promulgated by physiologists and will be established as ***preventive and promotive physiology***.

PHYSIOLOGY FOR MEDICAL RESEARCH

Physiology is the core subject of medical research. The inventions and discoveries in medical science and advances in medicine are mainly due to research contributions from physiology. Therefore, from its inception in 1901, the Nobel Prize in the field of medical sciences has been designated as 'Nobel Prize in Physiology' or 'Physiology and Medicine'. Many Nobel Prize winners in medicine starting from Emil Adolph Von Behring (1901), Sir Ronal Ross (1902), Prof. Finsen NR (1903), Prof. Ivan Petrovich Pavlov (1904) to Dr. Robert G. Edward (2010), John O'Keefe (2014) are physiologists or physicians who have worked in medical physiology or medical fields linked to physiology. Etiopathogenesis of the diseases and physiological basis of management are elucidated through research discoveries in physiology.

Scientist contributed

Prof. Behring was awarded **first Nobel Prize** in Physiology or Medicine, 1901, for his work on physiology of immunity and serum therapy, especially its application against diphtheria. This opened the path in the domain of medical therapy, a victorious weapon against illness and deaths. He developed quantitative methods for the bioassay of antisera and antitoxins.

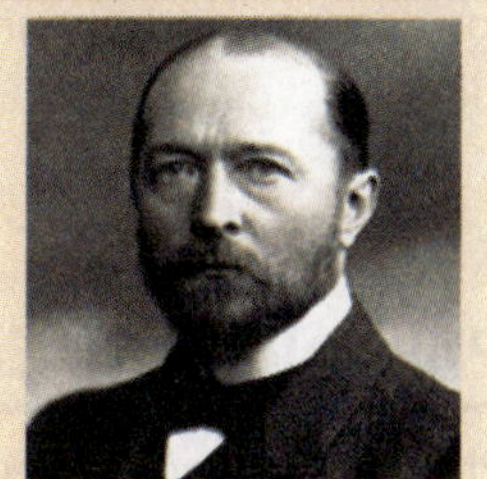

Emil Adolph Von Behring
(1854–1917)

Scientist contributed

The **Nobel Prize in Physiology or Medicine for the year 2010**, was awarded to Robert G. Edwards *for the development of in vitro fertilization*; Dr. Edward had worked extensively in the field of reproductive physiology and infertility for more than 4 decades.

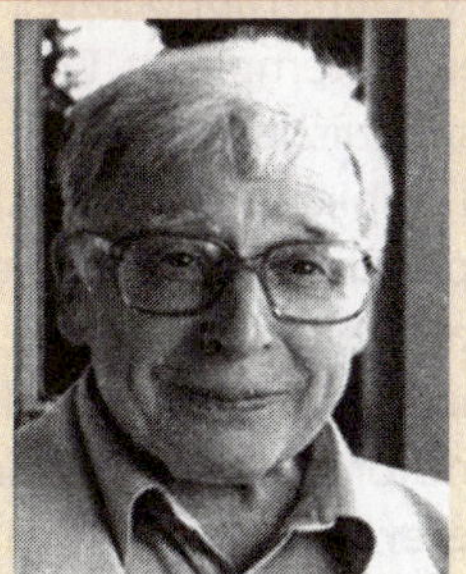

Robert G Edwards
(Born: 27 September 1925, Batley, United Kingdom)

Scientist contributed

The **Nobel Prize in Physiology or Medicine 2014** was divided, one half awarded to John O'Keefe, the other half jointly to May-Britt Moser and Edvard I. Moser *"for their discoveries in Neurophysiology that constitute a positioning system in the brain*. They studied the movements of rats and signals from nerve cells in the hippocampus, an area located in the center of the brain. In 1971 he discovered that when a rat was at a certain location in a room, certain cells were activated, and that when the rat moved to another location, other cells became activated. That is to say, the cells form a kind of internal map of the room.

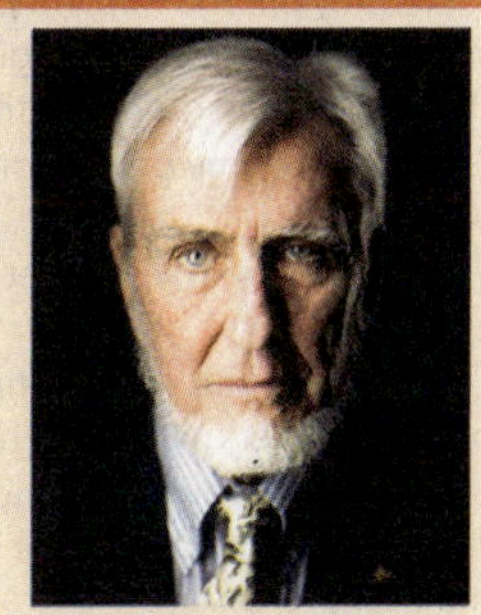

John O'Keefe
(Born: 18 November 1939, New York, NY, USA)

For Basic and Clinical Research

Research in basic and clinical physiology has contributed to enormous growth of clinical medicine. Basic research reveals the mechanism and pathophysiology of diseases, whereas clinical research unravels the management and prevention of diseases. Usually clinicians will not have enough interest and time for research. The *collaborative research* between physiology and clinical departments creates avenues for clinical research, ignites research interest in clinicians, improves research outlook, attracts extramural financial support from various funding agencies and yields more productive results. The ultimate objective of a medical research should be to reduce suffering, facilitate healing, cure the ailment, prevent the occurrence of disease and promote health. Physiologists should make efforts for larger participation of physician in research and ensure research to be more applied and clinical.

PHYSIOLOGY FOR INTEGRAL PROGRESS

Physiology for Ethics

Physiology teaches the ethics and values of life. Appropriate judgment and application of knowledge for healing the human suffering is true physiology. Ethics of medical practice was devised by **Hippocrates,** an ancient Greek physician. Hippocrates was a teacher at the School in the Health Temple at Cos, Greece. Writings of the group are distinguished by a high ethical tone, keen observation, logical application of existing ideas and cautious judgment. Hippocrates established the popular ethics of medical practice for physicians, which is commonly known as **'Hippocratic Oath'** that all physicians solemnly pledge at the time of obtaining their degrees to start medical practice [**Reference**: Jones WHS and Withington ET. *The works of Hippocrates*. 4 volumes. London, Heinemann: 1923].

Scientist contributed

'Hippocratic Oath' with modification is as follows.....

I solemnly pledge to consecrate my life to the service of humanity; I will give to my teachers the respect and gratitude that is their due;

I will practice my profession with conscience and dignity;

The health of my patient will be my first consideration;

I will respect the secrets that are confided in me, even after the patient has died;

I will maintain by all the means in my power, the honor and the noble traditions of the medical profession;

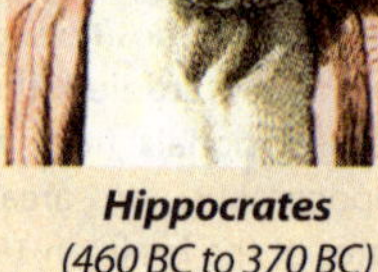

Hippocrates
(460 BC to 370 BC)

My colleagues will be my sisters and brothers;

I will not permit considerations of age, disease or disability, creed, ethnic origin, gender, nationality, political affiliation, race, sexual orientation, social standing or any other factor to intervene between my duty and my patient;

I will maintain the utmost respect for human life;

I will not use my medical knowledge to violate human rights and civil liberties, even under threat;

I make these promises solemnly, freely and upon my honor.

Physiology for Integral Knowledge

Physiology provides the knowledge to gain and maintain good health. Physiology teaches us how various organ-systems in the body work inter-dependently for maintaining an effective homeostasis. For example, respiratory system provides oxygen to the tissues of the body with the help of a central pump (the heart) that maintains a dynamic circulation, under the integrated control of neural and endocrine factors. In this process, no organ-system is big or small, as contribution of each organ leads to fulfillment of the primary objective of supplying blood, oxygen and nutrients to the body parts. Derangement of any of these participating systems leads to development of bodily dysfunctions. We should understand that this basic principle of a structured system of working is essential for creating a healthy environment and harmonious progress of an organization.

Physiology for Spiritual Progress

The fundamental aim of our terrestrial existence *is to attain perfection*; the perfection in physical growth, perfection in beauty, perfection in mind and intellect and perfection in inner disciplines. A progressive evolution of consciousness is spirituality. Inner progress is achieved by improvement in body physiology. For example, practice of pranayama not only improves breathing capacity and oxygenation of the body, but also strengthens the neural elements, metabolic functions and causes purification of mind and vital and enhances cognitive faculties. In human body, there are subtle physical centers such as spinal-cord center, heart center, throat center, pineal center, etc. and they are rich in different kinds of spiritual energies. Focusing the concentration on these centers releases the energy from the center that helps in purifying and enriching the mind and body. With knowledge in physiology it becomes easy concentrating and releasing energy from these centers. A physiologist having the holistic knowledge of working of the body and with true aspiration for progress is privileged for acquiring higher knowledge, force and consciousness. One will realize that learning and teaching physiology in its true essence is the best method to acquire peace of mind, release stress from the body, and establish contact with the higher consciousness, i.e., with the Divine.

Thus, *to study human physiology is an opportunity, to become a physiologist is a privilege, to encourage others to practice physiological means of health-promotion is a unique occasion, and to practice physiology for integral progress is the reality in life.*

CHAPTER SUMMARY

Physiology is the key subject in Medicine. Knowledge in physiology is fundamental in understanding all other subjects in medicine. Physiology provides the foundation for medical practice. Understanding physiology is central to obtain and maintain perfect health. Physiology is the basis for prevention of diseases and promotion of health. Physiology is the core of medical research. Learning physiology is crucial to the integral progress.

CHAPTER

2

Functional Organization of Human Body

Learning Objectives

On completion of study of this chapter, the student **WILL** be able to:

1. Understand the physiological organization of different systems of the body.
2. Say the general functions of each system.
3. Conceptualize the general integration of body systems.

NATURE OF ORGANIZATION

The organization of human body was studied first time systematically by **Leonardo da Vinci**, the great artist-philosopher-scientist of all the times.

Scientist contributed

Leonardo da Vinci
(1452–1519)

This picture of Leonardo has a very close resemblance with Sri Aurobindo and once he had commented on him as one of his past incarnation.

Leonardo left extraordinary drawings of physiological interest on body functions, muscle actions, and on heart valves, papillary muscles of ventricle and hydraulic operations in the cardiovascular systems. He had adequate knowledge on functioning of the human body. He had many paintings that are widely acknowledged and appreciated. Among them, commonly known are the paintings of Mona Lisa, The Last Supper and The Great Lady Anatomy. The painting of 'great lady anatomy' depicting the internal anatomical structures with details of some of the internal organs in a female (given below), is the first kind of scientific picture on the human anatomy and physiology.

Source: Leonardo da Vinci on the human body. Henry Schuman Publ., New York: 1952.

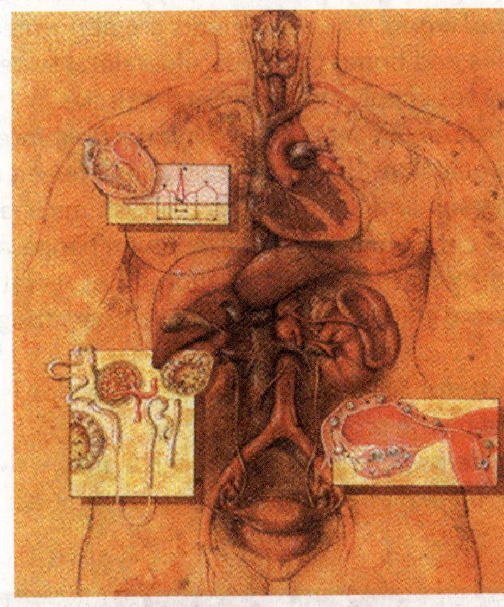

'The Great Lady Anatomy' painting of Leonardo da Vinci.

Unicellular vs Multicellular Organisms

Unicellular Organisms

In unicellular organisms such as ameba, the processes that sustain life are carried out by a single cell interacting with the environment around it. Therefore, unicellular organisms have simpler organization:

1. As they are surrounded by fresh water, the O_2 and soluble nutrients enter the cell by simple diffusion, and macromolecules of nutrients are ingested by phagocytosis.

2. Metabolic waste products, including CO_2 diffuse out of the cell into water, and undigested materials are removed by exocytosis.
3. The presence of contractile proteins in the cell enables it to move by pseudopodia away from noxious stimuli or towards food, and facilitates the movements in phagocytosis and exocytosis.
4. Reproduction is achieved by simple cell division, and no meeting of sexes is involved.

Multicellular Organisms

In multicellular organisms such as animal and man, the **cells** are organized into **tissues** (nerves, muscles, connective tissue, lymphoid tissue, epithelial tissue, blood etc.); and the tissues are organized into larger units known as **organs** (e.g. kidney, liver etc.). The tissues and organs are further organized into **functional systems** meant for performing various body functions.

Major Physiological Systems

The body systems can be broadly divided into:

1. The ***system for supplying nutrition to the body***, which is achieved by the gastrointestinal (GI) system.
2. The ***systems to support the body for locomotion and external works***. The movements are performed by the muscles and bones (the musculoskeletal system), and the nerves supplying the skeletal muscles.
3. The ***systems for internal communication, integration and regulation***: The communication between the cells and organs and control of organ systems is achieved by the circulating blood, gaseous exchange at tissue level through respiration, the hormones secreted from endocrine glands, and the neurons innervating the tissues.
4. The ***systems for reproduction***: Reproduction is accomplished by the reproductive organs.
5. The ***systems for excretion***: Though kidney is the major organ of excretion, lower parts of GI tract (colon, rectum, and anal canal) and skin also contribute to excretion of wastes from the body.

Thus, the **major body systems** are:

Musculoskeletal system: This system enables the body adopt posture against gravity, and move about in the environment. This is mainly for execution of works.

Gastrointestinal system: The GI system serves to ingest, digest, and absorb nutrients, water and electrolytes, and excrete undigested or unabsorbed waste matter.

Respiratory system: The respiration is responsible for delivering atmospheric oxygen to the blood, and excreting CO_2 produced by the cells of the body.

Blood: The blood serves as transport medium for conveying nutrients and oxygen to all the cells, and for delivering waste products from tissues to the organs that excrete them (the lungs and kidneys). Blood contains cells that take part in body defence mechanisms.

Cardiovascular system: The heart is the central pump that generates pressure for flow of blood in the blood vessels that serve as vehicular system for blood to flow.

Urinary system: The urinary system consisting mainly of kidneys, ureter and urinary bladder excretes waste products such as urea, uric acid and creatinine, and plays a major role in maintaining the *constancy of the composition* of the fluid immediately surrounding each cell (the extracellular fluid), which is referred to as the internal milieu.

Endocrine system: Hormones secreted by various endocrine glands serve mainly regulatory functions. They control metabolism, growth, development and reproductive functions.

Reproductive system: Reproductive organs and genital structures ensure maintenance of progeny and the species.

Nervous system: The nervous system is mainly for coordination, communication and regulation of body functions.

CHAPTER SUMMARY

The human body consists of various systems that are organized to perform their respective functions independently and interdependently. The major objectives of this systemic organization are to provide nutrition and energy for carrying out external works, provide support to the body for locomotion, execution and protection from environment, to control body activities, and to reproduce the offspring for continuation of the species.

CHAPTER 3

Principles of Homeostasis

Learning Objectives

On completion of study of this chapter, the student **MUST** be able to:
1. Define homeostasis.
2. Name the scientist who gave the concept of *milieu interior*, and the scientist who coined the term homeostasis.
3. Explain the feedback mechanisms of homeostatic regulation.
4. Give the examples of homeostatic regulations.
5. Understand that dysfunctions are mainly due to failure of homeostatic regulations.

The student **MAY** also be able to:
1. Describe the details of negative and positive feedback mechanisms.
2. Give a note on intracellular homeostasis.

Concept of Homeostasis

Homeostasis is ***defined*** as the maintenance of constancy of the internal environment of the body. In the nineteenth century, **Claude Bernard,** a French physiologist, was first to introduce the concept of ***milieu intérieur***, which means the internal environment of the body. He had following remarkable observations:

1. The volume and composition of the fluid are maintained constant, independent of the changes in the environment in which the animal lives.
2. He designated the fluid (ECF) in the body as the *internal environment*, to differentiate it from the external environment of the body.
3. He suggested that the ability to regulate internal environment is the major reason for humans and animals to live a normal life in spite of changes and challenges imposed on them by the external environment.
4. He noted the difference between intracellular and extracellular fluid and had proposed that the extracellular fluid is the internal environment of the body.

Extracellular Fluid as the Internal Environment

About 60% of the total body weight is water, which means a man weighing 70 kg has a total water content of about 42 liters, of which 28 liters is present inside the cells and 14 liters is present outside the cell. The electrolyte composition of the extracellular fluid roughly resembles that of seawater, which is rich in sodium and chloride, and poor in potassium. The intracellular fluid contains more potassium and less sodium-chloride.

Scientist contributed

Claude Bernard, a student of François Magendie (1783–1855) was a genius and great French physiologist of all time. He was the first scientist to introduce the concept of *milieu intérieur*, preservation of the internal stability despite changes in the external environment. This concept was later utilized to understand the mechanism of 'homeostasis'. He emphasized the concept of integrated interrelation between the parts of a living being. He demonstrated the glycogenic function of the liver, manifold digestive action of pancreatic juice, vasomotor mechanism (sympathetic control) for regulation of blood flow. Many important practical concepts have been derived from his studies on CO poisoning, asphyxia and anesthesia. He was the first to provide satisfactory explanation for the mechanism of action of any drug.

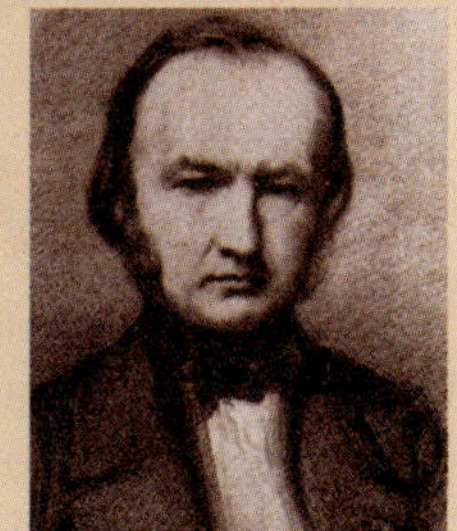

Claude Bernard
(1813–1878)

Source: Baillerie JB. Lessons of experimental physiology has applied medicine. Paris, 1855-56.

In 1929, an American physiologist **Walter Cannon** coined the term ***'homeostasis'*** *(homoios* means 'like'

Flowchart 3.1: Feedback mechanism of homeostatic regulation. Note, failure of feedback control leads to the dysfunctions or diseases.

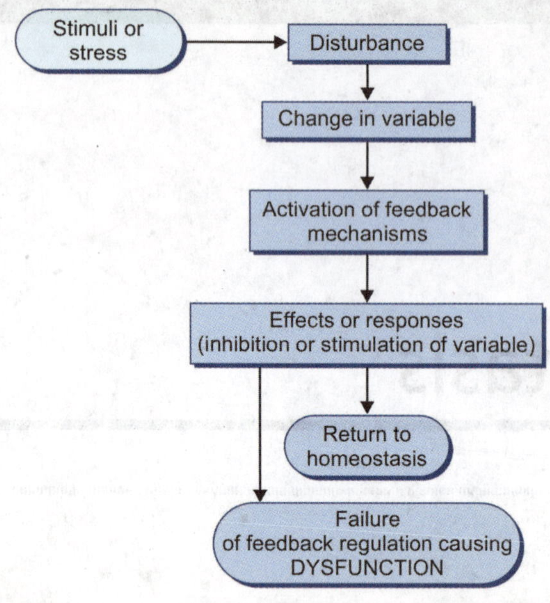

and *stasis* means 'standing still') to describe the phenomenon of the constancy of the internal environment. He described that the capacity of self-regulation is the cause for maintenance of steady states in the body, which occurs due to coordinated integration of various physiological mechanisms.

Scientist contributed

Walter Bradford Cannon was an American physiologist, Professor and Chairman of the Department of Physiology at Harvard Medical School. He coined the term *fight or flight response*, and he expanded on Claude Bernard's concept of homeostasis.

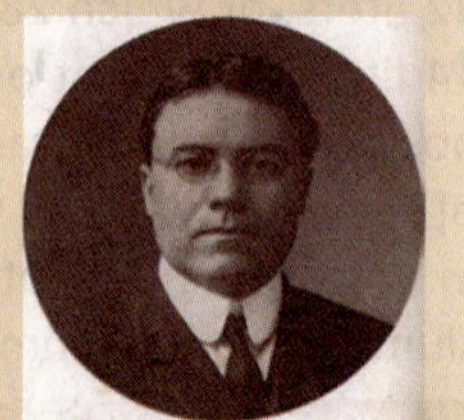

Walter Bradford Cannon
(1871–1945)

HOMEOSTATIC MECHANISMS

Homeostasis is the stability of the internal environment. It is not only the equilibrium of the internal environment as a whole, but also the balance of the composition and components of the environment and the physiological variables that influence the environment. Homeostasis of the composition of internal environment, especially of the body fluids, and various other body parameters that influence the environment, is the minimum requirement for smooth functioning of the body. Abnormal deviation from these homeostatic processes leads to bodily dysfunctions. Therefore, it is fundamental to know how the homeostasis of different physiological variables is achieved and how the abnormalities in these homeostatic regulations lead to various dysfunctions.

Feedback Mechanisms of Homeostatic Regulations

Homeostatic regulation is mainly achieved through the feedback mechanisms that operate to safeguard a set point already set for the physiological variable. The stimulus for feedback control is a change in the level of the variable, which is detected by the sensor (the receptors) that activate the feedback system which in turn triggers a response to bring the variable back to the normal range of the set point and restores homeostasis (Flowchart 3.1). There are two types of feedback regulations: The negative feedback and the positive feedback.

Negative Feedback

The negative feedback mechanism is the usual mechanism of homeostatic regulation. When the variable is raised above the set point, the negative feedback mechanism triggers processes that inhibit the formation of the variable (Flowchart 3.2) and when the variable is lowered below the set point, negative feedback system withdraws the inhibition to allow production of the variable. Thus, the negative feedback system provides the physiological basis for homeostatic regulation (detailed description is given below).

Positive Feedback System

In a positive feedback system, increase in the variable triggers processes that further increase the variable. Therefore, this control mechanism does not operate to provide homeostasis. Rather, positive feedback mechanism is a vicious cycle that terminates only when the stimulus applied to trigger is withdrawn or the process itself is self-terminated. Examples of positive feedback regulation are:

1. The ***parturition reflex initiated by oxytocin***: Towards term, when the head of the matured fetus presses on the uterine cervix, the cervical distension sends signal to posterior pituitary to release oxytocin. Oxytocin

Flowchart 3.2: Components of negative feedback regulation system.

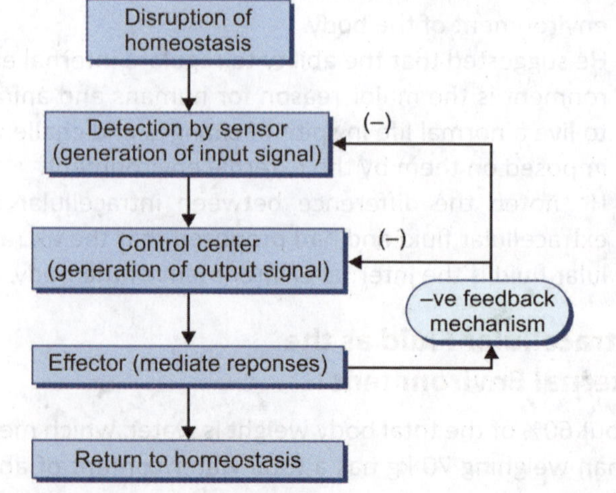

Flowchart 3.3: Hodgkin's cycle as an example of positive feedback mechanism. In this, opening of a set of Na^+ channels activates opening of subsequent sets of Na^+ channels (+ve feedback) that leads to depolarization of the cell.

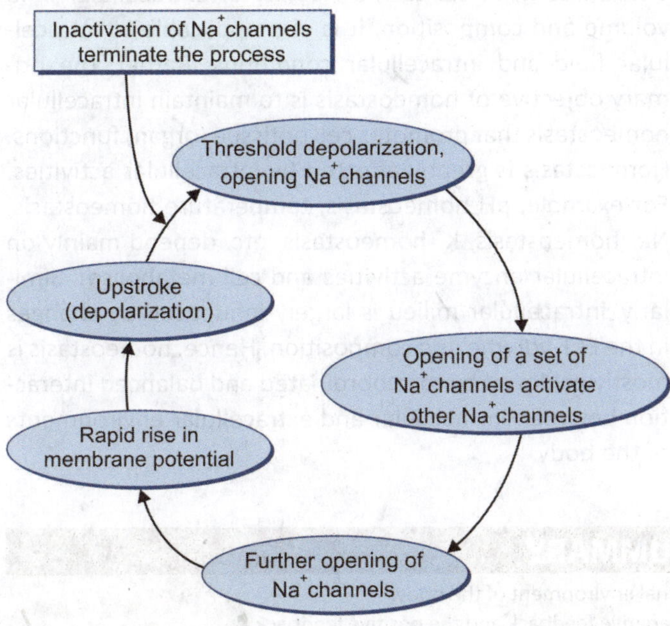

increases the excitability of myometrium and causes uterine contraction. Contraction of uterus further pushes the fetus onto the cervix, and cervical distension further increases oxytocin release that promotes uterine contraction, and the vicious cycle continues till the baby is delivered.

2. **LH surge:** This is increased luteinizing hormone (LH) secretion that leads to ovulation. Normally, estrogen inhibits LH secretion. But, before ovulation, estrogen provides positive feedback to LH secretion, which results in LH surge.
3. **The Hodgkin's cycle:** Sodium influx that causes upstroke (depolarization) of nerve or muscle action potential (Flowchart 3.3). Opening of few set of sodium channel provides positive feedback for opening of other sodium channels that results in massive sodium influx causing depolarization.
4. **Activation of digestive enzymes:** The activation of digestive enzymes pepsinogen and trypsinogen by pepsin and trypsin respectively.
5. **Enzyme cascade hypothesis of coagulation:** Activation of one clotting factor, which acts as an enzyme to activate the next clotting factor in the coagulation cascade.

Negative Feedback System

Negative feedback control system requires a sensor that detects the change in variable, a control center that receives input from the sensor and initiates command signal, and an effector that brings in responses according to the command signal directed from the control center (*see* Flowchart 3.2). Physiological variables sometimes require more than one homeostatic mechanism for their regulation. For example, control of arterial pressure involves pressure monitoring system, volume monitoring system, hormonal mechanisms, reflex regulation, autonomic control, etc.

The sensor: The sensor contains receptors that monitor the change of the variable and provide sensory signals to the control center of the changes detected. The examples are carotid sinus and aortic arch that contain baroreceptors in their wall and detect change in pressure in their lumen. They send signals to the control centers located in the medullary cardiovascular centers.

The control center: Usually, control centers are located in the central nervous system, especially in the brain. For example, centers for blood pressure regulation are located in medulla and the hypothalamus.

The effector: The effector is the target organ that carries out the command of the control center to achieve an effective response. For example, blood vessels and heart are the effector organs for blood pressure regulation. Depending on the rate of sympathetic and vagal discharges, the effector organs change their activities to achieve the target effect. When the deviation is the increase in the variable above the set point, the effector will be inhibited and inhibition continues until the variable is reduced to the normal set point. Reverse process is initiated when the variable is reduced below the set point (Application Box 3.1).

Application Box 3.1

Priorities in homeostatic controls: Life-saving regulatory mechanisms normally take precedence over those that are activated routinely. For example, regulation of body temperature on exposure to extreme weather gets priority over the control of water content of the body in natural conditions. Similarly, activation of withdrawal reflex in response to a noxious stimulus, which protects the body from injury, takes precedence over other somatic reflex and visceral reflexes.

Kidney Plays a Vital Role

The kidneys are important organ for the homeostasis of many physiological variables such as regulation of blood volume and blood pressure, pH balance, electrolyte composition of body fluids, and osmolarity of fluid compartments.

Examples of Homeostatic Regulations

Important examples of homeostatic regulations are control of pH, osmolarity, and water and electrolyte composition of the body fluids, regulation of solutes in the blood like blood sugar, balance of body weight, etc. Another example is the myotatic or stretch reflex that seeks to maintain muscle length. Details of few examples are given below:

Body temperature regulation: The temperature of the body is maintained within a narrow range of 96°F to 98.4°F. Increased temperature above normal is called as fever and below is called as hypothermia. When temperature is above normal, the body activates controlling mechanisms to increase heat loss through cutaneous vasodilation and sweating. When hypothermia develops, the body responds by decreasing heat loss through vasoconstriction and by increasing heat production through shivering.

Blood pressure regulation: The normal systolic pressure in adult is kept constant between 100 and 140 mm Hg and diastolic pressure between 60 and 85 mm Hg. Sustained rise in pressure is called hypertension, and fall in pressure is called hypotension that initiates many neural and humoral mechanisms to restore blood pressure (for details refer "Regulation of blood pressure".

Regulation of hormone secretion: Secretion of many hormones such as thyroxine, cortisol, etc. is regulated mainly by negative feedback mechanisms. Increase in hormone concentration in plasma inhibits their production and decrease in concentration facilitates their production mainly by altering the secretion of their regulating trophic hormones. This forms the basis of diagnosis of these hormonal disorders.

INTRACELLULAR HOMEOSTASIS

Though, traditionally homeostasis (constancy of internal environment) refers to the stability of extracellular fluid volume and composition, it is also applicable to intracellular fluid and intracellular conditions. Rather, the primary objective of homeostasis is to maintain intracellular homeostasis that promotes cell or tissue (organ) functions. Homeostasis is greatly affected by intracellular activities. For example, pH homeostasis, temperature homeostasis, Na^+ homeostasis, K^+ homeostasis, etc. depend mainly on intracellular enzyme activities and cell metabolism. Similarly, intracellular milieu is largely influenced by changes in the ECF volume and composition. Hence, homeostasis is mostly achieved by the coordinated and balanced interaction between intracellular and extracellular environments of the body.

CHAPTER SUMMARY

Homeostasis is ***defined*** as the maintenance of the constancy of the internal environment of the body.
Homeostatic regulation is achieved by two feedback mechanisms: The negative feedback and the positive feedback.

Negative Feedback

The negative feedback mechanism is the general mechanism of regulations in which if the variable is raised above the set point, the feedback mechanism triggers processes that inhibit the formation of the variable and if the variable is lowered below the set point, the feedback system withdraws the inhibition to allow production of the variable. Regulation of hormone secretion is the common examples.

Positive Feedback

In a positive feedback system, increase in the variable triggers the processes that further increase the variable. This process triggers a vicious cycle that terminates only when the stimulus applied to trigger is withdrawn or the process itself is self-terminated. Important examples of positive feedback regulation are parturition reflex initiated by oxytocin, LH surge during ovulation, The Hodgkin's cycle of sodium influx during depolarization of action potential, and enzyme activation in coagulation cascade.

Important to Know (Must Read)

1. Usually no **Long Questions** are asked from this chapter.
2. Homeostasis, Feedback mechanisms, Negative feedback system, may be the **Short Questions**.
3. In **Viva**, examiner may ask… Define homeostasis, Give examples of homeostasis, and What are the feedback mechanisms and give their examples.

CHAPTER

4

Cellular Organization and Intercellular Connections

Learning Objectives

On completion of study of this chapter, the student **MUST** be able to:

1. Give the structure and list the functions of cell membrane, organelles and nucleus.
2. Name various cytoskeletons and molecular motors of cell and give their functions.
3. Classify intercellular junctions and give their functions.
4. Describe the importance of gap junction in health and disease.
5. Classify cell adhesion molecules and give their functions.

The student **MAY** also be able to:

1. Give the details of composition of cell membrane and function of each constituent.
2. Describe the details of the structure, functions and dysfunctions of each organelle of the cell.
3. Explain the detailed structure, functions and dysfunctions of microfilaments, cellular motors and cell adhesion molecules.
4. Give the structure, functions and dysfunctions of intercellular junctions.

CELLULAR ORGANIZATION

The cell is the structural and functional unit of tissues. A cell consists of three fundamental structures: cell membrane, cytoplasm and nucleus (Fig. 4.1).

1. The **cell membrane** or the plasma membrane is the boundary in all animal cells that surrounds the *cytoplasm*, the fluid medium containing a variety of organelles.
2. In **cytoplasm**, *organelles* are bound by membranes similar to the structure of cell membrane. The organelles usually present in animal cells are mitochondria, ribosome, peroxisome, lysosomes, centrioles, endoplasmic reticulum and Golgi apparatus. Cytoplasm also contains filamentous *cytoskeletal structures* such as microfilaments, intermediate filaments and microtubules.
3. The **nucleus** is present at the center of the cell. In addition, there are many other proteins in the cells like actin and myosin that provide strength and mobility to the cell and also the mechanisms for adhesion to other cells.

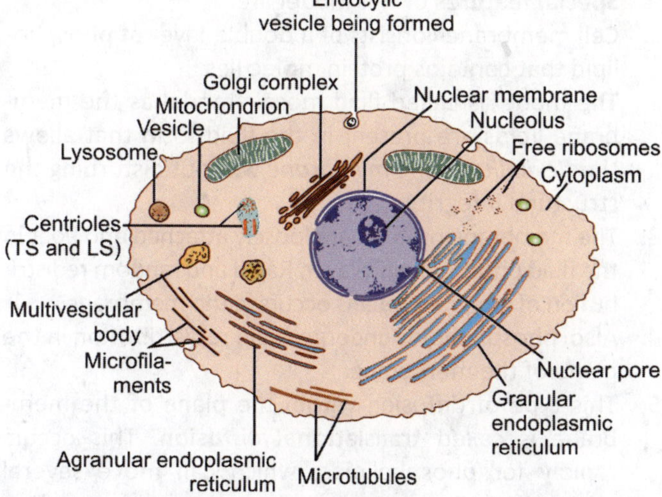

Fig. 4.1: Structure of a cell. Note the organization of various organelles and nucleus in the cell.

Cell Membrane

Cell membrane is the protective sheath of the cell. It exchanges materials between the cytoplasm and the external environment, facilitates interaction between cells and helps in anchoring the cells to each other.

Structure of Cell Membrane

The cell membrane is basically a double layer of lipid molecules having thickness of 7–10 nm, into which are inserted

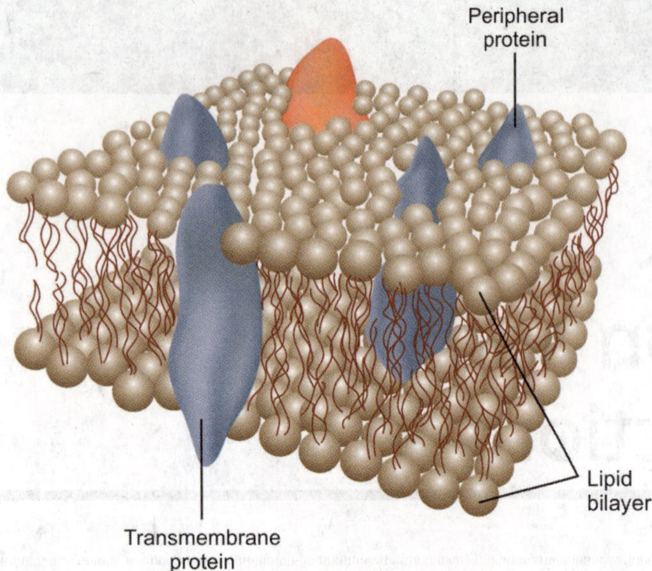

Fig. 4.2: Structure of a cell membrane (The Fluid Mosaic Model). Note the arrangement of lipid bilayers and proteins in the membrane.

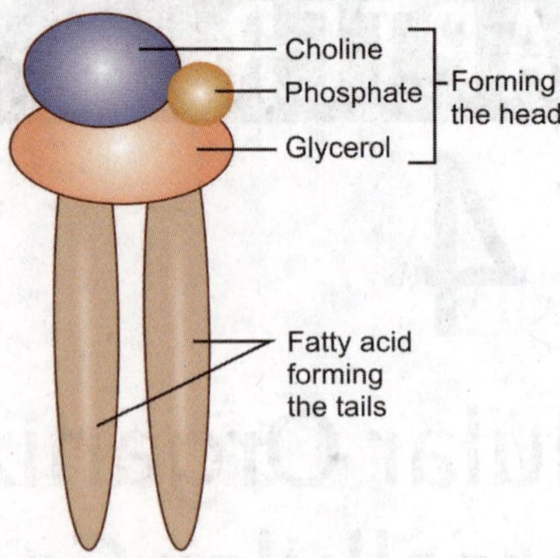

Fig. 4.3: Amphipathic nature of membrane lipid. Note that polar head is hydrophilic and nonpolar tail is hydrophobic.

or attached various protein molecules (Fig. 4.2). Lipids constitute about 45% of the dry weight of the membrane and protein constitutes about 50% and carbohydrate constitutes 5%.

Fluid-Mosaic Model of the Membrane

Though, many models for cell membrane have been described in the past, the widely accepted one is *Fluid-Mosaic Model* described by Singer and Nicolson in 1972.

Special features of this model are:

1. Cell membrane consists of a double-layer of phospholipid that contains protein molecules.
2. The model is called fluid mosaic model as the membrane lipids are present in the fluid form that allows the *flexibility of the membrane* without disturbing the structural integrity.
3. The membrane proteins are loosely attached and float in the fluid phospholipid bilayer. Rapid and random redistribution of integral proteins occurs in the membrane.
4. Also, phospholipids undergo rapid redistribution in the plane of the membrane.
5. This type of diffusion within the plane of the membrane is called **translational diffusion**. This occurs rapidly for phospholipids, which can move several micrometers per second.
6. The fluidity of the membrane is mainly dependent on the lipid composition of the membrane.

   Effect of temperature: In a lipid bilayer, the hydrophobic chains of fatty acids are highly aligned or arranged orderly to provide a rather stiff structure. When temperature increases, the hydrophobic side chains undergo a transition from its ordered gel or crystalline state to a more disordered liquid state. The temperature at which this disorder or melting occurs is called **transition temperature** (Tm). When the fatty acid chains are longer and more saturated, they interact more strongly with each other and cause higher values of Tm. As a result, higher temperature is required to increase the fluidity of the lipid bilayer having long chain and saturated fatty acids. Thus, *degree of unsaturation* determines the fluidity of the membrane.

Lipid Bilayer

The major lipids in the cell membrane are phospholipids, glycolipids and cholesterol.

1. The **phospholipids** are phosphatidylcholine, sphingomyelin, phosphatidylserine and phosphatidyl ethanolamine.
2. **Glycolipids** are generally found in the outer layer.

   Lipids are *amphipathic* ("amphi" means both) molecules as their head or polar region is hydrophilic and tail or nonpolar region is hydrophobic (Fig. 4.3). The globular or the head end contains phosphate or hydroxyl moieties that are positively charged and soluble in water. The tail end contains two chains of fatty acids that are insoluble in water. The arrangement is such that the hydrophobic tail ends are directed toward the center and the hydrophilic head is located to periphery of the membrane (as depicted in Figure 4.2). Thus, hydrophilic head of lipid molecules faces the aqueous phase from both inside and outside the cell. A similar bilayer arrangement is found in bile salts where they form spherical micelles.
3. **Cholesterol** is incorporated into the hydrophobic regions of the membrane, and serves to reinforce the lipid permeability barrier.

Application Box 4.1

Determinant of the fluidity of membrane: The fluidity of a membrane depends on the composition of lipids and the degree of unsaturation. The major determinant is its ***cholesterol-phospholipid ratio***. In eukaryotes, the ratio is about 1:1. Higher cholesterol content reduces the fluidity of the membrane.

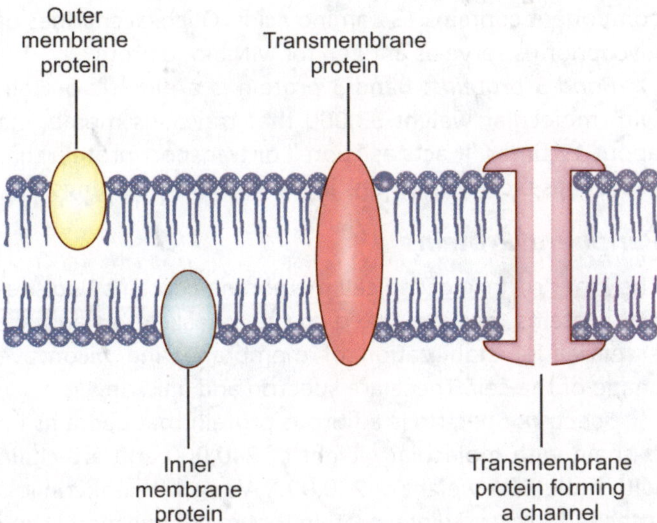

Fig. 4.4: Arrangement of proteins in the membrane. Note the presence of integral (or transmembrane) protein and peripheral (outer membrane and inner membrane) proteins. A membrane channel is formed by a transmembrane protein.

The individual phospholipid molecules can move freely within the specific layer (but not from one layer to another). Hence, the cell membrane is said to be fluid in nature (Application Box 4.1).

Functions of the Lipid Bilayer

The main function of the lipid bilayer of a cell membrane is to create a **permeability barrier** between the interstitial fluid and the cytoplasm. The permeability of a substance depends on whether it is lipid-soluble or water-soluble. *Lipid soluble substances* like oxygen and alcohol can pass easily through the cell membrane, whereas *water soluble substances* like urea and glucose cannot pass easily. Thus, lipid bilayer makes the membrane semipermeable.

Membrane Proteins

The protein content of biological membrane depends on the function of the membrane. For example, in the Schwann cell, the cell membrane is concerned with insulating the nerve axon, which is mainly the function of lipids. Therefore, protein constitutes less than 25 percent of the membrane. In membrane of mitochondria, which is involved in cell metabolism, 75 percent of the membrane is protein. However, average protein content of membrane is 50–60% of the membrane mass.

Membrane proteins are of two types: Integral proteins and peripheral proteins (Fig. 4.4).

Integral Proteins

Some membrane proteins that span the entire thickness of the membrane are known as integral proteins. They are also called **transmembrane proteins**. Some integral proteins penetrate only a portion of the membrane (Fig. 4.4), so that they are exposed either to the external environment of the cell (interstitial fluid) or to the cytoplasmic surface of the membrane (intracellular fluid). Some membrane proteins also move laterally within the membrane (e.g. membrane receptors can move to sites of endocytosis).

The **functions of integral membrane proteins** are as follows:

1. **Serve as channel proteins***:* Channels or pores are integral proteins through which water-soluble substances like glucose and electrolytes can diffuse across the cell membrane.
2. **Act as carriers:** Carrier proteins transport substances through cell membrane by facilitated diffusion; for example transport of glucose through glucose transporter.
3. **Serve as ion pumps:** Membrane proteins serve as pumps for active transport of ions across the membrane; for example Na^+–K^+ ATPase that pumps K^+ into the cell and Na^+ out of the cell against their concentration gradient.
4. **Serve as receptor and enzyme proteins:** Integral proteins that are present toward the outer half of the membrane usually serve as receptors and usually those on the inner half serve as enzymes. Membrane G proteins belong to this category of proteins.
5. **Antigenic functions:** Complex membrane proteins such as glycoproteins act as antigens on the surface of the cell; for example blood group antigens in the membrane of red cells.

Peripheral Proteins

Some protein molecules are inserted lightly in the outer or inner border of the membrane or are just bound to the surface of the membrane. Such proteins are called peripheral proteins.

They are of two types: Intrinsic and extrinsic proteins.

Intrinsic proteins: They are present on the inner surface of the membrane. They usually serve as enzymes or anchor proteins for cytoskeleton and other microfilaments that maintain cell shape.

Extrinsic proteins: They are present on the outer surface of the membrane. They serve as **cell adhesion molecules** for anchoring cells with basal lamina and with neighboring cells. They can be removed without disrupting the membrane.

Membrane Carbohydrates

The external surface of the cell membrane is loosely covered by a carbohydrate layer known as the cell coat or **glycocalyx.** These carbohydrates are usually oligosaccharides that are covalently linked to membrane proteins forming glycoproteins or lipids forming glycolipids. Some are also polysaccharide chains of proteoglycans, the integral membrane protein. Thus, the outer surface of the lipid bilayer is covered by a layer of glycoproteins and glycolipids.

Functions of the Glycocalyx

1. Glycocalyx serves as a **protective coat**. Carbohydrate is negatively charged and therefore prevents negative particles like protein molecules to interact between cells.

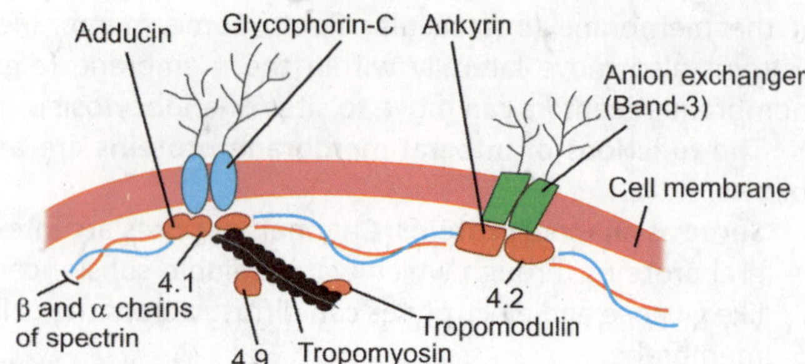

Fig. 4.5: Structure of red cell membrane. Note the presence of special proteins such as ankyrin, spectrin and adducin that provide plasticity (deformability) to the membrane, in addition to the presence of anion exchanger (band 3 protein) and glycophorin-C and other submembrane proteins.

2. Some of the transmembrane glycoproteins like selectins recognize and bind with specific oligosaccharides on other cell membranes, and therefore, permit **temporary cell-to-cell adhesion**. Such temporary adhesion occurs between neutrophils and endothelial cells at the site of inflammation. Stronger adhesion between cells is formed by integral membrane proteins such as integrins.
3. Some carbohydrate molecules serve as **receptors**.

Functions of Cell Membrane

1. Cell membrane **maintains a constant and distinctive intracellular environment**, which is essential for functioning of the organelles. For example, the intracellular fluid has lower concentration of sodium and chloride, low pH, but higher concentration of potassium, organic phosphates and magnesium.
2. Cell membrane **maintains cell volume** by actively transferring ions across it, especially by pumping sodium ions out of the cell.
3. In neurons and muscle cells, it maintains a **potential difference** between intracellular and extracellular surfaces, which enables cells to respond to various stimuli.
4. Cell membrane helps in **recognizing foreign cells or antigens** so that they can be destroyed by phagocytes.

Special Features of RBC Membrane

The red cell membrane is most extensively studied membrane. In addition to the general features of membrane described above, red cell membrane contains some special proteins such as integral and peripheral proteins.

Integral Proteins

Two special types of integral proteins are found in red cell membrane (Fig. 4.5). These are glycophorins and band-3 proteins.

Glycophorins: Glycophorins are glycoproteins that contain 60% carbohydrate and 40% protein. The carbohydrate component is oligosaccharide and the polypeptide component contains 131 amino acids. Oligosaccharides of glycophorins serve as antigen for MN blood group.

Band-3 proteins: Band-3 protein is a dimeric protein with molecular weight 93,000 that traverses membrane about 12 times. It acts as "pore" or transport protein that exchanges bicarbonate ions in the capillaries of lungs.

Peripheral Proteins

The inner surface of red cell membrane contains two special proteins that are linked to the cytoskeleton and are essential for stabilization of membrane and biconcave shape of the cell. These are spectrin and ankyrin.

Spectrin: Spectrin is a fibrous protein that contains an α-chain with molecular weight of 240,000 and a β-chain with molecular weight of 220,000. Along with ankyrin it is attached to cytoskeletal protein that maintains membrane integrity and cell shape.

Ankyrin: The cytoskeletal proteins are attached to spectrin through ankyrin. Ankyrin has molecular weight of 200,000. It has two domains: one bind with spectrin and other with N-terminal region of band-3 protein that extends into cytoskeleton (Application Box 4.2).

Application Box 4.2

***Diseases due to membrane protein defects*:** Disorders of red cells such as hereditary spherocytosis and elliptocytosis occur due to defects in the membrane proteins (for details, refer "Red Blood Cell").

Cell Organelles

The usually occurring organelles in animal cells are mitochondria, endoplasmic reticulum, Golgi apparatus, ribosome, peroxisome, lysosome and centriole. The red blood cell is the only living cell, which loses nucleus and most of its organelles such as mitochondria, ribosome and lysosome during maturation.

Mitochondria

Mitochondria are the "power house" of the cell. They are cigar-shaped organelles whose shape, size and number vary in different tissues of the body. They are most abundant in cells that have high rate of metabolism, as in liver, cardiac muscle, etc.

Structure

Mitochondria consist of two important components: Membranes and cristae.

Mitochondrial Membranes

Electron microscopy shows that each mitochondrion has two layers of membranes: the outer and inner membranes.

Outer Mitochondrial Membrane: This forms a continuous envelop of the organelle. Outer membrane consists mostly of phospholipids and cholesterol, and contains a specific membrane protein that forms *"porin"*. Porins are channels that permit substances with molecular weight of less than 10,000 to diffuse freely across the outer membrane.

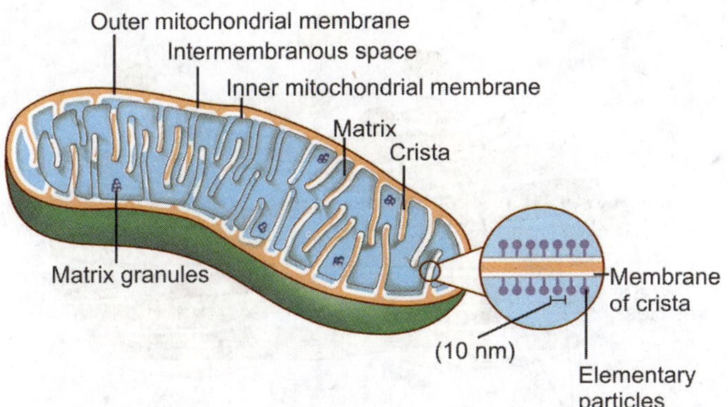

Fig. 4.6: Structure of mitochondria. Note that the cristae are infolding of inner mitochondrial membrane.

Inner Mitochondrial Membrane: It is rich in proteins, and the ratio of lipid to protein is 0.27 to 1. Hence, it is virtually impermeable to polar and ionic substances. The inner membrane is folded into multiple incomplete septa like structures called **cristae** (Fig. 4.6), which is rich in many enzymes like cytochromes b, C_1, C, a and a_3, NADH dehydrogenase, succinate dehydrogenase, electron transferring flavoproteins, carnitine-palmitoyl transferase, etc.

Important Note

Number of cristae: Number of cristae is more in resting state of mitochondrion, and decreases in the respiring state.

Mitochondrial Matrix

The region enclosed by the inner membrane is called **matrix**. An amorphous material fills the matrix, which contains enzymes involved in the Kreb's citric acid cycle and fatty acid oxidation (Table 4.1). Matrix also contains several strands of DNA, ribosomes and enzymes for synthesis of proteins coded in the mitochondrial genome.

Functions

The inner membrane contains the cytochromes of the electron transport system and the associated enzymes for oxidative phosphorylation. The TCA cycle takes place in the matrix. The initial breakdown of proteins, carbohydrates and fats occurs in the cytoplasm of the cell, and the final end product that enters the mitochondria as acetyl-CoA combines with oxaloacetate to from citric acid. The end products of the citric acid cycle (Kreb's cycle) are CO_2, H_2O and ATP.

Like most components of the cell, mitochondria have a short lifespan and are constantly renewed. As they have strands of DNA they are capable of self-replication as well as protein synthesis (Clinical Box 4.1).

Clinical Box 4.1

Mitochondrial diseases: The disease that affects mitochondrial energy transduction is called ***Luft's disease***. The abnormality of mitochondrial DNA leads to cellular dysfunction called as ***mitochondrial cytopathy syndrome***, which manifests with muscle weakness, degenerative lesions of the brain and high levels of lactic acid in blood. Mitochondria are also damaged by free radicals and affected in age-related degenerations.

Table 4.1: Mitochondrial enzymes.
A. Membrane enzymes
I. Enzymes of outer membrane
1. Cytochrome b_5 and b_5 reductase
2. Fatty acid CoA synthase
3. Phospholipase A
4. Nucleoside diphosphokinase
II. Enzymes of inner membrane
1. Cytochrome b, C_1, C, a and a_3
2. NADPH dehydrogenase
3. Succinate dehydrogenase
4. Electron transferring flavoproteins
5. β-OH-butyrate dehydrogenase
6. Carnitine palmitoyltransferase
7. All translocases
B. Enzymes in inter-membrane space
1. Adenylate kinase
2. Nucleoside diphosphokinase
3. Sulfite oxidase
C. Enzymes in the matrix
1. Pyruvate dehydrogenase complex
2. Citrate synthase
3. Isocitrate dehydrogenase
4. Malate dehydrogenase
5. Fatty acid oxidation system
6. Ornithine transcarbamylase
7. α-oxoglutarate dehydrogenase
8. Aconitase

Endoplasmic Reticulum

The endoplasmic reticulum (ER) consists of a network of anastomosing membranous ***tubules***, ***vesicles***, and flattened ***cisternae***. The membranes of ER are continuous with the outer membrane of nucleus and are also connected with Golgi apparatus (Fig. 4.7). ER is the site of the synthesis of proteins and lipids for the membrane of the cell and organelles, and secretory vesicles of the cytoplasm. They are of two types: rough ER and the smooth ER.

Rough Endoplasmic Reticulum

When surface of ER is studded with ribosome, the organelle is called rough ER (RER) or *granular ER* as it gives a "rough" or "granular" appearance to it. In some cells such as red blood cells, the ribosomes lie free in the cytoplasm. RER are present in more number in cells that are actively involved in protein synthesis like acinar cells of pancreas and neurons. In neurons, *the Nissl garanules are modified RER*.

Functions of RER

1. It is concerned with ***protein synthesis***. Therefore, it is abundant in cells of endocrine glands and cells secreting digestive enzymes.

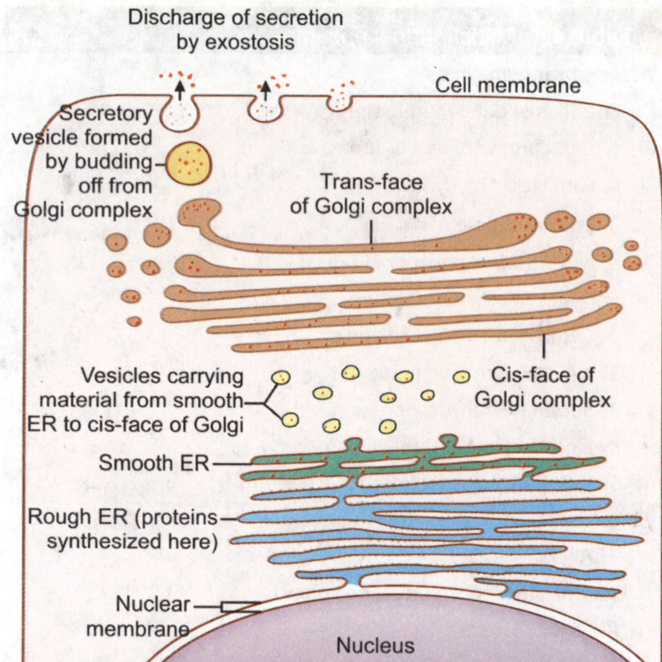

Fig. 4.7: Structure of endoplasmic reticulum (ER). Note that the inner part of ER is in continuity with the nuclear memberane and the outer part interacts with Golgi complex. Rough ER has numerous ribosomes on the membrane, and smooth ER has no ribosome on the surface.

2. It also plays some role in the conjugation of carbohydrates with proteins to form glycoproteins, a function which it shares with the Golgi apparatus.

Smooth Endoplasmic Reticulum

When ribosomes are not attached to the surface of ER, the organelle is called smooth ER (SER) or *agranular ER* as its surface has "smooth" or "agranular" appearance.

Functions of SER

1. It is concerned with the synthesis of lipids. Hence it is abundant in cells that synthesize cholesterol, steroid hormones and phospholipids.
2. In muscles, it is called sarcoplasmic reticulum, which is specialized for the storage of calcium ions that is released during excitation-contraction coupling.
3. SER is part of intracellular transport system as it is continuous with the RER and Golgi apparatus.
4. It is also the site for the detoxification or neutralization of hormones and toxic substances.

Golgi Apparatus

The Golgi apparatus (GA) is also known as Golgi complex or **dictyosome**. It is present in all cells and generally is located close to the nucleus. It appears as flat discs that are dilated peripherally and stacked together in a bunch as **stack of cisternae** (Fig. 4.8). Anatomically and functionally it is closely associated with endoplasmic reticulum. Functionally GA two main regions: cis and tranas. The region nearer to the nucleus is the **cis face** (***cis Golgi***)

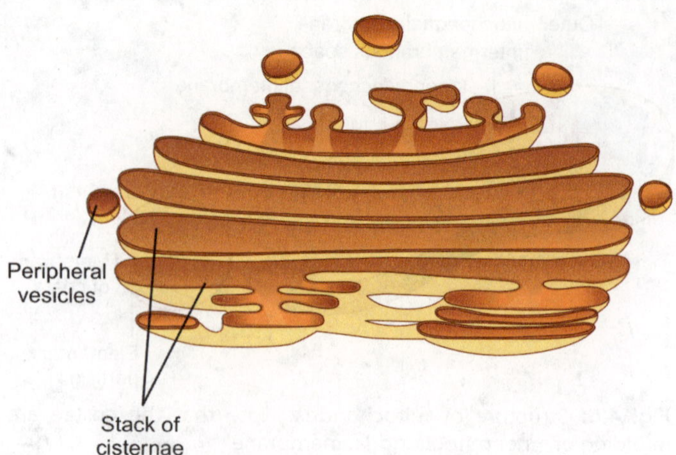

Fig. 4.8: Structure of Golgi complex. Note the structure mainly consisting of stack of cisternae.

and the region close to the membrane is the **trans face** (***trans Golgi***) (Fig. 4.7).

Major Functions of GA

1. It is the site for the **packaging of secretory products into the secretory granules**. Materials produced in rough ER travel through the lumen of smooth ER. Vesicles budding off from smooth ER transport material to cis-face of Golgi complex. Some proteins are phosphorylated here, and then pass to the trans-face, where they are packaged into the secretory vesicles (Fig. 4.7).
2. It is the site for the **incorporation of carbohydrates** into the newly synthesized proteins to form glycoproteins.
3. Lysosomal enzymes are formed in GA.
4. Transports material to other organelles and cell surface.

Lysosomes

Lysosomes are membrane-bound spherical organelles that contain a variety of ***hydrolytic enzymes*** meant for intracytoplasmic digestion. More than 40 different lysosomal enzymes (lysozymes) have been isolated. Some important lysozymes are listed in Table 4.2. Lysosomes are found in almost all animal cells except erythrocytes. They are particularly abundant in cells having high phagocytic activity such as neutrophils and monocytes.

Important Note

Absence of lysosomes: Lysosomes are present in all cells except RBC. They are prominently present in neutrophils.

In granulocytes, the lysosomes appear as cytoplasmic granules. Lysosomal activity of a cell tissue can be determined (Application Box 4.3).

Application Box 4.3

Marker for lysosomal activity: Acid phosphatase is used as a marker for lysosomal activity.

Table 4.2: Important lysosomal enzymes.

A. Proteolytic enzymes
1. Cathepsins (proteinases)
2. Collagenases
3. Elastase
B. Lipolytic enzymes
1. Lipases
2. Phospholipases
3. Fatty acyl esterases
C. Carbohydrate splitting enzymes
1. α-glycosidase
2. β-galactosidase
3. Hyaluronidase
4. Arylsulfatase
D. Nucleic acid hydrolyzing enzymes
1. Ribonuclease
2. Deoxyribonuclease
E. Other enzymes
1. Acid phosphatases
2. Catalase

During the process of phagocytosis, the **phagosome** that is formed by the cytoplasmic pseudopodia containing foreign body such as bacteria, viruses, etc. fuse with the lysosomes to from **phagolysosome** (Fig. 4.9) and lysosomal enzymes later digest these foreign organism. Therefore, lysosomes are known as ***autophagosomes.***

The interior of lysosome is acidic (pH is about 5) compared to its cytosolic exterior (pH of cytoplasm is about 7.2). Acidic interior of this organelle is due to the action of proton pump, the **H^+-ATPase**, present on the lysosomal membrane that pumps protons (H^+) from cytosol into the lysosomal interior against its electrochemical gradient. The lysosomal enzymes are **acid hydolases** as they function best in acidic pH.

Types of Lysosomes

There are three forms of lysosomes: Primary lysosomes, secondary lysosomes (endolysosome) and tertiary lysosomes (phagolysosome) (Flowchart 4.1).

Primary lysosomes: They are formed with hydrolytic enzymes synthesized by rough endoplasmic reticulum and packaged in the Golgi apparatus. They are generally referred to as *storage vacuoles*.

Secondary lysosomes: These are lysosomes fused with endosomes. Hence they are called ***endolysosome.***

Tertiary lysosomes: These are *autophagic vacuoles* or autophagosomes. They are formed by fusion of phagocytic vacuoles with primary lysosomes. Hence they are called ***phagolysosome***.

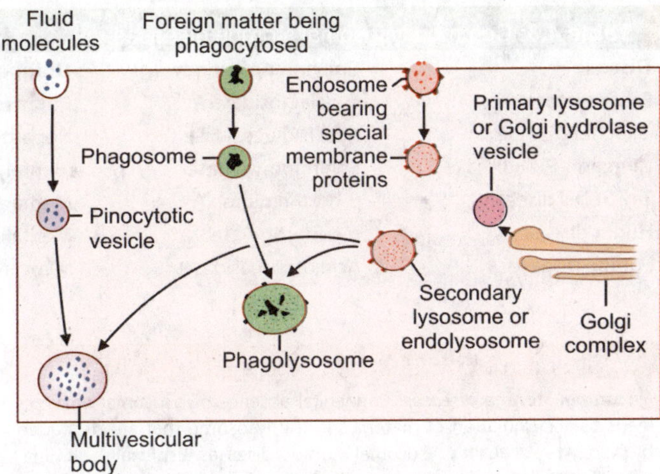

Fig. 4.9: Formation of primary lysosome, secondary lysosome and phagolysosome.

Flowchart 4.1: Types of lysosomes and their functions.

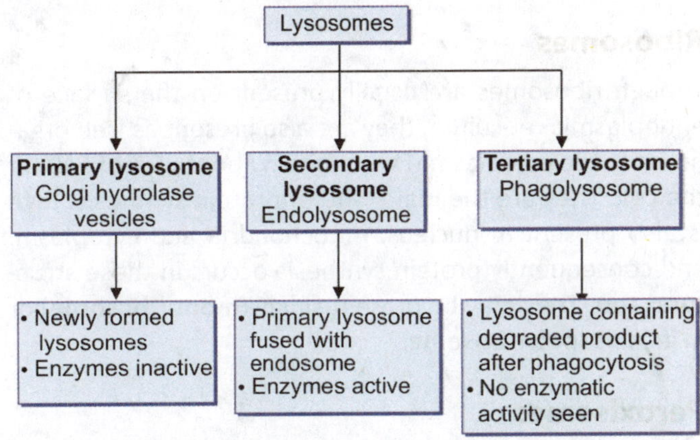

Important Note

Residual bodies: After the materials in phagosome have been digested by lysosome, some waste materials may be left. The undigestible remnants in the lysosomes are called as residual bodies.

Functions of Lysosome

1. Lysosomes contain many enzymes essential for **intracellular digestions**. Absence of these enzymes leads to various storage diseases (Clinical Box 4.2), as listed in Table 4.3.
2. Lysosomes kill and remove infective organisms and foreign bodies.
3. Acrosome, located on the head of spermatozoa is a specialized lysosome that contains many hydrolytic enzymes. Acrosome plays an important role in penetration of ovum by sperm.
4. **Autolysis:** When a cell is damaged or ruptured, the enzymes liberated within the cytoplasm digest the cytoplasmic contents, a process known as *autolysis*. The autolytic enzymes are mainly lysosomal enzymes.
5. Lysosomes remove intracellular products of metabolism from the cell.

Table 4.3: Common lysosomal storage diseases.

Disease	Enzyme deficiency	Unique features
Fabry disease	α-galactosidase A	Cutaneous angiokeratomas and hypohydrosis.
Gaucher disease	Acid β-glucosidase	Hepatosplenomegaly, and skeletal dysplasia.
Niemann-Pick disease	Sphingomyelinase	Mental retardation, seizures, lung failure.
Tay-Sachs disease	β-hexaminidase A	Mental retardation, macrocephaly and hypercusis in infants.
Hurler disease	α-L-iduronidase	Mental retardation, coarse facies, CVS involvement.
Pompe disease	Acid α-glucosidase	Myocardiopathy

Clinical Box 4.2

Lysosomal storage diseases: Congenital absence of lysosomal enzymes leads to accumulation of materials in the lysosome that are degraded by lysozymes, causing lysosomal storage diseases. Especially, elimination of certain substances from the cells of the body, e.g. glycogen, cerebrosides, gangliosides and sphingomyelin mainly depend on the activity of lysosomal enzymes. Therefore, in the absence of active lysosomes, intracellular accumulation of these substances interferes with normal cell function and produces diseases. Accumulation of partly digested cellular material is called ***inclusion bodies***.

Ribosomes

Though ribosomes are usually present on the surface of endoplasmic reticulum, they are also present as free organelles in the cytoplasm. They contain about 85% of RNA of the cell. They are the major site of protein synthesis. RNA is also present in nucleus, mitochondria and cytoplasm, and consequently protein synthesis occurs in these structures too. They may be present singly (**monoribosome**) or in groups (**polyribosomes**)

Peroxisomes

Peroxisomes are small spherical organelles having diameter of about 0.5 μ, and therefore denoted as **microbodies**.

Specialties of peroxisomes:

1. They are formed by budding from or by division of smooth endoplasmic reticulum. They are referred to as *subcellular respiratory organelles*. But, they do not have energy-coupled electron transport system.
2. They contain **oxidases** that promote oxidation of lipids (especially β-oxidation of long chain fatty acids) forming acetyl-CoA and hydrogen peroxide (H_2O_2), and **catalases** that liberate oxygen from H_2O_2. They protect the tissue from oxidative stress (Application Box 4.4)
3. With the help of **peroxins**, the protein chaperons, various proteins with specific signal sequence are directed to peroxisome. The membrane of peroxisome contains a number of specific proteins that transport substances between peroxisome matrix and cytosol.
4. Peroxisome matrix contains **more than 50 enzymes** that are involved in many metabolic reactions of lipids (long chain fatty acids, plasmalogen, cholesterol, bile acids) purines, amino acids and H_2O_2. Deficiency of enzymes leads to many diseases (Clinical Box 4.3)
5. Proliferation of peroxisome is caused by many synthetic products that act on receptors in the nuclei of cells, known as **peroxisome proliferation activated receptors** (PPARs). PPARs are members of nuclear receptor superfamily those on activation bind to DNA and produce changes in mRNA production. PPARs have extensive physiologic effects and affect many tissues and organs.

Application Box 4.4

Peroxisomes protect from oxidative stress (OS): H_2O_2, a potent oxidant produced during metabolic reactions is one of the agents for oxidative stress. H_2O_2 is destroyed by catalase, a peroxisomal enzyme, which is designated as an antioxidant for combating OS. Thus, peroxisomes protect cells from the toxic effects H_2O_2. Hence, increased catalase activity is one of the markers of OS.

Clinical Box 4.3

Diseases of peroxisomes: Peroxisomes may be abnormal or absent in inherited disorders

1. ***Zellweger syndrome***, which occurs due to mutations in the gene encoding certain proteins such as peroxins or peroxisomal enzymes. This syndrome is characterized by profound neurologic impairment, accumulation of very-long chain fatty acids, abnormalities in synthesis of bile acids and marked reduction of plasmalogens. The child usually dies within a year in this disorder.
2. Another similar genetic disorder is ***infantile Refsum disease***, which is less severe and only few proteins are affected.
3. ***Brown-Schilder's disease (Adenoleukodystrophy)*** occurs due to insufficient oxidation of very long chain fatty acids by peroxisomes. This is an autosomal recessive disease manifests with progressive degeneration of liver, kidney and brain.
4. ***Primary hyperoxaluria*** occurs due to defective peroxisomal metabolism of glycosylate derived from glycine.

Centrosomes

Centrosome is located close to the nucleus in eukaryotic animal cells. It is formed by two **centrioles** placed at right angle to each other that are present within the amorphous pericentriolar material. Centrioles are short cylindrical structures made up of microtubules placed in group of three (triplets) that run longitudinally in the wall of centrioles. There are nine sets of triplets arranged at regular intervals in the wall of each centriole (Fig. 4.10). The subunits of microtubules in centrosome are **γ-tubulins**. Centrosomes are ***microtubule-organizing center*** (MTOCs).

Functions

Centrosomes regulate chromosome movement during cell division. They duplicate themselves and move apart from each other to the poles of mitotic spindle to monitor the process of cell division.

Cytoskeleton

Cytoskeleton is an intracellular system of fibers that not only maintains the structural integrity of the cell, but also allows appropriate change in cell shape for cell mobility and participation of cell in various physiological activities. It consists of microfilaments, microtubules and intermediate filaments. These cytoskeletal elements are made up of different cell proteins (Table 4.4).

Microfilaments

All eukaryotic cells contain microfilaments that contribute to the maintenance of and change in cell shape and regulation of cell functions. These are long solid filaments (Fig. 4.11A) having diameter of about 7 nm. They are made up of **actin**. Actin is the most common cell protein that accounts for about 15% of total protein in the cells.

Actin in the globular form is called **G actin**, which is the unpolymerized actin subunit. G actin subunits polymerize to form the filamentous actin, referred to as **F actin**. In vivo, actin filaments polymerize and depolymerize. Also, polymerization occurs at one end of actin filament and depolymerization occurs at the other end.

Special characteristics:

1. Though microfilaments are well developed in muscle cells, they are present in almost all cells and better organized in cells that secrete granular content by exocytosis. For example, the developed contractile system in platelets consists of microtubules and extensive network of microfilaments.
2. Microfilaments help platelets to change shape and move granules from interior of cytoplasm to canaliculi for release of chemicals (*release reaction of platelet*).
3. In cells with microvilli on their epithelial surface, microfilaments extend into the microvilli.

Functions

1. Microfilaments are the major contractile fibers of the cell that help in change in cell shape and cell movement.
2. As microfilaments exhibit contractile phenomena within the cytoplasm, they help in phagocytosis, transport and secretion of cellular materials, cell contraction, cell discharge, movement of secretory granules, etc.

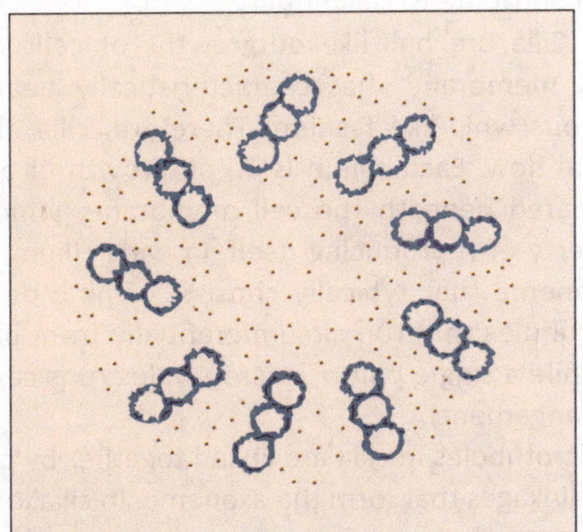

Fig. 4.10: Transverse section across a centriole. Note nine groups of tubules, each group having three microtubules.

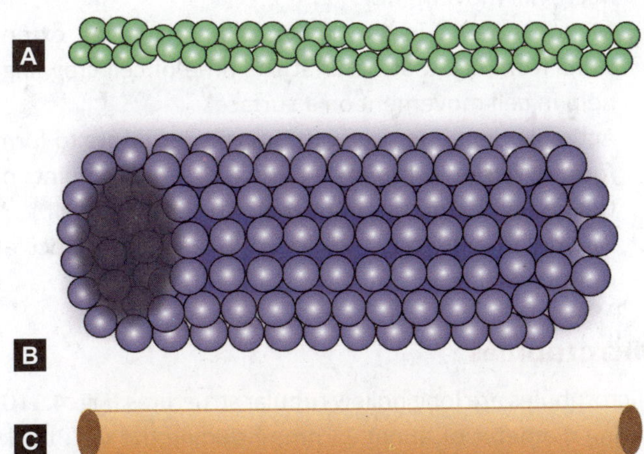

Figs. 4.11A to C: Structure of microfilaments (A), intermediate filaments (B) and microtubules (C).

Table 4.4: Protein subunit and diameter of cytoskeletal elements of cell.

	Microfilament	Intermediate filament	Microtubule
1. Shape	Double stranded helical arrangement	Tubular hollow	Long, non-branching
2. Diameter	7 nm	10 nm	25 nm
3. Basic protein units	Actin	Various proteins	Tubulin
4. Location in cell	– Forms a network adjacent to cell – Core of microvilli – Contractile elements of muscle	– Extend across cytoplasm connecting desmosome and hemidesmosome – The nuclear lamina – In skin epithelium as keratin	– Mitotic spindle – Core of cilia
5. Major functions	Essential element of contractile element of muscles	Provide mechanical strength and link cells together	Provides network for movement of organelles, Movement of cilia

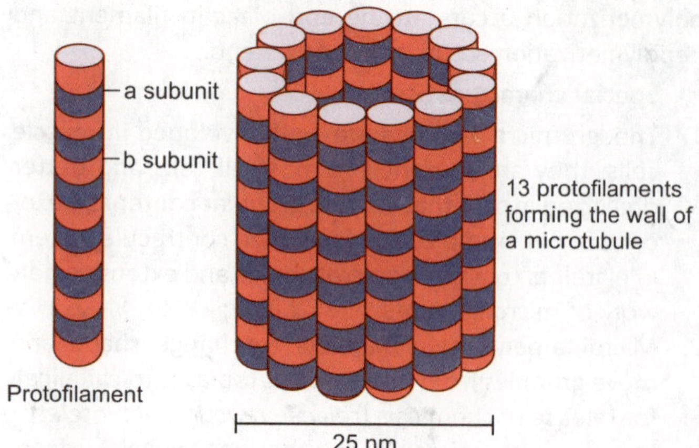

Fig. 4.12: Schematic representation depicting the formation of microtubule.

3. Filamentous actin helps in movement of chromosome and cell division.
4. Through anchoring proteins, F actin fibers attach to various cytoskeletal structures and interact with membrane bound proteins.
5. Microfilaments project into the microvilli present on the epithelial surface such as on the intestinal mucosa, and extend up to the tip of microvilli. They help in microvilli movement.
6. Microfilaments in the lamellipodia (lamellar extensions from cell that occur at the time of cell crawling) help in cell movement on a surface.
7. Actin filament interacts with **integrin receptors** to form ***focal adhesion complexes (FAC)***. FAC serve as points of traction with the surface over which cell pulls itself.
8. Microfilaments are also used by some molecular motors as tracks.

Microtubules

Microtubules are long hollow tubular structures (Fig. 4.11C) having diameter of about 25 nm, including the wall thickness. The inner cavity diameter of microtubules is about 15 nm. They are made up of subunits of globular proteins called **tubulins** that are arranged in a closely packed helical manner.

Tubulins in microtubules are of two types: α-**tubulin** and β-**tubulin**, except the tubulins in centrioles that are γ-tubulins. The α and β-tubulin subunits form heterodimers that aggregate to make tubular structures (***protofilaments***) of stacked rings. Each ring in microtubule usually contains 13 subunits (13 protofilaments) (Fig. 4.12).

Special characteristics:

1. A unique property of tubulin subunits is their *property of disaggregating (disassembly) and re-aggregating (assembly)*. Therefore, microtubules form a dynamic cytoskeletal framework of the cell. Microtubules are polar in nature with assembly predominating end (+ve end) and disassembly predominating end (–ve end). The process of assembly and disassembly may occur simultaneously.
2. Many drugs act by inhibiting microtubule assembly (Clinical Box 4.4)
3. Interaction with GTP facilitates microtubule formation.
4. Microtubule growth is temperature sensitive with cold conditions favoring disassembly.
5. In cells with cilia and flagella, microtubules extend into these structures.
6. Kinesin and dynein are microtubule-based molecular motors.

Functions

1. Microtubules serve as *cytosolic guide rails* for transport of substances within the cytoplasm or transport of secretory granules to the cell membrane. They help in transport of vesicles and organelles from one part of the cell to another.
2. They contribute to the maintenance of cell strength and cell shape.
3. They help in the formation of spindles that move chromosomes during mitotic cell division.
4. They are the pillars for structure and function of cilia.
5. They contribute to cell motility.

Cilia: Cilia are hair-like outgrowths of cells of the epithelial membrane that characteristically beat in a synchronous whip-like fashion. Therefore, cilia allow a directional flow. Each cilium is an outgrowth of a basal body situated beneath the cell membrane, which has the property of reproducing itself. In each cilium, there is an **axoneme** that typically consists of nine doublets of microtubules that run circumferentially from base to the tip while a single pair of microtubules runs centrally (9 + 2 arrangement).

1. All microtubules in cilia are linked together by protein cross-linkages that form the axoneme. In cilia, dyneins are present close to axoneme, called ***axnemal dyneins***.
2. The coordinated interaction between tubulins of axoneme and axonemal dyneins promotes ciliary movement.
3. Basal body is present at the base of axoneme, which has arrangement of microtubules in nine sets of triplets similar to that of arrangement in centriole.

Clinical Box 4.4

Cytotoxic drugs act by inhibiting microtubular functions: Many cytotoxic drugs act by inhibiting the microtubular activity. For example, anticancer chemotherapeutic agents such as *vincristine* and *vinblastine* promote disassembly of microtubules. Paclitaxel, another anticancer drug binds with microtubules and stabilize them against depolymerization. The stabilized microtubules function abnormally and do not undergo dynamic changes necessary for cell cycle completion. It prevents formation of mitotic spindles, and cells die. *Colchicine* inhibits microtubule assembly.

Intermediate Filaments

These are filamentous structures made up of various subunits (Fig. 4.11B). The average diameter of these filaments varies from 8 to 14 nm.

Functions:

1. They connect the nuclear membrane to the cell membrane and also membranes of cell organelles. Therefore, the major function of these filaments is to *integrate the organelles within the cytoplasm*.
2. They form supple skeletal network for the cell and *resist rupture of cell* from external pressure. In the absence of microfilaments, cells easily rupture. Blister formation in skin is common in humans when these filaments are absent or abnormal.
3. They are used as cell markers (Clinical Box 4.5)

Clinical Box 4.5

Intermediate filament proteins are cell markers: Proteins of intermediate filaments are cell specific. Therefore, they are frequently used as cellular markers. For example, cytokeratin is the marker of epithelial cells, whereas vimentin is the marker of fibroblast.

Molecular Motors

Molecular motors help in the movement of various cell parts, proteins and organelles within the cell cytoplasm. They are 100-kDa ATPases. They have two domains: The domain that attaches with cargo (the cell part to be moved) and the other domain attaches with microtubules or actin filaments. The domain attaching with microtubules or actin is the head part that contains ATPase, which causes hydrolysis of ATP to provide energy for movement of molecules. Molecular motors can be broadly divided into two categories: Microtubule-based and actin-based.

Microtubule-based Molecular Motors

Microtubule-based molecular motors make movement of molecules along the microtubules. They are mainly kinesin and dynein.

Kinesin

The *conventional kinesin* is a double-headed molecule that transports its cargo toward the negative terminal of microtubules. One head attaches with microtubule and the other head with the cargo. Some kinesins move cargo toward the positive terminal of microtubules. Other kinesins are involved in cell divisions such as mitosis and meiosis.

Dynein

Dynein is also a double-headed molecule. There are two types of dynein: Cytoplasmic form and axonemal form.

Cytoplasmic Dynein: It functions like that of conventional kinesin that moves cargo toward the negative terminals of microtubules.

Axonemal Dynein: Cilia and flagella contain dynein-based molecular motors that are axonemal type. Thus, these dynein molecules are responsible for beating cilia and flagella.

Actin-based Molecular Motors

Actin-based molecular motors make movement of molecules along the actin filaments. These are mainly **myosin I–V**. However, there are 18 types of myosins. In myosin II, the head binds with actin and pulls actin by bending the neck region. In myosin V, the heads of myosin molecules walk on the microfilaments one after another. Myosin molecules perform various functions like muscle contraction, contraction of intestinal villi, cell migration etc.

The Nucleus

Structure of Nucleus

All living cells in humans except red blood cells contain nuclei. Platelets are cellular fragments. Most cells are uninucleated and the nucleus is commonly located at the center of the cell as round, intensely stained structure. However, there are variations in the size, shape and location of the nucleus within the cell, especially in different types of leucocytes and muscle cells. Nucleus is bound by a bilayer nuclear membrane that surrounds the nucleoplasm. The nucleus contains nucleoplasm and nucleolus.

Nuclear Membrane

The nuclear membrane is a double-layered membrane (Fig. 4.13). The space between the two membranes is called **perinuclear cisterns**. In some cells, nuclear membrane is in continuity with the membrane of endoplasmic reticulum. There are circular openings in the nuclear membrane known as **nuclear pores** that serve as passages for the exchange of materials between the cytoplasm and the nucleoplasm, especially for the transport of mRNA and proteins. There are two **special transport proteins** in the nuclear membrane, known as *importins* and *exportins*

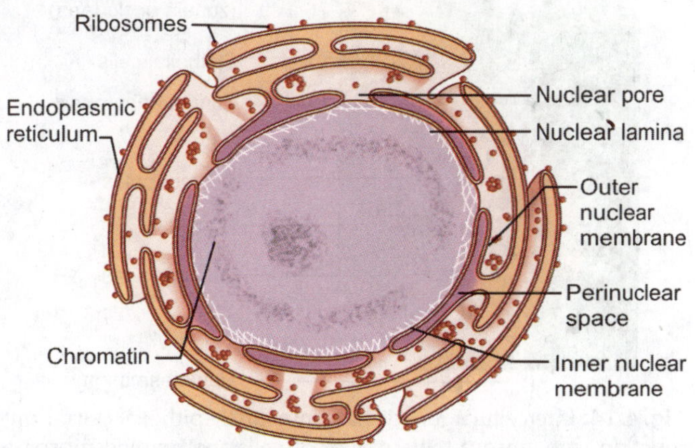

Fig. 4.13: Structure of nucleus and nuclear envelope.

that regulate transport of molecules across nuclear membrane. Another nuclear membrane protein known as **Ran**, plays organizing role in these transport mechanism.

Nucleoplasm

The nucleoplasm is the nuclear matrix, which is a gel like ground substance that contains genetic material in the form of DNA. When cell is not dividing the genetic material is present in the form of tangled mass called **nuclear chromatin** and when cell division begins, the tangled mass unwinds and appears as distinct strands known as **chromosomes**. The nuclear chromatin is made up of coiled strands of DNA, bound to large quantities of basic proteins (histones).

Nucleolus

The nucleus contains nucleolus, a patchwork of granules rich in RNA. There may be multiple nucleoli in a nucleus, especially in developing cells. Nucleoli synthesize ribosomes.

Functions of Nucleus

Nucleus regulates cell functions. It contains DNA that is responsible for transmission of hereditary features. It also contains RNA that is essential for protein synthesis. Nucleus is the main regulator of cell divisions. Details of the functions of DNA and RNA are discussed in the next chapter "Physiology of Genetics".

INTERCELLULAR JUNCTIONS

In tissues, junctions formed between the cells are called intercellular junctions or **intercellular connections**. The cells in tissues are usually held together by the extracellular matrix.

1. In connective tissues such as fibroblasts, cartilage and bones, the ***extracellular matrix*** is abundant, and therefore the cells are sparsely distributed within the substance of the matrix.

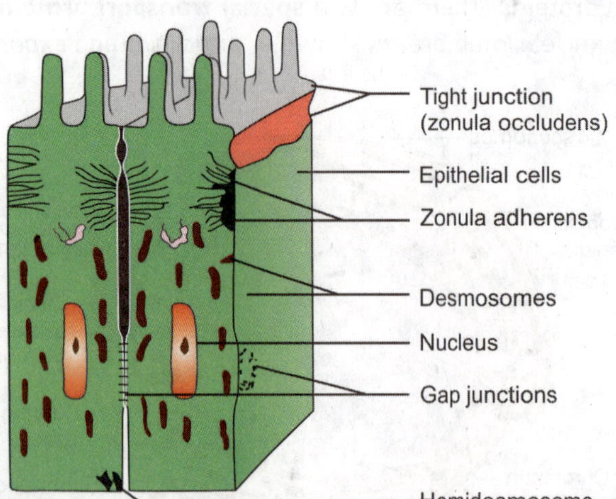

Fig. 4.14: Intercellular junctions in intestinal epithelial cells. Tight junctions are present toward apex of cells and hemidesmosome toward the base of the cell.

Table 4.5: Types of intercellular connections.

A. Junctions that tie cells together
1. Tight junctions
2. Anchoring junctions
a. Cell to cell anchoring junctions
– Desmosome
– Zonula adherens
b. Cell to basal lamina anchoring junctions
– Hemidesmosome
– Focal adhesion
B. Junctions that allow transfer of ions and small molecules
1. Gap junctions

2. In other connective tissues such as muscle, the cells are held together by **cell to cell adhesions**.
3. In epithelial tissues that line the free surfaces such as skin, and basement membrane of tubular structures and cavities of the body such as alimentary tract, kidney tubules and urinary bladder, the cells are bound tightly together by specialized **intercellular junctions** (Fig. 4.14).
4. In epithelial and connective tissues, the normal space between cells (intercellular space) is 20–25 nm. In epithelial tissues, the extracellular matrix is reduced to a thin layer known as the **basal lamina**.

Types

Functionally, **intercellular connections** or junctions are of two types: junctions that tie cells together and Junctions that allow transfer of ions and small molecules (Table 4.5).

Tight Junctions

Tight junctions are commonly found in the epithelium of the GI tract, nephrons, urinary tract, hepatobiliary tract, and choroid plexus. They are also called **zonula occludens**.

Special features of tight junctions:

1. Tight junctions are typically located toward the apical region of the cells (Fig. 4.15).
2. At tight junctions, the outer layer of the cell membrane of neighboring cells fuse with each other that obliterates the intercellular space close to their apical margin.
3. They are made up of ridges, half of which is contributed by both neighboring cells and each half is bound tightly to each other. Therefore, they practically form the barrier for transport of solutes and solvents from the lumen into the interstitial space and between cells.
4. They contain ion and water channels that make them selectively leaky, though the degree of leakiness varies in different epithelia.
5. The membrane proteins that contribute to formation of tight junctions belong to three main families: **occludin, claudins** and **junctional adhesion molecules** (JAMs).

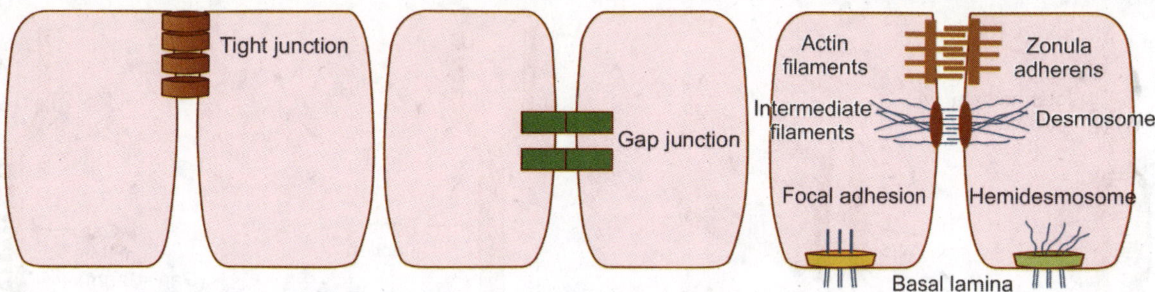

Fig. 4.15: Schematic representation and locations of specialized junctions connecting the cells.

6. Many other membrane proteins from cytosolic side interact with tight junctions.

Functions of Tight Junctions

1. In general, they form **selective permeability barrier** that prevent transport of macromolecules from the luminal fluid into the interstitial space. Thus, macromolecules pass only through the epithelial cell as vesicles (vesicular transport).
2. Due to the presence of leaky channels, small size water-soluble particles are permitted through tight junctions. However, the degree of permeability varies. For example, in the gut, Na^+ ions pass fairly freely, while in the urinary bladder, the passage for sodium is almost nil. Furthermore, the permeability of a substance through tight junctions can be increased, depending on the osmolality gradient across the epithelium. This forms the **paracellular transport** of solutes and solvents.
3. In the brain, tight junctions between endothelial cells of cerebral blood vessels contribute to the **effectiveness of blood-brain barrier**.
4. In the ciliary bodies, they form *blood-aqueous barrier* between the cells of inner non-pigmented epithelium.

Anchoring Junctions

Anchoring junctions are of two types: Cell to cell anchoring junctions and cell to basal lamina anchoring junctions.

Cell to Cell Anchoring Junctions

Cell to cell anchoring junctions are desmosome and zonula adherens.

Desmosomes

1. Desmosomes are the junctions characterized by ***focal thickening*** of two adjacent cell membranes (Fig. 4.15). The *thickened area* is the presence of dense layer of proteins on the cytoplasmic surface of the membrane.
2. Thickened area of two sides is separated by a gap of 25 nm.
3. ***Intermediary filaments*** from cytosol are attached to the thickened areas.
4. The intercellular space between the two membrane thickenings also contains filamentous cell adhesion materials such as **desmogleins** and **cadherins** (Fig. 4.16).

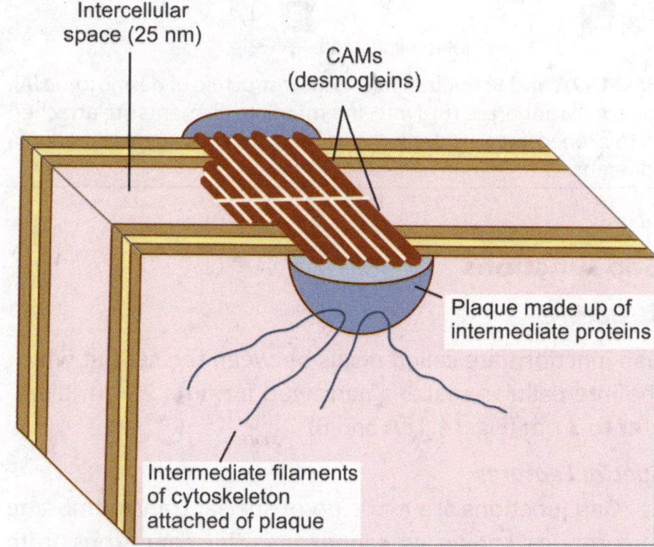

Fig. 4.16: Cell adhesion molecules (desmogleins and cadherins) in desmosomes.

5. Extracellular portions of many membrane proteins are also present in this space.

Zonula Adherens

Zonula adherens is located below the base of tight junctions (Figs. 4.17A and B). It is the *major site of attachment for intracellular microfilaments*. Cadherins are present in the intercellular space at this junction.

Cell to Basal Lamina Anchoring Junctions

Cell to basal lamina anchoring junctions are hemidesmosome and focal adhesion.

Hemidesmosomes

In appearance, they look like half of desmosomes, and therefore are called hemidesmosome. Microfilaments are attached to it intracellularly. In contrast to presence of cadherins and desmogleins in desmosome, hemidesmosomes contain integrins.

Focal Adhesions

Focal adhesions (focal spots) connect cell to the basal lamina. Intracellularly, they are associated with actin filaments. Therefore, they assist in cell movement.

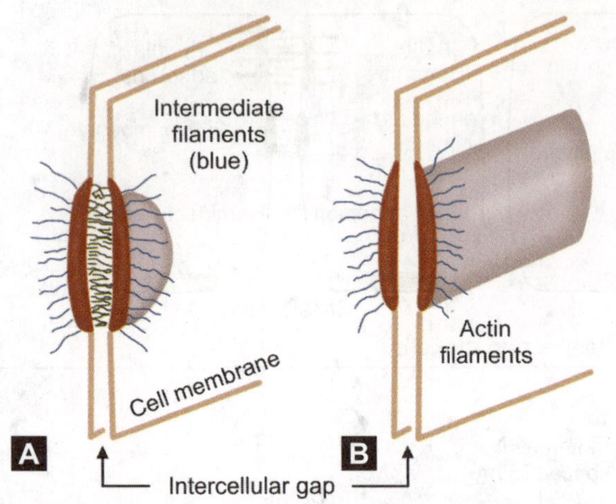

Figs. 4.17A and B: Electron microscopic structure of desmosome (A), and zonula adherens (B). Note, intermediate filaments are attached to thickened area in desmosome, and actin filaments in zonula adherens.

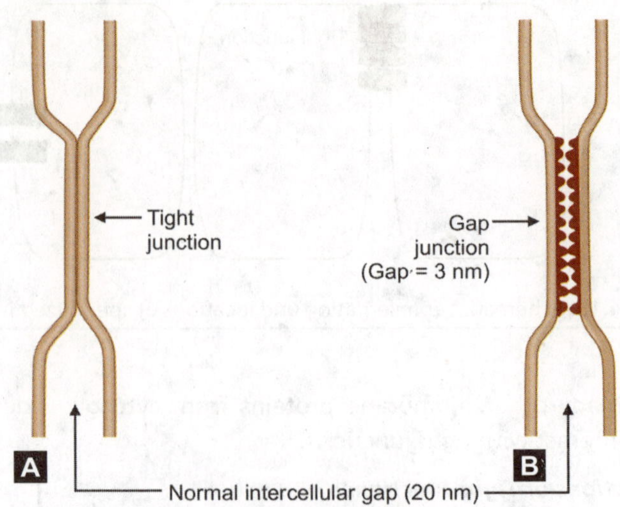

Figs. 4.18A and B: Gap of 3 nm between cells at gap junctions (B), and no gap between cells at tight junctions (A).

Gap Junctions

Structure

Gap junctions are called **nexus** between the cells at which the intercellular space is narrowed from its 25 nm diameter to 3 nm (Figs. 4.18A and B).

Special Features

1. Gap junctions are made up of special transmembrane proteins known as **connexons**. The connexons from the membrane of two adjacent cells are lined up with one another (Fig. 4.19A).
2. Each connexon is formed by six identical protein subunits called **connexins**. Connexin surrounds an aqueous channel and when connexon of adjacent cells are aligned, the aqueous channels of both cell membranes become a continuous one (Fig. 4.19B). This allows substances of adjacent two cells to pass through the channel without passing through the ECF. The diameter of the channel is about 2 nm.
3. As connexons of one cell membrane are aligned with the connexons of the adjacent cell membrane and they connect the cytoplasm of adjacent cells through their aqueous channels, water, ions, amino acids, sugars and hormones can pass from cell to cell through them.
4. As connexons keep the adjacent cell membranes at a fixed gap, the junction is named as "gap junctions".
5. There are 20 different connexon genes (Clinical Box 4.6).

Clinical Box 4.6

Mutation of connexon genes: In humans, there are about 20 different genes that code for connexin proteins. Mutation of these genes results in diseases that are specific for tissues. For example, mutation of a specific connexin gene that produces ***Charcot-Marie-Tooth disease***, exclusively affects peripheral neurons. Therefore, peripheral neuropathy is the outstanding feature of this disease.

Functions

1. **Electrical synapses**: As the pores of gap junction are larger than ligand-gated or voltage-gated channels, passage of substances is easier through them. Gap junctions easily allow ions to pass through and serve as *electrical synapses,* as they permit rapid propagation of electrical activity from cell to cell. Therefore, tissues with gap junctions between cells behave as **physiological syncytium** (Application Box 4.5).
2. Gap junctions also permit passage of organic solutes such as sugars and amino acids with molecular weight upto 1000 from cell to cell.
3. Chemical messengers and hormones are also exchanged between cells through gap junctions.

Regulation of Gap Junction Functions

Though transport of ions through gap junctions is not an active process, they do not just act as mere passive conduits. Their activities are regulated by intracellular calcium concentration and cytosolic pH. Increase in any of these parameters can prevent transport through gap junctions by closing their channels.

Application Box 4.5

Functional syncytium: Gap junctions are present abundantly in heart muscle. As they serve as electrical synapses, electrical impulses pass easily from cell to cell in cardiac muscle. Thus, stimulation of one muscle cell in heart results in activation of all muscle cells. This makes the ventricular and atrial muscle as functional syncytium. However, ventricular and atrial muscles are two separate functional syncytia as ventricles and atria are separated by non-conducting septa. Gap junctions are also present in visceral smooth muscles that conduct electrical impulses from cell to cell. Hence, visceral smooth muscles also have syncytial behavior.

Cell Adhesion Molecules

Cells are attached to each other and to the basal lamina by cell adhesion molecules (CAMs) that are present

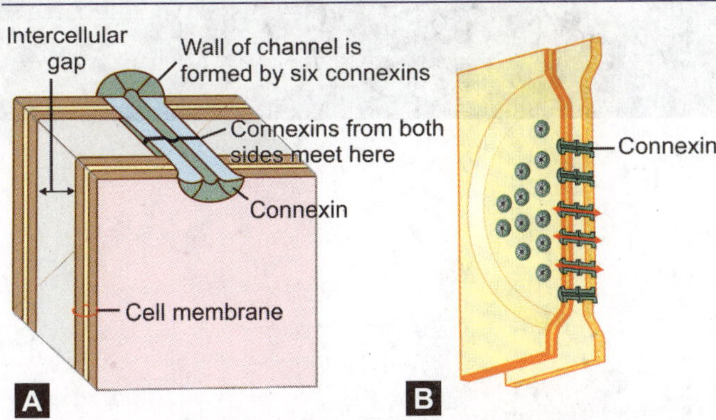

Figs. 4.19A and B: Structure of gap junction under electron microscope (A), and alignment of connexins in gap junctions (B).

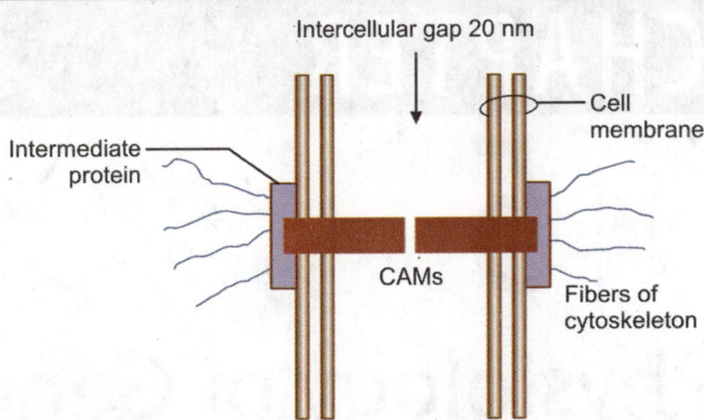

Fig. 4.20: Location of cell adhesion molecules (CAMs) between two cells.

abundantly at intercellular connections (Fig. 4.20). By their property of adhesions between the cells, they provide stability to the tissue.

Systems of Binding

They have both extracellular and intracellular bindings.

Extracellular Binding

Many of CAMs bind to membrane proteins called **laminins**. Laminins are cross-shaped large membrane molecules that have multiple receptor domains on the extracellular matrix. CAMs bind to these extracellular receptor domains.

Intracellular Binding

Cell adhesion molecules (CAMs) pass through the cell membrane to expose into the interior of the cell and attach with the cytoskeleton inside the cell. This intracellular binding of CAMs with cytoskeletal structures enhances strength of cell adhesions.

Nature of Binding

Cell adhesion molecules (CAMs) exhibit both homophilic and heterophilic bindings.

Homophilic Bindings

In homophilic bindings, CAMs attach with similar molecules present on the other cells.

Heterophilic Bindings

In heterophilic bindings, CAMs attach with different molecules of other cells.

Types of CAMs

Though there are confusions on classifying CAMs, they can be broadly categorized into four varieties: Integrins, IgG superfamily proteins, cadherins and selectins.

Integrins: Integrins are heterodimeric proteins that bind to various receptors.

IgG superfamily proteins: CAMs belonging to IgG superfamily are immunoglobulins.

Cadherins: These are calcium dependent molecules that mediate homophilic binding.

Selectins: They have carbohydrate binding domains, that resemble lectin-like structure.

Functions of CAMs

1. They zip cell to cell. Cell adherence is strengthened by CAMs.
2. For their attachment with cytoskeleton, they play role in cell movement.
3. Cellular signals are transmitted out of the cell or extracellular signals are transmitted into the cell via CAMs.
4. They play significant role in inflammation and wound healing.
5. CAMs prevent apoptosis. Loss of cellular contact from extracellular matrix due to defects in CAMs hastens the process of apoptosis.

CHAPTER SUMMARY

The cell is the structural and functional unit of tissues. A cell consists of cell membrane, cytoplasm and nucleus.

1. The cell membrane is the lipid bilayer that forms the boundary in all animal cells and is selectively permeable to the substances.
2. Cells are bound to each other by means of intercellular junctions and cell adhesion molecules. In the upper apical part are the tight junctions and in the base are hemidesmosome and focal adhesion. In the middle of the cells are desmosomes and gap junction. There are many other proteins in the cells like actin and myosin that provide strength and mobility to the cell and also the mechanisms for adhesion to other cells.
3. Gap junctions allow ions to pass from cell to cell much faster. Therefore, they are called electrical synapse. Gap junctions provide the physiological basis for syncytial nature of a tissue like, cardiac tissue.

Important to Know (Must Read)

1. **Long Questions** are usually not asked from this chapter.
2. Cell membrane, Mitochondria, Lysosomes, Cytoskeleton, Molecular motors, Gap junctions, CAMs, Intercellular junctions, may come as **Short Questions**.
3. In **Viva**, examiner may ask… cell membrane, cell organelles, cytoskeletal proteins, molecular motors, intercellular junctions and gap junctions, and cell adhesion molecules.

CHAPTER

5

Physiology of Genetics and Apoptosis

Learning Objectives

On completion of study of this chapter, the student **MUST** be able to:

1. Understand the basic principles of genetics, structure and functions of chromosomes, and functions of genes/DNA and RNA.
2. Appreciate the application genetics in medicine.
3. Understand the basic principles of recombinant DNA technology, polymerase chain reaction, cloning, mutation and blotting techniques.
4. Learn the genetic basis of cancer and gene therapy.
5. Understand the concept of apoptosis.

The student **MAY** also be able to:

1. Understand the mechanism of gene expression and protein synthesis.
2. Explain the process and importance of recombinant DNA technology, polymerase chain reaction and blotting techniques.
3. Describe different types of cancer genes, and the physiological basis of gene therapy.
4. Explain the mechanism and importance of apoptosis.

PHYSIOLOGY OF GENETICS

Physiology of genomics is a developing branch of medicine. It deals with the understanding of the concept of gene and gene therapy in the treatment of genetic disorders.

Genetics is the science of heredity, dealing with resemblances and differences of related organisms resulting from the interaction of their genes and the environment. Application of knowledge of genetics to understand the heritable basis of the diseases and to improve the management of diseases through gene intervention, is called **medical genetics**. Mendel's work in 1886 that hereditary characteristics are transmitted to offspring by separate units laid the foundation of genetics. Later, Johannied, the Danish botanist in 1909 termed these units as genes and, Morgan, the American geneticist established that the hereditary characteristics are transmitted on chromosomes.

Chromosomes

The term chromosome was coined by Waldeyer in 1888. Chromosomes transmit the genetic information from parents to offspring. There are 46 chromosomes in cells of all tissues except gametes that contain 23 chromosomes. Autosomes are present in somatic cells and sex chromosomes in gametes.

Structure of Chromosomes

Each chromosome consists of two chromatids that are connected at the centromeres (or kinetochore). Each chromatid is composed of two chromosomes (Fig. 5.1). Typically, the centromere is not midway between the two ends of chromatids. When chromatid has a short arm and a long arm, the chromosome is called ***submetacentric***. If two arms of the chromatid are of equal length, the chromosome is ***metacentric***, if one arm is too short the chromosome is ***acrocentric*** and if centromere lies at one end (each chromatid has only one arm), the chromosome is ***telocentric*** (Figs. 5.2A to D). Chromosomes are distinguishable only during mitosis. In the interphase (between successive mitoses), chromosomes elongate and assume the form of a long thread called **chromonemata** (Application Box 5.1). Though chromosomes are formed mainly by DNA, they also contain RNA, the basic protein histones, complex proteins, organic phosphorous compounds and inorganic salts.

Application Box 5.1

Karyotyping: Identification of each chromosome and mapping out the chromosomes is called karyotyping. Karyotyping is done for studying the morphology and number of chromosomes. Though karyotyping can be done in any nucleated cell, lymphocytes are preferred. The study is done by arresting the dividing cells in metaphase by colchicine and spreading them on glass slide and staining them with Giemsa stain. In many cases, chromosomal abnormalities can be correlated with specific diseases.

The DNA

Deoxyribonucleic acid (DNA) is found in bacteria, and in nuclei and mitochondria of all eukaryotic cells. DNA is the component of chromosome. Chromosome appears in pairs, except in germ cells. Chromosomes are made up of a mammoth molecule of DNA, which is about 2 m in length. However, DNA is accommodated in the nucleus as most part of it at intervals is wrapped around histone proteins to form **nucleosomes**. About 25 millions of nucleosomes are present in a nucleus. The complex of DNA and the histone protein is called **chromatin**. As cell division begins, acetylation of histone loosens the coiling and pairs of chromosomes become visible.

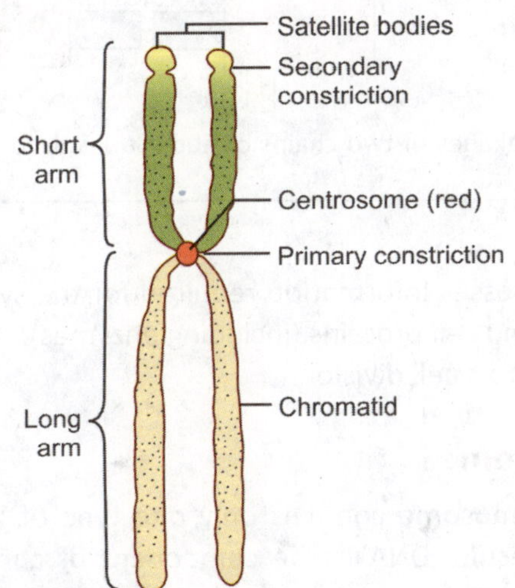

Fig. 5.1: Structure of a chromosome.

Important Note

DNA Content of a Cell: It has been estimated that total DNA content of a cell (all chromosomes put together) is represented by about 6×10^9 nucleotide pairs. Of these, 2.5×10^8 is present in Chromosome 1, which is the largest chromosome. The Y chromosome, which is the smallest chromosome, contains 5×10^7 nucleotide pairs.

DNA Nucleotides

A molecule of DNA is made up of two strands of polynucleotides linked together in the form of a double helix (Fig. 5.3). A nucleotide consists of a nitrogenous base, a sugar molecule (deoxyribose) and a phosphate molecule. In DNA, the nitrogenous bases are **purines** (adenine and guanine) and **pyrimidines** (cytosine and thymine). Nucleotides in DNA from a polymer of polynucleotides through covalent bonds between the sugar molecules. [Nitrogenous bases are often designated by their first letter i.e. *A* for adenine, *T* for thymine, *G* for guanine and *C* for cytosine]. The purine and pyrimidine bases encode **genetic message** (Application Box 5.2).

Application Box 5.2

The Genetic Message: The genetic message is encoded by purine and pyrimidine bases in the nucleotide chains of DNA. The amino acid sequence in the protein synthesized in the cell decides the text of the message. The RNA transfers the message form DNA blueprint to the ribosome where protein synthesis occurs. The proteins formed from DNA blueprint include all enzymes that control cell metabolisms.

Important Note

Gene and Proteins: A ***gene*** is defined as the amount of information necessary to specify a ***single protein*** molecule. Proteins determined by a single gene may divide to form different proteins with various physiological actions. Also, different mRNAs may form from a single gene that can guide formation of various proteins.

Double Helix Structure

In the double helix, the sugar phosphates form the backbone with all the bases being present inside the helical structure. Each nucleotide consists of a sugar deoxyribose,

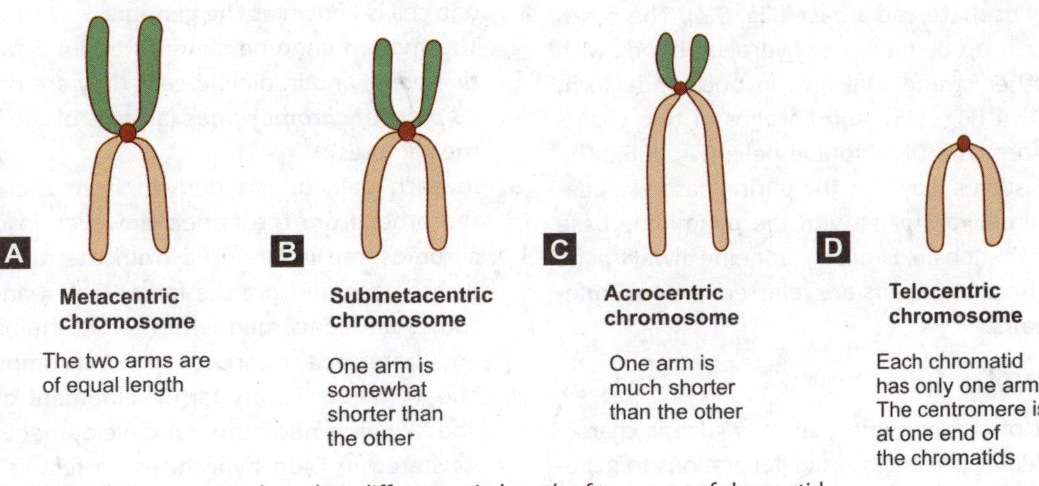

Figs. 5.2A to D: Types of chromosome, based on differences in length of two arms of chromatid.

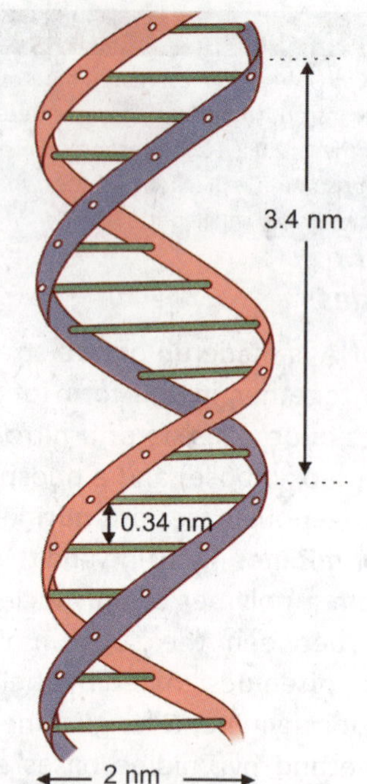

Fig. 5.3: Double helix structure of DNA molecule.

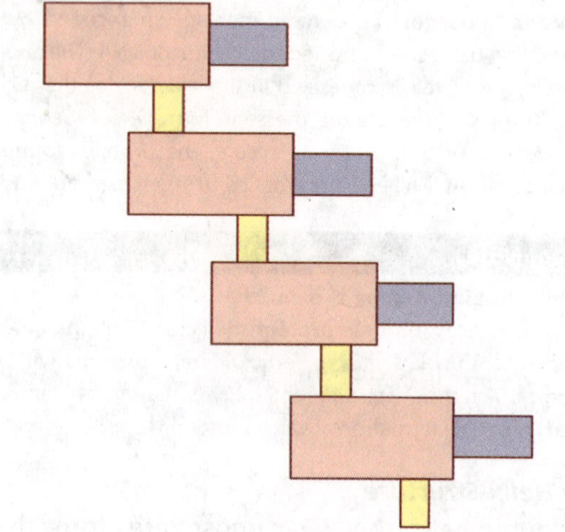
Fig. 5.5: Linkages of nucleotide to form one strand of DNA molecule.

a molecule of phosphate and a base (Fig. 5.4). The bases on one strand pair up by means of hydrogen bonds with bases on the other strand. Linkages in nucleotide form one strand of DNA (Fig. 5.5), and linkages of two chains of nucleotides form the DNA double helix (Fig. 5.6). The paring occurs in such a way that the purine base like guanine in one chain always pairs with the pyrimidine base cytosine in the other chain. Similarly, adenine always pairs with thymine. These base pairs are referred to as **complementary base pairs**.

Functions of DNA

1. DNA as part of chromosome transmits genetic characteristics (hereditary features) from generations to generations.

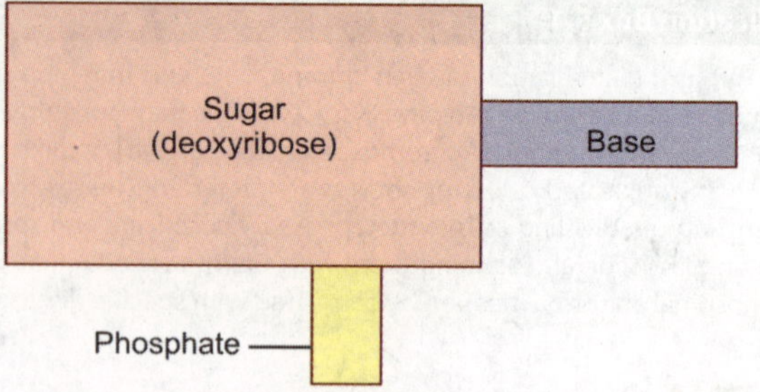

Fig. 5.4: Composition of a nucleotide. The base may be adenine, cytosine, guanine or thymine.

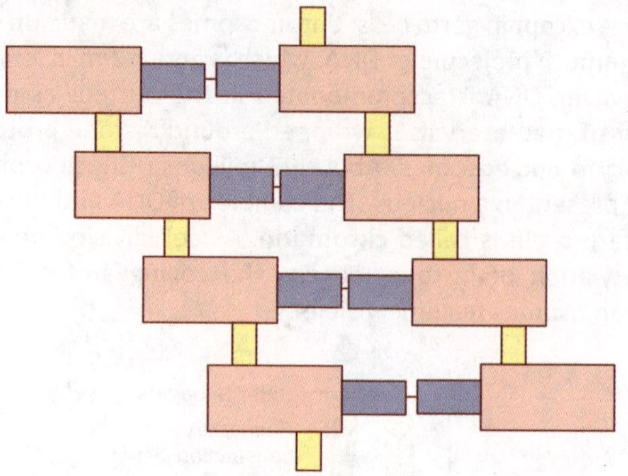
Fig. 5.6: Linkages of two chains of nucleotides to form the DNA molecule.

2. It possesses information required for the synthesis of RNA and cell proteins (including enzymes).
3. It controls cell division.

The Genome

Each chromosome contains only one type of long-chain DNA molecule. DNA is the component of chromosome that carries the **genetic message** (blueprint of heritable characteristics) of the cell (Refer, Application Box 5.2).

1. The total genetic information stored in chromosomes of a cell is known as **the genome.**
2. The **human genome** contains about *3 billion nucleotide pairs*, and in diploid cells they are organized into ***23 pairs of chromosomes*** (all cells of the body, except the gametes).
3. In each pair, one is derived from the mother and the other from the father. However, in males, the *X* chromosome is inherited from the mother, and the *Y* chromosome from the father. The *X* and *Y* chromosomes are concerned with the determination of sex, and therefore they are called **sex chromosomes**.
4. The *XX* are necessary for development of the female and *XY* pair is necessary for development of the male. As stated in **Lyon hypothesis**, in female, one of the two X chromosomes (paternal or maternal derived), is

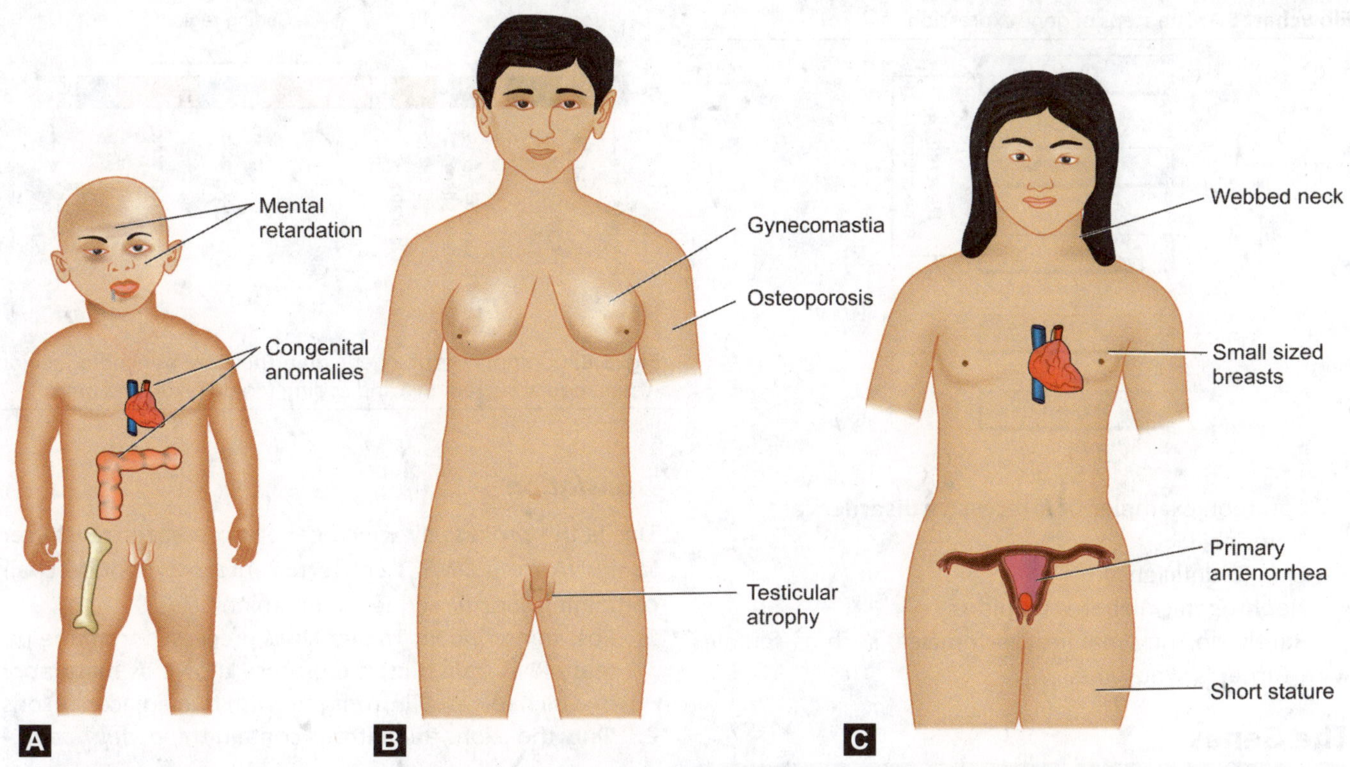

Figs. 5.7A to C: Clinical features of three important chromosomal abnormalities. (A) Down's syndrome; (B) Klinefelter's syndrome; (C) Turner's syndrome.

inactivated during embryogenesis. This inactivation is passed to all the somatic cells, while the germ cells in female remain unaffected. That means ovary will have always active X chromosome.

5. The inactive X chromosome in the somatic cells in female lies condensed in the nucleus and is called as **sex chromatin**. This phenomenon in females helps in **nuclear sexing** (Clinical Box 5.1).
6. Gametes (sperm and ovum) have half this number of chromosomes, and therefore are said to be **haploid cells**.
7. During fertilization of an ovum by a sperm, the diploid number is restored, so that each cell carries 23 chromosomes from each parent.

Clinical Box 5.1

Nuclear Sexing: Determination of sex by identification of sex chromatin in the nucleus of somatic cells is called nuclear sexing (Fig. 5.7). This is done for genetic female testing by preparing and staining the smears of squamous cells scrapped from oral cavity or by identifying ***Barr body*** attached to nuclear lobes in the circulating neutrophil, in females. A minimum of 30% cells positive for sex chromatin indicates the person as female genetically.

Chromosomal Disorders

Chromosomal abnormalities may be either due to the defect in autosomes or in sex chromosomes, and are accompanied by congenital abnormalities.

1. **Trisomy 21:** The commonest abnormality of autosomal chromosome is the presence of three instead of two chromosomes in the number 21 pair. The condition is known as trisomy 21. The resulting clinical condition is called ***mongolism***, or **Down's syndrome**, which is characterized by mental retardation, congenital anomalies and abnormal physical features (Fig. 5.7A).
2. **Turner and Klinefelter syndromes:** The common sex chromosomal abnormality in female is *Turner syndrome* in which one *X* chromosome is absent (i.e. *XO*), and in male is *Klinefelter syndrome* in which an extra *X* chromosomes is added (XXY). In these conditions, the subject is sterile, and has peculiar physical abnormalities. **Klinefelter's syndrome** that occurs in males, presents with gynecomastia, osteoporosis, and testicular atrophy (Fig. 5.7B). **Turner's syndrome** that occurs in females presents with short stature, webbed neck, small breast size and primary amenorrhea (Fig. 5.7C).
3. **X-linked Disorders:** An abnormal gene located in an autosome leads to an autosomal trait; whereas location of abnormal gene in a sex chromosome gives rise to sex-linked traits. However, all the known sex-linked genetic disorders are due to the defective genes located on one *X* chromosomes, and therefore they are called as *X*-linked disorders. Very few of them are *X*-dominant, but most are *X*-recessive. Therefore, *many X-linked disorders do not manifest in females* who have normal *X* chromosome allele. However, sex linked genetic disorders at all times manifest in males as they do not have normal neutralizing *X* allele.

Flowchart 5.1: The steps of gene expression.

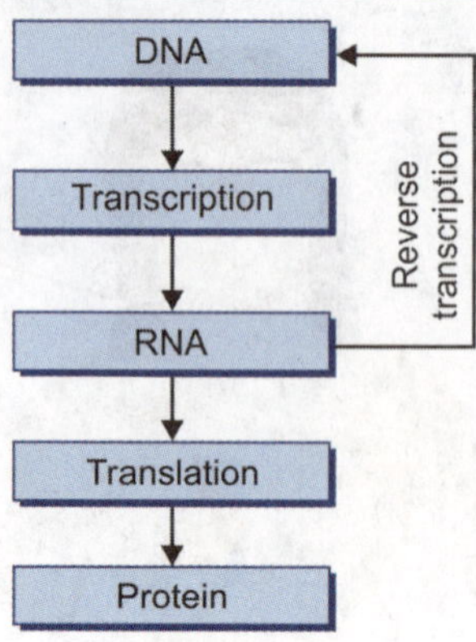

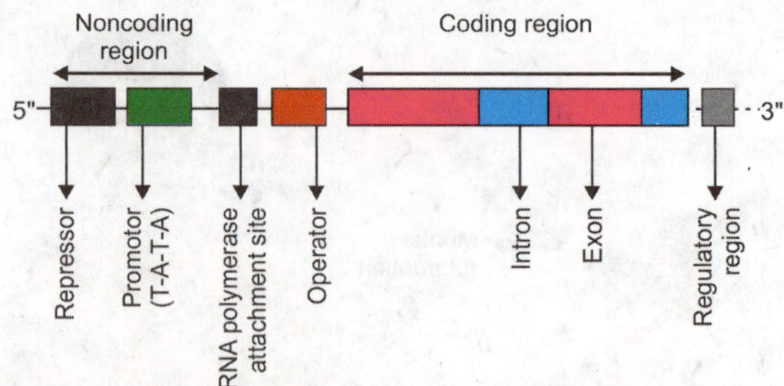

Fig. 5.8: Components of a gene unit. There are noncoding region (three regulatory regions) and coding region (exon and intron).

Common examples of ***X*-recessive disorders** are:

- Hemophilia
- G-6-PD deficiency
- Nephrogenic diabetes insipidus.

Rarely do they manifest in females, such as females with Turner 's syndrome.

The Genes

The gene is the functional unit of DNA. A gene is defined as the portion of DNA responsible for the production of a single RNA molecule. Each chromosome contains myriad of genes. The genes do not exercise their powers all the time. The inherent control mechanisms are such that only selected genes are switched on at any given time. Though, the DNA of each cell in a multicellular organism has same DNA sequence and same genetic capabilities, the difference between different cell types lies in the differences in genetic expression.

Gene Expression

The genetic expression of each cell type is selective, and therefore, the protein synthesis is different in different tissues. Genetic expression occurs in two broad steps: transcription and translation (Flowchart 5.1).

Transcription

Transcription is the process in which RNA is synthesized from DNA. In this process:

1. The genetic information stored in DNA is transferred to the RNA.
2. During the process of formation of RNA, the relevant part of the DNA double helix unwinds and exposes the gene unit, which is then copied.
3. The DNA strand that directs the synthesis of mRNA through complementary base pairing is called **template strand** (also called, coding strand or sense strand) and the other DNA strand is called **noncoding strand** or antisense strand.
4. The enzyme *RNA polymerase* carries out transcription by binding to a site on DNA called **promoter site**.

Translation

This is the process by which genetic message transferred to mRNA from DNA is converted into polypeptide chain containing specific sequence of amino acids.

1. Post-transcription: The mRNA is processed from the primary RNA transcript; the process known as **maturation** in which released introns join with two adjacent exons.
2. Only the exons and introns contain the *genetic code*.

Gene Unit

Each gene unit is organized into three components: regulatory DNA sequence (repressor, promoter and operator), exons and introns (Fig. 5.8). Out of these, introns are removed during post-transcriptional events and adjacent exons join. Regulatory DNA sequence plays major role in transcription.

The regulatory DNA sequences are non-coding sequences that ensure that the gene is transcribed at the right time and in the proper cell. There are three types of regulatory nucleotide sequences per gene.

1. The **promoter DNA sequence** that contains a sequence of Thymine-Adenine-Thymine-Adenine (T-T-T-A) nucleotides. This acts as the *recognition site* for the enzyme RNA polymerase to attach with nearby transcription *start site* before it can move forward to begin transcription of the exons and introns.
2. The promoter separates from the exons and introns by about ten nucleotides known as the **operator**. The operator should be free of attached molecules for the RNA-polymerase to reach the exons and introns.
3. A repressor nucleotide sequence located ahead of the promoter region is known as *5′ region*, which codes for a repressor protein. This protein under certain conditions attaches itself to the operator that prevents the RNA-polymerase from moving towards the structural gene. There is often another regulatory nucleotide sequence at the other end known as *3′ region*.

Exons are the DNA coding sequences that code for the formation of RNA.

Introns are DNA coding sequences inserted at intervals between segments of exons.

During the formation of RNA, both the introns and exons are transcribed, but the later one is translated into sequences of amino acids for the synthesis of a specific polypeptide within the ribosome.

Steps of Protein Synthesis

Protein synthesis occurs in *three major steps*.

1. **Transcription:** The two strands of DNA fiber separate from each other over the area bearing a particular cistron. Thus, the ends of the bases linked to the opposite strand become free. A molecule of mRNA is synthesized as a guide or a template. The code for the sequence in which amino acids are to be linked is passed on from DNA to mRNA (Fig. 5.9). This is called **transcription**, which occurs under the influence of *RNA polymerase*. The part of the mRNA strand that bears the code for one amino acid is called **codon**. The molecule of RNA now separates from the DNA strand and moves from nucleus to cytoplasm, where it attached with ribosome.
2. **Amino acid activation and translation:** On the ribosome, one side of tRNA attaches to amino acid, and on the other side bears a code for three bases (**anticodon**) that are complementary to the bases coding for its amino acid on mRNA. In the presence of enzyme *aminoacyl tRNA synthase*, amino acids react with ATP, get activated and attach with specific tRNA. Under the influence of the ribosome, several units of tRNA along with their amino acids become arranged along-side the strand of mRNA. In the sequence determined by the code on mRNA. This is called **translation**. Translation occurs in three steps:
   - **Initiation:** translation of mRNA with formation of initiation complex.
   - **Elongation:** elongation of polypeptide chain by sequential addition of amino acids to the growing end.
   - **Termination:** termination of polypeptide synthesis evoked by **nonsense codon**.
3. **Post-translational modification:** Post-translational modifications such as proteolytic degradation, hydroxylation, glycosylation, etc. make the protein more functional.

Regulation of Gene Expression

Gene expression is regulated by following mechanisms.

1. **Gene amplification:** Enhancement of gene expression can cause drug resistance. For example, amplification of the gene coding for dihydrofolate reductase causes development of drug resistance by cancer cells to chronic administration of methotrexate.
2. **Gene rearrangement:** This enhances the generation of antigen specific immunoglobulins.
3. **Regulation through transcription factors:** Transcription factor regulate interaction of protein with specific segments of DNA.

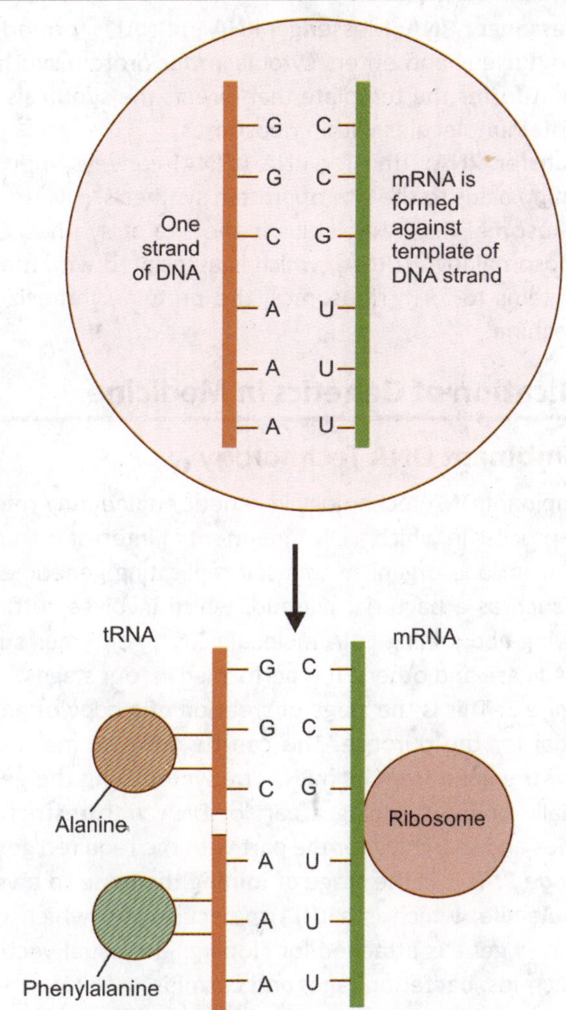

Fig. 5.9: Steps of protein synthesis. Transcription takes place in the nucleus (upper picture) and translation takes place in the cytoplasm (lower picture).

4. **Regulation through mRNA:** Modification of mRNA activity is the major mechanism of regulation of gene expression.

The RNA

Ribonucleic acid is made up of a single chain of polynucleotides (polymer of ribonucleotides). Unlike DNA, which is double stranded, the RNA has a single strand. RNA is present in the nucleus, cytoplasm, ribosome and to some extent in mitochondria.

RNA differs from a DNA strand in many aspects such as:

1. RNA chain is much shorter in length than the DNA chains.
2. The sugar-phosphate that forms the backbone contains ribose instead of deoxyribose.
3. The base thymine is replaced by uracil.

Types of RNA

There are three types of RNA and they have different functions.

1. **Messenger RNA:** Messenger RNA (mRNA) is formed in the nucleus and enters cytoplasm for protein synthesis. It forms the template that directs the synthesis of protein molecules within ribosomes.
2. **Transfer RNA:** Transfer RNA (tRNA) conveys specific amino acids to the site of protein synthesis.
3. **Ribosomal RNA:** Nucleolus is the site of synthesis of ribosomal RNA (rRNA), which is associated with many proteins to form ribosomes, the protein-synthesizing machine.

Application of Genetics in Medicine

Recombinant DNA Technology

Recombinant DNA technology in genetic engineering refers to the process in which a DNA fragment of interest is transferred from one organism to a self-replicating genetic element such as a bacterial plasmid, which involves cutting, modifying and joining DNA molecules using enzymes such as DNA ligase and others. It is performed in four stages.

Stage 1: This is the **stage of creation of a copy of gene** essential for the purpose. This can be done by making a copy of the gene from its mRNA, by synthesizing the gene artificially or by chopping a part of DNA with restriction enzymes and searching for the part with the required gene.

Stage 2: This is the **stage of joining the gene to a vector molecule,** which is a DNA molecule with which the generated gene is attached for cloning. The usual vectors are plasmids, bacteriophages and cosmids.

Stage 3: This is the **stage of introduction of vector DNA into the host cell** to produce *chimeric DNA* or recombinant DNA.

Stage 4: This is the **stage of cloning of chimeric DNA.** The chimeric DNA contained in a vector is introduced into bacterial cells by the process called *transfection*. The host cell allows multiplication of the chimeric DNA of the vector that leads to production of large number of identical target cloned DNA molecules. The cloned DNA is released form the vector by cleavage, which is isolated, characterized and used for different purposes.

Scientists contributed

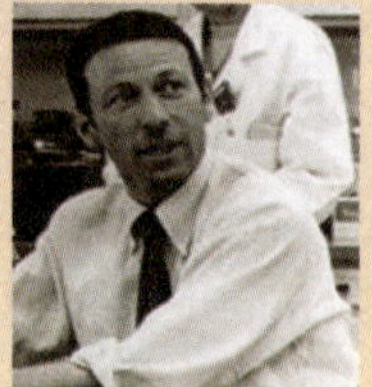

Paul Berg

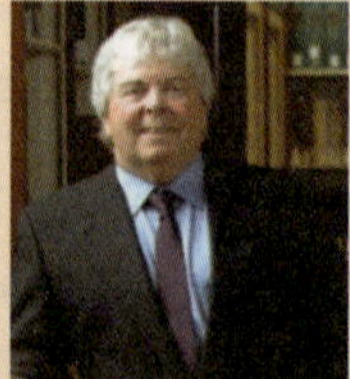

Herbert W Boyer

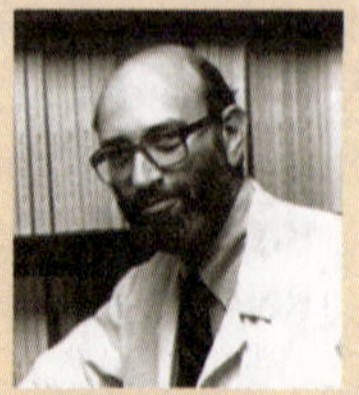

Stanley N Cohen

Invention of recombinant DNA technology—the way in which genetic material from one organism is artificially introduced into the genome of another organism and then replicated and expressed by that other organism—was largely the work of **Paul Berg** (born 1926, New York), **Herbert W Boyer** (born 1936, Pennsylvania), and **Stanley N Cohen** (born 1935, New Jersey), although many other scientists made important contributions to the new technology as well.

Uses of Recombinant DNA Technology

1. **Synthesis of hormones:** By recombinant DNA technology, hormones like insulin, growth hormone, erythropoietin etc, can be produced in large amount for therapeutic purposes.
2. **Laboratory diagnosis:** Diagnosis of diseases like AIDS has become simple by using recombinant DNA technology.
3. **Gene therapy:** It is useful in therapy for genetic defects.
4. **Use in forensic medicine:** DNA fingerprinting technique is useful in medicolegal cases.
5. **Use in agricultural purposes:** Recombinant DNA technology is used in generating genetically engineered plants to enhance the yield of crops.

PCR and Blotting Techniques

Polymerase Chain Reaction

Polymerase Chain Reaction (PCR) is a specific and very rapid method of amplifying a target DNA sequence. This involves denaturation of DNA (separation of double stranded target DNA into single strand by heating), cooling the single DNA strand and DNA amplification. The DNA amplification is achieved by formation of new DNA strand in the presence of enzyme DNA polymerase and the substrate deoxyribonucleotide triphosphate. PCR causes million fold amplification of target DNA.

Scientist contributed

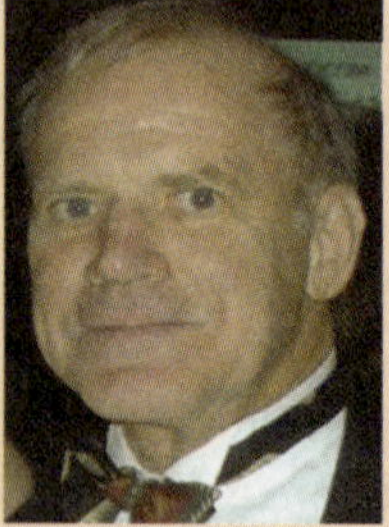

Kary Mullis
(Born 1944, North Carolina, USA)

Kary Mullis, PhD, who conceived PCR as a method to copy DNA and synthesize large amounts of a specific target DNA, was awarded the **1993 Nobel Prize in Chemistry.**

Uses of PCR

PCR is highly sensitive and can detect the presence of even a single molecule of DNA. PCR is used for quick diagnosis of AIDS, DNA fingerprinting and sex identification.

Blotting Techniques

Blotting techniques are methodical techniques used for the identification of a particular DNA, RNA or a protein. There are three techniques: ***southern blotting*** (for DNA), ***northern blotting*** (for RNA) and ***western blotting*** (for protein).

Southern blotting

In southern blotting, DNA is extracted from the cells like leucocytes) and cleaved into fragments by *restriction endonucleases*.

1. DNA extracted and fragments are separated and denatured.
2. The DNA fragments are transferred into a sheet of nitrocellulose paper from the agarose gel by blotting.
3. Then DNA fragments are fixed to the membrane usually by ultraviolet cross-linking.
4. The labeled DNA is formed by hybrid complexes.
5. Following the hybridization reaction, the membrane is washed and regions of hybridization are identified by autoradiography.

Southern blotting is used for ***DNA fingerprinting*** and for ***detection of mutant gene*** that causes diseases like cystic fibrosis.

Northern blotting

Northern blotting is similar to southern blotting except that the RNA is used instead of DNA. Northern blotting is used for analysis of gene expression in a particular tissue.

Western blotting

Western blotting is used for identification of specific proteins. First, the SDS polyacrylamide gel electrophoresis is performed for the protein mixture, and then the electrophoresed protein bands are transferred from SDS polyacrylamide gel to a nitrocellulose membrane. Afterward, probing is performed using a labeled antibody probe. Western blotting along with ELISA is a confirmatory test for HIV.

Cloning

Cloning means ***production of many identical copies of a molecule***. Generally, there are four types of cloning: Gene cloning, reproductive cloning, tissue cloning and embryo cloning.

Gene Cloning

Gene cloning, also referred to as ***DNA cloning*** or ***recombinant DNA technology*** is the process of transfer of a specific DNA fragment of one organism to a self-replicating genetic component of the cloning vector such as bacterial plasmid. Following transfer of the DNA fragment, the molecule is propagated in the host organism. Gene cloning is used widely in genetic engineering for *sequencing genomes* and in *gene therapy*.

Reproductive Cloning

Reproductive cloning is used to ***produce an animal having the same nuclear DNA*** from the existing animal. The *Broad methodology:*

1. The technique of reproductive cloning uses the principle of *somatic cell nuclear transfer*, in which genetic material from the adult donor cell is transferred to an egg from which the genetic material has been removed.
2. The new egg containing the DNA of the donor cell is allowed to divide by chemicals or electric current.
3. After attaining a suitable stage, the cloned embryo is transferred to the uterus of the host female where it grows into a complete fetus.

Reproductive cloning can be used to reproduce animals that are difficult to breed. The ***Dolly sheep*** is the first cloned animal (Roslin Institute in Edinburgh, Scotland, 1997).

Embryo Cloning

This is also called ***therapeutic cloning***, which refers to the production of human embryos for research purposes. The aim of this is not to create a cloned human being, rather to yield stem cells to study human evolution and disease treatments. Stem cells are extracted in the blastocyst stage of development, which can practically generate any type of cells in the human body. Stem cells are used to replace degenerating cells as in Alzheimer's disease, cancer, etc.

Tissue Cloning

This technique is called ***tissue culture***, in which cells are allowed to grow in a suitable medium. The cloned cells are used to study of the action of hormones, antibiotics and pharmaceutical products.

Mutation

Mutation refers to ***a change in the DNA structure of a gene***. Mutation is caused by mutagens, the factors that produce mutation. The known mutagens are X-rays, ultraviolet light, certain chemicals, etc. There are two major types of mutations: Point mutation and frame-shift mutation.

Point Mutation

In point mutation, one base pair of DNA replaces the other. This is of two types: transitions and transversion. ***Transition*** is the type of mutation in which one purine or pyrimidine is replaced by another purine or pyrimidine. In ***transversion*** type of mutation, a purine is replaced by pyrimidine or pyrimidine is replaced by purine.

Frame-shift Mutations

In this mutation, base pairs are either deleted or inserted into the DNA. Hence, this is also called ***deletion or insertional mutations***. The deletion or insertion leads to change in the frame of mRNA. Therefore, mRNA becomes unable to recognize that a new base is added or missing. However, translation continues and proteins formed have many altered amino acid sequence.

Mutation results in diseases such as sickle cell disease, phenylketonuria, cystic fibrosis, etc.

Genetic Screening

Genetic screening is detecting the ***genetic variations in a human being***. It is used for diagnosing diseases at various stages and for various purposes such as prenatal diagnosis, diagnosis of carrier states and prognostic diagnosis.

Prenatal Diagnosis

Prenatal diagnosis aims at identifying the health problems in the fetal stage and therefore has preventive values. This is performed by chorionic villus sampling, amniocentesis and pre-implantation diagnosis.

Diagnosis of Carrier States

A group of people carry and transmit the disease without suffering from it. The identification of such carrier people is important in preventing the spread of disease in the community. The examples of carrier states include sickle cell anemia, cystic fibrosis and phenylketonuria.

Prognostic Diagnosis

Some diseases like type II diabetes mellitus or Huntington's chorea that are present in childhood are likely to occur in genetically susceptible individuals when they become adult or middle aged. Genetic screening of such people to identify the susceptibility of the disease helps in preventing the disease to occur.

Genetic Basis of Cancer

Some cancers such as cancer of colon and female breast, retinoblastoma, leukemia etc. have hereditary predisposition. Defective DNA and chromosomal abnormalities are among the etiological factors in the genesis of cancers like acute myeloid leukemia and Burkitt's lymphoma. Ionizing radiations like exposures to ultraviolet rays produce cancer by causing mutagenesis (damaging the genetic constitution) of the individual.

Cancer Genes

There are genes that predispose to cancer and genes that prevent cancers. **Cancer producing genes** are oncogenes and defective P53 gene. **Genes preventing cancer** are tumor suppressor genes (or antioncogenes) and RB gene.

Oncogenes

Cancer causing genes are called oncogenes. There are more than 100 oncogenes have been described so far. The **proto-oncogenes** are normal genes that encode proteins controlling normal cell functions. Many factors stimulate conversion of proto-oncogenes to oncogenes. The factors that promote this conversion are:

1. **Chromosomal translocation:** In this, a part of chromosome is translocated to other chromosome. For example, an area of chromosome 8 in patients with Burkitt's lymphoma is translocated to either of the chromosome 2, 14 and 22.
2. **Missense mutation:** In this, amino acid sequence of proto-oncogene changes that helps the protein to convert into oncogene.
3. **Gene amplification:** Amplification of some of the genes to become oncogene has been implicated in the genesis of lung, breast, stomach and colon cancer.

Defective P53 Gene

Normally, stimulation of P53 gene results in formation of **P53 protein**. P53 protein serves as a transcription factor for many physiological functions that prevent malignancy. These are:

1. P53 protein activates genes that promote DNA repair.
2. It activates genes that arrest cell division.
3. It also stimulates genes that help apoptosis.

About *half of malignancies are associated with defects in P53 gene*.

Mutator Genes

Normally, damage to DNA is repaired by caretaker genes. Mutator gene is the faulty caretaker gene that has lost normal surveillance function and therefore helps in genesis of cancer.

Telomerase

Telomerase recognizes telomere in cell divisions. Cancer cells express more telomerase that promotes telomere lengthening and this helps in cancerous proliferation.

Genes preventing cancer

RB Gene

Retinoblastoma (RB) gene serves as cancer suppressor. Mutation or deletion of this gene results in retinoblastoma.

Tumor Suppressor Gene

These are also called **anti-oncogenes** that prevent genesis of cancer. More than ten such genes have been identified. These genes are inactivated by mutation. Thus, mutation causes cancer.

Gene Therapy

Hereditary disorders occur due to transmission of defective genes. Gene therapy aims at providing the correct copy of the gene concerned. This is achieved by:

1. **Gene replacement:** Replacement of a mutant gene with a normal gene
2. **Gene correction:** Correction of the specific bases of DNA

3. **Gene augmentation:** Insertion of a foreign DNA into the genome of a cell to rectify the genetic defect

Somatic Cell Therapy

In humans, somatic (nongametic) cells are used in the gene therapy as changes in these cells cannot be inherited.

The broad steps are:

1. Cells are isolated with the defective gene from the patient and grown in culture.
2. Grown cells are transfected with a remedial gene construct.
3. Transfected cells are then transfused back into the patients.

It is successfully tried in ***cystic fibrosis*** of the lung and ***severe combined immunodeficiency syndrome***. Without ADA (adenosine deaminase), the child develops SCID and dies of infection in the early childhood.

In cancer, gene therapy is very useful, in which oncogenic gene is inactivated by introducing a gene like tumor suppressor gene. This selectively kills the cancer cells.

APOPTOSIS

Apoptosis is the **programmed cell death**. Apoptosis is a Greek word meaning *'falling off'* or *'dropping off'*, first described 1972. It is a distinct process from necrosis. It is a form of coordinated and internally planned cell death, which is of greater significance in a variety of physiologic and pathologic conditions.

Apoptosis is the programmed cell death that has genetic control. **Genes of the own cells** play important role in this programmed cell death. Apoptosis is a natural process, and examples are:

1. Death of neurons in central nervous system during brain development and synapse formation is an example of apoptosis.
2. During fetal development, degeneration of many tissues like web in the fingers is other example.
3. Many blood cells like eosinophils undergo apoptosis.

Scientist contributed

For many years, the terms "apoptosis" and "programmed cell death" were not highly cited. What transformed cell death from obscurity to a major field of research were two things: the identification of components of the cell death control and effector mechanisms, and the linkage of abnormalities in cell death to human disease, in particular cancer. The 2002, **Nobel Prize in Physiology and Medicine** was awarded to **Sydney Brenner, Horvitz** and **John E Sulston** for their work identifying genes that control apoptosis. The genes were identified by studies in the nematode *C Elegans* and these same genes function in humans for apoptosis.

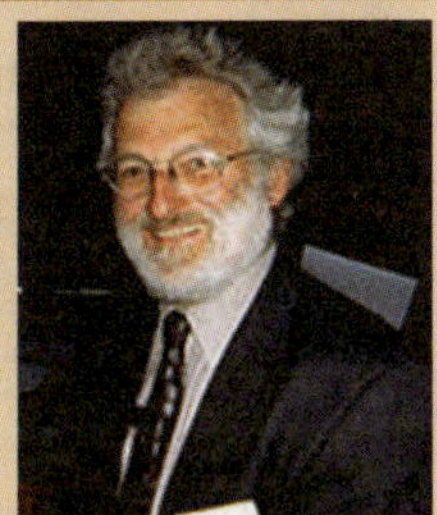

John E Sulston
(Nobel Prize, 2002, for pioneering research on apoptosis)

Mechanisms of Apoptosis

Stimuli

Activation of cysteine proteases in the cell called **caspases** triggers apoptosis. Normally, caspases are present in the inactive form in the cell, and stimulated by external and internal stimuli.

Internal stimuli: Mitochondria release cytochrome and a protein called *smac* that causes activation of the *caspase 9*, which induces apoptosis. In mitochondria, apoptosis inducing factor is located in the intermembrane space that migrates to nucleus and destroys DNA.

External stimuli: External stimuli are various ligands that bind with cell surface to activate apoptosis. One such factor is tumor necrosis factor that activates the enzyme *caspase 8*. Activation of caspase promotes DNA fragmentation and chromatin condensation.

Molecular Mechanisms of Apoptosis

Initiation of Apoptosis

Stimuli signaling programmed cell death act either on the cell membrane or intracellularly.

(a) Usually it is triggered by absence of stimuli that are normally required for normal cell survival such as absence of certain hormones, growth factors, cytokines, etc.
(b) Activation of receptors like receptors of TNF initiates programmed cell death.
(c) Intracellular stimuli may include heat, radiation, hypoxia, etc.
(d) Genetically programmed events.

Regulation of Apoptosis

Once apoptosis is initiated, certain intracellular proteins provide signal for the final programmed cell death, which actually determine the outcome. These **regulatory proteins** include the following:

(a) **BCL-2:** BCL-2 is a protein which is equivalent to CED-9, the cell death gene found in nematodes. BCL-2 is located in the outer mitochondrial membrane and control apoptotic process by binding to various cytosolic proteins. Usually it binds to BAX and BAD proteins that are known to promote apoptosis. It may also bind with BCL-XL protein that inhibits apoptosis. Another binding protein present in the cytosol is the pro-apoptotic protease-activating factor (apzaf-1), which is a mammalian counterpart of gene CED-4 of nematode. Thus, apoptosis depends on binding of BCL-2 with pro-apoptotic and anti-apoptotic proteins.
(b) **Other apoptotic regulator proteins:** Other regulator proteins of apoptosis are TP53 (p53) protein, caspases, BAX and certain viruses such as adenovirus, papilloma virus, hepatitis B virus, etc.

Flowchart 5.2: Major steps of apoptosis.

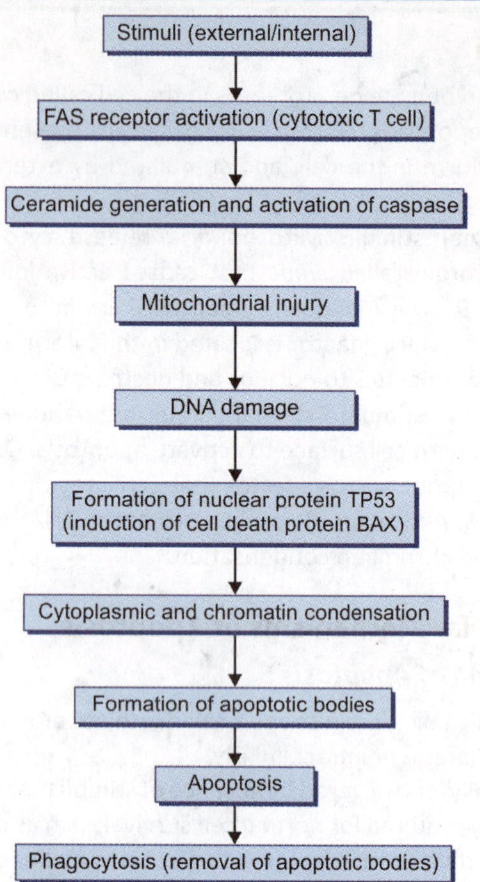

Steps of Apoptosis

Apoptosis occurs in following major steps (Flowchart 5.2).

(a) **FAS receptor activation:** CD 95 or FAS, the surface receptor present on cytotoxic T cells when comes in contact with the target cell, is activated. This leads to ***activation of caspases*** and subsequent proteolysis.

(b) **Ceramide generation:** Hydrolysis of sphingomyelin on the cell membrane generates ceramide. Ceramide causes mitochondrial injury.

(c) **DNA damage:** Damage by various agents and activated oxygen species like free oxygen radicals leads to apoptosis. DNA injury influences nuclear protein TP53 that induces the synthesis of cell death promoting protein BAX.

(d) **Cell shrinkage:** Cell reduces in size and cytoplasmic condensation occurs.

(e) **Formation of apoptotic bodies:** Apoptotic bodies are formed as described below.

(f) **Phagocytosis:** The dead apoptotic cells and their fragments are identified and engulfed by phagocytes.

Physiologic and Pathologic Processes

Apoptosis is a biologic phenomenon, which has both physiologic and pathologic processes.

Flowchart 5.3: Physiologic process of apoptosis, which occurs in three main steps.

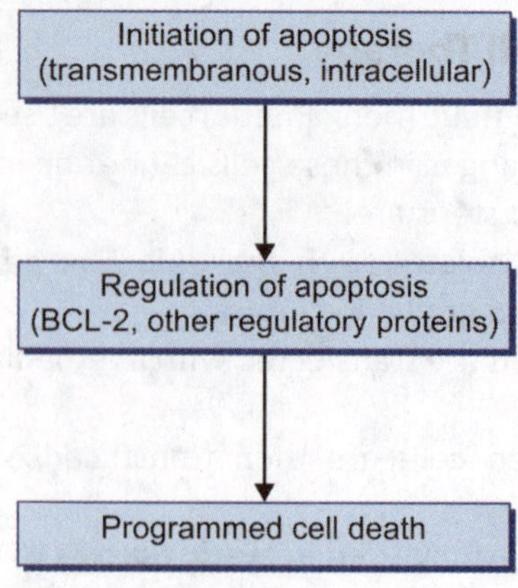

Physiologic Processes

Physiologic processes occur in three steps (Flowchart 5.3). They are influenced by many factors and examples are:

1. Physiologic involution of cells in hormone-dependent tissues such as endometrial shedding in menstrual cycles, regression of lactating breast after cessation of breast-feeding.
2. Normal shedding of intestinal epithelium.
3. Involution of the thymus after childhood.

Pathologic Process

Pathologic processes are initiated by following factors.

1. Tumor cell death on exposure to chemotherapeutic agents.
2. Transplant cell death by cytotoxic T cells that cause transplant rejection.
3. Cell death induced by viral infections as occurs in viral hepatitis.
4. Pathologic atrophy following withdrawal of stimuli. For example, prostatic atrophy after orchiectomy.
5. Cell death induced by radiation, hypoxia and thermal injury.
6. Degenerative diseases of CNS such as in Alzheimer's disease, Parkinson's disease, etc.

Changes in Apoptosis

Pathophysiologic Changes

Changes in apoptosis confuses with the changes in necrosis. **In necrosis**, cytoplasm is homogenously eosinophilic, and nuclear changes are pyknosis (condensation and clumping of nucleus), karyolysis (disintegration of the nucleus) and karyorrhexis (nucleus fragments into small bits and disperses into cytoplasm). In apoptosis, there is condensation of nuclear chromatin and cell fragments into apoptotic bodies that are phagocytosed by macrophages (Fig. 5.10).

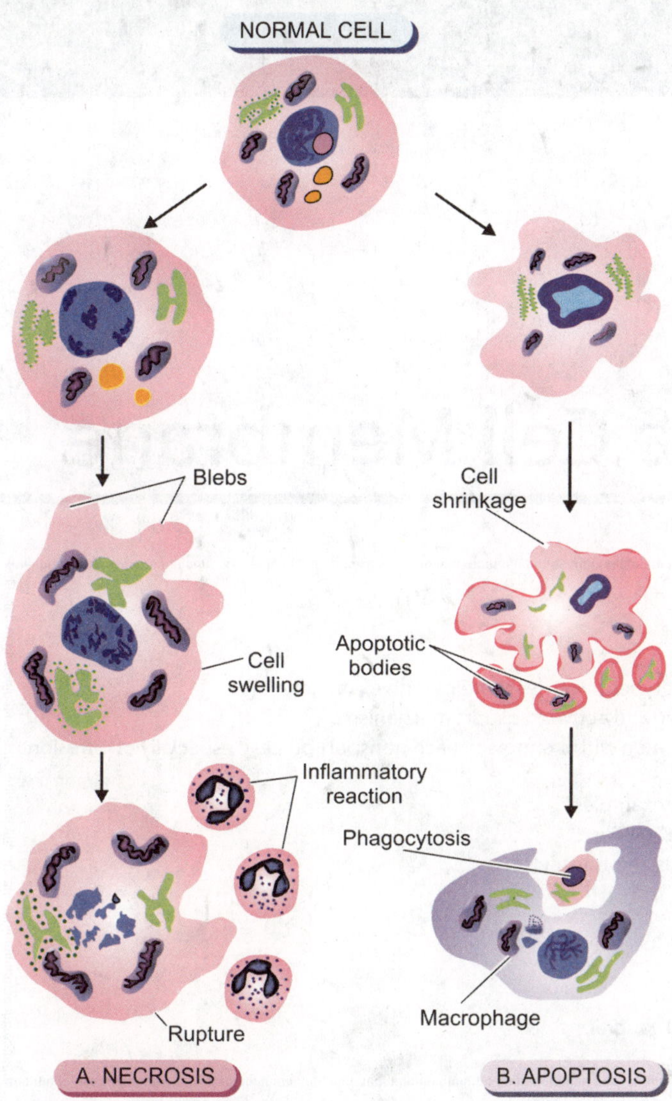

Fig. 5.10: Morphological changes in apoptosis. In necrosis, cytoplasm is homogenously eosinophilic, and nuclear changes are pyknosis, karyolysis and karyorrhexis. In apoptosis, there is condensation of nuclear chromatin and cell fragments into apoptotic bodies that are phagocytosed by macrophages. Inflammatory response around apoptosis is absent.

The characteristic changes in apoptosis include the following:

1. May involve single cells or a cluster of cells. The apoptotic cells become round or oval and reduce in size. The cytoplasm becomes **intensely eosinophilic** containing condensed or fragmented nuclear chromatin material. Typically, *inflammatory response around apoptosis is absent*.
2. Though cytoplasm is reduced, organelles remain almost normal.
3. Cell membrane convolutes with formation of membrane-bound spherical structures called **apoptotic bodies** that contain compacted organelles.
4. **Chromatic condensation** occurs around the periphery of nucleus.
5. **Phagocytosis** of apoptotic bodies occurs by macrophages.

Biochemical Changes

Biochemical changes include:

1. **Proteolysis** of cytoskeletal proteins.
2. Cross-linking of protein molecules.
3. Fragmentation of nuclear chromatin by *activation of nuclease*.
4. A glycoprotein molecule called **thrombospondin** and a phosphoprotein called **phosphatidylserine** appear on the outer surface of apoptotic bodies, which facilitate recognition by macrophages for phagocytosis.

Application

Identification of components of the cell death control and effector mechanisms and the linkage of abnormalities in cell death to human disease, in particular cancers, has unraveled the research for preventing the cell death. Understanding the concept of apoptosis has promising role in future regenerative medicine.

CHAPTER SUMMARY

Physiology of genomics is a developing branch of medicine. It deals with the understanding of the concept of gene and gene therapy in treatment of genetic disorders. Discovery of cancer genes (oncogenes) and genes preventing cancers has changed the concept and modality of treatment of malignancies. Understanding the concept of apoptosis has promising role in regenerative medicine.

Important to Know (Must Read)

1. **Long Questions** may be asked on 'Recombinant DNA technology and PCR' or 'Mechanism of Apoptosis' for PGs, but not for UGs.
2. Structure and function of DNA, protein synthesis, blotting techniques, cloning, genetic screening, gene therapy, and oncogenes, may be asked as **Short Notes/Questions** in exams.
3. In **Viva,** examiners usually ask on structure and functions of chromosomes, genome, chromosomal disorders, nuclear sexing, gene amplification, uses of recombinant DNA technology and PCR, types of cloning with examples, types of mutation, importance of genetic screening, types of oncogenes, tumor suppressor genes, types of gene therapy, and definition and changes in apoptosis.

CHAPTER 6

Transport Across the Cell Membrane

Learning Objectives

On completion of study of this chapter, the student **MUST** be able to:

1. Name common ion channels in the membrane; and name different types of carrier proteins with examples.
2. Classify transport processes and list the differences between passive and active transport mechanisms.
3. Describe the mechanism, factors affecting and physiological application with example of each transport process, especially of diffusion and osmosis.
4. Explain the primary and secondary active transport processes with examples.
5. Describe the structure, mechanism of action and functions of Na^+-K^+ ATPase.
6. Describe the mechanism and importance of endocytosis, exocytosis and transcytosis.

The student **MAY** also be able to:

1. Describe the gating of ion channels.
2. Describe types of patch clamping.
3. Explain the properties of facilitated diffusion.
4. Define the concept of osmole and application of osmosis in clinical conditions.
5. Describe other types of ATPases.

Fluid and electrolytes on either side of the cell membrane pass through the membrane by various means due to the presence of different channels and carrier molecules. Selective membrane permeability generates the difference in composition between intracellular and extracellular fluids. Transport of specific substances, like drugs, chemicals and hormones also influence cell functions.

Passage of substances through the membrane can be broadly divided into two categories:

1. **Direct passage without involvement of carrier molecules:** Cell membrane is a lipid bilayer. Hence, lipid-soluble substances, such as gases, fatty acids, alcohol, ketone bodies, aldehydes and many small-uncharged molecules pass through the membrane easily. Water molecules also pass through membrane easily.
2. **Passage through channels or carrier proteins:** Though water passes easily through the membrane, water-soluble substances, such as electrolytes, glucose and amino acids do not penetrate membrane readily. There are two major means through which these substances are transported across the cell membranes: through water channels formed by integral proteins, and by combination with carrier molecules in the cell membrane.

PROTEIN CHANNELS IN THE MEMBRANE

Proteins that constitute channels are selectively permeable. They are tubular structures that connect the exterior with the interior of cells. The permeability of channels depends on molecular size, shape and charge.

Types of Protein Channels

Broadly, they are of two types: ion channels and water channels.

Ion Channels

Ion channels are integral proteins that span the entire width of the membrane. Normally, they are formed by several polypeptide subunits.

Mechanism of working of ion channels:

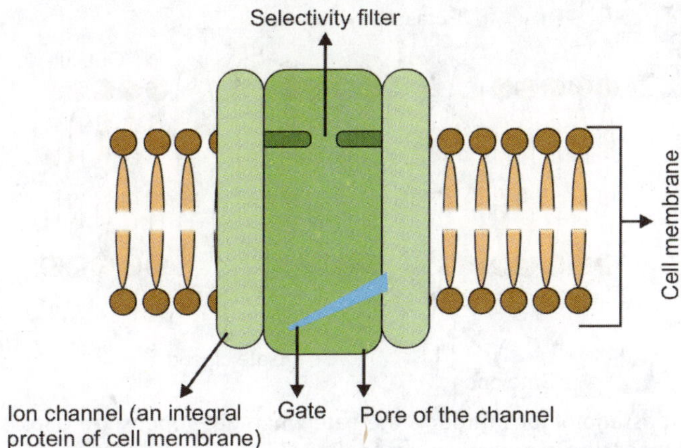

Fig. 6.1: A typical ion channel. Note the presence of selectivity filter and the gate.

1. Along the length of the integral protein, an **aqueous pore** is present, around which the polypeptide subunits are arranged. Ions pass through the aqueous pore from one side of the membrane to the other. Thus, ions cross the membrane *without entering through the lipid bilayer* of the membrane.
2. A polypeptide subunit forms **a gate** at one end of the channel that opens in response to a specific stimulus (Fig. 6.1).
3. Opening of the gate opens the channel and allows the ions to rapidly move (10^8 ions per sec) through the channel.
4. However, there is a **selectivity filter** that permits specific ions to pass through the channel. Therefore, *ion channels are often selective*.

Sodium and potassium channels are extensively studied membrane channels.

Sodium Channels

Sodium channels have been studied in detail among all the ion channels. It has subunits surrounding an aqueous pore of about 0.5 nm in diameter. The inner surface of the pore is negatively charged. It is selective for passage of sodium. Sodium channel is blocked by **tetrodotoxin**.

Potassium Channels

There are many types of potassium channels. They are about 0.3 nm in diameter. Potassium channels are blocked by *tetraethyl ammonium* or **4-aminopyridine**.

Calcium and Chloride Channels

There are various channels for Ca^{++} and for Cl^-. **Ca^{++} channels** can be voltage-gated, ligand-gated and stretch-sensitive (for details, refer to chapter 71). **Cl^- channels** are dimeric (have two pores) and pentameric (e.g. $GABA_A$ and glycine receptors). CFTR protein is a Cl^- channel.

Water Channels

Water channels are **aquaporins**. There are 13 types of aquaporins (for details, refer to 'Water reabsorption from kidney' in 'Renal Physiology').

Gating of Ion Channels

Some of the ion channels remain always open, and, therefore, they are referred to as ***nongated channels***. However, many ion channels open and close by gates. Ion channels are provided with gate on either side of the channel, and opening or closure of the gate regulates the movement of various ions through them.

There are three general mechanisms of gating: voltage-gating, ligand-gating and mechanical-gating.

Voltage-gating

Change in the membrane potential beyond a certain threshold value opens or closes the gate of the ion channels. Therefore, they are called ***voltage-gated channels***. For example, ion channels in excitable tissues, such as nerve and muscle are mainly voltage-gated channels like Na^+, K^+ and Ca^{++} channels. They are also present in pacemaker tissues in the heart and other organs. They are involved in generating and conducting action potentials.

Mechanism of gating:

1. The exact mechanism of voltage-gating is not known. It is proposed that alteration in membrane potential induces movement of some charged amino acids in helical segment of the channel protein that causes a *conformational change* of the channel protein, which in turn opens or closes the gate and allows the ions to pass through the channel rapidly.
2. For **Na^+ channels**, the gate is located on the outer end of the channel (Fig. 6.2A). The gate closes the outer opening of the channel when the cell is at RMP (–70 mV in nerve, –90 mV in muscle and –50 mV in pacemaker tissue). When inside becomes less negative, the gate opens and Na^+ influx occurs that leads to first, formation of local response and later, the genesis of action potential.
3. For **K^+ channels**, the gate is located on the inner end of the channel (Fig. 6.2B). The gate closes the cytoplasmic opening of the channel when the cell is at RMP. When interior becomes less negative and approaches towards positivity, more and more gates open and K^+ efflux occurs that leads to first, reversal of depolarization potential and later, the repolarization of action potential.

Important Note

Speed of opening of ion channel determines the slope of potential: Opening of K^+ channels is slower than the opening of Na^+ channels. Therefore, in action potential, the phase of repolarization, which is due to K^+ permeability, is less steep than the phase of depolarization.

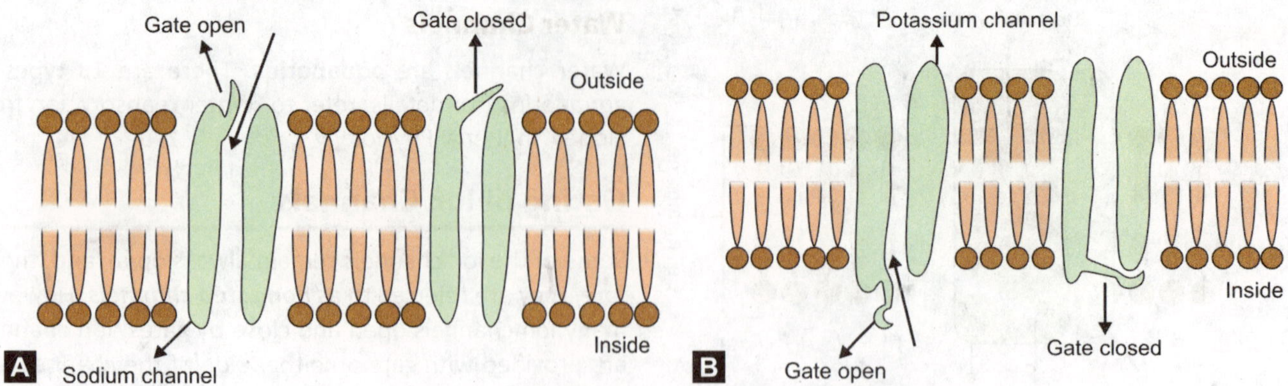

Figs. 6.2A and B: Gating mechanism of ion channel. Arrow indicates passage of ions through the gate when gate opens. (A) Gate is present on the outer side in sodium channel; (B) Gate is present on the inner side in potassium channel.

Ligand Gating

Interaction of the channel with a ligand (hormone or neurotransmitter) causes opening or closure of the channel. Hence, the channels are called ***ligand-gated channels***. As the ligand is a chemical agent, the gating is also called ***chemical gating***.

Mechanism of ligand gating:

1. The chemical agent binds with the specific receptor protein on the membrane and brings about conformational change in the protein that, in turn, directly or indirectly opens the channel.
2. **Nicotinic cholinergic receptor** channel in postsynaptic neuromuscular junction is a ligand-gated ion channel. Acetylcholine released at the nerve ending binds with these receptors and opens the ion channels that generate postsynaptic potential.
3. Acetylcholine at the parasympathetic endings binds with *muscarinic cholinergic receptors* on the membrane of GI smooth muscle cells and activates G protein, which, in turn, activates the enzyme that causes production of ***second messengers*** such as cyclic AMP or Ca^{++}. The second messengers activate enzymes like kinase that act on the ion channel by phosphorylation.
4. Other examples are the action of noradrenaline on β-adrenergic receptors on the smooth muscle cell.

Direct opening of channels: The receptor for the hormone or neurotransmitter may also be the channel itself, so that the action by the ligand is direct on the channel. For example, acetylcholine released at parasympathetic nerve endings acts on the receptor in the postsynaptic membrane in the cardiac pacemaker cells. This causes direct opening of K^+ channels in the pacemaker tissue and causes hyperpolarization that decreases the discharge rate of the pacemaker.

Mechanical Gating

Some of the channels are **mechanosensitive** and they respond to stretch. Examples are **ion channels in hair cells** in the cochlea and vestibular apparatus, and **stretch-sensitive channels** in the ventricular muscles. Stretch imparted on the membrane opens the channels.

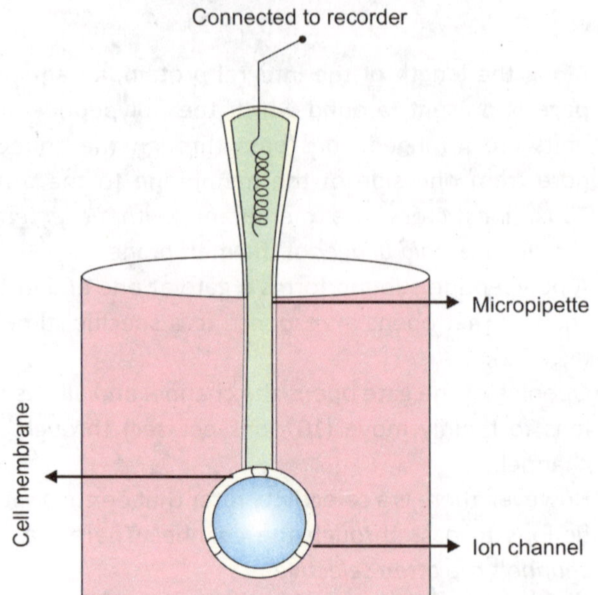

Fig. 6.3: Method of patch clamping (cell-attached patch). The micropipette records the activity of the channel in the membrane.

Patch Clamping

Latest information on membrane channels and carriers was gathered by application of a special technique known as ***patch clamp technique***. This is a very sensitive method as it can study the movement of ions by opening or closing of a single ion channel.

In this method:

1. A micropipette with tip diameter of about 1 µm is inserted into the membrane and suction is applied through the micropipette (Fig. 6.3).
2. By applying suction, a tiny patch of the cell membrane is sucked up, so that it seals the tip of the micropipette.
3. Such a small patch of membrane contains only a few channels, which helps to study them in detail.

Types of Patch Clamping

There are three types of patch clamping: cell-attached patch, whole-cell patch and inside-out patch.

Cell-attached patch: In this clamping, the patch of the membrane remains attached with the cell.

Whole-cell patch: In this type of clamping, the patch of the membrane provides access into the interior of the cell.

Inside-out patch: In this method, the patch of the membrane is pulled from inside of the membrane to the outside of the membrane.

However, the patch of the membrane is small enough to contain one or two channels. The channel characteristics can be studied by changing the chemical and electrical gradients across the membrane.

Uses of Patch-clamp Technique

1. The patch clamp technique is an essential tool for scientists studying the activity and behavior of ion channels in cell.
2. This helped to understand how defective regulation of ion channels underlies a host of diseases, including diabetes and cystic fibrosis.
3. Mechanisms of action of drugs that use or block ion channels such as Ca^{++} or K^{+} channels blockers were studied using this techniqu.

Scientists contributed

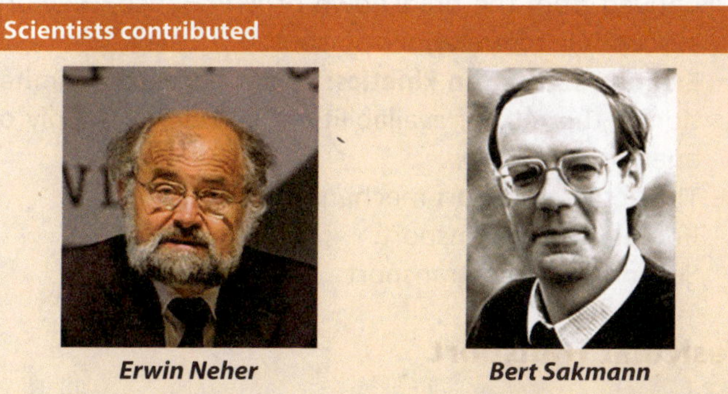

Erwin Neher ***Bert Sakmann***

The 1991 Nobel Prize in Physiology or Medicine was awarded to two German scientists, Erwin Neher and Bert Sakmann for creating the experimental measuring device that conclusively proved the existence and function of ion channels.

Neher and Sakmann Model

An extremely fine glass pipette with a very small opening is used to make contact with a tiny area, or patch, of the cell's outer membrane that will contain only a single ion channel. Applying a small amount of suction through the pipette forms a seal tight enough such that ions can only flow from the channel into the pipette. By fitting the pipette with a highly sensitive electrode, Neher and Sakmann could record ***every minute change in current produced*** as ions flow through the clamped channel into the pipette.

1. With their recording device, they showed how these channels function by opening up and closing in nerve cell membranes to allow certain ions through one at a time.

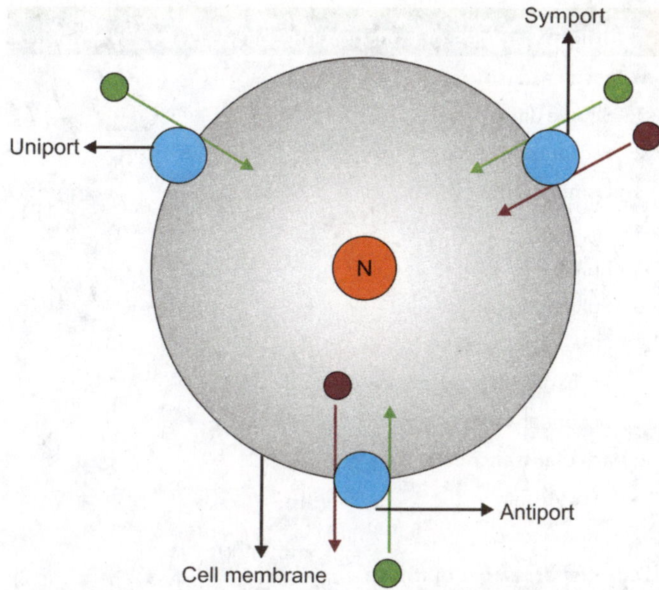

Fig. 6.4: Types of carrier proteins in the cell membrane. Uniport transports one substance, symport transports two substances in the same direction and antiport transports two substances in the opposite directions.

2. By altering the genes that encode ion channels and studying the consequences in cells allowed Neher and Sakmann to pinpoint the parts of the channel that open or close and that select which ions can pass through.

Types of Carrier Proteins

There are three different types of carrier proteins: Uniport, symport and antiport (Fig. 6.4).

Uniport: Uniport is the carrier protein that transports only one substance. For example, Na^{+} channels transport Na^{+} and K^{+} channels transport K^{+}.

Symport: Symport carriers transport two or more substances from one side of the membrane to the other ***in the same direction***. Transport of Na^{+} and glucose from the lumen of the intestine or kidney tubule into the epithelial cells through the same carrier protein is an example of symport mechanism. Such substances are said to be **co-transported**.

Antiport: Antiport carriers transport substances ***in opposite directions*** in which one substance is transported to the inside of the cell and other substance from inside the cell to the outside. Substances transported in opposite directions by one carrier are said to be **counter-transported**. Examples are:

1. A typical antiport carrier is the **sodium-potassium pump**, which is operated by Na^{+}-K^{+} ATPase. It actively transports 3 Na^{+} out of the cell, and 2 K^{+} into cells for each molecule of ATP hydrolyzed.
2. **Na^{+}-H^{+} exchanger** found in the proximal tubular cells of the nephron, for which the inward facilitated diffusion of Na^{+} is coupled with the outward diffusion of H^{+}.

Table 6.1: Types of transport processes.

A. Passive transports
1. Simple diffusion
2. Facilitated diffusion
3. Osmosis
4. Filtration
5. Bulk flow
6. Solvent drag
B. Active transports
1. Primary active transport
2. Secondary active transport
C. Vesicular transports
1. Exocytosis
2. Endocytosis
D. Transport across epithelia
1. Transcellular transport
2. Paracellular transport

Characteristics of Carrier-mediated Transport

Carrier-mediated transport systems exhibit ***two important properties***: Competition for the carrier protein and the saturation of the transport process.

Competitive inhibition: Presence of different molecules with similar structure *competes for the same carrier* ***protein*** for their transport, which results in competitive inhibition of the process. For instance, the presence of ketoses in intestinal content decreases the reabsorption of aldoses by the gut.

Saturation kinetics: The number of carrier proteins in a membrane is limited. Therefore, the rate of carrier-mediated transport reaches a maximum which is known as ***transport maximum*** or **Tm**. The Tm cannot be exceeded by increasing the concentration of the substance. Thus, the carrier-mediated transport exhibits saturation kinetics.

TRANSPORT PROCESSES

Types

Transport mechanisms through cell membrane can broadly be divided into three types: passive transport, active transport, and vesicular transport (Table 6.1). There is another process of transport called ***transport across epithelia***.

Special Features

Passive Transport

There are two common features of passive transport processes (Table 6.2). These are:

a. **Transport is downhill:** In passive transports, the substances pass through the membrane from both sides, however, net movement occurs down the electrochemical gradient;
b. **Transport does not require metabolic energy:** Passive transport does not require utilization of ATP.

Examples are simple diffusion, facilitated diffusion, osmosis, filtration, bulk flow and solvent drag.

Table 6.2: Differences between active and passive transport processes.

	Active transport	Passive transport
1. Nature of transport	Against electrochemical gradient	Along the gradient
2. Utilization of energy	ATP hydrolysis occurs	Not needed
3. Saturation kinetics	Is a feature	May not be present

Active Transport

Active transport differs from passive transport by its utilization of energy. The common features of active transport are (Table 6.2):

1. **Uphill transport:** Transport occurs against the electrochemical gradient of the substance.
2. **Requires energy:** Energy utilized for transport is derived from the breakdown of ATP. Hence, they are susceptible to metabolic poisons.
3. **Exhibits saturation kinetics:** This is because of limitation in the rate of availability of carriers or supply of energy.

The active transport mechanisms are:

1. Primary active transport.
2. Secondary active transport.

Vesicular Transport

This transport has no relation with the concentration gradient. However, it may utilize metabolic energy.

Vesicular transport mechanisms are:

1. Exocytosis.
2. Endocytosis.

SIMPLE DIFFUSION

Diffusion is the process of passive transport in which molecules move from the area of higher concentration to the area of lower concentration. In simple diffusion, molecules move due to their random movement. The examples of substances that pass through cell membranes by simple diffusions are transport of O_2, CO_2, urea, ammonia and ions. Across a membrane, diffusion of a molecule occurs when difference in concentration of the molecule exists on both sides of the membrane. The net movement of molecule ceases when the concentration of molecule on both sides becomes equal and a *diffusional equilibrium* is achieved.

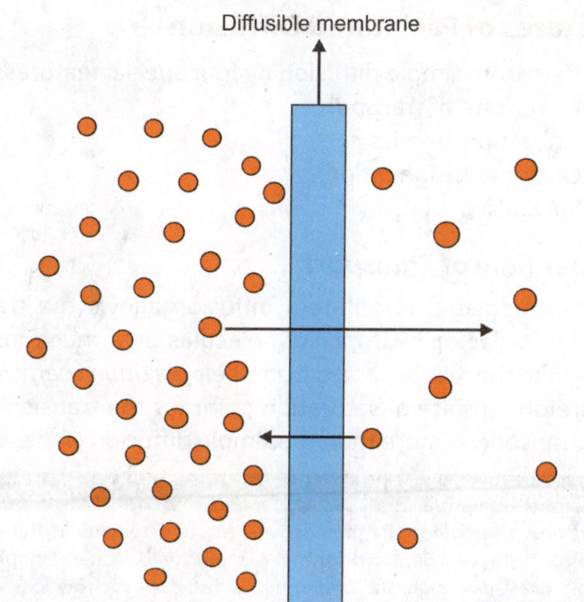

Fig. 6.5: Diffusion across the cell membrane. The molecules move in both directions, but the movement is more from higher to lower concentration of solutes. The length of arrow indicates the magnitude of movement of molecules.

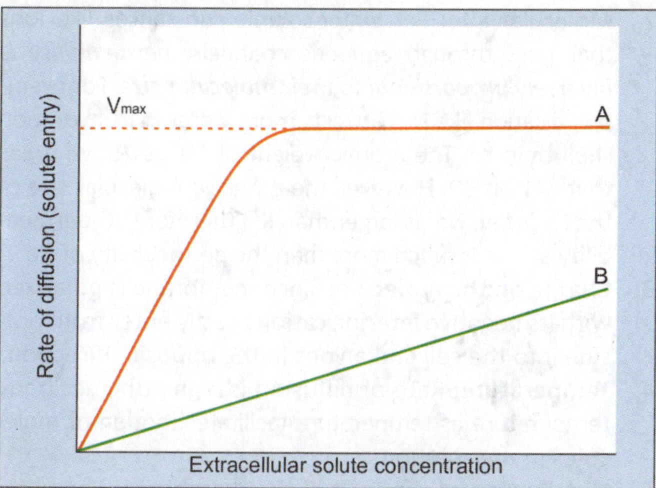

Fig. 6.6: Rate of diffusion (solute entry into the cell) by carrier mediated or facilitated diffusion (A) and simple diffusion (B). In simple diffusion, though a linear relationship exists between the rate of diffusion and concentration of solute throughout the process, total quantity of solutes transported is less due to slower rate of diffusion. In facilitated diffusion, though diffusion does not increase further after reaching V_{max} (maximum rate), the total amount of solutes transferred is more due to higher rate of diffusion.

Factors that Determine Rate of Diffusion

Factors determining the rate of diffusion across the cell membrane can be broadly divided into two categories: (a) properties of the substance and (b) the properties of the membrane.

Properties of the Substance

Properties of the substance that determine diffusion through membrane are mainly, (a) concentration and electrical gradients of the substance, and (b) permeability of the substance through the membrane.

Effect of Concentration and Electrical Gradients

The concentration or the **chemical gradients** of the substance is primarily responsible for the direction of transport of the substance (Fig. 6.5). The electrical potential difference **(electrical gradient)** also influences.

1. Normally, the cell membrane is polarized with the negative interior and positive exterior. Therefore, a positively charged molecule that diffuses from the outside to the negative interior is said to be moving ***along its electrical gradient***, and its diffusion from inside to the outside is said to move ***against its electrical gradient***.
2. Usually, substances move along both the electrical and chemical gradients (transfer along the ***electro-chemical gradients***). Electrochemical gradient is **mainly used for the ions**.
3. For gases, concentration gradient is expressed as *partial pressure*, and for water as *hydraulic pressure*.

Thermal energy contributes to random motion: In a liquid or gas, all particles are in constant and random motion due to ***thermal energy***. The *motion varies directly with temperature*. The motion is absent at absolute zero temperature. This random movement of particle provides the physical basis for diffusion of solutes and gas molecules in body fluids and across the cell membranes.

Unidirectional flux: When two liquids are separated by a semi-permeable membrane, the number of particles in the liquid striking a unit area from each side of the membrane at any given time is proportional to the concentration of the substance on that side. These particles succeed in passing through the membrane along the gradient, which is called ***unidirectional flux***.

1. Unidirectional flux is proportional to the **concentration of the substance** in the liquid.
2. Similarly, the unidirectional flux of the particles ***in the opposite side*** of the membrane is proportional to the *concentration of the substance on that side* of the liquid.
3. Hence, **net diffusion** is the difference between the opposing unidirectional fluxes.
4. Diffusion across the membrane ceases when the balance between the fluxes from both sides becomes zero.

A **distinguishing feature** of simple diffusion is the ***linear relationship*** between solute concentration and rate of diffusion (Fig. 6.6).

Permeability of the Substance

Permeability refers to the ease at which substances pass through the membrane.

The ***factors that determine the permeability*** are:

1. **Lipid-solubility:** As the membrane is a lipid bilayer, the permeability is *proportional to their lipid solubility* of the substance.

2. **Molecular size:** For water-soluble substances like ions that pass through aqueous channels, ***permeability is inversely proportional to their molecular size***. For example, a cation like Na^+ attracts more water in its hydration shell than K^+. The atomic weight of Na^+ is 23, whereas that of K^+ is 39. However, the effective molecular size of the hydrated Na^+ is larger than K^+. Therefore, K^+ permeability at rest is much more than the permeability of Na^+.
3. **Charge on the molecule:** Since membrane is polarized with its negative interior, cations easily enter from outside into the cell and anions in the opposite direction.
4. **Temperature:** Rate of diffusion is high at higher body temperature as temperature facilitates motion of molecules in the solution.
5. **Distribution of channels in the membrane:** The number of protein channels for the substance in the membrane determines the permeability of the substance through the membrane.
6. **Pressure gradient:** In addition to the electrochemical gradients of the substance, the fluid pressure gradient also contributes to the diffusion of the membrane. Diffusion is more from high pressure to low pressure, as the pressure causes greater number of molecule to hit the membrane.

Properties of the Membrane

In addition to the concentration gradient of the substance across the membrane, the **cross-sectional area** and **thickness** of the membrane influence diffusion. These factors are governed by **Fick's law of diffusion**. The rate of diffusion of a molecule through a membrane is proportional to the surface area (A) available for diffusion, and inversely proportional to the thickness of the membrane (T).

According to **Fick's law**, for a substance whose inside and outside concentrations are respectively C_i and C_0 mmol/l:

$$\text{Net Rate of Diffusion (J)} = \frac{-DA}{T} \times (C_i - C_0),$$

where D is the diffusion coefficient.

The minus sign indicates that the direction is down the concentration gradient. As thickness of biological membranes is fairly constant at 10^{-6} cm, D/T simplifies to the permeability coefficient 'P' of the membrane, and

$$\text{Flux} = -P \times A\,(C_i - C_0)$$

Facilitated Diffusion

When diffusion is facilitated by a carrier protein in the membrane, the process is called ***facilitated diffusion***. This is also called ***carrier-mediated diffusion*** as a carrier protein facilitates it. A typical example of facilitated diffusion is the transport of various sugars into red cells, adipose tissue, skeletal and cardiac muscles. Like simple diffusion, facilitated diffusion is also a downhill transport that does not require energy.

Features of Facilitated Diffusion

It differs from simple diffusion by four special features:
1. Faster rate of transport
2. Saturation kinetics
3. Competitive inhibition
4. Specificity.

Faster Rate of Transport

Carrier-mediated (facilitated) diffusion allows the transport of polar or hydrophilic molecules at a much faster rate than the rate expected from their *partition coefficient.* Therefore, inspite of saturation point for the transfer, the net transport is more than the simple diffusion (Table 6.3).

Important Note

Partition coefficient: Partition coefficient is the solubility of the substance in oil compared with the solubility in water. Lipophilic substances have high and hydrophilic substances such as ions and sugars have low partition coefficient. Therefore, hydrophilic molecules diffuse at a much faster rate through the membrane.

Saturation Kinetics

In simple diffusion, the rate of diffusion is proportional to the concentration of the substance and there is no saturation point. In facilitated diffusion, the ***number of carrier proteins*** available determines the rate of diffusion. When all the available binding sites on the carrier proteins are occupied, the system operates at the maximum capacity. This is called ***saturation point***. However, the rate of diffusion is faster in facilitated diffusion compared to simple diffusion, as there is no involvement of carrier protein in simple diffusion. Thus, the net diffusion in facilitated type is more than in simple type (*see* Fig. 6.6).

Competitive Inhibition

Many substances ***share same carrier protein*** for their transport. When more than one such substance are present on the same side of the membrane, they compete to bind with the carrier protein. Thus, one substance decreases the transport of the other. For example, transport of D-glucose across the epithelial membrane slows down once D-galactose is present along with it as they share same glucose transporter. Also, Na^+ and Ca^{++} compete for the *sodium-calcium cotransporter* on the membrane and excess presence of one inhibits the transport of the other. However, it should not be confused with sodium-calcium exchanger and sodium-glucose cotransporter.
1. It should not be confused with *sodium-calcium exchanger* that promotes the transport of both ions, in which increased concentration of one on one side of the membrane increases the transport of the other from opposite side of the membrane.
2. Also, this should not be confused with *carrier-mediated transport mechanisms by co-transporters* like sodium-glucose cotransporter that are essentially facilitatory for transport of more than one substance (Application Box 6.1).

Application Box 6.1

Salt is mixed with glucose in ORS: For example, presence of sodium in intestinal fluid increases the absorption of glucose from the gut content by the intestinal epithelial cells, which forms the physiological basis of adding sodium and glucose in equal proportion in the oral rehydration solution (ORS).

Specificity

The carrier proteins are specific for different molecules. For example, the carrier protein for protein does not transport cholesterol or fatty acid. However, specificity is not a rigid phenomenon as, more than one substance share the same carrier protein as for example, sodium-glucose co-transporter. Facilitated diffusion occurs through ion channels as occurs in sodium-glucose cotransport, in which glucose shares the sodium transport mechanism.

Factors Affecting Facilitated Diffusion

Factors that influence simple diffusion also affect facilitated diffusion as described above. However, the major factor is the **number of carrier proteins available** for the transport. Sometimes, facilitated diffusion is also operated by other factors like **hormones**. For example, transport of glucose by GLUT-4 into muscles and adipose tissue is insulin-dependent.

Table 6.3: Differences between simple diffusion and facilitated diffusion

	Simple diffusion	Facilitated diffusion
1. Mode of diffusion	No carrier molecule Involved	Carrier molecule involved
2. Saturation kinetics	No saturation kinetics, diffusion is linear	Has saturation kinetics. No increase in diffusion once saturation is reached
3. Competitive inhibition	Absent	Substances that share the same carrier protein compete for transport
4. Rate of diffusion	May be slow	Faster
5. Specificity	No specificity	Carrier protein may be specific

OSMOSIS

Definition: Osmosis is the process of movement of solvent from the solution with the lower concentration of solutes to the solution with higher concentration of solute, when both the solutions are separated by a semipermeable membrane.

Concept: Like solute particles, water (solvent) molecules are constantly influenced by thermal disturbance and, therefore, exhibit random movement (called ***thermodynamic activity of water***).

1. They pass through a semipermeable membrane, and their passage is proportional to the solvent molecules on that side.
2. If the membrane that separates two solutions of different solute concentrations is semipermeable, which allows the passage of solvent and not the solute particles, the solution with higher concentration solute will have lower thermodynamic activity of water, and vice versa.
3. Net water movement will, therefore, be from the *solution with a higher thermodynamic water activity to the solution with lower thermodynamic water activity*, i.e., from the side with lower solute concentration to the side with higher solute concentration (Figs. 6.7A and B).
4. Thus, the net flux of water (or solvent) through a semipermeable membrane from a solution of lower solute concentration to that of higher solute concentration is known as **osmosis**.

Osmotic Effectiveness of a Substance

A substance to maintain a stable osmotic pressure should be confined to one side of the membrane. Therefore, a

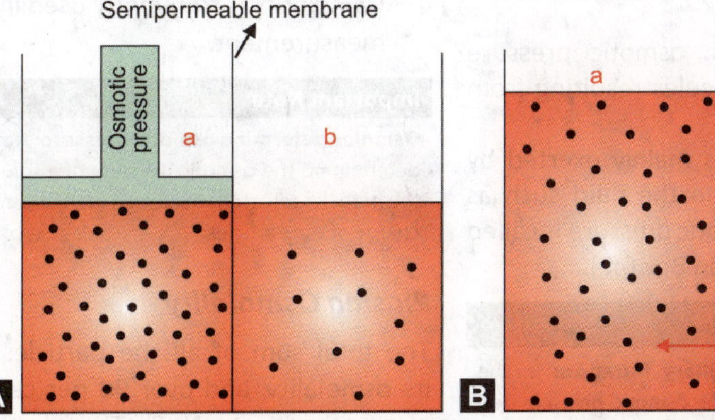

Figs. 6.7A and B: The process of osmosis. (A) Compartment 'a' containing more number osmotically active solutes is separated by a semipermeable membrane from compartment 'b' that contains less number of solutes (solute particles are represented by black dots). Solvent movement from 'b' to 'a' is prevented by application of osmotic pressure on 'a'. (B) Solvent (not the solute) moves from 'b' to 'a' (indicated by arrow mark) till osmotic equilibrium is reached, which results in increase in volume of 'a'.

substance like urea, which can diffuse readily across cell membrane, cannot impart sustained osmotic effects. Hence, urea is said to be ***osmotically ineffective***. Whereas a substance like glucose, which cannot freely diffuse through cell membrane because of its large molecular size, is osmotically active. However, glucose is not permanently osmotically effective as it is metabolized especially in blood, and, therefore, *its effect is not sustained*.

A better example of ***osmotically most effective*** substance is **plasma protein** as it is neither transferred from nor metabolized in the compartment. Other examples are various complex polysaccharides such as dextran. **Sodium chloride** is also osmotically effective even though Na^+ and Cl^- ions can diffuse through the cell membrane (Clinical Box 6.1).

Clinical Box 6.1

Normal saline is effective in hypovolemia: The application of osmotic effectiveness is important in the management of hypovolemia. A solution used to restore circulating blood volume should be the one whose active osmotic constituent remains within the circulation for a longer duration. Therefore, although 5 per cent glucose is isosmotic with plasma, it is usually not used to treat hypovolemia as it is rapidly metabolized, whereas 0.9% NaCl (the normal saline) is the satisfactory replacement for volume loss.

Osmotic Pressure

Osmotic pressure is the minimum pressure applied to the solution with higher solute concentration to prevent osmosis. When the membrane is impermeable to an osmotically active solute, osmotic flow of water ensues and continues into the side containing the solute until either the membrane bursts (*osmotic lysis* of cells), or some hydrostatic pressure prevents further osmotic flow. The *hydrostatic pressure necessary to prevent osmotic flow of water* is known as the **osmotic pressure** of the solution.

Osmotic pressure depends on the number of molecules or the ions dissolved in a solution rather than the nature of chemical composition.

1. In case of ***nondissociated solutes***, 1 gm mol wt of any substance shall contain similar number of molecules and, therefore, exerts similar degree of osmotic pressure (equal to 22.4 atmospheres).
2. In case of ***dissociated solutes***, osmotic pressure depends on the number of molecules resulting from the dissociation.

Osmotic pressure in body fluid is mainly exerted by osmotically active solutes dissolved in the fluid such as ***colloidal substances***. Hence, the osmotic pressure is called ***colloidal osmotic pressure*** (Application Box 6.2).

Application Box 6.2

Oncotic pressure determines rate of capillary filtration: In the plasma, the colloidal particles are proteins. The osmotic pressure due to presence of plasma proteins is called ***oncotic pressure***. The normal oncotic pressure is **25 mm Hg**. Oncotic pressure significantly contributes to filtration across the capillary membrane. Therefore, edema occurs in hypoproteinemia.

Terms Used in Osmosis

Mole

A mole (standard SI unit) is the molecular weight (MW) of a substance in grams, i.e. the gram molecular weight. For example, the MW of glucose is 180, so its mole is 180 gm; and for NaCl, the mole is 58.5 gm.

Osmole and Milliosmole

The concentration of osmotically active particles is usually expressed in osmoles (Osm). One **osmole** equals the gram molecular weight (i.e. one mole) of the substance divided by the number of freely moving particles each molecule liberates in solution. The **milliosmole** (mosm) is 1/1000 of 1 Osm.

1. If a solute is a ***non-ionizing compound*** like glucose, one osmole is equal to 1 mole of solute particle. Thus, 1 molar solution of glucose has a concentration of 1 Osm (1 osmole per liter).
2. If the solute is an ***ionizing compound*** like NaCl, each ion is an osmotically active particle. Therefore, in 1 molar solution of NaCl, NaCl would dissociate into Na^+ and Cl^- ions, so that each mole in solution would supply two osmoles of solute per liter of solution. Similarly, one mole of $CaCl_2$ would dissociate into Ca^{++}, Cl^- and Cl^-, and, thus, supplying 3 osmoles.

Osmolality and Osmolarity

Osmolality of a solution refers to the number of osmoles (number of osmotically active particles) dissolved in a kilogram of water. **Osmolarity** refers to the number of osmoles in one liter of plasma.

1. Unlike osmolality, the value in osmolarity is affected by the volume of other solutes in the solution.
2. Osmolarity is also affected by temperature.
3. Though osmotic pressure is determined by osmolality, the difference between osmolality and osmolarity is negligible.
4. Osmolarity is frequently used in physiology for its easy measurement.

Important Note

Osmoles determine osmotic pressure: Note that the important factor determining the osmotic pressure of a solution is the concentration of the particles released in solution (i.e. the osmoles), not the size, shape or charge of the particles.

Plasma Osmolality

The total sum of all the particles in plasma determine its osmolality, and over 90 per cent of the osmolality of plasma is due to NaCl. The plasma proteins contribute very little, even though their molecules are large in size. The **normal plasma osmolality is 290 mOsm per kg**, out of which 270 mOsm is due to the effect of NaCl.

Measurement of Osmotic Pressure

By Freezing Point Depression

Osmometers are used to measure osmotic pressure. The molar concentration of a solute in a solution determines the osmotic pressure, and also the vapor pressure and freezing point. A nonvolatile solute will depress both the vapor pressure and the freezing point in a predictable manner, which provides the basis for determining the osmotic pressure of a solution by osmometers. One mol per liter depresses the freezing point of water by 1.86°C. For human plasma, the average freezing point is –0.54°C, which corresponds to an osmolality of 290 mOsm/kg.

Tonicity

Tonicity refers to the osmolality of a solution in relation to plasma (same osmotic pressure or freezing-point depression as plasma).

Isotonic

Solutions, which have osmolality same as that of plasma, like 0.9% NaCl, are said to be *isotonic*.

Hypotonic

Solutions with lower osmolality are said to be *hypotonic*.

Hypertonic

Solutions with higher osmolality than that of plasma are said to be *hypertonic*.

The solution of 0.9% NaCl is isotonic, and, therefore, red cells do not change their shape and size in this solution. In hypotonic solutions, red cells undergo osmotic lysis due to endosmosis and in hypertonic solutions, they shrink due to exosmosis (Clinical Box 6.2).

Clinical Box 6.2

Hyperosmolal coma: In diabetes, increased plasma osmolality due to very high plasma glucose concentration causes shrinkage of cells. Especially, dehydration of brain cells leads to coma, which is an acute medical emergency. In chronic renal failure, very high urea and creatinine can cause encephalopathy.

A solution may be isotonic initially, but later becomes hypotonic if the osmotically active particles are transferred into the cell or metabolized. For example, 5% glucose solution is isotonic and remains so temporarily when infused intravenously. However, as glucose is rapidly metabolized, the net effect of infusion is like the infusion of a hypotonic solution. Therefore, infusion of ***normal saline** (0.9% NaCl)* ***is preferred in volume depletion***, as described above.

Using Van't Hoff Equation

The osmotic pressure produced by a concentration difference can be calculated by the Van't Hoff equation, which is: C × R × T, where p is the osmotic pressure (mm Hg), DC is the difference in the concentration of particles between the two solutions (mOsm/l), R is the natural gas constant (62 mm Hg × 1/mmol × °K), and T represents absolute temperature (°K).

Measuring Equivalent Hydrostatic Pressure

In experimental set up, osmotic pressure can be measured by measuring the hydrostatic pressure applied to prevent water from entering the solution with higher solute concentration.

OTHER TRANSPORT PHENOMENA

Filtration, Bulk Flow and Solvent Drag

Passage of water and solutes through capillary wall is the example of filtration and bulk flow. Capillary wall separates plasma from interstitial fluid. Water moves out of capillaries when the net hydrostatic pressure exceeds net osmotic pressure and from interstitial space into the capillaries when the net osmotic pressure exceeds the net hydrostatic pressure. This is called ***filtration***.

Filtration

Filtration is defined as the process by which fluid is forced through a membrane mainly because of the difference in hydrostatic and oncotic pressures on two sides.

Bulk Flow

When filtration results in movement of greater quantity of water, the process is called **bulk flow**.

Solvent Drag

During bulk flow of water, it carries with it, dissolved particles (solutes), a phenomenon known as ***solvent drag***.

Donnan Effect

Presence of nondiffusible ion on one side of the membrane affects the distribution of other ions to which membrane is permeable. This results in asymmetrical distribution of ions across the cell membrane.

Gibbs-Donnan Effect

The asymmetrical distribution of ions across the cell membrane at equilibrium has the following effects:

i. There will be an electrical difference across the cell membrane whose magnitude can be determined by **Nernst equation**.

ii. Because of presence of protein anions ($prot^-$) in the cells, there are more osmotically active particles in the cells than the interstitial fluid. This can lead to osmotic swelling and rupture, which is prevented by Na^+-K^+ pump that produces net movement of positive charge out of the cell and keeps the inside and outside of the cell in osmotic equilibrium. Thus normal cell volume and pressure depend on Na^+-K^+ pump.

Nonionic Diffusion

Ions are present either in undissociated (nonionic) or dissociated (ionic) form. In ionic form they can not be easily transported across the cell membrane as membrane is charged. However, in their undissociated (nonionic) form they diffuse through the membrane easily. This is called ***nonionic diffusion***.

1. Many ions in the body pass the membrane in undissociated form and then, they dissociate to their ionic form once they reach the other side of the membrane.
2. Nonionic diffusion occurs regularly along the epithelial membrane of kidney and GI tract.

ACTIVE TRANSPORT

The transport process that utilizes energy and occurs against the gradient is the active transport. By passive transport processes, the composition of intracellular fluid tends to equalize with that of composition of extracellular fluid. However, this should never happen practically, as it threatens cell volume and intracellular solute concentrations that are not compatible with life. Therefore, nature maintains inequality of fluid composition of intracellular and extracellular compartments by providing special transport mechanisms to the cell membrane that oppose these equilibrating transport processes. These transport processes are active processes. In these processes, substances are transported *against their chemical and electrical gradients*.

There are ***three common characteristics*** of active transport mechanisms:

1. **Uphill transport:** The transport occurs *against the electrochemical gradient* of the substance transported.
2. **Utilize metabolic energy:** Energy utilized for the active transport is derived from the breakdown of ATP. Therefore, mechanisms that prevent the supply of ATP hinder the active transport process. Especially, the process is susceptible to metabolic poisons.
3. **Exhibit saturation kinetics:** Like any carrier-mediated transport, this has also a saturation point for limitation in the rate of availability of carriers and the supply of energy.

   There are two types of active transports:

1. Primary active transport
2. Secondary active transport

Primary Active Transport

Primary active transport is the transport mechanism that directly utilizes metabolic energy for the transport process. The mechanism is operated by **ion pumps.** The features are:

1. In this process, the solute is transported *against its electrochemical gradients* with the help of energy.
2. The energy is derived from ATP.

Table 6.4: Types of ATPases, their location and functions.

Types	Example	Location in cell
P-type	Na^+–K^+ ATPase Ca^{++} ATPase H^+–K^+ ATPase	Plasma membrane Sarcoplasmic reticulum Plasma membrane
V-type	H^+ ATPase	Lysosomal membrane
F-type	Mitochondrial ATP synthase	Inner mitochondrial membrane
ABC transporters	CFTR protein	Plasma membrane
	MDR-1 protein	Plasma membrane

3. The ion pumps hydrolyze ATP to ADP and use energy in the third phosphate bond for the transport process. As the ion pumps hydrolyze ATP, these are also called ***ATPases***.
4. The commonly occurring ATPase is **Na^+–K^+ ATPase** or **Na^+–K^+ pump**.
5. Other common ATPases are Calcium ATPases, H^+-K^+ ATPase and H^+-ATPase.

They are ***classified*** into **P-type** (phosphorylation type), **V-type** (vacuolar type), **F-type** (energy coupling factor type) and **ABC transporters** (Table 6.4).

CFTR protein: Cystic fibrosis transmembrane regulator protein involved in genesis of cystic fibrosis; MDR-1 protein: multidrug resistance 1 protein that pumps atnicancer drug out of cancer cell that causes drug resistance in treatment of cancer.

Na^+–K^+ ATPase

Na^+-K^+ ATPase is present in all eukaryotic cells. This is an antiport that pumps K^+ into the cell and Na^+ out of the cell against their concentration gradients. This antiport transport system is primarily responsible for maintaining the high K^+ and low Na^+ concentration inside the cells.

Structure and its Functional Aspects

The Na^+-K^+ ATPase is a heterodimeric protein made up of two subunits: an α and a β subunit.

1. The α **subunit** is larger catalytic subunit with molecular weight of about 100,000 and β subunit is the smaller one (mol. wt. of about 55,000) of unknown functions.
2. At the **cytoplasmic side**, the α subunit has ATPase activity and binding sites for 3 Na^+, ATP and phosphate (Fig. 6.8).
3. At the **extracellular side**, α subunit has binding sites for 2 K^+ and ouabain.
4. Binding of three ions of Na^+ and an ATP molecule with the carrier on its intracytoplasmic surface causes hydrolysis of ATP giving rise to ADP and Pi.
5. The phosphate group is bound to an aspartic acid residue of the α subunit.
6. On activation, Na^+-K^+ ATPase pumps **three Na^+ ions out of the cell** and **two K^+ into the cell**. Na^+-K^+ pump

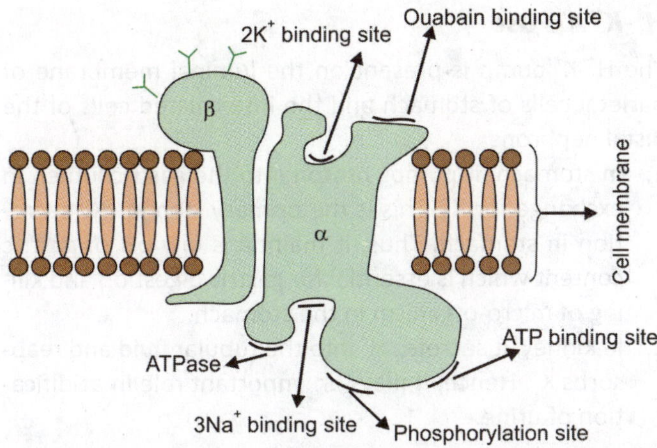

Fig. 6.8: Structure of Na^+-K^+ ATPase. It has a small β subunit and large α subunit. The extracellular surface of α subunit contains binding sites for two K^+ and ouabain, and intracellular surface has binding sites for three Na^+ and one ATP, a phosphorylation site and an ATPase site.

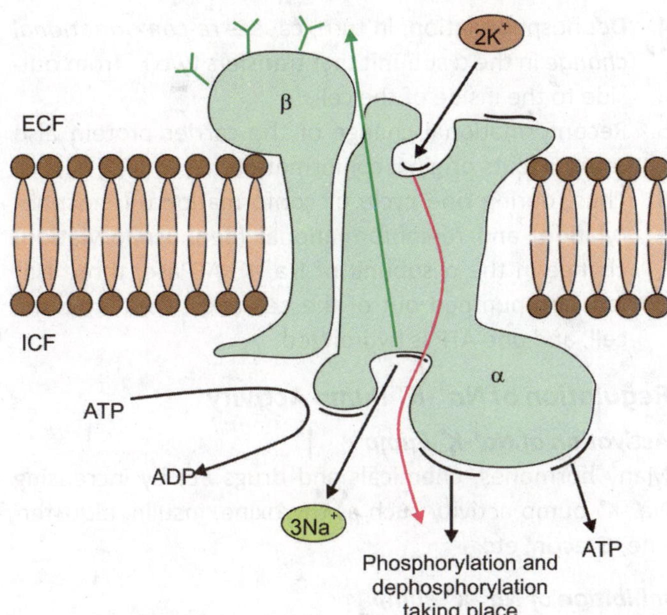

Fig. 6.9: Mechanism of action of Na^+-K^+ ATPase. Binding of three Na^+ and one ATP to their respective sites on α subunit activates ATPases that converts ATP to ADP. This causes phosphorylation of α subunit that changes its configuration and transfers 3 Na^+ to ECF. K^+ binds to K^+ binding site on the extracellular surface that causes dephosphorylation of α subunit and transfers two K^+ from ECF into the cell. Thus, three Na^+ are pumped out for entry of two K^+ into the cell, and one ATP is hydrolyzed.

catalyzed the hydrolysis of ATP to ADP, and uses this energy to pump three Na^+ out of the cell and two K^+ into the cell for each mole of ATP hydrolyzed. Therefore, Na^+-K^+ pump is an **electrogenic pump** as it forces net positive charge to out of the cell, and it has the coupling ratio of 3/2 (Application Box 6.3).

Application Box 6.3

Importance of electrogenic pump: Electrogenic pump creates the electrical potential across the membrane, which is the basic requirement in nerve and muscle fiber for transmitting electrical signal.

Functions

The Na^+-K^+ ATPase is a **P-type ATPase**, as the carrier protein is phosphorylated during the process. It pumps three Na^+ ions out of the cell and two K^+ into the cell. It serves many important cellular functions:

1. **Cytosolic ion concentration:** Na^+-K^+ pump opposes Na^+ to accumulate in the cell and K^+ to exit from the cell along their concentration gradient. Thus, Na^+-K^+ pump maintains high concentration of K^+ and low concentration of Na^+ in the cell.
2. **Cell volume:** By maintaining ion concentration on both sides of the cell, Na^+-K^+ pump regulates water movement across the cell membrane. This maintains intracellular water content and, therefore, the cell volume. Failure of Na^+-K^+ pump activity can lead to cell swelling and rupture.
3. **Protein synthesis:** The primary function of Na^+-K^+ pump is to maintain a high intracellular concentration of K^+, which is essential for protein synthesis.
4. **Resting membrane potential:** Na^+-K^+ pump also maintains resting membrane potential by maintaining ion gradients across the cell membrane.
5. **Hormone actions:** Na^+-K^+ pump mediates action of many hormones on the cell. Some important examples are thyroxine, aldosterone and insulin.

Scientist contributed

The Na^+-K^+ pump was discovered in 1957 by Danish physiologist **Prof Jens Christian Skou** of Aarhus University, who received the Nobel Prize for his discovery in 1997, which was the culmination of his four decades of research aimed at explaining the mechanism behind this vital motor of the cells. He received the **Nobel Prize in Chemistry** together with **Paul D Boyer** and **John E Walker** for his discovery of Na^+-K^+ ATPase

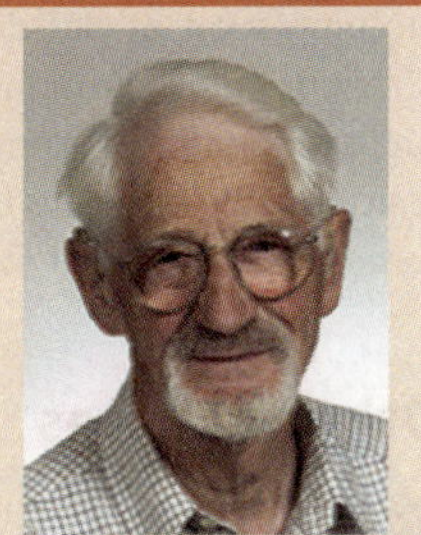

Jens Christian Skou
(Born: October 1918, Age 97 years)

Mechanism of Action

Being a P type ATPase, phosphorylation and dephosphorylation of the carrier protein lead to transfer of ions across the cell membrane.

1. Binding of three Na^+ and one ATP molecule to their respective sites on a subunit activates the enzyme ATPase that catalyzes the hydrolysis of ATP to ADP liberating high energy phosphate bond (**phosphorylation**).
2. This phosphorylation of α subunit by ATP causes ***conformational change*** in the carrier protein that transfers three Na^+ from inside to the outside of the cell (Fig. 6.9).
3. In the next step, two K^+ bind to the outer side of the α subunit, and this leads to the hydrolysis of the aspartic acid-phosphate bond (**dephosphorylation**).

4. Dephosphorylation, in turn, causes *re-conformational change* in the α subunit that transfers two K^+ from outside to the inside of the cell.
5. Reconformational change of the carrier protein also returns to its original conformation.
6. Thus, during one cycle of conformational (phosphorylation) and re-conformational (dephosphorylation) change in the α subunit of Na^+-K^+ ATPase, three Na^+ ions are pumped out of the cell and two K^+ into the cell, and one ATP is hydrolyzed.

Regulation of Na⁺-K⁺ Pump Activity

Activation of Na⁺-K⁺ Pump

Many hormones, chemicals and drugs act by increasing Na^+-K^+ pump activity such as thyroxine, insulin, aldosterone, G-actin, etc.

Inhibition of Na⁺-K⁺ Pump

Many hormones and chemicals act by decreasing Na^+-K^+ pump activity such as dopamine, digitalis, metabolic poisons like DNP (2,4 dinitrophenol), etc. (Clinical Box 6.3). Hypoxia and hypothermia inhibit Na^+-K^+ pump activity.

Clinical Box 6.3

Digitalis inhibits Na^+-K^+ pump: Cardiac glycosides like ouabain, or digitalis that are routinely prescribed in the management of heart failure inhibit Na^+-K^+ pump by binding to the external surface of the α-subunit and interfering with the hydrolysis of the aspartic acid-phosphate bond. This accumulates Na^+ inside the cell and prevents K^+ influx. Intracellular accumulation of Na^+ decreases Na^+ gradient from outside to inside. Calcium efflux through sodium-calcium exchanger in the membrane utilizes sodium gradient. Hence, decreased sodium gradient decreases calcium efflux causing increase in cytosolic calcium concentration that promotes myocardial contractility.

Other ATPases

Ca⁺⁺ ATPase

Other common example of primary active transport is the Ca^{++} pump, which is present in all cell membranes, membrane of endoplasmic reticulum, and sarcoplasmic reticulum in muscle cell.

Main features and functions Ca^{++} ATPase are:

1. This is a P-type ATPase.
2. The Ca^{++} pump present on the cell membrane actively transports calcium out of the cell, and, therefore, maintains a higher concentration of calcium in the ECF (10^{-3} molar) compared to inside the cell (10^{-7} molar).
3. The Ca^{++} pump present on the membrane of sarcoplasmic reticulum in muscle cell and endoplasmic reticulum in other cells transports calcium out of the cytoplasm into these organelles, and, therefore, maintains a low cytosolic concentration of calcium.
4. Also, it helps in storage of calcium in these organelles for ready availability of it at the time of need like muscle contraction.

H⁺-K⁺ ATPase

The H^+-K^+ pump is present on the luminal membrane of parietal cells of stomach and the intercalated cells of the distal nephrons.

1. In stomach, it pumps proton into the gastric lumen in exchange for K^+. This is the primary step in HCl secretion in stomach. Thus, it maintains low pH of gastric content which is essential for gastric digestion and killing of micro-organism in the stomach.
2. In kidney, it secretes H^+ into the tubular fluid and reabsorbs K^+. Hence, it plays an important role in acidification of urine.

H⁺ ATPase or Proton ATPase

The H^+ pump or **the proton pump** is located on the membrane of lysosome, endoplasmic reticulum and mitochondria.

In lysosome and endoplasmic reticulum: It is a **V-type ATPase**, named for its first discovery in the vacuoles and vesicles of the cells. It pumps H^+ (proton) from cytosol into these organelles. Thus, interior of these organelles become more acidic, which is needed for their physiological activities.

In mitochondria: Proton pump is also located in the inner mitochondrial membrane, but it is **F-type ATPase** in this organelle. Its main function is to synthesize ATP in mitochondria by utilizing energy stored in the proton gradient created by respiratory chain.

ABC Transporters

ATP-binding cassette (ABC) transporters belong to members of a superfamily of membrane transport proteins that bind to ATP. The main features are:

1. They have 12 membrane-binding domains.
2. They use energy derived from ATP for transporting a variety of compounds out of the cells, those include ions, steroids, peptides, bile acids, drugs and xenobiotics.
3. As drugs are transported out of the cells, they are known as ***MDR 1 protein (multidrug resistance 1 protein)***. Cells that usually express MDR proteins are liver, kidney and GI tract cells.
4. CFTR protein (cystic fibrosis transmembrane regulator protein), a chloride channel protein involved in genesis of cystic fibrosis also belongs to this superfamily of ABC transporters (Application Box 6.4).

Application Box 6.4

ABC transporters produce drug resistance in cancer cells: ABC transporters cause expulsion of cytotoxic drugs from cancer cells. This decreases effective concentration of drugs in the cells needed for killing cancer cells. Hence, cancer cells become resistant to anticancer chemotherapy. Examples are MDR 1 protein (multi-drug resistance-associated protein 1) and BCRP (breast cancer resistance protein).

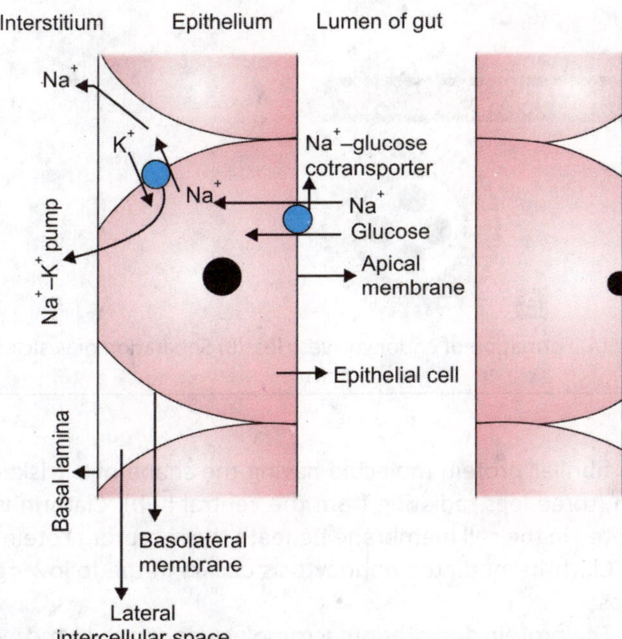

Fig. 6.10: Mechanism of secondary active transport. Na^+-K^+ pump located on basolateral membrane actively pumps sodium out of the cell that decreases cytosolic sodium and creates gradient for transport of sodium from lumen into the cell. The carrier protein (symport) that transports sodium also transports glucose into the cell. Thus, transport of glucose from lumen into the cell is the secondary active transport.

Secondary Active Transport

Many cells have several carrier mechanisms that transfer one solute against its concentration gradient by using the energy generated by gradient of another solute. Usually, Na^+ is the driver solute for most of these mechanisms. Energy created by Na^+ gradient is utilized for transport of other solutes. The Na^+ gradient is generated and maintained by Na^+-K^+ pump. Though the transport system by itself does not directly utilize energy, it depends on the function of Na^+-K^+ pump. Therefore, when the pump is inhibited by a blocking agent, transport process stops.

Typical example of secondary active transport is ***reabsorption of glucose from the kidney tubule or intestine***. The steps are as follows:

1. The primary active transport of Na^+ out of the basal and basolateral membranes of the proximal tubules of the nephron and the small intestine by Na^+-K^+ pump leads to decreased concentration of Na^+ in the cytosol of the epithelial cells.
2. This causes facilitated diffusion of Na^+ from the lumen into the cells.
3. The carrier protein that transfers Na^+ from the luminal fluid into the cell also transports glucose in the same direction (Fig. 6.10). Thus, the carrier protein is a **symport** that transports glucose simultaneously with sodium. The symport also transports amino acids and other solutes.

> **Important Note**
>
> **The carrier protein may also be an antiport:** The example of carrier protein being an antiport in secondary active transport is the counter-transporting hydrogen ion in the nephron out of the cell for bringing in sodium (Na^+-H^+ exchanger). Another example is Na^+-Ca^{++} exchanger in cardiac cell.

4. Since the transport depends on primary active transport of sodium by the Na^+-K^+ pump, it is known as a ***secondary active transport***.
5. As the carrier protein for secondary active transport system is an integral membrane protein *it exhibits competitive inhibition and saturation kinetics*. However, it differs from the usual carrier transport for its exclusive dependence on primary transport mechanism (the pump) and for transporting against its own electrochemical gradient.

VESICULAR TRANSPORT

The transport process that occurs by either fusion of vesicle or formation of vesicle is called as vesicular transport. Fusion of vesicle with the cell membrane occurs in **exocytosis** and formation of vesicle from the cell membrane occurs in **endocytosis**. Special utilities of vesicular transport are:

1. Macromolecules such as large protein molecules can not be transported by diffusion or active transport process. Therefore, they are transferred across the cell membrane mainly by vesicular transport.
2. Amino acids, sugars, waste products of metabolism, cellular secretions, hormones, neurotransmitters and organisms are transported by this mechanism.

Role of Vesicular Transport Proteins

In vesicular transport, formation and transport of vesicles are facilitated by some vesicular transport proteins. These proteins are: clathrin, coating proteins, dynamin and docking proteins.

Clathrin

Clathrin is a fibrillar protein located in the cell membrane beneath the receptor protein. There are two types of clathrins: AP-1 clathrin and AP-2 clathrin. **AP-1 clathrin** helps in transportation from Golgi apparatus to lysosome and **AP-2 clathrin** helps in transportation of endosomes.

Coating Proteins (COP)

There are two types of coating proteins: **COP I** and **COP II.** Coating proteins help in transportation of vesicles between endoplasmic apparatus and Golgi apparatus.

Dynamin

Dynamin helps in formation of vesicles from cell membrane, especially in clathrin-mediated endocytosis.

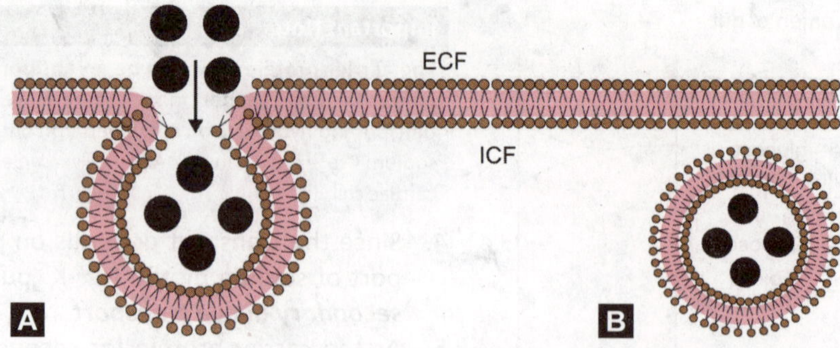

Figs. 6.11A and B: Constitutive endocytosis. It occurs in two major steps: (A) Formation of endocytic vesicles; (B) Separation of vesicles into the cytoplasm.

Docking Proteins

Before exocytosis of vesicles, docking of vesicles occurs. Docking proteins facilitate attachment of vesicle with membrane. Examples of docking proteins are **V snare protein** and **T snare protein** (For details, refer to the chapter 'Synaptic Transmission')

Types of Vesicular Transports

Vesicular transports are of three types: ***endocytosis, exocytosis*** and ***transcytosis***.

Endocytosis

Endocytosis is the process of transport in which a *substance is taken into the cell by means of vesicle formation*.

1. A region of plasma membrane is pinched off to form an endocytic vesicle that causes internalization of the substance to the cell.
2. The vesicle may contain fluid and dissolved solutes or particulate material.
3. The size of the vesicle varies from 0.1 µm to 2 µm.

Mechanisms of Endocytosis

Endocytosis occurs by two mechanisms: constitutive and clathrin-mediated.

Constitutive Endocytosis

Endocytosis by ***constitutive pathway*** occurs in almost all cells. It is called ***constitutive*** as the process occurs continually and does not require any specific stimulus. The steps are as follows:

1. The molecule or the substance makes contact with the cell membrane that invaginates to form an endocytic vesicle.
2. The non-cytoplasmic side of the membrane then fuses and the vesicle is pinched-off into the cytosol.

Thus, it occurs in *two major steps*: formation of vesicle and separation of vesicle from the membrane (Figs. 6.11A and B).

Clathrin-mediated Endocytosis

Clathrin-mediated endocytosis occurs at the specific site of the cell membrane where clathrin accumulates. **Clathrin** is a fibrillar protein molecule having the shape of a **triskelion** (three legs radiating from the central hub). Clathrin is located in the cell membrane beneath the receptor protein.

Clathrin-mediated endocytosis occurs in the following steps:

1. The protein and other macromolecules attach to *receptors* on the membrane surface. Receptors for these molecules are normally concentrated in small pits called ***coated pits***, beneath which are located fibrillar proteins called ***clathrin***. Contractile filaments like actin and myosin are also attached to the coated pits.
2. The attachment of the macromolecules to the receptors stimulates the invagination of the coated-pit, enclosing the molecule and a small portion of the ECF in the form of a vesicle. Clathrin molecule forms a geometrical array that surrounds the vesicle (Figs. 6.12A to C). Once the vesicle formation is completed, clathrin molecules detach from the vesicle and recycle to the membrane.
3. The endocytic vesicle detaches from the cell membrane.
4. Fusion of the endocytic vesicle with lysosomes that empty their acid hydrolases into the vesicle leading to the digestion of the substances in the vesicle.

Clathrin-mediated endocytosis internalizes not only various organisms, but also substances like growth factors and lipoproteins. Cell membrane also contains **caveoli**. Caveoli are membrane indentations coated with *caveolin*, the protein that facilitates endocytosis of proteins.

Scientist contributed

Discovery of receptor-mediated endocytosis: Anderson is responsible for two discoveries that changed our view of cell physiology: (1) receptor-mediated endocytosis in coated pits and coated vesicles (*Anderson et al., 1976; Anderson et al., 1977 a,b*); and (2) identification of caveolin, the protein that lines the surface of caveolae (*Rothberg et al., 1992*).

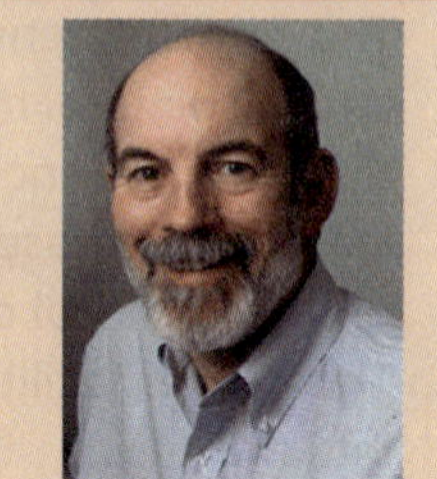

Richard GW Anderson
(1940–2011)

Types of Endocytosis

Endocytosis is of three types: phagocytosis, receptor-mediated endocytosis and pinocytosis.

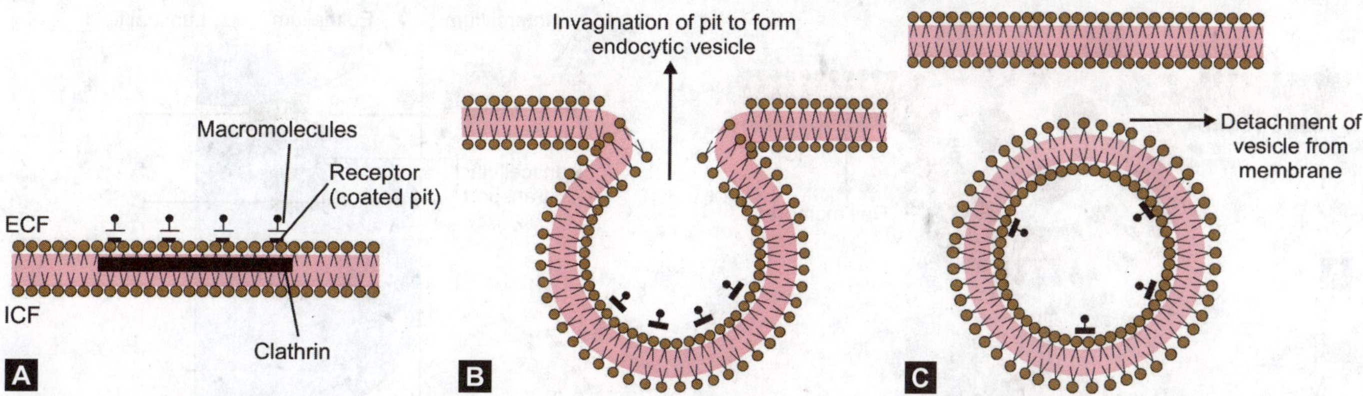

Figs. 6.12A to C: Mechanism of clathrin-mediated endocytosis. (A) Location of clathrin molecules and receptors for proteins and macromolecules in the cell membrane. (B) Attachment of macromolecules with receptors causes invagination of coated pit forming endocytic vesicle. (C) Detachment of vesicle from the membrane into the cell.

Phagocytosis

Phagocytosis, otherwise called ***cell-eating***, is the process of ingestion of large particles or microorganisms by specialized cells called ***phagocytes***. In this process, the phagocytic cells, such as macrophages engulf bacteria, foreign particles and tissue debris and digest them. The **phagocytic vesicles** vary from 1–2 µm in diameter. Phagocytosis occurs in three broad steps:

1. Attachment of the foreign molecule with cell membrane.
2. Engulfment of the foreign molecule in the form of endocytic vesicle.
3. Killing of the organism or degradation of the vesicular content.

Phagocytic cells include neutrophils, monocytes, macrophages and other cells of mononuclear phagocyte system (for details of phagocytosis, refer to Chapter on "White Blood Cells" in hematology section)

Receptor-mediated Endocytosis

Receptor-mediated endocytosis is an efficient process of endocytosis in which the extracellular molecule binds with the specific receptor on the cell membrane. Special features in this process are:

1. Receptors are concentrated at a depression on membrane called ***coated-pits***.
2. Once the external molecule attaches with receptor, the coated-pit pinches off from the membrane in the form of an ***endocytic vesicle*** causing rapid internalization of the molecule.
3. Hormones, growth factors, transport-proteins like transferrin, toxins, viruses, etc. enter cells by receptor-mediated endocytosis.

Pinocytosis

Pinocytosis is the ***fluid-phase endocytosis*** or 'cell drinking' by which substances in solution in extracellular fluid are internalized to the cell. It is a continuous process that occurs in most cells of the body. The stages in pinocytosis are the same as endocytosis except that the endocytic vesicle contains fluid instead of solid particles.

Exocytosis

Exocytosis is the process of export from the cell, which is reverse of endocytosis. By exocytosis, hormones, neurotransmitters, digestive enzymes and undigested foreign particles are released from cells. The steps of exocytosis are:

1. Before exocytosis, the molecules are synthesized in endoplasmic reticulum and packaged in Golgi apparatus to form the ***transport vesicles***.
2. The vesicles then move to the cell surface and fuse with the cell membrane
3. Release the content to ECF (Figs. 6.13A and B), which requires ATP and Ca^{2+}.

Emiocytosis is the term referring to exocytosis of specific hormones and granules.

Mechanism of Exocytosis

Exocytosis occurs in two pathways: ***constitutive*** and ***regulated***.

Constitutive Exocytosis

This type of exocytosis is seen in almost all cells. By this mechanism, some proteins are continuously secreted by the cells. For example, secretion of mucus by goblet cells of small intestine.

Regulated Exocytosis

In regulatory exocytosis, macromolecules that are stored in the vesicles fuse with cell membrane and release their content in response to specific extracellular stimulus. This is the major mechanism of rapid secretion of hormones, neurotransmitters and digestive enzymes in response to specific stimuli. This is also called ***non-constitutive exocytosis***.

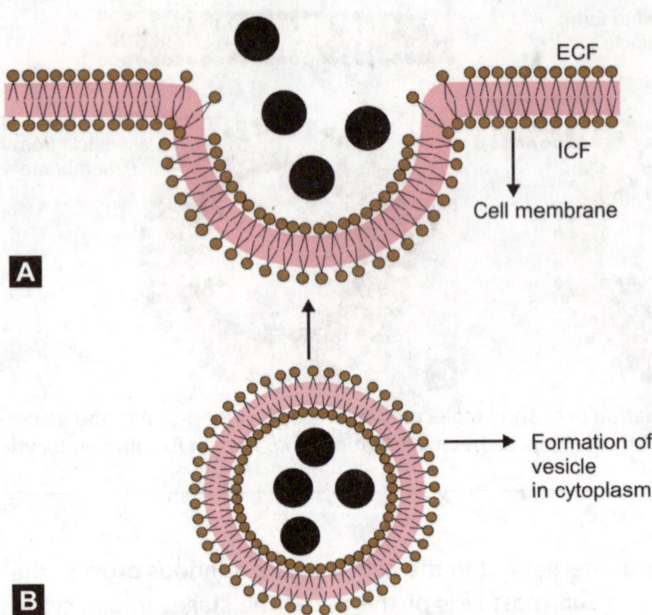

Figs. 6.13A and B: Constitutive exocytosis, which occurs in two major steps. (A) Formation of exocytic vesicles; (B) Fusion of vesicles with the membrane and discharge of its content into ECF.

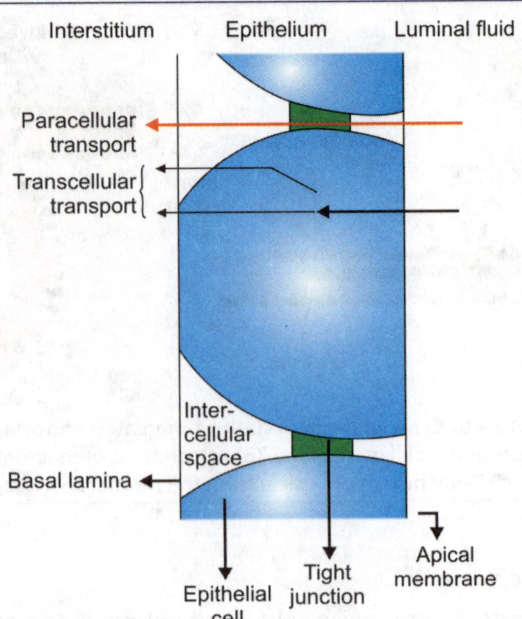

Fig. 6.14: Paracellular and transcellular transports. Paracellular transport occurs through the junction between the cells and transcellular transport occurs through the cell.

Transcytosis

When vesicular transport is limited within the cell, the process is called ***transcytosis*** or ***cytopemisis***. Vesicles are formed within the cell and transported in the cytoplasm.

TRANSPORT ACROSS THE EPITHELIA

Epithelium is a layer of cells present on the basement membrane. Two special features of epithelium make it permeable to various solutes.

1. First, the basolateral membrane contains active transport systems that creates gradient for transfer of ions from apical membrane, and various uniports and antiports that regulate exchange of other ions.
2. Second, tight junctions between cells allow selective ions to pass through and prevent large molecules like proteins to be transferred.

Thus, there are two mechanisms for transport across the epithelia:

a. **Transcellular transport** or transport through the cell i. e. from lumen through apical surface into the cytosol and from there through basolateral space or through basal membrane into the interstitial fluid.
b. **Paracellular transport**, which means transport through tight junctions between the cells bypassing the transport through cells (Fig. 6.14).

Reabsorption of sodium and glucose in kidney tubule and intestine is the example of transport across the epithelia.

Ultrafiltration through the glomerular capillary endothelium and Bowman's capsule epithelium is a special transport mechanism through epithelia. However, in ultrafiltration, transfer of substances occurs mainly due to the difference in pressures across the epithelium.

CHAPTER SUMMARY

Carrier Proteins

There are three different types of carrier proteins: uniport, symport and antiport.

Uniport : Uniport is the carrier protein that transports only one substance. For example, Na^+ channels transport Na^+ and K^+ channels transport K^+.

Symport: Symport carriers transport two or more substances from one side of the membrane to the other *in the same direction*. Transport of Na^+ and glucose from the lumen of the intestine or kidney tubule into the epithelial cells through the same carrier protein is the example.

Antiport: Antiport carriers transport substances *in opposite directions* in which one substance is transported to the inside of the cell and other substance from inside the cell to the outside. Examples of antiport are Na^+-K^+ pump and Na^+-H^+ exchanger.

Transport Processes

Broadly they are of 2 types: Passive transport and active transport

Passive Transports: Have two common features. 1. Transport is downhill (down the electrochemical gradient), and 2. Does not require metabolic energy (ATP is not utilized). Diffusion and osmosis are examples of passive transport.

Active Transport: Active transport utilizes energy. The common features are: 1. Uphill transport (against the electrochemical gradient); 2. Requires energy; and 3. Exhibits saturation kinetics.

The active transport processes are of two types: ***primary active transport***, and ***secondary active transport***. Na^+-K^+ pump is the prototype of ***primary active transport***. When a transport system by itself does not directly utilize energy, but depends on the function of a primary active pump (Na^+-K^+ pump), the process is called ***secondary active transport*** (SAT). Reabsorption of glucose from the kidney tubule or intestine is an example of SAT.

Vesicular Transport

The transport process that occurs by either fusion of vesicle or formation of vesicle is called ***vesicular transport***. Fusion of vesicle with the cell membrane occurs in **exocytosis** and formation of vesicle from the cell membrane occurs in **endocytosis**. Macromolecules such as large protein molecules that can not be transported by diffusion or active transport process are transported by vesicular transport. Amino acids, sugars, waste products of metabolism, cellular secretions, hormones, neurotransmitters and organisms are transported by this mechanism.

Important to Know (Must Read)

In final examination, **Long Questions** are asked on 'Passive transport processes (diffusion, facilitated diffusion, osmosis)' or 'Active transport mechanisms'.

Carrier proteins, facilitated diffusion, Gibb-Donnan effect, Na^+-K^+ pump, secondary active transport, exocytosis, endocytosis, are usually asked as **Short Note Question** in exams.

In viva, examiners usually ask about different types of ion channels in the membrane, types of gating of ion channels, patch-clamping, examples of uniport, symport and antiport, factors affecting diffusion, examples of facilitated diffusion, osmotic pressure, definitions of osmolality and osmolarity, definitions and examples of filtration, bulk flow and solvent drag, Donnan effect, structure and function of Na^+-K^+ ATPase, other ATPases, vesicular transport proteins, types of endocytosis and exocytosis with examples, definition of Transcytosis.

CHAPTER

7

Membrane Potential

LEARNING OBJECTIVES

On completion of study of this chapter, the student **MUST** be able to:

1. Understand the concept of resting membrane potential (RMP).
2. Explain the mechanism of genesis and maintenance of RMP.
3. Give the normal values of RMP of different excitable tissues and equilibrium potential of important ions.

The student **MAY** also be able to:

1. Explain the concept of Gibbs-Donnan Equilibrium.
2. Explain the concept of Nernst Equation
3. Explain the concept of Goldman-Hodgkin-Katz equation.
4. Give the principle of recording of RMP.

An electrical potential difference exists across the membrane of all living cells with the inside being negative in relation to the outside. This potential difference is called membrane potential as ions arrange themselves along the outer and inner surfaces of the cell membrane. At resting state of the cell, the membrane potential is called **resting membrane potential** (RMP). RMP is also called transmembrane potential. Special features of RMP are:

1. The RMP is different in different tissues (Table 7.1).
2. In a nerve cell, the RMP is –70 mV.
3. When the neuron is stimulated, membrane potential changes and inside of the cell becomes positive due to depolarization. The membrane potential during this state of activation is called *action potential*.
4. RMP plays an important role in ***deciding the degree and duration of action potential***, as the RMP is the level from where the phase of depolarization starts.
5. In some tissues like visceral smooth muscles, RMP is not stable (fluctuates).

Table 7.1: RMP of important excitable tissues.

Tissue/Cell	RMP (mV)
Neuron	–70
Skeletal muscle	–90
Cardiac muscle	–90

CONCEPTS AND PHYSIOLOGICAL ASPECTS

Membrane potential is mainly due to distribution of ions across the cell membrane, which results mainly from the **selective permeability** of the cell membrane to various ions at rest. However, this is influenced by various forces acting on the ion distribution. Understanding the following concepts help the students to learn the physiology of RMP.

1. Selective permeability of the cell membrane to various ions
2. Gibbs-Donnan equilibrium
3. Nernst equation
4. Goldman-Hodgkin equation.

Selective Permeability of the Membrane

The cell membrane is selectively permeable to ions and other solute particles. Some ions are highly permeable, some are less permeable and others are impermeable. The permeability mainly depends on the molecular weight and the radius of ions in their hydrated form (Table 7.2).

1. Though the ions like Na^+, K^+, Cl^- and HCO_3^- are diffusible through the membrane, the **permeability is more for K^+**.

Table 7.2: Molecular weight and radius of hydrated ions and other substances.

Ions/substances	Molecular weight	Radius
K^+	39	0.12
Cl^-	35.5	0.12
H_2O	18	0.12
Ca^{++}	40	0.15
Na^+	23	0.18
Urea	60	0.23
Glucose	180	0.38
Albumin	69,000	7.50

2. Though the particle size of K^+ is large (atomic weight 39) as compared to Na^+ (atomic weight 23), the permeability for K^+ is 500 to 1000 times greater than that for Na^+ for its effective radius.
3. The membrane is practically impermeable to intracellular proteins and organic phosphates.

Gibbs-Donnan Membrane Equilibrium

When two solutions containing ions are separated by a semipermeable membrane, at equilibrium, each solution will be electrically neutral. That means, the total quantity of cations will be equal to total quantity of anions. Also, the product of diffusible ions on one side of the membrane will be equal to product of diffusible ions on the other side of the membrane. This is called Gibbs-Donnan membrane equilibrium.

For example, two solutions A and B containing sodium and chloride ions are separated by a semipermeable membrane. Then, according to Gibbs-Donnan equilibrium, each solution should be electrically neutral (Fig. 7.1), which means:

$$(\text{cations})_A = (\text{anions})_A, \text{ and } (\text{cations})_B = (\text{anions})_B$$

or $$(Na^+)_A = (Cl^-)_A, \text{ and } (Na^+)_B = (Cl^-)_B$$

The product of diffusible ions on both sides will also be equal, which means,

$$(\text{diffusible cations})_A \times (\text{diffusible anions})_A = (\text{diffusible cations})_B \times (\text{diffusible anions})_B$$

or $$[(Na^+)_A \times (Cl^-)_A] = [(Na^+)_B \times (Cl^-)_B]$$

Thus, the ratio of diffusible ions will be:

$$\frac{(\text{Diffusible cations})_A}{(\text{Diffusible cations})_B} = \frac{(\text{Diffusible anions})_B}{(\text{Diffusible anions})_A}$$

or $$\frac{[Na^+]_A}{[Na^+]_B} = \frac{[Cl^-]_B}{[Cl^-]_A}$$

Thus, there will be equal and balanced distribution of ions at equilibrium. However, when a non-diffusible ions 'X' is added on one side (let us say, side A), then as per Gibbs-Donnan equilibrium principle, the distribution of diffusible ions will change to maintain electroneutrality of both sides (Fig. 7.2).

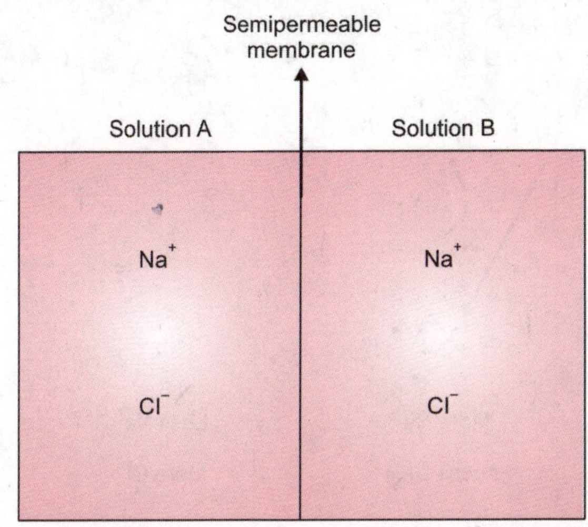

Fig. 7.1: Gibbs-Donnan equilibrium. Na^+ and Cl^- are equally distributed on both sides of semipermeable membrane, in solution A and B.

For both solutions to be electrically neutral:

$$(Na^+)_A = (Cl^-)_A + (X^-)_A, \text{ and } (Na^+)_B = (Cl^-)_B$$

Therefore, $(Na^+)_A + (Cl^-)_A + (X^-)_A > (Na^+)_B + (Cl^-)_B$

Also, for the product of diffusible ions on two sides to be equal,

$$(Na^+)_A \times (Cl^-)_A = (Na^+)_B \times (Cl^-)_B$$

Thus, $(Na^+)_A > (Na^+)_B$, and $(Cl^-)_A < (Cl^-)_B$

Consequently, there is unequal distribution of diffusible ions on both sides. Therefore, at equilibrium, Na^+ is more on the side which contains nondiffusible anions 'X' (side A) and Cl^- is more on the other side, i.e. B. However, their concentration ratios are equal.

Same analogy is applicable to intracellular fluid (ICF) and extracellular fluid (ECF). ICF contains non-diffusible anions like proteins and organic phosphate. Therefore, asymmetrical distribution of diffusible ions occurs across the cell membrane with cations being more inside than the outside. Therefore, at rest, interior of the cell is negative to the exterior [discussed below in genesis of membrane (potential)].

Nernst Equation

As described above, in accordance with Gibbs-Donnan equilibrium, asymmetrical distribution of diffusible ions occurs across the cell membrane with more cation (K^+) present inside. Therefore, K^+ will try to diffuse into the ECF from ICF, which is opposed by the electrical gradient, created by presence of non-diffusible anions inside the cell. Thus, finally equilibrium is reached between the concentration gradient and the electrical gradient resulting in diffusion potential ***(equilibrium potential)*** across the cell membrane.

The degree of this equilibrium potential is determined by Nernst equation:

$$E_{(m)} = \frac{RT}{ZF} \ln \frac{(\text{Conc})_i}{(\text{Conc})_o}$$

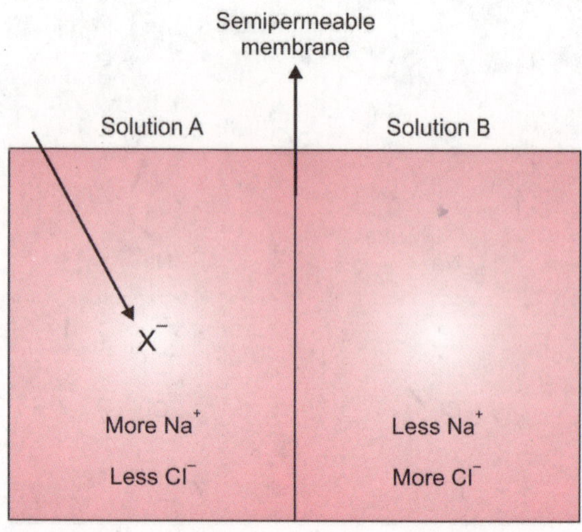

Fig. 7.2: When nondiffusible anion (X^-) is added to the solution A, more Cl^- is transferred to B to maintain balance of anion on both sides. Consequently, more Na^+ is transferred to solution A to maintain electroneutrality of both sides.

Where,

- $E_{(m)}$: Equilibrium potential (in millivolts) of the ions at which efflux and influx of the ions are equal
- R : The natural gas constant (8.316 joules/degree).
- T : The absolute temperature
- F : The faraday constant (Number of coulomb/mole of charge = 96,500 coulomb/mole)
- Z : The valency of the ion
- In : Natural logarithm
- $(Conc)_i$: The concentration of the ions in the intracellular fluid
- $(Conc)_o$: The concentration of the ions in the extracellular fluid

At normal body temperature (37°C), converting from the natural log to the base 10 log and replacing some of the constants with numerical values, the equation can be simplified to:

$$E_{(m)} = \pm 61 \log \frac{(Conc)_i}{(Conc)_o}$$

Thus, Nernst equation helps in calculating the equilibrium potential for each ion individually (Table 7.3).

Scientist contributed

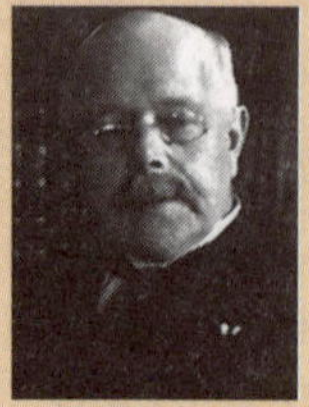

W H Nernst
(1864–1941)

Walther H Nernst, born in Briesen, West Prussia, on June 25, 1864, notable for the development of the ***Nernst equation*** and winner of **1920 Nobel Prize in chemistry**, was a major contributor to the study of membrane potential. He developed the Nernst equation to solve for the equilibrium potential for a specific ion. **Goldman, Hodgkin and Katz** furthered the study of membrane potential by developing the ***Goldman-Hodgkin-Katz equation*** to account for any ion that might permeate the membrane and affect its potential. The study of membrane potential utilizes electrochemistry and physiology to formulate a conclusive idea of how charges are separated across a membrane.

Table 7.3: Concentrations (mmol/L) of important ions in ECF and ICF and their equilibrium potential (EP) in a mammalian spinal motor neuron.

Ions	ECF	ICF	EP (mV)
Na^+	150	15	+ 60
K^+	5.5	150	–90
Cl^-	125	9	–70
HCO_3^-	21	5	–25
Calcium	2.5	10^{-4}	+130

Goldman-Hodgkin-Katz Equation

The magnitude of the membrane potential at any given time depends on the distribution of Na^+, K^+ and Cl^- and on the permeability of each of these ions. The role of different ions in the generation of membrane potential is accurately described by Goldman-Hodgkin-Katz (GHK) equation or also called **Goldman's constant field equation.**

$$V = \frac{RT}{F} \ln \frac{P_{K^+}[K^+]_o + P_{Na^+}[Na^+]_o + P_{Cl^-}[Cl^-]_i}{P_{K^+}[K^+]_i + P_{Na^+}[Na^+]_i + P_{Cl^-}[Cl^-]_o}$$

Where,

V : membrane potential,
R : gas constant,
T : absolute temperature,
F : Faraday constant,
In : natural logarithm
P_{K^+}, P_{Na^+} and P_{Cl^-} : permeabilities of the membrane to K^+, Na^+ and Cl^-, and $_i$ and $_o$ refer to inside and outside of the cell respectively.

Scientists contributed

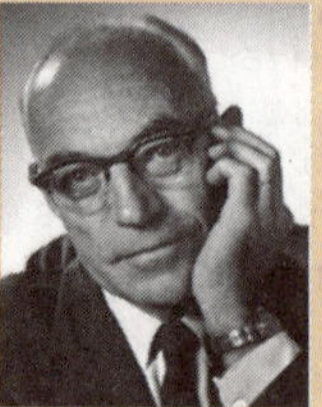

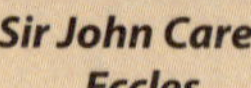

Sir John Carew Eccles

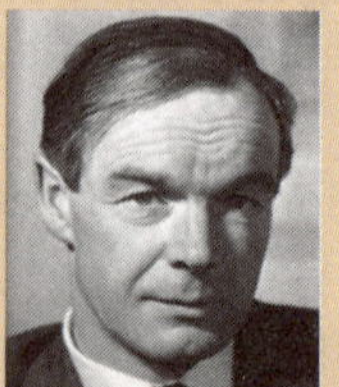

Alan Lloyd Hodgkin

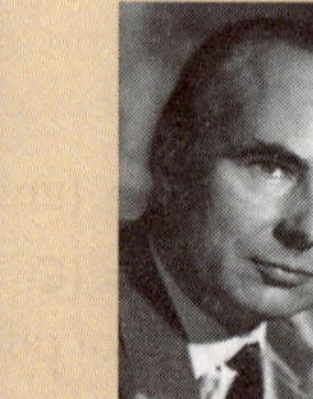

Andrew Fielding Huxley

The **Nobel Prize in Physiology or Medicine 1963** was awarded jointly to **Sir John Carew Eccles, Alan Lloyd Hodgkin and Andrew Fielding Huxley** "for their discoveries concerning the ionic mechanisms involved in excitation and inhibition in the peripheral and central portions of the nerve cell membrane".

Importance of Goldman Constant Field Equation

1. Important ions that generate membrane potentials in nerve and muscle fibers are sodium, potassium and chloride. The voltage of membrane potential is determined by the concentration gradient of each of these ions.
2. The relativity of importance of each ion in determination of the voltage depends upon the membrane permeability of individual ion.

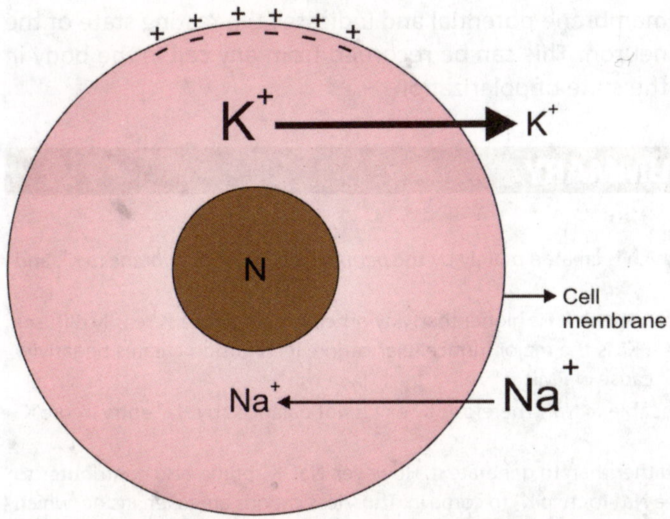

Fig. 7.3: Concept of the genesis of resting membrane potential (RMP). At rest, cell membrane is more permeable to K^+ than to Na^+. Hence, K^+ efflux is more than the Na^+ influx resulting in exit of more cations from the cell that creates relative negativity inside. This is the major cause of genesis of RMP. Direction and thickness of arrow indicate direction and magnitude of movement of ions. Size of letters for ions indicates their relative concentration in ECF and ICF.

3. Cation concentration from inside the membrane to outside is responsible for electronegativity inside the membrane. Due to concentration gradient, cations diffuse to outside of the cell leaving the non-diffusible anions inside the cell.

GENESIS OF RMP

Resting membrane potential (RMP) is the membrane potential at rest. In neurons, the RMP is –70 mV.

The RMP is created due to following factors.

1. **Permeability of the membrane to K^+:** Normally, K^+ is more inside and less outside the cell (*see* Table 7.3). Therefore, a concentration gradient exists for K^+ from inside to outside that facilitates K^+ to diffuse out of the cell. At rest, permeability of the membrane to K^+ is higher than any other ion. Therefore, K^+ easily diffuses out of the cell (Fig. 7.3), though this is opposed by the electrical gradient. As, K^+ is the major intracellular cation, its diffusion creates negativity inside the cell. The permeability of the membrane to K^+ is the major cause of RMP.
2. **Permeability of the membrane to Na^+:** At rest, ECF Na^+ is more than the ICF Na^+. Therefore, there is a concentration gradient for Na^+ from outside to inside, for which Na^+ diffuses into the cell. However, at rest membrane is less permeable to Na^+ (Fig. 7.3) than to K^+. Therefore, K^+ exit is not balanced by Na^+ entry (more K^+ goes out). Hence, interior of the cell remains relatively negative.
3. **Permeability to anions:** Exit of more cations from the cell should be accompanied by proportionate exit of anion to maintain electroneutrality. However, exit of K^+ (the cation) is not accompanied by exit of same amount of anions as permeability of anions at rest is also not same as that of K^+. Therefore, more negative ions remain inside.
4. **Role of Na^+-K^+ pump:** The role of Na^+-K^+ pump is to maintain RMP rather than to generate it. However, Na^+-K^+ pump also contributes to the genesis of RMP, as it is an electrogenic pump. It pumps out three Na^+ for two K^+ to come in. Therefore, it pumps more cations out of the cell and less into the cell. Thus, less cations are taken inside, which in other words, a relatively negativity is created inside (Application Box 7.1).

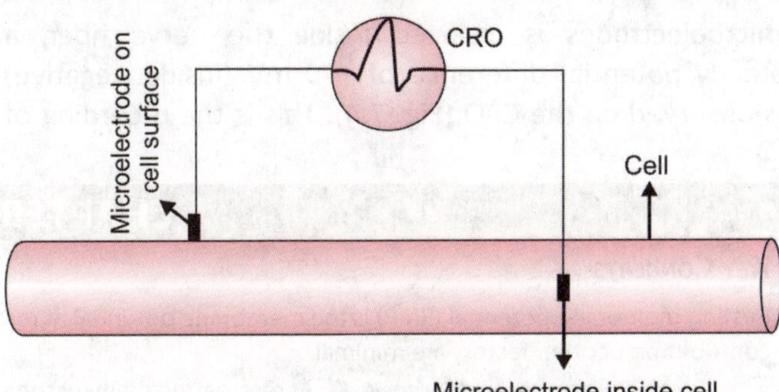

Fig. 7.4: Recording of membrane potential. (CRO: Cathode ray oscilloscope).

Application Box 7.1

Negativity is only along the membrane: It should be noted that the number of ions that are responsible for membrane potential is a very small fraction of the total number of ions actually present inside the cell. In the cell, the cations and anions are present in equal proportion except along the membrane. Therefore, negativity is created and maintained only close to the membrane.

Maintenance of RMP

K^+ diffusing out of the cell and Na^+ diffusing into the cell will come to halt once the concentration gradient ceases to exist for both the ions. However, that does not happen, as Na^+-K^+ ATPase helps in building the concentration gradient. It serves to pump back the Na^+ that diffuses into the cell and K^+ that diffuses out of the cell. Thus, Na^+-K^+ pump plays an **important role in maintaining RMP**.

Recording of Membrane Potential

The membrane potential is recorded like recoding of activity of any excitable tissue. This requires:

1. Microelectrodes
2. Electronic amplifiers
3. Cathode ray oscilloscope (CRO).

Basic Principle

Two microelectrodes are placed on the surface of a nerve fiber and connected to a CRO. When, one of the microelectrodes is inserted inside the nerve fiber, a steady potential difference of –70 mV (inside negative) is observed on the CRO (Fig. 7.4). This is the recording of membrane potential and indicates the resting state of the neuron. This can be recorded from any cell in the body in the state of polarization.

CHAPTER SUMMARY

Key Concepts

Resting membrane potential (RMP) is the membrane potential at rest, which is created mainly by the *permeability of the membrane to* K^+, and contribution of other factors are minimal.

1. *Permeability of the membrane to* K^+: At rest, permeability of the membrane to K^+ is higher than any other ion. Therefore, K^+ easily diffuses out of the cell, though this is opposed by the electrical gradient. As, K^+ is the major intracellular cation, its diffusion creates negativity inside the cell. The permeability of the membrane to K^+ is the major cause of RMP.
2. *Permeability of the membrane to* Na^+: At rest, membrane is less permeable to Na^+. Therefore, K^+ exit is not balanced by Na^+ entry (more K^+ goes out). Hence, interior of the cell remains relatively negative.
3. *Role of* Na^+-K^+ *pump:* The role of Na^+-K^+ pump is to maintain RMP rather than to generate it. However, Na^+-K^+ pump also contributes to the genesis of RMP, as it is an electrogenic pump. It pumps out three Na^+ for two K^+ to come in. Thus, less cations are taken inside, which in other words, a relatively negativity is created inside.

Important to Know (Must Read)

1. In examinations, when students are asked about the mechanism of RMP, promptly they answer the role of Na^+-K^+ pump, and this is wrong. They should answer that it is the permeability of the membrane to K^+ that mainly contributes to the genesis of RMP.
2. Resting membrane potential comes usually as **Short Note/Question** in final exam.
3. In **Viva**, examiners usually ask about the genesis of RMP, and sometimes about the application of Nernst equation, Gibbs-Donnan equilibrium, and Hodgkin-Katz equation.

CHAPTER

8

Body Fluids

Learning Objectives

On completion of study of this chapter, the student **MUST** be able to:

1. Give the normal values of total body water (TBW) as % of body weight in different age groups in males and females.
2. Gives the % distribution of body water in different body fluid compartments.
3. Name different body fluid compartments, total fluid present in the compartment and composition of ions in each compartment.
4. Give the characteristics of an ideal indicator used for measuring body fluid volumes.
5. Name the units of measurement, name the indicator used, give the basic principle and method of measurement of body fluid volume of different compartments.
6. Explain why dehydration is common and often severe in children.

The student **MAY** also be able to:

1. Describe details of methods of measurement of various body fluid compartments.

Functions of cells depend on fluids present both outside and inside the cells. Unicellular organisms float in water or air and exchange their nutrients, waste products and gasses through their body surface, i.e., the cell membrane. However, multicellular organisms, especially organisms with complex body systems have no direct access to their immediate environment, and therefore, they contact outer environment through interstitial fluid and transport systems of their body. Therefore, body fluid is compartmentalized into intracellular and extracellular fluids in complex organisms. The body compositions and distribution of fluid in different compartment are as follows:

1. The body composition of a normal adult male on average consists of 15% fat, 18% proteins, 7% minerals and 60% water.
2. The total body water (TBW) as percentage of body weight on average is about 60% in adult males, which is about 10% more than adult females (Table 8.1).
3. In infants and children, though TBW as percentage of body weight is more than in adults, their absolute water content is significantly less.
4. In elderly people in both the sexes, TBW is about 10% less than their adult counterparts.
5. In females, TBW is less than males due to relatively greater amount of adipose tissue (subcutaneous fat) in them.

Of total body water, about two-third is present in intracellular compartment and one-third in extracellular compartment (Table 8.2).

BODY FLUID COMPARTMENTS

Extracellular Fluid Compartment

Fluid present in the spaces outside the cell constitutes extracellular fluid (ECF) compartment. This includes plasma, interstitial fluid and transcellular fluid.

Plasma

Plasma is the fluid part of the blood. It constitutes about 25% of the ECF, which is about 5% of the total body weight (Table 8.3).

Volume of plasma can be calculated from blood volume and PCV (packed cell volume) as:

$$\text{Plasma volume} = \text{Blood volume} \times \frac{100 - \text{Hematocrit}}{100}$$

Blood Volume and Red Cell Volume

Blood volume is the plasma volume and blood cell volume. It is about 80 ml/kg of body weight or 8% of the total body weight.

Table 8.1: TBW as % of body weight.

Age	Males	Females
Infants	65–70	65–70
Children (upto 9 years)	60–65	59–62
10–17 years	58–60	55–58
18–39 years	58–64	48–55
40–59 years	52–58	45–50
60 years and above	50–55	42–48

Table 8.3: Distribution of ECF in a 70 kg adult male.

Compartment	% of ECF	% of BW	Volume	% of b.w.
Plasma	25	4–5	3.5 L	8
Interstitial and transcellular fluid	10.5	15	10.5 L	25

(BW: Body weight; b.w.: Body water).

Red cell volume is the volume occupied by the circulating red cells. It is determined by subtracting plasma volume from total blood volume. However, it is also calculated by injecting red cells tagged with radioactive isotopes such as ^{51}Cr, ^{59}Fe or ^{32}P. Fraction of red cell tagged is measured after proper mixing has occurred. Total blood volume is less in children (Clinical Box 8.1).

Clinical Box 8.1

Dehydration is common and rapid in children: Ratio of ECF volume to ICF volume is larger in infants and children than in adults. However, as the total volume of ECF is much smaller in children than in adults. In addition, the regulatory mechanisms for maintaining ECF volume are not well developed in infants and children. Therefore, dehydration is more common and occurs rapidly in these age groups.

Interstitial Fluid

It is ECF volume present in the space between the cells (ECF outside the vascular system). Interstitial fluid surrounds all cells except blood cells and includes lymph (lymph constitutes 2–3% of the total body weight). It is in constant motion throughout the body and is exchanged rapidly with the circulating blood.

1. Interstitial fluid volume is about 15% of body weight.
2. It can not be measured directly as substances used for it rapidly equilibrate with plasma.
3. It is calculated by subtracting plasma volume from ECF volume.

Transcellular Fluid

Transcellular fluid represents fluid in the lumen of structures lined by epithelium.

1. It includes fluid in the secretion of exocrine digestive glands, cerebrospinal fluid (CSF), pleural, peritoneal, synovial and pericardial fluids, intraocular (aqueous and vitreous humors) fluids, bile, luminal fluids of the gut and fluid in the cochlea and kidney tubules.

Table 8.2: Distribution of total body water (TBW) in ECF and ICF compartments in a 70 kg adult male.

Compartment	% of BW	% of b.w.	Volume
TBW	60	100	42 L
ECF	20	33	14 L
ICF	40	67	28 L

(BW: Body weight; b.w.: Body water).

2. The total transcellular fluid volume is 1.5% of body weight, which is about 1L.

Intracellular Fluid Compartment

Intracellular fluid (ICF) is the fluid contained within the cells of the body. It constitutes about two-thirds of total fluid of the body. It can not be measured directly. It is measured by subtracting ECF volume from total fluid volume.

MEASUREMENT OF BODY FLUID VOLUMES

General Principle

The volume of fluid compartment is usually measured by the **indicator dilution principle**, which is based on the following relationship:

$$C = \frac{A}{V} \text{ i.e., } \quad V = \frac{A}{C}$$

Where, A is the amount of a substance injected intravenously, V is the volume in which the substance is distributed and C is the final concentration attained.

Characteristics of an Indicator

1. Should be relatively easy to measure.
2. Should remain in the compartment being measured.
3. Should not change the fluid distribution in the compartment being measured.
4. Should be non-toxic.
5. Must mix evenly throughout the compartment being measured.
6. Should remain unchanged by the body during the mixing period or the amount changed must be known.

Principle of Measurement

Size of fluid compartment is measured by injecting a substance and then calculating the volume of fluid in which the test substance is distributed. This is called the **volume distribution** of the injected substance, which is equal to the amount injected divided by concentration of the substance in the sample.

If indicator ***leaves the compartment by excretion or metabolism*** during the time allowed for mixing, then calculation is done as follows:

$$\text{Volume distribution} = \frac{\text{Amount injected} - \text{Amount removed}}{\text{Final concentration of the substance}}$$

Measurement of ECF Volume

The ECF volume is difficult to measure, as the limit of this space is ill-defined, and few substances mix rapidly in all parts of the space while remaining exclusively extracellular.

Methods of Measurement

ECF volume is measured by volume distribution principle using inulin, a polysaccharide having molecular weight of 5200.

1. **Radioactive inulin** is prepared by substituting ^{14}C for one of the carbon atoms of the molecule. Radioactive inulin levels are easily determined by counting the samples with suitable radiation detectors.
2. Also **Cl^-** ($^{36}Cl^-$ and $^{38}Cl^-$), **^{82}Br, mannitol and sucrose** are used for measurement of ECF volume.
3. Cl^- is largely extracellular. Therefore, radioactive isotopes of Cl^- (**$^{36}Cl^-$ and $^{38}Cl^-$**) are used for the purpose. However, ECF volume determined by using Cl^- is *greater than actual volume* as some Cl^- is also present in intracellular fluid.
4. **^{82}Br, sulphate, thiosulphate, thiocyanate and ferrocyanide** are also used for measuring ECF volume. As these ions interchange with Cl^- in the body, they determine greater values for ECF.
5. **Mannitol and sucrose** have also been used to measure ECF volume.

Measurement of Plasma Volume

Plasma volume is measured by **two dilution methods**.

First Method: In the first method, the substance used neither leaves the vascular system nor penetrates red cells. Examples are:

i. ***Evans Blue Dye*** (T-1824) that remains bound to plasma proteins.
ii. ***Radio-iodinated human serum albumin*** (RISA) i.e. serum albumin labeled with radioactive iodine. It slowly escapes from circulation into the interstitial fluid. Suitable sample of injected solution and plasma samples obtained after injection are counted in a scintillation counter.
iii. ***Radio-iodinated gamma globulin and fibrinogen***. These substances generally do not leak out of the blood stream.

Second Method: In the second method, ***radio-isotopes of phosphorus (^{32}P), iron ($^{55,59}Fe$) and chromium (^{51}Cr)*** are used that penetrate and bind to red cells. Therefore, the red cells volume, i.e. volume occupied by all the circulating RBCs in the body can be measured by injecting tagged red cells intravenously. After thorough mixing has occurred, fraction of the RBCs that is tagged is measured.

Commonly used tag is ^{51}Cr, which is attached to the red cells by incubating in a suitable 'Cr' solution. Then, plasma volume is calculated by using the formula:

$$\text{Plasma volume} = \frac{100 - \text{PCV}}{100} \times \text{Blood volume}$$

(PCV is packed cell volume, which is practically the red cell volume).

Measurement of Interstitial Fluid Volume

Interstitial fluid volume *cannot be measured directly* as it is difficult to sample and no substance penetrates exclusively in this compartment. Substance that equilibrates in interstitial fluid also equilibrates in plasma. Therefore, the interstitial fluid volume is estimated as the ***difference between ECF volume and plasma volume***.

Measurement of ICF Volume

Intracellular fluid volume (ICFV) cannot be measured directly by dilution principle as no substance remains confined only to this compartment. It is determined indirectly by *subtracting ECF volume from total body water* (TBW). Thus, first **TBW is measured**.

Measurement of TBW

Measurement of TBW is performed by indicator dilution principle:

1. **Deuterium oxide** (D_2O, heavy water) is usually used as it has properties that are slightly different from H_2O. However, in equilibration experiments for measuring TBW, it gives accurate results.
2. **Tritium oxide** and **aminopyrine** can also be used for measuring TBW.

Measurement of red cell volume, plasma volume effective blood volume is described in next chapter.

IONIC COMPOSITION OF BODY FLUIDS

Basic Features

1. The distribution of electrolytes varies in body compartments.
2. Sum of the concentrations of the cations equals the sum of the concentrations of the anions in respective compartments. This makes the fluid in each compartment electrically neutral.
3. Na^+, Ca^{2+}, Cl^- and HCO_3^- are largely extracellular (Table 8.4) and K^+, Mg^{++}, organic phosphates (PO_4^{3-}) and proteins (prot$^-$) are mainly intracellular.
4. Essentially, almost all the K^+ in the body is in the exchangeable pool, whereas only 65%–70% of the body Na^+ is exchangeable. Solutes that are exchangeable are osmotically active.
5. Almost all of the body Ca^{++} (in bone) and most of the body Mg^{++} (in bone and cells) are nonexchangeable.

Table 8.4: Concentration (mmol/L of H_2O) of major ions in ECF (plasma) and ICF.

Ions	ECF	ICF
Na^+	145	12
K^+	5	140
Ca^{++}(ionized)	1.2	0.1 µmol/L
Mg^{++}	1.5	20
Cl^-	110	5
HCO_3^-	27	10
PO_4^{3-}	2	60

Units for Measuring Solutes

The number of molecules, electrical charges, or particles of a substance per unit volume of a particular body fluid is frequently expressed in **moles, equivalents or osmoles.**

Moles

The mole is the standard unit for expressing the amount of substances in the SI unit system. A mole is the gram-molecular weight of a substance, i.e. the molecular weight of a substance, in grams. Each mole (mol) consists of approx. 6×10^{23} molecules. Thus, 1 mole of KCl = 39 + 35.5 gm = 74.5 gm (i.e. sum of atomic masses of all the atoms in the molecule).

The **millimole** (mmol) is 1/1000 of a mole. Thus, 1 mmol of KCl = 74.5 mg.

The concepts are:

1. The concentrations of two different substances on the basis of number of grams per liter of solution do not indicate how many molecules of each compound are present. Therefore, concentrations in units of grams per liter are often used when the chemical structure of the solute is unknown.
2. When the structure of a molecule is known, concentrations are expressed as moles per liter. This provides a unit of concentration based upon the number of molecules of the solute in solution. Thus a solution containing 74.5 gm of KCl in 1 liter of solution is said to be one-molar (1M or 1 mol/L) solution of KCl.
3. Since 1 mole of any molecule will have the same number of molecules (6×10^{23}), 1M solution of KCl contains the same number of solute molecules per liter as 1M solution of glucose or any other substance.

Equivalents

The equivalent is the standard unit for expressing the solutes in the body which are in the form of charged particles. One equivalent (Eq) is 1 mole of an ionized substance divided by its valency. One mole of KCl dissociates into 1 Eq of K^+ and 1 Eq of Cl^-. One Eq of K^+ = 39 gm/1 = 39 gm; whereas 1 Eq Ca^{++} = 40 gm/2 = 20 gm. The milliequivalent (mEq) is 1/1000 of 1 Eq.

The **normality (N)** of a solution is the number of gram equivalents in 1 liter. Therefore, 1 N solution of hydrochloric acid (HCl) contains 1 + 35.5 gm/L = 36.5gm/L.

Osmolarity and Osmolality

The number of osmoles per liter of solution is called osmolarity, whereas the number of osmoles per kilogram of solvent is osmolality. Osmotically active substances in the body are dissolved in water. As the density of water is 1, osmolal concentration is expressed in ***osmoles per liter*** (Osm/L) of water. Details of osmole, milliosmole, osmolarity and osmolality are described in Chapter 6, under 'Osmosis'. Regulation of composition, osmolality and volume of body fluid and the related applied physiology are described in in chapter "Regulation of volume, osmolality and composition of body fluid compartments", in Volume II, Section 13 (Integrative Physiology).

pH of Body Fluids

The hydrogen ion concentration of body fluids is expressed as H^+ or pH (negative logarithm of H^+).

$pH = -\log_{10}[H^+]$.

1. When pK (K is the ionization or dissociation constant) of a buffer system is known, it is possible to determine the effective pH range of the buffer. Hence, pK = negative log of K (–log K) and is equal to the pH at which half of the acid molecules are dissociated and half are undissociated.
2. Blood pH is 7.35–7.45, at the range of H^+ conc. 20–126 mEq/L.
3. Acidosis refers to blood < 7.35 and alkalosis refers to blood > 4.45.

Concept and mechanism of pH-buffer system and acid-base balance are described in detail last section of the book "Integrative Physiology" in chapter 'Basic principle of acid-base homeostasis'.

CHAPTER SUMMARY

Key Concepts

1. Total body water (TBW) as percentage of body weight on average is about 60% in adult males, which is about 10% more than in females.
2. In infants and children, though TBW as percentage of body weight is more than in adults, their absolute water content is significantly less. Therefore, dehydration occurs faster and often may be fatal, if not treated early and adequately.
3. Measurement of body fluid volume id based on 'indicator dilution principle'.

4. K^+ is more in ICF (140 mmol/L of water) and less in ECF (5 mmol/L of water), where as Na^+ is less in ICF (12 mmol/L of water) and more in ECF (145 mmol/L of water).

Points to be Noted (Must Read)

1. Measurements of plasma volume, blood volume and ECF volume are usually asked in written examinations.
2. In **Viva**, questions from following topics/concepts are asked:
    - % of total body water in males and females in different age groups.
    - Principle of measurement of fluid volumes (indicator dilution principle).
    - Characteristics of an indicator.
    - Basic method of measurement of ECF and ICF.
    - Different isotopes/dyes used for measuring different fluid volumes.
    - Why is dehydration common in children?
    - Concept of moles, osmoles, equivalents, osmolality and osmolarity.

SECTION–2

Blood and Immunity

9. Composition and Functions of Blood and Plasma Proteins
10. Bone Marrow and Hemopoiesis
11. Red Blood Cells
12. Erythropoiesis
13. Destruction of Red Blood Cells
14. Hemoglobin and Blood Indices
15. Pathophysiology of Anemia and Polycythemia
16. Blood Groups and Physiological Basis of Blood Transfusion
17. White Blood Cells
18. Thymus, Lymphoid Tissues and Lymph
19. Physiology of Immunity
20. Platelets and Their Role in Hemostasis
21. Blood Coagulation

"The spirit shall look out through Matter's gaze
And Matter shall reveal the Spirit's face
Then man and superman shall be at one
And all the earth become a single life."

Sri Aurobindo (in 'SAVITRI')

CHAPTER 9

Composition and Functions of Blood and Plasma Proteins

Learning Objectives

On completion of study of this chapter, the student **MUST** be able to:

1. Define blood, and give the composition and functions of blood.
2. Name the layers of blood after centrifugation, name the cells present in buffy coat, and give uses of buffy coat preparation.
3. Give the normal value of blood volume in adults and children, and describe the methods of blood volume measurement.
4. Give the composition and functions of plasma.
5. Name the plasma proteins, give their normal values, and list the functions of plasma proteins.
6. Give the uses of fresh frozen plasma.

The student **MAY** also be able to:

1. Describe the determination of blood volume, plasma volume, and cell volume.
2. Give the importance of specific gravity and viscosity of blood.

Hematological investigations are commonly performed laboratory tests in medical practice because many bodily dysfunctions reflect through alteration in blood even in their early stage and hematological changes are reliable indices of the intensity and progress of the diseases. Moreover, blood is an easily accessible and readily available tissue sample for investigations, and many blood tests can be performed in physician's office. Therefore, examination of blood is common and an essential component in patient management. Therefore, a student of medicine should have adequate knowledge in physiology of blood.

Hematology is the study of physiology of blood and blood disorders. Study of ***blood physiology*** includes the study of different components of blood, their formation, their role in different body functions and dysfunctions, and ***study of blood disorders*** includes the pathophysiology of diseases of blood and their management, and pathological alterations in blood in other (non-hematological) diseases.

Blood examination reveals two fundamental aspects of hematology:

1. If the bone marrow is producing adequate number of mature cells of hematopoietic lineages
2. If development of each hematopoietic lineage is qualitatively normal.

Though investigations on peripheral blood by different blood counts and smear examination help to answer these two major questions, ***study of bone marrow*** provides a better picture of the disease and adds to hematological diagnosis.

BLOOD

Blood is **defined** as liquid connective tissue that fills the heart and blood vessels. The normal blood volume in an average adult is 5–6 liters, which accounts for about 8% of the body weight.

Composition of Blood

Blood consists of two components: cells and fluid. The **cellular component** comprises of different formed elements, and the **fluid component** is the plasma.

1. The **formed elements** are red blood cells (erythrocytes), white blood cells (leucocytes), and platelets (thrombocytes).
2. The **plasma** consists of about 55% of the total blood volume which is made up of water and solid particles.

When blood is collected in an anticoagulated tube and allowed to settle by centrifugation, ***three layers*** are

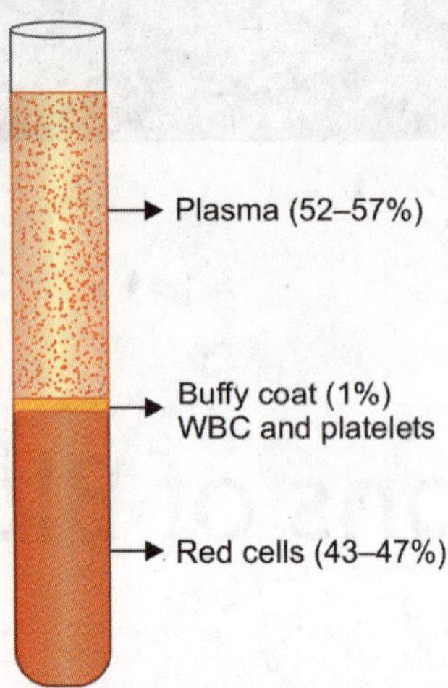

Fig. 9.1: Appearance of centrifuged blood. Note, about 1% of blood forms the buffy coat (present between plasma and red cell mass) that mainly contains WBC and platelets.

distinctly visible. The upper **plasma layer** is separated from lower **red cell mass** by a thin **buffy coat** (Fig. 9.1).

Buffy Coat

The thin middle layer that separates the upper plasma and lower red cell mass after centrifugation of blood is the buffy coat.

1. The buffy coat contains leucocytes and platelets.
2. In diseases, abnormal cells are found in the buffy coat like *LE cells* in systemic lupus erythematosus and atypical or *primitive blood cells* (atypical mononuclear cells, promyelocytes, metamyelocytes, blast cells, megakaryocytes etc.) in malignant or premalignant conditions (Clinical Box 9.1).

Clinical Box 9.1

Buffy coat preparation: The blood film may be prepared from buffy coat for the detection of the abnormal cells in blood. Also, ***buffy coat preparation*** is very useful for the detection of bacteria, fungi or parasites within neutrophils, monocytes or circulating macrophages.

Functions of Blood

1. **Respiratory functions:** Blood transports oxygen from lungs to tissues, and carbon dioxide from tissues to the lungs. Thus, by transporting gases blood serves an important function of respiration.
2. **Transport medium:** Blood acts as the transport medium for various hormones, chemical substances, nutrients, vitamins, etc. Hormones secreted from various endocrine tissues, and nutrients absorbed from GI tract circulate in blood and distribute to all tissues of the body. Thus, blood regulates growth and metabolism of the tissues.
3. **Temperature regulation:** Blood plays an important role in temperature regulation as it conducts heat from the interior of body to the surface through blood vessels. Temperature is continuously produced in the body. Blood absorbs this heat and transfers to the body surface. Therefore, vasoconstriction preserves body temperature and vasodilation facilitates heat dissipation from the body.
4. **Excretory function:** Blood helps in excretion of waste materials by transporting them from different parts of the body to the kidney.
5. **Water homeostasis:** Fifty-five percent of blood contains plasma and 92% of plasma contains water. Loss of water from body as occurs in diarrhea, vomiting, excessive sweating etc. results in decreased blood volume (hypovolemia). Persistent hypovolemia results in cellular dehydration. In response to hypovolemia, mechanisms are activated to increase the water content of blood that aims at maintaining cellular hydration. Thus, by maintaining blood volume, water homeostasis of the body is maintained.
6. **Acid-base balance:** Blood contains plasma proteins and hemoglobins. They (protein and Hb buffers) play important role in maintaining acid base balance of the body. Also, bicarbonate in blood buffers the acids.
7. **Immunity:** Blood forms a critical component of body immunity. It contains cells that play primary role in cellular immunity and also contains antibodies that play major role in humoral immunity. Blood also contains cells and chemicals that take part in nonspecific defenses of the body.
8. **Storage:** Blood is the storage site of electrolytes, nutrients, chemicals, hormones, etc.
9. **Body color:** Blood provides natural color to the body. In anemia and hypovolemia, body becomes pale.
10. **Nutritive functions:** Blood delivers all nutrients, such as glucose, lipids, proteins, vitamins, minerals, etc. to all tissues of the body for their utilization and storage.
11. **Oncotic pressure:** The albumin present in blood exerts osmotic pressure, known as oncotic pressure that controls capillary filtration and prevents edema formation (discussed more in 'functions of plasma proteins').

Blood Volume

The total blood volume can be roughly calculated as 70–80 ml/kg of body weight. In adult males, the total volume of blood is about 5 to 6 liters and in females about 4.5 to 5.5 liters. In children, though the absolute volume of blood present is significantly less than adults, the volume expressed per kg of body weight is more (80–90 ml/kg-BW). Blood volume is also expressed per square meter of body surface area, which is normally 2.8 lit/m^2 of the body.

Determination of Blood Volume

Blood volume is determined by determining the plasma volume and cell volume separately. The normal ratio of plasma volume to cell volume is 55:45.

Table 9.1: Composition of plasma.
1. Water (92%)
2. Solids or Solutes (8%): plasma proteins make 90% of solids
a. Inorganic
i. Anions: Chloride, bicarbonate, phosphates, sulphates, etc.
ii. Cations: Na^+, K^+, Ca^{++}, Mg^{++}, etc.
b. Organic
i. Colloids: Plasma proteins
ii. Crystalloids: Glucose, lipid, urea, uric acid, etc.

Measurement of Cell Volume

Cell volume is measured by measuring the **volume of red cells**. The volume of *leucocytes and platelets is ignored* as they constitute minor fraction of the total cell volume. Red cell volume is measured by radioactive isotope study.

Red cell volume

Red cell volume is the volume occupied by all circulating red cells.

1. It is usually calculated by subtracting plasma volume from total blood volume.
2. It is also directly calculated by injecting tagged red cell. The *radioactive isotope of chromium* is usually used as tag, though isotopes of iron (^{59}Fe) and phosphorous (^{32}P) are also used.
3. The commonly used chromium isotope is **^{51}Cr**, which is attached to red cells through incubation of cells in the chromium solution.

Determination of Plasma Volume

Plasma volume is usually measured by using dyes. The dye used is *Evans blue* (T-1824). Plasma volume is also measured by injection of serum albumin labeled with radioactive iodine. An average plasma volume is about 3.5 L (5% of the body weight of a 70 kg man).

Total blood volume is calculated by multiplying plasma volume with 100/(100 – hematocrit). (Hematocrit is to be determined). If hematocrit is 40 and plasma volume is 3.5 L, then blood volume will be:

$$3.5 \times \frac{100}{100-40} = 5.8 \text{ L}$$

Effective Blood Volume

Effective blood volume = the total blood volume – the volume that is sequestrated.

This means the volume which is present actually in the circulation that helps in perfusion of tissue. However, it is difficult to estimate the sequestered volume of blood in the visceral organs.

Specific Gravity and Viscosity of Blood

Specific gravity: Specific gravity or density of whole blood is approximately 1.050.

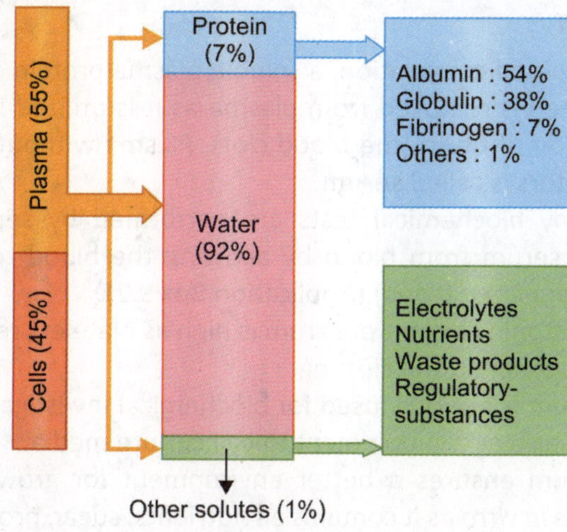

Fig. 9.2: Constituent of plasma. Note, 92% of plasma is water and 2% is solute.

1. This depends on the number of cells and composition of plasma.
2. Specific gravity is measured by the extent of light bending in a refractometer or as part of a test strip dipped into blood.
3. Usually, loss of water from blood as occurs in dehydration increases specific gravity.

Viscosity: Viscosity of blood or any liquid is a measure of resistance to flow.

1. Blood viscosity is 4 to 5 times that of water.
2. It is mainly due to the number of cells and macromolecules like proteins present in the blood.

PLASMA

Plasma is the fluid component of blood which constitutes about 55% of the total blood volume. The remaining 45% is constituted by cells (formed elements). If the **whole plasma** is to be used for investigations, blood is collected with anticoagulants (***anticoagulated blood***). Plasma can be stored for years for future investigations (Application Box 9.1).

Application Box 9.1

Fresh Frozen Plasma: In some conditions, plasma needs to be stored for years for future analysis, for which plasma is stored frozen below –20ºC. This is called fresh frozen plasma (FFP), which can be stored up to 7 years in a blood bank. However, to preserve clotting factors plasma should be frozen within 6 hours after collection. FFP is used for **plasmapheresis** (therapeutic plasma exchange).

Composition of Plasma

Plasma constitutes water and solids (Table 9.1). Water content of plasma is about 92% of the total plasma. The major solute (solid) content is the plasma proteins, which constitutes about 7% of the plasma and other solutes make up the rest 1% (Fig. 9.2).

Serum

During blood coagulation, a soluble plasma protein called fibrinogen is removed from plasma as it is utilized in the formation of fibrin (the blood clot). Plasma without clotting factors is called **serum**.

1. Many biochemical tests are performed by separating serum from blood by allowing the blood to clot (*coagulated blood*) (Application Box 9.2).
2. Serotonin content of serum is high as platelets release serotonin during clotting.
3. Serum is not only used for biochemical investigations, but also as a supplement to cell culture media.
4. Serum ensures a better environment for growth of cells *in vitro* as it contains all nutrients, sugar, proteins, hormones and other factors.
5. Fetal calf serum is used often for growth of human cells.

Application Box 9.2

Separating serum: Plasma is separated by centrifuging anticoagulated blood. The serum is separated from blood by ***allowing the blood to coagulate*** (serum = blood – fibrinogen and other clotting factors).

PLASMA PROTEINS

Plasma proteins are the major solute constituents of plasma. The normal plasma protein concentration is 6–8 g/ 100 ml of plasma.

Types of Plasma Proteins

Plasma proteins are of three types: albumin (4–5.5 g%), globulin (1.5–3 g%), and fibrinogen (0.3 g%). Plasma proteins are formed mainly in the liver.

Albumin

This is the major constituent of plasma proteins.

1. Albumin is formed in the liver.
2. It has half life of about 20 days and its molecular weight is 66000.
3. Being smallest in diameter among the plasma proteins, in kidney diseases with glomerular injury it appears early in urine (**albuminuria**).
4. In **kidney diseases**, albuminuria decreases plasma protein concentration that leads to **hypoalbuminemia.** Hypoalbuminemia also occurs in in **liver diseases** due to decreased formation of albumin. In such conditions, *decreased colloidal osmotic pressure* (oncotic pressure) of plasma results in **edema formation** (see below).

Globulin

This is formed in the liver, cells of reticuloendothelial system and plasma cells.

1. Globulins are divided into three categories: α (α_1, α_2), β (β_1, β_2) and γ.
2. The molecular weight of globulins is 90000–156000.
3. Globulins include different transport proteins like transferrin, ceruloplasmin, hemopexin, etc.
4. They form different lipoproteins in combination with lipids in plasma.
5. Antibodies (immunoglobulins) are γ-globulins that are formed by plasma cells.
6. The normal ***albumin-globulin ratio*** (AGR) is 1.5 to 2.5:1. In many diseases, AGR is altered. Detection of AGR helps in diagnosing and assessing the prognosis of some diseases.
7. **Albumin-globulin ratio** (AGR) is important (Clinical Box 9.2)

Clinical Box 9.2

Albumin-globulin ratio: The normal albumin-globulin ratio (AGR) is 1.5 to 2.5:1. In many diseases, especially in immunological and inflammatory diseases, AGR is altered. Detection of AGR helps in diagnosing and assessing the prognosis of some diseases.

Fibrinogen

The molecular weight is 340000. It is produced in the liver. It plays an important role in blood coagulation. It also contributes to the viscosity of plasma and determination of ESR.

Functions of Plasma Proteins

1. **Osmotic pressure:** Plasma proteins are osmotically active molecules, and the osmotic pressure of plasma due to plasma proteins is called ***oncotic pressure***. The normal oncotic pressure is 25 mm Hg. This pressure helps in maintaining volume of the vascular compartment. Oncotic pressure retains fluid in the vascular compartment and, therefore, ***prevents loss of fluid from capillaries into the interstitial tissue space*** (functionally, it opposes the action of hydrostatic pressure). Therefore, when oncotic pressure decreases due to hypoproteinemia as occurs in liver and kidney diseases, edema manifests due to escape of water into the interstitial tissue space. The oncotic pressure is due to the presence of albumin in the plasma.
2. **Viscosity**: Plasma protein contributes to about 50% of the viscosity of blood (red cells account for rest of the viscosity). The viscosity depends on the *molecular shape of the plasma protein*. This is why fibrinogen molecules that are elongated and fibrillar in shape contribute more to blood viscosity than albumin molecules that are ellipsoid in structure.
3. **Immunity**: Antibodies are plasma proteins (gamma globulins). Antibodies mediate humoral immunity that protects the body from infections, especially extracellular pathogens and from the effect of toxic substances.

4. **Coagulation**: Blood clotting depends on concentration of fibrinogen that forms fibrin thread, the final step in blood coagulation. Also, other clotting factors like prothrombin are plasma proteins.
5. **Transport:** Plasma proteins serve as carrier molecule for transport of various substances like hormones, drugs, metals, etc.
6. **Buffering:** Plasma proteins form an important buffering system of the body called ***protein buffers***. This helps in acid-base balance of the body.
7. **Protein store:** Plasma proteins serve as ***mobile protein reserve*** of the body, which can be utilized for tissue growth, especially in situations of protein depletion.
8. **Synthetic function:** Plasma proteins provide substrate for the synthesis of protein hormones like erythropoietin, etc. and various enzymes.
9. **Determination of ESR:** ESR mostly depends on the concentration of fibrinogen in the plasma. Fibrinogen facilitates ***rouleaux formation***, which in turn increases the rate of sedimentation of red cells. Therefore, conditions in which fibrinogen concentration is more like acute inflammations, ESR becomes more (Details of ESR are described in chapter "The Red Blood Cells").

Separation of Plasma Proteins

Plasma proteins can be separated by methods like salt separation, paper electrophoresis, Cohn's fractionation, ultracentrifugation, immunochemical analysis, etc. Determination of concentration of various fractions is useful for estimation of albumin-globulin ratio (AGR) and for diagnosis and prognosis of different diseases.

CHAPTER SUMMARY

Key Concepts

1. Blood is *defined* as liquid connective tissue that fills the heart and blood vessels. The normal blood volume in adults is 5 to 6 liters, which accounts for about 8% of the body weight.
2. Blood consists of two components: cells and fluid (plasma).
3. The **plasma** consists of about 55% of the total blood volume which is made up of water and solid particles.
4. When blood is collected in an anticoagulated tube and allowed to settle by centrifugation, ***three layers*** are distinctly visible. The upper **plasma layer** is separated from lower **red cell mass** by a thin *buffy coat*.
5. The **buffy coat** contains leucocytes and platelets. In diseases, abnormal cells are found in the buffy coat like *LE cells* in systemic lupus erythematosus and atypical or *primitive blood cells* (atypical mononuclear cells, promyelocytes, metamyelocytes, blast cells, megakaryocytes, etc.) in malignant or premalignant conditions.
6. Plasma without clotting factors is called **serum**. Many biochemical tests are performed by separating serum from blood by allowing the blood to clot.
7. There are three major plasma proteins: albumin, globulin and fibrinogen. Albumin is the main plasma protein that maintains oncotic pressure. Globulin is for immunity and fibrinogen is for blood clotting.

Important to Know (Must Read)

1. In examinations, usually long questions do not come from this chapter. However, Types and functions of plasma proteins, may come as a **Long Question**.
2. Determination of blood volume, types of plasma proteins, and functions of plasma proteins may be asked as **Short Notes/Questions** in exams.
3. In **Viva**, examiners invariably ask the definition of blood, composition of blood, functions of blood, composition of plasma and function of each constituent, importance of buffy coat, how are plasma and serum separated, fresh frozen plasma, types of plasma proteins, functions of plasma proteins.
4. When a student fails to answer the composition of blood and plasma, and functions of plasma proteins, it becomes difficult for examiner to give the pass mark.

CHAPTER 10

Bone Marrow and Hemopoiesis

LEARNING OBJECTIVES

On completion of study of this chapter, the student **MUST** be able to:

1. Name the types of bone marrow and give their functions.
2. Comprehend the basic cellular architecture of bone marrow.
3. Appreciate the importance of myeloid-erythroid ratio in bone marrow.
4. Define hemopoiesis and name the sites of hemopoiesis in different stages.
5. Understand the difference between medullary and extramedullary hemopoiesis.
6. Name the sites of hemopoiesis in different age groups.
7. Name the types of stem cells and give their properties.
8. Outline the steps of different series (erythropoiesis, leucopoiesis and thrombopoiesis) of hemopoiesis.
9. Describe regulation of hemopoiesis.

The student **MAY** also be able to:

1. List the indications of bone marrow biopsy.
2. Understand the need for bone marrow aspiration.
3. Draw and describe the cells in hemopoietic series.
4. Describe the cellular patterns in bone marrow biopsy.

BONE MARROW

Bone marrow is the site of normal hemopoiesis after birth. Hemopoiesis (or hematopoiesis) describes the formation of blood cells, which is an active process that must maintain normal number of blood cells in peripheral blood and also should be able to respond to the increased demands in situations like hemorrhage or infections. During fetal life, hemopoiesis mainly occurs in the spleen and liver, and subsequently in red bone marrow present in the medullary cavity of all bones. From childhood, red marrow is progressively replaced by fat tissues (yellow marrow). Therefore, normal hemopoiesis in adults is restricted to vertebrae, sternum, ribs, clavicles, pelvic bones, skull and ends of humerus and femurs.

Bone marrow contains a range of hemopoietic precursor cells and a storage pool of mature cells for their release into peripheral circulation. All blood cells are derived from the pluripotent stem cells, referred to as hemopoietic stem cells (HSCs). HSCs sustain life long production of all blood lineages. HSCs provide homeostasis of blood cells through their ability to generate the hundreds of millions of red cells, white cells and platelets needed every day.

Types of Bone Marrow

There are three types of bone marrow: red marrow, yellow marrow and white marrow.

Red Marrow

The red marrow is the active marrow and is red in colour. It consists of many blood vessels that contain sinusoidal capillaries (vascular sinuses), and the marrow stroma (Fig. 10.1).

Marrow stroma: The marrow stroma consists principally of a network of sinuses that originate at the endosteum from cortical capillaries and terminate in the collecting vessels that enter the systemic circulation. Hematopoiesis takes place in the ***intersinus spaces***. The trilaminar sinus wall contains three components:

1. Endothelial cells
2. Thin basement membrane
3. Adventitial reticular cells.

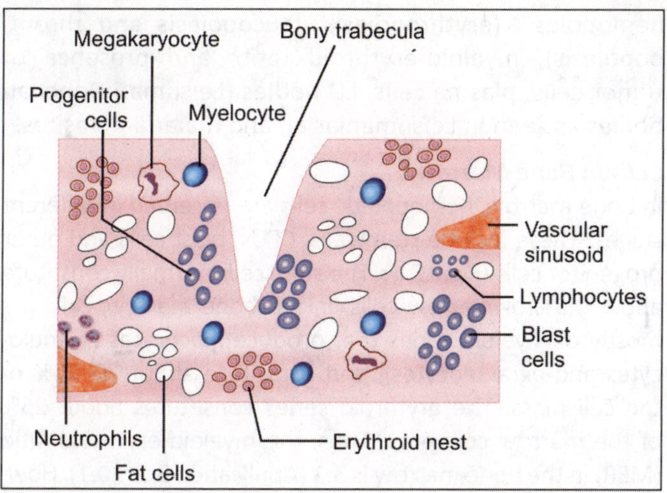

Fig. 10.1: Structural organization of bone marrow depicting different types of cells. Note the presence of blast cells, progenitor cells, megakaryocytes, myelocytes, and fat cells. Red cells develop from 'erythroid nests'.

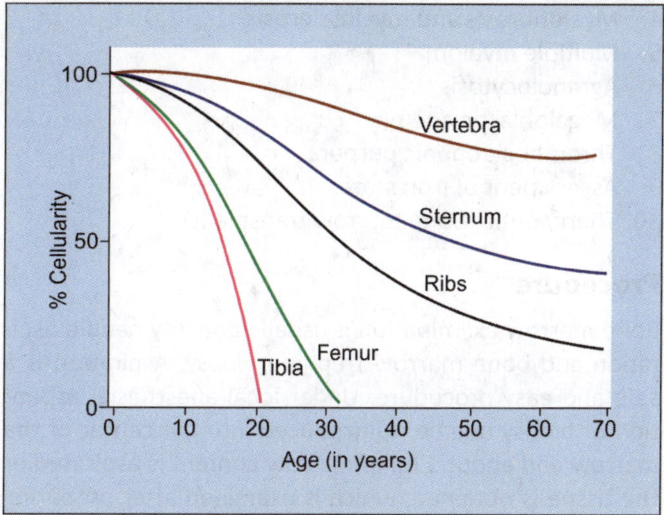

Fig. 10.2: Hemopoietic activity in adult life. Note, though the hemopoietic activity ceases in tibia and femur by third decade of life, it continues in vertebra, sternum and ribs.

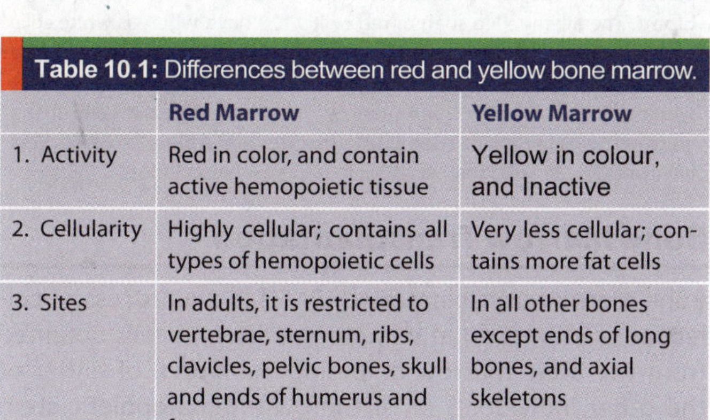

Table 10.1: Differences between red and yellow bone marrow.

	Red Marrow	Yellow Marrow
1. Activity	Red in color, and contain active hemopoietic tissue	Yellow in colour, and Inactive
2. Cellularity	Highly cellular; contains all types of hemopoietic cells	Very less cellular; contains more fat cells
3. Sites	In adults, it is restricted to vertebrae, sternum, ribs, clavicles, pelvic bones, skull and ends of humerus and femurs.	In all other bones except ends of long bones, and axial skeletons

The bone forming cells are present between the sinusoidal capillaries. The adventitial reticular cells are fibroblasts capable of transforming into adipocytes (fat cells). Endothelium and reticular cells are the sources of cytokines that profoundly influence hemopoiesis. All types of precursor cells (blast cells, progenitor cells, megakaryocytes) are present in the bone marrow trabeculae. Red cells are produced from the erythroid 'nests'.

Red bone marrow is present in almost all bones of the body at birth. However, with advancement of age red marrow is replaced by fatty tissue and slowly becomes inactive. At the age of 20–30 years, red marrow of long bones cease to produce cells, and active marrow is limited to the membranous bones like skull bones, vertebrae, ribs, sternum and pelvic and pectoral girdles (Fig. 10.2).

Yellow Marrow

The yellow marrow contains less blood vessels and more fat cells and fibro-fatty tissue. The yellow marrow does not participate in hemopoiesis. Fat cells replace hematopoietic cells in the bones of hands, feet, legs and arm at about age of 20 years. Fat occupies 50% of the space of red marrow in adult and further fatty degeneration continues slowly with aging. Yellow marrow can revert back to hemopoietically active red marrow when prolonged demand persists as occurs in chronic hemolytic anemia. Differences between red and yellow marrow are listed in Table 10.1.

White Marrow

In very old individuals, a gelatinous transformation of fat to a mucoid material occurs in bone marrow. This type of marrow in elderly persons is called white marrow.

Bone Marrow Examination

Bone marrow examination is indicated in complex hematological disorders and malignant hematological conditions that require detailed analysis of cellularity and activity of the marrow. The bone marrow examination is done for the following types of assessments:

1. Cellularity of the marrow (normocellualr, hypercellular or hypocellular)
2. Myeloid-Erythroid ratio
3. State of erythropoiesis, myelopoiesis and megakaryopoiesis
4. Number of lymphocytes (normal, increased or abnormal)
5. Plasma cells (normal or increased)
6. Other cells : Metastatic tumor cells, parasites (malaria, Leishmania Donovani, etc.), fungus or any other cells.
7. Iron stores evaluated by Persian blue reaction (normal, increased or decreased)

Indications for Bone Marrow Examination

Usual indications for bone marrow examination are:

1. Anemias: Aplastic anemia and refractory anemias
2. Aleukemic leukemia
3. Differentiation of leukemias

4. Myelofibrosis and myelosclerosis
5. Multiple myeloma
6. Agranulocytosis
7. Megaloblastic anemia
8. Thrombocytopenic purpura
9. Assessment of iron stores
10. Therapeutic (Bone marrow transplant)

Procedure

Bone marrow examination is usually done by needle aspiration and bone marrow trephine biopsy. Aspiration is a safe and easy procedure. Under local anesthesia, aspiration or biopsy needle is introduced into the center of the marrow and about 1 ml of marrow content is aspirated or the tissue is obtained, which is examined after preparing a stained smear. Staining is usually done by Romanowsky dyes or May-Grünwald-Giemsa stain. The usual sites of aspirations are sternum (sternal puncture), ileac crest and spinous process of vertebra.

Bone Marrow Needle Aspiration

The usual sites of aspirations are sternum, ileac crest and spinous process of vertebra (Clinical Box 10.1).

Clinical Box 10.1

Sites of marrow aspiration: Bone marrow aspiration is relatively an easy procedure. Commonly used needle is Salah Needle that has the provision of adjusting the depth of penetration into the marrow. The common sites of bone marrow aspiration are: sternum, posterior-superior iliac spine, iliac crest, anterior-superior iliac spine, and spinous process of lumbar vertebra. In infants, upper end of tibia is the deal site for marrow aspiration.

Sternal Puncture

This is the commonest procedure for bone marrow aspiration, especially in adults. The needle is introduced into the marrow cavity of mid-manubrium sterni.

Iliac Crest Puncture

The ileac crest, particularly the region of the posterior spine is the preferred site for bone marrow aspiration, especially in children. It is also done in adults.

Vertebral Puncture

Spinous process of vertebrae of the lumbar segments is preferred when sternal puncture fails to reveal proper cytology or when sternum is otherwise contraindicated for the process.

Bone Marrow Biopsy

Bone marrow biopsy is performed by biopsy needle. This is called ***trephine biopsy***. The sites of biopsy are same as for needle aspiration. Biopsy is more tedious and risky than aspiration.

Features of Marrow Smear

The examination of stained marrow smear is performed for assessing cellularity of the marrow, effectiveness of hemopoiesis (erythropoiesis, leucopoiesis and thrombopoiesis), myeloid-erythroid ratio, and presence of tumor cells, plasma cells, LD bodies (Leishman Donovan bodies as seen in Leishmaniasis), and malaria parasites.

Cells in Bone Marrow

In bone marrow, hemopoietic cells are observed in different stages. These include stem cells, CFUs, blast cells and other progenitor cells (Fig. 10.1). The stem cells normally constitute about 0.5% of marrow cells. In red bone marrow, cells are mostly of myeloid series that produce leucocytes (granulocytes and agranulocytes), and constitute about 70–75% of the cell mass. The erythroid series constitutes about 25% of the marrow cell mass. Thus, the myeloid-erythroid ratio (MER) in the bone marrow is 3:1 (Application Box 10.1). However, in the peripheral blood, red cells are much more than the white cells, *leucocyte-erythrocyte ratio* being 1:700.

Application Box 10.1

MER in bone marrow preserves leucocyte population in peripheral blood: The average life span of red cell is 120 days, whereas white cells stay in peripheral blood for few hours to few days. Therefore, to preserve white cell population in peripheral blood nature has provided more white cell precursors in bone marrow. This (more myeloid cells in the marrow) helps to replace adequate leucocytes in the blood as leucocytes have shorter life span than erythrocytes in circulating blood.

Bone Marrow Transplantation

Bone marrow transplantation (BMT) is the process of collection and infusion of hematopoietic stem cells obtained from the bone marrow or peripheral blood, of either of the other individuals or of the own hematopoietic stem cells (HSC).

Important Note

Sources of hematopoietic stem cells:
1. **Bone Marrow:** Bone marrow is the richest source of HSC.
2. **Peripheral Blood:** Few HSC are present in peripheral blood. They are mobilized into peripheral blood from bone marrow by administration of G-CSF or GM-CSF.
3. **Umbilical Cord Blood:** Collected following delivery. This is a rich source.

Scientist contributed

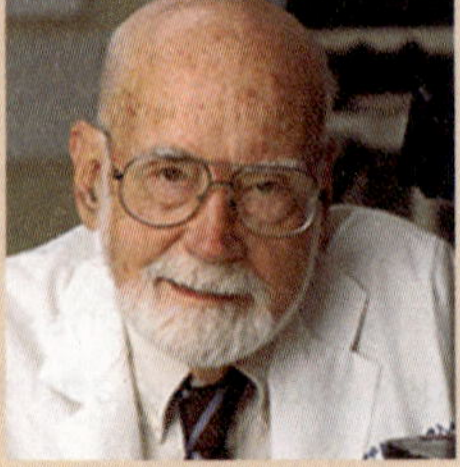
Dr E Donnall Thomas

Dr E Donnall Thomas received **Nobel Prize in Physiology and Medicine in 1990**, for Bone Marrow Transplantation. Dr. Thomas and his colleagues pioneered the successful use of bone marrow transplantation. This procedure replaces cancerous cells and stem cells damaged by chemotherapy and radiation with donated healthy cells that engraft within a patient's bone marrow. The discovery was a cure for leukemia and other blood cancers, and earned Thomas the 1990 Nobel Prize in physiology or medicine.

HEMOPOIESIS

Hemopoiesis is the process of formation (development, maturation and release) of blood cells. This is also called hematopoiesis. Blood cells are continuously destroyed in the body. Therefore, replacement of blood cells is also a continuous phenomenon and is an essential part of homeostasis of blood cells.

Scientist contributed

A Maximow is the first scientist to study the process of hemopoiesis. He studied the contribution of endothelium to blood regeneration (hemopoiesis). He especially studied the relation hemopoiesis with connective tissue and vascular endothelium.

Source: Maximow A. Relation of blood cells to connective tissues and vascular endothelium. Physiol Rev 1924; 4: 533-563.

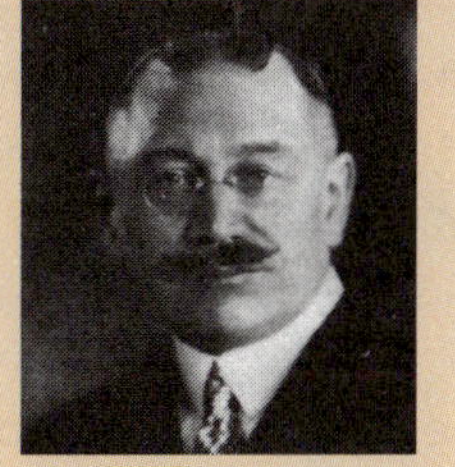

Alexander Maximow
(1874–1928)

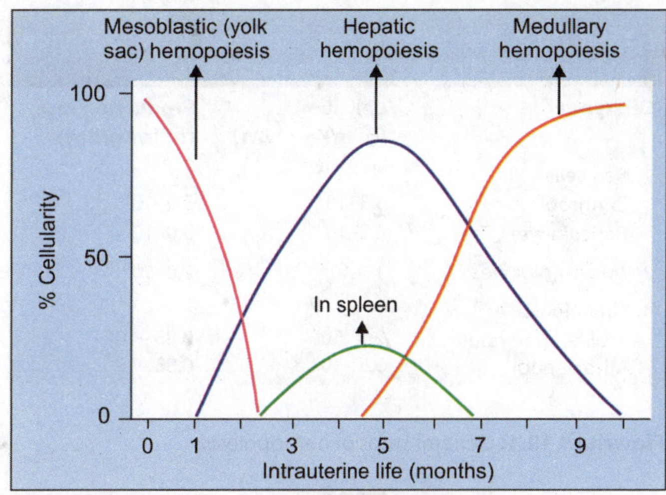

Fig. 10.3: Hemopoietic activity during intrauterine life.

Sites and Stages of Hemopoiesis

Location of hematopoiesis depends on the stage of hematopoiesis. During intrauterine life, hematopoiesis occurs first in the yolk sac, and later in the liver and spleen. After birth, hematopoiesis is confined to bone marrow. The environment in these organs (yolk sac, liver, spleen and bone marrow) where hematopoiesis takes place is called hematopoietic microenvironment. Hematopoiesis occurs in three stages: mesoblastic, hepatic and medullary.

Mesoblastic Stage

Mesoblastic stage is the stage of development of blood cells in the yolk sac and non-yolk sac regions during embryonic stage of intrauterine life. Yolk sac contains cells with multilineage differentiating capabilities that start functioning as early as second week of gestation. There are also few non-yolk sac regions that participate in hematopoiesis. Important among them are paraaortic splanchnopleura (PSP) and aorta-gonad mesonephros (AGM) regions. PSP region gives rise to B-cell progenitors and AGM region contains pleuripotent stem cells. Early lymphoid precursors have also been identified in the day-8 yolk sac. Also, lymphohematopoietic stem cells have been detected in vivo in the 9th day yolk sac.

Hepatic Stage

During second trimester of pregnancy, hemopoiesis takes place in the liver and spleen. This is called hepatic stage. In liver, hematopoiesis ***starts as early as 5th week of gestation***, which reaches its peak in 5th month and ceases at birth (Fig. 10.3). In spleen, hematopoiesis *occurs mainly in the second trimester* and the degree of hematopoiesis is quite less than that in the liver. Normally, *hematopoiesis does not occur in liver and spleen during post-natal life* (after birth). However, when the demand for blood cells is more than the rate of production, hematopoiesis does occur in liver and spleen.

Medullary Stage

Formation of blood cells in the bone marrow is called medullary hemopoiesis. Marrow cavities in the bone appear as early as ***5th month of fetal life***, and soon they become hemopoietic. In initial phase, bone marrow is the exclusive site for granulocytic and megakaryocytic proliferation, during which erythropoietic activity is confined to liver. Erythropoiesis in bone marrow occurs effectively towards the end of third trimester of pregnancy and then continues throughout life.

After birth, hemopoiesis stops in liver and gets confined only to the bone marrow. When hemopoiesis occurs in liver and spleen in postnatal life, is called extramedullary hemopoiesis. Extramedullary hemopoiesis after birth is always non-physiological (Application Box 10.2).

Application Box 10.2

Extramedullary hemopoiesis after birth is abnormal: Hemopoiesis in liver and spleen is physiological during intrauterine life. However, hemopoiesis in these organs or in any other organ (Extramedullary hemopoiesis) after birth is considered abnormal.

Rate of Medullary Hemopoiesis

Bone marrow is one of the largest organs in the human body. It produces about 6 billion cells (2.5 billion red cells, 2.5 billion platelets and 1 billion granulocytes) per kg of body weight per day in adolescents and adults. However, the rate of production is adjusted to the needs of day-to-day life. Different cell population and their rate of productions are listed in Table 10.2.

Sites of Medullary Hemopoiesis

Bone marrow is the sole site of erythropoiesis in human beings. In long bones, active marrow regresses rapidly after first decade of life and ceases to produce cells between 20–30 years of life (Fig. 10.2). Hemopoiesis continues to occur in active marrow of vertebrae, pectoral and

Table 10.2: The different cell population in bone marrow and their rate of production in the marrow.

Cell types	Cell number (cells/Kg of BW)	Production rate (cells/Kg/day)
1. Red cells Erythroblast Reticulocyte	 $5.3–10^{3}$ $8.2–10^{6}$	 $3.0–10^{9}$ $3.0–10^{9}$
2. Megakaryocytes	$15–10^{6}$	$2.0–10^{6}$
3. Granulocytes Proliferation pool Mitotic pool	 $2.1–10^{9}$ $5.6–10^{9}$	 $0.85–10^{9}$ $0.85–10^{9}$

Flowchart 10.1: General steps of hemopoiesis

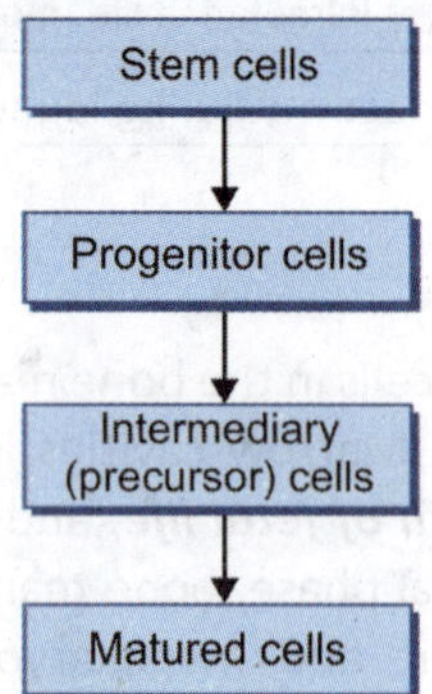

pelvic girdles, ribs, sternum and skull. However, with age the degree of hemopoiesis also decreases in these bones.

Steps of Hemopoiesis

Hematopoiesis occurs in the bone marrow from hematopoietic stem cells (Flowchart 10.1). The mother hematopoietic stem cell is the pluripotent stem cells (PPSC), also called as hemocytoblast. PPSC is the *multilineage stem cell* capable of producing two important groups of stem cells. These are myeloid stem cells and lymphoid cells. Lymphoid stem cells are unipotent stem cells (UPSC) that produce only lymphocytes, whereas myeloid stem cells are pluripotent in nature that from a group of different progenitor cells that are meant to produce red cells, granulocytes, monocytes and platelets. Thus, bone marrow contains two types of cells: stem cells and progenitor cells. In fact, stem cells develop into progenitor cells. The differences between these cells are listed in Table 10.3.

Table 10.3: Differences between stem cells and progenitor cells.

Characteristics	Stem cell	Progenitor cell
1. Proliferative potential	Large	Limited
2. Renewal potential	Adequate	Absent
3. Differentiation potential	Present	Present
4. Cells of origin	Unknown	Stem cells
5. Cytokine responsiveness	More	Less
6. Staining with rhodamine and Hoechst stains	Dim	Bright

Stem Cells

Properties

Stem cells in the bone marrow have two important properties: self renewal and differentiation.

Self Renewal

This is the property of duplicating themselves. That means they renew themselves and therefore physiologically they do not die and at the same time they proliferate into different lineage of cells. Due to self renewal, the bone marrow never goes out of stock for stem cells. Stem cell reserve in bone marrow remains always adequate.

Differentiation

This is the property of developing into specific lineage of cells. Due to the property of differentiation, stem cells differentiate into progenitor cells of various cell lines. Thus, different cell lineages are formed from stem cells that give rise to specific blood cells.

Scientist contributed

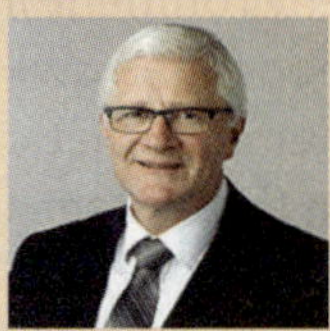
John Edgar Dick

Stem-cell scientists led by **Dr John Edgar Dick** was the first to study the details of properties and nature of stem cells. He has transformed the study of human hematopoiesis and leukemogenesis, with his development of methodologies for transplanting human bone marrow into immune-deficient mice, with resultant multilineage repopulation of murine bone marrow and other hematopoietic tissues. Using this approach, he has identified long-term repopulating human hematopoietic stem cells and generated mouse models of leukemia.

Types

There are two different stem cells: myeloid stem cells and lymphoid stem cells (Fig. 10.4).

Myeloid Stem Cells

Myeloid stem cells are pluripotent (tri-lineage) in nature that give rise to three types of different progenitor cells. These are erythroid progenitors that form erythroid series, the granulocytic progenitors that form granulocytes (neutrophil, eosinophil, and basophil), monocytic progenitors form monocytes, and megakaryocytic progenitors that form platelets.

Lymphoid Stem Cells

Lymphoid stem cells are unipotent stem cells (UPSC) that produce only cells of lymphocyte series.

Progenitor Cells

Progenitor cells develop from stem cells. Progenitor cells form colony forming units (CFUs) that give rise to different types of blast cells. ***Myeloid stem cells*** differentiate into CFU-GEMM, i. e. CFU for granulocyte, erythrocyte, megakaryocyte and monocyte. CFU-GEMM develops into three major CFUs (Fig. 10.4).

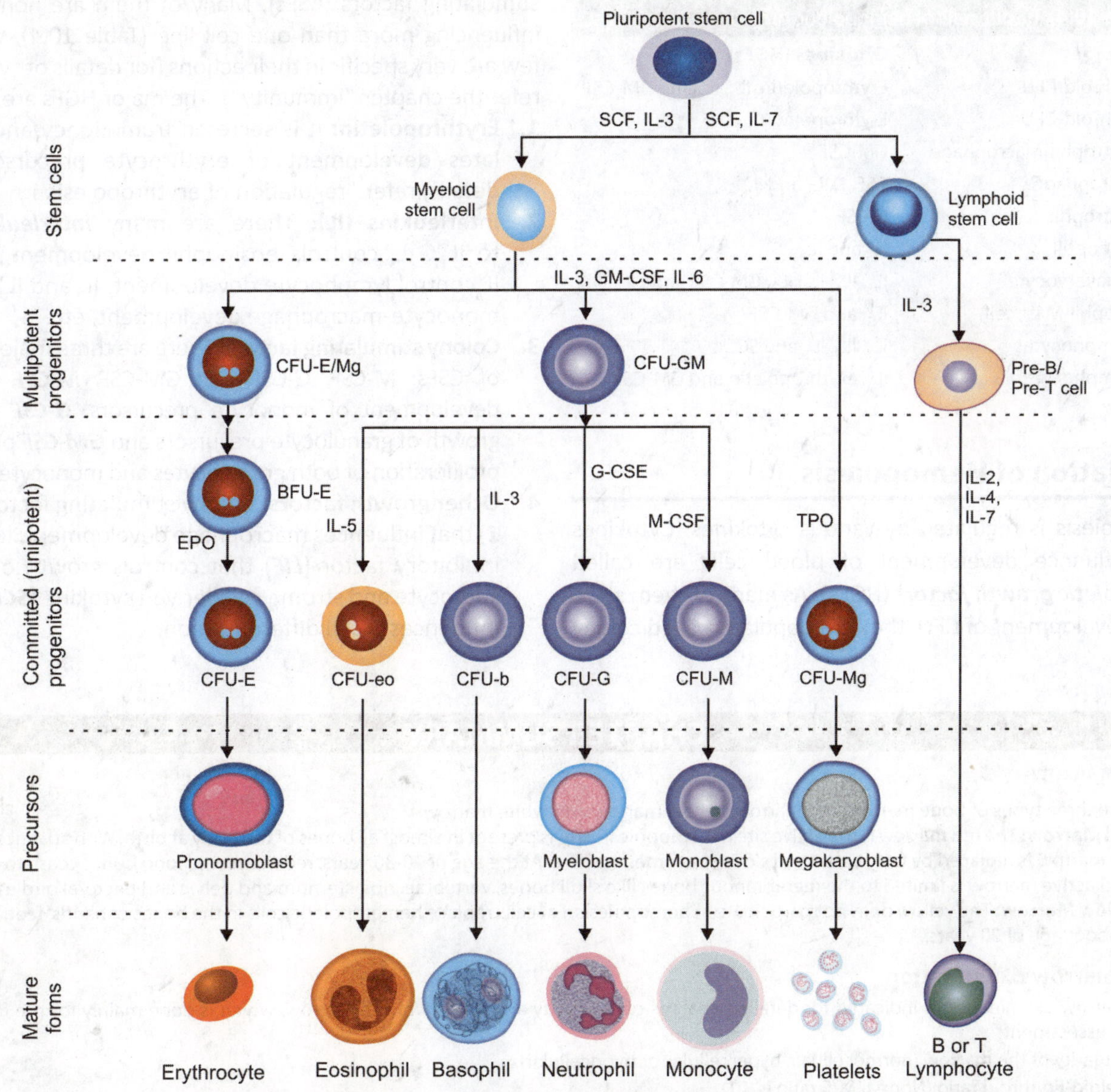

Fig. 10.4: Types and stages of hemopoiesis and major cytokines influencing them. (SCF: Stem cell factor, BFU: Burst-forming unit, CFU: Colony-forming unit, CSF: Colony-stimulating factor, GM: Granulocyte-monocyte, IL: Interleukins, EPO: Erythropoietin, TPO: Thrombopoietin).

1. **CFU-E:** CFU-E is the CFU for erythroid series that form ***proerythroblast***, which in turn develops into precursor cells of erythroid series.
2. **CFU-GM:** CFU-GM is the multilineage CFU that in turn forms CFU for granulocytes (***CFU-G***) and CFU for monocytes (***CFU-M***). CFU-G develops into ***myeloblast*** that differentiates into three lineage of granulocytes (neutrophil, eosinophil, and basophil). CFU-M develops into ***monoblast*** that differentiates into monocyte.
3. **CFU-Mega:** CFU-Mega differentiates into megakaryoblast that in turn forms platelets.

Types of Hemopoiesis

Hemopoiesis is broadly divided into three types: erythropoiesis, leucopoiesis and thrombopoiesis. Erythropoiesis is the development of red cells, leucopoiesis is the development of leucocytes and thrombopoiesis is the development of thrombocytes (platelets).

The PPSC diffentiates into five major blast cells (CFUs are excluded here) that give rise to five different cell lines (Fig. 10.4).

1. The ***proerythroblast*** that forms erythroid series for final development of red cells.
2. The ***myeloblast*** that differentiates into three lineages of granulocytes series (neutrophil, eosinophil, and basophil).
3. The ***monoblast*** that differentiates into monocytes.
4. The ***lymphoblast*** that develops into lymphocytes
5. The ***megakaryoblast*** that finally forms platelets.

Details of development of each cell line have been described in their respective sections.

Table 10.4: Target cells of hemopoietic growth factors (HGFs).

Cell lineage	Cytokines (HGFs)
1. Erythroid-BFU	Erythropoietin, IL_3, IL_4 and GM-CSF
2. Erythroid-CFU	Erythropoietin
3. Neutrophil-Macrophage	GM-CSF
4. Macrophage	CSF-1, IL_1 and IL_8
5. Neutrophil	G-CSF
6. Eosinophil	IL_5 and IL_3
7. Megakaryocyte	IL_3, IL_1, IL_6, IL_4, GM-CSF and LIF.
8. Basophil-Mast cell	IL_3, and GM-CSF
9. B lymphocytes	IL_7, IL_4, IL_5 and SCDC
10. T lymphocyte	IL_2, erythropoietin and GM-CSF

Regulation of Hemopoiesis

Hemopoiesis is regulated by various cytokines. Cytokines that influence development of blood cells are called ***hemopoietic growth factors*** (HGFs). As many of them stimulate development of CFU, they are popularly called colony stimulating factors (CSFs). Many of them are nonspecific, influencing more than one cell line (Table 10.4), whereas few are very specific in their actions (for details of cytokines, refer the chapter "Immunity"). The major HGFs are:

1. **Erythropoietin:** It is secreted from kidney and stimulates development of erythrocyte precursors (for details, refer "regulation of erythropoiesis').
2. **Interleukins (IL):** There are many ***interleukins***, IL_1 to IL_{11}. IL_5 controls eosinophil development, IL_2 and IL_4control lymphocyte development, IL_1 and IL_2 control monocyte-macrophage development, etc.
3. **Colony stimulating factors:** There are three major groups of CSFs: M-CSF, G-CSF and GM-CSF. ***M-CSF*** controls development of monocyte precursors, ***G-CSF*** controls growth of granulocyte precursors and ***GM-CSF*** promotes proliferation of both granulocytes and monocytes.
4. **Other growth factors:** Colony stimulating factor 1 (***CSF 1***) that influences macrophage development, leukemia inhibitory factor (***LIF***) that controls growth of megakaryocyte and stroma cell derived cytokine (***SCDC***) that influences B cell differentiation.

CHAPTER SUMMARY

Bone Marrow

There are three types of bone marrow: red marrow, yellow marrow and white marrow.

Red Marrow: The red marrow is the active site of hemopoiesis and is present in almost all bones of the body at birth. With advancement of age, red marrow is replaced by fatty tissue and slowly becomes inactive. At the age of 20-30 years, red marrow of long bones cease to produce cells, and active marrow is limited to the membranous bones like skull bones, vertebrae, ribs, sternum and pelvic and pectoral girdles.

Yellow Marrow: The yellow does not participate in hemopoiesis. Fat cells replace hematopoietic cells in the bones of hands, feet, legs and arm at about age of 20 years.

Bone Marrow Examination

Bone marrow examination is indicated for detailed analysis of cellularity and activity of the marrow, which is done mainly for the following types of assessments:

1. Cellularity of the marrow (normocellualr, hypercellular or hypocellular)
2. Myeloid-Erythroid ratio (Normal M/E ratio is 3:1)
3. State of erythropoiesis, myelopoiesis and megakaryopoiesis

Hemopoiesis

Hematopoiesis occurs in three stages: mesoblastic, hepatic and medullary.

Mesoblastic Stage: Mesoblastic stage is the stage of development of blood cells in the yolk sac and non-yolk sac regions during embryonic stage of intrauterine life.

Hepatic Stage: During second trimester of pregnancy, hemopoiesis takes place in the liver and spleen. This is called hepatic stage. In liver, hematopoiesis starts as early as 5th week of gestation, which reaches its peak in 5th month and ceases at birth. In spleen, hematopoiesis occurs mainly in the second trimester and the degree of hematopoiesis is quite less than that in the liver.

Medullary Stage: Formation of blood cells in the bone marrow is called medullary hemopoiesis. Marrow cavities in the bone appear as early as 5th month of fetal life, and soon they become hemopoietic. Erythropoiesis in bone marrow occurs effectively towards the end of third trimester of pregnancy and then continues throughout life.

Steps of Hemopoiesis

Hematopoiesis occurs in the bone marrow from hematopoietic stem cells that are pluripotent stem cells (PPSC). PPSC is the multilineage stem cell capable of producing two important groups of stem cells: myeloid stem cells and lymphoid cells. Lymphoid stem cells are unipotent stem cells (UPSC) that produce only lymphocytes, whereas myeloid stem cells are pluripotent in nature that from a group of different progenitor cells that are meant to produce red cells, granulocytes, monocytes and platelets.

Important to Know (Must Read)

1. Stages, types and regulation of hemopoiesis, may come as a **Long Question**.
2. Types of bone marrow, Stages of bone marrow, Stem cells, Regulation of hemopoiesis, Hemopoietic growth factor, may come as **Short Questions**.
3. In **Viva**, examiner may ask....types of bone marrow, structure of bone marrow, when hemopoiesis starts in different stages, medullary and extramedullary hemopoiesis, properties of stem cells, HGFs for different types of hemopiesis.

CHAPTER

11

Red Blood Cells

Learning Objectives

On completion of study of this chapter, the student **MUST** be able to:

1. Give the dimensions of red cell and normal red cell count in different age groups in males and females.
2. List the functions of red cells.
3. Give the list of abnormal forms of red cells and the common condition in which these abnormalities are observed.
4. Appreciate the importance of specialties of red cell membrane.
5. Understand the meaning of red cell fragility and give the causes of increased and decreased fragility of red cells.
6. Give the values of hematocrit in males and females and common conditions of variations in hematocrit.
7. Explain the mechanism of erythrocyte sedimentation rate (ESR), list the factors affecting ESR, give the values of ESR in males and females, and list the physiological and pathological variations in ESR.

The student **MAY** also be able to:

1. Understand the importance of special type of metabolism in red cell.
2. Leann the types of abnormal red cells in common conditions.

The red blood cells (or red cells) are named as **erythrocytes** as they appear red (*erythros* means red) in a stained smear of peripheral blood.

1. The red color of erythrocytes is due to the presence of hemoglobin that accounts for approximately 90% of weight of red cells.
2. In a stained smear, the central part of red cells is pale that gives the appearance of a halo and peripheral part is more red, as in these cells the center is thin and periphery is thick.
3. Red cells are the major cellular elements of blood and perform transport of oxygen from lungs to tissues, and carbon dioxide from tissues to the lungs.

STRUCTURE AND FUNCTIONS

Structure

The normal human red cell is a circular, non-nucleated and biconcave disc (Fig. 11.1). The surface area of the red cell is much greater than that of a sphere of the same size. Therefore, exchange of oxygen and carbon dioxide is maximal with the biconcave configuration of red cells.

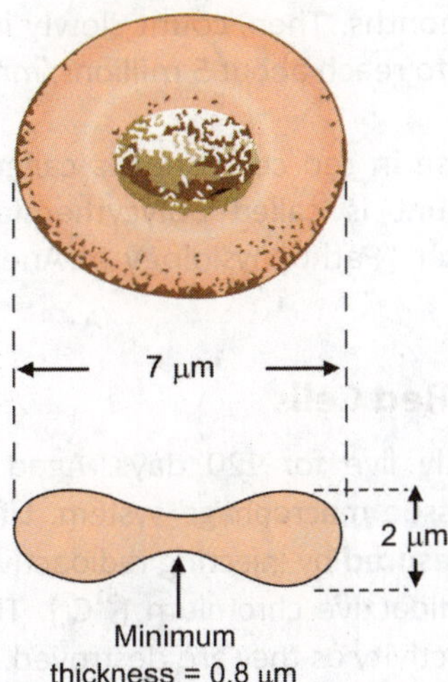

Fig. 11.1: Structure of a red cell. Note the biconcave dimension of red cell. The center is thin (minimum 0.8 µm), and periphery is thick (2 µm).

Red Cell Dimensions

Shape	:	Biconcave
Size	:	7.5 (7 to 8) µm in diameter

Thickness : 2 μm at the periphery and 1 μm at the center
Surface area : 140 μm^2
Volume : 87 μm^3 (78 to 94 μm^3)

The advantages of biconcavity of red cells:

1. When exposed to hypotonic environment, red cells withstand lysis to a greater degree as they swell to a larger extent to attain spherical shape before bursting. Thus, they do not easily lyse when blood becomes hypotonic.
2. It increases the surface area for exchange of gases (oxygen and carbon dioxide).
3. It helps in easy folding of red cells and therefore, facilitates their movement through the narrow capillaries.

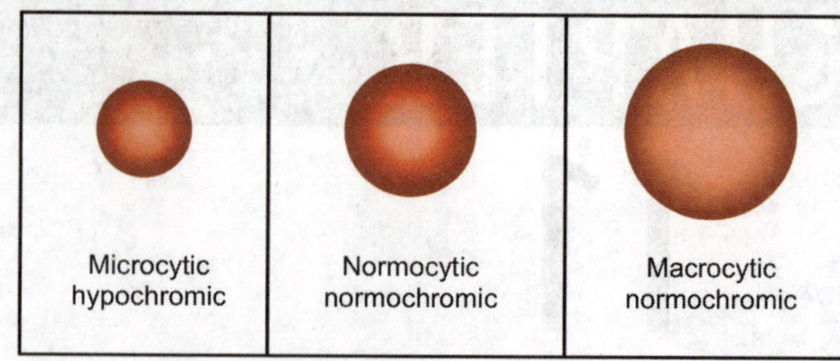

Fig. 11.2: Comparison of microcytic and macrocytic red cells with normocytic cell.
Courtesy: Figure 2.1, Essentials in Hematology and Clinical Pathology by Ramadas Nayak et al., 1st edition, 2012; Jaypee Brothers Medical Publishers (P) Ltd.

Red Cell Composition

Red cells are composed of water 62.5%, hemoglobin 35%, and other substances 2.5% that constitute glucose, lipids (cephalin, cholesterol and lecithin), proteins (glutathiones and albumin like insoluble proteins) and enzymes (glycolytic enzymes, carbonic anhydrase and catalase).

Red Cell Count

In adult males : 4.5–6 (average 5.2) millions per cu mm of blood
In adult females : 4–5.5 (average 4.7) millions per cu mm of blood
In newborns : 6–8 millions per cu mm of blood
In children : 3–5 millions per cu mm of blood

The count is more in infants mainly due to hemoconcentration. The count rapidly decreases to its lowest level at about 2–4 months. Then, count slowly increases from one year of life to reach about 5 millions/mm^3 at about 10 years.

The decrease in red cell count is called anemia and increase in count is called polycythemia (for details, refer the chapter "Pathophysiology of Anemia and Polycythemia").

Life Span of Red Cells

Red cells usually live for 120 days. Aged red cells are destroyed by tissue macrophage system. **Life span of red cells can be measured** by injecting radioactive iron or RBCs tagged with radioactive chromium (^{51}Cr). The tagged red cells lose radioactivity as they are destroyed. Complete disappearance of radioactivity gives the life span of red cells.

Abnormal Red Cells

Based on Size

Normocyte, Microcyte and Macrocyte

1. **Normocyte:** A normal red cell is called a normocyte, the volume of which is about 87 μm^3 (78–94 μm^3). Red cells are non-nucleated biconcave discs. The cell diameter is about 7.5 μm. The normal red cell is also called ***discocyte***, as it is a smooth, biconcave disc (Figs. 11.2 and 11.3A).
2. **Microcyte:** When the volume of red cell is less than 80 μm^3, is called a microcyte (Figs. 11.2 and 11.3B). ***Microcytosis*** occurs in conditions of decreased cell size like *iron deficiency anemia*.
3. **Macrocyte:** When the volume of red cell is more than 94 μm^3, is called a macrocyte (Figs. 11.2 and 11.3C). ***Macrocytosis*** occurs in conditions of increased cell size like *megaloblastic anemia*.

Anisocytes

This means the red cells are of different sizes. **Anisocytosis** is seen in different types of anemias (Fig. 11.3E).

Hypochromic Cells

Hypochromic red cells (hypochromia) are cells with pale appearance. **Hypochromia** occurs either due to decreased hemoglobin concentration as seen in iron deficiency or due to abnormal thinning of red cells. Usually the cells are microcytic.

Based on Shape

Poikilocytes

This means red cells are of different shapes. **Poikilocytosis** is usually seen when older cells are present in circulation (Fig. 11.3D).

Spherocytes

When red cells assume spherical shape, are called spherocytes (Fig. 11.3F). This is seen in conditions like **hereditary spherocytosis**.

Elliptocyte

When red cells assume oval shape with varying degrees of elliptical aberration, are called elliptocytes (Fig. 11.3G). **Elliptocytosis** occurs in hereditary elliptocytosis, thalassemia and iron deficiency anemia.

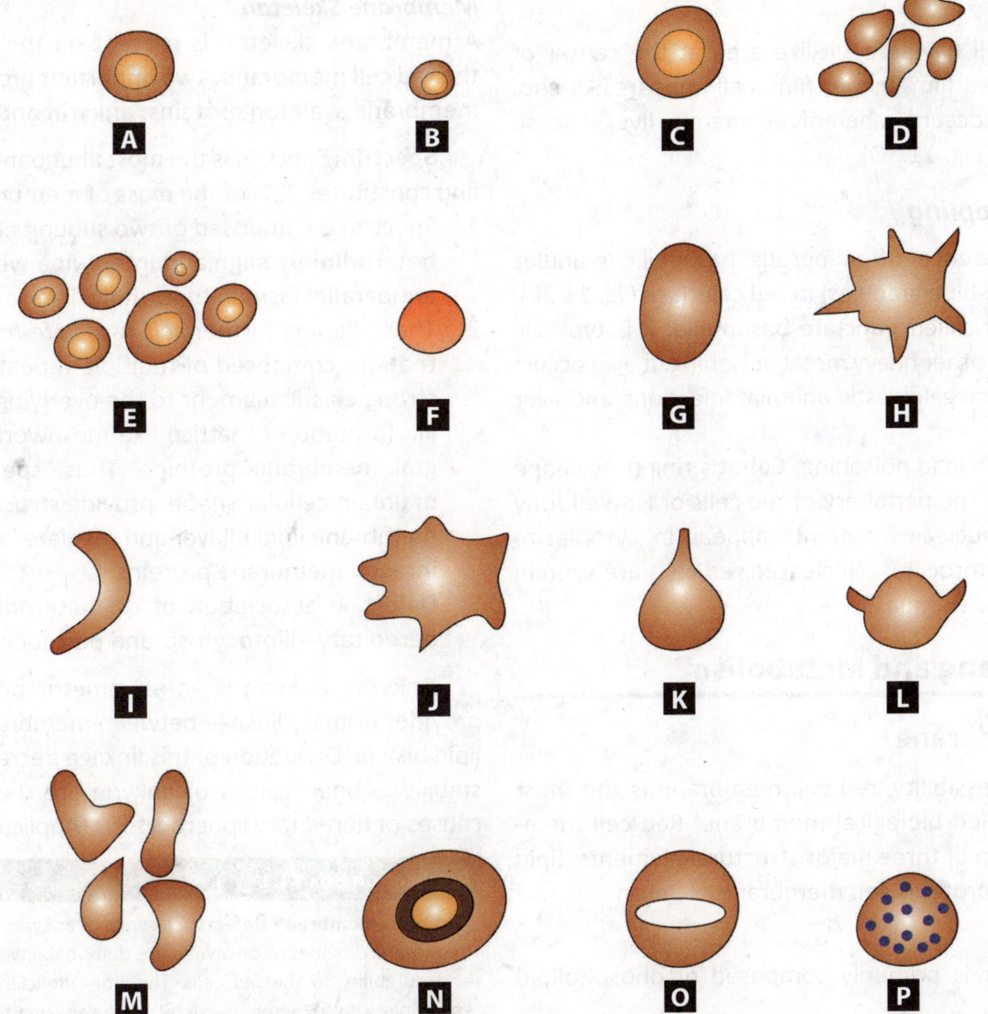

Fig. 11.3: Normal and abnormal red cells. (A) Normal red cell; (B) Microcyte; (C) Macrocyte; (D) Poikilocytes; (E) Anisocytes; (F) Spherocyte; (G) Elliptocyte; (H) Acanthocyte; (I) Drepanocyte (sickle cell); (J) Echinocyte (burr cell or crenated cell); (K) Dacryocyte; (L) Keratocyte; (M) Schistocytes (fragmented red cells); (N) Target cell; (O) Stomatocyte; (P) Basophilic stippling.

Acanthocyte

When a red cell has irregular shape with 2 to 10 hemispherically tipped spicules of variable length and diameter is called acanthocyte. **Acanthocytosis** is seen in abetalipoproteinemia, alcoholic liver disease and malabsorptive states (Fig. 11.3H).

Drepanocyte (Sickle Red Cells)

Drepanocyte is the red cell having *sickle shape* (Fig. 11.3I). **Drepanocytosis** is seen in sickle cell anemia.

Echinocyte (Burr Cells)

A "burr cell" or crenated red cell is an echinocyte (Fig. 11.3J). **Echinocytosis** occurs in uremia and liver disease.

Dacryocyte (Tear Drop)

When the red cell assumes the appearance of a tear drop, is called dacryocyte (Fig. 11.3K). **Dacryocytosis** occurs in myelofibrosis with myeloid metaplasia, thalassemia and myelophthisic anemia.

Keratocytes

Keratocytes are red cells having a pair of spicule. **Keratocytosis** usually occurs by mechanical damage or by removal of a Hinz body by pitting action of the spleen. 'Hamlet cells' and 'bite cells' are also used to describe keratocytes (Fig. 11.3L).

Schistocytes

Schistocytes are fragments of red cells (*see* Fig. 11.3M). They are smaller than red cells and they have sharp angles and spurs. **Schistocytosis** (red cell fragmentation) occurs in thalassemia, mechanical stress (microangiopathic hemolytic anemia, cardiac hemolytic anemia, etc.), and thermal injury (severe burns).

Target Cells

When a red cell has a central deeply stained round area in addition to its normal feature, the cell is called target cell (*see* Fig. 11.3N). Target cells are seen in chronic liver disease, obstructive jaundice, iron deficiency anemia and thalassemia.

Stomatocyte

This is a red cell having a slit-like area at the center of the cell in a dried film. In wet film, cell appears like cup. **Stomatocytosis** occurs in hemolytic anemia, liver disease and alcoholism (Fig. 11.3O).

Basophilic Stippling

This means presence of numerous basophilic granules (coarse and dark-blue granules) in red cells (*see* Fig. 11.3P). This condition is called **punctate basophilia**. It is typically seen in lead and other heavy metal poisoning. It also occurs in thalassemia, megaloblastic anemia, infections and liver disease.

Sometimes in lead poisoning, **Cabot's ring** (ring shape or figure of 8) at the periphery of red cells or **Howell Jolly bodies** (small nuclear fragments appear in cytoplasm) are found in erythrocytes. Nucleated red cells are seen in severe hemolytic anemia.

Cell Membrane and Metabolism

Red Cell Membrane

For its easy accessibility, red cell membrane is the most thoroughly studied biological membrane. Red cell membrane is made up of three major structural elements: lipid bilayer, integral proteins and membrane skeleton.

Lipid Bilayer

The lipid bilayer is primarily composed of phospholipid and cholesterol:

1. The lipid bilayer provides an impermeable barrier between cytoplasm and external environment.
2. It also helps to maintain a slippery exterior, so that the red cells do not stick to the vascular endothelium.

Integral Proteins

Integral proteins are embedded in the lipid bilayer. The important membrane proteins are *band-3 protein* (anion exchanger-1), the *glycophorins*, Rh D protein and various ion channels (Refer to Fig. 4.5; Chapter 4).

1. These proteins allow red cells to participate in wide range of functions including antigenic determination and cellular metabolism.
2. Band-3 is the major **anion-exchanger** (chloride-bicarbonate exchange) and also regulates metabolic pathways by sequestering key enzymes like enzymes of glycolytic pathways.
3. Glycophorins constitute more than 60% of negative surface charge of red cells; they modulate interaction between red cells and interaction of red cells to endothelium.
4. There are five different types of glycophorins: A, B, C, D and E. **Glycophorin-C** provides stability and shape to the red cell membrane, and its deficiency leads to elliptocytosis.

Membrane Skeleton

A membrane skeleton is present on the internal side of the red cell membrane. Two important proteins are part of membrane skeleton proteins: **ankyrin and spectrin.**

Spectrin: Spectrin is the most abundant skeletal protein and constitutes 75% of the mass of membrane skeleton.

1. Spectrin is composed of two subunits: α and β. The $\alpha\beta$ **heterodimers** align and intertwine with each other in antiparallel fashion to form flexible rod like structure.
2. These dimers further *self-associate to form tetramers* that are composed of multiple repeats and provide a strong elastic filament to the overlying cell membrane via formation of lattice-like meshwork linked to integral membrane proteins. Thus, spectrin molecules maintain cellular shape, provide ***structural support*** to membrane lipid bilayer and regulate lateral mobility of integral membrane proteins.
3. Defect in association of $\alpha\beta$ heterodimers results in hereditary elliptocytosis and poikilocytosis.

Ankyrin: Ankyrin is an asymmetric polar protein that provides primary linkage between membrane skeleton and lipid bilayer. Disruption of this linkage decreases membrane stability. Abnormalities of ankyrin are the most common causes of hereditary spherocytosis (Application Box 11.1).

Application Box 11.1

Common membrane defects: Presence of ankyrin and spectrin in the membrane provides biconcave shape, deformability, membrane stability and durability to the red cells. Therefore, deficiency of ankyrin and spectrin results in membrane defects like **spherocytosis, elliptocytosis and poikilocytosis,** etc. These defects also make the cells rigid so that the cells are destroyed prematurely.

Deformability of Red Cells

An important determinant of red cell survival is its deformability. Deformability is ascribable to the intrinsic deformability of the red cell membrane. When red cells become rigid, the viscosity of blood increases and cells are lysed while passing through the splenic pulp. The primary cause of decreased deformability is due to spherocytosis of the cell rather than stiffening of their membrane.

Metabolism of Red Cells

Red cells have no nuclei, mitochondria and ribosomes. Therefore, adequate synthesis of proteins and lipids does not occur in red cells.

1. Glucose is the primary fuel for red cells. Though enzymes for glycolysis are present, enzymes for TCA cycle are absent. ATP is formed by ***Embden-Mayerhoff pathway*** (EM pathway). The ***HMP shunt*** provides NADPH.
2. Glucose entry into the red cells occurs easily by facilitated diffusion, which is **independent of insulin** action. Red cells depend mostly on glucose metabolism for their energy supply.

3. 90% of glucose is oxidized by EM pathway and 10% by HMP shunt.

EM Pathway

Red cells metabolize glucose, usually by anaerobic glycolysis using EM pathway:

1. Two ATP molecules are generated by glycolysis through EM pathway.
2. 2, 3-DPG is produced in red cells. 2, 3-DPG influences oxygen affinity of hemoglobin and therefore, plays an important role in red cell function.
3. Hypoxia inhibits Kreb cycle and therefore, stimulates 2, 3-DPG formation, whereas, acidosis inhibits glycolysis and therefore, decreases 2, 3-DPG formation.

HMP Shunt

The enzyme in the red cell, glucose-6-phosphate dehydrogenase (G-6-PD) is the main enzyme for HMP shunt:

1. HMP shunt generates NADPH, keeps glutathione in reduced state, which is a strong reducing agent and prevents damage to the red cell.
2. Therefore, G-6-PD deficiency interferes with red cell functions (Clinical Box 11.1).

> **Clinical Box 11.1**
>
> **G-6-PD deficiency causes hemolysis:** In the absence of G-6-PD, an *inborn error of metabolism*, red cells are susceptible to the damages due to oxidation. Therefore, hemolytic anemia is common in G-6-PD deficiency. Especially, hemolysis is facilitated on exposure to antimalarial drugs, though these individuals are generally malaria resistant.

Functions of Red Cells

1. The most important function of red cell is to *transport oxygen* from lungs to the tissue. This is due to the presence of hemoglobin in the red cell which has high affinity for oxygen.
2. Hemoglobins also participate in *carbon dioxide transport* from tissues to lungs and maintenance of *acid base balance*.
3. Red cells contribute to *50% of viscosity of blood*.
4. Antigen on red cell membrane helps in *blood group classification*.

APPLIED ASPECTS

Red Cell Fragility

The tendency of the cells to hemolyze is called fragility of the cells. There are 2 types of fragility: mechanical and osmotic.

Mechanical Fragility

Lysis of red cells due to mechanical stress and strain is called ***mechanical fragility***. Red cell diameter is slightly less than the diameter of average capillaries. Therefore, when red cells pass through capillaries and splenic pulp, their membrane undergoes mechanical stress:

1. On average, a red cell passes about three lakh times though capillaries during its life span, which makes the cell more fragile.
2. Also, when red cells become older, the membrane becomes rigid. Increased membrane stiffness and mechanical stress make cell vulnerable to rupture.
3. Red cell membrane defects increase mechanical fragility.

Osmotic Fragility

Lysis of red cells on exposure to different osmotic solutions is called osmotic fragility. Osmotic fragility is defined as the ease with which the red cells are ruptured when they are exposed to hypotonic solutions. It assesses the integrity of red cell membrane. The **osmotic fragility test** helps in the diagnosis of anemia in which the physical properties of the red cells are altered. This test detects whether or not the red cells can easily be hemolyzed. The red cell membrane allows water to pass through while restricting solutes. This is called **osmosis**.

1. In an ***isotonic solution***, the solution of equal concentration as that of red cell content, the red cells remain intact. Such a solution has same tonicity with that of plasma. Examples are 0.9% NaCl, 5% glucose, 10% mannitol and 20% urea.
2. When suspended in **hypertonic solution**, a solution with more tonicity (> 0.9% NaCl), red cells shrink due to loss of water from them by *exosmosis*.
3. Red cells absorb water by *endosmosis*, when kept in **hypotonic solutions**, a solution with less tonicity (< 0.9% NaCl). Endosmosis results in hemolysis due to swelling and rupture of the cells (Clinical Box 11.2).

Interpretation: When the rate of hemolysis of red cells is increased, the osmotic fragility is said to be increased, and when the rate of hemolysis is decreased, the osmotic fragility is said to be decreased.

> **Clinical Box 11.2**
>
> **Shape of red cell determine hemolysis:** Increased osmotic fragility denotes decreased resistance of cells to rupture. As the resistance of the red cell membrane to rupture is related to its geometric configuration, ***red cells that are spherical demonstrate increased hemolysis***, whereas red cells that are ***flat like sickle cells demonstrate decreased hemolysis***.

Normal Value and Variations

Normally, osmotic fragility begins at 0.45 to 0.50 and completes at 0.30 to 0.33.

Conditions of Diminished Fragility

- Iron deficiency anemia
- Thalassemia
- Sickle cell anemia
- Obstructive jaundice
- Post-splenectomy

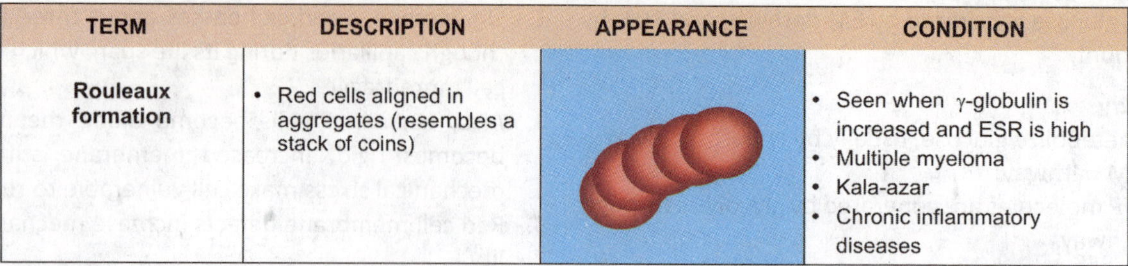

TERM	DESCRIPTION	APPEARANCE	CONDITION
Rouleaux formation	• Red cells aligned in aggregates (resembles a stack of coins)		• Seen when γ-globulin is increased and ESR is high • Multiple myeloma • Kala-azar • Chronic inflammatory diseases

Fig. 11.4: Rouleaux formation.
Courtesy: Figure 42.6, Essentials in Hematology and Clinical Pathology by Ramadas Nayak et al., 1st edition, 2012; Jaypee Brothers Medical Publishers (P) Ltd.

Conditions of Increased Fragility

- Hereditary spherocytosis
- Congenital hemolytic anemia
- Other conditions in which spherocytes are found in the blood.

Packed Cell Volume (Hematocrit)

Hematocrit is the fractional volume of blood that erythrocytes occupy. Hematocrit or packed cell volume (PCV) is the amount of packed red blood cells following centrifugation. When blood is centrifuged in a tube the red cells are packed together at the bottom of the tube by centrifugal force, as cells are heavier than the plasma. The hematocrit is a macroscopic observation by which the percentage volume of the packed red blood cells is measured. Hematocrit is therefore known as PCV.

1. PCV is a **reliable index of the red cell population.** It provides useful information about the red cell mass which is correlated with red cell count and their hemoglobin content.
2. These measurements (PCV, red cell count and Hb content) are essential for determination of **red cell indices** that help in detecting and classifying the various types of anemias.

Normal Value and Variations

Adult male : 46% (40–50%)
Adult female : 42% (37–47%)

Hematocrit decreases in conditions of decreased red cell count and **increases** in conditions of increased red cell count. When cells are deformed as occurs in spherocytosis or sickle cell disease, more plasma is trapped between the packed cells, which gives a ***false high result***.

Erythrocyte Sedimentation Rate

Red cells have the property of rouleaux (piling one on the other) formation (Fig. 11.4). The piled red cells are heavier than the individual red cells. Therefore, when whole blood is allowed to settle, sedimentation of erythrocytes is facilitated due to the presence of rouleaux. The ***rate at which the red cells fall*** (sediment), is known as the erythrocyte sedimentation rate (ESR).

> **Important Note**
> **Difference between ESR and PCV:** In hematocrit, packing of red cells is accomplished by centrifugation, where as in ESR, the columns of red cells settle by gravity.

Factors Affecting ESR

ESR depends on 3 major factors: (1) The shape and number of red cells, (2) Size of rouleaux, and (3) Plasma factors. Other factors also contribute.

Shape and Number of Red Cells

Shape of red cells: The most important factor determining ESR is the shape of red cells:

1. The **biconcave shape favors** rouleaux formation.
2. The alteration of shape of erythrocyte decreases rouleaux formation.
3. Therefore, **ESR is less** in hereditary spherocytosis and sickle cell anemia.

Red cell mass: Red cell mass contributed to blood viscosity.

1. **Increase in cell mass increases viscosity** of blood. Increase in viscosity *decreases ESR*.
2. Thus, **ESR decreases** in polycythemia and **increases** in anemia (except sickle cell anemia).

Size of Rouleaux

ESR depends on the mass of the falling particles, i.e. the size of rouleaux (the red cell aggregates). The larger the size of rouleaux, the faster is the fall. Therefore, the **factors that increase the size of rouleaux facilitate ESR**. Increase in red cell size without change in their shape increases the size of rouleaux.

Plasma Factors

The size and number of rouleaux mainly depends on the **fibrinogen** concentration of plasma. **Globulin** content of plasma also contributes:

1. In normal blood, red cells remain separate as they have negatively charged surface that tend to repel one another. When fibrinogen concentration increases

in plasma, **fibrinogen neutralizes the charges** on red cells, thereby removes the repelling forces. This facilitates rouleaux formation.

2. In some pathological conditions, in addition to fibrinogen, few other plasma factors called as **acute phase-reactants** increase in the blood. These phase reactants also neutralize the charges on the red cell surface and facilitate rouleaux formation. Therefore, ESR increases in **acute infections and noninfective inflammations**.
3. Rise in **C reactive protein** in the plasma in acute rheumatic fever is an example of such acute phase reactants.
4. In **malignancies and collagen diseases**, ESR increases due to rise in plasma level of globulin.

Other Factors

Body **temperature** and **plasma viscosity** affect ESR. Increased temperature increases ESR by decreasing viscosity. When, the medium for sedimentation (the plasma) becomes thicker, rate of sedimentation decreases.

Normal Values and Variations

ESR is usually measured by Wintrobe and Westergren methods. ESR is different in males and females.

In Wintrobe method:

Males : 0–9 mm/hr
Females : 0–20 mm/hr

In Westergren method:

Males : 3–5 mm/hr
Females : 5–12 mm/hr

Physiological Variations

1. Pregnancy: During pregnancy ESR increases due to increase in plasma fibrinogen content
2. During menstrual bleeding, ESR is more
3. ESR is more in parturition
4. Gender: ESR is more in female
5. Age: ESR is high in newborn and infant

Pathological Variations

Increase in ESR

1. Tuberculosis
2. Acute inflammations like cellulitis
3. Chronic inflammations like arthritis
4. Malignancy
5. All types of anemias except membrane abnormalities like hereditary spherocytosis and sickle cell disease
6. Collagen diseases like SLE
7. Chronic infections like chronic tonsillitis

Decrease in ESR

1. Polycythemia
2. Sickle cell anemia
3. Hypofibrinogenemia
4. Hereditary spherocytosis
5. Hyperviscosity syndromes

CHAPTER SUMMARY

Key Concepts

1. Red cells are anuclear biconcave discs. The cells are highly deformable due to presence of ankyrin and spectrin in the membrane skeleton.
2. Deformability of the red cells allows them to pass through capillaries and splenic pulp.
3. Change in shape and rigidity of the membrane make the red cells susceptible to hemolysis.
4. Also, biconcave shape and membrane plasticity help red cells to resist osmotic lysis (less osmotically fragile).
5. PCV (hematocrit) is a reliable index of red cell mass.
6. Negative charges on cell surface inhibit bigger rouleaux formation. In infection, inflammation, malignancy and collagen diseases, the inflammatory or abnormal proteins produced by the disease neutralize the negative charge and facilitate rouleaux formation. This increases ESR in these conditions, which is a marker of intensity of the disease.

Important to Know (Must Read)

1. In examinations, usually **Long Questions** do not come from this chapter.
2. Osmotic fragility, ESR, and hematocrit may be asked as **Short Notes** in exams.
3. Many questions are asked in **Viva** from this chapter. Examiners invariably ask the dimensions of RBC, why is RBC biconcave and what are the benefits of it, normal red cell count, and the conditions of increase and decrease in count, common abnormalities of red cells, basics of red cell metabolism, types of fragility and factors affecting them, importance of PCV, factors increasing and decreasing ESR, common conditions of increase and decrease in ESR.
4. When a student fails to answer the size and shape of normal red cells, basics of red cells, and normal red cell count, it becomes difficult for examiner to give the pass marks.

CHAPTER 12

Erythropoiesis

Learning Objectives

On completion of study of this chapter, the student **MUST** be able to:

1. Define erythropoiesis, give the stages and sites of erythropoiesis, and differentiate extramedullary from medullary erythropoiesis.
2. Describe different steps of erythropoiesis with the help of schematic diagram of cells.
3. Describe the details of regulation of erythropoiesis.
4. Give the source, mechanism of action and functions of erythropoietin, and regulation of erythropoietin secretion.
5. List the differences between red cells and reticulocytes.
6. Give the structure and normal count of reticulocyte and alteration in reticulocyte count in different conditions.
7. Understand the importance of reticulocyte response.

The student **MAY** also be able to:

1. Understand the concept of effective erythropoiesis.
2. Explain reticulocyte index.

The process of production of red cells is called ***erythropoiesis***. Red cells have a finite lifespan of about 120 days. The new cells are formed at a pace that replaces the cells destroyed. Bone marrow precisely replaces the cells lost by senescence, hemorrhage or destruction. **Red cell mass** in a normal man is 26–32 ml/kg and in women 23–29 ml/kg of body weight. The volume of red cells (red cell mass) in the body is maintained and regulated by the bone marrow.

SITES AND STAGES OF ERYTHROPOIESIS

Definition: Erythropoiesis is defined as the process of formation of red cells. This is an important component of hemopoiesis.

Stages of Erythropoiesis

There are **three stages** of erythropoiesis: mesoblastic, hepatic and medullary.

Mesoblastic Stage

During intrauterine life, erythropoiesis first takes place in the **mesoderm of yolk sac** and mesoderm of the body. This is called **mesoblastic stage**. During this stage, erythropoiesis is intravascular.

Hepatic Stage

From the 5th week of gestation, erythropoiesis takes place in the liver and spleen (**hepatic stage**).

Medullary Stage

From the 5th month of intrauterine life, the bone marrow starts forming red cells (**medullary stage**). However, erythropoiesis in bone marrow is very slow in second trimester.

1. **Medullary erythropoiesis** becomes more effective towards the end of third trimester (Refer to Fig. 10.3; Chapter 10). After birth, bone marrow becomes the sole site of erythropoiesis.
2. *Extramedullary erythropoiesis in postnatal life is always considered abnormal.*
3. Till adolescent period, marrow cavities of all bones are involved in erythropoiesis, after which erythropoiesis regresses in the limb bones.
4. After the age of 20–30 years, erythropoiesis is mostly limited to sternum, ribs, vertebrae, skull, pelvic and pectoral girdles (Refer to Fig. 10.2; Chapter 10).

Important Note

Extramedullary erythropoiesis after birth is abnormal: After birth, erythropoiesis occurs only in bone marrow. Extramedullary erythropoiesis in postnatal life is always considered abnormal.

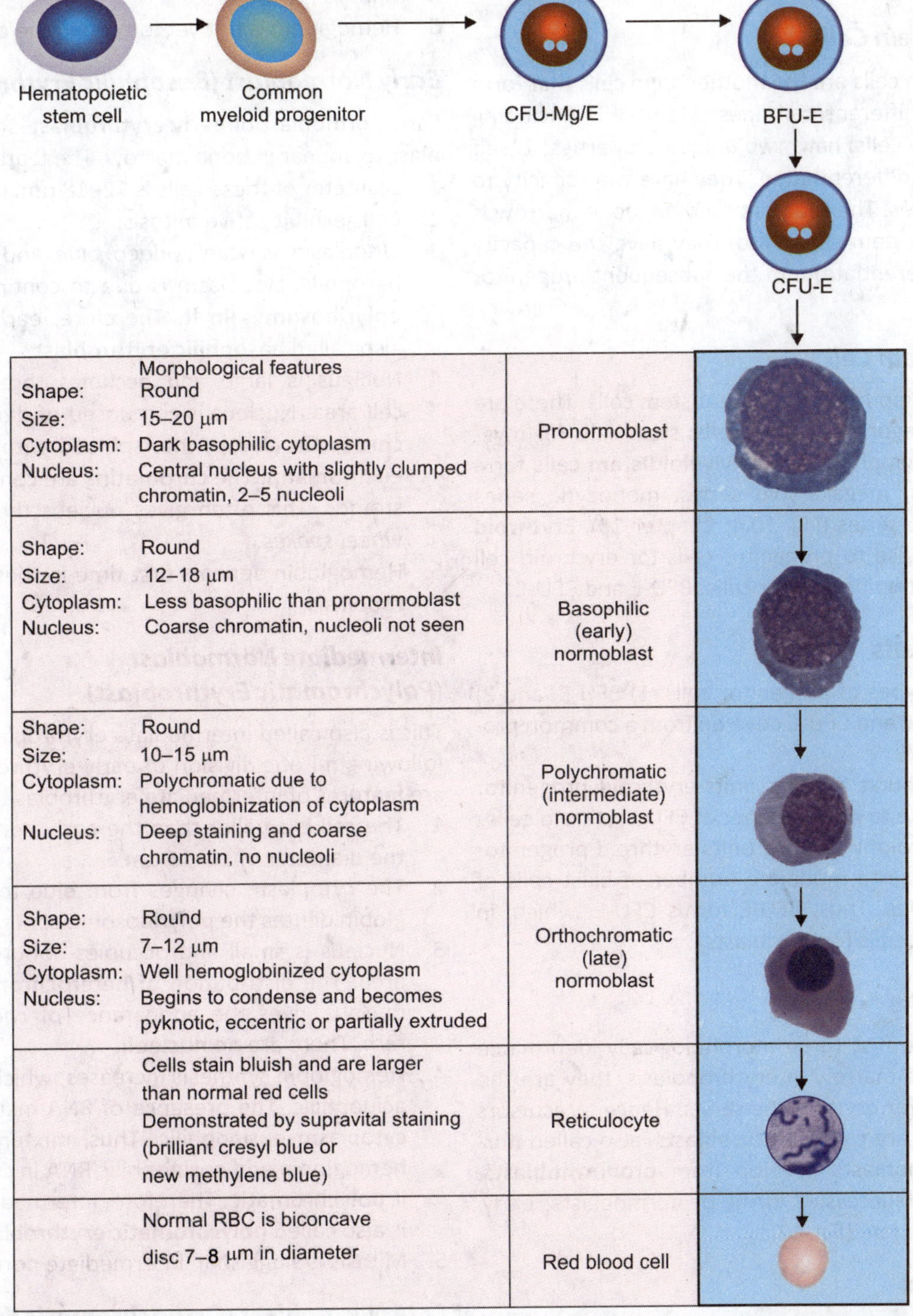

Morphological features		
Shape: Round Size: 15–20 μm Cytoplasm: Dark basophilic cytoplasm Nucleus: Central nucleus with slightly clumped chromatin, 2–5 nucleoli	Pronormoblast	
Shape: Round Size: 12–18 μm Cytoplasm: Less basophilic than pronormoblast Nucleus: Coarse chromatin, nucleoli not seen	Basophilic (early) normoblast	
Shape: Round Size: 10–15 μm Cytoplasm: Polychromatic due to hemoglobinization of cytoplasm Nucleus: Deep staining and coarse chromatin, no nucleoli	Polychromatic (intermediate) normoblast	
Shape: Round Size: 7–12 μm Cytoplasm: Well hemoglobinized cytoplasm Nucleus: Begins to condense and becomes pyknotic, eccentric or partially extruded	Orthochromatic (late) normoblast	
Cells stain bluish and are larger than normal red cells Demonstrated by supravital staining (brilliant cresyl blue or new methylene blue)	Reticulocyte	
Normal RBC is biconcave disc 7–8 μm in diameter	Red blood cell	

Fig. 12.1: Stages of erythropoiesis. (BFU: Burst forming unit; CFU: Colony forming unit; Mg/E: Megakaryoid/Erythroid).
Courtesy: Figure 39.1, Essentials in Hematology and Clinical Pathology by Ramadas Nayak et al., 1st edition, 2012; Jaypee Brothers Medical Publishers (P) Ltd.

Steps of Erythropoiesis

There are **four major cell-stages** or steps of erythropoiesis: ***stem cells, progenitor cells, precursor cells and mature cells***. Each stage has sub-stages. Red cells are formed from pluripotent hemopoietic stem cells, which give rise to committed stem cells. Committed stem cells form subsequent progenitor and precursor cells that finally produce reticulocyte and mature red cells (Fig. 12.1).

In general, during erythropoiesis, following cellular changes take place:

1. Cell size progressively reduces.
2. Size of nucleus and number of nucleoli decrease, chromatin material condenses and finally nucleus disappears.
3. Staining reaction of cytoplasm changes from deep basophilic to polychromatophillic (acidophilic plus basophilic) and finally to acidophilic type. This occurs mainly due to gradual reduction in quantity of RNA material.

Stem Cells

Pluripotent Stem Cells

Pluripotent stem cells are the mother stem cells that form stem cells for different cell lines. Stem cells (including committed stem cells) have two unique properties: 1. self renewal, and 2. differentiation. They have the capacity to renew themselves. Therefore, at no time, bone marrow is depleted of the stem cells. Also, they have the capacity to develop (differentiate) into the subsequent progenitor cells.

Committed Stem Cell

These cells develop from pluripotent stem cells. There are specific two categories of stem cells: stem cells for myeloid series and lymphoid series. **Myeloid stem cells** form erythroid series, megakaryoid series, monocytic series and granulocytic series (Fig. 10.4; Chapter 10). **Erythroid stem cells** give rise to progenitor cells for erythroid cell lines. There are two progenitor cells: BFU-E and CFU-E.

Progenitor Cells

There are two types of progenitor cells: 1) BFU-E, and 2) CFU-E. The BFU-E and CFU-E develop from a common progenitor CFU-Mg/E.

BFUs-E are burst forming units-erythroid progenitor cells that give rise to large number of CFU-erythroid cells.

CFUs-E are colony-forming units-erythroid progenitor cells that give rise to moderate number of blast cells of erythrocytic series. Thus, BFU-E forms CFU-E, which, in turn, forms blast cells (erythroblasts).

Precursor Cells

As blast cells are first to be morphologically identifiable cells in the bone marrow in erythropoiesis, they are the true precursors for erythrocytic series. Hence, precursors for erythrocytes are called **erythroblasts**, also called **normoblasts**. Normoblasts develop from **pronormoblasts**. There are three successive forms of normoblasts: early, intermediate and late (Fig. 12.1).

Pronormoblast

Pronormoblasts (**proerythroblasts**) are the first blast cells to appear in bone marrow and the **first identifiable cells of erythrocyte series**. Following are the characteristics of pronormoblast.

1. This is a large cell, having diameter of about 15–20 µm. Cell is irregularly rounded or slightly oval.
2. The cytoplasm is less in amount, occupies about 20% of the cell. Presence of ***high concentration of polyribosomes*** makes the cytoplasm intensely basophilic. Cytoplasm has *high content of RNA*, which indicates vigorous protein synthesis in the cell.
3. The nucleus is large and occupies 80% of the cell. It contains multiple nucleoli.
4. Mitosis is present.
5. Hemoglobin is not yet formed in the cell.

Early Normoblast (Basophilic Erythroblast)

Early normoblast or **early erythroblast** is the first erythroblast to appear in bone marrow. The features are:

1. Diameter of these cells is 12–18 µm.
2. Cells exhibit active mitosis.
3. Cytoplasm is scanty, deep blue and basophilic. The basophilic cytoplasm is due to continuation of many **polyribosomes** in it. Therefore, early normoblast is also called **basophilic erythroblast**.
4. Nucleus is large and occupies three-fourth of the cell area. Nucleus is composed of dark violet **heterochromatin clumps** interspersed with pink clumps of euchromatin. The **chromatins** are connected by linear strands. This often gives nucleus the *appearance of wheel spokes*.
5. Hemoglobin appears first time in these cells in erythropoiesis.

Intermediate Normoblast (Polychromatic Erythroblast)

This is also called intermediate erythroblast. This appears following mitotic division of early erythroblast. Following are features of intermediate erythroblast.

1. The cell is smaller than the early normoblast, having the diameter of 10–15 µm.
2. The cytoplasm changes from blue to pink as hemoglobin dilutes the polyribosome content.
3. Nucleus is small and occupies about half of the cell area. The distribution of **heterochromatin clumps** in nucleus gives the appearance of *checkerboard pattern*. There are **no nucleoli**.
4. Hemoglobin synthesis increases, which makes the cell acidophilic. The presence of RNA material makes the cytoplasm eosinophilic. Thus, mixture of acidophilic hemoglobin and eosinophilic RNA in cytoplasm makes it **polychromatic**. Therefore, intermediate normoblast is also called **polychromatic erythroblast**.
5. Mitosis is sluggish in intermediate normoblast.

Late Normoblast (Orthochromatic Erythroblast)

This is also called late erythroblast. This is produced by final mitosis in the erythropoietic series.

The features are:

1. This is smallest in the erythroblastic series (7–12 µm in diameter) and mitosis is absent.
2. Cytoplasm is deeply eosinophilic giving the appearance of an orthochromatic cell. Hence, this is also called **orthochromatic erythroblast**.
3. Nucleus is small and pyknotic at the beginning. Sometimes, dark nuclear chromatin materials are arranged in a typical pattern to give the appearance of a *cartwheel*. Finally, the pyknotic nucleus disintegrates.

4. Hemoglobin synthesis increases and almost completes in this stage.

Mature Cells

Reticulocytes

Reticulocytes are the immediate precursors of red cells. Therefore, they are also called **juvenile red cells**.

1. They are mature cells with full complement of hemoglobin.
2. They are slightly larger than red cells.
3. They have a network of reticular nuclear material. The reticular network is nothing but the remnants of disintegrated organelles, and especially of the nuclear fragments. Due to the presence of reticular network, the cells are called reticulocytes.
4. The reticulum is stained by **supravital stains**.
5. Hemoglobin synthesis continues to some extent in some reticulocytes. The reticulocyte count is 0–1 per cent of red cells in adults (details of reticulocyte are given below).

Erythrocytes

Erythrocytes are the final cells in erythropoiesis. They are biconcave discs. They have the diameter of about 7.5 µm (for details of red cells, refer to the previous chapter).

Duration of Erythropoiesis

The total period for erythropoiesis occurs in 7 to 9 days. It takes 5 to 7 days for progenitor cells to become reticulocytes and another 2 days for reticulocytes to become red cells.

REGULATION OF ERYTHROPOIESIS

There are many factors that effectively control erythropoiesis. In physiological conditions, total cell mass is maintained at its optimal size by the suitable adjustments in the rate of erythropoiesis.

Feedback Controls

In animals, spleen is the reservoir of red cells, but not in humans. Therefore, there is no specific origin of signals from a particular reservoir for the production of red cells and consequently, there is *no anatomical tissue feedback* for erythropoiesis. Hence, mechanisms controlling erythropoiesis can broadly be divided into two categories: the functional feedback and the end-product feedback.

Functional Feedback

The functional feedback is the feedback that originates from the tissues signaling the rate of their requirement which is normally served by red cells. Red cells supply oxygen to the tissues, and, therefore, **oxygen requirement of the tissue** is the major functional feedback for red cell production. *Erythropoietin is the chief mediator* of this functional feedback.

End-product Feedback

The end-product feedback is due to the products of red cell destruction. It is believed that the products released from red cell destruction (hemolysis) influence red cell production. This is supported by the observation that hemolytic anemia is associated with more erythroid hyperplasia and reticulocytosis than the hemorrhagic anemia of equal severity. However, the precise mediator of end-product feedback is not clearly identified, though in vitro studies have demonstrated the stimulatory effects of **hemin** on erythropoiesis.

Factors Controlling Erythropoiesis

The factors controlling erythropoiesis can broadly be divided into three categories: hormonal, dietary and others (Table 12.1).

Hormonal Factors

Erythropoietin

History

In 1906, French Professor Dr Paul Carnot and his associates suggested that hypoxia generates humoral factor capable of stimulating red cell production. In 1950, Kurt Ressmann provided strong support for existence of a hormonal mechanism, and few years later, it was named as erythropoietin. In 1957, Jacobson and coworkers found that the erythropoietin is produced by kidney.

Table 12.1: Factors controlling erythropoiesis.
A. Hormonal factors
1. Erythropoietin
2. Androgens
3. Estrogen
4. Thyroxine
5. Anterior pituitary hormones
– Growth hormone
– TSH, ACTH, LH, FSH, Prolactin
6. Corticosteroid
7. Interleukins
B. Dietary factors
1. Vitamins (vitamin B_{12}, folic acid, vitamin C)
2. Proteins
3. Minerals (iron, copper, cobalt and nickel)
C. Other factors
1. Intrinsic factor
2. Chemical factor
3. Environmental factor (hypoxia)
4. Drugs

Source

Erythropoietin is produced mainly by the **interstitial cells in peritubular capillary bed of kidney**. To some extent, it is also produced by juxtaglomerular cells and extraglomerular mesangial cells of kidney. Kidney secretes about 85% of erythropoietin (Application Box 12.1). The rest 15% comes from liver. The nonparenchymal cells (Kupffer cells) of liver and perivenous hepatocytes produce erythropoietin. There are also evidences that erythropoietin is produced in brain, uterus and oviducts.

Application Box 12.1

Renal disease causes anemia: As kidney is the major source of erythropoietin, chronic renal diseases that reduce renal mass significantly produce anemia. Anemia is also produced following nephrectomy. In such conditions, erythropoietin produced by liver fails to meet the normal demand of erythropoiesis as the amount secreted from liver is not adequate.

Structure

Erythropoietin is a *glycoprotein* containing 165 amino acids. There are four oligosaccharide chains attached with polypeptide chain. These oligosaccharide chains are necessary for the physiological activity of erythropoietin. Erythropoietin has molecular weight of 34,000 dalton.

Mechanism of Action

Erythropoietin acts on erythropoietin receptors that belong to ***cytokine receptor superfamily***. The receptor has *tyrosine kinase activity*. Binding of erythropoietin with its receptor initiates activation of a cascade of **serine and threonine kinases** that finally leads to activation of **JAK-2 protein**. Formation of JAK and other signaling proteins brings about changes in cell functions in a similar way to that of growth hormone.

Functions

Erythropoietin stimulates erythropoiesis in several ways:

1. It acts mainly on the **progenitor cells and early precursor cells**. It especially stimulates BFU-E and CFU-E to form pronormoblasts.
2. It decreases cell cycle length of precursor cells, and therefore, enhances mitosis.
3. It facilitates maturation of normoblasts.
4. It increases hemoglobin synthesis in normoblasts.
5. It acts on the stem cells to promote their transformation towards erythroid series.
6. It stimulates early release of immature erythrocytes (reticulocytes) into circulation.

Regulation of Erythropoietin (Ep) Production

Factors regulating Ep production can be divided into factors increasing and factors decreasing the production.

Factors that increase Ep production: Hypoxia, low blood volume, anemia, lung diseases and hormones like epinephrine, norepinephrine, androgen, thyroxine, prolactin, ACTH, etc. facilitate Ep production. Hypoxia stimulates erythropoiesis by increasing erythropoietin production. This is the mechanism of polycythemia that occurs at high altitude.

Factors that decrease Ep production: Estrogen inhibits erythropoiesis. Adenosine antagonist such as theophylline decreases erythropoietin secretion.

Metabolism

Ep is inactivated mainly in liver. The usual half-life of Ep in circulation is about 5 hours. However, if carbohydrate component, especially sialic acid residue of erythropoietin molecule is damaged (even partly), the half-life is shortened to 5 minutes.

Interleukins and GM-CSF

Interleukin 1, 3 and 5 that are produced mostly from T-cells act mainly on the stem cells to convert them to the progenitor cells. **GM-CSF** (granulocyte-macrophage colony-stimulating factor), which is produced from T-cells, endothelial cells, and fibroblasts stimulates production of committed stem cells.

Androgens

Androgens stimulate erythropoiesis. This is the major cause of higher red cell count in males than in females. Red cell count is same in both genders till puberty. Androgen stimulates erythropoietin production. Also, it directly stimulates erythropoiesis.

Estrogens

Estrogen inhibits erythropoiesis by inhibiting erythropoietin production and also by decreasing the response of stem cells to erythropoietin. Estrogen also decreases hepatic synthesis of globulin.

Thyroxine, Cortisol and Growth Hormone

1. Thyroxine stimulates erythropoiesis. Though the exact mechanism of thyroxine increasing red cell count is not known, it stimulates erythropoietin production.
2. Growth hormone increases the mitosis and maturation of erythroid precursors.
3. Cortisol produces mild erythrocytosis.

Dietary Factors

Iron

Iron is the raw material for synthesis of heme component of hemoglobin. Therefore, iron deficiency results in hypochromic microcytic anemia.

Vitamin B_{12} and Folic Acid

These two vitamins are necessary for maturation of red cell precursors as they promote DNA synthesis.

1. For synthesis of DNA, thymine is required and tetrahydrofolate is necessary for thymine synthesis, which is formed from folic acid.
2. Folate, after its absorption from intestine, becomes methyl-tetrahydrofolate in blood, which in the tissue

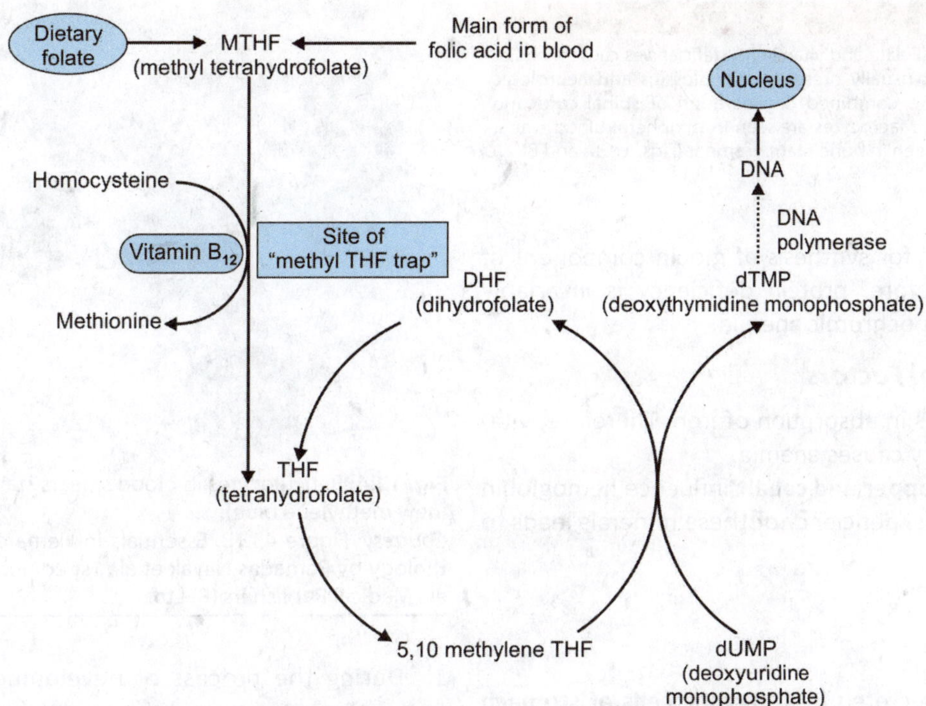

Fig. 12.2: Interaction and role of folic acid and vitamin B_{12} in DNA synthesis.
Courtesy: Figure 4.2, Essentials in Hematology and Clinical Pathology by Ramadas Nayak et al., 1st edition, 2012; Jaypee Brothers Medical Publishers (P) Ltd.

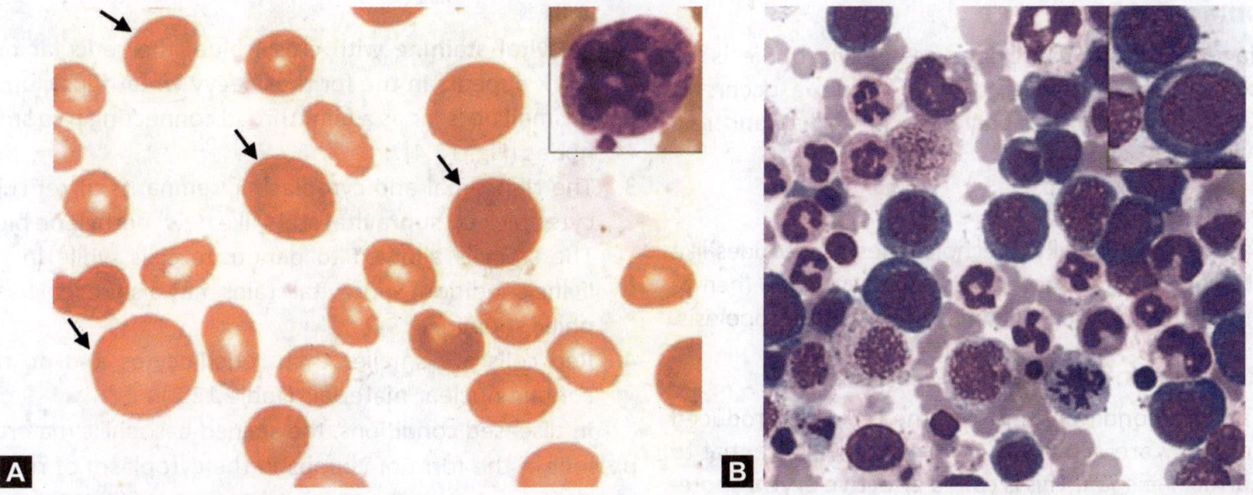

Figs. 12.3A and B: Megaloblastic anemia. (A) Peripheral blood smear demonstrates macrocytosis (larger red cells) and hypersegmented neutrophil (in the inset); (B) Bone marrow aspirate smear shows megaloblasts.
Courtesy: Figures 4.5A and B, Essentials in Hematology and Clinical Pathology by Ramadas Nayak et al., 1st edition, 2012; Jaypee Brothers Medical Publishers (P) Ltd.

becomes ***5,10-methylene tetrahydrofolate***, the active form of **tetrahydrofolate**. This ***promotes formation of deoxythymidylate from deoxyuridylate***, which is required for synthesis of DNA.

3. Therefore, folate deficiency leads to arrest of mitosis and chromosome division in the absence of DNA synthesis.
4. **Vitamin B_{12}** promotes conversion of **methyl-tetrahydrofolate** to its active **tetrahydrofolate** (THF) **form.** Methyl-THF accumulates in the cell, which is known as **methyl-THF trap**. Therefore, vitamin B_{12} deficiency also causes arrest of chromosomal division.
5. In fact, folic acid and vitamin B_{12} interact with each other for synthesis of DNA (Fig. 12.2).

Thus, in deficiencies of these two vitamins, megaloblasts are produced in the bone marrow instead of normoblasts (Fig. 12.3B). Therefore, the resulting anemia is called megaloblastic anemia (Clinical Box 12.1). Megaloblasts produce macrocytes that manifest as **macrocytic anemia** (Fig. 12.3A).

Clinical Box 12.1

***Megaloblastic anemia*:** Folate and vitamin B_{12} deficiencies cause megaloblastic anemia. Patient usually presents with glossitis and neurologic manifestation (subacute combined degeneration of spinal cord and peripheral neuropathy. Macrocytes are seen in peripheral blood smear and megaloblasts are seen in bone marrow smear (Figs. 12.3A and B).

Protein

Protein is essential for synthesis of globin component of hemoglobin. Therefore, protein deficiency is invariably associated with hypochromic anemia.

Other Nutritional Factors

1. **Vitamin C** helps in absorption of iron. Therefore, vitamin C deficiency causes anemia.
2. Minerals like **copper and cobalt** influence hemoglobin formation. Thus, deficiency of these minerals leads to anemia.

Other Factors

Intrinsic factor

Intrinsic factor is secreted from **oxyntic cells of stomach** along with hydrochloric acid. It helps in absorption of vitamin B_{12} **(extrinsic factor of Castle)** from terminal part of ileum. Therefore, intrinsic factor deficiency produces megaloblastic anemia (pernicious anemia).

Environmental Factors

Hypoxia due to any cause increases erythropoiesis by increasing erythropoietin production. Hypoxia occurs at high altitude, and is commonly seen in cardiac and respiratory diseases.

Drugs and Chemicals

Vasoconstrictor agents like catecholamines, nucleotides like cAMP, NAD, NADP, products of red cell destruction (hemolysates), cobalt salts and thyroxine stimulate erythropoiesis.

Effective vs Ineffective Erythropoiesis

Under normal conditions, most of the red cells produced in the marrow are actively alive or have the potential to live a normal life span. This is called **effective erythropoiesis**. However, a fraction of red cell production is ineffective with destruction of nonviable red cells either within the marrow or shortly after they are released into circulation. When percentage of production of these nonviable red cells is increased, the erythropoiesis is called **ineffective erythropoiesis**. Ineffective erythropoiesis is suspected when *reticulocyte count is normal despite erythroid hyperplasia of marrow*.

RETICULOCYTES

Structure

Reticulocytes are **juvenile red cells** in the bone marrow. They develop into mature red cells and few of them pass into circulation along with red cells.

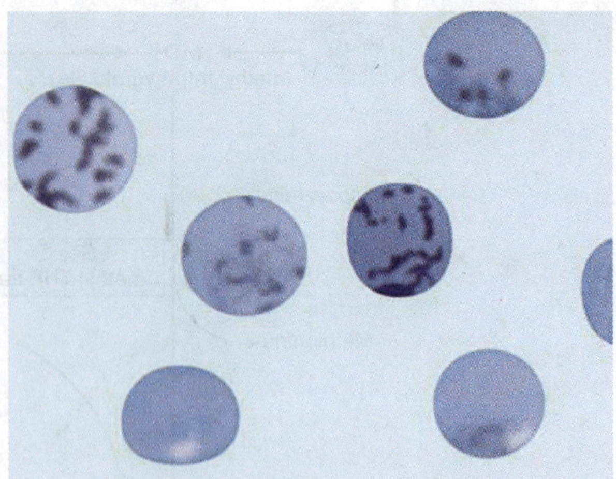

Fig. 12.4: Reticulocytes in blood smears stained by supravital dye (new methylene blue).
Courtesy: Figure 43.1B, Essentials in Hematology and Clinical Pathology by Ramadas Nayak et al., 1st edition, 2012; Jaypee Brothers Medical Publishers (P) Ltd.

1. During the process of development of cells in the erythrocytic series, the nuclei are lost but not the cytoplasmic RNA. Therefore, reticulocytes do not possess nuclei but contain a network of reticulum in the cytoplasm that represents the ***remnants of basophilic cytoplasm*** (the RNA material) of the precursor cells.
2. On **vital staining** with cresyl blue, the reticular network appears in the form of heavy wreath, or clumps of small dots, or as a faint thread connecting two small nodes (Fig. 12.4).
3. The ribosomal and cytoplasmic remnants of reticulocytes pick up **supravital stain** like new methylene blue. The stain is allowed to penetrate cells while in the living condition. Supravital stains may also reveal basophilic stippling.
4. Red cells are smaller than reticulocytes and do not contain nuclear materials (Table 12.2).

In diseased conditions, the stained basophilic materials present in the form of clumps in the cytoplasm of reticulocytes or red cells. They appear as discrete blue particles **(punctate basophilia)** (Refer to Fig. 11.4, Chapter 11). The *basophilic stippling* represents precipitation of RNA materials in the cytoplasm (Clinical Box 12.2).

Clinical Box 12.2

Punctate basophilia: Basophilic stippling is seen in red cells and reticulocytes in toxic conditions, such as heavy metal poisoning, especially in **lead poisoning**.

Development

Reticulocytes are produced in the bone marrow from late normoblast (orthochromatic erythroblast).

1. The nucleus is removed from the late normoblast to become reticulocyte.

Table 12.2: Differences between reticulocytes and red cells.

	Reticulocytes	Red cells
Size	8 μm	7.5 μm
Nuclear material	Present	Absent
Count	Very few (1% of red cells)	Plenty (5 million/mm^3)
MCHC*	Less	More

* MCH is same in both the cells

2. Reticulocytes lose their mitochondria and ribosomes, and basophilic tint to become mature red cells.
3. About 1% of circulating red cells is replaced everyday by newly formed red cells.
4. With the release of young red cells into the circulation, a few reticulocytes are also released. When the bone marrow sends out red cells at an increased rate, more reticulocytes are released. Thus, the ***number of reticulocytes in the peripheral blood is an index of erythropoiesis***, especially in anemia (Clinical Box 12.3).

Clinical Box 12.3

Reticulocytes indicate bone marrow activity: Reticulocytes are the immediate precursors of red cells. Therefore, when the demand for red cells in the body is increased, reticulocyte formation and release are also increased. Thus, reticulocyte count increases along with red cell count. Sometimes, the demand may be so high that nucleated red cells are also released from bone marrow.

Reticulocyte Count

The normal reticulocyte count in adult is 0–1% of the red cells. In newborns, the count is 2–6%. The number falls during the first year of life to less than 1% and then the level is maintained throughout life.

Reticulocyte Response

The reticulocyte count is performed to assess the ***therapeutic response of anemias to treatment*** in which the patient is deficient in one of the substrates essential for the synthesis of red cells. When therapy begins, new red cells are formed and released rapidly into the circulation before cells are fully matured. Therefore, many reticulocytes are also released with the release of young red cells. This results in increase in reticulocyte, which is called ***reticulocyte response***.

1. Reticulocyte response indicates a favorable response to treatment.
2. This is typically observed at the beginning of treatment for *pernicious anemia* and *iron-deficiency anemia*.

When vitamin B_{12} is administered as part of the treatment for pernicious anemia, the number of reticulocytes increases in the blood in the initial phase of treatment, which indicates that the patient is responding well to treatment. Similarly, when iron is given in the treatment of iron-deficiency anemia, reticulocyte number increases (Clinical Box 12.4).

Clinical Box 12.4

Reticulocyte count indicates response to treatment: As reticulocytes in the peripheral blood indicate a good response to therapy, reticulocyte count is carried out to ***assess the response of patient to the treatment*** in pernicious and iron-deficiency anemia.

Alteration in Reticulocyte Count

Reticulocytosis

Increase in reticulocyte count is called reticulocytosis. This is seen in various physiological and pathological conditions.

Physiological: Newborns and infants have higher count than adults. Count is more at high altitude.

Pathological: Hemolytic anemia, acute hemorrhage, during treatment for deficiency anemias (reticulocyte response), and any condition that stimulates bone marrow to produce red cells.

Reticulocytopenia

There is no physiological reticulocytopenia. Reticulocytopenia always indicates diseased state. It is seen in aplastic anemia, myxedema, hypopituitarism and leucoerythroblastic anemia.

Leucoerythroblastic Reaction

The **leucoerythroblastic reaction** is used to describe the presence of immature myeloid cells and nucleated red cells in the peripheral blood, which occurs often as a consequence of disturbance of the bone marrow architecture by abnormal tissues. This is seen in secondary carcinoma of bone, myelofibrosis, postsplenectomy states, thalassemia major and multiple myeloma.

Reticulocyte Count in Ineffective Erythropoiesis

Reticulocyte remains almost normal in ineffective erythropoiesis. In fact, ineffective erythropoiesis is suspected when *reticulocyte count is normal despite erythroid hyperplasia of marrow*.

Reticulocyte Index

Effective erythropoiesis is estimated by reticulocyte count, which is normally expressed as the % of red cells. However, it can also be expressed as the total number of circulating reticulocytes per unit of blood, i.e.:

Absolute reticulocytes = reticulocyte percentage × red cell count

To use reticulocyte % as a measure of the rate of red cell production, the % may be corrected for the hematocrit. This is called reticulocyte index or **corrected reticulocyte count**.

$$\text{Reticulocyte index} = \text{Reticulocyte \%} \times \frac{\text{Actual Hct}}{\text{Normal Hct}}$$

CHAPTER SUMMARY

Key Concepts

1. Erythropoiesis occurs in 3 stages in fetal life: mesoblastic (in yolk sac), hepatic (in liver and spleen) and medullary (in red bone marrow). After birth, erythropoiesis is completely medullary. Extramedullary erythropoiesis after birth is always considered abnormal.
2. In erythropoiesis, hemopoietic stem cells become progenitor cells that, in turn, form precursor cells. Hb appears in early normoblast and completes in late normoblast. Nucleus becomes pyknotic and extruded in late normoblast.
3. Erythropoietin secreted mainly from kidney is the primary regulator of erythropoiesis. Hypoxia, low blood volume, anemia, lung diseases and hormones, like epinephrine, norepinephrine, androgen, thyroxine, prolactin, ACTH, etc. facilitate Ep production, and, therefore, these factors/conditions stimulate erythropoiesis.
4. Reticulocyte has no nucleus, but contains RNA materials that make the reticular appearance in cytoplasm in supravital stain. Reticulocyte count is about 1% in adults.
5. Reticulocyte count increases when vitamin B_{12} is administered as part of the treatment for pernicious anemia. The response is called reticulocyte response. It is also seen when iron therapy is given in iron-deficiency anemia.
6. Reticulocyte count is an index of effective erythropoiesis, especially in anemia.

Important to Know (Must Read)

1. In examinations, 'steps of erythropoiesis and its regulation' usually comes as a **Long Question**. This is a common question, very often asked in final exam. A student must not miss it.
2. Erythropoietin, regulation of erythropoiesis, reticulocyte, and reticulocyte response, are usually asked as **Short Questions** in exams.
3. In **Viva**, examiners usually ask stages of erythropoiesis, medullary and extramedullary erythropoiesis, factors affecting erythropoiesis, regulation of erythropoiesis, source and functions of erythropoietin, role of folic acid and vitamin B12 in erythropoiesis, differences between red cells and reticulocyte, reticulocyte response, and causes of reticulocytosis and reticulocytopenia.

CHAPTER

13

Destruction of Red Blood Cells

Learning Objectives

On completion of study of this chapter, the student **MUST** be able to:

1. Say the lifespan of normal red cell.
2. Give the site and mechanism of red cell destruction.
3. Describe the fate of destroyed red cells.
4. List the common causes of hemolytic jaundice.
5. Explain why hemolytic jaundice is common in newborns.

The student **MAY** also be able to:

1. Give the physiological basis of hemolytic jaundice.

The average lifespan of normal red cell is 120 days. After red cells live their normal life, they become less active and more rigid, and get trapped by cells of reticuloendothelial system, especially by the macrophages in the liver and spleen. These macrophages engulf red cells by phagocytosis and release hemoglobin. Also, the rigid cells get ruptured while passing through narrow capillaries.

MECHANISMS OF DESTRUCTION

There are two mechanisms of red cell destruction: intravascular and extravascular (Fig. 13.1).

Intravascular Destruction

Red cells are destroyed in the circulation, when their cell membrane is breached. Normally, intravascular demise of red cell is less frequent. The causes are:

1. The membrane of older red cells becomes rigid and becomes susceptible to rupture during circulation inside the blood vessel.
2. If there is a defect in the membrane, hemolysis in circulation is facilitated.

   For example, in ***paroxysmal nocturnal hemoglobinuria***, complement complexes create holes in the red cell membrane that promotes intravascular hemolysis.
3. Intravascular destruction is also common in ***cardiac valve hemolysis*** and ***microangiopathic hemolytic anemia***.

Extravascular Destruction

Macrophages differentiate young and senescent red cells. They ingest older red cells.

Two important changes occur in senescent red cells that make them vulnerable to mechanical destruction or phagocytosis by macrophages:

1. Decreased deformability
2. Alteration in surface properties.

Decreased Deformability

Deformability of red cells helps them to easily pass through the narrow capillaries and splenic pulps. The ***biconcave shape*** and to some extent the ***viscosity of hemoglobin solution*** in the cell **facilitate the ability of red cells to deform**. Therefore, decreased deformability due to **change in shape** as occurs in spherocytosis or elliptocytosis, and **increased internal viscosity** as occurs in sickle cell or Hb-C disease, make the red cells vulnerable to lysis while passing through the splenic pulp.

Alteration in Surface Properties

Binding of antibodies or complement components to the surface of red cells, changes the chemical composition of the membrane. Especially, binding of **IgG** or **C_3** causes oxidation of membrane components. This is detected by macrophages that ingest red cells.

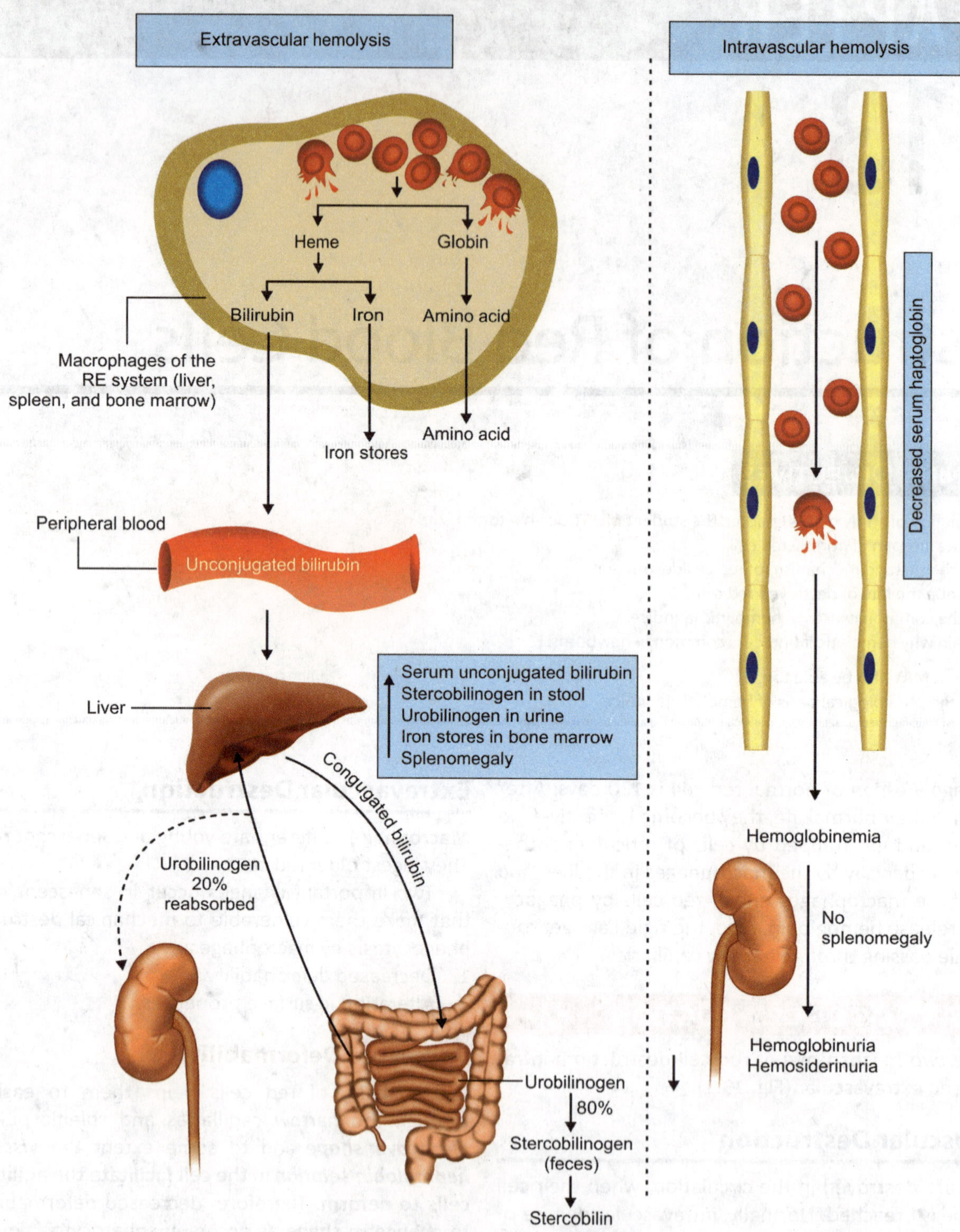

Fig. 13.1: Mechanism and consequences of extravascular and intravascular hemolysis.
Courtesy: Figure 5.2, Essentials in Hematology and Clinical Pathology by Ramadas Nayak et al., 1st edition, 2012; Jaypee Brothers Medical Publishers (P) Ltd.

FATE OF DESTROYED RED CELLS

Destruction of red cells causes release of Hb, which is then converted to heme and globin. Heme is converted to bile pigments. Fate of destroyed red cells depends on whether the cells were destroyed intravascularly or extravascularly.

Fate in Intravascular Destruction

Destruction of red cells in circulation releases Hb into plasma. In plasma, Hb binds with **haptoglobin** (Application Box 13.1). The Hb-haptoglobin complex is transported to liver, where the heme of Hb is converted to iron and **biliverdin** by *heme oxygenase*. CO is released during cleavage of heme by heme oxygenase. Biliverdin is further degraded to **bilirubin** (Fig. 13.1). Heme in the plasma binds with **hemopexin**, a plasma glycoprotein. When the capacity of hemopexin to bind with heme is saturated, heme binds with albumin to form **methemalbumin**.

Application Box 13.1

Plasma haptoglobin indicates hemolysis: In intravascular hemolysis, Hb-haptoglobin complex clears haptoglobin from plasma. Therefore, haptoglobin content of the plasma is decreased in hemolysis and the degree of decrease is apparently proportionate to the rate of hemolysis. Therefore, estimation of plasma haptoglobin level is an index of hemolysis.

Fate in Extravascular Destruction

In the phagocytic cells, red cells are degraded by lysosomes into lipids, protein and heme. Heme is catabolized to bilirubin, and protein and lipids are reprocessed in their catabolic pathways.

1. Bilirubin formed from destruction of red cells regardless of their site of destruction is finally excreted through bile into the GI tract. In the intestine, bilirubin is converted to ***urobilinogen*** by bacterial reduction. Urobilinogen is further converted to stercobilinogen and stercobilin that are excreted in stool (Fig. 13.1).
2. A small fraction of urobilinogen is absorbed from intestine and excreted through urine as urinary urobilinogen.

Important Note

Assessment of hemolysis: Estimation of fecal stercobilinogen and urinary urobilinogen content indicates the intensity of hemolysis as they are good markers of the rate of hemolysis.

HEMOLYTIC JAUNDICE

Hemolytic jaundice occurs from increased destruction of red cells or their precursors in the marrow, causing increased bilirubin production (Table 13.1). Jaundice due to hemolysis is usually mild because the healthy liver can excrete a bilirubin load of six times of its normal concentration. However, this does not happen in newborn. Hence, hemolytic jaundice is common in newborn (Clinical Box 13.1).

1. Heme is converted to **biliverdin** by *heme oxidase*, and biliverdin is converted to **bilirubin** by *biliverdin reductase* (Fig. 13.2).
2. Unconjugated bilirubin bound to albumin enters liver and get conjugated by the action of *glucuronosyltransferase*, to from **bilirubin diglucuronide**.
3. Following enterohepatic circulation, bilirubin is excreted through bile into intestine, where it is converted to **urobilinogen** by bacterial reduction.
4. A fraction of it is absorbed into blood from intestine and excreted in urine. Urobilinogen content of stool and urine indicates rate of hemolysis. As bilirubin is unconjugated, which is mostly bound to protein, there is no excretion of bilirubin in urine. Hence, hemolytic jaundice is called **acholuric jaundice**.

Table 13.1: Causes of hemolytic jaundice.

A. Inherited disorders
1. Spherocytosis, elliptocytosis
2. Glucose 6-PD deficiency
3. Pyruvate kinase deficiency
4. Sickle cell anemia
B. Acquired disorders
1. Microangiopathic hemolytic anemia
2. Paroxysmal nocturnal hemoglobinuria
3. Spur cell anemia
4. Immune hemolysis
– Warm and cold antibodies
– Hemolytic diseases of newborn
– Incompatible blood transfusion
5. Drug-induced (rifampicin, probenecid)
6. Burn

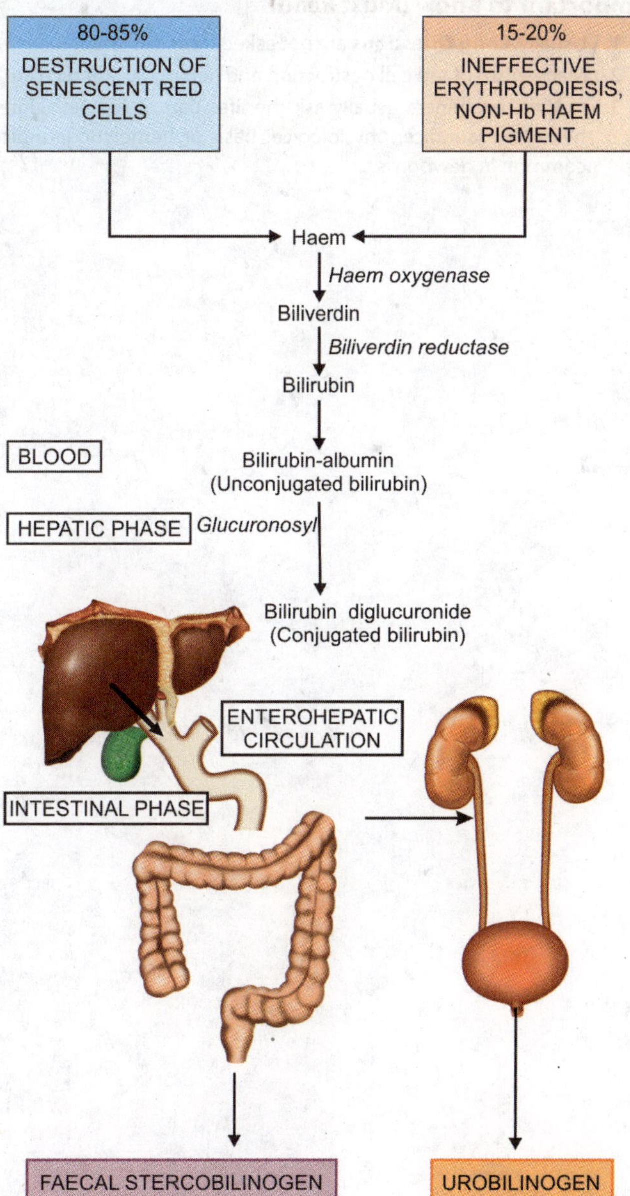

Fig. 13.2: Metabolism of bilirubin (hepatic phase and intestinal phase) and pathophysiology of hemolytic jaundice.

5. Increased fecal stercobilinogen can cause **dark-brown colored stool**.
6. The plasma bilirubin is usually less than 6 mg% and liver function tests are usually normal. For details, refer Chapter 41 "Functions of liver and pathophysiology of jaundice" in GI System.

Clinical Box 13.1

Hemolytic jaundice is common in newborn: Normally, healthy liver can excrete a bilirubin load of six times of its normal concentration. However, in newborn as hepatic enzyme systems are not well developed, the bilirubin metabolism is not effective. Hence, hemolytic jaundice is common in them, especially in premature deliveries.

CHAPTER SUMMARY

Key Concepts

1. Red cells after their life span of 120 days (senescent red cells) are destroyed intravascularly or picked up and phagocytosed by the cells of reticuloendothelial cells (extravascular destruction).
2. Bilirubin released from macrophages enters liver for metabolism, and from there it enters intestine, where it is converted to stercobilinogen and excreted in feces.
3. About 20% of bilirubin enters kidney and excreted as urobilinogen.
4. Levels of stercobilinogen and urobilinogen indicate the rate of hemolysis.
5. Excess of hemolysis causes bilirubin accumulation, leading to hemolytic jaundice.

Important to Know (Must Read)

1. Usually, **Long Questions** are not asked from this chapter.
2. Mechanism of red cell destruction and hemolytic jaundice are usually asked as **Short Questions**.
3. In **Viva**, examiners usually ask the life span of red cells, fate of red cells, mechanism of hemolysis, bilirubin metabolism, causes of hemolytic jaundice, physiological basis of hemolytic jaundice, laboratory tests to detect hemolysis, and why hemolytic jaundice is common in newborns.

CHAPTER 14

Hemoglobin and Blood Indices

Learning Objectives

On completion of study of this chapter, the student **MUST** be able to:

1. Give the structure of Hb and the steps of Hb synthesis.
2. Classify Hb, and give the structure of normal and common abnormal Hb.
3. Give the normal values of Hb in males and females and list the functions of Hb.
4. List the common physiological and pathological alterations in Hb concentration.
5. Name the various Hb complexes and common conditions in which they are formed.
6. Name the various blood indices, give their formulas for calculation, give their normal values and name common conditions of their alterations.

The student **MAY** also be able to:

1. Explain the importance of glycated Hb.
2. Appreciate the use of blood indices in classification of anemia.
3. Describe the fate of Hb.

HEMOGLOBINS

Hemoglobin (Hb) is a conjugated protein present in red blood cells and it constitutes more than 90% of the dry weight of these cells. It transports oxygen from the lungs to the tissues, and carbon dioxide from tissues to the lungs. Hb also serves to destroy the nitric oxide molecule, which is physiologically important.

1. Oxygen affinity of Hb is an important property of Hb.
2. This affinity increases with oxygenation that makes the oxy-Hb dissociation curve sigmoid-shaped.
3. The oxy-Hb releases proton and deoxy-Hb binds proton.
4. The concentration of Hb within red cells of human beings is very high (34 g/dl), which increases its ability to carry adequate oxygen.

Structure and Synthesis of Hb

Hb is synthesized in the precursors of red cells during their development in the bone marrow. It appears in the early normoblast stage and attains maximum concentration in the late normoblast stage.

Structure

Hb is made up of **heme** and **globin.**

Heme

Heme is a complex molecule made up of a series of ***tetrapyrrole rings***, terminating in *protoporphyrin*, with a central iron atom. Following destruction of red cells, the components of hemoglobin undergo metabolic degradation (Flowchart 14.1).

1. The ***iron part of heme is recycled*** and used up again in the hemoglobin synthesis.
2. The only component of Hb that ***cannot be recycled is protoporphyrin***, which forms *bilirubin*.

Globin

This is a protein substance that consists of **two pairs of polypeptide chains**. Each amino acid chain is attached to a heme moiety to form a single hemoglobin molecule. After the degradation of hemoglobin, the globin component breaks down into its amino acid constituents that are recycled for hemoglobin synthesis.

Flowchart 14.1: Fate of hemoglobin.

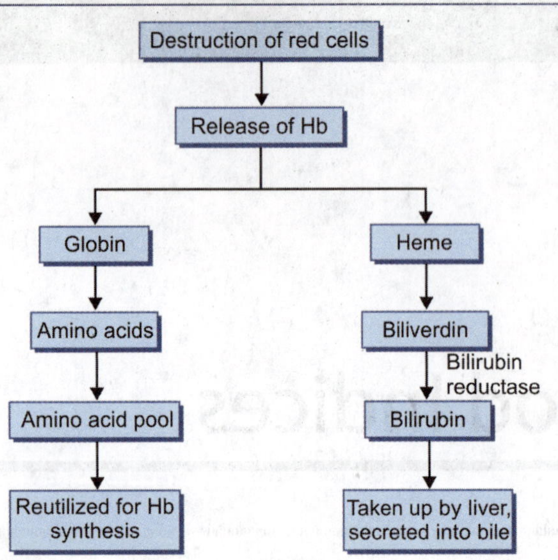

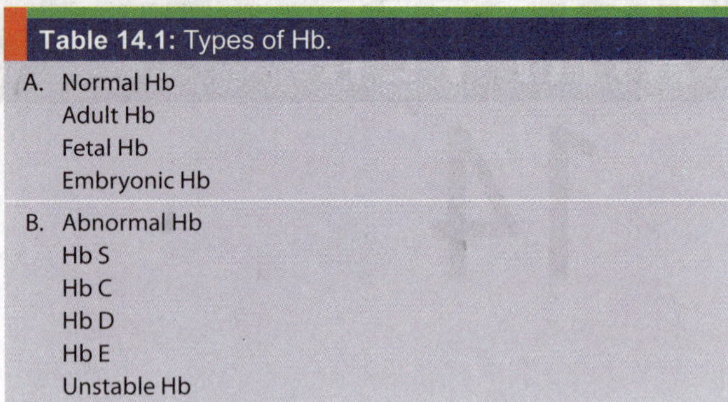

Table 14.1: Types of Hb.

A.	Normal Hb Adult Hb Fetal Hb Embryonic Hb
B.	Abnormal Hb Hb S Hb C Hb D Hb E Unstable Hb

Synthesis of Hb

Formation of Hb requires heme and globin. Heme is formed in mitochondria and globin in ribosomes.

1. **Succinyl-CoA,** an intermediary product of TCA cycle combines with **glycine** to form α-***amino-β-ketoadipic acid*** with the help of pyridoxal phosphate, which in turn forms **α-amino-δ-levulinic acid** (ALA) in the presence of *ALA synthase* (Flowchart 14.2).
2. ALA is converted to porphobilinogen, which forms protoporphyrin-IX.
3. Ferrous iron is introduced into protoporphyrin-IX and in the presence of *heme synthase*, heme is formed.
4. Globin, the protein component formed by ribosome combines with heme to form hemoglobin.

Important Note

Iron and protein are needed: As iron and amino acids are raw materials for synthesis of heme and globin, iron and protein deficiencies lead to hemoglobin deficiency.

Types of Hemoglobin

Hemoglobins can be broadly divided into normal and abnormal types (Table 14.1).

Normal Hemoglobins

Adult Hemoglobins

Adult Hb are of two types: Hb A and Hb A_2.

Hemoglobin A (Hb A)

Hb A is the major Hb and comprises about 97% of hemoglobin of adult red cells. It consists of two α and two β chains with the structural formula $\alpha_2\beta_2$. Hb A is detected in small amount in the fetus as early as the eighth week of intrauterine life. During the first few months of post-natal life, Hb A replaces Hb F and the adult pattern is fully established in 6 months.

Flowchart 14.2: Steps of hemoglobin synthesis.

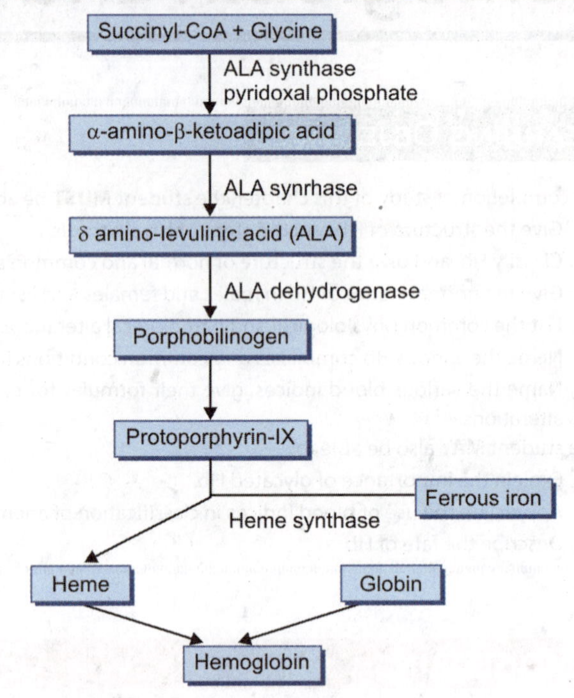

Hemoglobin A_2 (Hb A_2)

This is the minor hemoglobin in the adult red cells. It has the structural formula of $\alpha_2\delta_2$. Hb A_2 is present in very small amounts at birth and reaches the adult level of 3% during the first year of life. Its concentration increases in some anemias.

Fetal Hemoglobin (Hb F)

Hb F is the major hemoglobin in intrauterine life. It has the structural formula of $\alpha_2\gamma_2$. Hb F accounts for 70 to 90% of hemoglobin at term. It then falls rapidly to 25% in one month, and 5% in six months. The adult level of 1% is not reached in some children until puberty. Hb F concentration in adults increases in some types of anemia, hemoglobinopathies, and sometimes in leukemia.

Hemoglobin Bart's (Hb Bart's)

This is the minor hemoglobin present in fetal life. It consists of 4 gamma (γ) chains, γ_4. Hb Bart's concentration increases in fetal life in thalassemia.

Embryonic Hemoglobins

These hemoglobins are confined to the very early stages (embryonic stage) of development. There are 3 embryonic hemoglobins:

1. **Gower Hb 1:** It consists of 2 zeta and 2 epsilon chains ($\zeta_2\varepsilon_2$).
2. **Hb Gower 2:** It consists of 2 alpha and 2 epsilon chains ($\alpha_2\varepsilon_2$)
3. **Hb Portland:** It consists of 2 zeta and 2 gamma chains ($\zeta_2\gamma_2$).

Abnormal Hemoglobins

There are **four clinically important abnormal hemoglobins**: Hb S, Hb C, Hb D, and Hb E. These are present in different hereditary hemoglobinopathies.

1. The most commonly encountered hemoglobin is **Hb S** which consists of $\alpha_2\beta_2$, but in the beta chain, valine is substituted for glutamic acid at the sixth position.
2. Hb S is present in sickle cell anemia.

Unstable hemoglobins: Unstable hemoglobins are hemoglobin variants that undergo denaturation, and precipitate in the red cells as ***Heinz bodies***. Unstable hemoglobins are present in some form of congenital non-spherocytic hemolytic anemia.

Normal Values, Functions and Variations

Normal Values

Adult males: 14 to 18 (16 ± 2) g/dL of blood
Adult females: 12 to 16 (14 ± 2) g/dL of blood

In newborns, hemoglobin concentration is normally 16 to 22 g/dL, which occurs mainly due to hemoconcentration. It decreases to 9 to 14 g/dL at about two to four months of age. By ten years of age, the normal hemoglobin concentration will be 12 to 14 g/dL. There may be a slight decrease in hemoglobin level after 50 years of age.

Functions of Hb

Hemoglobin serves **three important functions**.

1. It transports oxygen from lungs to the tissues by forming oxyhemoglobin and carbon dioxide from tissues to lungs by forming carbaminohemoglobin. When fully saturated, 1g of hemoglobin carries 1.34 ml of oxygen. Thus, **oxygen carrying capacity** of blood can be calculated easily if the value of blood hemoglobin concentration is known. For example, if Hb is 15 g%, 100 ml of blood will carry 15 × 1.34 = 20.7 ml of oxygen.
   - Iron component of Hb is essential for the primary function of the hemoglobin; i.e., the transport of oxygen.
   - When reduced hemoglobin is exposed to oxygen at increased pressure, oxygen is taken up at the iron atom until each molecule of hemoglobin has bound four oxygen molecules, one molecule at each iron atom. This is not a true oxidation-reduction reaction, and therefore, combination of hemoglobin with oxygen is known as ***oxygenation***.
   - The oxygen molecules combine with hemoglobin to form **oxyhemoglobin.**
   - Hemoglobin returning with carbon dioxide from tissues is called **reduced hemoglobin.**
2. Hemoglobin acts as a **buffer** in maintaining blood pH.
3. Hb serves to destroy physiologically important nitric oxide molecule.
4. It imparts red color to the blood. Erythrocytes look red due to the presence of hemoglobin in them, which is a red pigment.

Variations in Hb Concentration

Conditions that Decrease Hb Concentration

Physiological

Children have values lower than that in adults and **women** have values lower than that in males. Hb is less during **pregnancy** due to hemodilution.

Pathological

Hb is less in different types of **anemia** (for details, see next chapter). However, relative decrease in Hb concentration occurs in different pathological **conditions that produce hemodilution** like excess ADH secretion as occurs in pituitary tumors.

Conditions that Increase Hb Concentration

Physiological

Hb level is high at **high altitude** that occurs due to *hypoxia*. Hb is more in **newborns**. In **excessive sweating**, relative increase in Hb occurs due to hemoconcentration.

Pathological

Hb concentration increases in **conditions that produce hemoconcentration** like severe diarrhea, vomiting etc; and **conditions that produce hypoxia** like congenital heart disease, emphysema, etc. It may also be due to **polycythemia vera** (for details, see next chapter).

Hemoglobin Ligands (Complexes)

Besides its binding with oxygen to form **oxyhemoglobin** (and release of oxygen from hemoglobin to form **reduced or deoxygenated Hb**), Hb combines with other chemicals and gases to form **Hb-complexes**, some normally and some abnormally. Some commonly encountered complexes are nitrosohemoglobin, carbaminohemoglobin, carboxyhemoglobin, methemoglobin, sulfhemoglobin, cyanmethemoglobin and glycosylated and glycated hemoglobins.

Nitrosohemoglobin

Nitric oxide (NO) is a physiologic ligand of Hb.

1. NO stimulates a cytosolic heme protein, *guanylate cyclase* to from cyclic GMP that mediates many physiological

activities including vasodilation, inhibition of platelet aggregation and macrophage cytotoxicity.
2. Hb and myoglobin rapidly react with NO and prevent guanylate cyclase activation.
3. Binding of Hb with NO destroys NO and forms nitrosohemoglobin by formation of nitrosyl heme.
4. Especially, ***stroma-free Hb*** inactivates NO. Therefore, stroma-free Hb as occurs in hemoglobinemia causes vasoconstriction.

Carbaminohemoglobin

Carbon dioxide (CO_2) is a physiologic ligand of Hb.
1. Binding of CO_2 with Hb leads to formation of carbaminohemoglobin.
2. CO_2 combines with globin, not with heme.
3. It helps in transport of CO_2 from tissues to lungs.

Carboxyhemoglobin

Carboxyhemoglobin, also called *carbomonoxyhemoglobin* is formed when heme iron of Hb combines with carbon monoxide (CO).
1. Hemoglobin has a much greater affinity for CO than for oxygen. Hb binds with CO about **200 times more** strongly than it binds oxygen.
2. Therefore, it readily combines with CO even when CO is present in low concentration.
3. However, formation of carboxyhemoglobin is **reversible**, which means, once CO is removed from the blood, the hemoglobin combines back with oxygen.
4. Carboxyhemoglobin is found in very low concentrations in normal persons.
5. In **smokers, its concentration is high**, ranging from 1 to 10 g/dL. Therefore, tissue oxygenation is impaired in smokers.

Methemoglobin

Methemoglobin is Hb in which iron has been oxidized from ferrous to ferric state.
1. Methemoglobin is not capable of reversibly binding with oxygen. Therefore, in methemoglobinemia oxygen carrying capacity is grossly reduced.
2. Normally, its concentration is very low.
3. But, its formation increases in the presence of certain chemicals or drugs.
4. However, the formation of methemoglobin can be **reversible**.

Cyanmethemoglobin

Cyanmethemoglobin (**hemiglobincyanide**) is formed by the action of cyanide anion (CN^-), for example potassium cyanide (KCN^-). However, the combination is **reversible**.
1. **Hemiglobin** is the hemoglobin in which the iron has been oxidized by cyanide to the ferric state.
2. **Hemiglobincyanide** is the methemoglobin bound to cyanide ions.

Sulfhemoglobin

Sulfhemoglobin is formed on exposure to some toxic agents, usually sulfur-containing drugs and chemicals.
1. In sulfhemoglobin, the iron is in ferrous state, but oxygen affinity is about **100 times lower** than the normal Hb.
2. Sulfur is not attached with iron, rather is bound to porphyrin ring.
3. Once sulfhemoglobin is formed, it is **irreversible** and ***remains throughout the life of the carrier RBC***.

Glycosylated or Glycated Hemoglobin

In our body, glucose gets attached to protein by enzymatic and nonenzymatic processes and hemoglobin being the major protein in circulation undergoes the same too. The resulting structure is called glycosylated hemoglobin. This is a natural physiological process of body.
1. The fraction of HbA, known as **HbA1c** is of actual clinical interest.
2. In HbA1c, glucose is attached to terminal valine in β chain.
3. In normal individuals, glycosylated Hb (HbA1c) is present in very less concentration, less than 4% of total Hb. The normal HbA1c is 4 to 5.6%, and 5.7 to 6.4% is prediabetes.
4. As per WHO criteria, if HbA1c is 6.5% or more, it is considered abnormal (Clinical Box 14.1).
5. Its concentration increases in conditions in which blood glucose is chronically elevated like diabetes mellitus, Cushing's syndrome, hyperthyroidism, etc.
6. As per ADA (American Diabetic Association) criteria:

Clinical Box 14.1

Glycated Hb (HbA1c) indicates persistent hyperglycemia: When blood glucose is chronically elevated for more than three months, glycated Hb is formed. Therefore, instead of fasting blood glucose, emphasis is given on estimation of glycated Hb. Thus, glycosylated Hb is ***an index of chronic hyperglycemia*** in diabetic subjects.

In Oxidative Stress

Currently, the term **glycosylation** is not used. The process is called **glycation of proteins**. The resulting hemoglobin is called **glycated hemoglobin**.
1. This nomenclature has been used recently to differentiate the nonenzymatic glycation from enzymatic glycosylation of proteins that occurs normally in the ribosome-Golgi complex.
2. Glycation requires two factors, increased level of sugars and increased level of free radicals that promote this type of addition in order to gain neutrality.
3. Hence, glycated hemoglobin has recently been considered to reflect the **degree of oxidative stress** (Clinical Box 14.2).

Clinical Box 14.2

Importance of Glycated Hb: As noted above, glycated Hb is measured to detect the degree of hyperglycemia that is harmful to the body and it is also a measure of degree of oxidative stress. Oxidative stress is a potent inducer of aging.

Applied Physiology

Hb Destruction

Hb destruction occurs with destruction of red cells. When red blood cells are destroyed in the tissue macrophage system, or in the circulation, hemoglobin is degraded into heme and globin. Globin returns to the body's metabolic pool where its amino acids are subsequently reutilized (Flowchart 14.1). The porphyrin ring of heme is cleaved by the microsomal enzyme, heme oxidase, yielding ***biliverdin***. The biliverdin is further reduced to form **bilirubin** by biliverdin reductase (Refer to Fig. 13.2, Chapter 13). Therefore, excess hemolysis leads to jaundice (**hemolytic jaundice**) and hemoglobinuria (Application Box 14.1).

Application Box 14.1

Tissue Hypoxia and ARF: The primary function of hemoglobin is to carry oxygen from lungs to the tissues. Therefore, hemoglobin deficiency causes tissue hypoxia. The major effects of anemia are due to tissue hypoxia. In hemolysis, hemoglobin is released into blood (hemoglobinemia) and is filtered in the renal tubules to appear in the urine **(hemoglobinuria)**. In the tubules, hemoglobin forms casts that block the renal tubules and cause *acute tubular necrosis* (acute renal failure). Hemoglobinemia also exerts osmotic effect and increases blood viscosity that affects cardiac output and alters dynamics of blood flow.

Hemoglobin Estimation

Hemoglobin estimation is the most frequently ordered laboratory test in clinical practice. It is performed as routine investigation in outpatient departments and also as a bedside test in hospital patients. It is mandatory to assess the hemoglobin status of a patient prior to any surgical intervention. As it is more convenient, estimation of hemoglobin is preferred to the total RBC count to detect anemia. **Anemia** is said to be present when the hemoglobin level in blood is below the lower limit of the normal range for the age and gender of the individual (for details of anemia, refer to the next chapter).

BLOOD INDICES

The values of hemoglobin, PCV and total RBC count are used to calculate red cell volume and red cell hemoglobin content and concentration. These are called **red blood cell indices.** The commonly estimated blood indices are:

1. Mean cell volume (MCV)
2. Mean cell hemoglobin (MCH)
3. Mean cell hemoglobin concentration (MCHC)

The MCV defines the volume or size of the average RBC, the MCH defines the weight of hemoglobin in the average RBC, and the MCHC defines the hemoglobin concentration or color of the average RBC.

Other direct quantitative measurements of red cell indices are the **mean corpuscular diameter** (MCD) and **red cell distribution width** (RCDW). Determination of these indices is of considerable clinical importance and is widely used in the classification of anemia.

Mean Corpuscular Volume

Mean corpuscular volume (MCV) is the average volume of an RBC expressed in femtoliters (1 fL = 10^{-15} L). If the PCV and the number of red cells per liter are known, MCV is calculated by dividing the volume of red cells per liter by the number of red cells per liter.

$$\text{MCV (fL)} = \frac{\text{Hematocrit (\%)} \times 10}{\text{RBC count in millions/mm}^3}$$

Where the factor 10 is introduced to convert the hematocrit reading (in %) from volume of packed red cells per 100 ml to volume per liter. For example, if the hematocrit reading is 40%, and the red cell count is 5 millions, then MCV is calculated as:

$$\text{MCV} = \frac{40 \times 10}{5} = 80 \text{ fL.}$$

Normal value: The MCV in normal adults is between 78 and 96 fL.

Applied aspect: The MCV is the **index of the size of red cells**. It depicts whether the red cells are microcytic, normocytic or macrocytic. If the MCV is less than 78 fL, the red cells are considered ***microcytic*** and if greater than 96 fL, they are considered ***macrocytic***.

Mean Corpuscular Hemoglobin

The mean corpuscular hemoglobin (MCH) is the average weight of hemoglobin content in an RBC expressed in picograms (1 pg = 10^{-12} g). It is calculated by dividing the hemoglobin content of 1 liter of blood (in g/L) by the number of RBCs in 1 liter.

$$\text{MCH (pg)} = \frac{\text{Hb (g/dL)} \times 10}{\text{RBC count in millions/mm}^3}$$

For example, if the hemoglobin content is 14 g/dL, and the RBC count is 5 millions:

$$\text{MCH} = \frac{14 \times 10}{5} = 28 \text{ pg.}$$

Normal value: The normal range for MCH is 27 to 33 pg. It may be as high as 50 pg in macrocytic anemia, or as low as 20 pg or less in hypochromic microcytic anemia.

Mean Corpuscular Hemoglobin Concentration (MCHC)

The mean corpuscular hemoglobin concentration (MCHC) is the average hemoglobin concentration per unit volume of packed red cells. It is expressed as g/dL, or percent.

$$\text{MCHC (\%)} = \frac{\text{Hb (g/100 ml)}}{\text{PVC/100 ml}} \times 100$$

For example, if the hemoglobin concentration is 15 g/dL and hematocrit is 45%:

$$\text{MCHC} = \frac{15}{45} \times 100 = 33.3\%.$$

Normal value: The normal range of MCHC is between 33 and 37 g/dL (or %).

Applied aspect: MCHC above 40% indicates malfunctioning of the instrument or error in the calculation of the manual measurements used, as an MCHC of 37% is near the upper limits for hemoglobin solubility, thus limiting the physiologic upper limit of the MCHC. In hypochromic anemias, the hemoglobin concentration is reduced and values as low as 20% to 25% are not uncommon.

Color Index (CI)

This is the ratio of hemoglobin percent and RBC percent.

$$CI = \frac{\text{Hb percent}}{\text{RBC percent}}$$

100% of Hb = 14.8 g/100 ml.

100% of RBC = 5 millions/mm^3.

Normal value: The normal range of CI is between 0.85 and 1.10.

CI less than 0.85 indicates hypochromic anemia.

CHAPTER SUMMARY

Key Concepts

1. The normal hemoglobins are HbA and HbA$_2$. Hb A constitutes 97% of total Hb, it has the structure of two α and two β chains with the structural formula $\alpha_2\beta_2$.
2. Main function of Hb is the transport of oxygen from lungs to tissues and CO_2 from tissues to lungs.
3. Hb in males is 14 to 18 g%, and in females is 12 to 16 g%.
4. Persistent elevation in blood glucose manifests in increased HBA1c. If HBA1c is more than 6.5%, it is considered abnormal.
5. Blood indices (MCV, MCH and MCHC) are useful in classification of anemia.

Important to Know (Must Read)

1. In examinations, usually **Long Questions** are not asked from this chapter.
2. Structure of Hb, functions of Hb, abnormal Hb, all types of hemoglobin complexes, and all blood indices are usually asked as **Short Questions** in exams.
3. In **Viva**, examiners usually ask types of Hb, structure of Hb, normal values of Hb in males and females, conditions of increased and decreased Hb, broad steps of Hb synthesis, major steps of Hb degradation, Hb complexes and their clinical significance, importance of HbA1c, normal values and significance of all blood indices. These questions are very common in oral exam and students are expected to answer these questions related to Hb.

CHAPTER

15

Pathophysiology of Anemia and Polycythemia

LEARNING OBJECTIVES

On completion of study of this chapter, the student **MUST** be able to:

1. Define anemia and polycythemia.
2. Classify anemia, and give the common causes of each category of anemia.
3. Give the salient blood picture of common types of anemia.
4. List the types and causes of polycythemia.

The student **MAY** also be able to:

1. Explain the causes and salient blood picture of iron-deficiency anemia, spherocytosis, sickle-cell anemia and thalassemia.
2. Briefly describe the blood picture and bone marrow picture of polycythemia vera.

Alterations in red cell count are grouped into two major types, anemia (erythrocytopenia) and polycythemia (erythrocytosis). Anemia is the decreased red cell mass and polycythemia is the increased red cell mass.

1. As anemia decreases oxygen-carrying capacity of blood, it is usually expressed in terms of hemoglobin concentration of blood, and the clinical features of anemia are primarily due to tissue hypoxia and hypoxia-induced compensatory mechanisms.
2. Polycythemia is better expressed in terms of hematocrit percentage because the clinical features of it are primarily due to the size of red cell mass and the degree of viscosity.
3. Though, defining strictly, polycythemia is the increase in all formed elements of blood, it usually refers to increased red cell mass as red cells are the major constituents of blood.

ANEMIA

Anemia is defined as decreased red cell count or hemoglobin content of blood.

1. Detection of anemia is usually performed by estimating hemoglobin content of blood.
2. It can also be done by performing either total RBC count of blood or by estimating packed cell volume (hematocrit).
3. Clinically, anemia is detected by assessing the degree of paleness usually by looking at the lower palpebral conjunctiva or nail beds.
4. Detection of morphological type of anemia depends on various blood indices (as described in the previous chapter).

Classification

Anemias can be classified either morphologically or etiologically. **Common causes** of anemia are:

1. Inadequate supply of nutrients resulting in deficiency anemias (deficiency of iron, vitamins and proteins)
2. Aplasia of bone marrow
3. Anemia associated with chronic diseases
4. Anemia associated with renal failure
5. Anemia due to inherited diseases (e.g. thalassemia)
6. Anemia due to blood loss

However, they are best **classified etiologically** into ***two broad groups*** as decreased red cell production and increased red cell destruction (Table 15.1).

Morphological Classification

Morphologically, anemia are classified into hypochromic microcytic, normochromic, microcytic and macrocytic normochromic types (Refer to Fig. 11.3, Chapter 11).

Hypochromic Microcytic Anemia

MCV, MCH, and MCHC are below normal. Such subnormal red cell indices correspond to **microcytosis** and **hypochromia** of red cells in the blood film (Figs. 15.1A and B). Micronormoblasts are seen in bone marrow examination. This occurs due to the result of a defect in red cell formation in which hemoglobin synthesis is impaired to a great extent.

The common examples are:

i. ***Iron-deficiency anemia*** in which there is inadequate iron for the formation of the heme component of the hemoglobin, and
ii. ***Thalassemia*** in which the formation of the globin component of hemoglobin is defective.

Table 15.1: Classification of anemia.

A. Decreased red cell production
1. Stem cell failure - Aplastic anemia - Anemia of leukemia
2. Progenitor cell failure - Pure red cell aplasia - Chronic renal failure - Chronic diseases
3. Precursor cell failure - Megaloblastic anemia - Iron-deficiency anemia - Thalassemia - Hemoglobinopathies
B. Increased red cell destruction or loss
1. Acquired causes - Acute blood loss - Hypersplenism - Micro- and macroangiopathic - Antibody-mediated
2. Hereditary causes - Membrane defects - Enzyme defects - Globin defects

Normochromic Normocytic Anemia

MCV, MCH, and MCHC are within the normal range. Size and hemoglobin concentration of the red cells are normal in the blood film. It usually occurs in following conditions:

i. Substantial blood loss(*blood loss anemia*),
ii. Hemolysis (*hemolytic anemia*) and
iii. Impairment of red cell production by bone marrow failure or chronic renal failure (*aplastic anemia*).

Macrocytic Normochromic Anemia

The MCV is above the upper limit of the normal. It corresponds to **macrocytosis** of red cells in the blood film. The red cells are usually normochromic, though they are macrocytic. Megaloblasts are seen in bone marrow examination (Fig. 15.2). Howell Jolly body, hypersegmentation of neutrophils, basophilic stippling are also seen (Refer to Fig. 12.3, Chapter 12). The typical example of this type of anemia is ***megaloblastic anemia*** that occurs due to deficiency of vitamin B_{12} or folic acid.

Etiological Classification

Blood Loss Anemia

Anemia due to blood loss mainly occurs due to acute hemorrhage or chronic hemorrhage.

Acute hemorrhage: Anemia due to acute hemorrhage depends on the extent of blood loss and the time that has lapsed since bleeding.

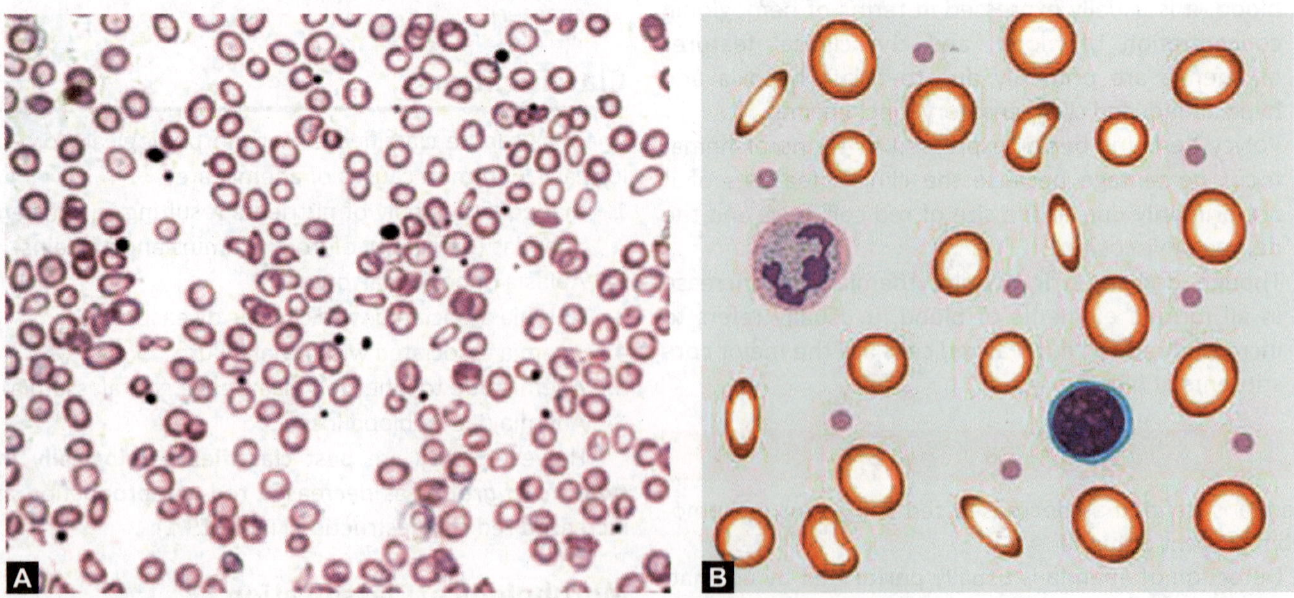

Figs. 15.1A and B: Microcytic hypochromic anemia. (A) Peripheral blood smear (note microcytosis); (B) Schematic picture of the smear (note presence of microcytes with hypochromia).
Courtesy: Figures 3.3A and B, Essentials in Hematology and Clinical Pathology by Ramadas Nayak et al., 1st edition, 2012; Jaypee Brothers Medical Publishers (P) Ltd.

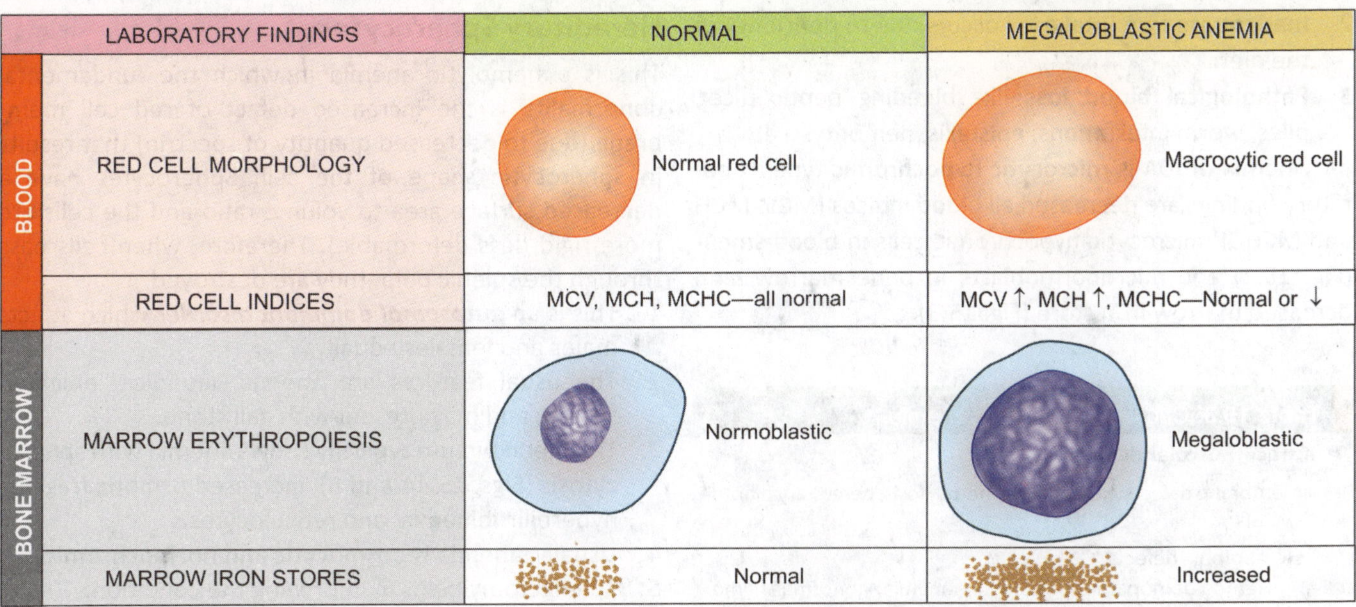

Fig. 15.2: General laboratory findings in macrocytic anemia, compared with the normal report.

Table 15.2: Causes of aplastic anemia.

1. Acquired conditions:
   i. Chemicals: Benzene, DDT and pentachlorophenol
   ii. Drugs:
      - anticancer drugs (cyclophosphamide, busulphan, methotrexate, 5-fluorouracil, daunorubicin)
      - antibiotics (chloramphenicol)
      - diuretics (acetazolamide)
      - anti-inflammatory (phenylbutazone)
      - anticonvulsant (carbamazepine, hydantoin)
   iii. Radiation of bone marrow
   iv. Viral infections: Epstein-Barr virus, hepatitis (non-A, non-B)
2. Hereditary conditions:
   i. Fanconi anemia
   ii. Shwachman syndrome
3. **Idiopathic** (commonest, 65% of all causes)

1. In acute blood loss, usually there is a reduction in the total blood volume. Therefore, hemoglobin in the residual blood is normal.
2. However, when the compensatory mechanisms set in to expand the blood volume, hemodilution decreases hemoglobin content.
3. Therefore, estimation of hemoglobin after few hours of acute blood loss does not assess the actual degree of anemia.

Chronic hemorrhage: Chronic hemorrhage occurs mainly in gastrointestinal, genitourinary and respiratory tract diseases.

1. **Gastrointestinal blood loss:** Peptic ulcer, hemorrhoids, hiatus hernia, carcinoma of the stomach and colon, esophageal varices, chronic aspirin ingestion, ulcerative colitis, hookworm infestation, etc.
2. **Respiratory diseases:** Respiratory diseases that produce epistaxis, hemoptysis as occurs in pulmonary tuberculosis or bronchogenic carcinoma produce anemia.
3. **Genitourinary diseases:** Diseases that cause hematuria and hemoglobinuria produce anemia.
4. **Diseases of genital tract:** In females, loss of blood from genital tract like menstrual disorders (menorrhagia, metrorrhagia) and uterine pathologies produce anemia.

Aplastic Anemia

Aplastic anemia is the anemia due to impaired red cell production. Marrow examination shows a near absence of hematopoietic precursor cells. The common causes of aplastic anemia are listed in Table 15.2.

Hemolytic Anemia

Hemolytic anemia results from increase in the rate of red cell destruction. Defects causing premature red cell destruction may be divided into two broad categories: intracorpuscular, and extracorpuscular (Table 15.3).

Common Anemias

Iron-deficiency Anemia (IDA)

This is the commonest form of anemia in the developing countries. It usually occurs due to deficiency of iron in the diet. There are three major factors in the pathogenesis of IDA.

1. **Increased physiological demand** for iron as occurs in pregnancy, lactation, growing children. Therefore, in these groups, extra iron should be available in the diet; otherwise IDA occurs.

2. **Inadequate iron intake**, as occurs due to deficiency in the diet.
3. **Pathological blood loss** like bleeding peptic ulcer, piles, worm infestations, epistaxis, hemoptysis etc.

Anemia of IDA is **microcytic hypochromic** type. Laboratory findings are decreased all blood indices (MCV, MCH and MCHC), microcytic hypochromic cells in blood smear (Fig. 15.1) and micronormoblasts in bone marrow, and dcreased marrow iron store (Fig. 15.3).

Table 15.3: Causes of hemolytic anemia.

A. Intracorpuscular defects
1. Membrane defects: hereditary spherocytosis, hereditary elliptocytosis
2. Hemoglobin defects: i. Hemoglobinopathies: Sickle cell anemia, abnormal hemoglobins like, Hb-C, Hb-E, Hb-D, etc., unstable hemoglobin disease. ii. Thalassemia: Thalassemia major and minor
3. Enzyme defects: Deficiency of pyruvate kinase and glucose-6 phosphate dehydrogenase.
B. Extracorpuscular defects
1. Acquired: i. Immune mechanisms: Warm and cold antibodies, hemolytic diseases of newborn, incompatible blood transfusion, drug induced anemia. ii. Non-immune mechanisms: Cardiac hemolytic anemia, March-hemoglobinuria iii. Drug-induced iv. Infections v. Burn etc.
2. Hereditary

Hereditary Spherocytosis

This is a hemolytic anemia in which the fundamental abnormality is the increased defect of red cell membrane (due to decreased quantity of spectrin) that results in spherocytic shape of the cell. Spherocytes have a decreased surface area to volume ratio and the cells are more rigid (less deformable). Therefore, when cells pass through the splenic pulp, they are destroyed.

1. This is an ***autosomal dominant disorder*** which affects males and females equally.
2. The usual features are anemia, jaundice, enlarged spleen, and may present with gall stone.
3. The blood picture typically shows anemia with spherocytosis (Figs. 15.4A and B), increased osmotic fragility, hyperbilirubinemia, and reticulocytosis.
4. Usually, anemia is **normocytic and normochromic**.
5. Splenectomy helps in improving the condition.

Sickle-cell Anemia

This is a hereditary disorder in which red cells contain an abnormal hemoglobin called **Hb S.** Hb S is the hemoglobin in which *glutamic acid is replaced by valine at the 6th position of beta chain*. In the deoxygenated state, conformational changes induced by Hb S makes the cell more rigid and deformed to take the shape of a sickle (Fig. 15.5). Therefore, cells undergo **intravascular hemolysis**.

1. Diagnosis is usually made by **sickle test** (demonstrating sickling of red cells when the blood is mixed with freshly prepared solution of a reducing agent like sodium metabisulphite) (Figs. 15.6), **hemoglobin solubility test** (relative insolubility of reduced Hb S in phosphate buffer), and **hemoglobin electrophoresis**.

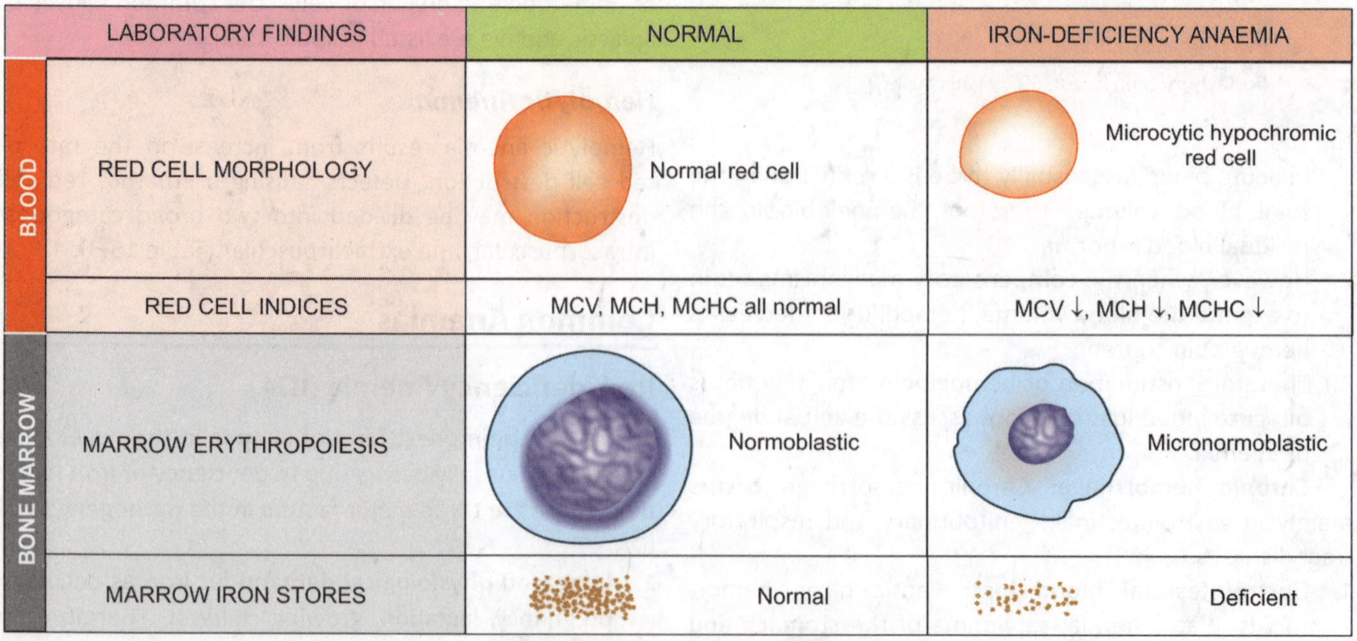

	LABORATORY FINDINGS	NORMAL	IRON-DEFICIENCY ANAEMIA
BLOOD	RED CELL MORPHOLOGY	Normal red cell	Microcytic hypochromic red cell
BLOOD	RED CELL INDICES	MCV, MCH, MCHC all normal	MCV ↓, MCH ↓, MCHC ↓
BONE MARROW	MARROW ERYTHROPOIESIS	Normoblastic	Micronormoblastic
BONE MARROW	MARROW IRON STORES	Normal	Deficient

Fig. 15.3: Iron deficiency anemia. Note microcytic hypochromic red cells in peripheral blood smear and micronormoblasts in bone marrow with decreased iron store.

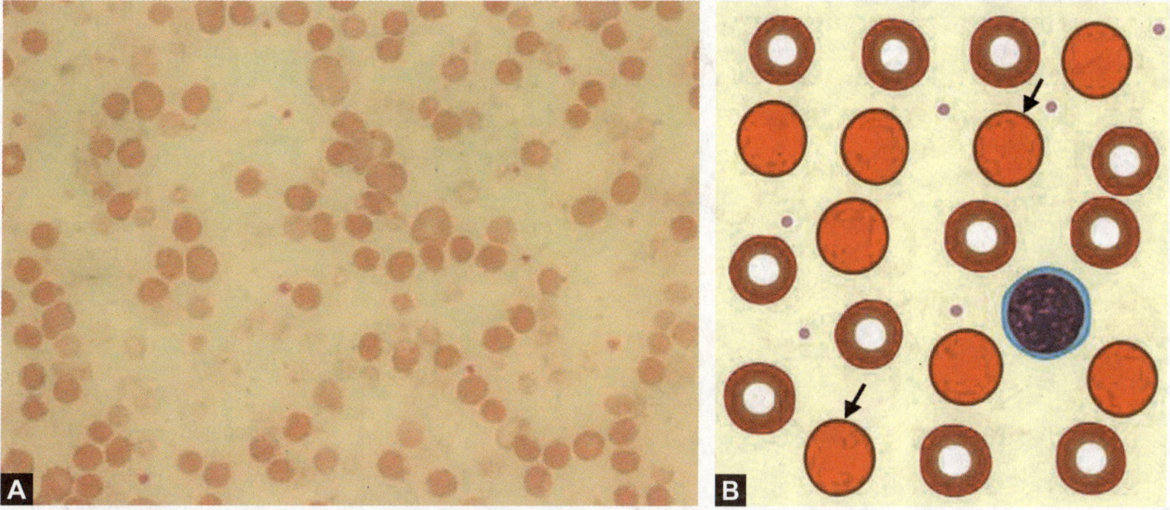

Figs. 15.4A and B: Picture of peripheral blood smear showing numerous spherocytes in hereditary spherocytosis (A). Note the presence of many spherical red cells (indicated by arrows, in the schematic picture B).
Courtesy: Figures 6.3A and B, Essentials in Hematology and Clinical Pathology by Ramadas Nayak et al., 1st edition, 2012; Jaypee Brothers Medical Publishers (P) Ltd.

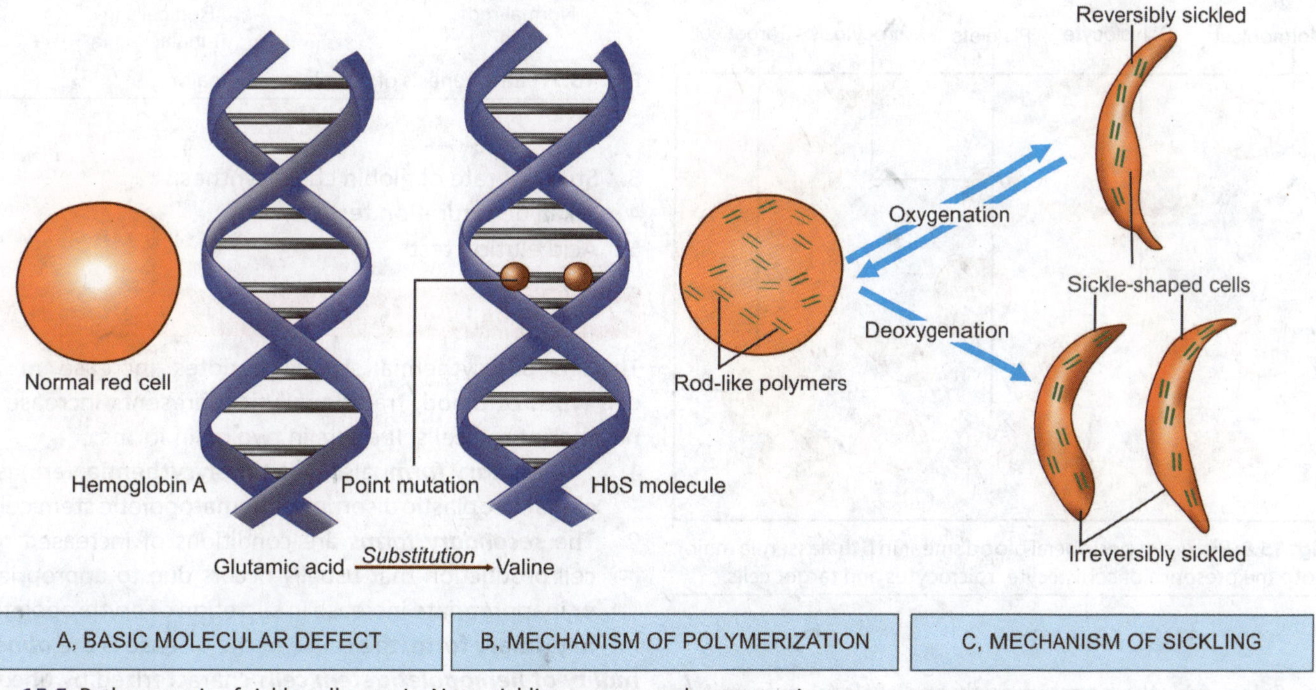

Fig. 15.5: Pathogenesis of sickle cell anemia. Note, sickling occurs on deoxygenation.

2. Hyposplenism is usually associated, due to micro-infarctions in spleen. Autosplenectomy may occur.
3. The anemia is usually **normochromic** and **normocytic**.

Thalassemia

Thalassemia is a genetically determined heterogenous group of commonest *monogenic disorder* in which the rate of **synthesis of one or more types of hemoglobin polypeptide chain is decreased**. Thus, there are two major classes of thalassemia: α thalassemia and β thalassemia, in which α and β globin genes are involved respectively. This causes decrease in the respective polypeptide chain of hemoglobin (Fig. 15.7).

β *thalassemia*

In **β thalassemia** (failure to synthesize β chain), which is more common, there is excess α chain production that damages red cell precursor and red cells.

1. There are many homozygous and heterozygous, and major and minor forms of the disease.
2. In **β thalassemia major**, anemia develops in first few months of life and becomes progressively severe.

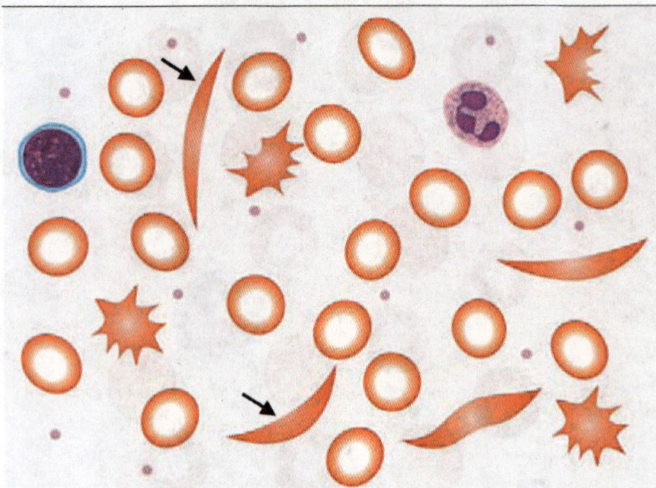

Fig. 15.6: Examination of peripheral blood smear in sickle-cell anemia. Note the red cells in sickle shape.
Courtesy: Figure 8.4B, Essentials in Hematology and Clinical Pathology by Ramadas Nayak et al., 1st edition, 2012; Jaypee Brothers Medical Publishers (P) Ltd.

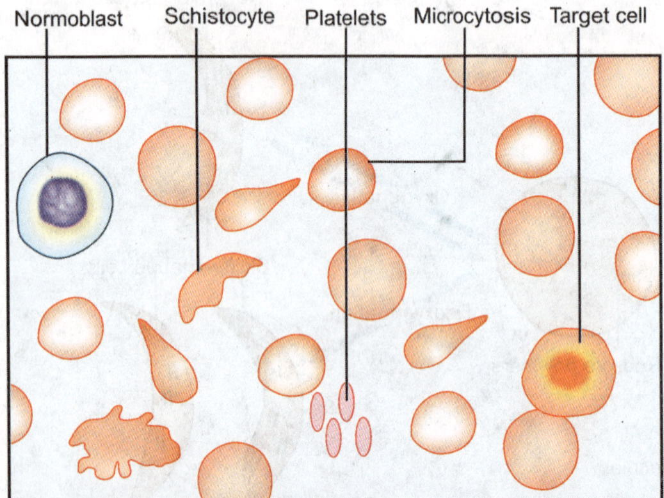

Fig. 15.8: Picture of peripheral blood smear in β thalassemia major. Note the presence of schistocyte, microcytes and target cells.

3. Splenomegaly, hepatomegaly and skeletal deformities are common.
4. Though anemia is usually *microcytic and hypochromic*, all forms and combinations are not uncommon (Fig. 15.8).

α-thalassemia

Anemia of **α-thalassemia** (failure to synthesize α chain) is more *hemolytic* than dyserythropoietic.

The thalassemias are **diagnosed** by:

1. Hemoglobin electrophoresis
2. Demonstration of **Hb-H inclusions** (in the absence of sufficient alpha chains, excess of beta or gamma chains aggregate to form Hb-H)

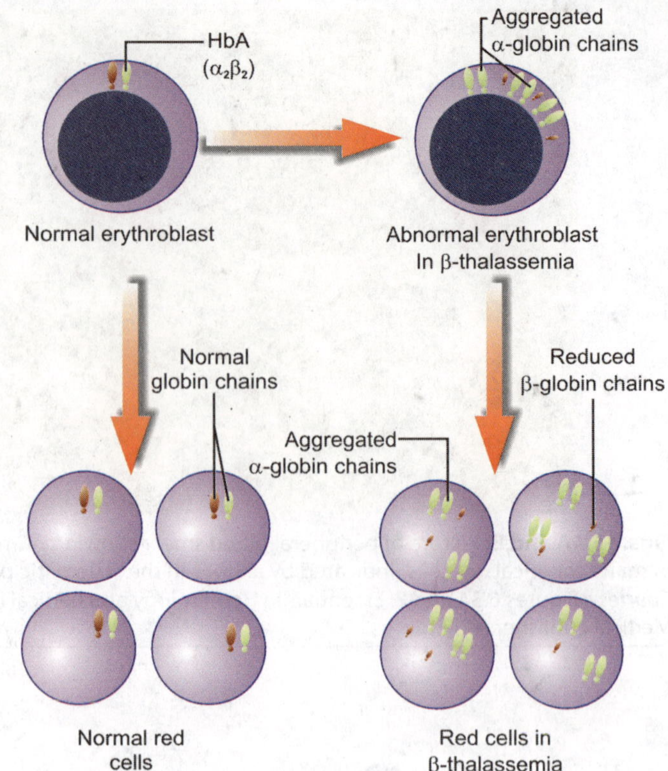

Fig. 15.7: Pathogenesis of β thalassemia major.

3. Study of rate of globin chain synthesis
4. Alkali denaturation test
5. Acid elution test

POLYCYTHEMIA

Though polycythemia strictly denotes increase in all cell types of blood, traditionally it represents increase in number of red cells. It exists in two main forms:

1. The ***primary form***, also called **polycythemia vera,** is a clonal neoplastic disorder of hematopoietic stem cells.
2. The ***secondary forms*** are conditions of increased red cell production that usually occurs due to appropriate or inappropriate increase in secretion of erythropoietin.

In primary form, the cause of the disease is the ***abnormality of hemopoietic stem cells*** characterized by uncontrolled proliferation of cells of erythroid, granulocytic and megakaryocytic series, resulting in increase of all forms of formed elements of blood. Thus, ***primary polycythemia*** is appropriate for the primary form.

In secondary forms, the cause of the disease is ***excess erythropoietin secretion*** that results in increase in red cell production (mostly without increase in granulocytes and platelets). Thus, ***secondary erythrocytosis*** is more appropriate than secondary polycythemia for the secondary forms.

Types of Polycythemia

Polycythemia is broadly divided into ***three forms*** (Table 15.4). The **primary form** is the *polycythemia vera*. The **secondary**

forms are secondary to other conditions or diseases. The ***relative or apparent polycythemia*** is not true polycythemia, but a spurious increase in red cells due to dehydration.

Polycythemia Vera

Polycythemia vera is an **abnormality of hematopoietic stem** cell in which a single stem cell is transformed into a cell that has a selective growth advantage that gradually becomes the major source of marrow precursors.

1. Disease commonly starts in 6th decade of life, and usually presents with headache, plethora (a ruddy complexion), pruritus, thrombosis and GI bleeding. For plethoric appearance of patients, the disease is also called **polycythemia rubra vera**.
2. Bone *marrow is characteristically hypercellular* with involvement of all lineages.
3. Erythrocyte count is usually very high. Leucocytosis with absolute neutrophilia and thrombocytosis are common.
4. The disease is treated by ***phlebotomy*** (removal of about 500 ml of blood in 2 to 4 day's time).
5. *Myelosuppressive drugs* like hydroxyurea and busulfan are also prescribed to inhibit marrow activity.

Table 15.4: Types of polycythemia.

A. Primary polycythemia
– Polycythemia vera
B. Secondary polycythemia (secondary erythrocytosis)
1. Appropriate increase in erythropoietin secretion (proportionate to the degree of tissue hypoxia) – High altitude – Congenital heart disease with right to left shunt. – Chronic pulmonary diseases – Chronic smokers – Enzyme deficiency in red cells
2. Inappropriate increase in erythropoietin secretion – Renal tumors, renal cyst, hydronephrosis – Liver tumors (mainly hepatocarcinoma) – Brain tumors (cerebellar hemangioma) – Endocrine disorders (pheochromocytoma, virilizing ovarian tumors, Bartter syndrome)
C. Apparent (relative) polycythemia
– Dehydration – Redistribution of body fluid

CHAPTER SUMMARY

Key Concepts

1. Anemia can be classified of morphologically and etiologically. Morphologically, anemias are classified into hypochromic microcytic, normochromic microcytic, and macrocytic normochromic types.
2. The commonest cause of anemia in the Indian subcontinent is nutritional deficiency anemia, especially the iron-deficiency anemia (IDA).
3. IDA manifests with microcytosis and hypochromic red cells in peripheral smear.
4. The next common anemia is megaloblastic anemia that occurs due to vitamin B_{12} deficiency. In this, macrocytosis is seen in peripheral smear, and megaloblasts in bone marrow smear.
5. Polycythemia vera occurs due to hemopoietic stem cells producing more erythroid lineage, resulting in excessive production of red cells.

Important to Know (Must Read)

1. In examinations, classification of anemia with causes and blood picture may come as a **Long Question**.
2. Types of anemia, megaloblastic anemia, iron-deficiency anemia, thalassemia and polycythemia are usually asked as **Short Questions** in exams.
3. In **Viva**, examiners usually ask about types of anemia, causes of anemia, peripheral blood picture in common anemias, like IDA and megaloblastic anemia, and definition and types of polycythemia.
4. As anemia is common in India, questions are frequently asked from this chapter, and the student is expected to answer these questions.

CHAPTER

16

Blood Groups and Physiological Basis of Blood Transfusion

Learning Objectives

On completion of study of this chapter, the student **MUST** be able to:

1. List the uses of blood groups, classify blood groups and give the physiological basis of blood grouping.
2. Describe the agglutinogens, agglutinins in ABO system, give % distribution of ABO blood groups in population and understand the mechanism of inheritance of ABO blood groups.
3. Define Landsteiner's law and give its physiological basis.
4. Describe the antigens and antibodies in Rh system, and the mechanism of Rh incompatibility.
5. Give the etiology, features, physiological basis of treatment and prevention of erythroblastosis fetalis.
6. Understand the concept of universal donor, universal recipient, and major and minor cross matching.
7. List the usual hazards of blood transfusion.

The student **MAY** also be able to:

1. Explain the role of H antigen in ABO typing.
2. Appreciate the importance of Bombay blood group.
3. Name the anticoagulants used for blood collection and list the changes in red cells following storage of blood.
4. Name the common diseases associated with various blood groups.
5. List the indications of blood transfusion and learn the procedure of transfusion.

BLOOD GROUPS

Human red cells contain numerous surface structures that are recognized as antigens by the immune system of the individual who does not possess them. These surface structures are called **blood group antigens**. Based on the presence of antigens on red cell membrane, usually corresponding antibodies are absent in the plasma of that individual. This forms the physiological basis of blood groups and principle of blood transfusion:

1. The blood group antigens are called **agglutinogens** and the antibodies against them are called **agglutinins** as the reaction between them results in clumping or agglutination of red cells.
2. There are more than 30 known blood group systems in our blood containing about 400 antigens (Table 16.1).
3. Many of them have *cold antibodies* that do not react at body temperature. Therefore, only few of them are immunologically active.
4. The blood group systems that are most important for blood transfusion are ABO and Rh systems.
5. Other major blood group systems that have medical and medicolegal importance are MNS, Lewis, Duffy, Kell, P and Lutheran systems.

Uses of Blood Groups

Red cells have traditionally been considered as less active cells that contain mainly hemoglobins. However, they play important role in many physiological processes of the body due to the presence of antigens on their surface:

1. Characterization of red cell antigen and antibodies forms the basis of **compatibility testing for blood transfusion**. When the blood group of an individual is known, in emergency situations, blood can be transfused immediately with the suitable blood. Therefore, ABO and Rh blood groups are usually displayed in the identity cards of individuals.
2. The blood group antigens have provided the scientific basis for ***understanding hemolytic diseases*** of the newborn and autoimmune hemolytic anemias.

Table 16.1: Blood group systems, their genes and total antigens.

Blood groups	Genes	Total antigens
ABO	ABO	4
Rh	RHD, RHCE	45
MNS	GYPA, GYPB	40
P	P1	1
Lutheran	LU	18
Kell	KEL	22
Duffy	FY	6
Kidd	HUT11	3
Lewis	FUT3	3
Lewis like	–	3
Diego	SLC4A1	7
Cartwright	ACHE	2
Xg	XG	1
Li	–	2
Scianna	SC	3
Dombrock	DO	5
Colton	AQP1	3
Landsteiner-Wiener	LW	3
Chido-Rodgers	C4A, C4B	9
H	FUT1	1
Kx	XK	1
Gerbich	GYPC	7
Cromer	DAF	10
Knops	CR1	5
Indian	CD44	2
Er	–	2

3. Blood group antigens play a critical role in ***susceptibility to infections*** by malaria parasites, bacteria and viruses. Also, few blood groups provide resistance to some diseases (see above).
4. Red cell antigens are also ***associated with clinical disorders***. Absence of certain red cell antigens is associated with specific dysfunctions, and certain inherited and acquired diseases are associated with alteration of red cell antigen expression. These associations have led to understanding of pathophysiology of these pathologic processes.
5. Medicolegal experts take the help of characterization of red cell antigen and antibodies in establishing the identity of the father in cases of ***disputed paternities*** (and also to identity the mother in cases of disputed maternity).
6. Specific blood groups have been reported to be associated with ***human behaviors***. Therefore, blood groups are believed to contribute to the personality of the individual.

ABO System

ABO system was the first blood group system to be known (described in 1901):

1. This is the most important system in transfusion medicine, as ABO agglutinogens are highly antigenic.
2. Physiologically, it is most significant of all blood group systems, because of natural occurrence of A and B antibodies in the plasma of individuals who lack corresponding antigen on their red cells.
3. In addition, transfusion of incompatible ABO blood groups instantly leads to serious consequences.

ABO Agglutinogens

In ABO system, in essence there are **two antigens**, the ***antigen A*** and the ***antigen B***. A antigen has two sub-types, **A and A_1**. The genes for antigens for ABO system are ***ABO genes located on chromosome 9***.

Occurrence

These antigens are present on the **membrane of red cells**:

1. They are also found in other tissues like salivary gland, testes, lungs, kidney and pancreas. Therefore, they are secreted in minute quantity in saliva, pancreatic secretion and seminal fluid.
2. Some individuals, especially blood group O, secrete blood group H antigens in saliva and other body fluids; they are called **H secretors** (*see* below, role of H antigen).

Time of Appearance

ABO antigens are present since fetal life. They *first appear at sixth week of intrauterine life*. At birth, the concentration is about one-fifth of concentration in adults. Concentration rises slowly to reach a significant level at puberty and **reaches maximum at 15–17 years of life** (Application Box 16.1). Therefore, for collection of blood for blood transfusion, the *age of the donor should be minimum of 15 years*.

Application Box 16.1

Donor's age should be above 15 years: Concentration of ABO antigens rises gradually and reaches its significant level at 15–17 years. Therefore, for collection of blood for blood transfusion, the age of the donor should be minimum of 15 years.

Chemical Nature

Blood group antigen A and B are complex ***oligosaccharides***. There is difference in their terminal sugars. For agglutinogen A, terminal sugar is ***N-acetylgalactosamine***, and for agglutinogen B, terminal sugar is ***galactose***.

Blood Groups Based on Antigens

Based on the presence or absence of A and B antigens on the red cell membrane individually or in group, four blood groups have been described.

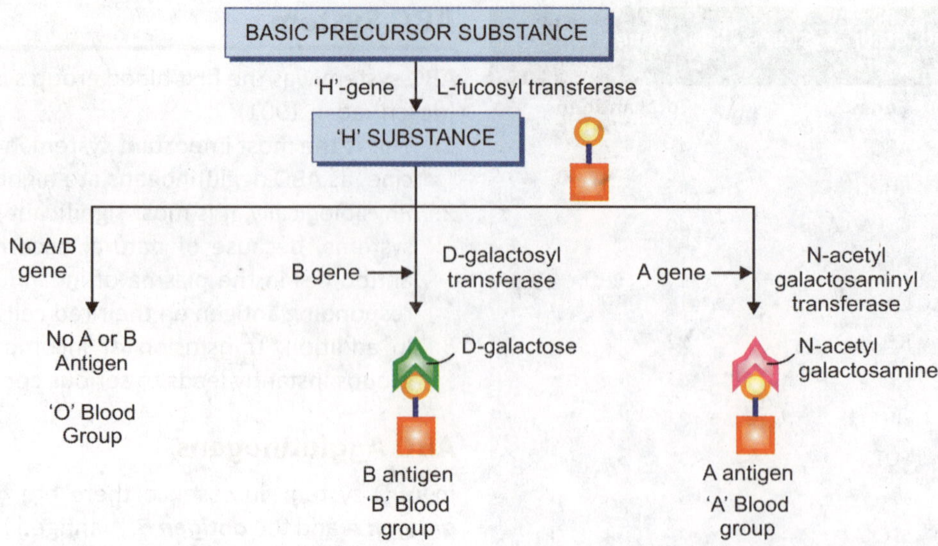

Fig. 16.1: Role of H gene in the formation of A and B antigens.
Courtesy: Figure 58.1, Essentials in Hematology and Clinical Pathology by Ramadas Nayak et al., 1st edition, 2012; Jaypee Brothers Medical Publishers (P) Ltd.

Group A	: Antigen A is present
Group B	: Antigen B is present
Group AB	: Both A and B antigens are present
Group O	: Neither A nor B antigen is present

Subtypes

As A antigen has two sub-types, A and A_1, the group A is subdivided into two groups: the **group A_1** containing A and A_1 antigens, and **group A_2** containing A antigen alone. Similarly, the AB blood group is subdivided into A_1B and A_2B blood groups.

Distribution

In the Indian population, the approximate distribution of the ABO blood group is as follows:

A : 27%
B : 31%
AB : 8%
O : 34%

In the A blood groups, A_1 is 75% and A_2 is 25%.

Role of H Gene and H Antigens

The expression of A and B antigens are dependent on the presence of H genes. Most of the individuals are homozygous for the H gene. The sequence of events in the formation of A and B red cell antigens is:

1. A and B red cell antigens are glycoproteins and their formation starts with **basic precursor substances** (Fig. 16.1).
2. Basic precursor substance is first converted to **H substance** (by transferase) under the influence of **H gene.**
3. H substance is partially converted under the influence of **A and B genes** (and specific transferase) into **A and B antigens**. Some of the H substance remains unconverted.
4. Since O group individuals do not have A and B genes, neither A nor B antigen is formed, and these have only H substance (H remain unchanged). A, B and H antigens may be detected in the saliva and other body fluids also. Such individuals are called ***secretors***, while the remaining without it are ***non-secretors***.

Important Note

Secretors and Nonsecretors: The individuals who secrete A, B and H antigen substances in the saliva and other body fluids **are called secretors and those who do not are called nonsecretors.**

Bombay Blood Group

In 1952, Bhende, Bhatia and Deshpande discovered a new blood group called as Bombay blood group (Phenotype Oh). These individuals **lack the H gene**, and therefore the *basic precursor substance can not be converted into H substance*. This in turn results in **failure to form A or B antigen**. When their blood sample is tested for routine AB grouping, they will be labeled as blood group O. However, their serum contains anti A and anti B and anti H antibodies. These individuals therefore, **should be transfused with only Bombay blood group**.

ABO Agglutinins

In ABO system, agglutinins are of **two types: anti-A (α) and anti-B (β).** The α agglutinin has *two subtypes*, α **proper and $α_1$**.

Occurrence

These antibodies are found in plasma. Usually, specific antibodies are formed against a particular antigen, when they are exposed to that antigen. But, blood group antibodies are ***naturally occurring antibodies*** as they are formed without prior exposure to the antigens and are present in the blood of individuals in whom the respective antigens are absent. However, the mechanism of development of blood group antibodies (as naturally occurring) is not known.

Time and Mechanism of Appearance

Anti-A and anti-B agglutinins are not formed during fetal life and are absent at birth. They *appear in the second week of neonatal life* and increase very slowly in concentration to attain the **peak level at about 10 years of life**:

1. The exact mechanism of formation of agglutinins in the absence of their corresponding agglutinogen is not clearly known. It has been proposed that ***intestinal bacteria and food contain antigens*** similar to that of blood group agglutinogens. Therefore, when the baby starts eating and food gets absorbed from intestine, antigens are absorbed into the blood.
2. As these antigens are recognized as *non-self antigens* by the body's immune system, they stimulate antibody production.
3. However, these antigens are present in very low concentration and antibodies against them are produced very slowly; therefore, antigen-antibody reaction does not occur (Application Box 16.2).
4. Moreover, antigens are removed by phagocytic cells.

Application Box 16.2

ABO incompatibility does not cause hemolytic diseases of newborns: ABO antigens are also expressed in other tissues, and therefore, ABO compatibility is of significant consideration in organ transplantations. However, in newborns, ABO incompatibility rarely causes clinical hemolytic disease because antibodies against A and B antigens are predominantly IgM that do not cross the placenta during fetal life, and antigens A and B are not well developed at birth.

Chemical Nature

The α and β agglutinins are globulins and belong to **Ig M category**. Therefore, they do not cross the placenta. They function efficiently at low temperature, i.e. between 5° to 20° C. Therefore, they are called **cold antibodies.**

Agglutinins Against Blood Groups

Antibodies are directed against the antigens:

1. The individuals with ***blood group A antigen*** on the red cell membrane do not have anti-A antibody, rather possess **anti-B antibody** in their plasma.
2. Persons with ***blood group B*** do not contain anti-B, rather have **anti-A antibody** in their plasma (Table 16.2).
3. Individuals with ***blood group AB do not have any antibody***.
4. Individuals with ***blood group O*** have both the **anti-A and ant-B antibodies** in their plasma.

These facts were first noted and described by **Karl Landsteiner** in 1900, and his theory is popularly known as **Landsteiner's law.**

Table 16.2: Occurrence of antigens and antibodies in ABO system.

Blood groups	Antigen (on RBC)	Antibody (in plasma)
A	A	Anti-B
B	B	Anti-A
AB	A and B	Nil
O	Nil	Anti-A and anti-B

Scientist contributed

Karl Landsteiner discovered ***isoagglutinin in human blood*** in 1900, leading to recognition of human blood groups and success of blood transfusion. The principle of presence or absence of agglutinogen and agglutinin in red cells and plasma in various blood groups is popularly known as Landsteiner Law. He received **Nobel Prize in Physiology or Medicine in 1930.**

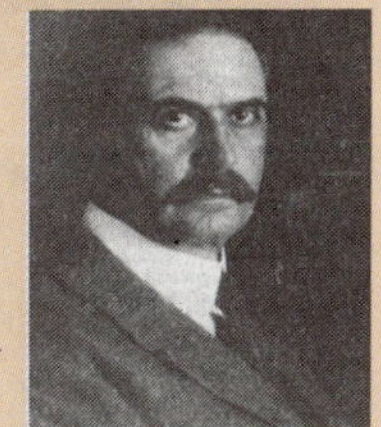

Karl Landsteiner
(1868–1943)

Landsteiner's Law

This law states that if a particular agglutinogen is present on the red cell membrane of an individual, the corresponding agglutinin must be absent in his plasma. Conversely, if the agglutinogen is absent in the red cells, the corresponding agglutinin must be present in the plasma. This law holds good for ABO system. However, the second part of the law does not apply for Rh and many other blood group systems as there are no naturally occurring agglutinins in these systems.

Antigen and Antibodies for ABO Blood Groups

Thus, in ABO system, **blood group A** has antigen A on the red cell membrane and anti-B antibody in the plasma, **blood group B** has antigen B on the red cell membrane and anti-A antibody in the plasma, **blood group AB** has both antigens A and B on the red cell membrane and no antibodies in the plasma, and **blood group O** has no antigens on the red cell membrane and possesses both agglutinins anti-A and anti-B in the plasma (Table 16.2).

Blood Grouping

Blood grouping is performed by suspending the red cells of the person's blood group to be checked in the anti-A and anti-B antisera that are commercially available. If the agglutination (clumping of red cells, as checked under the microscope) is present, red cells contain that particular antigen (Fig. 16.2)

Inheritance of ABO Blood Groups

Blood groups are genetically determined. Normally, presence of a blood group antigen is a dominant characteristic. Therefore, the antigen is present in the phenotype irrespective of the genotype (Table 16.3).

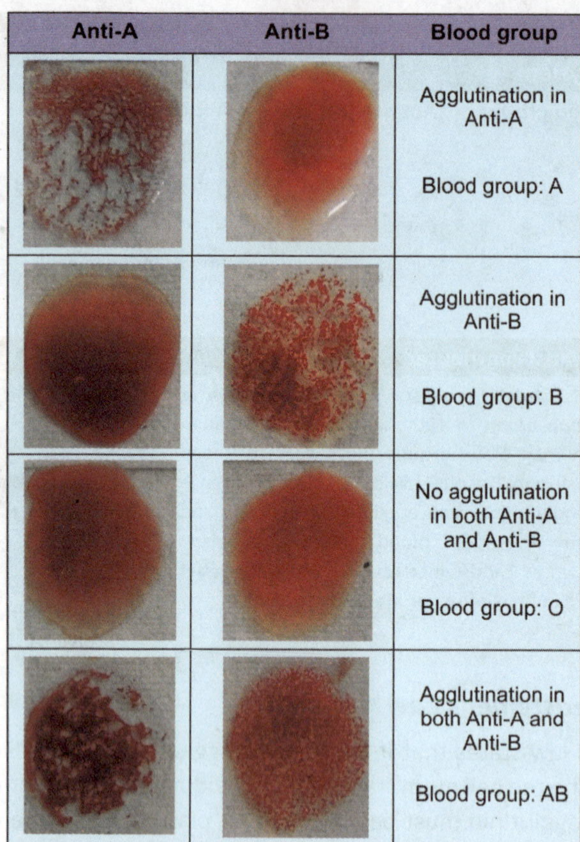

Fig. 16.2: Method of blood grouping.
Courtesy: Figure 58.2, Essentials in Hematology and Clinical Pathology by Ramadas Nayak et al., 1st edition, 2012; Jaypee Brothers Medical Publishers (P) Ltd.

There are **three types of genes**: O, A and B. Therefore, a person can have any of the six possible genotypes: OO, OA, OB, AA, BB, and AB. Gene O is genetically not important. Therefore, the respective phenotype may be **A or B or AB or O** (Clinical Box 16.1). For example, if blood group of one parent is A and other parent is B, then there is possibility of child having any of the four blood group of ABO system (Fig. 16.3).

Clinical Box 16.1

Disputed paternity: The knowledge of inheritance of blood group is useful to solve the cases of disputed paternity. When the blood group of a child and the mother is known, it can be told whether the man in suspicion could have been the father of the child or not. However, blood group can never prove that a particular man is the father of a particular child. This is because the blood group of the man can be one out of several other possible men. Therefore, determination of blood group gene only helps to identify, not confirms the identity. MNS system is more useful in this regard.

Rh System

The Rh (Rhesus) system is the second most important blood group system in transfusion medicine. This was first described in *Rhesus monkeys* in 1940 by **Landsteiner and Weiner**; hence it is called Rh system (for Rhesus). First, it was discovered that injection of red cells of Rhesus monkey into rabbit results in development of antibody against rhesus red cells, later it was found that rabbit serum containing anti-Rhesus antibody agglutinate human red cells. This led to the discovery of Rh system in humans.

Table 16.3: ABO phenotypes and their possible genotypes.

Phenotype (blood group)	Genotype
A	AA, AO
B	BB, BO
AB	AB
O	OO

Parents: Father — Mother
Phenotype: A — B
Genotype: AO — BO
Gamates: A, O — B, O
Offspring
Genotype: AB, AO, OB, OO
Genotype: AB, A, B, O

Fig. 16.3: Inheritance of ABO antigen.

Rh Antigens

In Rh system, there are six antigens, but there are no naturally occurring antibodies. The antigens are C, D, E, c, d and e. Out of these *six antigens*, immunologically most active is the **D antigen**:

1. Thus, in Rh system, there are two blood groups: **Rh positive** (D antigen present) and **Rh negative** (D antigen absent).
2. The gene for Rh antigen is the RHD and RHCE genes that are located on ***chromosome 1***.
3. The antigens of Rh system participate in cation transport and membrane integrity of red cells.
4. Rh antigens are membrane proteins found in red cell membrane, not in any other tissues.

Inheritance

Rh antigen is inherited as dominant gene:

1. In Indian population, 95 to 98% are Rh +ve and 2 to 5% are Rh –ve.
2. Rh +ve individual may have homozygous (DD) or heterozygous (Dd) genotypes. Usually, 60% of Rh +ve individuals have Dd genotype and 40% have DD genotype. The genotype of Rh –ve person is dd.
3. If one of the parents is homozygous positive and the other is homozygous negative, all offsprings will be heterozygous positives (Fig. 16.4).

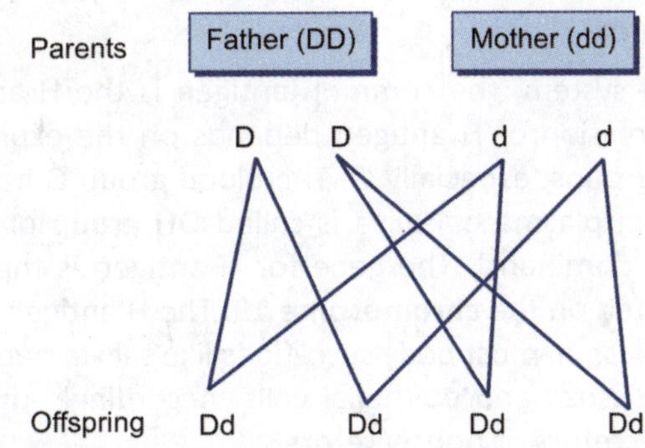

Fig. 16.4: Inheritance of Rh antigen.

4. Similarly, if the father and mother are homozygous negatives, all offsprings will be homozygous negatives, and when one of the parents is heterozygous positive and the other homozygous negative, 50% of offsprings will be heterozygous positive and 50% will be homozygous negatives.

Rh Antibody

The antibody in the system is called ***anti-D antibody***, which is produced only when an Rh negative individual receives the Rh positive blood:

1. These antibodies develop very slowly in the first encounter, but form rapidly following subsequent encounters. Rh antibody is of ***Ig G type***, which can cross placental barrier.
2. Hence, if antibodies are present in mother's blood, can be transferred to the fetus.
3. Rh antibody is best reactive at body temperature, and therefore, designated as **warm antibody**.

Rh Incompatibility

Rh incompatibility occurs when an Rh negative individual receives Rh positive blood.

1. Normally, when an Rh negative person receives Rh positive blood, there will be no immediate reactions as Rh negative individual does not normally has anti-Rh antibody.
2. However, the donor's red cells induce an immune response in the recipient to synthesize anti-Rh antibodies, which takes about *two to four months to reach a significant titer*. However, by that time the donor's red cells die their natural death within 120 days. The anti-Rh antibody cannot produce any harm to the recipient's red cells because the Rh negative recipient's red cells contain no Rh antigens.
3. But, if the same Rh negative person who has already received a Rh positive blood before, receives a second Rh positive transfusion later, the anti-Rh antibodies are synthesized in large amount immediately by the memory cells. This antibody reacts against the donor cells and causes reactions of mismatch transfusion.
4. Thus, the Rh negative individual can safely receive Rh positive blood once in life time.

The similar Rh incompatibility occurs in pregnancies when Rh negative mother bears Rh positive fetus, which leads to **erythroblastosis fetalis**. The first child does not suffer. However, subsequent pregnancies carry risk for the fetus. The disorder is called erythroblastosis fetalis.

Erythroblastosis Fetalis

Etiopathogenesis

This is a **hemolytic disease of the newborn** which occurs due to Rh incompatibility when an Rh negative mother carries Rh positive fetus during pregnancy:

1. Usually, no reaction occurs in the first pregnancy. However, at the time of delivery **during placental separation**, a small amount of fetal blood leaks into the maternal circulation. This induces formation of anti-Rh agglutinins in the mother.
2. Therefore, in subsequent pregnancies, the anti-Rh agglutinin from mother, which is predominantly IgG type crosses placenta to enter into fetal circulation and causes hemolysis.
3. In third and subsequent pregnancies, the degree of hemolysis becomes severe.

Clinical Features

The features are mainly due to hemolysis. Hemolysis leads to anemia, extramedullary hemopoiesis and neonatal hyperbilirubinemia. If the hemolysis is severe, the fetus may die *in utero* or if the fetus is born alive, he may have the following features:

1. **Anemia:** Anemia is proportionate to the degree of hemolysis.
2. **Hemolytic jaundice:** Occurs due to hemolysis. Serum bilirubin level may be more than 25 mg% in severe cases.
3. **Generalized edema:** Edema occurs in the whole body due to anemia and hypoproteinemia. This is called **hydrops fetalis**.
4. **Kernicterus:** This is a neurologic syndrome with major motor deficits that occurs due to the ***deposition of bilirubin in the basal ganglia.*** Hyperbilirubinemia occurs due to hemolysis. Basal ganglia have more affinity for bilirubin. However, bile pigments cannot cross the blood-brain barrier (BBB) in adults. Therefore, *hemolysis in adults does not produce kernicterus*. As BBB is not fully developed in fetuses, infants and children, in them bilirubin enters brain and gets deposited in the basal ganglia. Therefore, ***hemolysis in infancy and early childhood causes kernicterus***. The dysfunctions mainly manifests in the form of motor dysfunctions.
5. **Extramedullary hemopoiesis:** Due to severe anemia, extramedullary hemopoiesis occurs, for which **erythroblasts** (nucleated red cells) are released into the blood. Erythroblasts are seen in plenty in peripheral smear. Hence, the disease is called erythroblastosis fetalis.

Treatment

About 50% of the fetuses and newborns with erythroblastosis fetalis have mild hemolysis and do not require treatment. In severe cases, the major modalities of treatment are intrauterine fetal transfusion, exchange transfusion and phototherapy:

1. **Intrauterine fetal transfusion:** If the disease is diagnosed in fetus and found to be severe, the treatment is intrauterine fetal transfusion. Presently, the fetal transfusion is carried out by intraperitoneal route, which has replaced the direct intravascular fetal transfusion.
2. **Exchange transfusion:** The treatment of newborns with severe anemia, jaundice and hydrops is exchange transfusion soon after birth. Exchange transfusion removes sensitized red cells, bilirubin and maternal antibody from the plasma. A *double-volume exchange transfusion* (2 x 80 ml/kg) replaces 90% of the infant's blood volume with antigen negative red cells. Blood chosen for exchange should be ABO negative, Rh negative and cross-matched against mother's blood.
3. **Phototherapy:** Intensive phototherapy is very effective in reducing serum bilirubin level (Clinical Box 16.2).

Clinical Box 16.2

Phototherapy for neonatal jaundice: Bilirubin in excess is toxic to the body, especially it produces neurotoxicity. However, on exposure to light bilirubin becomes nontoxic, which is the physiological basis of phototherapy. Bilirubin, on exposure to light undergoes structural and configurational isomerization and photo-oxidation. These changes in bilirubin make it less toxic and less lipophilic products that are excreted efficiently without hepatic conjugation. Therefore, phototherapy is the primary treatment for unconjugated hyperbilirubinemia in newborns. *Neonatal jaundice* is mainly hemolytic and unconjugated.

Prevention

Erythroblastosis fetalis is prevented by administering a single dose of anti-Rh antibodies in the form of Rh immunoglobulin during the postpartum period following the first delivery. The disease can also be prevented by **passive immunization** of the mother with a small dose of Rh immunoglobulins during pregnancy.

Other Blood Group Systems

MNS System

The MNS system of blood group was first described in 1927 (MN in 1927; S in 1947). This system has three antigens: M, N and S. The antigens are expressed in red cells and endothelial cells of renal capillaries. The MNS antigens are major contributor for negative charges on the red cell membrane. The common phenotypes are M, N, MN and S. This system is helpful for **solving the paternity dispute**. MNS groups are also useful for *anthropological and genetic studies*.

H System

In the H system, the common antigen is the H antigen. The expression of H antigen depends on the expression of ABO groups, especially O. The blood group O having H antigen in plasma or saliva is called **OH group** or **Oh** (if H is not dominant). The gene for H antigen is the FUT1 (H), located on the **chromosome 19**. The H antigen is present in plasma, most body secretions like saliva, sweat and semen, tissues and epithelial cells. Accordingly they are called **secretors** or **nonsecretors**.

Lewis System

The Lewis system was described in 1946. This system has two antigens: Le^a and Le^b. These are not truly red cell antigens as they are produced in the plasma and then are absorbed into the red cells. Antigens are also present in body secretions and lymph. The gene for antigen Le^a is FUT3(Le) gene located in **chromosome 19**. The antigens of Lewis system serve as receptor for Helicobacter Pylori. The antibodies are of the IgM type. They do not cross the placental barrier and therefore, do not cause hemolytic disease of the newborn.

Ii System

Ii system was first described in 1956. There are two antigens in the Ii system, the 'I' and the 'i' antigens. The antigens are present in plasma, red cells, lymph and secretions. The Ii system differs from other blood groups in several ways:

1. At birth the I antigen is poorly developed, but red cells of fetus and neonate are rich in the i antigens.
2. There is gradual changeover from i to I antigen in the first two years of life.
3. In conditions like hemoglobinopathies, red cells show increased i antigens without any decrease in I antigens.

Pl System

The Pl system or also called P system was first described in 1927. There are three antigens in this system: P_l, P and P^k. The genes for these antigens are Pl genes that are located on **chromosome 22**. These antigens are distributed in red cells, platelets, lymph and fibroblasts. P_l antigen is ***associated with parasitic infections***.

Duffy System

This system was described in 1950. There are three blood group antigens in this system: the Fy^a, Fy^b and Fy^3. The genes for these antigens are FY genes that are located on ***chromosome 1***. These antigens serve as receptors for pro-inflammatory chemokines like IL-8. This system has three blood groups: Fya, Fyb, and Fyab. A close relationship between Duffy blood group and malaria has been well established. The Fyab blood groups is resistant to Plasmodium Vivax, whereas the Fya and Fyb are susceptible to vivax malaria. This is because, Fya and Fyb antigens serve as receptors for plasmodium if present separately on the red cell mambrane, and thus ***increase their entry into the red cells***.

Kidd System

This system was described in 1951. There are three antigens in this system: the Jk^a, Jk^b and Jk^3. The genes for these antigens are Jk (HUT11) genes that are located on ***chromosome 18***. The antigens are specifically present on the red cell membrane (and in no other tissues). They are responsible for ***delayed hemolytic transfusion reactions***.

Kell System

The Kell system was described in 1946. In this system, the common antigens are: K, k, Kp^a and Kp^b. There are two sets of genes for these antigens: KEL and XK. The KEL genes are located on ***chromosome 7*** and are expressed in red cells, bone marrow and fetal liver. The XK genes are located on ***X chromosome*** and are expressed in red cells, skeletal and cardiac muscles and neural tissues. People having K +ve blood group (containing K antigen on the red cell membrane) are ***susceptible to chronic granulomatous diseases***.

Lutheran System

The Lutheran system was described in 1951. There are three blood group antigens in this system: the Lu^a, Lu^b and Lu^3. The genes for these antigens are LU genes that are located on ***chromosome 19***. The antigens are distributed in red cells, brain, heart, kidney, lung, pancreas, placenta and skeletal muscles. In addition to *antibody recognition*, they play possible role in *cell adhesion*, *receptor function* and *intercellular signaling*.

Blood Group-associated Diseases

There are diseases that are prevalent in different blood groups. There are diseases that occur in the absence or alteration of blood groups (Table 16.4).

Table 16.4: Blood group-associated diseases.

A. Diseases due to occurrence blood groups	
Group A	: Carcinoma of salivary glands, stomach colon, rectum, uterus and ovary; ITP; coronary thrombosis, pernicious anemia
B	: E coli UTI, gonorrhea
O	: Peptic ulcer, rheumatoid arthritis, typhoid fever, von Willebrand disease
Le	: Sjögren syndrome
Fya/b	: Vivax malaria
K	: Chronic granulomatous diseases
Rh –ve	: Autoimmune hemolytic anemia
Ii	: Hemoglobinopathies
B. Blood group associated with disease resistance	
P_I/P^k	: E coli pyelonephritis
Fyab	: Plasmodium vivax malaria
C. Absence of antigen associated with diseases	
Rh_{null}	: Hereditary stomatocytosis, hemolytic anemia
Kx	: Hereditary Acanthocytosis
D. Diseases associated with alteration of antigens	
Weak AB	: Leukemia, Hodgkin disease, aplastic anemia
Weak Rh, K	: Autoimmune hemolytic anemia
Weak MN	: Bacterial infection, preleukemia, leukemia
Acquired A	: Myelogenous leukemia
Acquired B	: Bacterial infections, GI lesions
Acquired K	: Enterococcus faecium infection
Acquired Jk^b	: E. faecium and micrococcus infections

PHYSIOLOGICAL BASIS OF BLOOD TRANSFUSION

Transfusion of whole blood or a component of blood is common in medical practice. The common is the transfusion of whole blood or red cell concentrates that are required for the treatment of acute hemorrhage or severe anemia. However, one should be careful for the possibility of transmissions of infectious diseases like HIV and hepatitis, and other hazards of transfusions, when transfusion is given frequently.

Indications for Transfusion

1. **Acute blood loss:**
   - Whole blood is preferred.
2. **Chronic anemia:**
   - Packed red cells are preferred to whole blood.
3. **Bone marrow failure:**
   - Leukemia
   - Aplastic anemia
   - Bone marrow infiltration by neoplastic cells.

   In bone marrow failure, fresh blood and specific blood components are required. Red cells are administered along with granulocytes to resist against infections.
4. **Purpura:**
   - Platelet transfusion is preferred.
5. **Clotting factor deficiencies:**
   - Fresh frozen plasma is preferred. In hemophilia, cryoprecipitate (rich in factor VIII and fibrinogen) is given.
6. **Preparation for surgery and during surgery:**
   - If the patient is anemic, blood is transfused prior to surgery. During major surgeries, blood transfusion is routinely administered. Loss of 500 ml of blood is usually tolerated during surgery in a patient with normal Hb prior to surgery. If blood loss is expected to be more than this, transfusion is always planned.
7. **Burns:**
   - Plasma rich in protein is lost from the burn surface. This is corrected with plasma and colloids. If anemia is severe, packed red cells are transfused.
8. **Anemia:**
   - Usually, blood transfusion is not required in chronic stable anemia. In hemoglobinopathies like thalassemia and sickle cell anemia, blood transfusion is

the cornerstone of the treatment. Repeated and multiple transfusion in thalassemia and sickle cell disease not only aim to improve Hb content, but also to inhibit erythropoiesis so that defective cells are not produced. However, **transfusional hemochromatosis** limits usefulness of this treatment.

Procedure of Blood Transfusion

The first step in any transfusion is the identification of a **healthy and appropriate donor**. **Blood grouping** for Rh and ABO types of both recipient and the donor, and **cross-matching** of blood of both recipient and the donor are the next important steps in all blood transfusions to ensure safety and compatibility. In mismatch transfusion, agglutination (clumping) of red cells occurs in recipient's blood leading to acute hemolysis, which may be life threatening. Therefore, a suitable transfusion should always include:

i. Selection of appropriate donor
ii. ABO and Rh typing
iii. Cross matching
iv. Antibody screening of the patient (to detect the presence of clinically significant antibodies).

Selection of Appropriate Donor

Healthy donors free from transfusion-transmissible diseases should be identified for blood transfusion:

1. Ideally, the age of the donor should be 18 years or above and should not be above 60 years. Donor should be voluntarily willing to donate blood.
2. The hemoglobin status of the donor should be estimated. There should be minimum of 12 g% Hb in female, and 13 g% Hb in male donors.
3. Donor must be screened for AIDS, hepatitis, lymphomas, and protozoal organisms like malaria, filaria, etc.

ABO and Rh Typing

The two major blood group systems for transfusion are ABO and Rh systems. ABO incompatibility causes immediate reactions and may even kill the persons. The Rh incompatibility causes delayed reactions. Therefore, ABO and Rh compatibility must be ensured before any transfusion. The concept of **universal donor and recipient** helps in this process.

Universal Donor

The **blood group O negative** (O group and Rh –Ve) persons are considered to be the universal donor because their red cells contain no antigens. Therefore, their blood cells on transfusion to any individual do not cause agglutination reaction. Hence, blood group O –Ve can be given to any individual (Clinical Box 16.3).

Universal Recipient

Individuals having **blood group AB positive** (AB group and Rh +Ve) are considered to be the universal recipient because their plasma contains no antibodies. Therefore, they can safely receive blood from any one as they do not cause agglutination reaction against any blood cells.

Clinical Box 16.3

Cross-matching is a must before transfusion: Though technically the concept of universal recipient is true, transfusion of blood based on this concept alone may not provide full assurance of compatibility always as there are many other minor blood group systems. Therefore, prior to blood transfusion ***cross-matching should always be done*** to eliminate the possibilities of any form of mismatching. However, in an emergency condition, this concept may be used in selecting the donor, if the blood groups of donor and recipient are known without waiting for the report of cross-matching.

Cross-matching

There are two types of cross-matching: major and minor.

Major Cross-matching

In major cross-matching, the cells of the donor are directly matched against the plasma of the recipient:

1. As it is important to ensure that antibodies present in the recipient's plasma do not harm the donor's red cells, this cross-matching is called *major cross-matching*.
2. The ABO agglutinogens are **highly antigenic** and produce agglutination even in low concentration. Therefore, though donor's red cells are less in quantity than the recipient, they produce agglutination reactions.
3. ABO agglutinins do not react highly, as they are ***cold antibodies***. Moreover, donor's agglutinin is diluted in large volume of recipient's plasma; hence not capable of inducing agglutination reaction.
4. Therefore, it is important to match **donor's agglutinogen (red cells) against recipient's agglutinin (plasma)**.

Minor Cross-matching

In minor cross-matching, the donor's plasma is checked against the red cells of the recipient:

1. It is called minor cross-matching, because it is not very important to assess the reactivity of donor's agglutinin against recipient's cells.
2. This is because; small volume of the donor's plasma is diluted in a large volume of the recipient's plasma.
3. Therefore, the agglutinin titer of donor's plasma falls to such a low level after transfusion that they are unlikely to damage the red cells of the recipient.
4. However, for full compatibility, minor cross-matching should also be performed.

Antibody Screening of the Patient

The patient who receives transfusion, his serum should be screened for various antibodies like autoantibodies that may react against the donor's cells and cause hemolysis. Therefore, it is ideal to do the antibody screening of the patient.

Blood Collection and Storage

Collection of Blood

Venipuncture is done to collect blood:

1. Ideally, not more than 350 ml of blood is collected from a single donor at a time.
2. From antecubital vein, blood flows freely into a collecting bottle or bag that contains anticoagulant.
3. The usual collection time is 7–10 min.
4. The blood mixes with 50 to 70 ml of **anticoagulant consisting of citrate, phosphate and dextrose (CPD).** ***Disodium hydrogen citrate*** is used instead of trisodium citrate as anticoagulant, because this favors fall of pH which is required for survival of red cells.
5. BP and heart rate are monitored after collection, especially before they get up from the supine posture.
6. Normally, some degree of diaphoresis, bradycardia, hypertension and dizziness accompany this bleeding.
7. Donors are advised not to go for work for rest of the day and should also avoid exercise.
8. They are also advised not to donate blood for at least next three months.

Autologous Donor Blood

When the donor is the recipient himself, the blood collected is called autologous donor blood and the transfusion is called autologous transfusion:

1. Autologous transfusion was not practiced before. However, AIDS epidemic has increased the necessity and importance of autologous transfusion in transfusion medicine.
2. This can be done prior to a planned surgery.
3. The Hb of the person should be more than 12.5 g%.
4. Blood is collected every 72 hours upto 72 hours prior to surgery or till the Hb level has not gone below 11 g%.
5. Usually 2 to 4 units of blood of 250 ml each can be collected. Then, the same blood (recipient's own blood) is used during surgery.

Storage of Blood

Blood is stored in the blood bank at **4°C.** Stored blood for transfusion should ideally be used within 2 weeks of storage. However, blood should not be used if it is stored for more than 3 weeks, because gross hemolysis occurs after this period.

Red Cell Changes during Storage

Red cells undergo rapid changes during storage in simple citrate solutions even at 4° C. During cold storage, the changes that occur are mainly due to reduction of metabolism of cells. The changes are:

1. Increase in sodium and decrease in potassium concentration in the red cells. This occurs due to decreased active transport of ions across the cell membrane. At low temperature, **Na^+-K^+ pump activity is grossly decreased.** This results in net increase in the total base and water of the cell. The inhibition of Na^+-K^+ pump increases intracellular sodium concentration that causes water to enter the cell by endosmosis.
2. Cells swell and become more spherocytic. This results in spontaneous hemolysis. Leucocytes and platelets almost totally disappear within 24 to 48 hours of storage.
3. The ATP content in the cell decreases and inorganic phosphate concentration increases. This is due to imbalance between phosphorylation and dephosphorylation processes in the cell.

Changes in Stored Blood after Transfusion

1. Within 24 hours of transfusion, the cell metabolism greatly increases. Consequently, the sodium is extruded from the cells and the potassium is drawn back into the cells.
2. The volume, shape, and fragility of the red cells come back to normal within 24 to 48 hours.
3. Red cells show 80 % of survival 24 hours after transfusion if the transfusion is given within 14 days of storage of the blood. But the survival rate greatly decreases if the blood is stored for more than 2 weeks.
4. Therefore, it is advisable to use blood ideally within 14 days of storage, though blood can be used upto 21 days.
5. Blood should never be used after 30 days of storage.

Hazards of Blood Transfusion

Blood transfusion, even in ideal condition carries risks of adverse reactions. Mostly, transfusion reactions occur due to human error:

I. **Due to Mismatched Transfusion:** When an incompatible blood is transfused, the mismatched transfusion reaction occurs immediately. The reaction is primarily due to agglutination of donor's red cells followed by their hemolysis. This is called **acute hemolytic transfusion reactions.** Usually it occurs due to ABO incompatibility. The severity of the reaction depends on the degree of hemolysis. The complications of mismatched transfusion are:
   1. Shivering and fever (***febrile reactions***) occur usually
   2. Hemoglobinemia and ***hemoglobinuria***
   3. Hemolytic jaundice
   4. ***Acute renal failure.***

   Renal failure occurs due to:
   - i. hemoglobin casts blocking the renal tubules and damaging the tubules,
   - ii. release of toxic substances from the lysed red cells cause renal vasoconstriction, and
   - iii. circulatory shock.

5. *Hyperkalemia* (due to release of potassium ions from red cells). This may cause cardiac arrest in diastole.

II. Due to Faulty Techniques of Giving Blood: Due to wrong method of transfusion, following complications may arise:

1. **Thrombophlebitis:** This is a common complication in those who receive repeated transfusions.
2. **Air Embolism:** Air enters the venous circulation and gets lodged at the outlet of the right ventricle and blocks the flow of blood to the lungs. Death may occur in severe cases. Use of plastic bags has reduced this complication.

III. Due to Massive Transfusion: This occurs when more than 10 units of blood are given within 24 hours or when the total blood volume is exchanged within 24 hours. This leads to **circulatory overload**. Cardiac arrhythmias and even sometimes cardiac arrest occur due to high potassium level in the stored blood.

IV. Febrile Reaction: The patient feels cold and may get rigor due to rise in body temperature. This occurs mainly due to presence of pyrogens in the transfusion apparatus.

V. Allergic Reactions: This is less frequent and is characterized by itching, erythema, nausea, vomiting, and in severe cases may cause anaphylactic reactions.

VI. Transmission of Diseases:

1. Hepatitis
2. Malaria
3. AIDS
4. Syphilis.

CHAPTER SUMMARY

Key Concepts

1. Blood group of an individual depends on presence or absence of a specific blood group antigen on the surface of red cell (RBC membrane).
2. If a blood group antigen is present on the surface of red cell, the corresponding antibody must be absent in his plasma. However, if a blood group antigen is absent on the surface of red cell, the corresponding antibody may (or may not be) present in his plasma. This is called Landsteiner's law.
3. In ABO system, the agglutinogens are highly antigenic. Therefore, for compatible blood transfusion, blood grouping and cross-matching must be done before the transfusion.
4. In major cross-matching, cells of the donor are matched against the plasma of the recipient.
5. Blood group AB positive is the universal recipient, and O negative is the universal donor.
6. For, blood is collection, disodium hydrogen citrate is the preferred anticoagulant, as it ensures low pH, which facilitates red cell survival.
7. Erythroblastosis fetalis occurs in Rh incompatibility when a mother with Rh negative blood group bears the fetus with positive blood group during pregnancy. It is treated by exchange transfusion and prevented by passive immunization with anti-D antibody.

Important to Know (Must Read)

1. In examinations, 'Physiological basis of blood grouping of ABO system' comes as a **Long Question**.
2. Landsteiner's law, ABO agglutinogens, ABO agglutinins, inheritance of blood group, Rh incompatibility, erythroblastosis fetalis, cross matching, universal donor and recipient, changes in red cells following storage, and hazards of blood transfusion are usually asked as **Short Questions** in exams.
3. In **Viva**, examiners usually ask about types of blood groups, uses of blood groups, Landsteiner's law, ABO agglutinogens, ABO agglutinins, H antigens, Bombay blood group, inheritance of blood group, Rh incompatibility, causes, features, treatment and prevention of erythroblastosis fetalis, types and importance cross matching, universal donor and recipient, method of blood collection, how to store blood in blood bank, changes in red cells following storage, and hazards of blood transfusion, and common diseases prevalent in various blood groups.
4. As blood groups have general and special interest in medicine, a student is expected to answer these questions.

CHAPTER

17

White Blood Cells

LEARNING OBJECTIVES

On completion of study of this chapter, the student **MUST** be able to:

1. Classify leucocytes, and give the percentage of different leucocytes in blood.
2. Give the steps of leucopoiesis.
3. Give the general life history of leucocytes.
4. Describe the structure and functions of leucocytes, and list the common causes of decrease and increase of each type of leucocyte.
5. Explain the mechanism of phagocytosis and killing of organisms by neutrophil.
6. List the components of mononuclear-phagocyte system (MPS).
7. Understand the general role of leucocytes in defence mechanisms of the body.
8. Define and classify leukemia.

The student **MAY** also be able to:

1. Describe the role of eosinophil in allergy.
2. Explain the role of MPS in defense of the body.
3. Briefly describe different types of leukemia.

GENERAL INTRODUCTION

Leucocytes or white blood cells perform the defense functions of the body. There are two series of leucocytes: **myeloid series and lymphoid series**. Each cell line has separate pathway of development from distinct primitive cells (Fig. 17.1):

1. The *myeloid series matures into granulocytes and monocytes*. The **granulocytes** are neutrophils, eosinophils and basophils.
2. The *lymphoid series matures into lymphocytes*.

Though monocytes and lymphocytes have some granules, they are not usually visible with commonly used stains. Therefore, monocytes and lymphocytes are traditionally classified under **agranulocytes** (Table 17.1). The leucocytes of granulocytic series develop from myeloblasts that are virtually agranular cells. During the process of development, the precursor cells synthesize proteins and store them in cytoplasmic granules. The enzymes of granules take part in killing organisms:

1. Granulocytes exhibit active motility and migrate to the site of inflammation by amoeboid movement to kill organisms by phagocytosis.
2. Neutrophils are highly amoeboid and phagocytic, and kill a variety of microorganisms, especially bacteria. Therefore, neutrophils are considered as *first line of defense* against acute bacterial infections.
3. Monocytes are also actively phagocytic and are considered as *second line of defense* against infections, especially in chronic and parasitic infections.
4. The eosinophils and basophils are specialized to participate in *allergic inflammatory responses*.
5. Lymphocytes are involved in *immunological responses*:

Life of leucocytes: In general, leucocytes have ***three phases*** in their life: marrow phase, circulatory phase and tissue phase.

1. In the **marrow phase**, they develop from progenitor cells where they proliferate and grow into mature leucocytes and get released into circulation.
2. In the **circulatory phase**, they circulate for few hours before entering into tissues where they live a longer period of their life.
3. In the **tissue phase**, they enter the tissues. In the tissue, monocytes become macrophages that take part in nonspecific defenses of the body as a component of mononuclear phagocyte system.

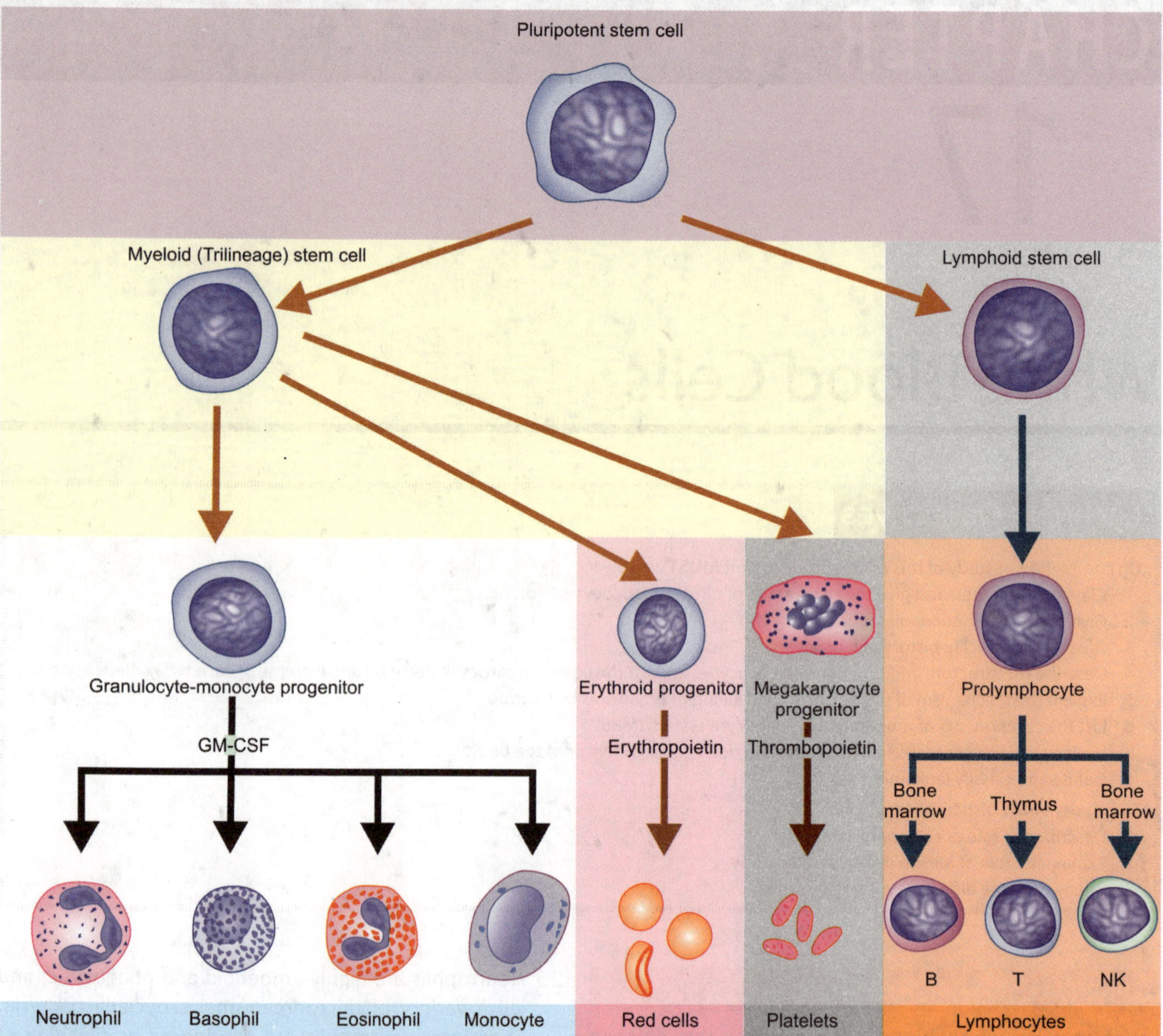

Fig. 17.1: Development of leucocytes. Note, Granulocyte and monocytes develop from myeloid stem cells, and lymphocytes develop from lymphoid stem cells.

Table 17.1: Types of leucocytes and their distribution in peripheral blood as DLC and absolute count.

Leucocytes	Percentage (DLC)	Absolute count (per cu mm)
A. Granulocytes		
1. Neutrophils	50–70	2000–2750
2. Eosinophils	1–4	40–440
3. Basophils	0–1	20–80
B. Agranulocytes		
1. Monocytes	2–8	1500–4000
2. Lymphocytes	20–40	500–800

Usually, life span is 6 to 10 days in the marrow phase, 6 to 8 hours in the circulatory phase and 4 to 5 days or more in tissue phase (Flowchart 17.1)

LEUKOPOIESIS

Leukopoiesis is the development of leucocytes.

Stages of Leukopoiesis

The pluripotent stem cells in the bone marrow give rise to committed stem cells. The committed stem cells in the bone marrow are broadly of two types: The **myeloid stem cells** and **lymphoid stem cells**. The stem cells for lymphoid series form lymphocytes.

The stem cells for myeloid series are ***trilineage stem cells*** that form stem cells for three series of blood cells:

1. Erythroid series for red cells,
2. Megakaryocytic series for platelets and
3. Stem cells for granulocyte-monocyte series.

Flowchart 17.1: Life span of leucocytes (granulocytes and monocytes) in different phases.

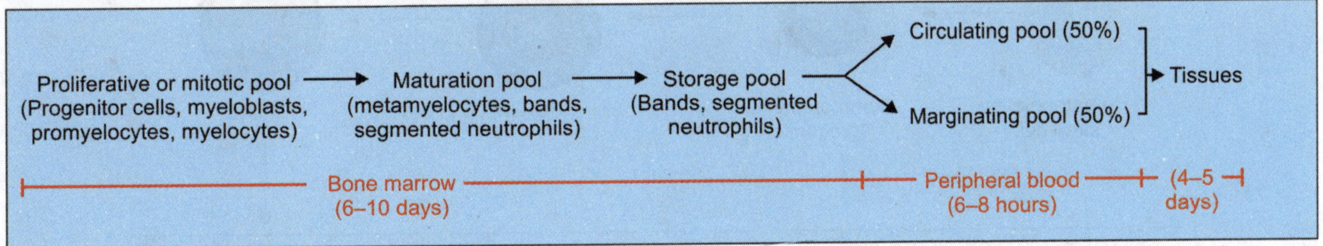

Flowchart 17.2: Details of stages in leucopoiesis.

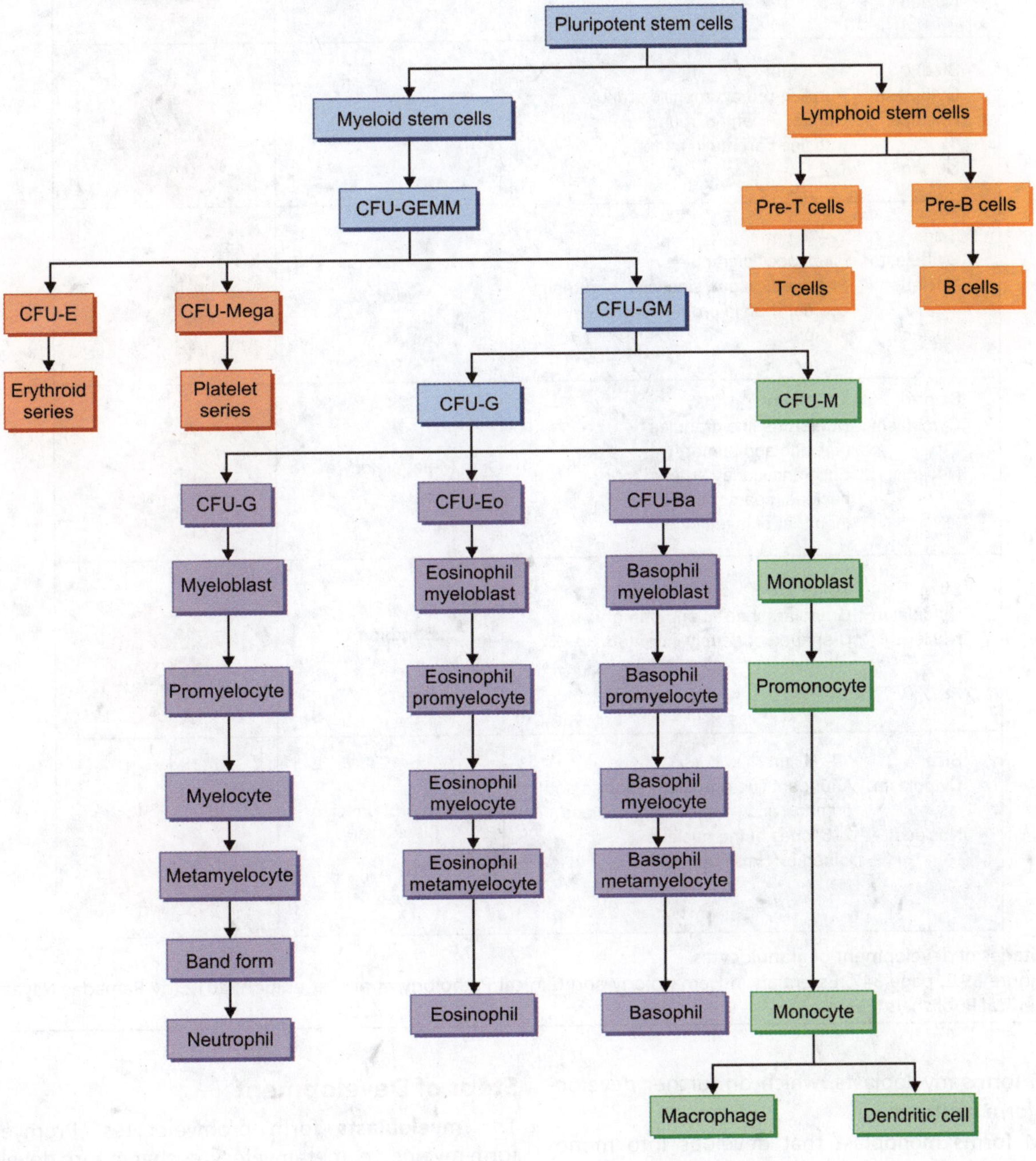

- Pluripotent stem cells
  - Myeloid stem cells → CFU-GEMM
    - CFU-E → Erythroid series
    - CFU-Mega → Platelet series
    - CFU-GM
      - CFU-G
        - CFU-G → Myeloblast → Promyelocyte → Myelocyte → Metamyelocyte → Band form → Neutrophil
        - CFU-Eo → Eosinophil myeloblast → Eosinophil promyelocyte → Eosinophil myelocyte → Eosinophil metamyelocyte → Eosinophil
        - CFU-Ba → Basophil myeloblast → Basophil promyelocyte → Basophil myelocyte → Basophil metamyelocyte → Basophil
      - CFU-M → Monoblast → Promonocyte → Monocyte
        - Macrophage
        - Dendritic cell
  - Lymphoid stem cells
    - Pre-T cells → T cells
    - Pre-B cells → B cells

The stem cells for granulocyte-monocyte of myeloid series give rise to three categories of ***progenitor cells*** (colony forming units or CFUs): CFU-GM, CFU-Eo and CFU-Bas (Flowchart. 17.2):

1. **CFU-GM** is the phagocytic series progenitor cell that on further differentiation from CFU-G (for neutrophils) and CFU-M (for monocytes).
2. The CFUs form ***blast cells.***

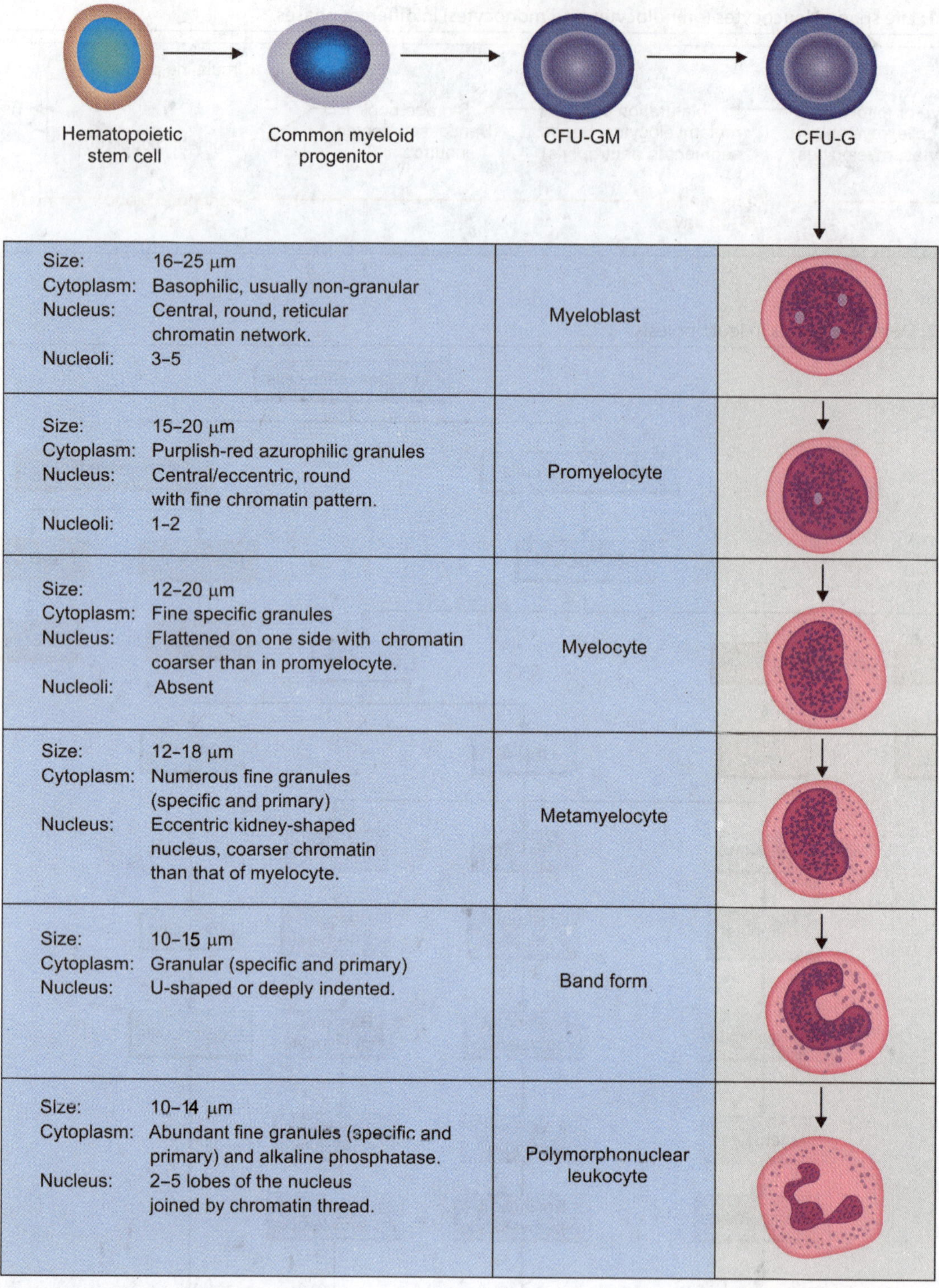

Fig. 17.2: Stages of development of granulocytes.
Courtesy: Figure 39.2, page 347, Essentials in Hematology and Clinical Pathology et al.; 1st edition, 2012, by Ramadas Nayak; Jaypee Brothers Medical Publishers (P) Ltd.

3. CFU-G forms myeloblasts, which on further development form neutrophils.
4. CFU-M forms monoblast that develops into monocytes.
5. CFU-Eo forms eosinophil-myeloblast that develops into eosinophils.
6. CFU-Bas forms basophil-myeloblast that develops into basophils.

Steps of Development

The **myeloblasts** form promyelocytes. Promyelocytes form myelocyte, metamyelocytes that in turn develop into mature leucocytes (Fig. 17.2).

Colony-forming Units

Colony forming units (CFUs) are progenitor cells that develop from committed stem cells. There are different

CFUs for different cell lines (as described above). However, they possess the properties of stem cells and can not be distinguished morphologically.

Blast Cells

These are earliest precursor cells of leucocyte development that are *morphologically distinguishable*:

1. The blast cells for neutrophils are **myeloblasts**, for eosinophil are eosinophil-myeloblasts, and basophils are basophil-myeloblasts, for monocytes are **monoblasts** and for lymphocytes are **lymphoblasts**.
2. The blast cells are large cells (16–20 μm) with large nucleus containing multiple nucleoli.
3. The nucleoli are prominent features of blast cells and are the sites of assembly of ribosomal proteins and r-RNA.
4. The cytoplasm is scanty.
5. Cells are actively mitotic.

Myeloblasts: The earliest precursor cells for neutrophils are myeloblasts. They have scanty blue cytoplasm with 5–10 nucleoli in a large nucleus. There are separate myeloblasts for eosinophils (eosinophil-myeloblasts) and basophils (basophil-myeloblasts).

Monoblasts: These are the blast cells for monocytes. As they resemble myeloblasts morphologically, they are also called myelomonoblasts.

Lymphoblasts: These are blast cells for lymphocytes. They have fewer nucleoli. Nuclear chromatins are clumped.

Promyelocytes and Promonocytes

The promyelocytes and promonocytes develop from myeloblasts and monoblasts respectively:

1. The cells are also large and cytoplasm is granular.
2. Nucleus is round and condensed and contains less nucleoli.
3. Cells are mitotic.
4. **Promonocytes** are larger cells (larger than myeloblasts) that on further development form monocytes, the ***largest cells*** in peripheral blood.
5. The **promyelocytes** are also larger cells and contain large population of **peroxidase-positive granules**. The granules are large in size having diameter of about 500 nm.

Neutrophilic Myelocytes

Myelocytes have diameter of about 12–20 μm:

1. They contain round concentric nucleus. Nucleoli are absent.
2. Cells show some degree of mitosis. About *three cell divisions* occur in this stage of maturation.
3. The characteristic feature of this stage is appearance of **peroxidase negative specific granules**.
4. The granules are usually spherical (about 200 nm) or rod shaped.
5. The peroxidase positive granules are less than peroxidase negative granules. This is because, with each mitotic division, peroxidase positive granules are reduced whereas peroxidase negative granules continue to be formed.

Metamyelocytes

The diameter of metamyelocyte is 12–18 μm. The cells are nondividing (**no mitosis**) and have mixed granule populations.

Neutrophils

Neutrophils developed from metamyelocytes are **juvenile neutrophils** (band forms) that further grow into **matured neutrophils** (segmented neutrophils) (Fig. 17.2).

Regulation of Leukopoiesis

Leucopoiesis is mainly regulated by cytokines (for details of cytokines, refer 'Immunity'), especially, colony stimulating factors (CSFs), interleukins and tumor necrosis factors (TNFs). T lymphocytes, monocytes, fibroblasts, endothelial cells, liver and kidney are the major sources of hemopoietic growth factors (HGFs) (Fig. 17.3). Types, sources and functions of HGFs are listed in Table 17.2.

Interleukins

IL-1, IL-6 and IL-3 promote maturation of stem cells. IL-5 helps in development of eosinophil, and therefore, IL-5 is also called eosinophilic growth factor. IL-3 and IL-4 facilitate development of basophils. IL-2 inhibits myelopoiesis.

Colony-stimulating Factors

There are different colony stimulating factors (CSFs). The important CSFs that influence leucopoiesis are GM-CSF, G-CSF and M-CSF.

GM-CSF: This is the granulocyte-monocyte colony stimulating factor (GM-CSF), secreted by fibroblasts, vascular endothelial cells, monocytes and T lymphocytes. GM-CSF stimulates differentiation and proliferation of pluripotent stem cells into committed cells. GM-CSF also helps in differentiation of CFU into granulocyte and monocyte precursors and their further development into mature cells. It synergizes with IL4 to produce dendritic cells.

G-CSF: This is the granulocyte colony stimulating factor. It is produced by monocytes, endothelial cells and fibroblast. It helps in development and functions of granulocytes.

M-CSF: This is the monocyte colony stimulating factor. This is also called CSF-1. It is produced by fibroblasts, endothelial cells and macrophages. It promotes proliferation of monocytes and macrophages, and also stimulates functions of monocytes.

Tumor Necrosis Factor

Tumor necrosis factors (TNFs) help in proliferation and differentiation of stem cells.

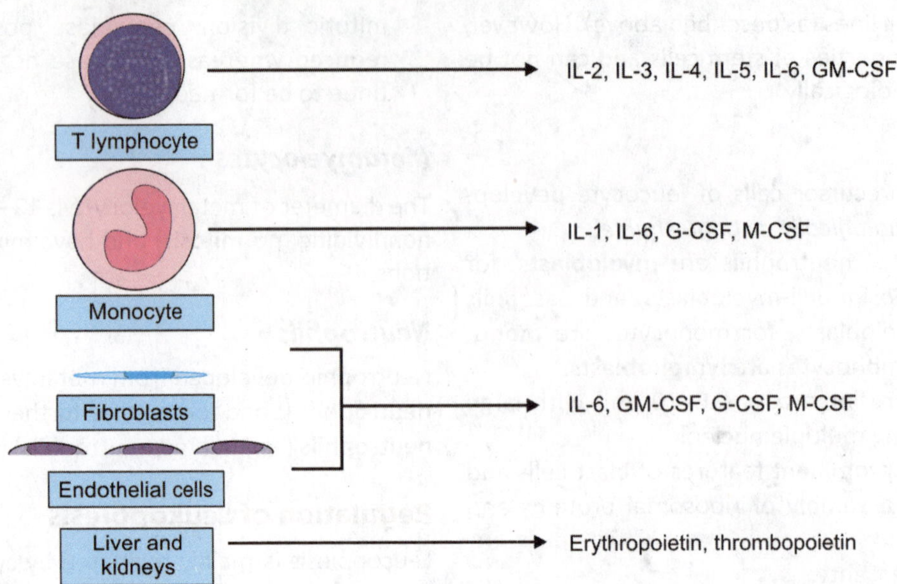

Fig. 17.3: Sources of major hemopoietic growth factors (HGFs).

Table 17.2: Major hemopoietic growth factors their sources and actions.

Sl. No.	Growth factor	Sources	Actions
1.	Interleukin-1 (IL-1)	Activated macrophages	Mediates synthesis and release of acute phase proteins by liver cells, synthesis of other cytokines
2.	Interleukin-2 (IL-2)	T lymphocytes	Growth factor for activated T cells
3.	Interleukin-3 (IL-3)	T lymphocytes	Growth factor for hematopoietic stem cells
4.	Interleukin-6 (IL-6)	T lymphocytes monocytes/ macrophages	Growth factor for B and T lymphocytes mediates acute phase response
5.	C kit ligand (CSF) (Stem cell factor)		Acts with other growth factors to stimulate pluripotent stem cells
6.	GM-CSF	T cells, fibroblasts, endothelial cells	Multilineage growth factor for factor for neutrophils, monocytes/ macrophages,
7.	G-CSF	Monocytes/macrophages, fibroblasts	Lineage restricted growth factor for neutrophils
8.	M-CSF	Monocytes/macrophages, fibroblasts, endothelial cells	Lineage restricted growth factor for monocytes and macrophages
9.	Erythropoietin	Kidneys and liver	Lineage restricted growth factor for erythrocytes
10.	Thrombopoietin	Kidneys and liver	Lineage restricted growth factor for platelets

Life History of Leukocytes

Leucocytes have mainly three phases in their life: The marrow phase, the circulation phase and the tissue phase (Fig. 17.4).

Marrow Phase

This is the phase of development in bone marrow, hence also called **development phase**. Marrow phase has two pools: mitotic pool and maturation pool.

Mitotic Pool

The development from myeloblasts to myelocytes is the phase of mitotic pool, as cells undergo mitosis in these stages.

Maturation Pool

This is the phase of maturation of metamyelocytes into mature cells. Cells do not undergo mitosis in these stages.

Duration of Leucopoiesis: From myeloblast to matured leucocytes, the process of development usually takes 10 days. About 5 days are spent in the mitotic pool (development upto myelocytes) and another five days are utilized in the maturation pool (development from metamyelocyte to the mature cells).

Circulation Phase

The matured cells are released into circulation and remain in circulation for few hours before they enter the tissues (**circulation pool**):

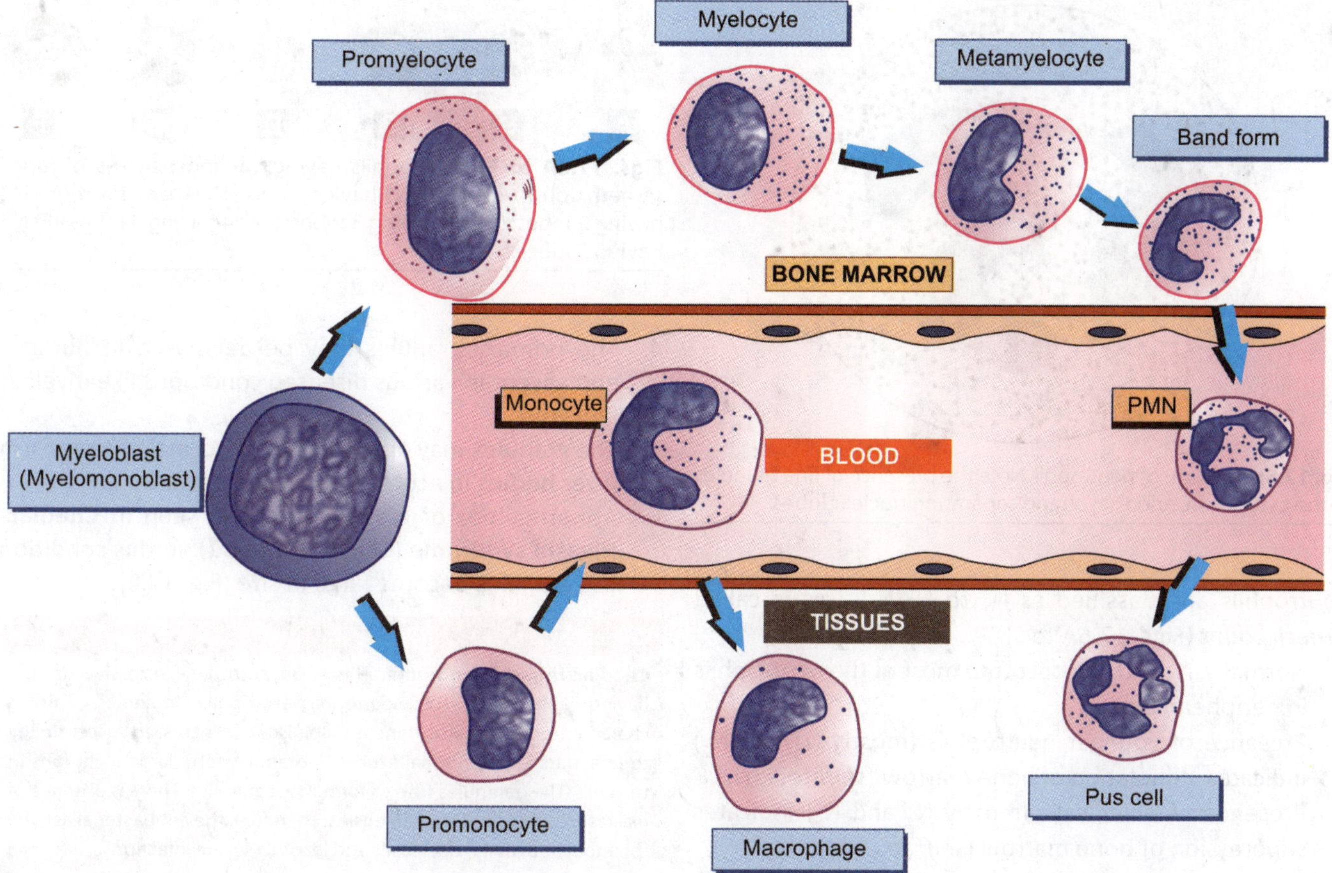

Fig. 17.4: Life cycle of leucocytes. Note three phases of life cycle in bone marrow, blood, and tissues.

1. At rest, many leucocytes especially neutrophils, adhere to the endothelial lining of blood vessels, which is called **margination pool** of leucocytes (Application Box 17.1).
2. In addition, leucocytes actually circulate in the blood (the **active circulation pool**).

Application Box 17.1

Disruption of margination causes leucocytosis: Leucocytes adhere to inner lining of blood vessel, called margination. In exercise and other conditions of increased hemodynamics, the leucocytosis occurs mainly due to disruption of margination of leucocytes.

Tissue Phase

After their activities in circulation, leucocytes enter the tissues. This is called ***tissue pool*** of leucocytes. Granulocytes live for few days in the tissues (Application Box 17.2), whereas monocytes remain for a longer period. In the tissues, monocytes are transformed into **tissue macrophages** that remain for many years.

Application Box 17.2

Apoptosis of leucocytes: Apoptosis is the programmed cell death. This is a physiologic phenomenon of elimination of mature cells from the body. Biochemically, apoptosis occurs due to internucleosomal DNA fragmentation, and morphologically, by nuclear and cytoplasmic condensation. The apoptotic cells are phagocytosed by macrophages. Senescent neutrophils and eosinophils undergo apoptosis.

NEUTROPHILS

Neutrophils are most prevalent leucocytes in blood. They provide the **major defense against acute pyogenic infections**. Neutrophils exhibit ameboid movements. In infections, they migrate to the site of microbial invasion in response to chemical factors. They ingest organisms and kill them. Thus, in neutropenia, body is vulnerable to bacterial infections.

Structure

Neutrophils are common granulocytes. The major identifying features of neutrophils are:

1. The average size of neutrophils varies between 10–14 µm.
2. The cytoplasm of neutrophils contains **fine pink colored granules**.
3. The nucleus is usually **multilobed** and the lobes are connected by thin strand (Fig. 17.5). Nucleus may contain **Barr body** (Application Box 17.3).

It is not known why the segmentation of nucleus of neutrophil occurs. The nucleus of **juvenile neutrophil** is single lobed (*band form*), whereas in mature neutrophils the number of lobes increases with age.

Arneth count: The oldest neutrophils may have 6 or 7 lobes in their nucleus. Based on the nuclear lobes

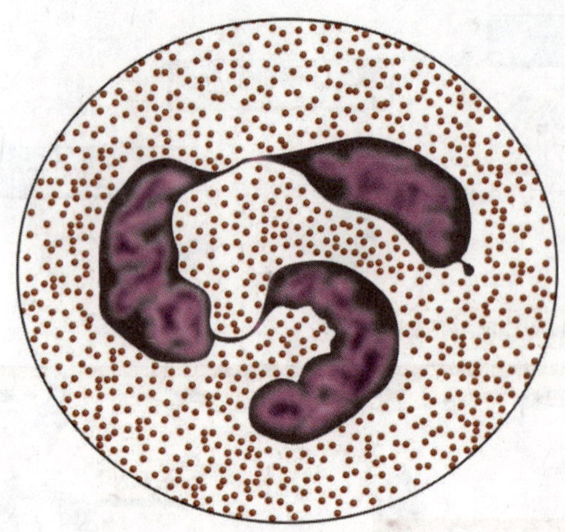

Fig. 17.5: Structure of neutrophil. Note the presence of fine granules in the cytoplasm, and thin strand separating nuclear lobes.

neutrophils are classified as N_1 to N_6/N_7. This is called ***Arneth count*** (Figs. 17.6A to F).

1. Normally, N_2 and N_3 constitute most of the neutrophils in peripheral blood.
2. Presence of younger neutrophils (mostly N_1 and N_2) indicates stimulation of bone marrow (*shift to left*).
3. Presence of older cells (mostly N_4 and N_5) indicates suppression of bone marrow (*shift to right*).
4. Hypersegmented nucleus of neutrophils is typically seen in megaloblastic anemia that occurs due to folate and vitamin B_{12} deficiency (Figs. 17.7A and B).

Application Box 17.3

Sex determination: In females, sex chromatin is present in about 30% of neutrophils as a drumstick appendage attached to the nuclear lobe. Drumstick appendage of chromatin is about 1 µm in length attached to the nucleus by a thin chromatin strand. Presence of this chromatin appendage indicates 2X chromosomes. Thus, it helps in determination of gender of the individual.

Granules of Neutrophils

Neutrophils have **four types of granules**: primary or azurophilic granules, secondary or specific granules, tertiary granules and secretory granules. Primary granules are formed during granulopoiesis, whereas other granules are formed at later stages. The granular contents are determined by the time of their appearance in the leucopoiesis.

Primary Granules

These are *peroxidase positive granules*. They are also called **azurophilic granules**:

1. In addition to myeloperoxidase, they contain lysosomal enzymes and elastase, proteinase and α-1 antitrypsin.
2. They also contain antimicrobial proteins like cathepsin-G, defensins and bactericidal-permeability increasing proteins.
3. Contents of azurophil granules also cause tissue destruction during inflammation.

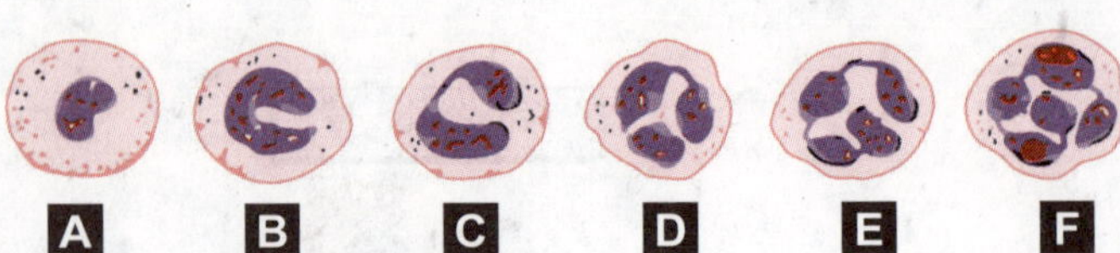

Figs. 17.6A to F: Neutrophils having varying degrees of lobes (Arneth Count). (A and B) N1 having single lobe (band form); (C) N2 having 2 lobes; (D) N3 having 3 lobes; (E) N4 having 4 lobes; (F) N5 having 5 lobes.

4. The primary granules may be decreased in number and absent in various diseased conditions like myeloid leukemia.
5. The granules may also become abnormal as they form **Auer bodies** in acute myeloid leukemia.
6. Abnormalities of granules are also seen in **Chediac-Higashi syndrome** (Clinical Box 17.1). In this condition the granules become large in size (Fig. 17.8).

Clinical Box 17.1

Chediac-Higashi syndrome: This is an autosomal recessive disease having abnormality of neutrophil azurophilic granules. This is characterized by occulocutaneous albinism and increased susceptibility to infection. The abnormal azurophil granules form large inclusions in the cells. The garanules fuse to form megagranules. There is absence of elastase, cathepsin-G and defensins. Therefore, the antibacterial activity (phagocytic activity) decreases and leads to severe infections.

Secondary Granules

By definition, secondary granules do not contain peroxidase (peroxidase negative):

1. They are also called **specific granules**.
2. The secondary granules contain lactoferrin, gelatinase, lysozyme, vitamin B_{12} binding protein and other proteins.
3. Lysozyme is microbicidal and lactoferrin is antibacterial.
4. About 16% granules contain only lactoferrin, 24% contain only gelatinase and 60% contain both.
5. In inflammatory responses, gelatinase containing granules are more readily released than the other granules.
6. The number of specific granules may be decreased in different conditions. The granules may disappear and nuclear lobes may become big giving spectacular appearance in **Pelger-Huet anomaly**. Morphologically, abnormalities of specific granules are **Alder-Reilly anomaly** and **May-Hegglin anomaly** (Fig. 17.8).

Tertiary Granules

Tertiary granules contain gelatinase, alkaline phosphatase and cytochrome-b. The alkaline phosphatase is located on the luminal side of the granule membrane. The low ***leucocyte alkaline phosphatase score is associated with chronic myeloid leukemia***.

Secretory Granules

These are secretory vesicles and different from azurophilic and specific granules. They contain CD3, phospholipase and tyrosine kinase. Toxic granulations occur in severe infections (Clinical Box 17.2).

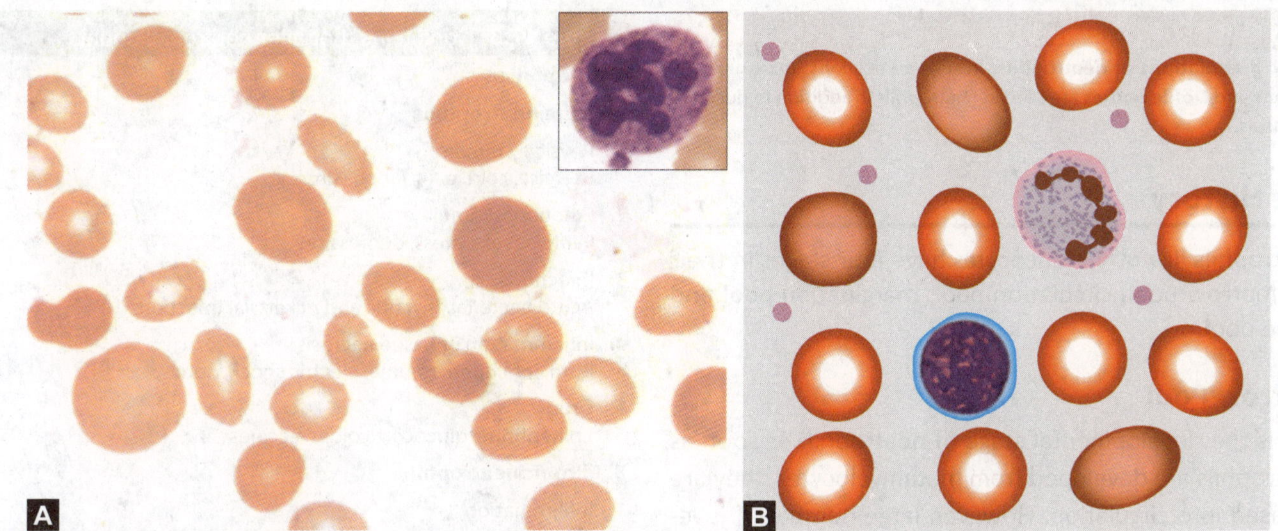

Figs. 17.7A and B: Hypersegmented neutrophil in megaloblastic anemia (in the inset), as shown in original peripheral blood smear (A) and drawn picture of the smear (B).
Courtesy: Figures 4.5A and B, Essentials in Hematology and Clinical Pathology by Ramadas Nayak et al., 1st edition, 2012; Jaypee Brothers Medical Publishers (P) Ltd.

	Mode of inheritance	Characteristic morphology	Appearance of leukocyte	Functional abnormalities
Pelger-Hüet anomaly	Autosomal dominant	Lack of neutrophil nuclear segmentation beyond 2 lobes		Nil
Alder-Reilly anomaly	Autosomal recessive	Large lilac inclusions in cytoplasm of all leukocytes.		Nil
May-Hegglin anomaly	Autosomal dominant	Large basophilic inclusions in all leukocytes. Giant platelets and thrombocytopenia		Abnormal bleeding due to thrombocytopenia
Chediak-Higashi anomaly	Autosomal recessive	Large gray blue granules in cytoplasm of monocytes and granulocytes. Defective lysosomal granules		Poor chemotaxis. increased susceptibility to pyogenic infections. Bleeding tendency
Chronic granulomatous disease of childhood (CGD)	X-linked Autosomal recessive	Normal appearance but defective function		Deficient NADPH oxidase, with absent H_2O_2 production. Phagocytosis and killing of organisms is impaired

Fig. 17.8: Qualitative dysfunctions of neutrophils.
Courtesy: Figure 19.3, Essentials in Hematology and Clinical Pathology by Ramadas Nayak et al., 1st edition, 2012; Jaypee Brothers Medical Publishers (P) Ltd.

Clinical Box 17.2

Toxic granulations of neutrophils: In severe infections, **toxic granulations** and **Döhle bodies** are seen in neutrophils in addition to nuclear pyknosis.

Life History

Neutrophils like other leucocytes have four stages in their life: marrow pool, circulation pool, margination pool and tissue pool.

Marrow Pool

This is the developmental stage of neutrophil. As soon as neutrophils are developed from metamyelocytes, they are released into circulation. However, large number of juvenile neutrophils are present in bone marrow, which constitutes marrow pool of the cell. This ***serves as the reservoir for peripheral neutrophils.***

Circulation Pool

In peripheral blood, about 50% of neutrophils are present in circulation pool that actually circulate in the blood. Rest, 50% remains in the margination pool.

Margination Pool

About 50% of the neutrophils in the blood remain adhered (marginated) to endothelial lining of the blood vessels. This is called margination of leucocytes. Neutrophils present in the margination pool serve as the immediate source for circulation pool. In fact, any factor that causes disruption of margination increases neutrophil count and causes acute leucocytosis.

Tissue Pool

After their usual life in circulation for about 6–8 hours, neutrophils enter tissues where they live for about 4 days.

Neutrophil Count

Normally, neutrophils constitute 50–70% of the total leucocytes in the peripheral blood:

1. The neutrophil count in the blood is maintained due to the balance between **neutrophilopoiesis** that releases neutrophils into circulation and the **shift of neutrophils into marginated and tissue pools**.
2. In circulation, many neutrophils adhere to endothelium called **margination**.
3. Margination is due to firm attachment of neutrophils to endothelial lining, which is mediated by ***selectins***, polypeptides that contain sugar binding site.
4. Temporary release of neutrophils from marginated pool also accounts for increase in count of neutrophils.
5. Neutrophil count alters in various conditions (Table 17.3).

Table 17.3: Conditions that alter neutrophil count.

Conditions
Neutrophilia
A. Acute neutrophilia
1. Physical stimuli Exercise, cold, pain, labor, surgery
2. Emotional stimuli Panic, severe stress, depression
3. Infections Acute bacterial, mycotic and rickettsial infections
4. Inflammation or tissue necrosis Burn, infarction, trauma, electric shock, gout
5. Drugs Epinephrine, glucocorticoids, vaccines
B. Chronic neutrophilia
1. Inflammation Pancreatitis, myositis, colitis, rheumatoid arthritis
2. Endocrine disorder ACTH excess, thyroid storm
3. Tumors Gastric, renal, bronchial and hepatic tumors
4. Blood diseases Chronic hemolysis, meyloproliferative diseases
Neutropenia
A. Decreased neutrophil production
1. Congenital, e. g. Kostmann syndrome
2. Infections: Typhoid and paratyphoid fevers
3. Drugs: Chloramphenicol, phenylbutazone, phenytoin
4. Aplastic anemia
B. Increased neutrophil destruction
1. Parasitic infections: Malaria, kala azar
2. Viral infections: Measles, influenza
3. Hypersplenism
4. Autoimmune diseases: SLE, Felty syndrome

Functions

Neutrophil is actively phagocytic. They contain many antimicrobial and bactericidal chemicals in their granules (*see* above). Therefore, neutrophils are capable of ingesting and killing microbial organisms. During inflammation due to acute bacterial infections, neutrophils soon migrate to the site of infection and kill the organisms. Hence, neutrophils are considered as the first line of defense against acute bacterial infections. Neutrophils provide major nonspecific defense against invasion of pyogenic organisms. Consequently, neutropenia predisposes body to pyogenic infection.

Neutrophil Phagocytosis

Phagocytosis is the process of ingestion and killing of microbes or a foreign substance by a phagocyte. Actively phagocytic cells are neutrophils, monocytes and macrophages. Steps of phagocytosis include chemotaxis, diapedesis, adherence, ingestion and killing (Fig. 17.9).

Chemotaxis

Chemotaxis is the process of migration of neutrophils to the site of infection. The bacterial invasion triggers acute inflammatory response:

1. The chemical substances are released from the site of inflammation or infection by the infecting organisms or inflammatory cells.
2. These chemical factors attract neutrophils to the site of infection. Consequently, they are called **chemotaxins** (*taxin* means movement; chemical that produces movement is a chemotaxin) or ***chemoattractants*** or ***chemotactic factors***.

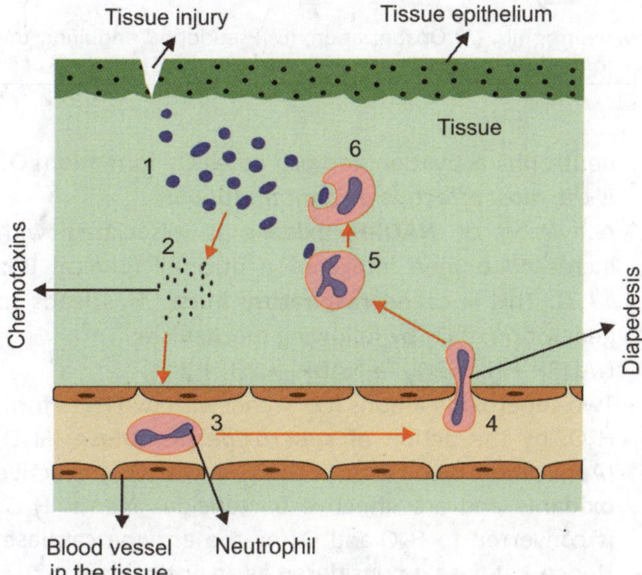

Fig. 17.9: General steps of phagocytosis by neutrophil. (1) Invasion of organism into the tissue; (2) Release of chemotaxins from organism and injured tissue; (3) Chemotaxis; (4) Diapedesis; (5) Opsonization and adherence; (6) Ingestion and killing.

3. Chemotaxins are usually the microbial products or chemicals secreted from leucocytes or chemicals released from damaged tissue.
4. Complement proteins, especially C5a and C3 also act as chemotaxins.
5. During chemotaxis, neutrophils change their shape and become highly ameboid.
6. Also, the bone marrow is stimulated in response to plasma factors and more neutrophils are produced.

Diapedesis

The neutrophils must enter the tissue from their circulation pool to kill organisms at the site of inflammation in the tissue. The process, by which neutrophils pass through the capillary endothelial cells to reach the invader in the tissue, is called diapedesis. The activated neutrophils first marginate (**margination and pavementing**) adhere tightly to endothelial lining (**rolling and adhesion**) with the help of L-selectins and then by their ameboid movement they squeeze through the space between endothelial cells (**emigration and diapedesis**) (Figs. 17.10A to D).

Opsonization and Adherence

The process by which the bacteria are made tasty to the phagocyte is called opsonization. In this process, antigen is coated by opsonins. The chemicals that facilitate the process of opsonization are called **opsonins**:

1. **IgG antibody** and complement proteins (C5a, C3b) are known high-quality opsonins.
2. Bacteria coated by opsonins bind to the receptor on the neutrophil membrane. The attachment of membrane of phagocyte to the membrane of microbe is called ***adherence***.

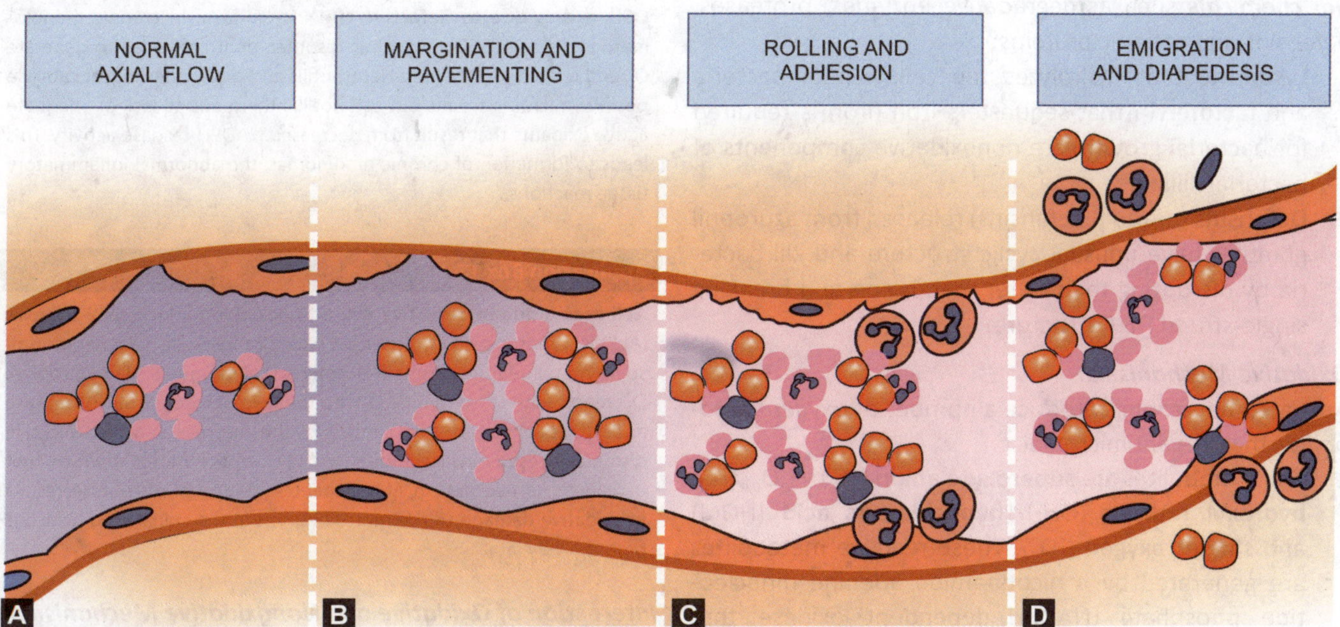

Figs. 17.10A to D: Details of diapedesis of neutrophils. It occurs in three phases: margination and pavementing, rolling and adhesion, and emigration and diapedesis.

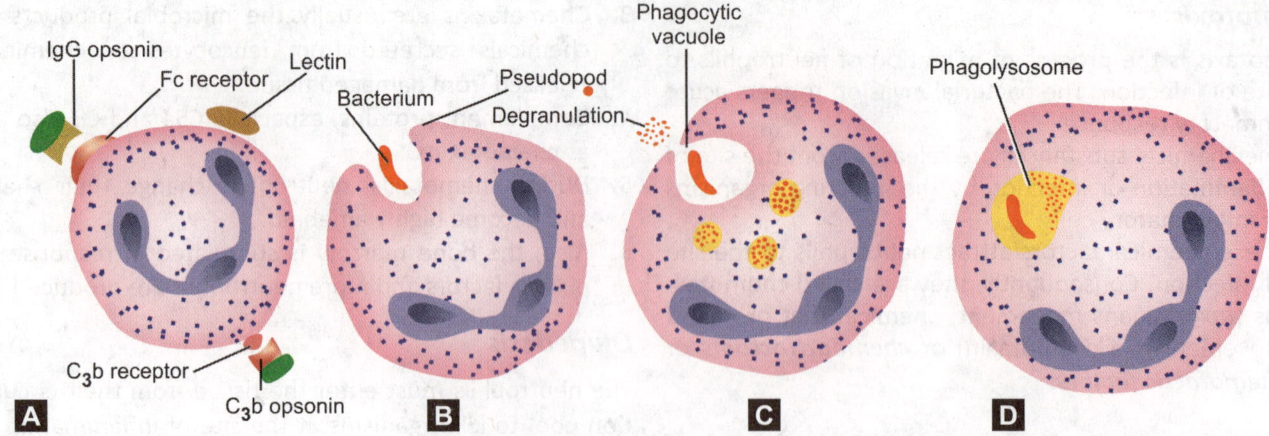

Figs. 17.11A to D: Details of opsonization, endocytosis and killing by neutrophils. (A) Opsonization; (B) Pseudopod engulfing the opsonized particle; (C) Phagocytic vacuole formation; (D) Phagolysosome formation.

3. Opsonization facilitates the process of adherence (Fig. 17.11A).

Ingestion (Endocytosis)

Adherence facilitates motor activity of neutrophils. The membrane of phagocyte extends projections from both the sides to encroach on to the microbe (Fig. 17.11B). These extensions are called pseudopodia. Pseudopodia finally surround the microbe and form phagocytic vesicle (Fig. 17.11C). The phagocytic vesicle fuses with the lysosome to form ***phagolysosome*** (Fig. 17.11D).

Killing

The bactericidal (killing of bacteria) mechanisms can broadly be divided into two types: nonoxidative and oxidative.

Nonoxidative Mechanisms

Neutrophil granules contain a wide variety of ***antibacterial chemicals*** such as degradative enzymes, proteases, defensins and cationic proteins:

1. **Lysozyme** that hydrolyzes the cell wall of bacteria and **lactoferrin** that sequesters iron (iron is required for bacterial growth) are nonoxidative components of bacterial killing.
2. **Defensins** (α and β defensins) released from azurophil granules have unusual cyclic structure and kill bacteria by disrupting their outer membrane and breaking single-strand DNA structure.

Oxidative Mechanisms

Activated neutrophils produce a number of *oxygen metabolites* that are antimicrobial.

1. The metabolites are **superoxide anion** (O_2^-), H_2O_2, **free hydroxyl radicals** (OH·), **hypochlorous acid** (HOCl) and **singlet oxygen** ($'O_2$). These reactive metabolites are generated by a nicotinamide adenine dinucleotide phosphate (NADPH)-dependent oxidase that reduces molecular oxygen to O_2^-. The oxidase is quiescent in resting neutrophils and is stimulated following neutrophil activation and promotes O_2^- formation. ***O_2^- is the most effective oxidant metabolite***.
2. Activation of **NADPH oxidase** is associated with increased oxygen intake of neutrophil (Clinical Box 17.3). This is called **respiratory burst**. This leads to generation of O_2^- by following mechanism:
$NADPH + H^+ + 2O_2 \rightarrow NADP^+ + 2H^+ + 2\,O_2^-$
Two **superoxide anions** (O_2^-) react with two H^+ to form H_2O_2 by the action of ***superoxide dismutase*** (SOD) (Application Box 17.4). Both O_2^- and H_2O_2 are **active oxidants** and are effective bactericidal agents. H_2O_2 is converted to H_2O and O_2 by the enzyme **catalase**. Hence, catalase is considered as an **antioxidant**.
3. **Myeloperoxidase**, the enzyme of primary granules facilitate conversion of Cl^- to HOCl, which is also a potent oxidant.

Clinical Box 17.3

CGD occurs due to defective NADPH-oxidase: In chronic granulomatous disease (CGD), a genetic disorder, neutrophils fail to generate O_2^- and related metabolites. Neutrophils and monocytes ingest catalase positive microorganisms but can not kill them due to lack of adequate active oxidants that result from decreased NADPH-oxidase activity. This leads to formation of chronic granulomas, the abnormal inflammatory tissue reactions.

Application Box 17.4

ALS occurs due to defective dismutase: Amyotrophic lateral sclerosis (ALS) is a motor system disease in which progressive degeneration of spinal motor neurons results in atrophy of skeletal muscles (amyotrophy). O_2^- reacts with H^+ to form $H_2O_2$with the help of cytoplasmic dismutase and $H_2O_2$is converted to H_2O and O_2 by the enzymes catalase. Defective dismutase results in accumulation of O_2^- in the motor neurons that damages the neurons. In ALS, genetic mutation of dismutase results in oxidative damage to the motor neurons in the spinal cord, which is progressively fatal.

Interaction of Oxidative and Nonoxidative Mechanisms

Nonoxidative mechanism facilitates the activity of oxidative mechanism for bacterial killing. The protease enzymes

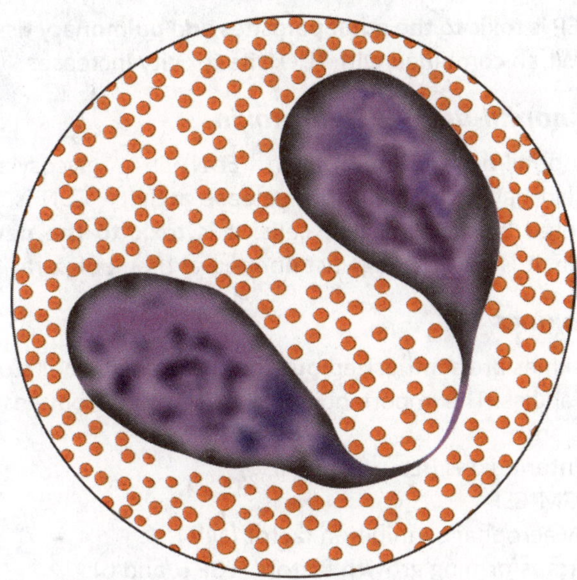

Fig. 17.12: Structure of eosinophil. Note the presence of brick red coarse granules in the cytoplasm, and spectacular nuclear lobes.

of primary granules and collagenase enzymes of secondary granules produce a **killing zone** around the activated neutrophil by locally damaging the inflammatory tissue, which helps the oxidant metabolites to promote their bactericidal properties. However, in diseases like rheumatoid arthritis, this becomes detrimental due to destruction of larger quantity of host tissue.

Applied Aspects

Chemotaxis and phagocytosis require active movements of neutrophil. When neutrophil is activated, its **cytosolic calcium concentration** increases that promotes contraction of microfilaments, microtubules and myosin-1 filaments. This increases the ameboid movement and activity of neutrophils. **Neutrophil hypomotility**, a ***primary phagocytic dysfunction*** of neutrophil, decreases phagocytic activity. There are about 15 primary disorders of neutrophil function.

EOSINOPHILS

Eosinophils are known for their protective function **against allergy** including asthma, and helminthic parasite infections. Like neutrophils, eosinophils produce *proinflammatory mediators*:

1. Eosinophil-specific granule proteins are toxic for many mammalian cells and parasitic larvae.
2. In addition, **cytokines** produced by eosinophil such as leukotrienes and PAF, aid to their defense functions.
3. Eosinophils have short life span in circulation, whereas they **live longer in tissue**. They are primarily tissue dwelling cells. There are 100 eosinophils in tissue to 1 eosinophil in peripheral blood.
4. Eosinophils are present in the epithelia of respiratory, gastrointestinal and genitourinary tract.

Table 17.4: Eosinophil-derived chemicals.

A. Granule derived chemicals
1. Major basic protein
2. Eosinophil cationic protein
3. Eosinophil peroxidase
4. Eosinophil-derived neurotoxin
5. Lysophospholipase
6. Phospholipase D
7. Arylsulphatase
8. Acid phosphatase
9. Catalase
10. Histaminase
11. Hexoseaminidase
B. Cytokines (may or may not be stored in granules)
1. GM-CSF
2. TGF-α and TGF-β
3. Macrophage inhibition factor (MIF)
4. IL_{1-6}, IL_8 and IL_{12}
5. Tumor necrosis factor (TNF- α)
C. Lipid-derived chemicals
1. Leukotriene C
2. Platelet activating factor
3. PGE_1 and PGE_2
4. Thromboxane B_2

5. Their production and function are mainly influenced by **IL-5**. IL-5 also stimulates production and function of basophils that are closely related to eosinophils.

Structure

Eosinophils are granular leucocytes having the size same as that of neutrophils. However, the **granules are coarse and brick red** in color in blood smear stained by Leishman stain. Moreover, the **nucleus is usually bilobed** and the lobes are separated by a thick strand. This gives eosinophil nucleus an appearance of a pair of ***spectacles*** (Fig. 17.12). The granules are plenty, and sometimes encroach uopn the nucleus.

Chemicals Secreted by Eosinophils

Eosinophil secretes various chemicals that mediate many physiological activities. These chemicals may be divided into three categories: chemicals secreted from granules, cytokines, and lipid-derived chemicals (Table 17.4). The last two groups of chemicals are secreted from many other cells, whereas chemicals secreted from granules are eosinophil specific.

Eosinophil Granular Contents

The granules of eosinophil contain following major chemicals:

1. Major basic protein
2. Eosinophil cationic protein
3. Eosinophil-derived peroxidase
4. Eosinophil-derived neurotoxin
5. Cytokines
6. Other chemicals

Major Basic Protein

Major basic protein (MBP) is major ***toxic product*** of eosinophil. It is toxic against many intestinal parasites and their larvae such as:

1. Schistosomula (a larva of *S. mansoni*, which is an intestinal parasite, blood fluke) and the larva of *Ancylostoma duodenale* (hookworm)
2. *Ascaria lumbricoid* (roundworm)
3. *Toxocara canis*
4. *Wuchereria banccrofti* (filarial larva)
5. *Trichinella spiralis*
6. *Strongyloides stercoralis* (threadworm).

Eosinophil adheres with the IgG coated larva and this adherence results in secretion of MBP from eosinophil into the integument of the larva that causes damage to the larval tissue.

- MBP is also *toxic to pneumocytes and epithelial cells of respiratory tract*.
- MBP also makes the bronchial tree **hyper-responsive to bronchoconstrictors**.
- Therefore, these worm infestations are usually associated with respiratory symptoms like bronchial asthma (Clinical Box 17.4).
- Eosinophil peroxidase (EP) and MBP activate platelets, basophils and mast cells.
- Basophils also contain MBP, but the concentration is only 2% of eosinophils.

Clinical Box 17.4

Asthma like symptoms occurs in worm infestations: MBP released from eosinophil granules to kill worms, Is also toxic to lungs. MBP makes the bronchial tree hyper-reactive to bronchoconstrictors. Therefore, these worm infestations are usually associated with respiratory symptoms like bronchial asthma.

Eosinophil Cationic Protein

Eosinophil cationic protein (ECP) is rich in arginine.

- Though ECP has 66% structural homology with eosinophil-derived neurotoxin (EDN) and 31% homology with pancreatic ribonuclease, its ribonuclease activity is less compared to the ribonuclease activity of EDN.
- ECP is **toxic to helminthic parasites and tracheal epithelium**.
- ECP along with EDN produces **neurotoxicity**.

Eosinophil Peroxidase

Eosinophil peroxidase (EP) is a *heme containing protein*.

- It has 68% homology with neutrophil myeloperoxidase and other peroxidases.
- EP is **toxic to the adult parasites and pulmonary tissue**.
- When combined with H_2O_2, its toxicity increases.

Eosinophil-derived Neurotoxin

Eosinophil-derived neurotoxin (EDN) is a glycosylated protein having striking **ribonuclease activity**. EDN is also secreted by mononuclear cells. It is **toxic to the neural tissue**. It is not toxic against nonneural tissue of parasites.

Cytokines

Cytokines are synthesized outside the granules but stored in granules. The important cytokines secreted from eosinophils are:

1. Interleukins (IL_{1-6}, IL_8 and IL_{12})
2. GM-CSF
3. Macrophage inhibition factor (MIF)
4. Transforming growth factors (TGF α and β)
5. Tumor necrosis factor-α.

TGF-α mediates the important role of eosinophil in wound healing. Many of the cytokines like interleukins such as IL_5, IL_3 and GM-CSF act in autocrine fashion as eosinophil growth factor. MIF plays a role in the genesis of adult respiratory distress syndrome.

Other Chemicals

Lysophospholipase constitutes 10% of eosinophil proteins. The enzymes secreted from eosinophils like **phospholipase D, arylsulphatase-B, acid phosphatase, catalase and histaminase** are other granular proteins that take part in ***eosinophil-mediated inflammatory reactions*** and ***killing of parasites***.

Functions

Like neutrophils, eosinophils migrate into the tissues. There are selective chemoattractants for eosinophils such as **eosinophil chemotactic factor of anaphylaxis** (ECF-A). ECF-A in humans is a tetrapeptide that facilitates tissue accumulation of eosinophils. Eosinophils exhibit endothelial cell adhesion and chemotaxis to migrate into the tissues. Eosinophils participate in two important defense mechanisms of the body:

1. Against helminthic infections
2. Against allergy.

In Helminthic Infections

Eosinophils attack intestinal parasites especially the larva of S. mansoni, Trichinella spiralis, Toxocara canis, N. brasilensis, Fasciola hepatica, roundworms and hook worms:

1. They attack the larva opsonized by IgG, IgE and complements. First, eosinophils attach themselves to the larva, which activates the eosinophils.
2. Within about 3 hours of this adherence, the activated eosinophils secrete proteins from their granules onto surface of the larva.

Table 17.5: Causes of eosinophilia and eosinopenia.

A. Eosinophilia
1. Helminthic infections – Ascariasis (roundworm) – Filariasis – Toxocariasis – Ancylostomiasis (hookworm) – Stongyloidiasis – Trichinosis – Schistosomiasis – Fascioliasis – Echinococcosis
2. Allergic diseases
– Bronchial asthma – Allergic rhinitis – Atopic dermatitis – Urticaria – Food allergy – Hay fever
3. Drug reactions (drug allergy)
4. Eosinophilic leukemia
5. Tropical pulmonary eosinophilia
6. Addison's disease
7. Eosinophilia-myalgia syndrome
B. Eosinopenia
1. Glucocorticoid therapy
2. Cushing's syndrome
3. Aplastic anemia
4. Drug-induced agranulocytosis

3. Once, the tegument is breached, eosinophils crawl under it and secrete toxic mediators that destroy the tissues of larva and phgocytose the larva or larval fragments.
4. In this process, degranulation of eosinophils occurs.

In Allergy

In allergic condition like bronchial asthma, eosinophils play a major role in pathogenesis:

1. Bronchial hyper-reactivity is correlated with eosinophilia and airway eosinophil content.
2. Inhibition of airway eosinophilia by glucocorticoid has been reported to cause improvement in bronchial hyper-responsiveness and asthmatic symptoms.
3. Though, glucocorticoid causes eosinopenia by eosinophil apoptosis, the main mechanism is the inhibition of production of IL_5 and IL_3 from type 2 helper cells (T_4 lymphocytes).
4. It is not clear whether eosinophils prevent allergy and therefore eosinophilia occurs in allergy or eosinophilia in allergy aggravates the situation.
5. However, recruitment of eosinophil at the site of allergic inflammation is accompanied by increase in number of activated T cells and monocytes.

Table 17.6: Differences between basophils and mast cells.

	Basophils	**Mast cells**
Origin	Bone marrow	Bone marrow
Cells in blood	Present	Absent
Normal residence in connective tissue	No	Yes
Life span	Few days	Few months
Growth factor	IL-3	SCF
Major secretion	Histamine, IL-4,	Histamine, heparin
Receptors for	IgE, IgG	IgE

6. It has been proposed that asthma is an eosinophil-mediated disease driven by type-2 helper lymphocytes that secrete IL_5 and IL_3.

Alterations in Eosinophil Count

The normal eosinophil count is 2–4% in differential count (by examining blood smear), or 40–440 per µl of blood in absolute count (by hemocytometry). When eosinophil count is more than normal, called eosinophilia and less than normal, called eosinopenia (Table 17.5).

BASOPHILS AND MAST CELLS

Basophils are least frequent granulocytes. They account for less than 0.5% of leucocytes in blood. Though they recruit into tissues in response to immunological and inflammatory reactions, unlike eosinophils they ordinarily do not reside in the tissue. Though basophils and mast cells resemble functionally, they are not identical (Table 17.6):

1. Mast cells are derived from blood precursors, but they mainly reside in the connective tissues, particularly beneath the epithelial surfaces and around the blood vessels, where they live a longer period.
2. Basophils and mast cells have high-affinity receptors for IgE on their surface.
3. As IgE is a reagin antibody, these cells mediate many allergic responses of the body.
4. Basophils and mast cells also contribute to protect host responses associated with IgE production.

Structure

Basophils

Identifying features of basophils are (Fig. 17.13):

1. They have the same diameter as of neutrophils (10–14 µm).
2. The nucleus is usually less segmented and often appear 'S' shaped.
3. Nuclear chromatin shows marked condensation.

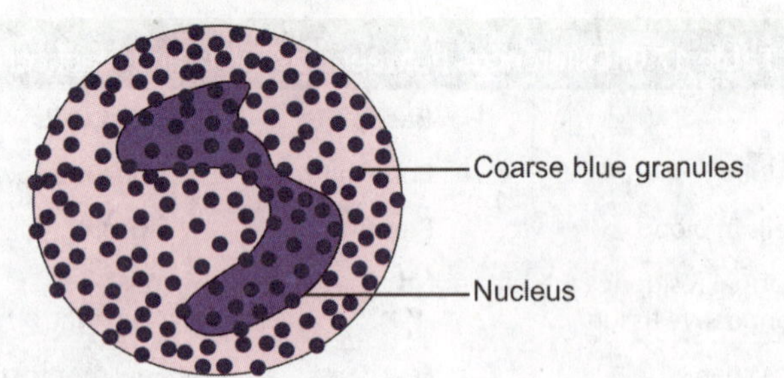

Fig. 17.13: Structure of basophil.

4. The granules are large in size and oval or round in shape, and more in number. As cell is heavily studded with granules, nucleus is often not visible. Granules are surrounded by membranes and contain dense particles called **Chracot-Lyeden crystals**.
5. Cytoplasm contains glycogen deposits, mitochondria, free-ribososmes and few lipid bodies.

Basophil granules secrete histamine, chondroitin sulphate, tryptase, carboxypeptidase A, cathepsin G, leukotrienes, eosinophil chemotactic factor of anaphylaxis (ECF-A), neural protease and MBP.

Mast Cells

Mast cells that remain in the tissues are round or elongated cells with nonsegmented nucleus. Granules are numerous, but smaller in size. There are many cytoplasmic filaments, numerous lipid bodies and no glycogen deposits. **Mast cell granules** secrete histamine, heparin, chondroitin sulphate, carboxypeptidase, cathepsin, ECF-A and neural protease. There are two types of mast cells: **mucosal mast cells** (mast cell present in the mucosa) and **connective tissue mast cell.**

Differences between Basophils and Mast Cells

Though there are functional homology between basophils and mast cells, there are many differences between them (Table 17.6).

Functions

Basophils and mast cells are mainly involved in allergic reactions. During allergy, these cells release the content of their granules. Mediators such as histamine released by degranulation produce antimicrobial and anti-host effects. The usual stimulus for basophil and mast cell degranulation is an allergen, which should ideally cross-link IgE molecule bound to the surface of basophils or mast cells via its high affinity Fc receptor for IgE.

Role in Acute Allergic Reactions

Basophils and mast cells have receptors for Fc region of IgE:

1. IgE binds to membrane of these cells and initiate degranulation. This leads to release of **histamine.** Acute allergies such as acute rhinitis, urticaria, food allergy etc are mediated by this mechanism.
2. However, massive release of histamine produces immediate hypersensitivity reactions, also known as **anaphylaxis**. Anaphylaxis is acute systemic allergic reaction that occurs in conditions like injections of penicillin or xylocaine anesthesia in sensitive individuals.
3. In anaphylaxis, histamine released from basophils and mast cells cause vasodilation and inhibition of cardiac output that lead to acute hypotension.

Role in Chronic Allergic Reactions

Basophils and mast cells also contribute to late-phase reactions. In chronic allergic conditions such as bronchial asthma, basophils and mast cells are recruited to the site of allergy. Especially, mast cells secrete cytokines that attract leucocytes, eosinophils and basophils, which in turn mediate chronic allergy. This mechanism of pathogenesis of late-phase reaction is termed as **mast cell-leucocyte cascade**.

Role in T-cell Dependent Responses

Activation of mast cells in the affected tissues along with infiltration of basophils occurs in a variety of T-cell dependent immunological responses. T-cells secrete growth factors for basophils and mast cells.

Role in Host Defense

Basophils and mast cells play critical role in host resistance to some viral, bacterial and parasitic infections. These cells increase in conditions like chicken pox, small pox and tuberculosis.

Normal Count

Normal basophil count is 0–1%, and absolute count is 20–80 per µl of blood. Mast cells are normally not found in blood. Increase in basophil count is called basophilia and decrease in count is called basopenia (Table 17.7).

Mastocytosis

Secondary increase in mast cell count usually occurs in allergic conditions like asthma, and connective tissue disorders like rheumatoid arthritis. However, primary increase in mast cell number occurs in a group of systemic disorders combinely called as **systemic mastocytosis**. Depending on the degree of mastocytosis, the condition has been classified into 4 categories:

Category I: Indolent mastocytosis as seen in urticaria pigmentosa.

Category II: Mastocytosis with meyloproliferative disorder.

Category III: Aggressive mastocytosis i.e., lymphadenopathic mastocytosis with eosinophilia.

Category IV: Mast cell leukemia.

Table 17.7: Alteration in basophil count.

A. Basophilia
1. Allergic and inflammatory conditions – Ulcerative colitis – Erythroderma – Urticaria – Drug and food hypersensitivity
2. Infections – Chicken pox – Small pox – Influenza – Tuberculosis
3. Endocrinal disorders – Myxedema (hypothyroidism) – Diabetes mellitus
4. Iron deficiency
5. Basophilic leukemia
6. Polycythemia
B. Basopenia
1. Cortisol therapy
2. Cushing's syndrome
3. Hyperthyroidism
4. Ovulation
5. Hypersensitivity reactions

MONOCYTES AND MACROPHAGES

Monocyte is the largest leucocyte in the peripheral blood. After spending life in blood, monocytes enter the tissues, where they are transformed into macrophages:

1. Monocytes and macrophages are mononuclear phagocytes.
2. In the tissues, they play an important role in nonspecific defense against microbial invasion.
3. The tissue macrophage system was previously called as ***reticuloendothelial system*** (the term has become obsolete). Presently, this is known as **mononuclear phagocyte system**.
4. Monocyte is the **second line of defense against** microbial infections.

Monocytes

Morphology

Monocytes are the largest blood cells. The identifying features are:

1. The diameter of monocytes varies between 12–25 µm.
2. The nucleus occupies half of the cell and remains eccentrically. Cytoplasmic-nuclear ratio is 50:50.
3. Often the nucleus is reniform (kidney shaped), but may be horse-shoe shaped, round or irregular (Fig. 17.14).

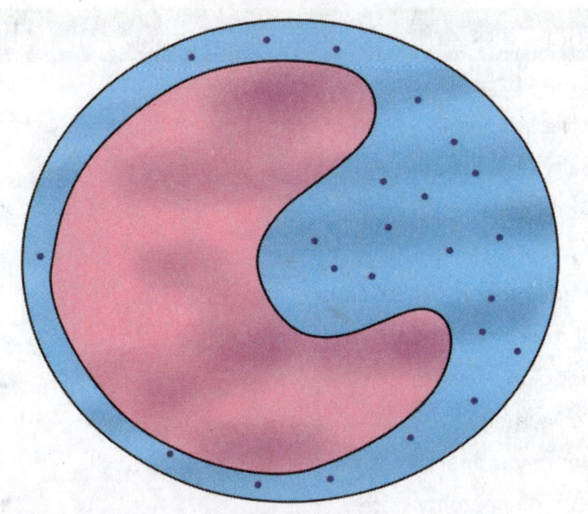

Fig. 17.14: Structure of monocyte.

4. There are characteristic fine nuclear chromatin net connecting small chromatin clumps. This gives the nucleus a **non-homogenous** or **stringy appearance**.
5. Cytoplasm is abundant and ground glass in appearance.
6. Though monocyte is traditionally classified as agranular leucocytes, fine pink-purple granules are present in about 40% of cells. Sometimes, large azurophil granules are also seen in monocytes. The monocyte granules contain hydrolytic enzymes such as acid phosphatase, lysozymes, etc. However, alkaline phosphatase is absent.

Monocytes have a number of receptors on its surface such as Fc receptors for IgG, IgA and IgE, receptors for complements, cytokines, and hormones like insulin, glucocorticoid and angiotensin. Monocytes and macrophages express HLA class II and their receptors on their surface that help in antigen presentation.

Functions

1. **Phagocytosis and microbial killing:** Monocyte is an active phagocyte:
   - It exhibits ***motility and chemotaxis***.
   - The presence of various ***surface receptors*** enhances their phagocytic activity by facilitating the recognition of various host-derived factors including immunoglobulins, complements, and integrins.
   - The receptors also *identify various sugar units* on microbial membranes.
   - The organisms once phagocytosed, are destroyed by **oxidants** produced by NADPH oxidase, nitric oxide synthase, and intracellular hydrolytic enzymes.
   - Monocyte also ***kills intracellular pathogens*** like viruses, and parasites.
   - Monocyte is the **second line of defense** against infections.
2. **Antigen presentation:** Monocyte is an important ***antigen presenting cell*** (APC):

Table 17.8: Causes of alteration in monocyte count.

A. Monocytopenia
1. Aplastic anemia
2. Hairy cell leukemia
3. Septicemia
B. Monocytosis
1. Acute monocytic leukemia
2. Chronic myelomonocytic leukemia
3. Hodgkin's disease
4. Polycythemia vera
5. Hemolytic anemia
6. Postsplenectomy state
7. Cytomegalovirus infection
8. Collagen diseases
9. Malaria
10. Kala azar
11. Glucocorticoid therapy
12. Chronic idiopathic monocytosis

- Partially digested product of the antigen (Ag) combines with the MHC II molecules produced by APC, and MHC + Ag complex expresses on the surface of APC.
- Lymphocytes, especially T cells are activated when they come in contact with MHC + Ag present on the APC surface.
- This is the first step in the activation of cellular immunity.

3. **Release of cytokines:** Monocyte secretes various chemokines that carry out different physiological functions:
   - Monocyte produces ***IL-1 and IL-6*** that are essential for coactivation of immunological responses.
   - Monocyte secretes ***TNF-α and interferons*** that facilitate killing of viruses and other microbial organisms.
   - Monocyte also secretes various ***growth factors*** like GM-CSF, M-CSF and erythroid colony potentiating factor that promote leucopoiesis and erythropoiesis, and transforming growth factors (TGF), PDGF and fibroblast growth factors (FGF).
   - Monocytes by secreting ***complement factors*** augment the local tissue defense responses.
   - Monocyte releases various ***enzymes*** like collagenase, elastase, plasminogen activator, etc. that participate in wound healing and tissue remodeling.

Life Span

Monocytes in circulation have a wide range of half life between 10–72 hours. Then, they enter the tissues where they live few weeks to months. The average life in tissues is three months. In tissue, they are transformed into **tissue macrophages**. If there is tissue infection or inflammation, within few hours monocytes migrate to the site of injury. However, initially the monocyte numbers are less than neutrophils. If inflammation persists for more than 12 hours, monocytes predominate over neutrophils.

Table 17.9: Distribution of cells of mononuclear phagocyte system.

A. In blood – Monocytes
B. In bone marrow – Monoblasts – Promonocytes
C. In tissues – Kupffer cell in liver – Osteoclasts in bone marrow – Alveolar macrophages in lungs – Histiocytes in connective tissue – Microglia in brain – Red pulp macrophages in spleen – Macrophages in lymph nodes and thymus – Messangial cells in kidney – Dendritic cells/histiocytes in skin – Type A cells in synovium
D. In body cavities – Pleural macrophages – Peritoneal macrophages
E. In inflammatory tissues – Epitheloid cells – Multinucleate giant cells

Normal Count

Normal monocyte count is 2–8%, and the average absolute count is 400/μl of blood. Increase in count is called monocytosis and decrease in count is called monocytopenia (Table 17.8). The monocyte count is more in neonates and infants, which is about 1000/μl of blood. Men tend to have slightly higher monocyte count than women. However, in adults count more than 800/μl of blood is considered as monocytosis.

Macrophages

Monocytes after their life span in blood enter tissues and transform into **tissue macrophages**. They form **mononuclear phagocyte system** in various tissues (Table 17.9) (Also, refer Fig. 19.2, Chapter 19):

1. Macrophages are capable of cell division and resident or noninflammatory macrophages in the tissue are self-sustaining.
2. The exact mechanism of differentiation of monocyte to macrophages is not known. However, on becoming macrophage there is increase in cell size, number of cytoplasmic granules and vacuoles, and increase in heterogeneity of the cell shape.

3. The average diameter of macrophages varies from 25 to 50 µm.
4. The nucleus is fusiform or reniform and is eccentrically placed with one or two nucleoli in it.
5. Cytoplasm contains multiple large azurophil granules.
6. They contain all the surface receptors that are present in monocytes.
7. In chronic tissue inflammations, macrophages are converted into **multinucleated giant cells** that are highly phagocytic and microbicidal.

Dendritic Cells

Few monocytes are transformed into highly specialized mononuclear cells called dendritic cells:

1. They play important role in antigen processing and presentation to the T cells.
2. They are specialized in antigen capture, rather than in phagocytosis. Thus, they are specific ***antigen presenting cells***.
3. However, unlike macrophages, dendritic cells lack receptors for immunoglobulins, complements and colony-stimulating factors, and specific granules in cytoplasm. Therefore, they are weakly phagocytic.
4. They are present in blood and bone marrow, where they account for about 0.1 to 1% of total mononuclear cells.
5. They are also present as Langerhans cells in skin, interdigitating cells in thymic medulla, and interstitial cells in the lung and heart.

LYMPHOCYTES

Lymphocytes are a heterogeneous group of cells with characteristic morphology. Lymphocyte is the only leucocyte that has different varieties of cells both morphologically and functionally. Structurally, lymphocytes are divided into two groups: small and large lymphocytes.

Structure

Small Lymphocytes

Small lymphocytes are same in size to that of red cells. They constitute 35% (20–50%) of total lymphocytes. The identifying features are:

1. The cells are 6–9 µm in diameter.
2. They have ovoid or kidney shaped nucleus with densely packed nuclear chromatin. Nucleus is usually eccentrically placed and occupies about 90% of the cell area (Fig. 17.15A).
3. There is a thin rim of bluish cytoplasm that does not contain granules.

Large Lymphocytes

Large lymphocytes constitute 65% (50–80%) of total lymphocytes. The identifying features are:

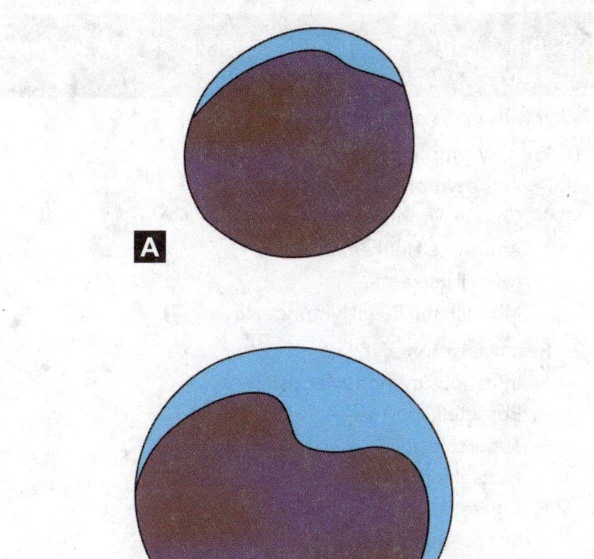

Figs. 17.15A and B: Structure of small lymphocyte (A), and large lymphocyte (B).

1. The cells are 10–15 µm in diameter (Fig. 17.15B).
2. The nucleus is homogenous and compact with dense nuclear chromatins. Nucleus is usually oval or kidney shaped and eccentrically placed.
3. The cytoplasm is navy blue in colour and usually does not contain granules. However, about 3% of large lymphocytes contain coarse pink granules (5 to 15 granules per cell). These granular lymphocytes are usually NK or T cells.

Normal Count and Functions

Normal lymphocyte count is 20–40% of total leucocytes. The absolute count is 500–8000 per cu mm of blood. Increase in count is called **lymphocytosis** and decrease in count is called **lymphocytopenia** (Table 17.10).

Functionally, lymphocytes are divided into three categories: B cells, T cells and NK cells. B cells on stimulation are transformed into **plasma cells** that secrete antibodies. B cells mediate humoral or antibody-mediated immunity. T cells mediate cellular or cell-mediated immunity. NK cells mediate natural and nonspecific immunity. Details of lymphocyte functions are discussed in the chapter "Immunity".

Summary of Blood Cells

To summarize, blood cells are formed elements of blood. Erythrocytes are anuclear cells having diameter of 7 to 8 µm that are primarily meant for transport of oxygen from lungs to the tissues. Leucocytes are of various sizes and they mainly play role in defence mechanisms. Platelets are anuclear and smaller cells (cellular fragments) that principally participate in homeostasis (Table 17.11).

Table 17.10: Causes of lymphocytosis and lymphocytopenia.
A. Lymphocytosis
1. Primary lymphocytosis – Acute lymphocytic leukemia – Chronic lymphocytic leukemia – Adult T-cell leukemia – NK-cell leukemia – Monoclonal B-cell lymphocytosis
2. Reactive lymphocytosis – Infectious mononucleosis – Bordetella pertusis – Tuberculosis – Postsplenectomy – Cigarette smoking – Septic shock – Drugs
B. Lymphocytopenia
1. Acquired lymphocytopenia – Aplastic anemia – AIDS – Hepatitis – Glucocorticoid therapy – Typhoid fever – Systemic lupus erythematosus
2. Inherited lymphocytopenia – Severe combined immunodeficiency states – Wiskott-Aldrich syndrome – Immunodeficiency with thymoma – Cellular immunodeficiency with immunoglobulins

LEUKEMIA

Definition and Concept

Leukemia is defined as a malignant neoplasia of hemopoietic cells in which there is abnormal proliferation of leucocytes and their precursors resulting in appearance of abnormal and immature cells in the peripheral blood associated with very high leucocytosis, and infiltration of tissues by leukemic cells.

1. There is increased infiltration of bone marrow by the proliferating leukemic cells.
2. The total leucocyte count is usually very high, except in subleukemic or aleukemic form of leukemia.
3. Usually, the proliferation involves leucoytic series.
4. Occasionally, erythroid precursors or megakaryocytes may also be involved in the disease process.

Types

Leukemia is classified into two main categories: myeloid (myelocytic) and lymphocytic leukemia. These two varieties are subclassified into acute and chronic types.

Acute Leukemias

Acute Lymphoblastic Leukemia

Acute lymphoblastic leukemia (ALL) is primarily a disease of children and young adults:

1. This constitutes 80% of **childhood acute leukemias**. It rarely occurs in adults.

Table 17.11: Summary of the formed elements in blood.

Name	Count	Features	Functions
A. Red blood cells (erythrocytes)	5.4 million/mm^3 in males; 4.8 million/mm^3 in fcmales.	7–8 µm diameter, biconcave discs, without a nucleus, life span about 120 days.	Transport oxygen and carbon dioxide.
B. White blood cells (leukocytes)	4000–11,000/mm^3.	Live for a few hours to few days.	Kill pathogens (body defence).
Neutrophils	50–70% of all WBCs.	10–14 µm diameter; nucleus is multilobed, connected by thin strands of chromatin; cytoplasm has fine, pink granules.	Phagocytosis of organisms (first line of defence).
Eosinophils	1–4% of all WBCs	10–14 µm diameter; nucleus is bilobed; coarse brick-red granules in cytoplasm.	Combat the effects of histamine in allergic reactions, kill parasitic worms.
Basophils	0–1% of all WBCs	10–14 µm diameter; nucleus is bilobed or irregular in shape; Large cytoplasmic granules are deep blue-purple.	Release heparin, histamine, and serotonin in allergic reactions that promote overall inflammatory response.
Lymphocytes	20–40% of all WBCs	Small lymphocytes are 6–9 µm in diameter; large lymphocytes are 10–14 µm in diameter; nucleus is round or slightly indented; cytoplasm forms a clear rim around the nucleus.	Mediate immune responses.
Monocytes	2–8% of all WBCs.	12–25 µm diameter; nucleus is oval or kidney-shaped or horseshoe-shaped; cytoplasm turbid in appearance.	Phagocytosis (after transforming into tissue macrophages).
C. Platelets (thrombocytes)	150,000–400,000/mm^3	2–4 µm diameter, cell fragments, no nucleus.	Form platelet plug in hemostasis (temporary hemostatic plug).

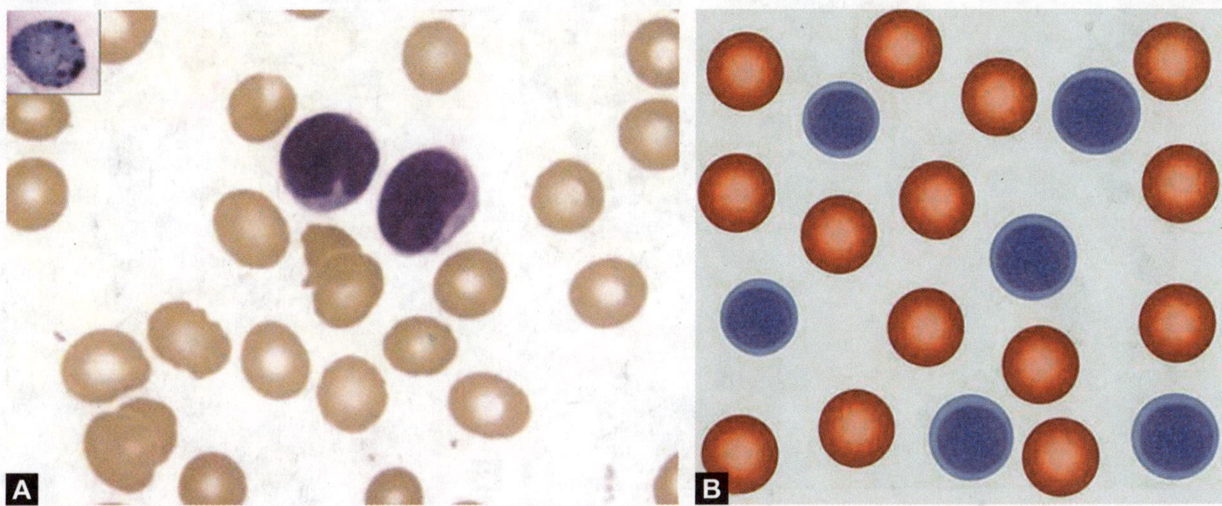

Figs. 17.16A and B: Peripheral blood film picture of acute lymphoblastic leukemia (ALL). Note the presence of many lymphoblasts. *Courtesy*: Figures 22.1A and B, Essentials in Hematology and Clinical Pathology by Ramadas Nayak et al., 1st edition, 2012; Jaypee Brothers Medical Publishers (P) Ltd.

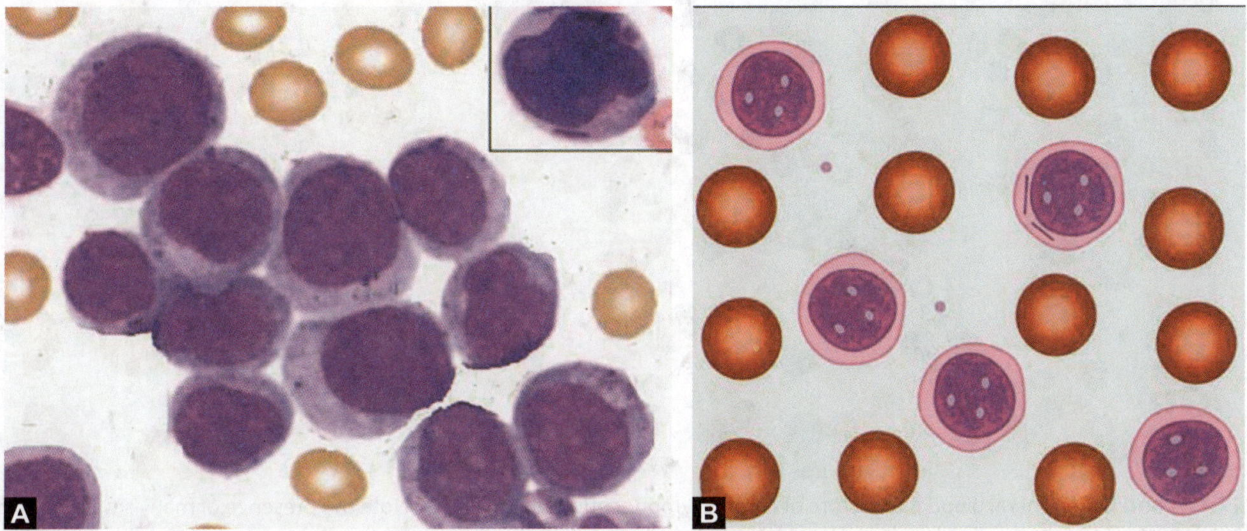

Figs. 17.17A and B: Peripheral blood film picture of acute myeloblastic leukemia (AML). Note the presence of many myeloblasts. *Courtesy*: Figures 23.1A and B, Essentials in Hematology and Clinical Pathology by Ramadas Nayak et al., 1st edition, 2012; Jaypee Brothers Medical Publishers (P) Ltd.

2. The most common mode of presentation is with symptoms of anemia or hemorrhage, infective lesions of the mouth and pharynx, fever, prostration, headache and malaise.
3. Generalized ***lymphadenopathy, splenomegaly*** and ***hepatomegaly*** are common and occur due to infiltration of organs by leukemic cells.
4. The typical blood picture is of ***anemia and thrombocytopenia***, with a moderate or marked ***increase in white cells***, the majority of which are blast cells '**lymphoblasts**' (Figs. 17.16A and B).

Acute Myeloblastic Leukemia

Acute myeloblastic leukemia (AML) primarily affects **adults between the ages of 15 and 40 years**. It constitutes only 20% of childhood leukemias:

1. The presentation is like that of ALL, but lymphadenopathy and hepatosplenomegaly is not common.
2. Blood picture presents anemia, thrombocytopenia, and moderate to high leucocytosis.
3. More than 60% of leucocytes in the peripheral blood are blast (**myeloblast**) cells (Figs. 17.17A and B).

Chronic Leukemias

Chronic Myeloid Leukemia

Chronic myeloid leukemia (CML) accounts for about 20% of all cases of leukemia. It is primarily a disease of **adults between the ages of 30 to 60 years** with the peak incidence in the 4th and 5th decades of life.

1. Onset is usually slow with nonspecific features like anemia, weight loss, weakness, and easy fatigability.

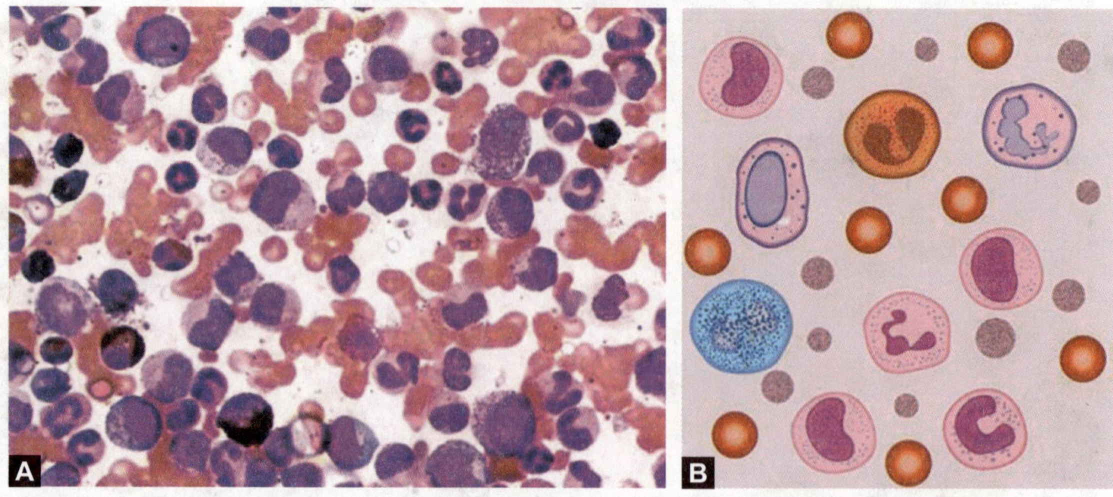

Figs. 17.18A and B: Peripheral blood film picture of chronic myeloid leukemia (CML). Note the presence of many myelocytes and metamyelocytes.
Courtesy: Figures 26.3A and B, Essentials in Hematology and Clinical Pathology by Ramadas Nayak et al., 1st edition, 2012; Jaypee Brothers Medical Publishers (P) Ltd.

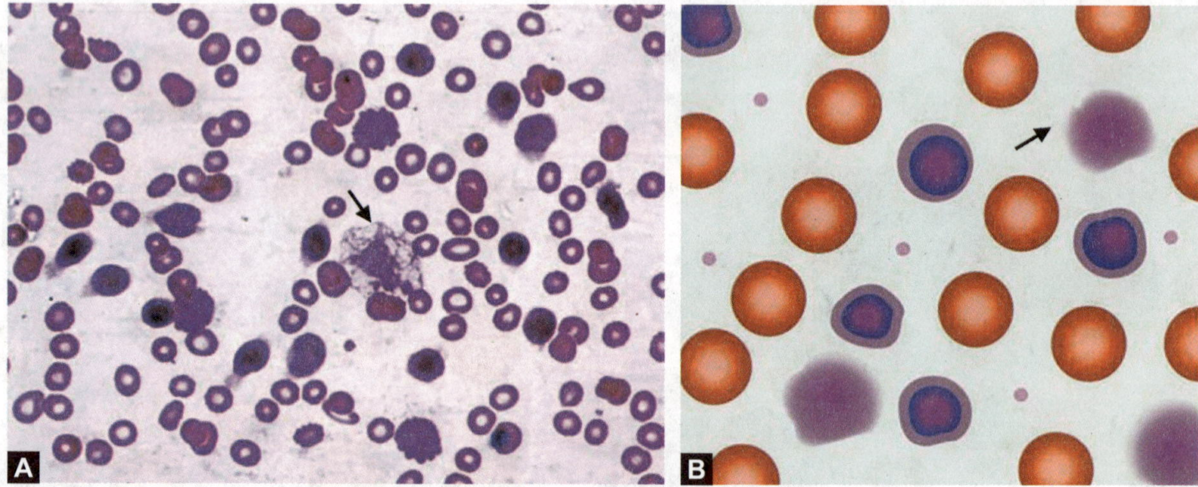

Figs. 17.19A and B: Peripheral blood film picture of chronic lymphocytic leukemia (CLL). Note the presence of many small lymphocytes.
Courtesy: Figures 27.1A and B, Essentials in Hematology and Clinical Pathology by Ramadas Nayak et al., 1st edition, 2012; Jaypee Brothers Medical Publishers (P) Ltd.

2. **Splenomegaly** *is the outstanding physical sign*. Hepatomegaly may be present, but lymph node enlargement is rare.
3. **Markedly elevated total leucocyte count** usually more than one lakh cells per cubic mm of blood is seen commonly.
4. **Neutrophils, myelocytes and metamyelocytes** constitute most of the circulating cells (Figs. 17.18A and B).
5. Blasts cells are present rarely except in the blastic crisis.

Chronic Lymphocytic Leukemia

Chronic lymphocytic leukemia (CLL) is the most indolent of all leukemias. It occurs typically in **persons over 50 years**:

1. Males are affected twice as frequently as females.
2. Patients present with nonspecific symptoms.
3. **Lymphadenopathy** *is the outstanding physical sign.*
4. Hepatosplenomegaly may be present.
5. Mild to severe increase in leucocyte count is seen.
6. More than 90% of leucocytes are mature lymphocytes (Figs. 17.19A and B).

CHAPTER SUMMARY

Key Concepts

1. In leucopoiesis, granulocytes and monocytes develop from myeloid stem cells and lymphocytes develop from lymphoid stem cells. Major hemopoietic growth factors are GM-SCF and interleukins.
2. Development of leucocytes in bone marrow occurs in 6 to 10 days (marrow phase), they spend 6 to 8 hours in peripheral blood (circulation phase), and then enter tissues (tissue phase).

3. Neutrophils are highly phagocytic cells, and are the first line of defense against acute pyogenic infection.
4. Eosinophils and basophils defend the body against allergy.
5. Monocytes are phagocytic, and defend the body against chronic infections. Monocytes enter the tissue to become tissue macrophages (Mononuclear phagocyte system)
6. Lymphocytes participate in immunity.
7. Leukemia is the malignancy of leucocyte precursor cells. ALL occurs in children, AML in young adults, CML in adults and CLL in elderly.

Important to Know (Must Read)

1. In examinations, 'Steps and regulation of leucopoiesis' and 'Development, life history, structure and functions of neutrophils' come as **Long Questions**.
2. Regulation of leucopoiesis, Life history of leucocytes, Types and fund functions of neutrophil granules, Phagocytosis by neutrophil, Oxidative mechanism of killing by neutrophils, Role of eosinophil in allergy, Functions of monocytes, and Leukemias, are usually asked as **Short Questions** in exams.
3. In **Viva**, examiners usually ask… the steps of leucopoiesis, hemopoietic growth factors controlling leucopoiesis, structure and function of each leucocyte, conditions that increase and decrease each leucocyte, role of neutrophil in acute defence, steps of phagocytosis, types of killing by neutrophil, definition and types of leukemia, and which leukemia is common in which age.
4. As TLC and DLC are routine and very useful hematologic investigations, questions on WBCs are very common in all exams (practical, theory and viva). Students are supposed to answer these questions well.

CHAPTER 18

Thymus, Lymphoid Tissues and Lymph

Learning Objectives

On completion of study of this chapter, the student **MUST** be able to:

1. Name the lymphatic tissues of the body.
2. Give the structure and functions of thymus.
3. Give the structure and functions of lymph node.
4. Give the structure and functions of spleen.
5. Give structure and functions of other lymphoid structures.
6. Composition, circulation and function of lymph.

The student **MAY** also be able to:

1. Describe the role of various lymphatic tissues in defence of the body.
2. Explain the development of lymphocytes in thymus.
3. Describe the lymphatic circulation.

THYMUS

The thymus is the organ usually not seen by most students and teachers as it is rudimentary in adults. The thymus is located in the superior mediastinum (Fig. 18.1). At birth, the thymus weighs 10–15 grams, which increases to 30–40 grams at puberty. Subsequently, much of the organ is replaced by fat and is atrophied in adults. The thymus is important as it produces T lymphocytes throughout life.

Structure

The thymus consists of right and left lobes that are joined together by fibrous tissue. Each lobe has a connective tissue capsule, which has septa passing inwards from the capsule that subdivide the lobe into a larger number of **lobules.**

1. Each lobule is about 2 mm in diameter. It has an outer **cortex** and an inner **medulla** (Figs. 18.2A to C).
2. Both the cortex and medulla contain cells of two distinct lineages. The medulla of adjoining lobule is continuous.
3. The thymus has a rich blood supply. It does not receive any lymph vessels, but gives off efferent vessels.

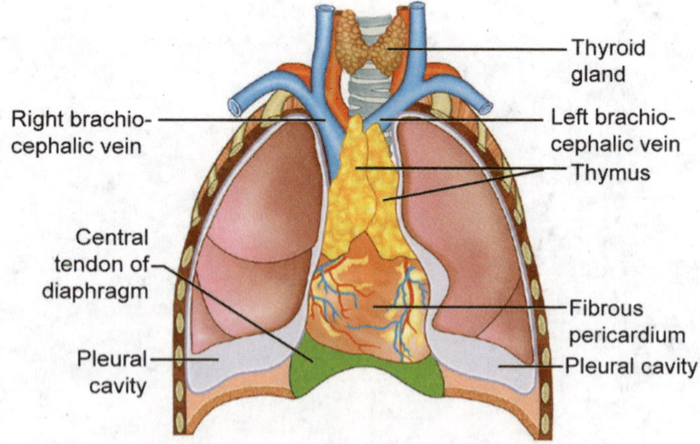

Fig. 18.1: Location of thymus in the mediastinum.

Epithelial Cells

Epithelial cells are called **epitheliocytes**. Seven types of epitheliocytes are recognized.

1. **Type 1** epitheliocyrtes line the inner aspect of the capsule, the septa, and blood vessels. These are the cells forming the partial haemothymic barrier mentioned above.
2. **Type 2 and type 3** cells are present in the outer and inner parts of the cortex respectively.

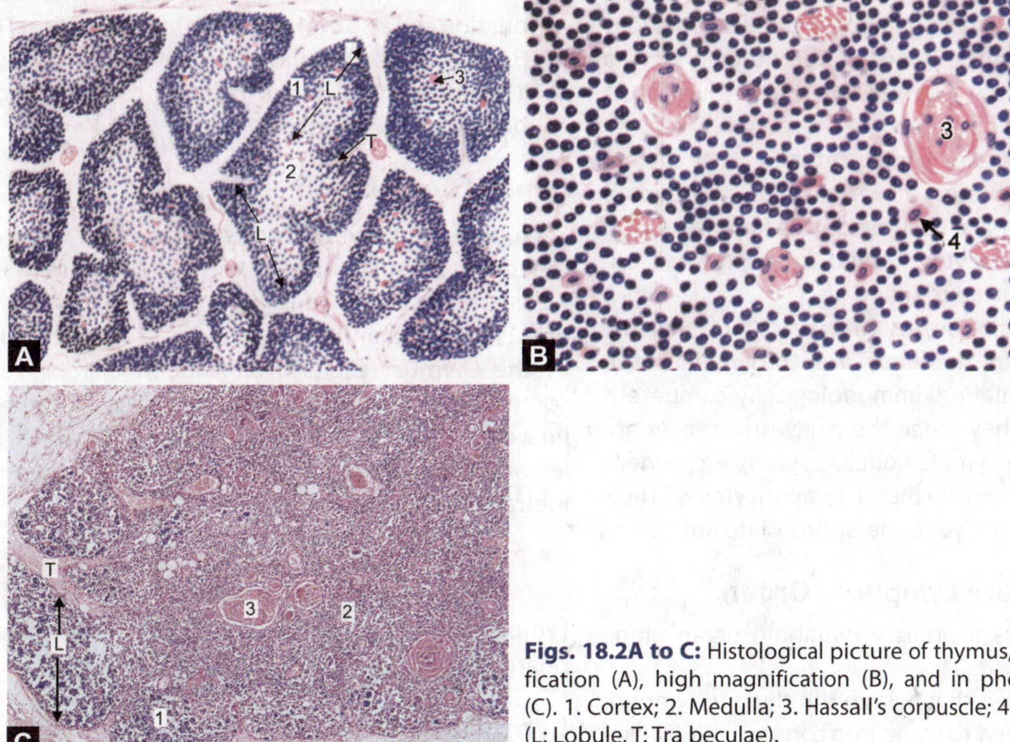

Figs. 18.2A to C: Histological picture of thymus, in low magnification (A), high magnification (B), and in photomicrograph (C). 1. Cortex; 2. Medulla; 3. Hassall's corpuscle; 4. Epithelial cell; (L: Lobule, T: Tra beculae).

3. **Type 4** cells lie in the deepest parts of the cortex, and also in the medulla. They form a network containing spaces that are occupied by lymphocytes.
4. **Type 5** cells are present around corpuscles of Hassall.
5. Cortical epitheliocyts are also described as ***thymic nurse cells***. They destroy lymphocytes that react against self-antigens.

Lymphocytes of the Thymus

Lymphocytes of thymus are called **thymocytes**.

1. In the medulla of each lobule also contains lymphocytes (medullary thymocytes), but these are less densely packed than the cortex (cortical thymocytes). Consequently, the epithelial reticulum is more obvious in the medulla than in the cortex.
2. As thymocytes divide they pass deeper into the medulla.
3. Thymocytes leave the thymus by passing into blood vessels and lymphatics.

Macrophages

Apart from epithelial cells and lymphocytes the thymus contains a fair number of macrophages that are part of mononuclear phagocyte system (MPS). The **subcapsullar macrophages** are highly phagocytic. Macrophages present more deeply are **dendritic cells.**

Corpuscular Hassall

These are small rounded structures present in the medulla of the thymus.

1. Each corpuscle has a central core formed by epithelial cells that have undergone degeneration. These cells ultimately form a pink staining **hyaline mass.**
2. Around this mass there is a wall formed by concentrically arranged epithelial cells.
3. The central mass of the corpuscle may also contain degenerating macrophages.

Functions of the Thymus

T cell develops from pre-T cell. The thymus is the site for T cell development. The **epithelial cells** play an important role in the development of bone marrow-derived pre-thymic cells into mature T cells (discussed below). Though thymus is reduced to a very small structure in adults, and in the atrophic adult thymus, cortex is mainly replaced by adipose tissue, the less cellular medulla remains apparently normal (Clinical Box 18.1).

Clinical Box 18.1

Effects of thymectomy: Thymectomy in young animals leads to lymphocytopenia, increased susceptibility to infections, atrophy of lymphatic tissues, failure to reject transplanted organs and suppression of delayed hypersensitivity reactions. Thymectomy in young animals leads to depletion of T cells and immunodeficiency within few months. These findings depict the importance of thymus in development of T cells in childhood and maintenance of T cells in adult life.

Role in Lymphopoiesis

The role of the thymus in lymphopoiesis is significant.

1. Stem cells from bone marrow that reach the superficial part of the cortex divide repeatedly to form smaller lymphocytes.

2. It has been proposed that during these mitoses, the DNA of the lymphocytes undergoes numerous random mutations, as a result of which different lymphocytes acquire the ability to recognize a very large number of different proteins and to react to them.
3. As it is not desirable for lymphocytes to react against the body's own proteins, all lymphocytes that would react against them are destroyed. It is for this reason that 90% of lymphocytes formed in the thymus are destroyed within three to four days.
4. The remaining lymphocytes that react only against proteins foreign to the body are thrown into the circulation as circulating, immunologically competent T lymphocytes. They lodge themselves in secondary lymph organs like lymph nodes, spleen, etc. where they multiply to form further T lymphocytes of their own type when exposed to the appropriate antigen.

Thymus as a Primary Lymphoid Organ

Thymus is regarded as a primary lymphoid organ along with bone marrow.

1. It has been observed that, within the thymus, lymphocytes are not allowed to come into contact with foreign antigens, because of the presence of the ***blood-thymic barrier***. It has also been stated that because of this thymocytes do not develop into large lymphocytes or into plasma cells, and do not form lymphatic nodules.
2. Recently, it has been postulated that the medulla of the thymus (or part of it) is a separate "compartment". After thymocytes move into this compartment they probably come into contact with antigens presented to them through dendritic macrophages. Such contact may be necessary step in making T lymphocytes competent to distinguish between foreign antigens and proteins of the body itself.
3. The proliferation of T lymphocytes and their conversion into cells capable of reacting to antigens, probably takes place under the influence of hormones produced by epithelial cells of the thymus. T lymphocytes are also influenced by direct cell contact with epitheliocytes. **Hormones** produced by the thymus may also influence lymphopoiesis in peripheral lymphoid organs. This influence appears to be specially important in early life, as lymphoid tissues do not develop normally if the thymus id removed.
4. Thymectomy has much less influence after puberty as the lymphoid tissues have fully developed by then.

Thymic Hormones

A number of hormones produced by the thymus have now been identified as follows:

1. **Thymulin:** Thymulin enhances the function of various types of T cell, specially that of suppressor cells.
2. **Thymopoietin:** Thymopoietin stimulates the production of cytotoxic T cells. The combined action of thymulin and thymopoietin allows precise balance of the activity of cytotoxic and suppressor cells.
3. **Thymosin:** ***Thymosin α-1*** stimulates lymphocyte production and also the production of antibodies. ***Thymosin β-4*** is produced by mononuclear phagocytes.
4. **Thymic humoral factor** controls the multiplication of helper and suppressor T cells.

Clinical Correlation

Enlargement of thymus is often associated with a disease called **myasthenia gravis**. In this condition there is a great weakness of skeletal muscles. In many such cases the thymus is enlarged and there may be a tumor in it. **Removal of the thymus** results in considerable improvement in some cases. Thus, myasthenia gravis is now considered to be a disturbance of the immune system, in which, antibodies are produced against these proteins rendering them ineffective (autoimmune disease).

LYMPHATIC TISSUES

Lymphatic system consists of lymphatic vessels and lymphatic tissues.

Lymphatic Vessels

When circulating blood reaches the capillaries, part of its fluid content passes into the surrounding tissues as tissue fluid. Most of this fluid reenters the capillaries at their venous ends. Some of it is, however, returns to the circulation through a separate system of lymphatic vessels (usually called lymphatics). The fluid passing through the lymphatic vessel is called **lymph**.

1. The smallest lymphatic (or lymph) vessels are lymphatic capillaries that join together to form larger lymphatic vessels.
2. The largest lymphatic vessel in the body is the thoracic duct, which drains lymph from the greater part of the body.
3. The thoracic duct ends by joining the left subclavian vein at its junction with the internal jugular vein (Fig. 18.3).

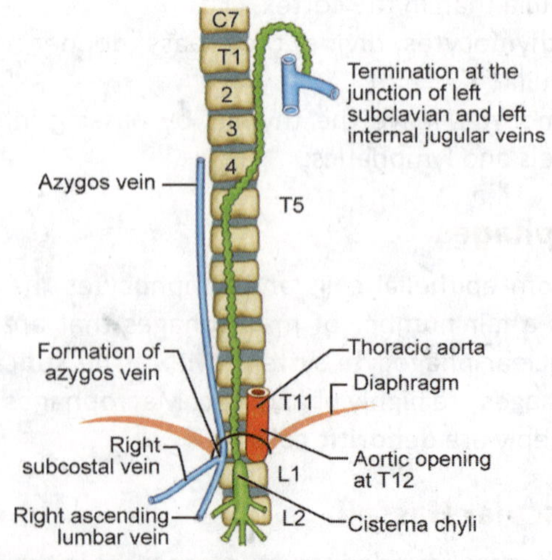

Fig. 18.3: Origin, course and termination of thoracic duct.

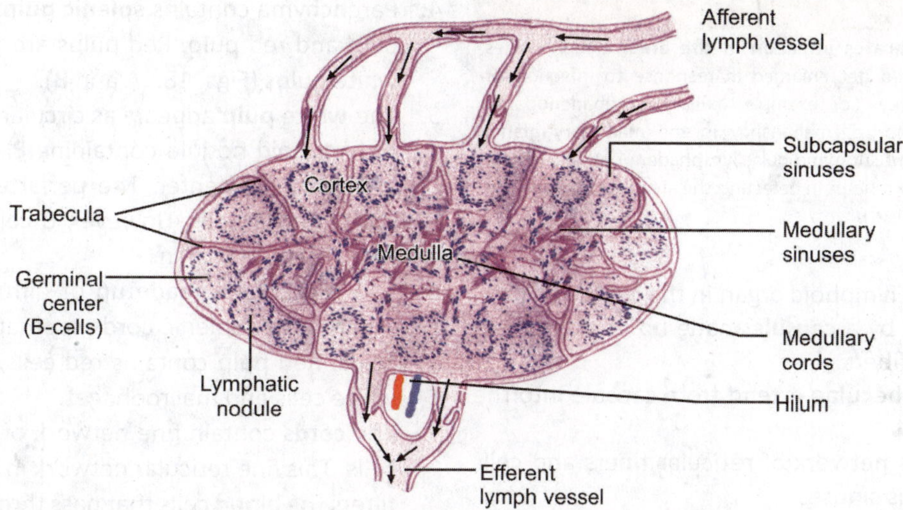

Fig. 18.4: Normal lymph node. Note the presence of germinal centers for B cells in the cortex.
Courtesy: Figure 11.4, Basic Histology, 1st edition, 2016, by V Subhadra Devi; Jaypee Brothers Medical Publishers (P) Ltd.

4. On the right side there is the right lymphatic duct that has a similar termination.

Lymphoid Tissues

Lymphoid tissue may be broadly classified as: Diffused lymphoid tissue and dense lymphoid tissue.

Diffused Lymphoid Tissue

Diffused lymphoid tissue consists of **diffusedly arranged lymphocytes and plasma cells** in the mucosa of large intestine, trachea, bronchi and urinary tract.

Dense Lymphoid Tissue

It consists of an aggregation of lymphocytes arranged in the form of **nodules**. These nodules are found either as discrete encapsulated organs or in close association to the lining epithelium of the gut. Dense lymphoid tissue can therefore be further divide as:

1. **Discrete lymphoid organs:** these include ***thymus, lymph nodes, spleen, and tonsils***.
2. **Mucosa associated lymphoid tissue (MALT):** small numbers of lymphocytes may be present almost anywhere in the body, but significant aggregations are seen in relation to the mucosa of the respiratory, alimentary and urogenital tracts. These aggregations are referred to as MALT.

   Mucosa associated lymphoid tissue in the respiratory system: in the respiratory system the aggregations are relatively small and are present in the walls of the trachea and large bronchi. The term bronchial associated lymphoid tissue (BALT) is applied to these aggregations.

   Mucosa associated lymphoid tissue in the alimentary system: This is also called gut associated lymphoid tissue (GALT) and includes Payer's patches of ileum, adenoids (located in the roof of pharynx), lingual tonsils in posterior 1/3rd of tongue, palatine tonsils and lymphoid nodules in vermiform appendix.

Note: Thymus and bone marrow are **primary lymphoid organ** while others are secondary lymphoid organ.

Lymph Node

Lymph nodes are small encapsulated organs present in the pathway of lymphatics. They are found usually in groups, especially in neck, submandibular region, axilla and inguinal regions.

1. They have afferent and efferent lymphatics. **Afferent lymphatics** penetrate the capsule and join the sinus inside.
2. **Trabeculae** extend from capsule into the stroma in the node.
3. **Stroma** is made up of reticular lymphoid tissue arranged in outer cortex and inner medulla (Fig. 18.2A and B).
4. **Cortex** has lymphatic nodules or follicles with definite germinal centers.
5. Each follicle has central pale area that represent *germinal center* and surrounding little darker area representing *B cell area* of the node.
6. The *T cell area* is present in the **paracortex**, the junction between cortex and medulla (Fig. 18.4).
7. **Medulla** has lymphoid cells arranged in strands forming medullary cords.
8. Lymph flows from afferent lymphatics to subcapsular sinus, and then along trabeculae to the **cortical and medullary sinuses**, and exits via **efferent lymphatics** at the hilus.
9. Thus, lymph nodes filter the lymph that flows through it (Clinical Box 18.2). Lymph nodes also assist in processing of lymphocytes that takes place in the germinal centers.

Clinical Box 18.2

Lymphadenopathy indicates infection in the area: Lymph nodes draining a particular area get enlarged in response to infection or inflammation in the area. For example, axillary lymphadenopathy indicates infection, tumor or malignancy in the mammary gland, especially in females, and submandibular lymphadenopathy in throat infections. Thus, clinically it helps in detecting the area of pathology.

Spleen

Spleen is the largest lymphoid organ in the body.

1. It is surrounded by a **capsule** made up of elastic and smooth muscle fibers.
2. A number of **trabeculae** extend from capsule into the organ.
3. **Stroma** contains network of reticular fibers and cells and many venous sinuses.
4. Parenchyma contains **splenic pulps** made up of white pulp and red pulp. Red pulps are present around the white pulps (Figs. 18.5A and B).
5. The **white pulp** appears as circular patches. It consists of lymphoid nodule containing B cells, central artery and germinal center. The periarteriolar lymphocytes are mainly T cells. However, B cells slightly predominate T cells in spleen.
6. The **red pulp** is made up of diffuse lymphoid tissue organized as splenic cords separated by venous sinusoids. Red pulp contains red cells, lymphocyte, other white cells and macrophages.
7. The **cords** contain fine network of reticular fibers and cells. This fine reticular network in the splenic red pulp filters the blood cells that pass through it. The arrangement of splenic circulation (open and closed circulation) in the red pulp and location of the sinusoids help in filtering senescent and abnormal cells (Fig. 18.6).
8. The aged and defective cells are easily detected and destroyed in the pulp. Otherwise also blood cells are trapped in the splenic pulp (Clinical Box 18.3).

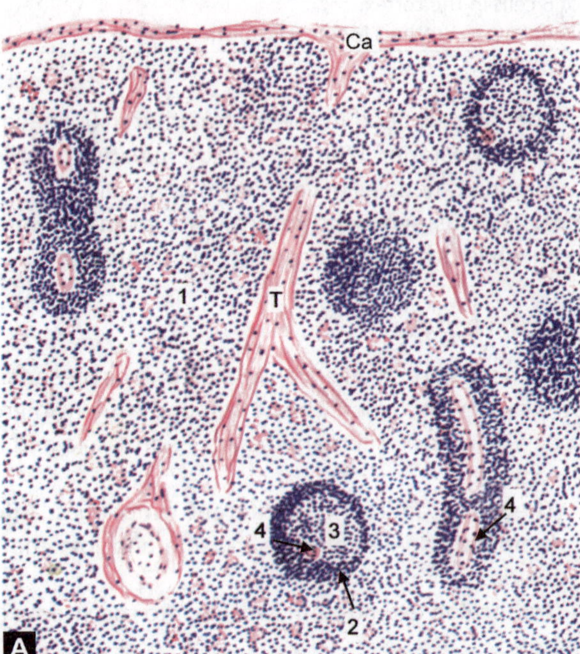

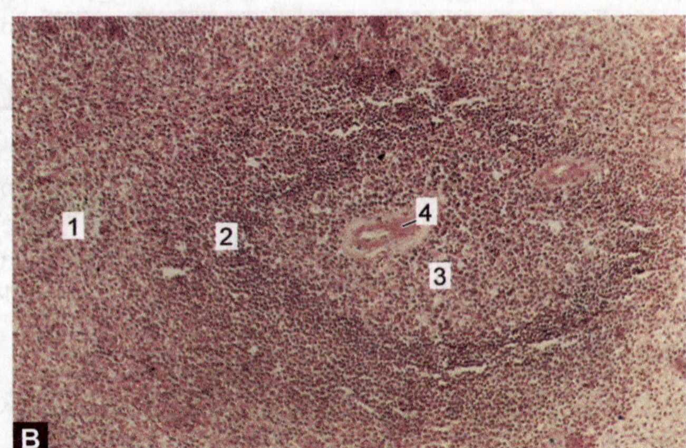

Figs. 18.5A and B: Histological picture of spleen, in low magnification (A), and in photomicrograph (B). (1: Red pulp; 2: White pulp; 3: Germinal center; 4. Arteriole; Ca: Capsule; T: Trabeculus).

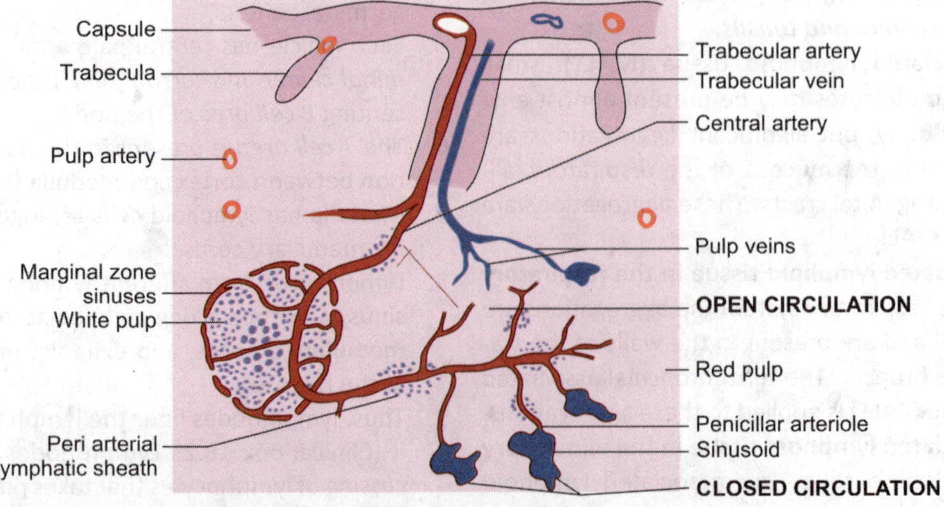

Fig. 18.6: The splenic circulation. Note the location of sinusoids that filter cells.

Clinical Box 18.3

Size of spleen determines blood cell count: As aged and defective cells are detected and destroyed in the pulp, invariably, ***splenectomy leads to increased cell count and splenomegaly results in decreased count of all cell lines.***

Functions of Spleen

1. Spleen plays important role in **immunity** (Clinical Box 18.4). Macrophages in spleen help in **phagocytosis** of pathogens or antigens. Spleen is the site for **production of B and T cells**. Germinal centers in the spleen helps in development of lymphocytes. Spleen also helps in **production of antibodies**.
2. Spleen removes **old and abnormal red cells, white cells and platelets**. Cells of MPS detect these senescent and abnormal cells and remove them from blood.
3. Spleen helps in **hepatic stage of hemopoiesis** during intrauterine life. Extramedullary hemopoiesis takes place in spleen in postnatal life in pathological conditions.
4. Spleen acts as an important **reservoir of blood** in mammals.
5. Macrophages in spleen **recycle iron**, which has been released from destroyed red cells. This iron is reutilized for synthesis of hemoglobin.

Clinical Box 18.4

Splenomegaly indicates general infections or pathology: Spleen detects abnormal cells and kills them. Therefore, splenomegaly is a common feature of many lymphomas and leukemias. Also, in chronic parasitic infections like malaria and kala azar, spleen is enlarged as spleen fights against such abnormalities. Degree of splenomegaly and consistency of spleen is important for a physician to asses the nature and progress of the disease.

Mucosa-associated Lymphoid Tissue

As discussed significant aggregation of lymphocytes seen in relation to the mucosa of the respiratory, alimentary and urogenital tracts are refereed as **mucosa-associated lymphoid tissue** (MALT). The total volume of MALT is more or less equal to that of the lymphoid tissue present in lymph nodes and spleen. Mucosa associated aggregations of lymphoid tissue have some features in common as follows:

- These aggregations are in the form of one or **more lymphatic follicles** (nodules) having a structure similar to nodules of lymph nodes. ***Germinal centers*** may be present. Diffuse lymphoid tissue (termed the **parafollicular zone**) is present in the intervals between the nodules. The significance of the nodules and of the diffuse aggregations of lymphocytes is the same as already described in the case of lymph nodes. The nodules consist predominantly of B, while the diffuse area consists of T lymphocytes.
- These **masses of lymphoid tissue** are present in very close relationship to the lining epithelium of the mucosa in the region concerned, and lie in the substantia propria. **Larger aggregations** extend into the submucosa. Individual lymphocytes may infiltrate the epithelium and may pass through it into the mucosa.
- The aggregations are not surrounded by a capsule, nor do they have connective tissue septa. A supporting network of reticular fibers is present.
- As a rule these masses of lymphoid tissue do not receive afferent lymph vessels, and have no lymph sinuses. They *do not therefore, serve as filters of lymph*. However, they are **centers of lymphocyte production**. Lymphocytes produced here pass into lymph nodes of the region through efferent lymphatic vessels. Some lymphocytes pass through the overlying epithelium into the lumen.

Mucosa-associated Lymphoid Tissue in Respiratory System

In the respiratory system the aggregations are relatively small and are present in the walls of the trachea and large bronchi. The term bronchial associated lymphoid tissue (BALT) is applied to these aggregations.

Mucosa-associated Lymphoid Tissue in Alimentary System

This is also called gut associated lymphoid tissue (**GALT**). In the alimentary system examples of aggregations of lymphoid tissue are tonsils, Peyer's patches and lymphoid nodules in vermiform appendix.

LYMPH AND LYMPHATIC CIRCULATION

Lymph is a transudate from blood and contains the same proteins, but in smaller amounts and in different proportions. Suspended in lymph there are cells that are chiefly lymphocytes. Most of these lymphocytes are added to lymph as it passes through lymph nodes, but some are derived from tissues drained by the nodes. Large molecules of fat (chylomicrons) that are absorbed from the intestines enter lymph vessels. After a fatty meal these fat globules may be so numerous that lymph become milky (is called **chyle**). Under these conditions the lymph vessels can be seen easily as they pass through mesentery.

Functional Anatomy

Lymphatics drain lymph from different tissues of the body and empty the same into the subclavian veins at their junctions with internal jugular veins.

1. Lymphatic vessels typically begin as blind tubular bulbs (**lymphatic bulbs**) that drain into meshwork of interconnected lymph vessels. For example, in the intestine, villous lacteals are lymphatic bulbs.

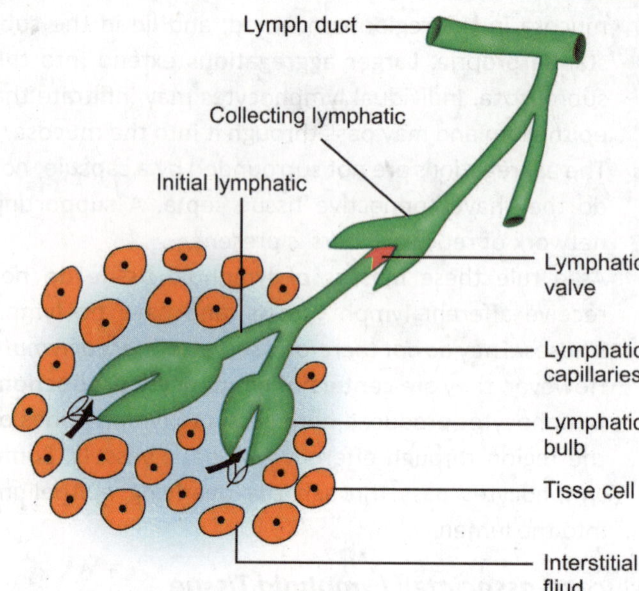

Fig. 18.7: The lymphatic drainage system. Note, there is no valve in initial lymphatics, but the valves are present in collecting lymphatics. Black arrows indicate the direction of flow of fluid movement into lymphatic bulb.

2. Tissue fluid enters into the bulbs that in turn drain to interconnected lymph vessels and then from these vessels into tubular lymphatic vessels and the larger lymphatic vessels (Fig. 18.7).
3. Lymphatic vessels coalesce into increasingly larger vessels.
4. Larger vessels are surrounded by contractile cells similar to that of smooth muscles of blood vessels.
5. Lymph nodes are interposed in the path of lymphatics.

> **Important Note**
>
> **Organs with no lymphatics:** Lymphatics are absent in bone, teeth, cartilage, placenta and CNS.

Types of Lymphatics

Lymphatics are of two types: Initial lymphatics and collecting lymphatics.

Initial Lymphatics

Initial lymphatics are lymphatic bulbs and interconnected vessels (lymphatic capillaries).

Lymphatic capillaries differ from vascular capillaries in several ways:

1. No basal lamina (or scanty basal lamia) under the endothelium.
2. Junctions between endothelial cells are open.
3. No fenestrations in endothelium (non-fenestrated)
4. Tight junctions (tight intercellular connections) are absent

Initial lymphatics ***lack valves and smooth muscles*** in their walls. Tissue fluid enters into them through gaps or loose junctions between the endothelial cells present in their linings. Movement of fluid in them is facilitated by **contraction of organs** in which they are present and the contraction of arterioles and venules with which they are often associated. They drain into collecting lymphatics.

Collecting Lymphatics

Collecting lymphatics are tubular and larger lymphatics.

1. They have valves and smooth muscles in their walls.
2. They **exhibit peristaltic contraction** that propels lymph in forward direction.
3. Lymph flow is further facilitated by skeletal muscle contraction, negative intrathoracic pressure (during inspiration), and suction effect created by higher velocity of flow in veins into which the lymphatics drain.
4. Unidirectional flow of lymph is maintained by presence of valves in the larger lymphatic ducts.
5. Substances that increase lymph flow are called **lymphagouges**. Usually, agents that increase capillary permeability also act as lymphagogues.

Table 18.1: Composition of lymph.

1. Proteins: 2–6 mg% (more in liver)
2. Lipids: Intestinal lacteals contain more lipid
3. Carbohydrate: Less than plasma
4. Clotting factors: Lymph draining from liver mainly contains clotting factors.
5. Cells: Mainly lymphocytes and few monocytes
6. Ions: Sodium, potassium, calcium, chloride, sulfates, phosphate
7. Water

Formation and Composition of Lymph

Lymph is formed from tissue fluid. Therefore, essentially it is a **modified tissue fluid** (Table 18.1). It is formed by transcapillary exchange and exchange between tissue fluid and lymphatic ducts. Lymph flow is much slower (1 mL/min in thoracic duct) than blood. Its colloidal osmotic pressure is less than that of plasma. Presence of more lipid gives milky color to the lymph, hence called **chyle**.

Functions of Lymphatic Circulation

1. Extra amount of fluid left in the tissue space by capillary filtration is taken up by lymphatics and returned back to circulation. Thus, lymphatics **prevent accumulation of excess free fluid** in the interstitial space (prevent edema formation), and at the same time *contribute to water content of plasma* to some extent.
2. In liver and intestine, a significant quantity of protein enters into interstitial space. This protein is returned to circulation via lymphatics. This accounts for 25 to 50% of circulating protein in the blood. Thus, lymphatics **maintain protein content of plasma**.

3. Long-chain fatty acids, cholesterol and fat-soluble vitamins absorbed from intestine are transported to circulation via lymphatics.
4. Mononuclear phagocytes in lymph nodes remove bacteria and pathogenic organisms from lymph draining from the organ. Thus, they play **protective function** (Clinical Box 18.5).

Clinical Box 18.5

Lymphadenopathy: Specific Lymph nodes draining from the **site of infection and inflammation are usually enlarged** during the active phase of the disease process**. Enlarged lymph nodes (lymphadenopathy)** in a particular part of the body provide clinical clue to the physician to locate the site of infection. For example, enlarged submandibular lymph glands indicate infection in the throat

CHAPTER SUMMARY

Key Concepts

1. Thymus is a primary lymphoid organ involved in T cell development.
2. Lymph node, spleen and associated lymphatic tissue are secondary lymphoid organs where the lymphocytes reside and mature.
3. Spleen is the site of destruction of old and abnormal blood cells.
4. Splenomegaly and lymphadenopathy indicates infection or proliferation of abnormal cells in general.

Important to Know (Must Read)

1. In examinations, **Long Questions** do not come from this chapter.
2. Functions of thymus, functions of spleen, composition and functions of lymph, & lymphatic circulation may come as **Short Questions** in exams.
3. In **Viva**, examiners may ask… hormones secreted from thymus, how T cells are developed in thymus, functions of thymus, spleen and lymph node, composition of lymph, and design of lymphatic circulation.

CHAPTER

19

Physiology of Immunity

LEARNING OBJECTIVES

On completion of study of this chapter, the student **MUST** be able to:

1. Classify immunity and give examples for each.
2. Classify lymphocytes and give their functions.
3. List the nonspecific defence mechanisms, and list the functions of NK cells.
4. List the cells of mononuclear phagocyte system.
5. Understand how inflammation and fever defend the body from microorganism.
6. Name the primary and secondary lymphoid organs and outline the general principles of immunity.
7. Describe the mechanism of cellular and humoral immunity.
8. Name the antibodies and give their functions.
9. Name the complements and give their functions.
10. Explain the mechanism of immunological tolerance.
11. Give the physiological basis of rejection of organ transplants and the prevention of its rejection.
12. Classify immunological disorders and give one example of each disorder.
13. Correlate the dysfunctions in AIDS to the pathophysiological problems.

The student **MAY** also be able to:

1. Explain the role of mononuclear cells, inflammation and fever in immunity.
2. Describe the role of complement system in immunity.
3. Explain the role of antibody in immune responses.
4. List different types of immunotherapy and describe importance of monoclonal antibodies in immunotherapy.
5. Understand the pathophysiology of immunodeficiencies.

The process of defense of the body against harmful elements that threaten our normal health is the immunity. Our environment is rich in varieties of infectious microbes, such as bacteria, viruses, fungi, protozoa and multicellular parasites. When these organisms enter the body they multiply, and if their growth and multiplication are unchecked, they produce disease in the host and eventually they may even kill the host. Therefore, the living beings require quick and continuous mechanisms to kill and remove the pathogens from their body.

1. Adequacy of the defense systems mainly depends on the **activities of immune mechanisms**.
2. Mammalians are endowed with various defense mechanisms that can broadly be divided into **specific and non-specific defenses**.
3. The specific defense mechanisms of the body are collectively known as **immunity**.
4. The immune responses greatly depend on the site of infection and the type of infecting organism (pathogen).

CLASSIFICATION OF IMMUNITY

The ability of the body to defend against invading agents is called immunity. The invader may be a living organism or a nonliving substance.

Immune responses broadly involve **two steps**:

1. Recognition of pathogen or the foreign material,
2. Reactions or responses to eliminate it. The responses are called **immune responses** (Table 19.1).

Table 19.1: Types of immunity.

A. Innate (nonadaptive) immunity
1. Nonspecific defenses
2. Relatively specific defense by NK cells
B. Acquired (adaptive) immunity
1. Naturally acquired
a. Active immunity (usually through infections)
– Cellular immunity
– Humoral immunity
b. Passive immunity (transfer of antibody from mother)
– Ig G via placenta
– Ig A via breast feeding
2. Artificially acquired
a. Active immunity
– Vaccination (antigens in vaccines are immunogenic but not pathogenic, stimulate immune responses and produce memory cells).
b. Passive immunity
– I.V. injection of antibodies such as anti-D immunization of Rh –ve mother.

Largely, immune responses are of **two types**:

1. Innate or nonadaptive response (Innate immunity).
2. Acquired or adaptive response (Acquired immunity).

Scientist contributed

Paul Ehrlich a German physician and scientist worked in the fields of immunology, and antimicrobial chemotherapy. He invented the precursor technique to Gram staining bacteria. The methods he developed for staining tissue made it possible to distinguish between different types of blood cells, which led to the capability to diagnose numerous blood diseases. He was awarded **Nobel Prize in Physiology or Medicine** in 1908 for his pioneering work on humoral immunity.

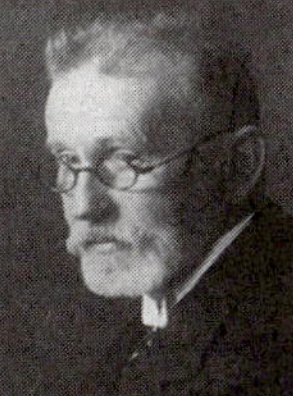

Paul Ehrlich
(1854–1915)

Innate immunity: Innate immunity is mostly ***nonspecific***:

1. It include phagocytosis, inflammation, release of cytokine and antibacterial peptides from phagocytes and inflammatory cells, activation of complement system, etc.

Scientists contributed

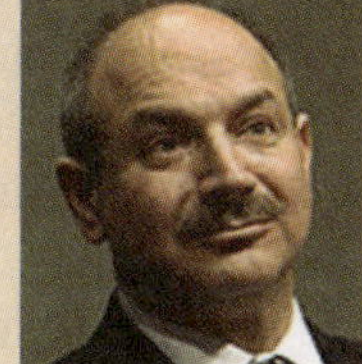

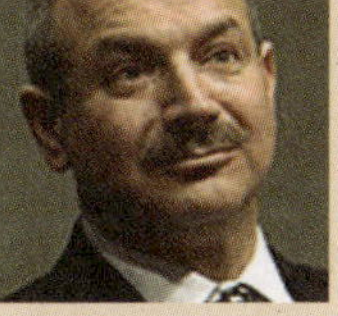

Bruce A Beutler

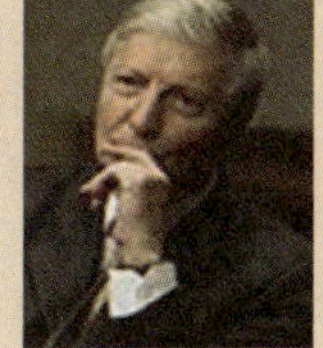

Jules A Hoffmann

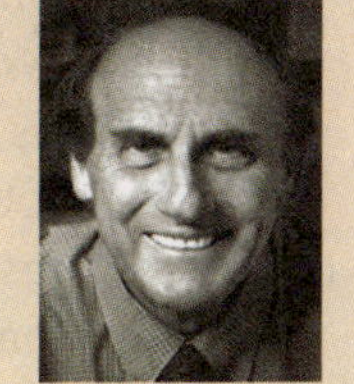

Ralph M Steinman

The **Nobel Prize in Physiology or Medicine 2011** was divided, with one half jointly to **Bruce A Beutler and Jules A Hoffmann** for their discoveries concerning the activation of **innate immunity**, and the other half of the prize was given to **Ralph M Steinman**, for his discovery of the dendritic cell and its role in **adaptive immunity**.

2. Though, highly developed in mammals, this is also the major mechanism of immunity in invertebrates and plants.

Acquired immunity: Vertebrates, especially mammals are gifted with acquired immunity in which specific set of lymphocytes are activated with specific antigens and eliminate antigens by ***specific mechanisms*** (specific immunity).

NONSPECIFIC DEFENSE SYSTEM (Innate Immunity)

Non-specific defense systems include the skin and mucous membrane (mechanical factors and chemical factors), antimicrobial mechanisms (interferons and complements), natural killer cells, phagocytosis, inflammation and fever. Thus, nonspecific defence mechanisms are:

1. Mechanical defense
2. Chemical defense
3. Defense by NK cells
4. Defense by phagocytic cells
5. Defense by inflammation and fever

Mechanical Defense

Skin and epidermis: Skin and epidermis are the most important and natural defense barriers of the body. They form the partition between the body and the external environment that immediately checks the entry of organisms into the body. Therefore, *loss of skin as occurs in burns leads to infection* and septicemia.

Mucous membranes: Mucous membrane also forms the physical barrier for the organisms and prevents their entry into the body. Wherever there is no skin on the body surface, mucous membrane covers the body, especially the surface of ***body cavities*** such as oral cavity, nasal cavity etc. Mucous membrane ***mechanically traps*** the organisms and ***secretes chemicals*** that inhibit the organisms.

Mucus: Mucus is secreted from glands located in the mucosal epithelium. Mucus, by virtue of its physical property traps microorganisms, especially in the respiratory, gastrointestinal and genitourinary tracts.

Hairs: Almost all openings (entry points) of the body such as nostrils, ears, eyes, anus, urethra and vagina (in females) are guarded by hairs. They filter microorganisms and prevent their entry into the body.

Cilia: Cilia also filter microorganisms. They are present in mucous membranes. They remove dust and microbes from upper respiratory tract. Along with mucus they also trap microbes.

Tear: Tear is secreted from lacrimal apparatus. It washes the microbes and dilutes the chemical substances produced by microbes.

Saliva: Saliva washes microbes from the oral cavity and keeps the mouth and teeth clean. It also contains antimicrobial chemicals.

Urine: During micturition, urine comes out of the urinary tract forcefully. Therefore, urine flow washes microbes from urinary tract.

Defecation: During the act of defecation, fecal matter is forcefully evacuated from the rectum and anal canal. Thus, along with fecal matters microbes are washed from lower GI tract.

Chemical Defense

Acidic pH of Skin: Acidic pH of skin inhibits growth of micro-organisms.

Bactericidal Substance of Sebum: Sebum is the secretion of the glands in the skin. It contains bactericidal substances like ***unsaturated fatty acids*** that kill microbes.

Chemicals in Body Secretions: Antimicrobial substances like ***lysozyme*** secreted in saliva, tear, sweat and other body secretions inhibit growth of micro-organisms.

Acidic pH of Stomach and Vagina: Strongly acidic pH of gastric secretion kills many micro-organisms and also destroys toxins in the stomach. Low pH of vaginal secretion also prevents entry of microbes into the body.

Complement Proteins: There are different complement proteins in plasma that are activated in response to entry of microorganisms into the body. They help in destroying the organisms by facilitating ***opsonization and phagocytosis***. They also participate in immunity (refer 'complement system').

Interferons: These are chemicals secreted from activated lymphocytes, etc., These are usually antiviral substances that kill viruses.

Defense by NK Cells

NK Cells

NK cells or **natural killer cells** are third category of lymphocytes that are neither B nor T cells:

1. They have the ability to kill a wide variety of micro-organisms and tumor cells.
2. They do not mature in thymus.
3. Unlike B and T cells, they lack surface antigen receptors.
4. They carry surface molecules **CD2, CD16, and CD56**, but negative for T cell marker CD3.
5. These are ***large granular lymphocytes*** (Fig. 19.1).
6. They constitute about **15% of total lymphocytes** in the body.
7. They are present in the spleen, lymph nodes, bone marrow and blood.
8. They take part in natural or innate immunity.
9. They recognize antibody coated target cells and kill them by ***antibody-dependent cell-mediated cytotoxicity*** (ADCC), which works more effective against viruses and tumour cells.

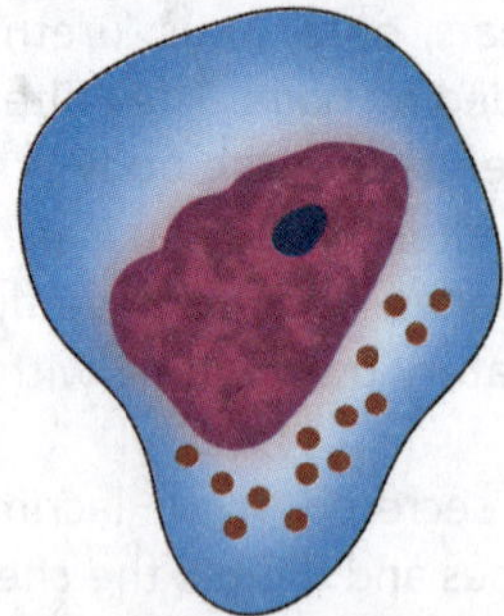

Fig. 19.1: NK Cell. Note the cell is large and cytoplasm is granular. *Courtesy*: Figure 29.3, Essentials in Hematology and Clinical Pathology by Ramadas Nayak et al., 1st edition, 2012; Jaypee Brothers Medical Publishers (P) Ltd.

Mechanism of Killing

NK cells **kill microbes** by following mechanisms:

1. **Osmotic lysis** by incorporating perforins into the surface of the microbes.
2. They release interferons that **activate phagocytosis** and immunity.
3. They possess Fc receptors that allow them to **kill antibody coated viruses.**
4. Kill by *antibody-dependent cell-mediated cytotoxicity* **(ADCC)**, especially the viruses and tumour cells.

Special Features: NK cells **differ from other lymphocytes** by following characteristics:

1. They do not require prior sensitization to kill microbes.
2. They do not involve major histocompatibility complex (MHC) antigen for killing micro-organisms.
3. They are the first line of defense against viral infections.
4. They are also active against tumor cells, especially malignant cells.
5. They usually attack cells that do not display proper markers.

Defense by Phagocytic Cells

Role of Granulocytes and Mononuclear Cells

Granulocytes (neutrophils, eosinophil and basophil), monocytes and macrophages kill micro-organisms by **phagocytosis**:

1. **Phagocytosis** is the process of ingestion of microbes or foreign cells or solid materials by a phagocyte. Phagocytes are **neutrophils, monocytes and macrophages** (scavenger cells). Monocytes transform themselves into macrophages in the tissue.
2. There are **two types** of macrophages: the wandering macrophages and fixed macrophages. The macrophages that are mobile in the tissues are called **wandering macrophages**.
3. The **fixed macrophages** are present in specific tissue sites in the body. These macrophages are mononuclear cells, and therefore this system of phagocytes is called as **mononuclear phagocyte system** (MPS). Previously, this system of cells was known as *reticuloendothelial system*, but they neither are reticular in appearance nor have endothelial origin. Therefore,

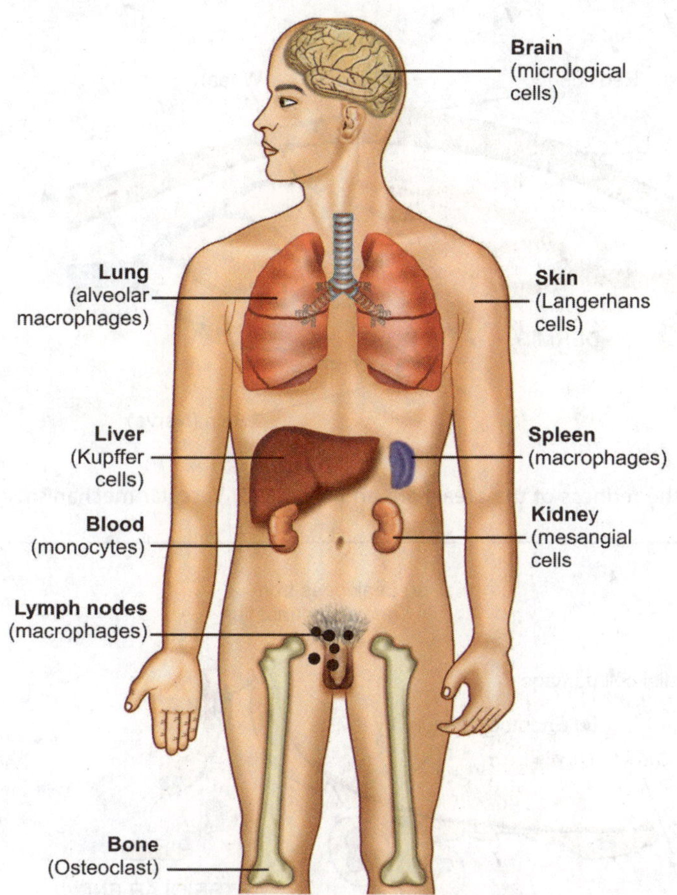

Fig. 19.2: Cells of mononuclear phagocyte system.

the term reticuloendothelial system is obsolete. The important examples of MPS include the following (Fig. 19.2):

a. Kupffer cells of the liver
b. Alveolar macrophages in the lungs
c. Microglia of brain
d. Tissue macrophages in the spleen and lymph nodes
e. Osteoclasts in bone
f. Mesangial cells in kidney
g. Histiocytes in connective tissues
h. Langerhans cells in the skin

Scientist contributed

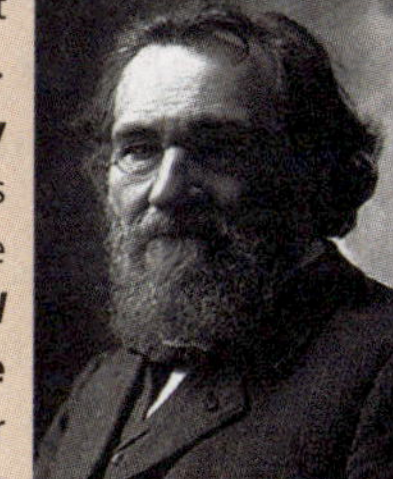

Élie Metchnikoff

Élie Metchnikoff was a Russian zoologist best known for his pioneering research n immunology. In particular, he is credited with the **discovery of phagocytes** (macrophages) in 1882. This discovery turned out to be the major defence mechanism in innate immunity. He and ***Paul Ehrlich*** were jointly awarded the **1908 Nobel Prize in Physiology or Medicine** "in recognition of their work on immunity". He established the concept of cell-mediated immunity, while Ehrlich described humoral immunity. Their works are regarded as the foundation of the science of immunology. In immunology, **Élie Metchnikoff** is given an epithet the "**Father of natural immunity**".

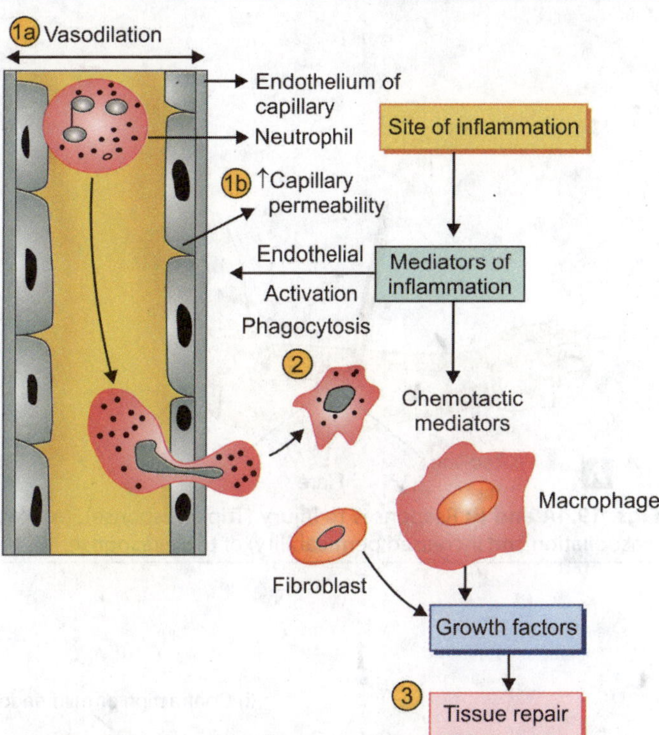

Fig. 19.3: Steps of inflammation. [1a: Vasodilation that increases blood flow to the area; 1b: Increased capillary permeability; 2: Phagocytosis by neutrophil; 3: Tissue repair (after few days) by macrophage and fibroblast that secrete growth factors].

Mechanism of phagocytosis includes chemotaxis, margination, adherence, ingestion, and digestion and killing (For details, refer "Neutrophil" Chapter 17, Figs. 17.11 to 17.13).

Defense by Inflammation and Fever

In the process of inflammation, microorganisms are killed by the chemicals released from the inflammatory cells, and also by phagocytes.

Inflammation

The response of the tissue to injury is known as inflammation. This is a defensive response of the body against the tissue injury. It is characterized by appearance of **four features** in sequence at the site of injury:

1. Rubor (redness)
2. Dolor (pain)
3. Calor (increased temperature)
4. Tumor (swelling).

The fifth component of inflammation is the *functiolesia*, the loss of function of the injured part of the body. Inflammation helps in killing the organisms and disposing them off. It also destroys toxins released by microbes, and helps in tissue repair. Thus, inflammation restores tissue homeostasis.

Stages of Inflammation

There are **three stages of inflammation**: vasodilation and increased permeability, phagocyte migration and phagocytosis, and tissue repair (Fig. 19.3).

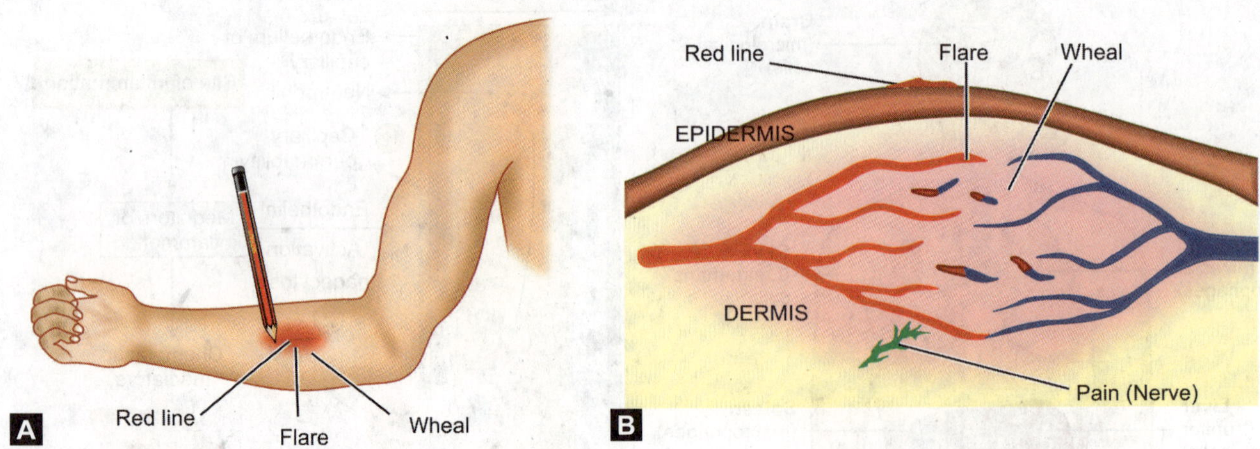

Figs. 19.4A and B: Responses to injury (Triple response). (A) Note the redness of the area, flare and wheal; (B) Vascular mechanisms (vasodilation and increased permeability) of triple response.

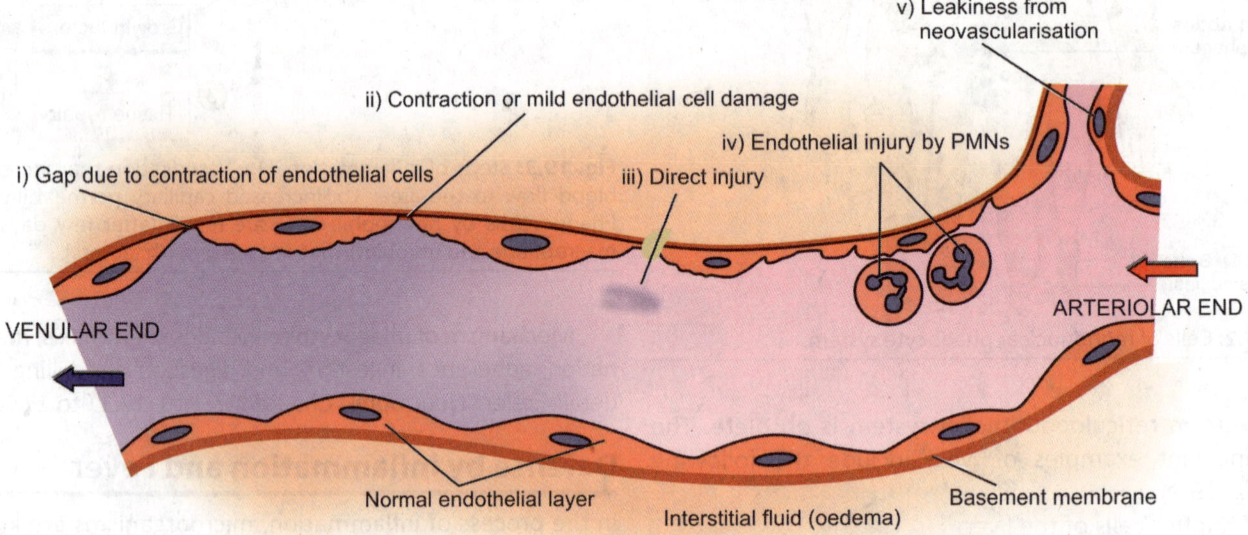

Fig. 19.5: Mechanisms of increased vascular permeability in acute inflammation. Note that contraction of endothelial cells increases the gap between them that facilitates permeability.

Vasodilation and Increased Permeability

Vasodilation occurs immediately following injury, which allows more blood to flow to the site of injury. This causes **redness of the area** (Figs. 19.4A and B). This is followed by increased permeability which allows fluid to escape into the tissue that causes **local swelling** (wheal), and also permits antibodies and phagocytes to enter the injured area:

1. Vasodilation and increased capillary permeability are produced by **histamine** released from mast cells, basophils, and platelets, **bradykinin** formed in the blood and in tissues from plasma kininogen and tissue kininogen respectively, **prostaglandins** released from damaged cells, and **complement proteins** formed by activation of complement system.
2. Contraction of vascular endothelial cells at the site of injury increases the gap between the cells that facilitats vascular permeability (Fig. 19.5).
3. The arteriolar dilation increases further blood flow that causes ***increased local temperature*** (calor) and ***flare*** i.e., spread of redness to the surrounding area, the phenomenon called **triple response** (Figs. 19.4A and B).

Phagocyte Migration and Phagocytosis

Within minutes to hours of inflammation, phagocytes appear at the site of injury. The first to appear is **neutrophil,** followed by **monocyte and macrophage** (Application Box 19.1):

1. Phagocytes reach the site of injury by **diapedesis and chemotaxis** (for details, refer Figs. 17.12 and 17.13, Chapter 17).
2. As the inflammatory response continues, **phagocytes die** in the process of killing the microbes.
3. Within few days, the dead phagocytes and damaged tissue cells form viscous fluid called **pus**. Usually, over a period of days pus is absorbed.

4. The pus that cannot be drained out from the region of inflammation slowly forms **abscess** (localized accumulation of pus).

Application Box 19.1

Alteration in cell count indicates nature of inflammation: As neutrophils first participate in inflammation, neutrophilia indicates acute inflammation or infection. As inflammation continues, monocytes and macrophages take part in phagocytosis. Therefore, monocytosis is the feature of chronic inflammation.

Tissue Repair

Tissue repair is the healing stage in inflammation. This is facilitated by migration of fibroblasts, macrophage and epithelial cells to the site of injury that repair and restore the epithelium by secreting growth factors. Tissue plasmin promotes migration of keratinocytes that aid to the healing process. Proliferation of collagen produces scar.

Role of NF-$_{k}$B

Recent evidences suggest that a transcription factor, called **nuclear factor kappa B ($_{K}$B)** (NF-$_{k}$B), plays an important role in inflammation:

1. Normally, NF-$_{k}$B is bound to another cytoplasmic protein called I_kB_α, and this binding keeps NF-$_{k}$B in an inactive state.
2. Viruses and cytokines that induce inflammation separate NF-$_{k}$B from I_kB_α. NF-$_{k}$B then migrates to nucleus and attaches with the DNA.
3. This induces the transcription of genes for formation of various chemicals that participate in inflammation.
4. Thus, NF-$_{k}$B stimulates synthesis and secretion of mediators of inflammation (Application Box 19.2).

Application Box 19.2

Cortisol acts through NF-$_{k}$B: Anti-inflammatory drugs like cortisol increase the production of I_kB_α in the cell, and therefore, prevent the activation of NF-$_{k}$B.

Systemic Response to Inflammation

Cytokines produced during inflammation induce systemic responses. The major change is the increase in **acute phase reactants** (APRs) in plasma. APRs are plasma proteins whose concentration increases at least by 25% in response to acute inflammations.

These **acute phase proteins** are mainly synthesized by liver. The important APRs are:

1. C-reactive protein (CRP)
2. Orosomucoid protein
3. Fibrinogen
4. Haptoglobin
5. Serum amyloid protein A
6. C_3 complement protein

The first to appear in acute inflammation is CRP. In many acute conditions, the **plasma level of high-sensitive CRP (hsCRP)** is an important marker of inflammation (Clinical Box 19.1). However, CRP concentration decreases rapidly within first week of the onset of the disease. The fibrinogen concentration increases slowly and remains elevated for 2 to 3 weeks. Increase in ESR in acute inflammation is due to increased level of fibrinogen that neutralizes the negative charges on the red cell surface.

Clinical Box 19.1

hsCRP is a prognostic marker: Estimation of ultrasensitive-CRP (us-CRP) has recently been used for diagnosis, and assessing the prognosis of inflammatory diseases and coronary artery disease.

Inflammatory Cells and Cytokines

Cells for acute inflammation: Neutrophils, eosinophils and basophils.

Cells for chronic inflammation: Monocytes, macrophages, lymphocytes and plasma cells.

These cells kill organisms by phagocytosis and also by secreting cytokines. Many of the mediators of inflammation are secreted by the inflammatory cells.

Fever

Fever is one of the protective phenomena of the body against infections:

1. Increased body temperature as occurs in acute infections and inflammations, ***prevents growth of microorganisms***.
2. Fever also facilitates the ***actions of interferon*** and different body ***enzymes*** that inhibit the growth of many microorganisms.
3. Therefore, unless very high and deleterious, fever should not be brought down immediately by antipyretics.

Contribution of Toll-like Receptors

Innate immunity in Drosophila is mainly due to the presence of a receptor protein called **'Toll'**. The toll binds with fungal antigens that activates of genes coding for antifungal proteins. A large number of **toll like receptors** (TLRs) are found in mammals including human beings. TLR4, one of these proteins, binds to bacterial polysaccharides and to CD14. It is proposed that this binding initiates intracellular events that activate transcription of genes for a variety of proteins ***required for innate immune responses*** (Application Box 19.3).

Application Box 19.3

Microbial functions require TRLs: Functions of many microorganisms are linked to TLRs:

1. Bacterial lipopolysaccharide produced by gram negative organisms is the cause of septic shock.
2. TLR2 mediates the response against microbial lipoproteins.
3. TLR6 cooperates with TLR2 in recognizing certain peptidoglycans.
4. TLR5 recognizes a molecule known as flagellin in bacterial flagella.
5. TLR9 recognizes bacterial DNA.

Pattern Recognition Receptors: TLRs are referred to as pattern recognition receptors (PRRS) AS they organize and respond to the molecular patterns expressed by pathogens. Few PRRs such as nucleotide-binding oligomarization protein domain (**NOD proteins**) may be intracellular. NOD 2 has recently been identified as the product of a candidate gene involved in inflammatory bowel disease and Croh'n disease.

SPECIFIC DEFENSE MECHANISMS (Acquired Immunity)

Acquired immunity is broadly divided into two categories: the cellular (cell mediated) immunity, and humoral (antibody mediated) immunity.

Cellular Immunity: Cell mediated immunity is due to the presence of **cytotoxic T cells** (killer cells) in the body:

1. These cells develop and proliferate in response to a particular antigen (or a specific organism) and kill that organism (or destroy that antigen).
2. This immunity is particularly effective against ***intracellular organisms*** like *viruses, parasites and fungi, cancer cells, tumor cells, and transplanted tissues.*

Humoral Immunity: Humoral immunity is due to the presence of **antibodies in the body**:

1. Antibodies are formed by plasma cells. Plasma cells are developed from activated B cells in response to antigen.
2. This immunity works mainly against ***extracellular organisms*** such as bacteria and the antigens dissolved in the body fluids.

Though pathogens stimulate activation of a particular immune mechanism predominantly, often they provoke both cellular and humoral immunity simultaneously.

Development of Immunity

Development of immunity is the development of lymphocytes. Immunity develops naturally in the body, but is activated in response to an antigen, which is generally an infective organism or a nonliving substance:

1. A specific antigen stimulates the development of a specific set of lymphocyte.
2. Functionally, lymphocytes are of three types: **B cell, T cell and NK cell.**
3. NK cell (described earlier) is mostly involved in relatively nonspecific defenses of the body.
4. The major sites of lymphocyte development are the **primary lymphoid organs**. In these organs, lymphocytes differentiate from their precursors that originate from the bone marrow, and proliferate and mature into functionally potent cells. In mammals, *T cells mature in the thymus*, and *B cells mature in the bone marrow and fetal liver*. Thus, **thymus, bone marrow and bursal equivalents** are the primary lymphoid organs.
5. After their maturity, they circulate in blood and migrate to **secondary lymphoid organ** where they reside.

Flowchart 19.1: General outline of the development of immunity. T4 cells induce development of both cellular and humoral immunity.

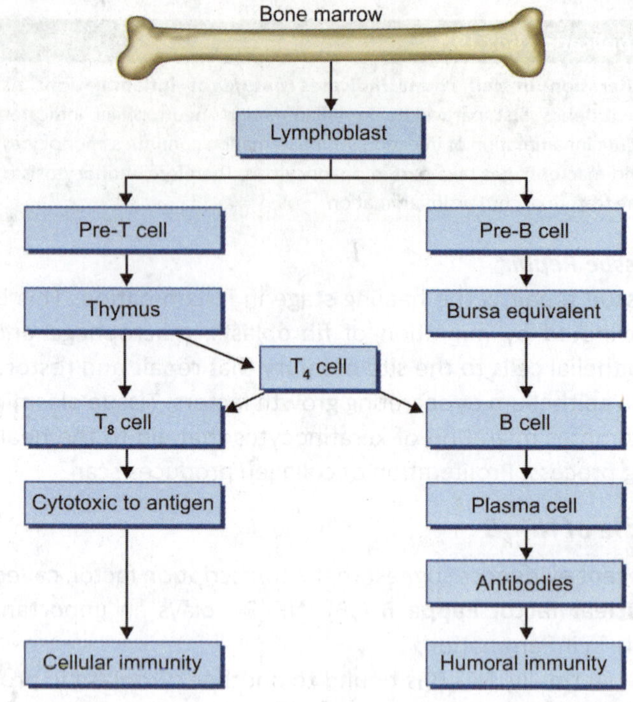

Secondary lymphoid organs are **lymph nodes, spleen and gut associated lymphoid organs.**

T cells develop in thymus, and B cells in bursal equivalents. The general outlines of development of immunity are summarized in Flowchart 19.1. For details of lymphoid tissues (thymus, lymph node, spleen, and other lymphoid tissues), and their functions, especially their role in immunity, refer the previous chapter. Distribution of T and B cells in different lymphoid tissues is depicted in Table 19.2.

Development of Bursa: B cells develop in bursa. In the birds, lymphoid tissue is present in bursa of Fabricius, which is located near the cloaca:

1. This bursa helps in development and processing of **B lymphocytes**, where pre-B cells develop into B cells. Therefore, these cells are called bursa-dependant cells or B cells.
2. However, in mammals there is no such bursa, but they have ***bursa equivalents***. The bursal equivalent issues are ***bone marrow and fetal liver***.

Development of Gut-Associated Lymphoid Organs: Lymphatic tissues are present at many places in GI tract starting from oral cavity to colon:

1. ***Tonsils*** (palatine, lingual and nasopharyngeal) that are present in the oral cavity and pharynx contain lymphatic follicles.
2. Lymphoid tissues are present extensively in the form of ***Payer's patches*** along the entire wall of intestine in the submucosal layer.

Table 19.2: Distribution of T and B cells in various lymphatic tissues of the body.

Lymphoid tissue	T cell (%)	B cell (%)
Thymus	100	0
Bone marrow	10	90
Spleen	45	55
Lymph node	60	40
Blood	80	20

3. Vermiform appendix is rich in lymphatic tissue.
4. Lymphatic tissues are also present in colon.
5. These lymphatic structures in GI tract provide immunity to body by killing organisms, parasites and larvae that try to enter blood from intestinal lumen.

Development of T Cells

Mechanism of Development

Development of T cells takes place in thymus. Hence, they are called thymus-dependent or T cells:

1. The stem cells or precursor cells that migrate to thymus before they mature into competent lymphocytes in the thymic environment are called **pre-T cells**. The lymphocytes that develop from pre-T cells are called T cells.
2. It is not clearly known whether the migration of prethymic (pre-T) cells is selective or random, and whether they are multipotent or destined to from only T cells.
3. Experimental evidences suggest that migration of stem cells into thymus is not a random process, but results from chemotactic signals that are periodically emitted from the thymus. **β_2-microglobulin,** a component of MHC-I molecule is putative chemoattractant for pre-T cells.
4. Though experimental evidences suggest that stem cells destined for thymus express CD7, a marker of T cells, they are multipotent in nature. However, in the thymic environment they develop only into T cells.
5. In the thymus, epithelial cells, macrophages and interdigitating cells are rich in MHC class II antigens. These cells are important in the differentiation of pre-T cells into T cells.
6. The most important among them is the **epithelial cell**. Specialized epithelial cells in the peripheral areas of cortex are called **thymic nurse cells**. The thymic nurse cells are pockets of thymocytes (cortical and medullary) that secrete IL-7, which supports differentiation and proliferation of pre-T cells.

Steps of Development

Stem cells (pre-T cells) first colonize in the subcapsular cortical region of the thymus. Then, they develop into large actively proliferating **lymphoblasts** that possess the property of self-renewal:

1. Lymphoblasts differentiate and proliferate into **Pre-T cells**.
2. Pre-T cells develop into **T cells**.
3. Pre T cells become **Naïve T cells**, that further proliferate to form **T immunoblasts** (Fig. 19.6).
4. There are ***2 types of T immunoblasts***. One set expresses $CD8^+$ on the surface that develops into $CD8^+$ cells (T_8 cell, or cytotoxic T cell) and the other set expresses $CD4^+$ on the surface that develops into $CD4^+$ cells (T_4 cell, Helper T cell).
5. As cells mature, they migrate to the medulla, and mature T cells leave thymus via postcapillary venules located at the corticomedullary junction, and also via lymphatic vessels.
6. After processing and development in the thymus, the mature T cells migrate into the lymph nodes, spleen, bone marrow, other tissues and blood.
7. T cells participate in cell-mediated or cellular immunity.

Changes during Development

During their processing (differentiation and proliferation) in the thymus, they undergo **two morphological and chemical changes** that confer on them the ability to recognize and kill the antigens. These changes are formation of specific receptors and synthesis of chemokines:

1. **Formation of specific receptors on T cells**
   The receptors to recognize the particular antigen are formed on T cell surface (Fig. 19.7), and are called **T cell receptors** (TCR). There are four types of polypeptides for TCR: α, β, γ and δ. However, only two sets are present in TCR. The combinations are either $\alpha\beta$ or $\gamma\delta$. Accordingly, TCR are either **$\alpha\beta$ TCR** or **$\gamma\delta$ TCR**. The T cells with $\alpha\beta$ TCR are called ***$\alpha\beta$ T cells***, and T cells with $\gamma\delta$ TCR are called ***$\gamma\delta$ T cells***. 95% of circulating T cells are $\alpha\beta$ T cells and only 5% are $\gamma\delta$ T cells.
2. **Synthesis of chemokines to kill antigens**
   The cells acquire capacities to from various chemokines that are capable of killing invading organisms. Important chemokines are lymphotoxin and interferons.

Types of T Cells

There are three types of T cells: the helper T cells (T_4 cells), cytotoxic T cells (T_8 cells), and memory T cells.

Helper T Cells (T_4 Cells)

The helper T cells are called T_4 cells as they contain CD4 protein on their cell surface. They are known as helper or **inducer cells** as they assist in induction of both cellular and humoral immunity. There are two sets of helper T cells: **Type 1 helper cells** (T_H1 cells) that assist in cellular immunity and **type 2 helper cells** (T_H2 cells) that assist in humoral

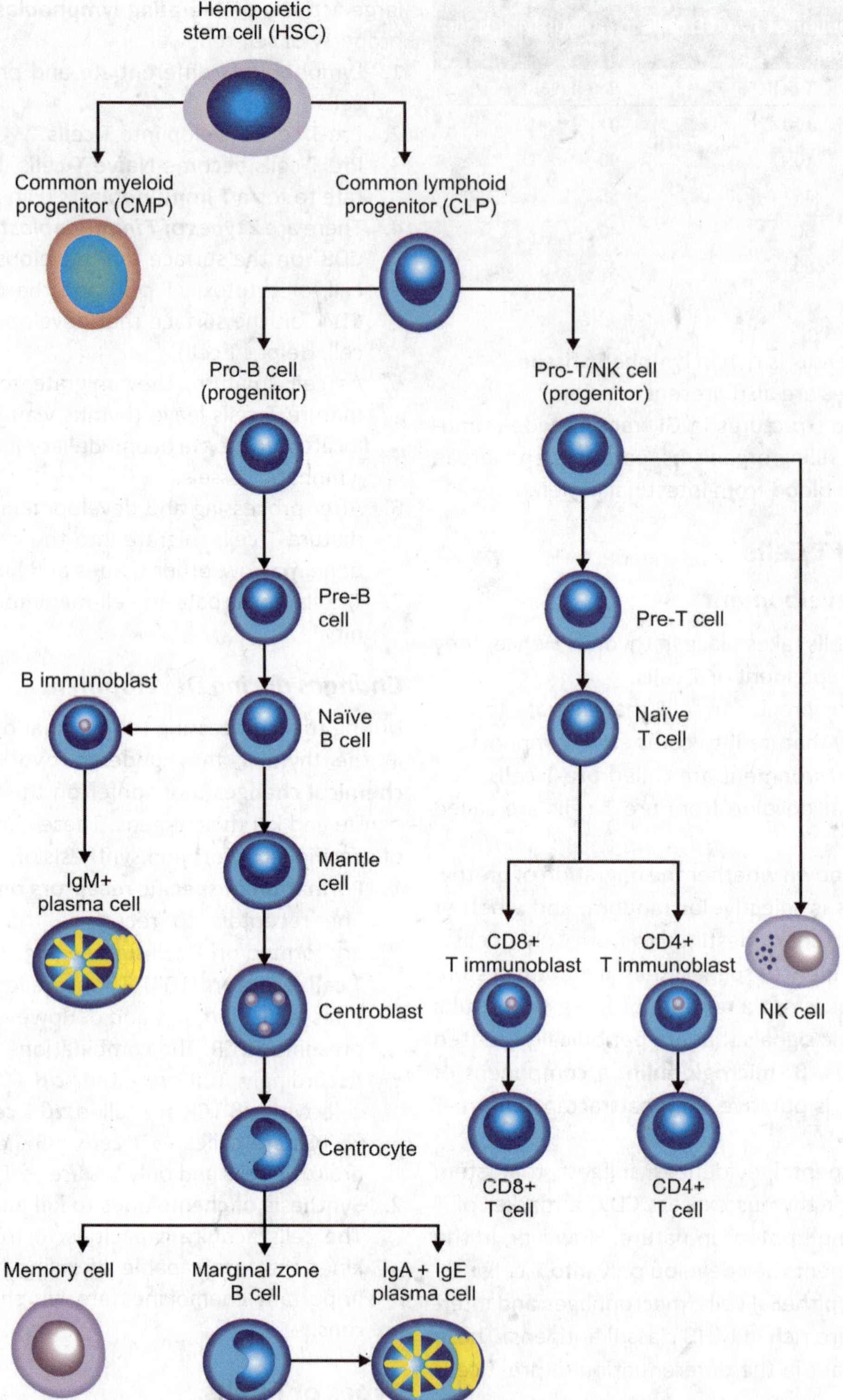

Fig. 19.6: Details of the development T cells and B cells.
Courtesy: Figure 29.2, Essentials in Hematology and Clinical Pathology by Ramadas Nayak et al., 1st edition, 2012; Jaypee Brothers Medical Publishers (P) Ltd.

immunity. Activated T_H1 cells secrete IL-2 and γ-interferon, and T_H2 cells secrete IL-4, IL-5, IL-6 and IL-10 (Fig. 19.7).

Cytotoxic T Cells

These are called **T_8 cells** as they contain CD8 protein on their cell membrane. They are called cytotoxic or **killer cells** as they kill invading organisms by producing cytotoxicity. They are sometimes also referred to as **suppressor T cells** (T_S).

Memory T Cells

A small subset of T cells remains in the tissue as memory T cells. These cells remember the initial immunologic insult,

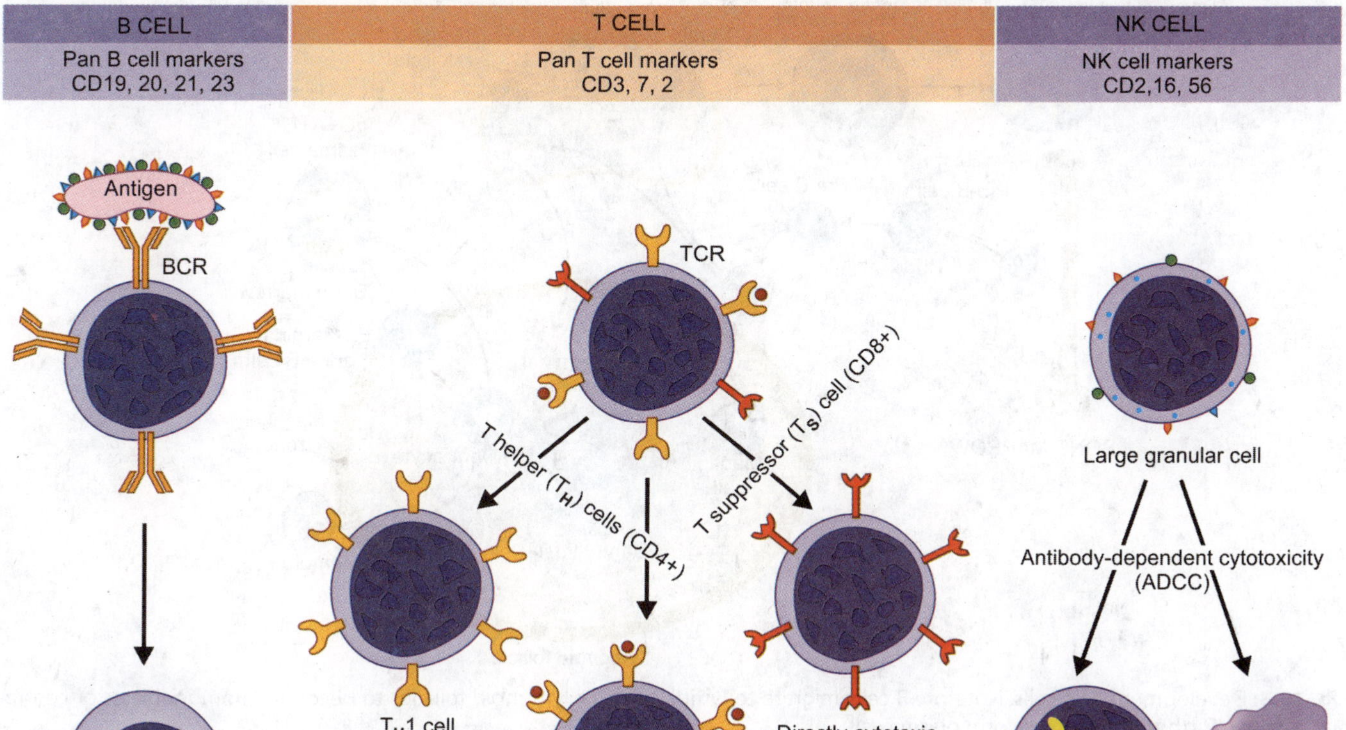

Fig. 19.7: Development of receptors on T cells, and functions of T cell, B cell and NK cell. (BCR: B cell receptor; TCR: T cell receptor).

and on subsequent exposure to same challenges they are activated immediately without presentation of antigen by antigen presenting cells (*see* below) and proliferate to millions of T cells that instantaneously fight to eliminate the antigens. Memory T cells ***live a very long life***, may be the entire life of the individual. Therefore, similar antigenic exposure at any time during the life of the person induces prompt and focused cell-mediated immune response.

T Cell Receptor

The T cell receptor (TCR) complex consists of seven polypeptide chains:

1. In the majority of (95%) of T cells, α and β chains form the antigen-binding site of TCR ***(αβ TCR)***.
2. Each of these chains has a variable and a constant region similar to immunoglubulins.
3. The α and β chains are linked together by a disulfide bond to form α-β complex which is composed of five polypeptide chains.
4. The variable regions of α and β chains bind antigen while CD3 converts this antigen recognition into intracellular activating signals.
5. In a minority of T cells, γ and δ polypeptide chains are present instead of α and β chains ***(γδ TCR)***.

TCR Gene Arrangement

The genetic structure of TCR bears resemblance to that of immunoglobulin. The TCR β chain gene is located on **chromosome 7** and TCR α chain gene is on chromosome 14:

1. Although all somatic cells contain T cell receptor gene in germ line configuration, **rearrangement occurs only in T cells.**
2. The TCR β gene consists of variable (V), diversity (D), joining (J) and constant (C) regions.
3. One segment each from V, D and J regions join together with deletion of intervening sequences. The rearranged gene is transcribed into mRNA. Rearrangement of other peptide chain occurs similarly.
4. As there are a number of V, D and J segments which code for amino acid sequences in variable region, it is possible to generate T cell receptor with different antigen specificities by various combinations during rearrangements.
5. Rearrangement of TCR β gene precedes the rearrangement of TCR α gene.

T Cell Ontogeny

Progenitor T cells from the bone marrow are transported to thymus where they undergo maturation. During maturation,

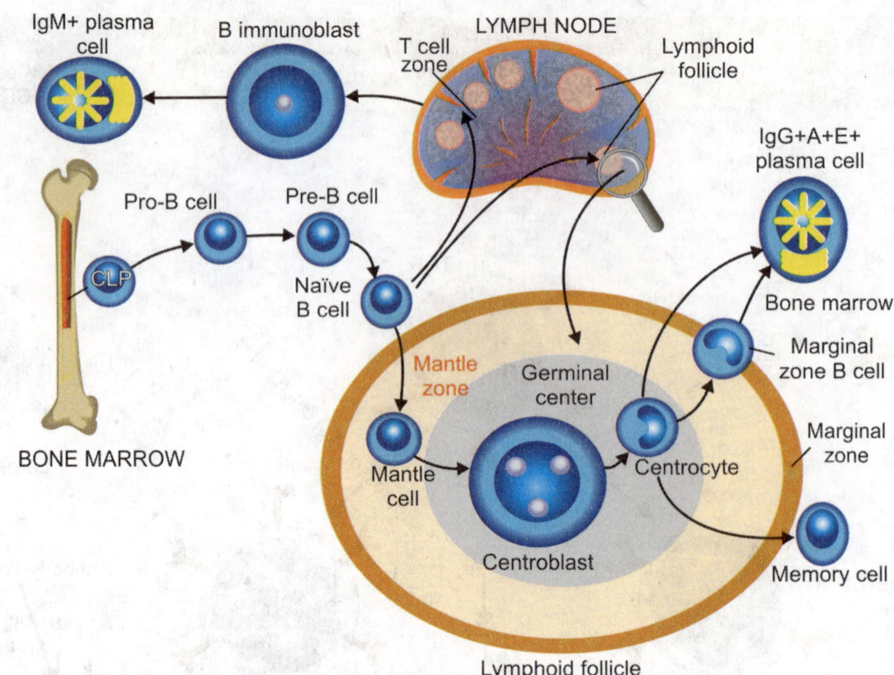

Fig. 19.8: Development of B cells. Note pre B cells migrate to lymph node or lymphoid follicles to become B immunoblasts or centroblasts, which further transform to form plasma cell.
Courtesy: Figure 29.1, Essentials in Hematology and Clinical Pathology by Ramadas Nayak et al., 1st edition, 2012; Jaypee Brothers Medical Publishers (P) Ltd.

there is rearrangement of TCR genes, expression of some cell surface proteins, and acquisition of ability to distinguish self antigen from foreign antigens:

1. Initially immature cortical thymocytes express CD7, TdT and cytoplasmic CD3 (cCD3).
2. Those T cells which subsequently are going to form α and β polypeptides ($\alpha\beta$ TCR), first rearrange TCR β gene followed by TCR α gene.
3. Expression of $\alpha\beta$ TCR occurs in association with expression of CD3 on surface of cells.
4. Initially both CD4 and CD8 antigens are acquired, but with further maturation cell retains either CD4 or CD8 antigen.
5. $CD4^+$ cells are called as helper or inducer T cells whereas $CD8^+$ cells are called cytotoxic T cells.
6. The mature T cells are released from thymus, circulate in peripheral blood and are transported to peripheral lymphoid organs.

Development of B Cells

The lymphocyte precursors that enter the bursa equivalents like fetal liver and bone marrow in mammals form B cells. They are called B cells as they develop in the bursa equivalent tissues (hence, bursa-dependent cells or B cells):

1. In the birds, a lymphoid tissue is present near the cloaca (the **bursa of Fabricius**) help in development and processing of B lymphocytes, where pre-B cells develop into B cells. However, in mammals there is no such bursa, but they have **bursa equivalents**.
2. During their development in bursa equivalent structures, **B cells acquire characteristic surface molecules**. They ***acquire receptors*** to recognize antigen and receptors for various cytokines, and most importantly the ***genes for immunoglobulin synthesis***. First, the ***gene rearrangement*** occurs for heavy chain and then the gene rearrangement occurs for light chain of immunoglobulins.
3. Pre B cells become **Naïve B cell**, that transform into **Mantle Cell, Centroblast and Centrocyte**. Centrcytes mature into ***plasma cell*** or transform to ***memory B cells*** (*see* Fig. 19.6)
4. Each B cell lineage is committed for making only one specific antibody against a specific antigen. This is the central theme of clonal selection theory of antibody production.
5. Pre B cells once mature in bursa equivalents migrate to lymph nodes, bone marrow, blood and other tissues like lymph nodes and lymphoid follicles.
6. In these structures (bone marrow, lymph nodes and lymphoid follicles), they further process to become **B immunoblasts** or **centroblasts**, those under on specific immunologic stimulation undergo further transformation to form **plasma cells** (Fig. 19.8).
7. Plasma cells produce large quantities of antibodies. Plasma cells are not normally found in blood. Antibodies formed by plasma cells kill or neutralize antigens.
8. A small set of B cells form **memory B cells** that on subsequent exposure to an antigen get readily converted into effective B cells (plasma cells) to carry out immuno-

logical functions. The memory B cells persist in the body for many years. Therefore, similar antigenic exposure in future induces prompt and heightened humoral immunological responses.

Antigens

Definition

Antigens are living organisms or substances that on entry into the body induce specific immunological reactions. Antigens have two important properties: immunogenicity and reactivity:

1. **Immunogenicity** is the ability to provoke an immune response i.e., to stimulate the production of specific antibody or proliferation of specific T cells or both.
2. **Reactivity** is the ability of the antigen to react specifically with an antibody or a cell or both.
3. An antigen that possesses both the properties is defined as a **complete antigen**.
4. An antigen that has the reactivity but lack immunogenicity is called **partial antigen** or a **hapten**.

Nature of Antigen

Antigens may be the entire micro-organism like a bacterium or a virus, or a part of the organism like capsule of the virus, flagella of bacteria or the cell wall of the organism. The antigen may also be a nonmicrobial substance, such as pollen, egg white, transplanted tissue or incompatible blood cells.

Chemical Nature: Antigens are large complex molecules. Usually, they are protein in nature. However, nucleoproteins, glycoproteins, or large polysaccharides also behave as antigens. Usually T cells respond to protein antigens, whereas B cells respond to proteins and non-protein antigens.

Antigenic Determinant

Specific portion of an antigen that triggers the immunological reaction is called antigenic determinant or **epitope**. Usually an antigen possesses many antigenic determinants, each of which induces production of a specific antibody or proliferation of a specific set of T lymphocytes.

MHC Antigens

Major histocompatibility complex or MHC antigens are self-antigens that help in identifying and rejecting the foreign antigens:

1. They are also called ***HLA antigens*** (human leucocyte associated antigens), as they were first identified on the membrane of leucocytes. However, afterward they were found to be present on the surface of all the body cells except in red cells (remember, red cells contain blood group antigens).
2. Like blood group antigens they are chemically glycoproteins. They are made up of α **and** β **subunits**.
3. Though MHC antigens are responsible for rejection of transplanted tissues, their normal function is to identify the foreign antigens and present them to the T cell for induction of cellular immunity.
4. The *recognition of an antigen* is the first and foremost step in the process of activation of immunological responses, especially for initiation of cellular immunity.

Types of MHC Antigens

There are two types of MHC antigens: type 1 or MHC I, and type 2 or MHC II antigens.

MHC I antigen: MHC I antigens are present on the cell membranes of all body cells except red cells. MHC I is made up of three α and one β subunits.

MHC II antigen: MHC II antigens are present on the surface of antigen presenting cells (APCs), thymus cells and activated T cells. MHC II is made up of two α and two β subunits.

Mechanism of Action of MHC Antigens

The proteins in the cells are continuously broken down to their peptide fragments. MHC I molecules pick up the peptide fragments containing 8–10 amino acids, whereas MHC II molecules pick up peptides containing 13–17 amino acids:

1. When a peptide fragment of a self protein is picked up by the MHC antigen and expressed on the surface of the APC along with MHC proteins, T cells ignore it.
2. However, when the peptide fragment is of a foreign protein, T cells recognize it and get activated that induce cell- mediated immunological responses.

Significance of HLA Antigens

1. They are important as histocompatibility antigens in organ transplantation.
2. HLA antigens play a major role in recognition of foreign antigens and in immunity.
3. In transfusion medicine, they are responsible for autoimmunization against platelet antigens and refractoriness to platelet transfusion, febrile transfusion reactions and graft versus host disease.
4. A relationship exists between presence of some HLA antigen and susceptibility to certain diseases.
5. HLA antigen typing can also be used for paternity testing.

Recognition of MHC-Ag Complex by TCR

The MHC protein-Antigen complex on the surface of the APCs binds to appropriate receptor on T cells. Therefore, receptors on the T cell should recognize a wide variety of protein complexes (Figs. 19.9A and B). As discussed above, TCR is made up of α and β subunits that form heterodimers to recognize the MHC proteins and the antigen fragments with which they are combined. These cells are called $\alpha\beta$ T cells. Details of TCR recognition of antigen presented by APCs are discussed below. About 10% of

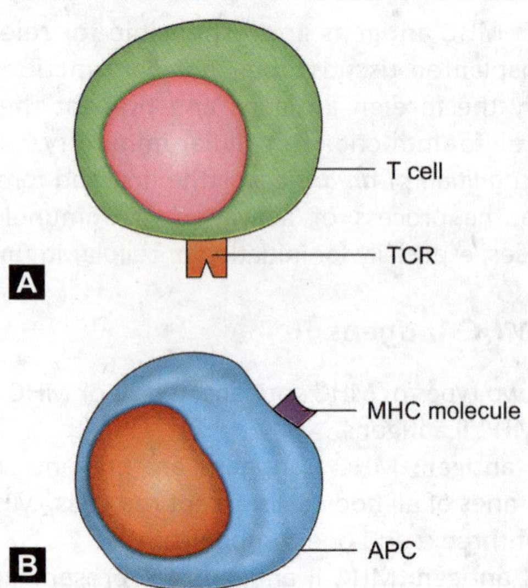

Figs. 19.9A and B: (A) T cell receptors (TCR); (B) Major histocompatibility complex (MHC) molecule expressed on the surface of antigen presenting cell (APC).

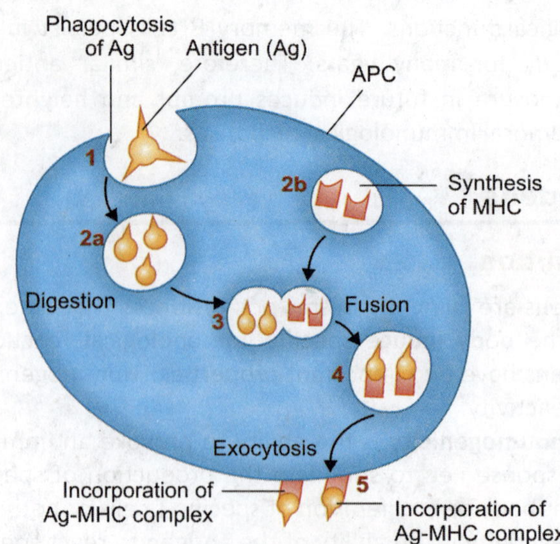

Fig. 19.10: Steps of antigen processing and presentation by antigen presenting cell (APC). (1: Phagocytosis of antigen (Ag); 2a: Partial digestion of Ag into its peptide fragments IN THE vesicle; 2b: Synthesis of MHC-II molecule; 3: Fusion of vesicles containing Ag fragments and MHC molecules; 4: Single vesicle containing antigen fragments attached to MHC molecules; 5: Incorporation of MHC-Ag complex on the membrane of APC during exocytosis).

circulating T cells are αδ T cells. These T cells are prominent in the mucosa of the gastrointestinal tract. The αδ T cells form a link between the innate and acquired immune systems, and help in secretion of cytokines.

CELLULAR IMMUNITY

Cell mediated immunity is mediated by **T cells**. Cellular immunity is particularly effective against ***intra-cellular organisms*** like *viruses, parasites and fungi, cancer cells, tumor cells, and transplanted tissues*. This immunity is induced following entry of an antigen into the body. However, antigen directly does not induce cellular immunity unless presented appropriately to the T cells. The antigen is recognized and processed by the antigen presenting cells (APCs) and then presented to the immunocompetent lymphocytes that are activated and proliferated to destroy the antigen.

Steps of Cellular Immunity

Mechanism of cellular immunity includes following steps:

1. Antigen recognition, processing and presentation
2. Activation and proliferation of T cells
3. Elimination of the invader

Antigen Recognition, Processing and Presentation

There are different varieties of antigens but human body has the ability to recognize each of them. This recognition ability is innate, which develops without prior exposure to the antigen. The precursor stem cells of lymphocytes differentiate into millions of different T and B cells. Each T or B cell type has the ability to respond to a particular antigen. On entry into the body, antigens bind with an appropriate receptor present on the B cell surface and activate the B cells:

1. However, for activation of T cell to occur the antigen should be processed and presented by the APCs to the appropriate receptors on the T cell.
2. The cells that process and present antigens to the T cells are called antigen presenting cells (APCs).
3. APCs include **macrophages**, **dendritic cells** and **B cells.**
4. APCs are present in more numbers specifically at locations that are the usual sites for antigen entry into the body like skin, and mucous membrane of respiratory, gastrointestinal and genitourinary tracts.

Steps of Antigen Presentation

There are **five major steps** in antigen presentation: ingestion of antigens, digestion of antigen, fusion of vesicles, binding of peptide fragments to MHC molecule, and incorporation of antigen-MHC complex into the cell membrane of APC (Fig.19.10):

1. **Ingestion of the antigen:** Antigens are ***ingested by APCs*** by the process of **endocytosis.**
2. **Digestion of the antigen and formation of vesicles:** Following phagocytosis, antigen is digested partially by the lysosomal enzymes and form ***phagosome*** within the cytoplasm of APCs. The phagosomal vesicles contain peptide fragments of antigens. Simultaneously, MHC II molecules are formed in the cell (***MHC vesicles***).
3. **Fusion of vesicles:** The phagosomal vesicles containing peptide fragments of antigen combine with the vesicles containing MHC II molecules. These two vesicles merge to form single vesicle.

4. **Binding of peptide fragments with MHC II molecules:** Following fusion of vesicles, antigen fragments bind with MHC II molecules. The fused vesicles containing MHC II and peptide fragments (***MHC-Ag complex***) undergo exocytosis.
5. **Incorporation of antigen-MHC complex into the cell membrane of APC:** During the process of **exocytosis**, the peptide fragments (antigens)–MHC-II complex ***get incorporated into the cell membrane of APC***:

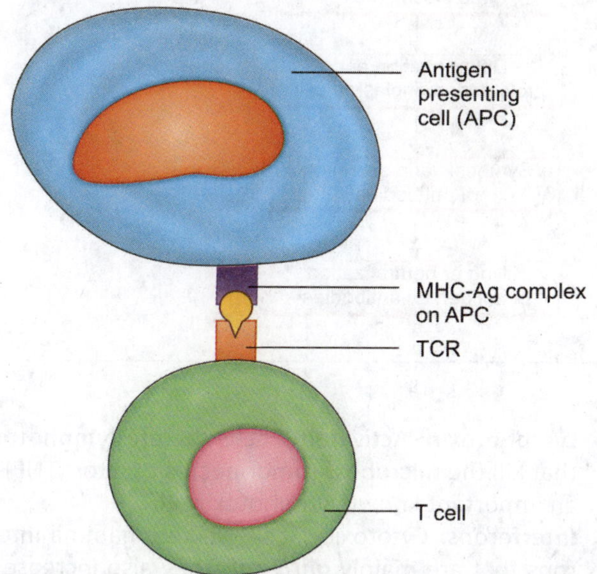

Fig. 19.11: Recognition of antigen by T cell. Note, MHC-Antigen complex attaches with T cell receptor for recognition of the antigen and induction of immunity.

– An APC containing the MHC-antigen complex migrate into the lymphatic tissue or circulate in the blood.
– When APC containing this MHC-Ag complex comes in contact with a particular T cell, the complex attaches with T-cell receptor (Fig.19.11).
– Consequently, the T cell gets activated that triggers cell mediated immunity.

Immunologic Synapse

For antigen recognition, antigen presenting cell (APC) presents the antigen to T cell. T cell receptors are surrounded by adhesion molecules. Proteins bind to complementary proteins in the APC when the two cells transiently join. The junction between T cell and APC is called immunologic synapse. The activity at this synapse permits the T cell activation to occur. It is now generally accepted that two signals are necessary to produce activation. One is produced by the binding of the digested antigen to the T cell receptor. The other is produced by the joining of the surrounding proteins in the synapse. If the first signal occurs but the second does not, the T cell is inactivated and becomes unresponsive.

Activation and Proliferation of T Cells

The cell-mediated immunity depends on the activation of T cells by a particular antigen. An activated T cell undergoes differentiation and proliferation into the ***effector T cells***, which eliminates the antigen. Activation of cellular immunity involves ***two steps***: activation of T cells and proliferation and differentiation of T cells (Fig. 19.12).

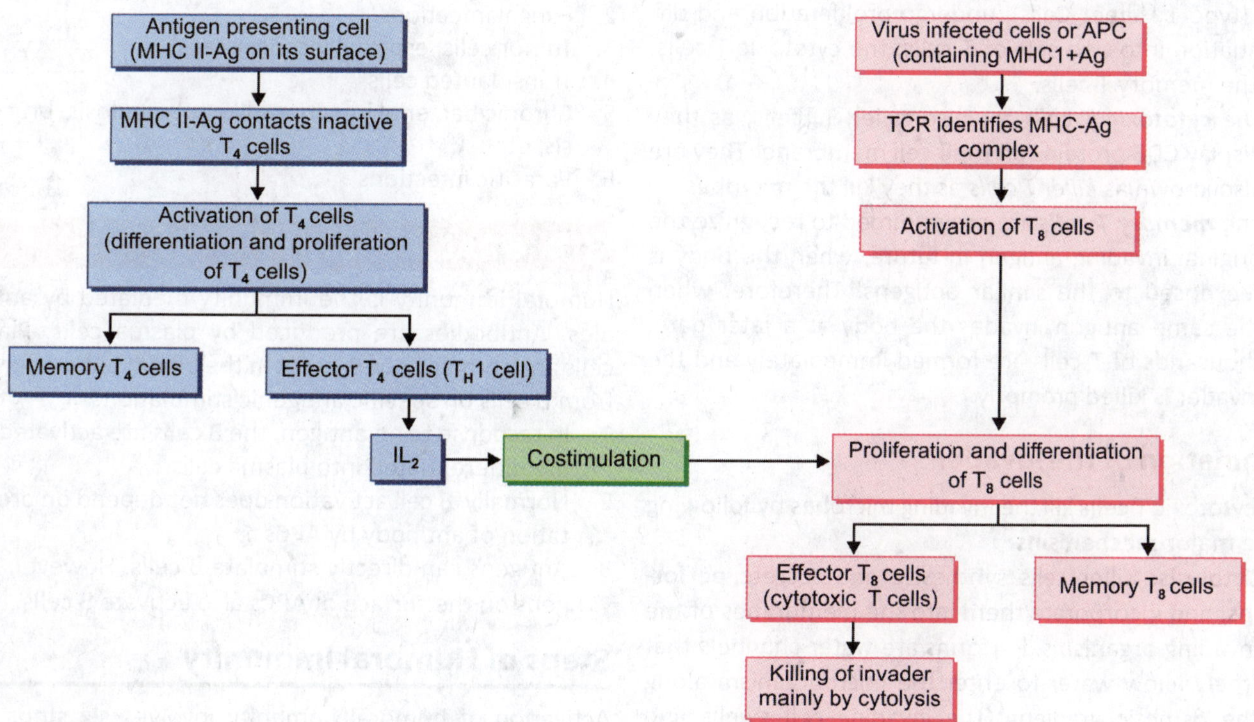

Fig. 19.12: Mechanism of cellular immunity.

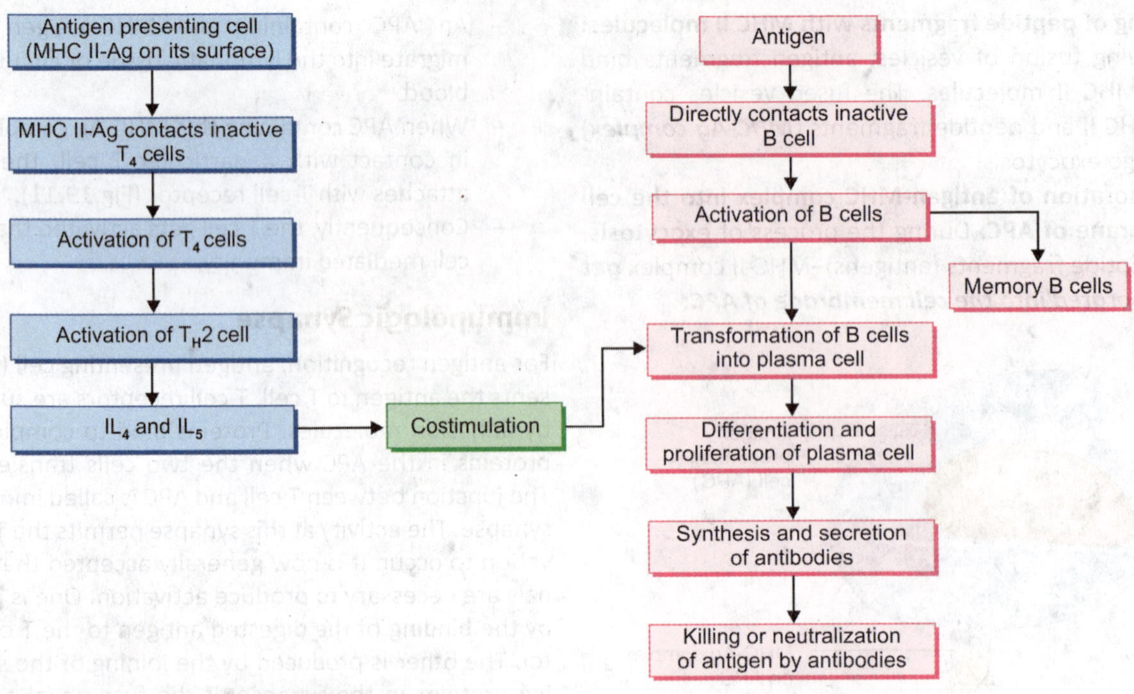

Fig. 19.13: Mechanism of humoral immunity.

Activation of T Cells

There are receptors on the T cell surface, known as TCR. When TCRs come in contact with MHC-antigen complex located on the surface of the APCs, T cells are activated (*see* Fig. 19.11). This is the first step in induction of cellular immunity.

Proliferation and Differentiation of T Cells

The activated T cells with proper costimulation by inducer cells (type 1 Helper Cells), undergo proliferation and differentiation into two sets of T cells: the cytotoxic T cells, and the memory T cells:

1. ***The cytotoxic T cells*** are also called T_8 cells, as they display CD8 proteins on their cell membrane. They are also known as *killer T cells* as they kill the microbes.
2. The ***memory T cells*** are programmed to recognize the original invading antigen in future, when the body is reexposed to the similar antigens. Therefore, when the same antigen invades the body at a later date, thousands of T cells are formed immediately and the invader is killed promptly.

Elimination of the Invader

The cytotoxic T cells kill the invading microbes by following **three major mechanisms**:

1. **Cytolysis:** Killer cells synthesize and secrete **perforins**, and incorporate them into the membranes of the invading organisms. Perforins are water channels that freely allow water to enter the microorganism along the osmotic gradient. The invading cell swells and finally undergoes **osmotic lysis.**
2. **Lymphotoxin:** Activated T cells secrete **lymphotoxins** that kill the microbes. Tumor necrosis factor (TNF)-β is an important known lymphotoxin.
3. **Interferons:** Cytotoxic T cells secrete gamma-interferons that are mainly ***antiviral***. They also increase the phagocytic activity of neutrophils and macrophages by promoting opsonization.

Cellular immunity is activated mainly against intracellular pathogens and tumor cells, as in:

1. Viral infections
2. Fungal infections
3. Tumor cells, especially cancer cells
4. Transplanted cells
5. Chronic bacterial infections like tuberculosis, brucellosis, etc.
6. Parasitic infections

HUMORAL IMMUNITY

Humoral immunity is the immunity mediated by antibodies. Antibodies are produced by plasma cells. Plasma cells are normally not present in the blood, but are formed from B cells on specific antigenic stimulation:

1. In response to an antigen, the B cells are activated and are differentiated into plasma cells.
2. Normally, B cell activation does not depend on presentation of antibody by APCs.
3. Antigens can directly stimulate B cells. However, antigens on the surface of APCs also activate B cells.

Steps of Humoral Immunity

Activation of humoral immunity involves **six steps** (Fig. 19.13):

1. Presentation of antigen
2. Activation of B cells
3. Differentiation of B cells into plasma cells
4. Proliferation of plasma cells and antibody production
5. Killing of the invaders by antibodies that include activation of complement system
6. Formation of memory B cells and subsequent immunological responses

Presentation of Antigen

Antigen presenting cells in humoral immunity include B cells themselves. Therefore, antigen presentation through APCs is **not a must** for induction of humoral immunity. However, antigen combined with MHC II molecules on the surface of APC (Ag-MHC complex) may also be presented to B cells.

Activation of B Cells

When an antigen binds directly to the receptors present on the surface of the B cells, the B cells are activated. B cells are also activated when they come in contact with MHC-antigen complex presented by the APCs:

1. This process of activation is accentuated by the **costimulation from type 2 helper cells**.
2. T_H2 cells stimulate B cell by secreting IL-2, IL-4, and IL-5.
3. Activated B cells form plasma cells and memory B cells.

Differentiation of B Cells into Plasma Cells

The activated B cell enlarges in size that undergoes complete transformation to become plasma cell. This is not a simple differentiation as occurs for T cells in cellular immunity:

1. The cell is transformed completely in structure and function.
2. Plasma cell has larger cytoplasm containing numerous rough endoplasmic reticulums.
3. The enlarged B cell appears almost like a **lymphoblast,** called **B immunoblasts** (*see* Figs. 19.6 and 19.8). Therefore, sometimes this differentiation is called as **blast transformation**. Co-stimulation by T helper cells (T_H2 cells) facilitates the process of transformation.

Proliferation of Plasma Cells and Antibody Production

Activated B cells are differentiated into plasma cells. Plasma cells then undergo proliferation to form millions of plasma cells. Plasma cells **secrete a large quantity of antibodies**:

1. A specific antigen stimulates activation of specific B cells that undergo proliferation of a selective clone of plasma cell.
2. This is called *clonal selection* of plasma cell.
3. Specific clone of plasma cells produce specific antibodies.

Killing of the Invaders

Antibodies attack antigens and kill organisms (destroy antigens) by following mechanisms:

1. **Neutralizing antigen:** Antibodies neutralize the antigens. For example, antigens detoxify the bacterial toxins and prevent them to induce immunological reactions.
2. **Immobilization of microbes:** Antibodies ***prevent the motility of bacteria*** thereby inhibit their spread to the surrounding tissue.
3. **Activation of complement system:** Antibodies (antigen-antibody complex) ***activate the classical pathway of complement system*** by activating C1 (for details, see below) and complements kill organisms.
4. **Precipitation of antigens:** Antibodies cause ***agglutination and precipitation*** of antigens. By this mechanism, soluble antigens become insoluble. Insoluble antigens are easily phagocytosed by phagocytic cells.
5. **Facilitation of phagocytosis:** Antibodies enhance phagocytosis by ***opsonizing the antigen***. Opsonization is the process by which microbes or antigens are made tasty to phagocytes for ingestion by coating antigen with opsonins like antibody, complement proteins, etc.
6. **Providing immunity to newborns:** IgG antibody can easily cross placenta and enter fetal circulation from the maternal blood. Thus, it provides immunity in newborns. IgA antibody from the maternal milk also provides immunity to the newborn.

Formation of Memory B Cells and Subsequent Immunological Responses

A small subset of activated B cells differentiates into **memory B cells**. However, this differentiation is not like blast transformation. Memory B cells normally remain inactive, unless stimulated by the similar antigens. They respond quickly and vigorously to the same antigens on subsequent exposures. The immunological responses on second and subsequent exposures to antigen are much more in intensity and duration than on first exposure. This is called **secondary immunological response** (see below). These memory B cells live a longer life, may be the life of the individual.

Types of Humoral Immune Responses

There are two types of immune responses: the primary response, and the secondary response.

Primary Response

When antigen enters into the body for the first time, the immune response induced is called primary response:

1. The antibodies are ***formed slowly*** with a latent period of about four days to four weeks.
2. The concentration of antibodies rises gradually and attains a smaller peak (Fig. 19.14).

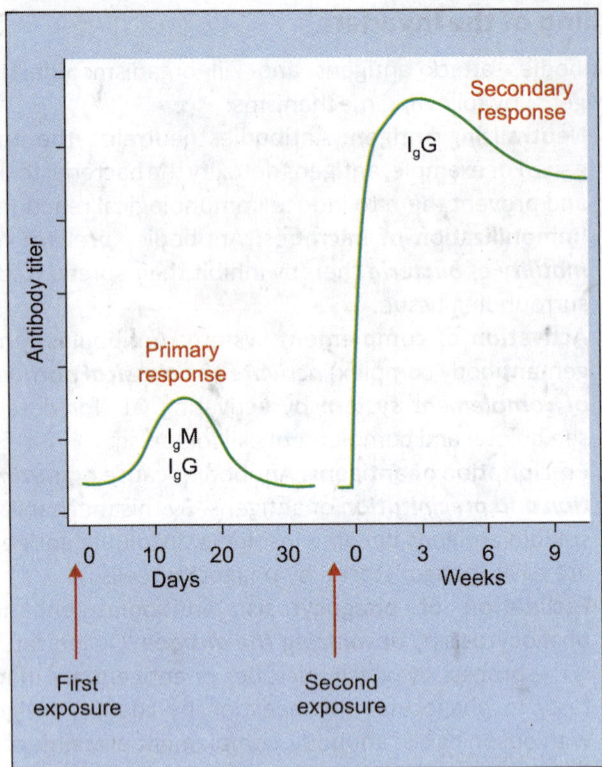

Fig. 19.14: Primary and secondary immunological responses.

3. Though **IgM and IgG** antibodies contribute to the primary response, the response is ***mainly due to IgM***.
4. Also, antibody titer in primary response returns back to normal within few days to weeks.

Secondary Response

When the same antigen enters the body for the second time, the immune response triggered is the secondary response:

1. It occurs speedily and intensely, which is due to the **immunological memory**.
2. Persistence of memory B and T cells help in carrying out the secondary response.
3. Antibodies are formed rapidly. Therefore, concentration of antibody rises fast (fast rising slope) and reaches a greater peak (*see* Fig. 19.14).
4. Antibody titer falls very slowly and never returns to normal, rather remains elevated for a longer duration. The antibodies in the secondary response are primarily of IgG type.

Complement System

There is a group of plasma proteins designated as complement proteins as they complement the effects of antibodies in destroying antigen. These proteins constitute the complement system:

1. Though there are more than 30 complement proteins, eleven are categorized in this system and are designated as C1–C9. C1 is further divided into C1q, C1r, and C1s (thus, total is 11).
2. These are a system of plasma enzymes that are normally present in the inactive form.
3. Once activated, they exert their immunological and inflammatory actions and boost the humoral immune mechanism.

Mechanisms of Activation of Complement System

There are **three mechanisms** of complement activation: classical pathway, alternative pathway and mannose-binding lectin pathway.

Classical Pathway

In this process, C1 binds with immunoglobulin attached to an antigen. This binding triggers a sequence of events that activates other complement proteins:

1. The mechanism of activation of complements is similar with the activation of intrinsic pathway of blood coagulation (the enzyme cascade theory), in which one activated protein activates the other protein (*see* Fig. 19.15).
2. Once, antigen-antibody complex activates C1, activated C1 (C1a) activates C2 and C4. Activated C2 and C4 (C4b, and C2a) activates C5, which (C5a) in turn activates C6, C7, C8, and C9.
3. These activated complement proteins kill microorganisms and facilitate inflammation by **following mechanisms:**
   - C3a, C4a, and C5a: Promote ***phagocytosis*** by facilitating chemotaxis, releasing histamine from mast cells, and causing arteriolar dilation.
   - C3b: Promote ***opsonization*** (makes the bacteria tasty to the phagocytes).
   - C5b, C6, C7, C8, and C9: Cause ***cytolysis*** of the microbes.

The activated complements incorporate perforins (pore-forming molecules) into the membranes of microbes. This results in transport of ions and water into the microbes through the pores, which finally result in ***osmotic lysis*** of microbes.

Alternative Pathway

This is also called **properdin pathway** as the key protein in the plasma for this pathway is the **properdin**. In this system, a circulating protein called **factor-1**, recognizes the polysaccharide unit present on the surface of microorganisms (but not in the normal mammalian cells). The interaction of factor-1 with the polysaccharide on microbes triggers a reaction that activates C3 and C5. Once C3 is activated, it activates other complement proteins (*see* Fig. 19.15).

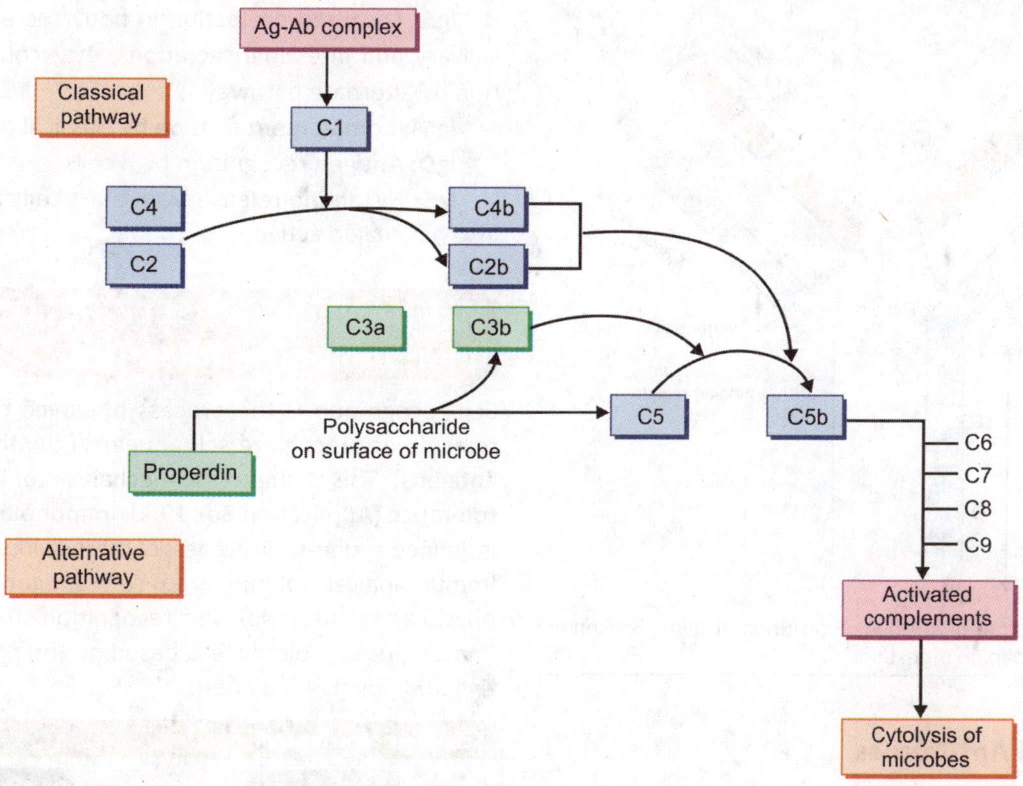

Fig. 19.15: Pathways of activation of complement system.

Table 19.3: Characteristics of antibodies.

	Characteristics	IgG	IgA	IgM	IgD	IgE
1.	Structure	Monomer	Monomer	Pentamer	Monomer	Monomer
2.	Heavy chain	$\gamma_1, \gamma_2, \gamma_3, \gamma_4$	α_1, α_2	μ	δ	ε
3.	Additional chain	Nil	J, SC	J	Nil	Nil
4.	Molecular weight	150	160-385	900	180	190
5.	Plasma level (mg %)	1000	200	120	03	02
6.	Half life (days)	21	06	05	03	02
7.	Complement activation	Yes	Yes	Yes	No	No
8.	Transfer through placenta	Yes	No	No	No	No

Mannose-binding Lectin Pathway

The plasma protein lectin binds with mannose group on the surface of bacteria, which activates complement proteins.

The complement system **activates B cell**, and thus serves as the link between innate and acquired immunity. Following apoptosis, complement proteins help in disposing the debris.

Antibodies

Antibodies are immunoglobulins (Ig). Ig binds specifically with the **antigenic determinant** of the antigen. This binding triggers the production of further antibodies. Binding of antigen with Ig is like the key fitting into the lock. There are specific antigen receptors on B cells. Binding of specific antigen with the specific receptor on B cell, results in production of specific antibody.

Types of Antibodies

There are **five types of antibodies**: IgG, IgA, IgM, IgD, and IgE (Table 19.3). They are produced in response to specific stimuli (specific antigens). A specific clone of B cells that are activated by specific antigenic stimulus produce specific antibody, i.e. monoclonal antibody (details, given below). The concentration of IgG in plasma is maximum (1000 mg%), followed by IgA (200 mg%), IgM (120 mg%), IgD (3 mg%), and IgE (0.05 mg%).

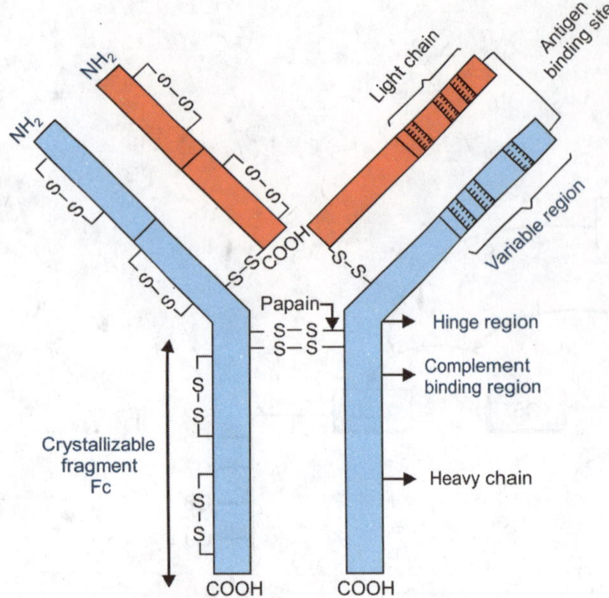

Fig. 19.16: Structure of antibody (immunoglobulin). Broken line indicates site of papain digestion.

Structure of Antibodies

Most antibodies have four polypeptide-chains. The two of them are **heavy (H) chains** and the other two are **light (L) chains** (Fig. 19.16):

1. The two H chains are identical to each other and contain about 450 amino acids, which may be either of α, γ, μ, δ and ε chains. The two L chains consist of about 220 amino acids. The polypeptides in L chain are κ and λ chains that are same in all antibodies. L chains are also identical to each other.
2. There may be some additional polypeptide chains in certain antibodies.
3. Antibodies are glycoproteins and their carbohydrate residue is attached to the heavy chains.
4. Disulfide bonds bridge the L and H chains. H chains are attached to each other at the middle by disulfide bonds. At this point, H chains display flexibility. Therefore, this region of H chain is called **hinge region**.
5. The tip of H and L chains is called **variable region**, as this region is different for each type of antibody. The variable region contains **antigen binding site.** This part of antibody recognizes and specifically attaches to a particular antigen.
6. The flexibility at hinge region allows the antibody to bind to two antigenic determinants (of antigens).
7. The rest of the H and L chain is called **constant region**, as this part of antibody is same in all types of antibodies.

Functions of Antibodies

Different antibodies play different role in immunological responses:

IgG: Complement fixation by classical pathway

IgA: Localized protection in body secretions like tear, salivary and intestinal secretions, etc.; complement fixation by alternate pathway

IgM: Complement fixation by classical pathway

IgD: Antigen recognition by B cells

IgE: Histamine release from mast cells and basophils; also has reagin activity

MECHANISMS OF SELF-RECOGNITION (Immunological Tolerance)

Self recognition is the process by which own MHC proteins do not recognize self antigens (identify only foreign antigens). This is due to the mechanism of **immunological tolerance** (Application Box 19.4). Immunological tolerance is defined as unresponsiveness of the individual to an antigen. Immunological tolerance to self antigen provides the physiological basis for self recognition. Development of immunological tolerance is based on the process of negative and positive selections.

Scientists contributed

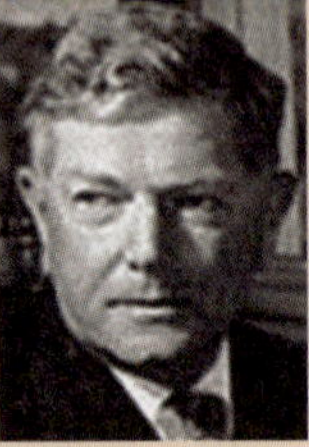

FM Burnet

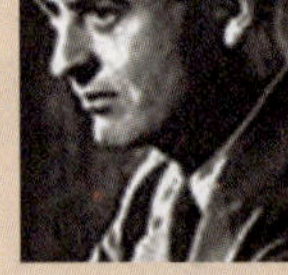

PB Medawar

The **Nobel Prize in Physiology or Medicine for the year 1960** was awarded to Australian scientist **Sir Frank Macfarlane Burnet** and Brazilian scientist **Sir Peter Brian Medawar** for their discovery of the mechanism of acquired immunological tolerance.

Negative Selection

During the process of development of T cells in thymus, cells with TCR that recognize peptide fragments of self proteins are eliminated while cells with TCR that do not recognize peptide fragments of self proteins are retained. This occurs either due to **deletion** (the self-reactive T cells undergo apoptosis) or **anergy** (the self-reactive T cells remain unresponsive to immunologic stimulation).

Clonal Deletion

During embryonic life, the clone of T cell and B cells containing receptors that react against self antigens are selectively removed from the body during their thymic and bursal development, so that they are not available in postnatal life to react against self antigens. These self reactive lymphocytes undergo apoptosis.

Clonal Anergy

The self-reactive clone of T and B cells those remain alive during post-natal life loose the capacity to be activated in response to self antigens. This is because they loose the activity of their receptors and lymphokine systems to react against self antigens, which may be due to the **immune suppression** of these cells by body's self regulating systems. This state of idleness is called clonal anergy.

Positive Selection

Immunological tolerance is also achieved by positive selection in which the T cells that are capable of recognizing self-MHC molecules during their thymic development survive and those that do not recognize undergo apoptosis. The T cells recognize MHC- self antigen complex as the self antigens and do not react against them.

Application Box 19.4

Fetal tolerance: Though fetus that grows in the mother's uterus is genetically a different organ (fetal graft) and foreign tissue immunologically, is not rejected during pregnancy like rejection of a transplanted organ. This is an example of **immunological tolerance**, called as fetal tolerance. Fetal tolerance is due to four mechanisms:

1. During the formation of placenta, trophoblast cells that separate the mother and fetus do not express MHC I and II antigens, and therefore, loose their immunogenicity. Instead, placenta expresses, HLA-G a nonpolymorphic antigen. Therefore, antibodies against fetal tissue do not develop.
2. Placenta has Fas ligand on its surface which attaches to the T cells. This attachment causes apoptosis of T cells that are supposed to react against fetal tissue.
3. Alpha fetoprotein (AFP) that is formed during fetal development causes suppression of T and B cells that react against fetal graft.
4. High level of progesterone during pregnancy is believed to suppress immunity against fetal tissue.

APPLIED PHYSIOLOGY

Organ Transplantation

Tissue or organ transplantation involves replacement of an injured or diseased tissue or organ by a new tissue or organ. Sometimes, it is required for the treatment of debilitating diseases like renal failure, liver failure, etc. Commonly transplanted organs are skin, kidney, bone and liver. However, the transplanted tissue is rejected as the recipient develops an immune response against the transplanted organ, which is a foreign tissue to him:

Scientists contributed

The **Nobel Prize in Physiology or Medicine for the year 1990** was awarded to American transplant surgeon **Joseph E Murray** and **E Donnall Thomas** for their discoveries concerning organ and cell transplantation in the treatment of human disease.

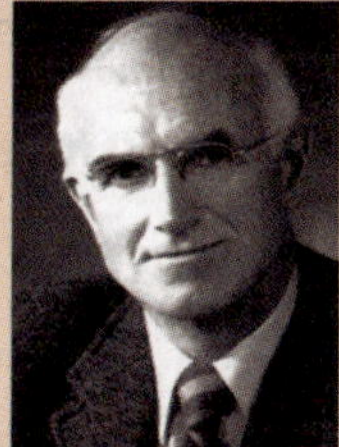

Joseph E Murray
(1919–2012)

1. **Transplant rejection** is due to the *activation of cellular immunity*.
2. The immune system recognizes the transplanted tissue as a foreign organ and initiates a series of immunological reactions that finally rejects the tissue.
3. The rapidity at which the transplanted tissue is rejected depends on degree of matching of MHC antigen (HLA antigen) of donor with the HLA antigen of the recipients.

Types of Transplants

1. **Autograft:** Transplantation of a tissue from one part of the body to another part of the same individual is called autograft. The best example is the skin graft on a burnt or scarred surface of the patient by taking a flap of skin from other part of his body. Autografts are never rejected.
2. **Isograft:** Transplantation of organs between the genetically identical individuals. The best example is the transplantation of ***tissues from the identical twin***. Isograft is also not rejected.
3. **Allograft:** This is the transplantation of organs between individuals of the same species, but with different genetic background. The example is transplantation from an individual other than identical twin. Allograft is rejected. If the graft is taken from the very close relations, rejection occurs slowly.
4. **Xenograft:** This is a transplant from or between different species. For example, transplantation of organ between animal and man. Commonly used xenograft is the physiological dressing using animal skin over severe burn surfaces. Xenograft is rejected fast.

Prevention of Transplant Rejection

A number of treatments are available to prevent rejection of a transplanted organ. These are:

1. **Immunosuppressive drugs:** The commonly used drug is ***azathioprine***. This is a purine antimetabolite that kills T lymphocytes. However, the individual on azathioprine *is susceptible to severe infection* because of immunosuppression.
2. **Glucocorticoid therapy:** Glucocorticoids have strong immunosuppressive activity. They inhibit proliferation of cytotoxic T cells by inhibiting the production of interleukin 2 (IL-2) from T_4 cells.
3. **Antilymphocyte globulins:** These are monoclonal antibodies produced against T lymphocytes. They inhibit T cell activity.
4. **Antibiotics:** Antibiotics usually used for the prevention of transplant rejection are cyclosporine, tacrolimus and rapamycin. ***Cyclosporine*** is a fungal extract and ***tacrolimus*** is an antibiotic of fungal origin. They prevent T cells from transcribing the IL-2 gene by preventing dephosphorylation of NF-AT, a transcription factor.

Rapamycin prevents activation of IL-2 receptor from producing T cell differentiation and proliferation.

5. **Monoclonal antibodies:** They prevent activation and proliferation of T cells.

Monoclonal Antibodies

Monoclonal antibodies are antibodies prepared from a single clone of B or plasma cells. They are used for immunotherapy of different diseases or to prevent rejection of transplanted tissue. They are obtained by fusing a B cell with a tumor cell that produces antibodies in large quantity.

Method of Production

An animal is immunized by injecting a particular antigen. The animal is then sacrificed and the **antibody producing cells** are extracted from the spleen of the animal:

1. The antibody producing cells are fused to the **myeloma cells** that are obtained from B lymphocyte tumor in a patient suffering from multiple myeloma.
2. Fusion of myeloma cell with antibody producing cell results in formation of a **hybridoma** which grows to become an antibody producing tumor.
3. The fused cells (hybridoma cells) are separated and every single cell is allowed to form a clone of cells.
4. The single clone of hybridoma cells produce specific antibody consisting of heavy or light chains of spleen cell or of myeloma cells. These are called monoclonal antibodies.

Uses of Monoclonal Antibody

Monoclonal antibodies are used in a wide variety clinical spectrum:

1. For measurement of drug level in patient's blood.
2. Diagnosis of allergic diseases, hepatitis, sexually transmitted diseases, etc.
3. Detection of cancer in the early stage.
4. Preparation of vaccines.
5. Prevention of transplant rejection.
6. Treatment of autoimmune diseases.

Scientists contributed

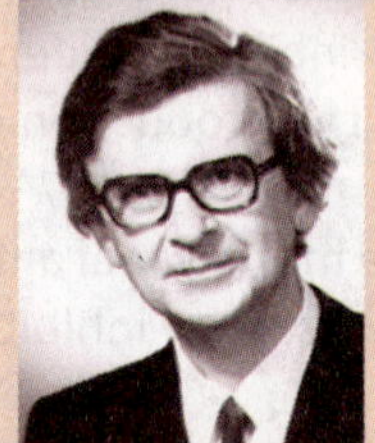
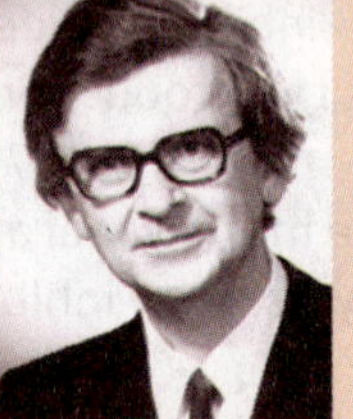

Niels K Jerne

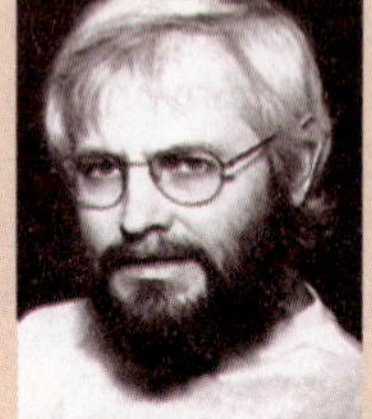

Georges JF Köhler

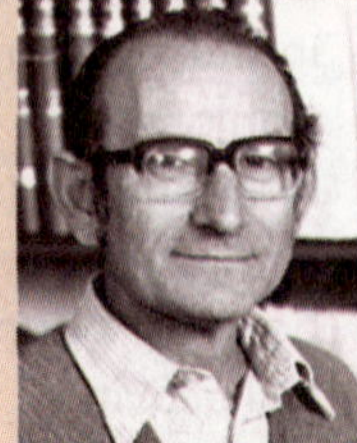

César Milstein

The **Nobel Prize in Physiology or Medicine 1984** was awarded jointly to **Niels K Jerne, Georges JF Köhler and César Milstein** "for theories concerning the specificity in development and control of the immune system and the discovery of the principle for production of monoclonal antibodies".

Immunotherapy

Immunotherapy is the treatment that aims at induction of the immune system of an individual. This is called **immunostimulation** or *immune enhancement*. This is especially helpful for the treatment of different malignant diseases. There are different types of immunotherapies: cellular immunotherapy, cytokine therapy, antibody therapy and adjuvant therapy.

Cellular Immunotherapy

Cells that have anti-tumor activity are injected into the blood of the cancer patient. These cells destroy the malignant tumor cells:

1. Patient's own inactive cytotoxic T cells or NK cells are used for this purpose.
2. In practice, these cells are removed from the blood of the patient and cultured with IL-2, which activates them.
3. These activated cells are called as lympokine-activated killer cells (**LAK cells**). LAK cells are then transfused into the patient's blood.

Cytokine Therapy

Different cytokines (see below) can be used in the treatment of different diseases. The best example is **interferon**. Interferons are especially used for the treatment of viral infections or malignancies. **Interleukin-2** is also used for the treatment of cancer.

Antibody Therapy

Monoclonal antibodies are extensively used for the treatment of malignancies or for preventing transplant rejection.

Adjuvant Therapy

Adjuvant is a compound, which is introduced with an antigen to enhance immune responses nonspecifically against the antigen. This was first discovered by Freund, hence called **Freund's adjuvant**:

1. Adjuvants may be **complete adjuvants** like tubercular bacilli and gram negative bacilli or **incomplete adjuvants** like aluminum hydroxide, aluminum phosphate, mineral oil, etc.
2. Adjuvants nonspecifically stimulate lymphocytes and macrophages.
3. However, adjuvants may cause delayed hypersensitivity reactions.

Immunological Disorders

Allergy

This is a hyper-reactive response of the body to an antigen which is usually tolerated by others. There are two types of allergies: the local allergy and the systemic allergy (anaphylaxis).

Local Allergy

When allergic reactions are limited to an area of the body, are called localized allergy. Examples are swelling of the lips, eczema, hives, urticaria, etc.

Systemic Allergy

When allergic reaction is generalized (affects systemic functions), is called systemic allergy or **anaphylaxis**. For example, anaphylactic reaction that occurs due to injection of penicillin or xylocaine in sensitive individuals. Anaphylaxis is an acute medical emergency, which may results in shock, called **anaphylactic shock**.

Scientist contributed

The **Nobel Prize for the year 1913 for Physiology or Medicine** was awarded to the Staff of Professors of the Caroline Institute, **Charles Richet, Professor of Physiology** in the Medical Faculty, Paris, for his work on anaphylaxis.

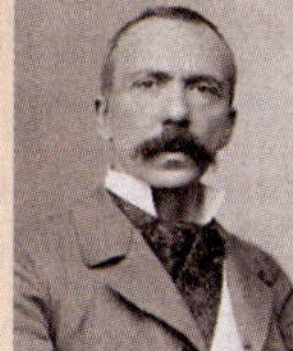

Charles Richet
(1850–1935)

Hypersensitivity Reactions

There are four types of hypersensitivity reactions:

Type I Reaction or Anaphylaxis

In this reaction, the individual over-reacts to a sensitized allergen. Usually it occurs on re-exposure. But in highly sensitive individual, it occurs on first exposure:

1. The antigen-antibody complexes release **histamine and slow-releasing substance A** from mast cells and basophils.
2. Histamine produces bradycardia and rapid vasodilation leading to **acute hypotension**.
3. Myocardial contractility is also inhibited resulting in reduced cardiac output. It is an acute medical emergency, which requires prompt medical support.

Type II Reaction or Cytotoxic Reaction

This reaction is caused by IgG or IgM antibody, which is ***directed against antigen present on person's red cells***. Incompatible blood transfusions, hemolytic diseases of newborn and autoimmune hemolytic anemias are examples. This causes **acute hemolysis** and requires early medical intervention.

Type III Reaction or Immune Complex Disease

In this reaction, the antigen and antibodies form complexes that escape phagocytosis. These **immune complexes *are deposited on the basement membrane*** of the blood vessels. They activate complements and induce inflammation. Examples are glomerulonephritis, systemic lupus erythematosus (SLE) and rheumatoid arthritis.

Type IV Reaction or Cell Mediated Reaction or Delayed Hypersensitivity Reactions

These reactions are *mediated by macrophages* that are activated by T cells.

1. Allergens (antigens) are taken up by APCs and presented to T cell.
2. This causes proliferation of T cells, some of which migrate to the location of allergen entry into the body. There, they secrete **cytokines** that activate macrophages and induce inflammatory reactions.
3. The appropriate example is the **skin test for tuberculosis**.

Autoimmune Diseases

Normally, the immune system does not react against self proteins. However, in some conditions, immune system fails to neglect self antigens and triggers immune reaction against body's own antigens. This results in autoimmune diseases:

1. This may be due to the *persistence of T cells or B cells that are active against self antigens*. Especially, failure of the process that removes antibodies against self antigens leads to formation of **autoantibodies** (Clinical Box 19.2). Thus, B cells produce antibodies against self antigens.
2. The common examples are SLE, rheumatoid arthritis, insulin-dependent diabetes mellitus, myasthenia gravis, Grave's disease, etc.
3. Autoantibodies may ***eliminate the receptors or activate the receptors***. For example, in myasthenia gravis, antibodies are formed against nicotinic cholinergic receptors that destroy the receptors, whereas in Grave's disease, antibodies formed against TSH receptors activate the receptors.

Clinical Box 19.2

Antibodies may cross-react: Sometimes autoantibodies may cross-react against the normal tissues and produce autoimmune diseases like **rheumatic heart disease**. Streptococcal pharyngitis that occurs in childhood stimulates formation of antibodies against streptococcal antigens, which cross-react against cardiac and joint tissues later producing rheumatic heart disease and arthritis. Another example is **Goodpasture syndrome**, in which antibodies formed against alveolar basement membrane cross react against glomerular basement membrane, resulting in pulmonary hemorrhage and glomerulonephritis.

Immunodeficiency States

Immunodeficiency diseases may be broadly classified into two categories: congenital or primary and acquired or secondary.

Congenital Immunodeficiency Syndromes

There are list of diseases in which severe combined immunodeficiency (SCID) occurs due to defects in development in either cellular or humoral immunity:

1. **Autosomal recessive SCID:** In this syndrome, stem cells (pre-T cells) in thymus fail to develop into mature T cells. Therefore, severe deficiency occurs in the cellular immunity.
2. **X-linked SCID:** In this disease, pleuripotent stem cells fail to develop into progenitor cells of lymphoid series. Therefore, severe deficiency occurs in the development of both humoral and cellular immunity.
3. **X-linked agammaglobulinemia:** In this defect, pre-B cells fail to develop into B cells. Therefore, severe deficiency of humoral system of immunity ensues.
4. **MHC class II deficiency:** Deficiency of MHC II antigen leads to deficiency of CD4 cells. Thus, both cellular and humoral immunities fail to develop.

Acquired Immunodeficiency Syndrome (AIDS)

AIDS occurs due to infection by human immunodeficiency virus (HIV). HIV is a ***retrovirus*** that binds to CD4 protein on the surface of helper cells and **decreases number of circulating T_4 cells**:

1. As helper cells are required for induction of both cellular and humoral immunities, HIV infection causes severe immunodeficiency state that *predisposes the individual to all type of serious infections and malignancies*. Consequently, the disease becomes a dangerous as cancer.
2. The usual **clinical features** are fever, lymphadenopathy, sore throat, diarrhea and weight loss.
3. Oral candidiasis, anogenital herpes simplex infection, *Pneumocystiis carinii* pneumonia, cryptococcus meningitis and cytomegalovirus infections are common.
4. Finally, the patient dies due to secondary infection or cancer.
5. The commonest malignancy is ***Kaposi's sarcoma***.
6. The disease is transmitted by blood, semen, or vaginal secretions or through breast feeding. The usual mode of transmission is sexual contact.
7. Though there is no definite treatment, **interferon, azathioprine and protease inhibitors** are used to reduce the severity. Efforts have been made recently to develop vaccines to prevent AIDS.

Cytokines

Cytokines are a group of hormone like substances that usually act in a paracrine fashion to control immunological responses. They are secreted from activated lymphocytes, macrophages, endothelial cells, glial cells, etc. They are classified into: interleukins, tumor necrosis factors (TNF), interferons, transforming growth factors (TGF) and GM-CSF (Table 19.4).

Interleukins

There are different types of interleukins. However, physiologically important interleukins are **IL-1 to IL-13:**

1. They are produced by macrophages, activated T cells, APCs, NK cells, mast cells and other somatic cells.
2. They assist in proliferation of B and T cells, activation of leucocytes, lymphopoiesis, erythropoiesis, thrombopoiesis and leucopoiesis.
3. The specific interleukins have specific functions. For example IL-1 produces fever, induces anorexia, increases neutrophil count and decreases lymphocyte count. Though it increases capillary permeability, it produces hypertension.

Tumor Necrosis Factors (TNFs)

There are two types of TNFs, TNF-α, and TNF-β. **TNF-α** is produced by activated macrophages. It acts like interleukin-1. It produces vascular thrombosis and tumor necrosis. **TNF-β** is produced by activated type 1 helper cells. The physiological effects are same as TNF-α.

Interferons (IFN)

There are three types of IFNs: IFN-α, IFN- β, and IFN-γ.

IFN-α: This is produced by macrophages, neutrophils, and other somatic cells. It prevents growth of viruses (antiviral). It also activates macrophages and NK cells, and induces the expression of type I MHC on all somatic cells.

IFN- β: Same as IFN-α.

IFN-γ: Secreted by activated type 1 helper cells and NK cells. It induces expression of MHC I on all somatic cells and MHC II on APCs. It activates macrophages, neutrophils and NK cells. It stimulates cellular immunity. It is also antiviral.

GM-CSF

Functions of GM-CSF have been discussed in detail in 'leucopoiesis'.

Table 19.4: Source and important functions of common cytokines.

Cytokines	Source	Cell target	Functions
IL1	Macrophage and monocyte Fibroblasts, endothelial cells Some epithelial cells	All cells	Activation of cellular immunity, activation of inflammation, and hemopoiesis, expression of adhesion molecules, Emigration of nutrophils and macrophages, role in fever and shock, hepatic production of acute ohase protein

Contd...

IL2	T_H1 cells	T cells	Stimulates cellular immunity, NK cells and macrophages
IL3	T cell	Progenitor cells	Activates hemopoiesis
IL4	T_H2 cells, mast cells, basophils and eosinophils	B cells	Stimulates humoral immunity, activates monocytes, IgE class switching
IL5	T_H2 cells, mast cells and eosino-phils	Eosinophil	Stimulates eosinophil development
IL6	T_H2 cells, fibroblast Monocytes and macrophages, Same as IL1	T and B cells Epithelial cells Hepatocytes, Monocyte/ Macrophage	Differentiation and growth of T and B cell, Hepatic production of acute phase proteins (ARP), activation of lymphocytes
IL8	Monocyte/ Macrophages T cells, Nutrophil, Fibroblasts, Endothelial cells Epithelial cells	Nutrophil Basophil T cells Monocyte Macrophages Endothelial cells	Chemotaxix of neutrophils and basophils, induces migration of Nutro-phil, Macrophages and T cells Stimulates release of histamine from basophils stimulates angiogen-esis
IL11	Osteoblasts, fibroblasts		Stimulates hemopoiesis and production of ARP
IL12	Macrophage and B cell Dendritic cells and nutrophils	T cell NK cells	Stimulates synthesis of IFNγ, activates T_H1 cell induces formation of T helper cells and killer cells Promotes CTL cytolytic activity, increases IFNγ production, decreases production of IL17
IL17	$CD4^+$ T cells	Fibroblast Endothelial cells	Increases secretion of other cytokines migration of nutrophils and monocytes
TNFα	T cell, B cells, NK cell Monocyte/ Macrophages Mast cells, basophils, eosinophils	All cells except RBC	Hepatic production of acute phase proteins, Systemic features (fever, shock), anoxia), expression of endothelial adhesion molecule Enhanced leukocyte toxicity, Induction of proinflammatory cytokines
TNFβ	B cells and T_H1 cells		Promotes inflammation
IFNα and β	Virally infected cells		Kill viruses
IFNγ	T_H1 cells, NK cells	All cells	Activation of macrophage and NK cells, inhibition of TH2 cells Stimulates secretion of Igs by B cells, Differentiation of T helper cells
TGFβ	T cell, B cells, and Mast cells		Suppresses immunity
GM-CSF	T cell, B cells, NK cell and Macrophages		Stimulates granulopoiesis and monocyte production
Mcp-1	Fibroblasts, smooth muscle cells, Blood mononuclear cells	Monocytes Macrophages NK cells, T cells	Chemoattractant for monocytes, T cells, NK cells Stimulates release of histamine from basophils
Eotaxin	Alveolar cells, Myocardium	Eosiniphil, baso-phil	Chemoattractant for eosiniphil, basophil Induces allergic pulmonary diseases
PF-4	Platelet Megakaryocytes	Fibroblasts Endothelial cells	Chemoattractant for fibroblasts inhibitory to haematopoietic precur-sors and endothelial cell proliferation

(TH1 cells: Type 1 helper cell; TH2 cells: Type 2 helper cell; TNF: Tumor necrosis factor; IFN: Interferon; TGF: Transforming growth factor).

CHAPTER SUMMARY

Key Concepts

1. Nonspecific immune mechanism (innate immunity) is mainly due to NK cells, phagocytosis by mononuclear phagocyte system, inflammatory cells, and chemicals present in skin and mucous membrane.
2. T cell (T8 cell or cytotoxic T cell) is for cellular immunity, which is mainly targeted against intracellular pathogens like viruses, parasites and fungi, cancer cells, tumor cells, and transplanted tissues.
3. B cell is for humoral immunity mediated by antibodies, which is mainly targeted against extracellular pathogens like bacteria.
4. Type 1 helper cell induces cellular immunity and type 2 helper cell induces humoral immunity.
5. Complement system activates B cells, and also helps in nonspecific immunity.
6. Monoclonal antibodies help in transplant rejection and used in immunotherapy.

Important to Know (Must Read)

1. In examinations, 'Mechanism of cellular immunity', 'Mechanism of humoral immunity', 'Mechanism of defense by phagocytic and inflammatory cells' and 'Development of T and B lymphocytes' usually come as **Long Questions**.
2. NK cells, Inflammation, Phagocytosis, Mononuclear phagocyte system, Development of T cell, Development of B cell, Types and functions of T cells, T cell receptor, MHC antigens, Immunoglobulins, Cellular immunity, Humoral immunity, Immune responses, Antigen presenting cells, Mechanism of antigen presentation by APCs, Complement system, Monoclonal antibodies, Immunological tolerance, Immunotherapy, Prevention of transplant rejection, Immunodeficiency states, AIDS, Autoimmunity, and Cytokines are usual **Short Questions** in exams.
3. In **Viva**, examiners may ask any questions from the topics listed as short notes. In addition, classification of immunity, types of antibodies and their functions, and all immunological disorders, may be asked.

CHAPTER

20

Platelets and Their Role in Hemostasis

Learning Objectives

On completion of study of this chapter, the student **MUST** be able to:

1. Define hemostasis and list the major steps of hemostasis.
2. Give the steps of thrombopoiesis and briefly describe its regulation.
3. Describe the structure (cytoskeletal systems and granules) of platelet and correlate the structure with platelet functions.
4. Appreciate the properties of platelet, especially platelet adhesion, aggregation and release reaction.
5. Explain the role of platelet in hemostasis, with special reference to the role in temporary hemostatic plug formation.
6. List the causes of thrombocytosis and thrombocytopenia.
7. List the platelet function tests.
8. Understand common platelet dysfunctions.

Student **MAY** also be able to:

1. Describe the role of platelets in hemostasis.
2. Describe platelet function test.
3. Describe the physiological basis of common platelet dysfunctions, especially ITP.

DEFINITION AND CONCEPT

Hemostasis is defined as the process of **arrest of bleeding** while maintaining blood in a fluid state within the vascular system.

Hemostasis is the mechanism by which loss of blood from vascular system is prevented by a complex interaction of vessel wall, platelets and plasma proteins. This happens broadly in two stages: primary and secondary.

Primary hemostasis: This is the initial stage during which vascular wall and platelet interact to limit the blood loss from damaged vessel. This is also called ***temporary hemostasis***, as platelet plug alone cannot stop bleeding for a longer duration.

Secondary hemostasis: A stable fibrin clot is formed from clotting factors by enzymatic reactions. This is also called ***definitive hemostasis***, as formation of clot in the vicinity of platelet plug finally stops bleeding.

Although formation of blood clot is needed to arrest blood loss, ultimately blood clot needs to be dissolved to resume the normal blood flow, and the process of dissolution of clot is called **fibrinolysis.**

Bleeding occurs when blood vessels are damaged. The vascular injury initiates a series of events in sequence that finally forms clot at the site of injury and prevents loss of blood from the body. Thus, hemostasis is a life-saving process that maintains homeostasis of blood volume.

Steps of Hemostasis

Hemostasis occurs in **three stages**: vasoconstriction, temporary hemostatic plug formation, and blood coagulation (Flowchart 20.1).

Vasoconstriction

Immediate response of blood vessel to injury is vasoconstriction.

1. This occurs due to the contraction of vascular smooth muscle in response to injury.
2. It instantaneously decreases loss of blood and also helps in platelet plug formation (*see* below).
3. Contraction of vascular smooth muscle to injury is initially a mechanical response (***stretch-induced contraction***).

Flowchart 20.1: Mechanism of hemostasis.

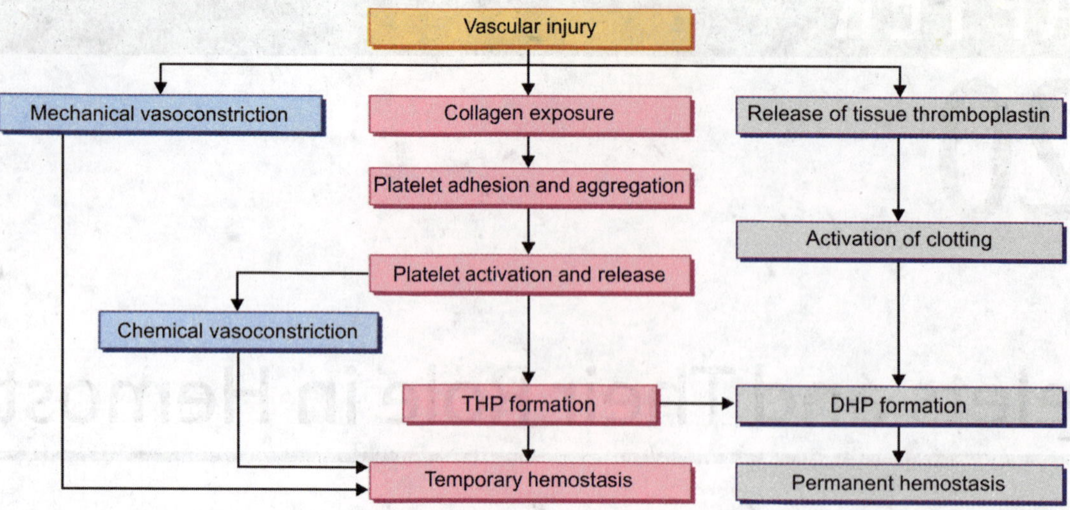

(THP: Temporary hemostatic plug; DHP: Definitive hemostatic plug).

4. However, later vasoconstriction is maintained and potentiated by secretion of ***vasoconstrictor substances*** like serotonin from the activated platelets.

Temporary Hemostatic Plug Formation

Formation of **platelet plug** at the site of injury is called *temporary hemostatic plug*. This occurs due to three properties of platelets: adhesion, aggregation, and release reaction (secretion) (Fig. 20.1).

1. The initial response of platelet to vascular injury is the change in shape of platelets and its increased surface adhesiveness to the injured vascular endothelium. This is called **adhesion.**
2. Platelets also stick to each other (aggregate) at the site of the injury. This is called **aggregation**.
3. Simultaneously, platelets are also activated to release a number of chemicals (**release reaction or secretion**) that further facilitate vasoconstriction, adhesion and aggregation.

The whole process finally results in formation of a platelet plug that arrests bleeding temporarily. As platelet plug is not a stable one, the plug is called **temporary hemostatic plug (or primary hemostatic plug)**, and the process is called *temporary hemostasis*. This is also called ***primary hemostasis*** as this is the first step in hemostasis that occurs very quickly and stops bleeding instantaneously.

Blood Coagulation

Immediately following injury, the clotting mechanism of blood is initiated. This results in formation of blood clot at the site of injury that stops bleeding.

1. The formation of blood clot occurs in and around the platelet plug and the plug formed is a stable one. Therefore, this plug is called a **definitive hemostatic plug (or secondary hemostatic plug)**.

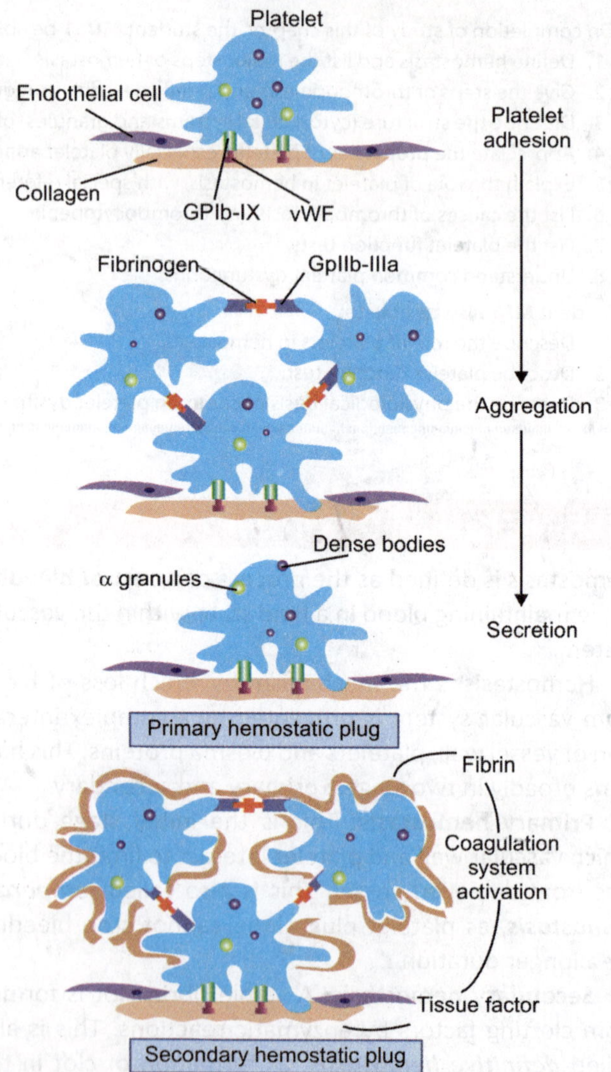

Fig. 20.1: Steps in hemostasis. Note that primary (temporary) hemostatic plug formation is the function of platelet that occurs in three stages (adhesion, aggregation and release reaction). *Courtesy*: Figure 33.8, Essentials in Hematology and Clinical Pathology by Ramadas Nayak et al., 1st edition, 2012; Jaypee Brothers Medical Publishers (P) Ltd.

2. This process is also called ***secondary hemostasis*** as this step follows the primary hemostasis.
3. Blood coagulation is initiated by the vessel injury that releases tissue factors and exposes collagen of the vessel wall (for details, see the next chapter).

THROMBOPOIESIS

The development of platelets is called **thrombopoiesis** or *thrombocytopoiesis*. Platelets are the smallest formed elements of blood. They are anuclear fragments of **megakaryocytes**. Megakaryocytes are the giant cells in the bone marrow: The major steps of thrombopoiesis are summarized in Flowchart 20.2.

Flowchart 20.2: Stages of thrombopoiesis.

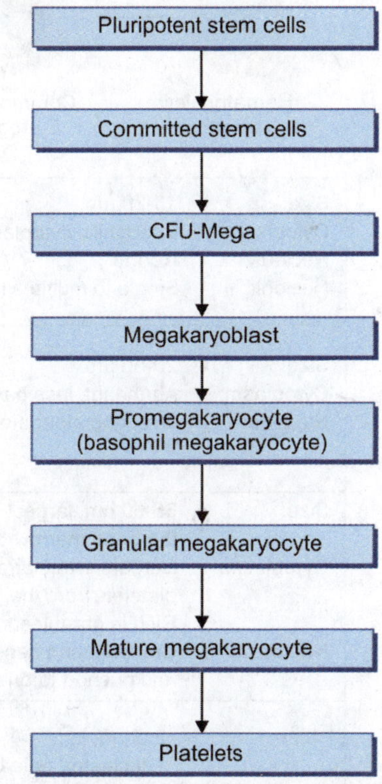

(CFU-Mega: Colony forming unit of megakaryocyte).

Stages of Development

Thrombopoiesis occurs in **three broad steps** (Figs. 20.2):

1. **Formation of megakaryoblast** from hemopoietic stem cells (Pluripotent stem cells, Committed stem cells and CFU-Mega).
2. **Megakaryopoiesis**: This is formation of megakaryocyte (Promegakaryocyte, basophil megakaryocyte, granular megakaryocyte and mature megakaryocyte) from megakaryoblast.
3. **Formation of platelets** from megakaryocytes

Stem Cells

Platelets develop from myeloid stem cells that form CFU-Mega, which in turn develop into megakaryoblast (for details, refer 'Hemopoiesis').

Megakaryoblasts

Megakaryoblasts are the ***first identifiable cells*** of the thrombopoietic series in the bone marrow. Their size is more than 15 µm. The cytoplasm is basophilic and nucleus is multilobed.

Megakaryocytes

Megakaryocytes grow in three stages: promegakaryocyte, granular megakaryocyte, and mature megakaryocyte.

Promegakaryocytes

The cells are bigger than megakaryoblast (size more than 20 µm).

1. Cytoplasm is basophilic and contains *few azurophilic granules* around the centrosome.
2. The nucleus is **horse-shoe shaped**.
3. This is also called ***basophil megakaryocyte***.

Granular Megakaryocytes

The cells are very big having the size between 25 and 50 µm.

1. Cytoplasm is acidophilic and contains numerous **azurophilic granules** around the centrosome.
2. The nucleus is irregular or horse-shoe shaped.

Mature Megakaryocytes

These are the **largest cells** in bone marrow. The characteristic features are:

1. These are **polyploid bone marrow cells** (ploidy means DNA content; diploidy means double amount of DNA; polyploidy means increased amount of DNA in the nucleus). Megakaryocyte has large nucleus, which is polyploid.
2. The cells are still **bigger in size** (more than 25 to 50 µm).
3. Cytoplasm contains numerous **granules of different kinds**. Four types of granules have been described in megakaryocyte: α-granules, dense granules, lysosomal granules, and myeloperoxidase granules.
4. Most of the proteins and granules of megakaryocyte determine the characteristic of platelets. When the need for platelet increases, the megakaryocytes increase in size, number and ploidy, and the opposite effects occur when the demand decreases.
5. Granules are present around the centrosome.
6. The nucleus is reduced in size.

Platelets

Megakaryocytes form platelets by ***pinching off bits of cytoplasm*** and ***extruding them into the circulation*** (Figs. 20.2). On average, each megakaryocyte produces about 1,000 to 3,000 platelets. Normally, platelet production per day is about 35,000 to 45,000 per microliter of blood.

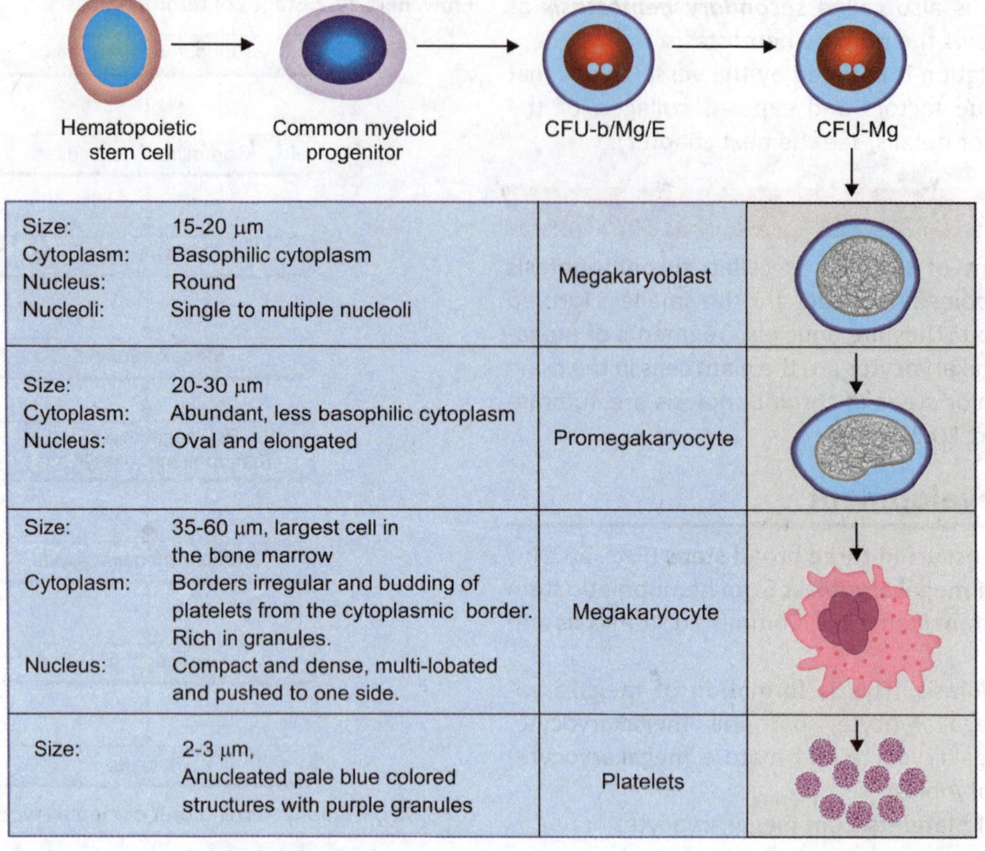

Figs. 20.2: Stages of thrombopoiesis. Note, megakaryopoiesis has 4 stages.
Courtesy: Figure 39.3, page 348, Essentials in Hematology and Clinical Pathology et al. 1st edition, 2012, by Ramadas Nayak; Jaypee Brothers Medical Publishers (P) Ltd.

Regulation of Thrombopoiesis

The production and release of platelets from bone marrow remains normally constant. The production of platelets is enhanced by removal of platelets from blood (*thrombocytopheresis*) and decreased by transfusion of platelets. This indicates that a **feedback regulatory mechanism** exists for platelet production. Thrombopoietin, interleukins and GM-CSF control thrombopoiesis.

Thrombopoietin

The endogenous thrombopoietin is a short-lived polypeptide, produced mainly from liver parenchymal cells. To some extent, it is also formed in kidney. However, the naturally occurring thrombopoietin for medical uses is very less. Therefore, commercial thrombopoietin have been synthesized by recombinant technology for use in thrombocytopenic conditions. Recombinant thrombopoietins have half-life of 20–40 hours. They are produced by E. coli. Thrombopoietin **stimulates differentiation and proliferation of megakaryocytes**.

Interleukins

Interleukin-1, interleukin-3, interleukin-6, and interleukin-11 stimulate platelet production. They do not stimulate thrombopoietin release.

GM-CSF

GM-CSF is produced by monocytes, T lymphocytes, fibroblasts, and endothelial cells. It stimulates erythropoiesis, granulopoiesis, and thrombopoiesis.

Life History

Platelets have the half-life of about 4 days. They survive in circulation for about 8–12 days. The aged platelets are removed from circulation by reticuloendothelial systems. **Spleen** plays an important role in destruction of platelets. Therefore, platelet count increases after splenectomy and decreases in splenomegaly.

STRUCTURE AND FUNCTIONS

Structure

Platelets are small, anucleate cell fragments adapted to participate in hemostasis. By their membrane properties they adhere to damaged blood vessels and aggregate with each other. Though the cells are small, platelets have developed cellular structures (Fig. 20.3)

1. They have highly developed **cytoskeletal system** suited for their functions.
2. They have specialized **canalicular system**.

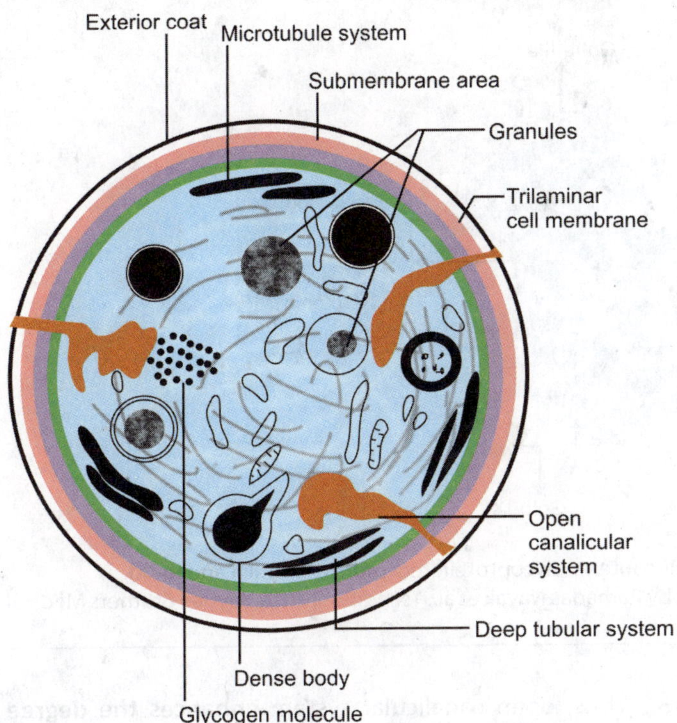

Fig. 20.3: Ultrastructure of platelet. Note the presence of open canalicular system, dense tubular system, and alpha and dense granules.

3. They have developed membrane systems. When activated, they change their shape due to change in activity of membrane structure and cytoskeleton. This helps in release of chemicals from its granules.
4. They contain extensive microtubules and microfilaments and **numerous granules**. Frequently, they change their shape with very long and thin processes extending out from their body called as **filopodia**.

Dimensions

Platelets are small, granulated, spherical, or oval bodies having diameter ranging from 1.5 to 3.0 µm. The size of platelets is approximately one-third to one-fourth of red cells. However, there is considerable variation in size of platelets even in the same individual. Few platelets may have diameter more than half the diameter of red cells (> 4 µm).

Cell Membrane

Cell membrane is covered by an **exterior glycocalix *coat*** that consists of **glycoproteins** including glycoprotein receptors, glycolipids, and mucopolysaccharides.

1. Platelets have negative charge on their surface due to presence of sialic acid residues attached to the exterior coat. This ***prevents the resting platelets to attach to each other*** or to the negatively charged endothelial cells.
2. The cell membrane is a **trilaminar unit** consisting of a bilayer of phospholipids in which cholesterol, glycolipids, and glycoproteins are embedded.
3. *Glycoproteins aid to prevent adherence of platelets to the normal vascular endothelium*.
4. However, **glycoprotein receptors** help in adhesion and aggregation of platelets.
5. Platelets have **receptors** on their cell membrane for collagen, ADP, von Willebrand factor (vWF), and fibrinogen.

Membrane Glycoproteins

The cell membrane contains integral membrane glycoproteins (Gp) (Fig. 20.4), which play an important role in hemostasis. Important platelet membrane glycoproteins and their functions are as follows:

Gp Ib-IX-V: This is a constitutively active receptor that mediates vWF dependent adhesion of platelets to subendothelial collagen.

Gp IIb/IIIa: On activation, serves to bind fibrinogen and thus mediates aggregation. Also, this is the receptor for vWF, fibronectin, and thrombospondin.

Gp Ia-IIa: Constitutively active receptor for collagen and mediates platelet adhesion independent of vWF.

Cytoskeletal Systems

Cytoskeletal system of platelets can be broadly divided into membrane and cytoplasmic cytoskeletal systems.

Membrane Cytoskeleton

An elongated tetramer of ***spectrin molecule*** is present in the cell membrane, which is connected to the ends of actin filaments that are situated close to the cell membrane and membrane of open canalicular system.

1. **Filamin 1** (actin binding protein) ***interacts with membrane glycoprotein and actin*** present below the membrane. Filamin 1 also connects these proteins (membrane glycoprotein and submembrane actin filaments) to the transmembrane spectrin network, and this ***provides stability*** to the membrane and discoid shape of the platelets.
2. Other membrane proteins include **talin, vinculin, and vimentin**. Membrane cytoskeleton plays important role in **platelet spreading** following their adhesion to the vascular endothelium.

Cytoplasmic Cytoskeleton

Cytoplasm contains a well-developed contractile system, which consists of an **extensive network of microtubules** and **microfilaments**.

Microtubules

There is a sub-membrane microtubular system consisting of many microtubules that are arranged beneath the membrane.

1. Microtubules are made up of α **and** β **tubulins.**
2. Cytosolic motors like *dynein and kinesin filaments* are also associated with microtubules.
3. Microtubules **provide stability to the membrane and support the discoid shape** of the cell.

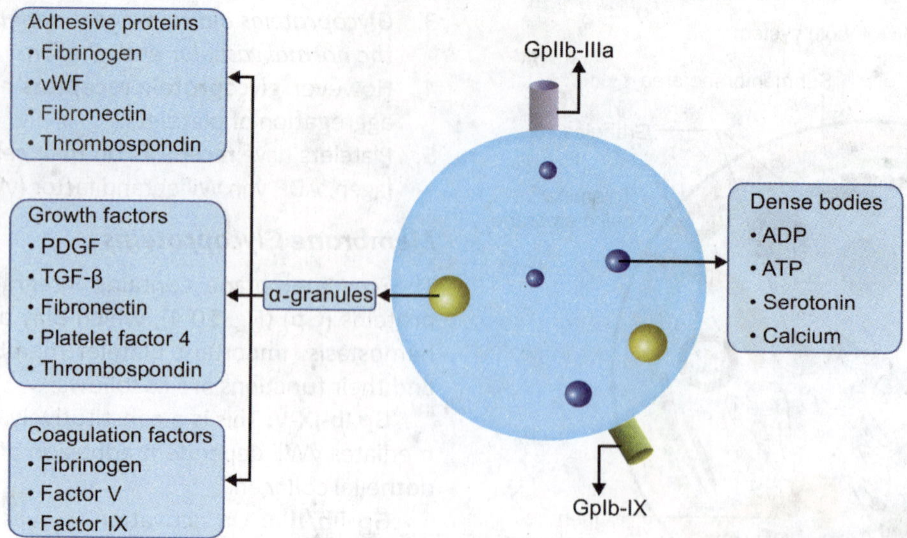

Fig. 20.4: Cellular constituents of platelet. Note the granules and their content. Glycoprotein receptors (GpIIb-IIIa and Ib-IX). *Courtesy*: Figure 33.1, Essentials in Hematology and Clinical Pathology by Ramadas Nayak et al., 1st edition, 2012; Jaypee Brothers Medical Publishers (P) Ltd.

Microfilaments

Platelet microfilaments consist mainly of **actin molecules** that polymerize into microfilamentous bundles. There are also few myosin filaments attached to actin filaments.

1. Actin and myosin filaments constitute **contractile system** in platelets.
2. The microfilament system is not prominent in the resting cells. However, when platelets are activated and they change their shape, microfilament bundles become more extensive.
3. They form the major contractile system of the cell that helps to **change the shape of platelets** and discharge their granular content to the exterior through canaliculi (**cell release**).

Cellular Systems

There are two developed cellular systems in platelets that help in platelet functions: open canalicular system and dense tubular systems (*see* Fig. 20.3).

Open Canalicular System

There are many canaliculi in the platelets that open to the exterior.

1. The open canaliculi are extensive invaginations of cell membrane deep into the cytoplasm that form the conduits for discharge of contents of granules.
2. Presence of numerous canaliculi in platelet eliminates the dependence of the cell for its chemical release solely on the *migration of granules to the periphery* for their fusion with cell membrane for exocytosis, as the granule-movement toward the interior of the cell and fusion of the granules with the canalicular membrane ***facilitates the process of release*** of chemicals from platelet granules.
3. Thus, open canalicular system **enhances the degree and rate of platelet release** (*see* below).

Dense Tubular System

This a closed system of channels formed by ***residual endoplasmic reticulum*** that are less extensive than canalicular system.

1. This system is found close to the open canalicular system.
2. They sequester the ionized calcium.
3. The membrane of tubular system contains *peroxidase activity*, and the interior contains **calreticulin**, a calcium binding protein that helps in **calcium accumulation**.
4. Release of calcium from dense tubular system **facilitates platelet release.**

Cytoplasmic Organelles

Cytoplasmic matrix contains microfilaments, structured filaments, and microtubules. Interspersed in the matrix are various types of granules and electron dense bodies. Organelles are mainly mitochondria. Sometimes Golgi apparatus is found.

Platelet Granules

Platelet contains numerous peroxisomes, mitochondria, lysosomes, and granules. Activation of platelet leads to discharge of content of granules that facilitate the process of hemostasis. The granules of platelets are of **two types**: the alpha granules and dense granules (Fig. 20.4).

Alpha granules: The alpha granules are abundant in platelets. About 50–80 granules are present per platelet. They are about 200 nm in diameter. They contain various chemicals (Table 20.1).

Dense granules: There are about 3–8 dense granules per platelet. They are also called **dense bodies**. They have diameter of about 20–30 nm. They contain chemicals like serotonin, ADP, calcium, ATP, etc.

Table 20.1: Contents of platelet granules.
A. Contents of alpha granules
1. von Willebrand factor
2. Thrombospondin
3. β-Thromboglobulin
4. PDGF (platelet derived growth factor)
5. PAF (platelet activating factor)
6. Platelet factor 4 (platelet phospholipid)
7. Fibronectin
8. Plasminogen
9. Platelet fibrinogen
10. Proaccelerin
11. α_2-Plasmin inhibitor
12. α_1-Protease inhibitor
13. Coagulation factors V and XI
14. Tissue plasminogen activator (tPA)
B. Contents of dense granules
1. Serotonin
2. ADP
3. Calcium
4. ATP
5. Pyrophosphate

Properties of Platelets

Platelets have **three unique properties**: adhesion, aggregation, and activation and release.

Adhesion

Platelets easily adhere to the damaged vascular endothelium. This is called platelet adhesion. Platelets have the tendency to stick to the exposed collagen of the injured vessel wall. *Adhesion is facilitated by von Willebrand factor.* However, platelets do not adhere to the normal vessel wall.

Role of membrane proteins: This means binding of platelets to non-endothelial surfaces, particularly subendothelium which is uncovered following vascular injury. **von Willebrand factor** mediates adhesion of platelets to subendothelium via GpIb on the surface of platelets (Clinical Box 20.1).

Clinical Box 20.1

Deficiency of membrane proteins causes bleeding disorder: Congenital absence of glycoprotein receptor GpIb **(Bernard-Soulier syndrome)** or of von Willebrand factor in plasma **(von Willebrand's disease)** causes defective platelet adhesion and ***bleeding disorder***.

Aggregation

Platelets not only stick to the injured vessel wall but also to each other. The property of platelets to stick to each other is called platelet aggregation. Fibrinogen and GpIIb-IIIa

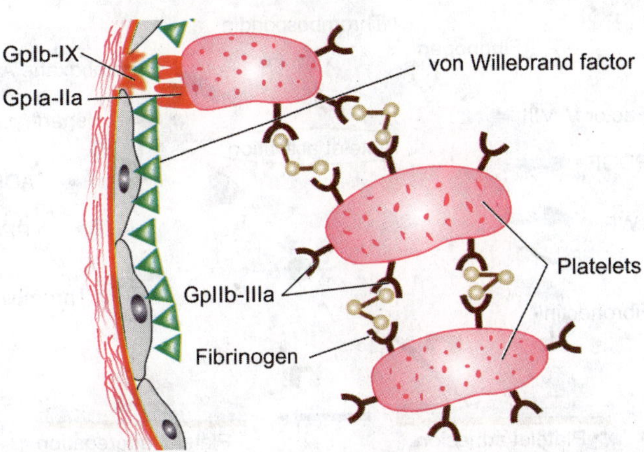

Fig. 20.5: Mechanism of platelet aggregation. Note, vWF facilitates adhesion of platelet to vascular endothelium, whereas fibrinogen and GpIIb-IIIa facilitated aggregation of platelet to each other.

mainly promote aggregation of platelet to each other (Fig. 20.5). *Also, thrombin, ADP and PAF promote platelet aggregation.*

Activation and Release (Secretion)

Platelets are activated when they bind to collagen or to each other.

1. The activation is facilitated by **thrombin and ADP.**
2. Platelets normally circulate as round to oval disc like structures. With activation platelets undergo shape change, i.e. they become more spherical and form **pseudopodia**. This shape change is due to recognition of microtubules and contraction of actomysin of microfilaments.
3. The activated platelets change their shape and discharge their granular contents (Fig. 20.6). The discharge of the granular content to the exterior through open canalicular system is called **platelet release** (*see* below).
4. The release reaction (secretion) is facilitated by chemicals released from platelet granules.

Functions of Platelets

In addition to their important role in hemostasis (described below), platelets serve many other functions of the body. Important functions of platelets are as follows:

1. **Temporary hemostasis:** Platelets prevent bleeding by forming plugs at the site of injury (temporary hemostatic plug). Platelets also promote vasoconstriction by producing serotonin that helps in hemostasis.
2. **Blood coagulation:** Platelets contribute to blood coagulation by releasing platelet factor 4, and synthesizing clotting factors V and XI.
3. **Clot retraction:** Platelets promote clot retraction, which is essential for stabilization of clot.
4. **Thrombolysis:** Platelet controls fibrinolysis.

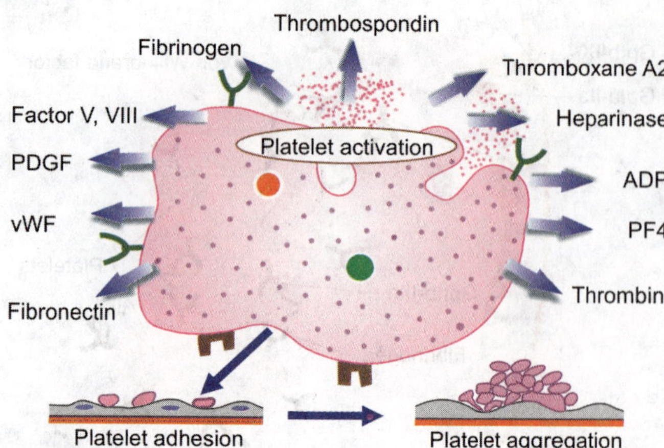

Fig. 20.6: Mechanism of platelet activation and release (Secretion). Note, the aggregated platelets are activated to discharge (release) their content.

5. **Phagocytosis:** Platelets phagocyteose smaller molecules like immune complexes and viruses.
6. **Storage and transport:** Platelets synthesize, secrete, and transport many chemical substances (as listed in Table 20.1)
7. **Vascular growth:** Platelets help in growth of vascular endothelium by secreting platelet-derived growth factor (**PDGF**). PDGF is also produced by macrophages and endothelial cells. PDGF is synthesized in three forms: PDGF-AA, PDGF-BB, and PDGF-AB (containing either of the two polypeptide chains A or B).

Normal Count and Variations

Normal count of platelet is 1.5–4 lakhs/mm^3 of blood.

Thrombocytopenia

Thrombocytopenia is defined as the platelet count less than 1.5 lakhs/mm^3 of blood.

1. However, significant bleeding occurs when platelet count decreases below 50,000/mm^3 of blood. Therefore, platelet count below 50,000/mm^3 of blood is called **critical count.**
2. Thrombocytopenia occurs in idiopathic thrombocytopenic purpura (ITP), aplastic anemia, hypersplenism, acute leukemia, cytotoxic chemotherapy and radiation (Table 20.2).
3. About 70% of platelets released from bone marrow are present in circulation and 30% are sequestered in spleen.
4. Therefore, splenectomy usually causes thrombocytosis and hypersplenism invariably causes thrombocytopenia.

Thrombocytosis

Thrombocytosis commonly occurs in polycythemia vera, chronic myeloid leukemia, iron deficiency anemia, splenectomy, chronic infection, surgery, and following acute hemorrhage.

Table 20.2: Variations in platelet count.

A. Thrombocytosis
1. Essential thrombocythemia
2. Other myeloproliferative diseases like polycythemia rubra vera, CML, etc.
3. Familial thrombocytosis
4. Acute blood loss
5. Iron deficiency
6. After splenectomy
7. Malignancies
8. Drugs: vincrisitine, epinephrine
9. After surgery
10. Chronic infection
B. Thrombocytopenia
1. Hereditary thrombocytopenias like Fanconi anemia, Alport syndrome, May-Hegglin anomaly, etc.
2. Hypersplenism
3. Idiopathic thrombocytopenic purpura (ITP)
4. HIV infection
5. Aplastic anemia
6. Massive transfusion of stored blood
7. Drugs: Heparin, quinidine, quinine, rifampicin, etc.
8. Acute leukemia
9. Cytotoxic chemotherapy
10. Irradiation of bone marrow

ROLE OF PLATELET IN HEMOSTASIS

Hemostasis is the **arrest of bleeding**. Hemostasis occurs in two major steps: temporary hemostasis and definitive hemostasis. Following injury to blood vessels, platelets aggregate at the site of injury and seal the opening in the vascular tree. This is the first and important step in prevention of bleeding, which is called **temporary hemostasis**. Simultaneously, mechanisms of coagulation of blood are also activated that form blood clot, the processes combinely known as **definitive hemostasis** (refer Flowchart 20.1).

Though platelet is essential for temporary hemostasis, it also contributes to **blood coagulation and clot retraction**. Platelet also controls **thrombolysis**.

Role in Temporary Hemostasis

Immediate hemostasis following vascular injury is achieved by formation of platelet plug (also called, **platelet thrombus**) at the site of injury. As platelet thrombus can be washed away, unless supported by a clot, this is called **temporary hemostatic plug**. Temporary hemostatic plug formation depends on adhesion, platelet aggregation, and release reaction.

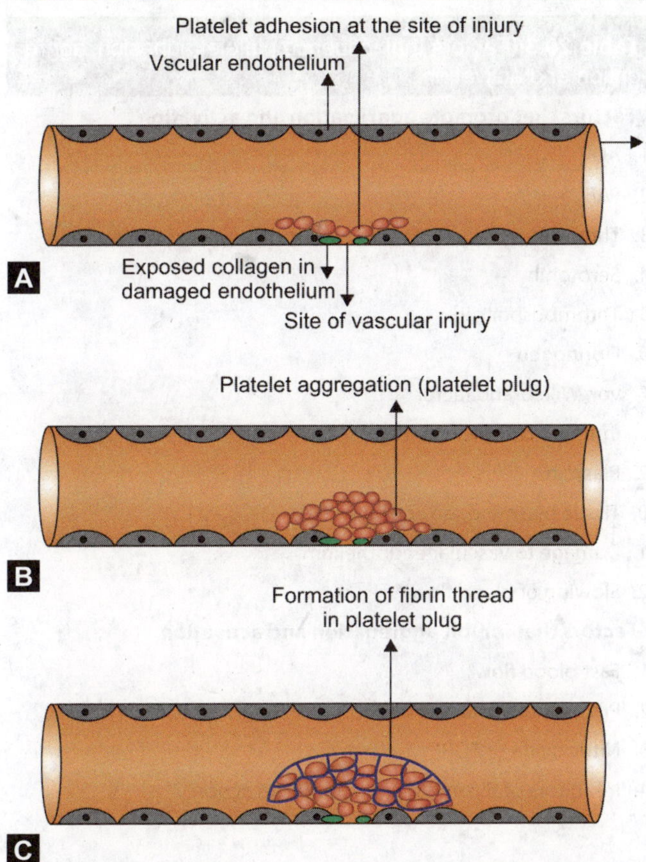

Figs. 20.7A to C: Role of platelet in hemostasis. (A) Platelet adhesion at the site of vascular injury. Note, exposed collagen of damaged vascular endothelium promote adhesion; (B) Platelet aggregation; (C) Formation of fibrin threads in and around the aggregated platelets (definitive plug formation).

Platelet Adhesion

The damage to blood vessel exposes underlying portion of the vessel wall that are normally concealed from the circulatory platelets by intact lining of the endothelium. Platelets have high affinity to adhere to the exposed vascular wall, which is called platelet adhesion (Fig. 20.7A). Especially, exposed **collagen** and **von Willebrand factor** in the injured vessel wall attract platelets as platelets have receptors for them on their cell membrane. However, platelet adhesion is also controlled by following factors:

1. **Depth and degree of injury:** Deeper and extensive the injury more is the platelet aggregation. This occurs due to release of more quantity of platelet activating factors from the tissue.
2. **Site of injury:** Injury in mucocutaneous vascular bed depends more on platelet for hemostasis, whereas injury of vascular beds in muscles and joints rely more on coagulation mechanism. Platelet aggregation is more in mucocutaneous tissue.
3. **Age of the individual:** As composition of vessel wall changes with age, platelet aggregation alters with age of the individual. In elderly individuals, the aggregation is less.
4. **Hematocrit:** Increased number of red cells increases platelet aggregation by forcing the platelets to the periphery of the blood stream. This is because red cells disproportionately occupy the axial region of the blood in the blood vessels pushing the leucocytes and thrombocytes to the vessel wall. Therefore, in anemia efficiency of platelet plug formation is less.
5. **Speed of blood flow:** When blood flow is faster, platelets do not get adequate time to interact with vessel wall. Also, the force tending to pull platelet from vessel wall and from another platelet is more in fast flow that prevents platelet adhesion and aggregation. Thus, sluggishness of blood flow facilitates platelet adhesion.
6. **Size of blood vessel:** This determines the number of platelets passing through the vessel at a given time that influences platelet adhesion to vessel wall.

Platelet Aggregation

Platelet adhesion is immediately followed by platelet aggregation at the site of injury (Fig. 20.7B). **Fibrinogen, GpIIb-IIIa,** and **thrombin** promote platelet aggregation. Simultaneously, platelets are activated, and activated platelets release chemicals from their granules (refer Fig. 20.5). These chemicals, especially **ADP** and **platelet activating factor** (PAF) further facilitate platelet aggregation (Clinical Box 20.2). Thus, accumulation of more platelets at the site of vascular injury facilitates the process of temporary hemostatic plug (platelet thrombus) formation. Then, formation of clot is initiated (Fig. 20.7C)

Clinical Box 20.2

Use of ADP inhibitors: ADP facilitates platelet thrombus formation. There are ADP receptors on the surface of platelets. In human beings, three types of ADP receptors have been identified on platelet membrane: $P2Y_1$, $P2Y_2$, and $P2X_1$. ADP released from dense granules during platelet activation binds with ADP receptors on platelet membrane and facilitates platelet aggregation that promotes platelet thrombus formation. Therefore, inhibitors of ADP (ADP receptor antagonists that prevent platelet aggregation) have been clinically tried in the prevention of myocardial infarction and stroke that occur due to platelet thrombus obstructing blood flow to the concerned tissues.

Important Note

Use of antiplatelet drugs such as aspirin: Aspirin inhibits platelet aggregation by inhibiting the membrane enzyme cyclooxygenase (Flowchart 20.3). Cyclooxygenase facilitates thromboxane A2 formation that facilitates platelet aggregation and causes vasoconstriction. Therefore, **dispirin** (soluble aspirin) is used in ***treatment and prevention of myocardial infarction and stroke***. Steroids inhibit phospholipase.

Platelet Activation and Release

Adhesion of platelets to damaged vascular endothelium activates the platelets. Polymerization of microfibrillar actin occurs in activated platelets that results in pseudopodia or spicules formation. Platelets are also activated by ***tissue factors and chemicals*** released from granules of the platelets, especially **PAF**. Thrombin and ADP also promote activation.

Flowchart 20.3: Synthesis of thromboxane A2, that promotes platelet aggregation. Note, aspirin inhibits cyclooxygenase.

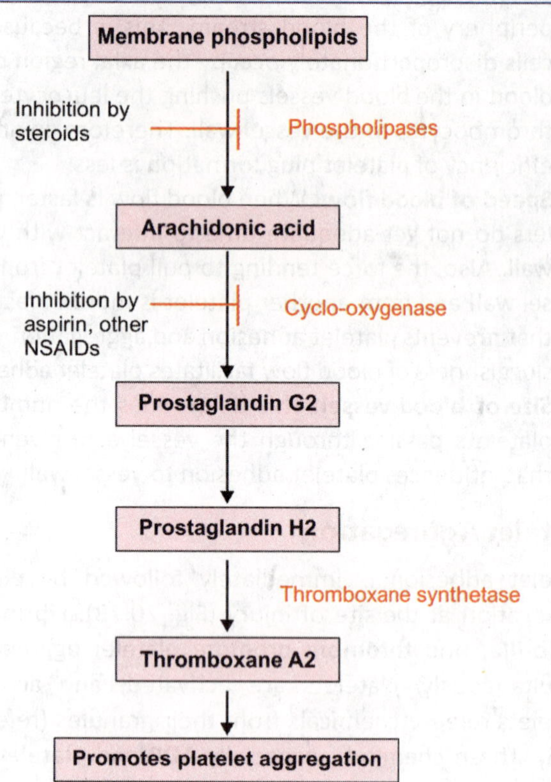

The activated platelets release various chemicals from their granules to the exterior via canalicular system; the process is called **release reaction** or **platelet release (secretion)**. Following are the possible mechanisms of platelet release.

Through Platelet Activating Factor

Platelet adhesion activates platelets. Activation of platelet is facilitated by PAF, a cytokine secreted from neutrophils, monocytes and platelets.

- PAF is a phospholipid produced from membrane lipids. PAF acts via G-proteins and activates phospholipase-C and diacylglycerol (DAG).
- DAG increases cytoplasmic calcium by promoting calcium release from dense tubular systems that are present close to open canaliculi.
- Calcium causes contraction of microfilaments that helps in movement of granules to the open canalicular system.
- Membranes of granules fuse with the membranes of canaliculi and the contents of granules are released into the canaliculi by exocytosis.
- From canaliculi, chemicals are transferred to the exterior of the cell. During this process, platelets change their shape and exhibit movement.

Through Thromboxane and Serotonin

Formation of DAG (as described above) activates the enzyme phospholipase A_2, which converts membrane phospolipid into arachidonic acid.

Table 20.3: Factors that influence platelet adhesion, aggregation and activation.

A. Factors that promote aggregation and activation
1. ADP
2. PAF
3. Thrombin
4. Serotonin
5. Thrombospondin
6. Fibrinogen
7. von Willebrand factor
8. Immune complexes
9. Plasmin
10. Tissue plasminogen activator (tPA)
11. Damage to vascular endothelium
12. Slowing of blood flow
B. Factors that inhibit aggregation and activation
1. Fast blood flow
2. Prostacyclin (PGI_2)
3. Nitric oxide or EDRF
4. Inhibitors of thrombin generation and action

- Arachidonic acid is converted to endoperoxides by cyclooxygenase. Endoperoxides in turn form **thromboxane A_2** ($TX\text{-}A_2$).
- $TX\text{-}A_2$ is a potent vasoconstrictor and also promotes platelet aggregation (Flowchart 20.3).
- **Serotonin** released from platelet produces vasoconstriction and promotes hemostasis.

Through Thrombospondin and Thrombonectin

Thrombospondin and thrombonectin released from platelet granules facilitate the activity of contractile system and further promote exocytosis of granules and release of their content to the exterior.

Normally, platelet thrombus formation is prevented due to the balance between the factors that promote and inhibit platelet adhesion, aggregation and activation (Table 20.3). Alteration in this balance, even without vascular injury leads to intravascular platelet thrombus formation resulting in tissue infarction.

Other Hemostatic Functions

Role in Blood Coagulation

Activation of platelet leads to increased **platelet coagulant activity**.

1. Platelet factor 4 (PF4) acts as a cofactor for blood coagulation (see next chapter).
2. Platelet synthesizes **coagulation factors V and XI**.
3. Platelet phospholipids present on the platelet surface accelerate the formation of Va, VIIIa, and XIa. Va is essential for conversion of prothrombin to thrombin.

Flowchart 20.4: Procoagulant activity of platelet. Platelets provides surface for activation of few clotting factors.

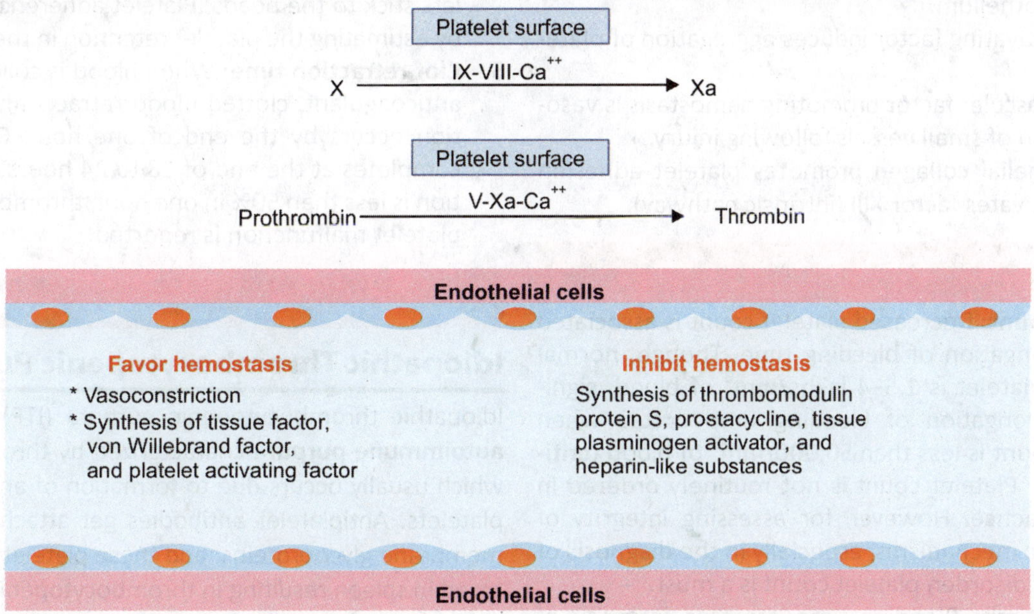

Fig. 20.8: Role of blood vessel in hemostasis. Note the factors produced by endothelial cells that promote and inhibit hemostasis.

4. They also facilitate the conversion of X to Xa and prothrombin to thrombin (Flowchart 20.4). Thus, platelets **accelerate thrombin formation**.

Role in Clot Retraction

If platelets are present in the clot in a test tube, within minutes to hours, the clot contracts, extruding a very large fraction of serum. This is called clot retraction.

1. The platelet filopodia extends into fibrin clot and fibrin strands tug with filopodia. Thus, shrinkage of platelet with contraction of filopodia causes internalization of fibrin that causes clot retraction.
2. In vivo, the phenomenon akin to clot retraction is the **consolidation of the thrombus**, which not only firmly **seals the opening in the injured vessel**, but also **facilitates wound healing**.
3. Clot retraction also *prevents the process of thrombolysis*.
4. Platelet deficiency prolongs the clot retraction time.

Role in Thrombolysis

Role of platelet in fibrinolysis is complex. Both **profibrinolytic and antifibrinolytic actions** of platelets have been demonstrated.

1. ***Thrombospondin, tPA, and plasmin that are profibrinolytic*** are synthesized and released by platelets.
2. However, antifibrinolytics like ***plasminogen activator inhibitor-1 and a$_2$-antiplasmin*** are also secreted from platelets.
3. Platelets by causing clot retraction decrease the efficiency of thrombolysis.
4. It appears that *antifibrinolytic effects of platelets predominate over their profibrinolytic effects* in vivo as platelet rich thrombus is known to resist thrombolysis.

Role of Vascular Wall in Hemostasis

Vascular endothelium plays an important role in hemostasis. Endothelial cells of blood vessel synthesize certain substances that are inhibitory and substances that have facilitatory influence on hemostasis (Fig. 20.8).

Inhibitors of Hemostasis

Endothelial cells synthesise certain substances which have inhibitory influence on hemostasis. These include;

- Thrombomodulin
- Protein S
- Heparin-related substances
- Prostacyclin (PGI2)
- Tissue plasminogen activator (tPA).

Thrombomodulin: Binding of thrombomodulin to thrombin causes activation of protein C. Protein C inactivates factors V and VIII and is a potent inhibitor of coagulation.

Protein S: Protein S is a cofactor for protein C. deficiency of protein C or protein S is associated with tendency toward thrombosis.

Heparin: Heparin-like substances on the surface of endothelial cells potentiates the action of antithrombin.

Prostacyclin: Prostacyclin, a prostaglandin synthesized by endothelial cells, induces vasodilation and also inhibits platelet aggregation. Endothelial cells also synthesize tissue plasminogen activator, which converts plasminogen to plasmin, and activates fibrinolytic system.

Promoters of Hemostasis

Certain factors synthesized by endothelial cells promote hemostasis. These are tissue factor, von Willebrand factor and platelet activating factor.

1. Tissue factor or thromboplastin activates extrinsic system of coagulation.

2. von Willebrand factor mediates adhesion of platelets to subendothelium.
3. Platelet activating factor induces aggregation of platelets.
4. Another vascular factor promoting hemostasis is vasoconstriction of small vessels following injury.
5. Subendothelial collagen promotes platelet adhesion an also activates factor XIII (intrinsic pathway).

PLATELET FUNCTION TESTS

1. **Platelet count:** Decreased platelet count is associated with prolongation of bleeding time. Though, normal count of platelet is 1.5–4 lakhs/mm^3 of blood, significant prolongation of bleeding time occurs when platelet count is less than 50,000/mm^3 of blood (**critical count**). Platelet count is not routinely ordered in clinical practice. However, for assessing integrity of hemostatic mechanisms, especially in the diagnosis of a bleeding disorder, platelet count is a must.
2. **Bleeding time:** Bleeding time assesses integrity of platelets. Bleeding time is routinely assessed before any surgery or dental procedures. It is prolonged in thrombocytopenia and thrombasthenia. **Thrombasthenia** is a condition in which platelet count is normal but functionally platelets are abnormal.
3. **Platelet aggregation tests:** Ability of platelets to aggregate is assessed with the help of **aggregometer**. In this test, an aggregating agent is added to a suspension of platelets in plasma and the response is measured turbidometrically as a change in transmission of light through the suspension.
4. **Platelet adhesiveness test:** Platelet's ability to adhere to glass surface is measured in this test. Anticoagulated blood is allowed to pass at a constant rate through a plastic tube containing glass beads, during which platelets stick to the beads. Platelet adherence is measured by estimating the platelet retention in the tube.
5. **Clot retraction time:** When blood is collected without anticoagulant, clotted blood retracts and 50% retraction occurs by the end of one hour. Clot retraction completes at the end of 18 to 24 hours. When retraction is less than 50% in one hour, thrombocytopenia or platelet malfunction is reported.

COMMON PLATELET DYSFUNCTIONS

Idiopathic Thrombocytopenic Purpura

Idiopathic thrombocytopenic purpura (ITP) is a **primary autoimmune purpura** characterized by thrombocytopenia which usually occurs due to formation of antibody against platelets. Antiplatelet antibodies get attached to platelet membrane glycoproteins, and these platelets are phagocytosed in spleen resulting in thrombocytopenia (Fig. 20.9).

It occurs in two forms: childhood ITP and adult ITP.

Childhood ITP: Childhood ITP is common but less severe and occurs equally in both genders that usually resolves spontaneously in six months.

Adult ITP: Adult ITP is less common and occurs predominantly in females.

1. The **common feature** of the disease is ***bleeding*** that usually occurs spontaneously. Skin is the commonest site of hemorrhage, exhibiting ***petechiae or ecchymoses***. Bleeding occurs from mucus membranes in the form of ***epistaxis*** (bleeding from the nose), or bleeding-gums.
2. **Diagnosis** is made by demonstrating thrombocytopenia, anemia, and anti-platelet antibodies in the patient.

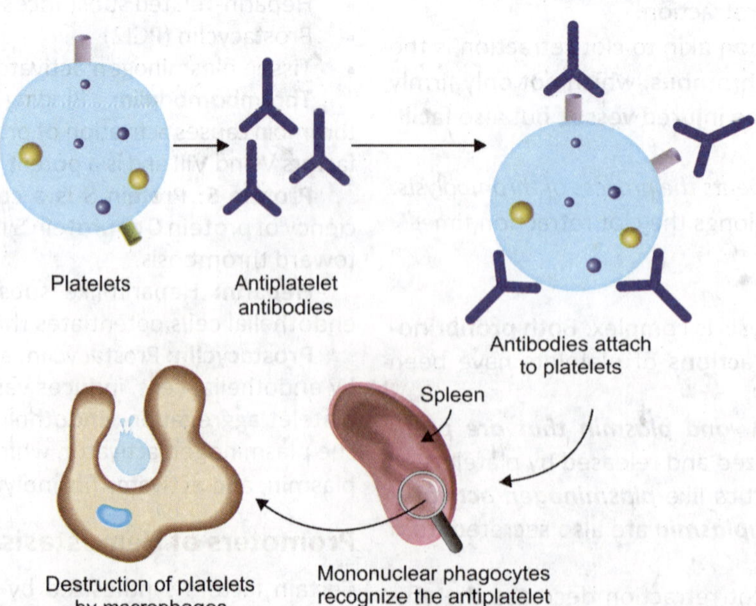

Fig. 20.9: Pathogenesis of ITP. Note that platelets having antiplatelet antibodies on their surface are destroyed in spleen.
Courtesy: Figure 35.1, Essentials in Hematology and Clinical Pathology by Ramadas Nayak et al., 1st edition, 2012; Jaypee Brothers Medical Publishers (P) Ltd.

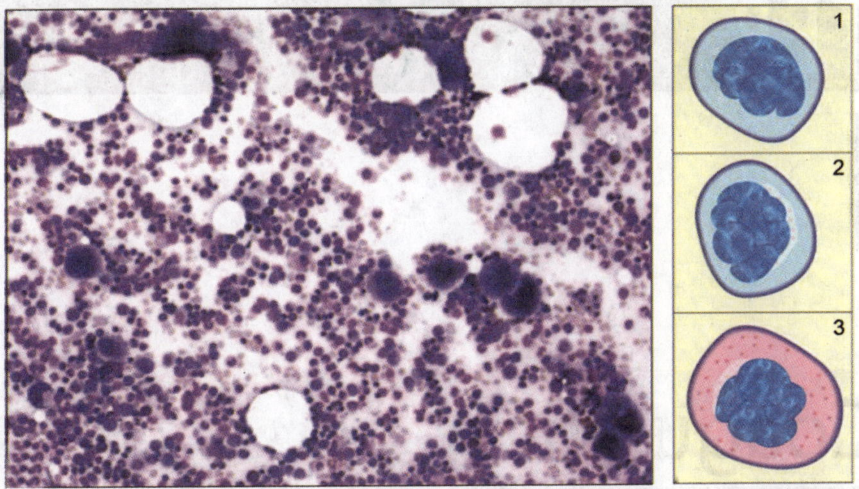

Fig. 20.10: Bone marrow smear in ITP. Note increased number of megakaryocytes.
Courtesy: Figure 35.2, page 302, Essentials in Hematology and Clinical Pathology by Ramadas Nayak et al., 1st edition, 2012; Jaypee Brothers Medical Publishers (P) Ltd.

Increased numbers of megakaryocytes are seen in bone marrow smear (Fig. 20.10).

3. The **treatment** consists of administration of corticosteroids, and splenectomy.

Thrombocytopenia in Pregnancy

Thrombocytopenia is common during pregnancy and usually asymptomatic.

1. A form, called as **gestational thrombocytopenia** that occurs during late gestation (count may be less than 70,000/cu mm of blood in last trimester) and resolves following delivery, but causes excessive bleeding during parturition.
2. Another form is **associated with preeclampsia**.
3. Pregnancy-induced hypertension (PIH) and thrombocytopenia (platelet count less than 50,000/cu mm of blood) have lower prognostic value.

Neonatal Autoimmune Thrombocytopenia

Sometimes, neonatal autoimmune thrombocytopenia (NATP) occurs in newborns and platelet count is less than 50,000/cu mm of blood in this condition. It may be associated with ***autoimmune hemolytic anemia***. Antibodies are demonstrated against ***platelet specific alloantigens***. It is more severe when the mother has ITP. NATP is treated by platelet transfusion, steroid and immunoglobulins.

CHAPTER SUMMARY

Key Concepts

1. Platelets are subcellular elements produced by pinching off from megakaryocytes.
2. Though platelets are small in size, they have highly developed membrane and cellular cytoskeletal system, open canalicular system, alpha and dense granules, and membrane glycoproteins. All these cellular specializations help in platelet functions: adhesion, aggregation, activation, and secretion.
3. Primary hemostasis (temporary hemostatic plug formation) is the first and important step in hemostasis, which mainly depends on platelets. Therefore, platelet deficiency leads to bleeding
4. Platelet also paly role in clotting by activating few clotting factors and promoting clot retraction.
5. Splenomegaly causes thrombocytopenia as platelets are destroyed in spleen.
6. Platelet count less than 50,000 per cu mm of blood is called critical count, as bleeding is significant below this count.

Important to Know (Must Read)

1. In theory examination, "Role of platelets in hemostasis", "Steps and regulation of thrombopoiesis", and "Structure, properties and functions of platelets" may come as **Long Questions**.
2. Temporary hemostatic plug, properties of platelets, thrombopoiesis, platelet granules, cytoskeletal and canalicular systems of platelets, functions of platelets, and platelet function tests may come as **Short Questions** in exams.
3. In **Viva**, examiners may ask... platelet count, functions of platelets, causes of thrombocytopenia and thrombocytosis, mechanism of temporary hemostatic plug formation, specialities of platelet structure, properties of platelets, steps of thrombopoiesis, regulation of thrombopoiesis, chemicals secreted from platelet granules, mechanism of platelet adhesion, mechanism of aggregation, mechanism of platelet release, causes and features of ITP, and platelet function tests.

CHAPTER

21

Blood Coagulation

LEARNING OBJECTIVES

On completion of study of this chapter, the student **MUST** be able to:

1. Name the clotting factors.
2. Describe the mechanisms (intrinsic and extrinsic) of blood coagulation.
3. Understand the importance of clot retraction.
4. Explain the anticlotting mechanism (process of fibrinolysis).
5. Appreciate the physiological basis of use of fibrinolytic agents in coronary artery disease and stroke.
6. List the anticoagulants.
7. List the investigations for detection of defects in temporary and definitive hemostatic plug formation.
8. Enumerate the common abnormalities of coagulation.

The student **MAY** also be able to:

1. Describe various clotting factors.
2. Describe the mechanism of action and uses of anticoagulants.
3. Understand the pathophysiology of common abnormalities of coagulation, such as DIC, hemophilia and von Willebrand disease.
4. Describe the physiological basis of investigations of bleeding disorders.

INTRODUCTION

Coagulation of blood is a vital physiological process, as hemorrhage is detrimental to life. Blood is maintained in a fluid state in the vascular compartment, yet swiftly coagulates to seal a vascular injury. Failure to form clot results in hemorrhage or thromboembolic phenomenon. Immediately following vascular damage, platelet plug (**temporary hemostatic plug**) formation occurs at the site of injury that immediately stops bleeding. However, unless associated with definitive hemostatic plug, hemorrhage continues as platelet thrombus is not a stable plug. The **definitive hemostasis** is the coagulation of blood, the process which is simultaneously activated along with the activation of platelets. Coagulation of blood occurs due to activation of clotting factors (coagulation proteins) that are normally present in their inactive form in plasma.

Clotting Factors

Coagulation of blood depends on a series of chemical reactions involving clotting factors. There are known 12 **clotting factors** (Table 21.1) that were depicted earlier as factors I to XIII (factor VI absent). Later, few more were added to the list.

Scientist contributed

In 1905, **Paul Morawitz** was the first scientist who systematically assembled coagulation factors into the scheme of coagulation and demonstrated that, in the presence of calcium and thromboplastin, prothrombin (II) was converted to thrombin, which, in turn, converted fibrinogen (I) into a fibrin clot. This theory persisted for 40 years until the discovery of factor V.

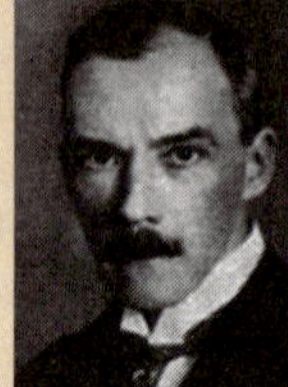

Paul Morawitz

Factor I

Factor I is the **fibrinogen**.

1. It is a dimeric glycoprotein with molecular weight of 340,000. Each of the two subunits consists of three chains: **Aα, Bβ and** γ. The A and B fibrinopeptides are separated by action of thrombin.
2. The genes for three chains of fibrinogen are found in the ***chromosome 4*** at q23–q32.

Table 21.1: Clotting factors.

Factor I	:	Fibrinogen
Factor II	:	Prothrombin (α2 - globulin)
Factor III	:	Tissue thromboplastin
Factor IV	:	Calcium ion
Factor V	:	Proaccelerin
	:	Factor VI does not exist
Factor VII	:	Proconvertin
Factor VIII	:	Antihemophilic factor [antihemophilic globulin (AHG) or antihemophilic factor A].
Factor IX	:	Christmas factor (antihemophilic factor B)
Factor X	:	Stuart-Prower factor,
Factor XI	:	Plasma thromboplastin antecedent (antihemophilic factor C)
Factor XII	:	Hageman factor, contact factor
Factor XIII	:	Fibrin stabilizing factor (Laki-Lorand factor)
HMW-K	:	High-molecular weight kininogen (Fitzgerald factor)
Pre-K	:	Prekallikrein (Fletcher factor)
Ka	:	Kallikrein
PL	:	Platelet phospolipid
Inhibitors		
	:	Protein C
	:	Protein Z
	:	Thrombomodulin
	:	Antithrombin III
	:	Tissue factor pathway inhibitor
	:	Protein Z-dependent protease inhibitor

3. Fibrinogen is present in plasma and α-granules of platelet.
4. Its plasma concentration is **2000–4000 µg/ml.**
5. Its half-life in plasma is 3–5 days.
6. **Fibrinogen is converted to fibrin** by IIa (thrombin) and is stabilized by physical contact with XIIIa (activated fibrin-stabilizing factor).
7. Fibrin forms the *structural meshwork that transforms the loose platelet plug into a solid hemostatic plug*.
8. Fibrinogen is an ***acute phase reactant*** and is synthesized by liver.
9. Its concentration is greatly increased in ***acute inflammations***.
10. IL-6 stimulates fibrinogen synthesis.

Factor II

Factor II is **prothrombin**, a vitamin K-dependent coagulation protein primarily synthesized in liver.

1. It is a single chain zymogen with molecular weight 72,000 and plasma half-life of about 60 h.
2. Its plasma concentration **is 100–150 µg/ml.**
3. The gene for human prothrombin is located on ***chromosome 11*** close to the centromere.
4. **Prothrombin is activated to thrombin** by Xa (activated Stuart-Prower factor).

   In clotting mechanism, **thrombin has many functions**, such as:

   1. It converts fibrinogen to fibrin monomers by removing fibrinopeptides A and B from fibrinogen. Fibrin monomers then form fibrin polymers (clot).
   2. It is a potent activator of platelets.
   3. It activates procarboxypeptidase B that inhibits plasmin-mediated fibrinolysis.
   4. It has also anticlotting activity. It binds to cofactor thrombomodulin on endothelial cells that allows protein C to be activated.
   5. It has growth factor and cytokine like activities that play a role in inflammation, wound healing and atherosclerosis.

   Inhibitors of thrombin: The primary inhibitor of thrombin in plasma is **antithrombin III**. Heparin cofactor II also inhibits thrombin.

Factor III

Factor III is a tissue factor, known as **tissue thromboplastin** (TPL).

1. It is a membrane protein containing 263 amino acids.
2. The gene for factor III is located on ***chromosome 1***.
3. Though TPL is not expressed normally in the cells in close contact with flowing blood, it is expressed in many extravascular tissues and in the adventitia of blood vessels.
4. It is an important physiological **initiator of extrinsic pathway for blood coagulation**.
5. When blood comes in contact with TPL following extravasation of blood from the injured vessel, circulating factor VII binds with TPL and gets rapidly converted to VIIa, an active protease that converts X to Xa. This initiates the process of coagulation.

Factor IV

Factor IV is **calcium**. Calcium acts as a cofactor in many steps of intrinsic and extrinsic pathways of blood coagulation, especially for **conversion of X to Xa** and **prothrombin to thrombin**.

Factor V

Factor V is **proaccelerin**.

1. This is a large glycoprotein with molecular weight 333,000 and plasma half-life of about 12h.
2. The gene for factor V is located in chromosome 1 at q21–q25.
3. The primary function of factor V is to **activate prothrombin to thrombin**, though it also participates in activation of Xa.
4. The acidic regions of factor V contain high aspartic and glutamic acid residues that are important in activating factor II. Sulfation of factor V potentiates its activity.

Factor VII

Factor VII is also called **proconvertin**. It is among the vitamin-K-dependent clotting factors.

1. It consists of single chain polypeptide.
2. It has the half-life of about 3.5 h, which is shortest amongst procoagulant factors.
3. The gene for factor VII is located on ***chromosome 13***.
4. It is activated by the tissue factor and inhibited by tissue factor pathway inhibitor (TFPI).
5. The primary function is to **activate X to Xa**. It also activates IX to IXa.

Factor VIII

Factor VIII is **antihemophilic factor**.

1. The gene for factor VIII is located on the ***X chromosome*** at q28. It is synthesized in liver.
2. Its half-life is 8 to 12 h when it is associated with vWF. The half-life is reduced when concentration of vWF is reduced in plasma. Therefore, ***deficiency of vWF also reduces the level of VIII***.
3. Factor VIII is activated by thrombin or Xa and the activation results in its release from vWF.
4. The main function of VIIIa is to **activate X to Xa**.

Factor IX

Factor IX is also called **Christmas factor** or **anti-hemophilic factor B**.

1. It is synthesized in liver dependent on vitamin K.
2. It has the half-life of 18–24 h.
3. The gene for factor IX is located on the tip of long arm of ***X chromosome***. Therefore, hemophilia B is a sex-linked disorder.
4. Factor IX is activated by XIa or VIIa-TF complex.
5. Along with cofactor VIIIa, it **activates factor X**. This activity is physiologically expressed on the surface of platelets and evidences suggest that platelets have receptors for IXa.

Factor X

Factor X is known as **Stuart-Prower factor**.

1. It is a vitamin K-dependent polypeptide synthesized by liver.
2. It has molecular weight of 59,000 and plasma half-life of 34 to 40 hours.
3. The gene for factor X is located on the ***chromosome 13*** in close proximity to factor VII gene.
4. Activation of Factor X is the target of both intrinsic and extrinsic pathways of coagulation.
5. It is activated by IXa of intrinsic pathway and VIIa of extrinsic pathway.
6. The primary function of factor Xa is the **conversion of prothrombin to thrombin**. It has also *mitogenic activity* for smooth muscle cells. It possesses receptor mediated *proinflammatory activity*.
7. Factor Xa is inhibited by antithrombin III (AT-III), which is accelerated by heparin. TFPI also inhibits Xa.

Important Note

Naming of Stuart-Prower Factor: Factor X deficiency was described in 1957 in a **woman named Prower** and **a man Stuart,** in whose blood the defects in blood clotting were observed. Later the clotting factor was identified and named after the patients.

Factor XI

Factor XI is known as **plasma thromboplastin antecedent** or **antihemophilic factor C**.

1. Factor XI, XII, HMW kininogen, and prekallikrein are some times called ***contact factors***.
2. Factor XI is synthesized in liver.
3. The gene for factor XI is located on ***chromosome 4*** at q32–35.
4. Factor XI is activated by factor XIIa, the process which is accelerated by HMW kininogen.
5. The major function of factor XIa is to **convert IX to IXa**.
6. It is inhibited by plasma protease inhibitors, such as α_1-trypsin inhibitor, C1-esterase inhibitor, α_2-plasmin inhibitor and AT-III.

Factor XII

Factor XII is known as **Hageman's factor**.

1. This is also called ***glass factor*** or ***contact factor***.
2. The gene for factor XII was located on ***chromosome 5***.
3. Factor XII is activated when it comes in contact with negatively charged surface. This is called ***contact activation***. HMW kininogen and prekallikrein facilitate the process.
4. XIIa **promotes the conversion XI to XIa**.

Scientists contributed

Oscar D Ratnoff and Joan E Colopy worked in the field of blood coagulation. In 1955, Ratnoff and Colopy identified a patient named **John Hageman** with a Factor XII deficiency that died from a thrombotic event and not a bleeding disorder. The factor was named as Hageman's factor.

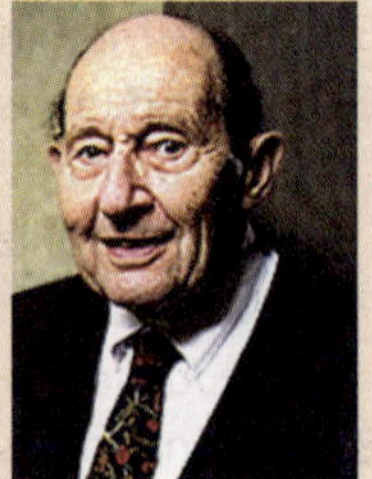

Oscar D Ratnoff

Factor XIII

Factor XIII is known as **Laki-Lorand factor**. As it causes stabilization of fibrin thread, it is also called ***fibrin-stabilizing factor***.

1. It is a glycoprotein consisting of A and B subunits.
2. It has molecular weight of 320,000 and half-life of about 10 days.
3. The B chain is not active enzymatically. The A chain (XIII-A) is a member of transglutaminase family, which contains 731 amino acids with molecular weight of 83,000.

4. In addition to its presence in plasma, it is also found in platelets, monocytes and macrophages.
5. The plasma XIII contains both A and B chains, and the cellular XIII contains only A chain.
6. The gene for A chain is located on ***chromosome 6*** and the gene for B chain is located on ***chromosome 1***.
7. Thrombin causes cleavage of A and B subunits of XIII that causes exposure of active site on A chain. This activates XIII to XIIIa. The XIIIa cross-links α and β chains of fibrin to **stabilize the fibrin plug**. In XIIIa deficiency, though clot formation occurs, hemostasis becomes inadequate.
8. It also promotes wound healing and tissue repair. It helps in maintenance of pregnancy.

HMW Kininogen

High molecular weight kininogen is also called ***Fitzgerald factor***.

1. It is a nonenzymatic cofactor that circulates in complex with factor XI and prekallikrein. It is a contact factor for coagulation.
2. The gene for HMW kininogen is located on ***chromosome 3***.
3. Its plasma half-life is 150 h.
4. It is synthesized by liver.
5. In addition to its **nonenzymatic function in contact activation**, it acts as a **thiol protease inhibitor**.
6. It is cleaved by **prekallikrein to bradykinin**, a potent vasodilator.

Prekallikrein

Prekallikrein is also called ***Fletcher factor***. It is a contact factor for coagulation.

1. The gene for prekallikrein is located on ***chromosome 4***.
2. It has half-life of 35 h in plasma. It is synthesized by liver.
3. It circulates as a complex with factor XI and HMW kininogen.
4. It causes ***contact activation of blood coagulation***.
5. Along with HMW kininogen and factor XII, it participates in *inflammatory response*.

Scientist contributed

Prekallikrein was initially described by **Dr Hathaway et al,** in 1965 after encountering a Kentucky family who exhibited strikingly abnormal APTT results, but showed no bleeding symptoms. The family appeared to have a hereditary deficiency in an unknown coagulation factor, later named ***Fletcher factor*** after the family (Fletcher family).

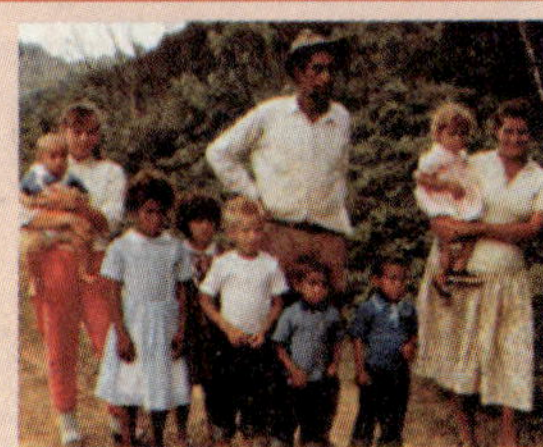

The Fletcher family

Thrombomodulin

Thrombomodulin is a ***cellular cofactor for thrombin***.

1. It is a transmembrane protein with molecular weight of 78,000.
2. The gene for thrombomodulin is located on ***chromosome 20***.
3. It independently cleaves many clotting factors, such as II, V and VIII.
4. When thrombin binds with thrombomodulin, the complex is localized to endothelial cell surface, which, in turn, causes 2000-fold **activation of protein C**.
5. Thus, thrombin in complex with thrombomodulin is ***converted from procoagulant to anticoagulant***. However, in the complex form, thrombomodulin does not cleave factors II, V and VIII.
6. Thrombomodulin also increases the action of thrombin to activate TAFI (thrombin-activable fibrinolysis inhibitor).

Protein C

Protein C is a vitamin K-dependent protein. However, unlike other vitamin K-dependent proteins (factors II, VII, IX and X), it is ***not a procoagulant***.

1. It regulates clotting by inactivating Va and VIIIa.
2. The gene for protein C is located on ***chromosome 2***.
3. It has molecular weight of 59,000 and half-life of about 6 h.
4. It is activated by thrombomodulin.

Protein S

Protein S is a single-chain glycoprotein cofactor synthesized primarily in liver. It is also synthesized by endothelial cells, megakaryocytes, Leydig cells and osteoblasts.

1. It has molecular weight of 75,000 and half-life of about 42 hours.
2. The gene for protein S is located on ***chromosome 3***.
3. Protein S acts as a cofactor for protein C. It forms a complex with protein C that **inactivates Va and VIIIa**. Thus, it is an important component of ***anticlotting mechanisms***. However, it does not require proteolytic activation for its activity.
4. It has also its independent anticoagulant activity by virtue of its ability to compete with factor Xa for binding with factor Va.

Protein Z

Protein Z is synthesized in liver. It has half-life of about 60 hours. The gene for protein Z is located on chromosome 3. Function of protein Z is ***similar to that of protein S***.

Tissue Factor Pathway Inhibitor (TFPI)

TFPI is a single chain polypeptide with molecular weight of about 35,000.

1. It is mainly synthesized by endothelial cells of blood vessels.
2. The gene for TFPI is located on ***chromosome 2***.
3. It has three protease inhibitor domains. It **inhibits factors Xa and VIIa**.

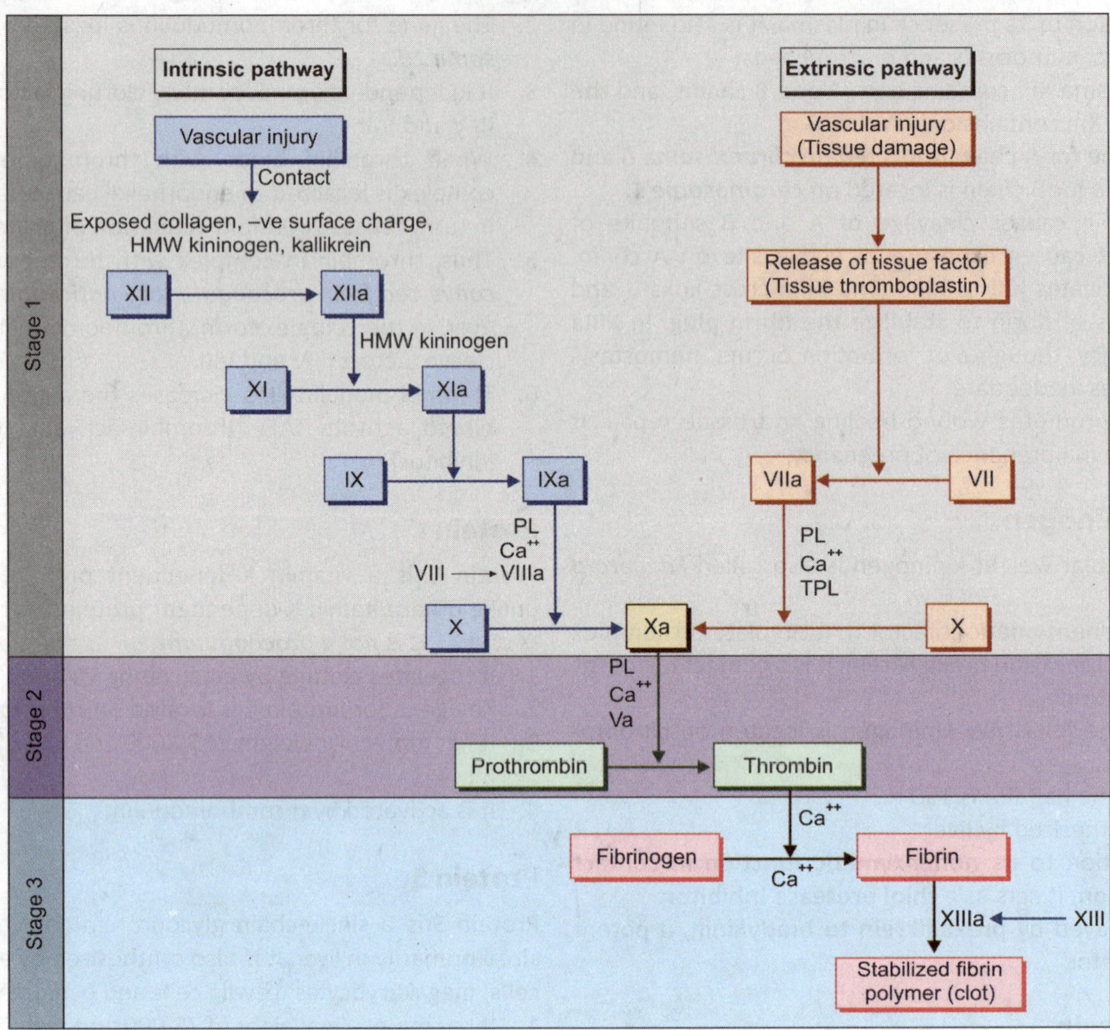

Fig. 21.1: Mechanism of blood coagulation. (TPL: Tissue thromboplastin; PL: Platelet phospholipids).

Antithrombin III (AT-III)

AT-III is member of a large family of serine protease inhibitors, known as *serpins*.

1. The gene for AT-III is located on ***chromosome 1***.
2. It **inhibits thrombin, Xa and IXa,** which is facilitated by heparin.
3. Factor VIIa is normally resistant to the action of AT-III. However, VIIa complexed with tissue factor is inhibited by AT-III in the presence of heparin.

MECHANISM OF BLOOD COAGULATION

Blood coagulation occurs in **three major stages** (Fig. 21.1):

Stage 1: Activation of Stuart-Prower factor (formation of prothrombin activator)

Stage 2: Formation of thrombin from prothrombin

Stage 3: Formation of fibrin from fibrinogen

Activation of Stuart-Prower Factor (Factor X)

Activation of Stuart-Prower factor or factor X is the key to blood coagulation. Factor Xa is called ***prothrombin activator*** as it activates prothrombin to form thrombin. Therefore, this process is also called ***prothrombin activation***. This is achieved by **two pathways**: the intrinsic pathway and the extrinsic pathway (Fig. 21.1).

Intrinsic Pathway

Intrinsic mechanism of prothrombin activation occurs in **four steps**:

Step 1 (Activation of XII)

Activation of intrinsic pathway starts with ***contact of Hageman factor with a negatively charged surface*** or ***exposed collagen*** of the injured vessel wall.

1. High molecular weight **(HMW) kininogen and kallikrein** act as cofactors to facilitate the activation of factor XII.
2. Exposed collagen stimulates platelet adhesion and aggregation before initiating blood coagulation.

Step 2 (Activation of XI)

Activated XII (XIIa) converts XI to its active form (XIa). This step is accelerated in the presence of ***HMW kininogen***.

Step 3 (Activation of IX)

XIa then converts IX to IXa, which is accentuated by VIIa. ***Calcium*** accelerates this process.

Step 4 (Activation of X)

Final step in activation of prothrombin activator is activation of X. IXa causes activation of X to Xa, the activated Stuart-Prower factor. The ***membrane phospholipid, calcium and activated factor VIII*** act as cofactors for the activation of Stuart-Prower factor.

Formation of VIIIa is crucial in Stage 1

Formation of VIIIa is the **key to the process of activation of X**. Factor VIII circulates as a **complex with vWF**.

1. Separation of VIII from vWF activates VIII.
2. Activation of VIII is ***facilitated by Xa and thrombin***, the factors that are the consequences of formation of VIIIa.
3. Thus, activation of factor VIII and further activation of clotting mechanism become a vicious cycle.

Enzyme Cascade Hypothesis

In the intrinsic system of blood coagulation, activation of one clotting factor **acts as an enzyme for the activation of next factor** that leads to sequential activation of subsequent factors in a series of steps. Therefore, the intrinsic process of blood coagulation is called ***enzyme cascade hypothesis***.

Extrinsic Pathway

Extrinsic pathway of blood coagulation occurs in **three steps**.

Step 1 (Release of TPL)

Key to the clotting mechanism is the release of ***tissue thromboplastin*** (TPL) from the injured tissue. As TPL is the **tissue factor** which is viewed as extrinsic to circulating blood, this system of blood coagulation is called ***extrinsic system of clotting***.

Step 2 (Activation of VII)

TPL converts factor **VII to its active form (VIIa)**. This is ***the key step in extrinsic mechanism***. VIIa directly activates not only X (Stuart-Prower factor), but also IX (Christmas factor). Thus, it also influences intrinsic mechanism of activation of factor X.

Step 3 (Activation of X)

VIIa converts **X to Xa**. This process is accelerated in the presence of ***calcium, platelet phospholipid and TPL***.

Note: Though there are intrinsic and extrinsic systems of blood coagulation, recently it is believed that these two systems do not operate independently, and all the clotting factors are interrelated for homeostasis.

Formation of Thrombin from Prothrombin

This is the **second stage** of blood coagulation in which activated Stuart-Prower factor (Xa) converts **prothrombin to thrombin**, in the presence of ***platelet phospholipid, calcium and activated factor V (Va).*** Factor Va acts as cofactor for acceleration of this process. Therefore, it is also called ***proaccelerin*** or ***accelerator globulin***.

Important Note

Thrombin formation occurs rapidly: Factor II is **prothrombin**, a vitamin K-dependent protein formed in liver. Prothrombin forms **thrombin**, which is basically a proteolytic enzyme having molecular weight of 34,000 dalton. It is formed rapidly and in large amount as both intrinsic and extrinsic mechanisms stimulate its formation.

Functions of Thrombin in Blood Coagulation

1. It converts ***fibrinogen to fibrin monomers*** by removing fibrinopeptides A and B from fibrinogen. Fibrin monomers then form fibrin polymers (clot).
2. It activates ***formation of prothrombin activator*** by stimulating the activation of VIII, V, and XIII. Thus, it provides *positive feedback* to the coagulation process.
3. It is a potent ***activator of platelets***.
4. It **activates procarboxypeptidase B** that *inhibits plasmin-mediated fibrinolysis*.
5. It has also an **anticlotting activity**. It binds to cofactor thrombomodulin on endothelial cells that allows protein C to be activated. Thus, thrombin balances the coagulation and anticoagulation processes in the body.
6. It helps in **repair of vessel wall**. It has growth factor and cytokine-like activities that play role ***in inflammation, wound healing and atherosclerosis***.

Inhibitors of thrombin: The primary inhibitor of thrombin in plasma is **antithrombin III**. ***Heparin cofactor II*** also inhibits thrombin.

Formation of Fibrin from Fibrinogen

This is the final stage of blood coagulation in which **thrombin acts as an enzyme** to convert fibrinogen to fibrin. In this process, first, the fibrin monomers are formed and afterward, they are polymerized to fibrin thread (blood clot). This occurs in **three steps**:

1. Proteolysis of soluble fibrinogen
2. Polymerization of fibrin monomers
3. Stabilization of fibrin polymer

Proteolysis of Soluble Fibrinogen

Fibrinogen has **three domains**: two peripheral (D) domains and one central (E) domain.

1. Thrombin binds with central domain and proteolytically ***releases two fibrinopeptides A and B*** from aminoterminals of Aα and Bβ chains of each fibrinogen molecules.
2. Release of fibrinopeptides leads to the formation of **fibrin monomer** (Flowchart 21.1).

Flowchart 21.1: Mechanism of fibrin stabilization.

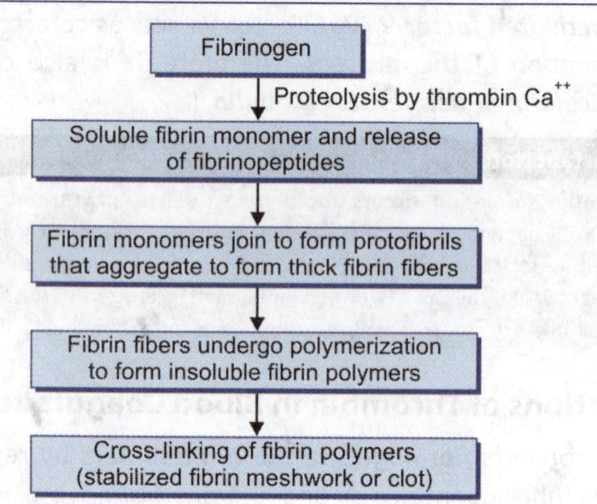

Polymerization of Fibrin Monomers

Fibrin monomers join to form **protofibrils**.

1. About 15 to 20 protofibrils aggregate to form **thick fibers of fibrin**.
2. Protofibrils also branch out to form into a meshwork of interconnected thick fibrin fibers. This is called ***polymerization of fibrin monomers***.
3. Thrombin initiates the process of polymerization and simultaneously activates XIII.
4. XIIIa completes the process of polymerization.

Stabilization of Fibrin Polymer

Fibrin stabilizing factor **(XIIIa) stabilizes the fibrin polymers** by cross-linking them.

1. XIII is converted to XIIIa by thrombin.
2. **Calcium acts as a cofactor** for this conversion.
3. ***Covalent cross-linking*** of fibrin polymers provides adequate strength to the fibrin thread and to the fibrin meshwork.
4. The stabilized fibrin meshwork is the blood clot.
5. Red cells and platelets are trapped inside the fibrin meshwork to give the volume to the clot.

Clot Retraction

The clotted blood consists of fibrin meshwork containing red cells and platelets trapped within the clot. ***Fibrin threads spread in all directions*** and adhere to the endothelial wall. When blood is allowed to clot in a test tube, the *fibrin mesh spreads all around* trapping all the serum within it. However, within minutes to hours, clot shrinks expressing serum out of it. This phenomenon is called ***clot retraction***.

1. The process of clot retraction is believed to occur in vivo that causes **consolidation of thrombus** (intravascular clot).
2. Clot retraction is the **function of platelets**.
3. For effective clot retraction to occur, normally functioning **platelets must be present in adequate number**.
4. Retracted clot decreases the efficiency of thrombolysis (fibrinolysis). Therefore, a ***thrombus rich in platelets is resistant to fibrinolytic agents***.

Mechanism of Clot Retraction

The platelets form spicules (**filopodia**) that extend along the fibrin threads.

1. Fibrin strands tug with the filopodia. Also, protofibrils of thick fibrin strand get embedded within the filopodia by the action of membrane cytoskeleton.
2. Later, platelets shrink with contraction of their filopodia. This causes **internalization of fibrin within the contracted platelets**. Thus, retraction of clot occurs.
3. ***Thrombin and calcium*** accelerate clot retraction.
4. ***Glycoprotein IIb/IIIa*** receptors on platelets facilitate clot retraction.

Functions of Clot Retraction

A retracted clot is a **consolidated and stable thrombus**, which not only firmly seals the opening in the injured vessel, but also has other functions. The functions of retracted clot are as follows:

1. Retracted clot (thrombus) strongly seals injured vessel.
2. It facilitates wound healing.
3. It prevents thrombolysis.

Prolongation of Clot Retraction Time

Normally, clot retraction begins within thirty seconds after clot formation. However, the process of retraction is very slow. About 50% retraction occurs at the end of one hour and completes in 18 to 24 hours.

1. Clot retraction time is said to be prolonged when **retraction is less than 50%** at the end of one hour.
2. In **Glanzmann thrombasthenia**, deficiency of IIb/IIIa receptors results in inhibition of clot retraction that causes prolongation of clot retraction time.
3. **Platelet deficiency** also prolongs the clot retraction time.

ANTICLOTTING MECHANISM (Fibrinolysis)

Tendency of blood to clot in vivo is prevented by naturally occurring anticlotting mechanisms. Thus, there is a balance between clotting and anticlotting mecahnisms.

1. In our body, normally, there is a low level of activation of coagulation factors. This results in a **basal coagulation** of blood. The basal coagulation may be due to minor injuries to blood vessels that occur during normal daily activities (**normal vascular stress**). However, coagulation process proceeds only when enough thrombin is generated in response to a significant vascular injury.

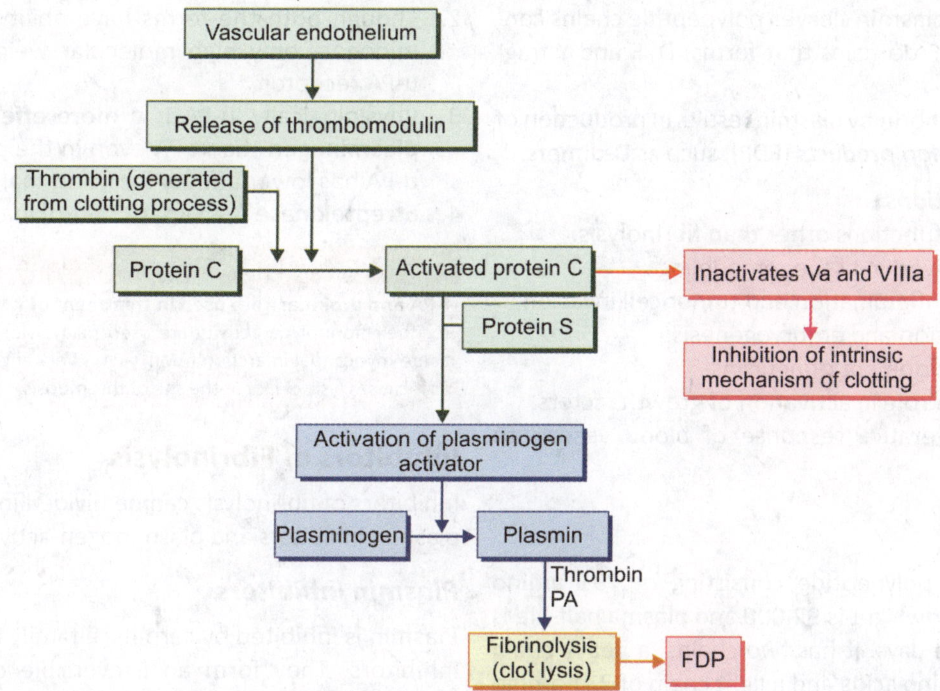

Fig. 21.2: Anticlotting (fibrinolysis) mechanism. [PA: Plasminogen activators (t-PA, u-PA); FDP: Fibrin degradation product]. Note, fibrinolysis occurs in three major steps: activation of protein C, activation of plasmin and fibrinolysis.

2. Moreover, the basal coagulation is balanced by the activity of **basal anticoagulation**, which is evidenced by the presence of ***low levels of protein C and tissue plasminogen activator activity*** in normal individuals.

Anticlotting mechanisms include **three naturally occurring systems**:

1. Presence of naturally occurring anticoagulants in the blood
2. Interaction between thromboxane A_2 and prostacyclin
3. An important role played by vascular endothelium.

Mechanism of Fibrinolysis

The process of blood coagulation automatically initiates the anticlotting mechanisms so that intravascular clot does not spread beyond the site of injury. Fibrinolysis occurs in three steps:

1. Activation of protein C
2. Activation of plasmin
3. Fibrinolysis

Activation of Protein C

Thrombin which is produced by clotting mechanism acts as an enzyme to activate protein C to its active form. The anticlotting mechanism activated by thrombin can also be initiated by **thrombomodulin**, a hormone secreted from endothelial cells of blood vessel. Thrombomodulin activates protein C (Fig. 21.2).

Activation of Plasmin

Activated protein C **inactivates the inhibitors of plasmin activator**. This, in turn, activates plasminogen activator, which promotes formation of **plasmin** from plasminogen. Activated protein C along with its cofactor protein S also **inactivates Va and VIIIa** into their respective inactive forms. This aids in prevention of coagulation.

Fibrinolysis

Plasmin acts as an enzyme to cause fibrinolysis (lysis of clot).

1. This process is facilitated by cofactors thrombin, tissue-type plasminogen activator and urokinase-type plasminogen activator.
2. Fibrin is degraded by plasmin to **fibrin degradation products** (FDP) (Clinical Box 21.1). The details of fibrinolysis by plasmin are given below.

Clinical Box 21.1

FDP level indicates the rate of fibrinolysis: Activation of clotting process as occurs in DIC activates the anticlotting mechanism (fibrinolysis). Fibrinolysis causes accumulation of FDP in plasma, which is subsequently excreted in urine. Hence, measurement of FDP in urine is an index of rate of fibrinolysis as well as intravascular coagulation.

Functions of Plasmin

Functions of plasmin can be broadly divided into two categories: Fibrinolytic actions and nonfibrinolytic actions.

Fibrinolytic Actions

Plasmin cleaves both fibrinogen and fibrin.

1. Plasmin initially cleaves α and β chains within the D domain of fibrinogen that releases Aα and Bβ fragments.

2. Subsequently, plasmin cleaves polypeptide chains connecting D and E domains that forms, D, E and Y fragments.
3. Degradation of fibrin by plasmin results in production of ***fibrin degradation products*** (FDP), such as **D-dimers.**

Nonfibrinolytic Actions

Plasmin has many functions other than fibrinolysis:
1. Plasmin is involved in tissue remodeling.
2. Plays a role in inflammation and tumor cell invasion.
3. Controls ovulation and embryogenesis.
4. Regulates development of neurons.
5. Plasmin plays a role in activation of growth factors.
6. Helps in proliferative response of blood vessels to injury.

Plasminogen

Plasminogen is a polypeptide consisting of 791 amino acids. Its molecular weight is 92,000 and plasma half-life is approximately two days. It has two chains: a heavy chain containing 560 amino acids and a light chain of 231 amino acids. Plasminogen is synthesized mainly in liver.
1. The gene for plasminogen formation is located on ***chromosome 6***.
2. Activation of plasminogen occurs from cleavage by **plasminogen activators** of the bond between arginine and valine at 560 and 561 positions respectively.
3. Thus, plasminogen is converted into plasmin, an active protease.

Plasminogen Activators

There are two major endogenous plasminogen activators: the tissue plasminogen activator and urokinase.

Tissue Plasminogen Activator (t-PA)

t-PA is a polypeptide having 527 amino acids and molecular weight 72,000. The gene for t-PA is located on ***chromosome 8***. It is synthesized primarily by endothelial cells. The half-life of t-PA is very short, about 5 minutes.
1. Thrombin, histamine, bradykinin, epinephrine, ADH, acetylcholine and gonadotropins control the secretion of t-PA.
2. Though, normally t-PA is a poor plasminogen activator by itself, in the presence of fibrin, its activity increases enormously.
3. Fibrin facilitates t-PA activity by increasing affinity of t-PA for plasminogen (Clinical Box 21.2).

Urokinase and Streptokinase

Urokinase plasminogen activator (u-PA) is a glycoprotein consisting of 411 amino acids. The gene for u-PA is located on ***chromosome 10***. It is formed by endothelial cells, macrophages and renal epithelial cells.
1. It exists in **two forms**: high molecular weight u-PA (molecular weight of 54,000) and low molecular weight u-PA (molecular weight of 33,000).
2. Though both the forms have ability to activate plasminogen, only high molecular weight u-PA binds to u-PA receptor.
3. Physiologically, **u-PA is a more effective activator of plasminogen** than t-PA even in the presence of fibrin. u-PA has lower affinity for fibrin than t-PA.
4. **Streptokinase** is a variant of urokinase.

Clinical Box 21.2

t-PA and urokinase are used in treatment of AMI: t-PA and urokinase for their fibrinolytic activity are used for lysis of intracoronary clot in acute myocardial infarction (AMI). t-PA is very effective for this purpose as it causes lysis of clot at the site of thrombosis.

Inhibitors of Fibrinolysis

Inhibitors of fibrinolysis can be divided into two categories: plasmin inhibitors and plasminogen-activator inhibitor.

Plasmin Inhibitors

Plasmin is inhibited by serpins, a family of serine protease inhibitors. They form an irreversible complex with the active site serine of the target protease.
1. α_2-**antiplasmin** is a serpin peptide containing 452 amino acids. Though it is synthesized by liver and kidney, it is a constituent of α-granules of platelet.
2. α_2-**macroglbulin** is a ***nonserpin plasmin inhibitor***, formed by endothelial cells and macrophages.

Plasminogen-Activator Inhibitors (PAI)

There are two PAIs: PAI-1 and PAI-2.
1. ***PAI-1*** is single chain polypeptide containing 402 amino acids, secreted by liver, monocytes, endothelial cells and adipocytes. This is the most important and **rapidly acting physiologic inhibitors of t-PA and u-PA.**
2. ***PAI-2*** is secreted by placenta, monocytes and tumor cells. It is less effective than PAI-1 in inhibiting plasminogen activators.

Plasmin Generation Defects

Fibrinolytic Deficiency

Fibrinolytic deficiency is usually due to **plasminogen deficiency**. There are **two types** of congenital plasminogen deficiencies: **type 1** and **type 2**.

In **type 1 plasminogen deficiency**, both concentration and function of plasminogen are reduced.

In **type 2 plasminogen deficiency**, though the concentration of plasminogen is normal its function is reduced.

The patient with plasminogen deficiency exhibits repeated episodes of thrombophlebitis, intracranial and mesenteric venous thrombosis, and pulmonary embolism (Application Box 17.1). Mutation in plasminogen activators also results in decreased fibrinolysis.

Enhanced Fibrinolysis

This usually occurs due to congenital or acquired *loss of fibrinolytic inhibitor activity*.

1. ***Deficiency of*** α_2**-antiplasmin** is a common cause. The patient presents with bleeding diathesis. In **promyelocytic leukemia**, bleeding occurs due to high level of plasmin generation and deficiency of α_2-antiplasmin.
2. **Acquired** α_2**-antiplasmin deficiency** may be seen in liver disease, DIC, nephritic syndrome and thrombolytic therapy.

Application Box 17.1

Pregnancy is a hypofibrinolytic state: In pregnancy, overall fibrinolytic activity is reduced. This leads to increased fibrin deposition, as suggested by increased D-dimer levels. The PAI levels also increase in pregnancy. The hemostatic and fibrinolytic imbalance is increased in preeclampsia and eclampsia. This predisposes to intravascular thrombosis..

Regulation of Blood Coagulation

Blood coagulation at the site of injury is a life saving process as it prevents loss of blood volume. However, once the clot (fibrin-platelet plug) is formed, the process of clotting must be terminated to avoid thrombotic occlusion in the adjacent normal areas of blood vessel. If clotting remains unchecked, coagulation of blood can spread to the entire vascular tree with modest procoagulant stimulus.

Coagulation in a normal blood vessel or circulation is highly dangerous. Fluidity of blood and absence of thrombosis (intravascular clot) are important physiological states that are essential for normal circulation and blood supply to tissues of the body.

The balance between coagulation and anticoagulation is due to play of various **regulatory mechanisms**, as listed below:

1. **Dynamism of blood flow:** Flow of blood is a dynamic process. When the rate of blood flow decreases, as occurs in vascular stasis, intravascular coagulation is facilitated. Thus, continuous and dynamic flow of blood should be maintained to prevent intravascular coagulation.
2. **Role of vascular endothelium:** Vascular endothelium plays an important role in restricting coagulation process to the site of injury.
   - Damage to vascular endothelium initiates the clotting mechanism by exposing its collagen and negatively charged particles.
   - Once adequate hemostasis is achieved, **thrombomodulin**, a hormone secreted by endothelial cells of blood vessel prevents further blood coagulation by activating protein-C-protein S complex.
   - Also, protease inhibitors AT-III and tissue factor pathway inhibitor are expressed on the surface of the endothelial cells.
   - Endothelial cells also inhibit platelet activation by releasing prostacyclin and EDRF that inhibit platelets (Refer to Fig. 20.11, Chapter 20).
3. **Heparin-antithrombin-III system:** Heparin is a naturally occurring anti-coagulant, secreted from mast cells and basophils. Heparin acts by activating the antithrombin III activity. Heparin-antithrombin III complex **prevents activation of clotting factor IX, X, XI and XII.**
4. **Negative feedback by thrombin:** Thrombin, which is a major mediator of blood coagulation, initiates the process of **anticlotting mechanism** (fibrinolysis). Thus, coagulation is an autoregulatory process.
5. **Role of liver:** Many ***coagulation factors*** are plasma proteins, **formed mainly in the liver**. Therefore, in liver diseases, clotting time is prolonged. Also, liver plays an important role in preventing intravascular coagulation by ***removing activated clotting factors*** from blood. This hepatic clearance of activated clotting factors is accelerated when clotting is spontaneously activated.
6. **Role of platelets:** In addition to its role in primary hemostasis, platelets contribute to coagulation in various ways.
   i. Following platelet activation, **platelet phospholipids** (platelet factor 3 and 4) released to their surface act as cofactors to accelerate the formation of Va, VIIIa and XIa. Cofactors Va and VIIIa are rapidly localized to the membrane of activated platelet.
   ii. Also, factor IXa formed by VIIa-tissue factor complex binds to the platelet surface. This leads to the formation of IXa-VIIa complex on the platelet surface, following which factor X is recruited from the plasma to the platelets and is activated to Xa on platelet membrane. Thus, ***platelet plays an important role in* activation of factor X**, which is a crucial step in blood coagulation. Thus, major clotting reactions occur in close interaction with platelets (Refer to Fig. 20.8, Chapter 20).
   iii. As platelets adhesion and aggregation are localized at the injured vessel wall, platelets help in **restricting clotting reactions** to the site of injury.

ANTICOAGULANTS

Anticoagulants prevent blood from clotting. They are mainly used:

1. For collection of blood sample for laboratory investigations
2. For preserving blood for transfusion
3. For anticoagulation therapy

Anticoagulants for Blood Collection

Anticoagulants are added to the blood sample especially during collection of blood by venipuncture, when whole anticoagulated blood is required for laboratory investigations. Though several anticoagulants are available for the purpose, commonly used are **EDTA, trisodium citrate, double oxalate, sodium fluoride,** and **heparin.**

1. While EDTA is used frequently for hematologic tests, citrated blood is used for coagulation studies and for preserving blood in the blood bank.

2. Use of heparin and fluoride (oxalated) is limited for the determination of blood gases and pH, and plasma glucose respectively.

EDTA (Ethylenediamine Tetra-acetic Acid)

The sodium and potassium salts of EDTA are the commonly used and most powerful anticoagulants.

1. It acts by its **chelating effect on the blood calcium**. It inactivates calcium by forming insoluble complex with it. As calcium is an important cofactor for blood coagulation, chelation of calcium prevents blood to clot.
2. The chelating effect of EDTA is achieved at a concentration of 1.2 mg of the anhydrous salt per ml of blood.
3. Excess EDTA irrespective of its salts, affects both red cell and leucocyte morphology by causing shrinkage and degenerative changes. Therefore, ***EDTA in excess*** of 2 mg/ml of blood results in ***decrease in PCV and increase in MCHC***. Platelets also swell and disintegrate causing an ***artificially high platelet count***, as the platelet fragments are large enough to be counted as normal platelets.

Sodium Citrate

Trisodium citrate is the commonly used anticoagulant in coagulation studies. It is prepared as 0.106 M solution of trisodium citrate in distilled water and then sterilized.

1. It **prevents coagulation by inactivating calcium ions**.
2. For coagulation studies like *determination of prothrombin time or partial thromboplastin* time, 9 volumes of blood are added to 1 volume of sodium citrate solution (9 : 1).
3. It is also used in *collection of blood for estimation of ESR by Westergren method*, where 4 volumes of venous blood are added to 1 volume of the sodium citrate solution (4 : 1).

Double Oxalate

As this anticoagulant contains ammonium and potassium oxalates, is called ***double oxalate***. Potassium oxalate alone causes shrinkage of red cells whereas ammonium oxalate increases their volume. Hence, double oxalate is also called ***balanced oxalate***.

1. It is prepared as the solution containing 1.2% ammonium oxalate and 0.8% potassium oxalate. Usually, 0.25 or 0.5 ml of the double oxalate solution is taken in a penicillin bottle and evaporated in an oven or in an incubator and then kept for collecting blood.
2. The oxalates form an **insoluble complex with the calcium** in the blood, and thereby prevent coagulation.

Sodium Fluoride

Sodium fluoride is used mainly for collecting blood specimen *for plasma glucose estimation*. Fluoride is an **inhibitor of glycolytic enzymes** and thus prevents loss of glucose. However, as fluoride is not a strong anticoagulant, it is mixed with the oxalate.

Oxalates

Oxalates of sodium, potassium, ammonium or lithium act as anticoagulant. They form **insoluble complexes with calcium**.

Heparin

Heparin is a natural constituent of blood. Sodium, lithium, potassium and ammonium salts of heparin are commercially available.

1. It prevents coagulation for approximately 24 hours by neutralizing thrombin. It **facilitates action of antithrombin III**. Thus, it ***prevents formation of fibrin from fibrinogen***.
2. Usually, it is used at a concentration of 10–20 IU per ml of blood.
3. It is commonly used for osmotic fragility test, blood gas determination and pH assays.
4. It is also commonly used in anticoagulation therapy and in preventing blood coagulation during animal experiments.

Anticoagulants for Treatment (Anticoagulation Therapy)

Anticoagulants are used for **treatment or prevention of thrombosis** (intravascular clots). They are usually required for:

1. Management of thrombotic diseases like venous thromboembolism
2. Placement of mechanical heart valves as heart valve prosthesis is associated with risk of thromboembolism
3. Prevention of thromboembolism in chronic nonrheumatic atrial fibrillation
4. Prophylaxis after attacks of cerebral ischemia
5. Management of ischemic heart disease
6. Peripheral vascular diseases
7. Placement of central venous catheters.

Anticoagulants used in anticoagulation therapy are of two types: **oral** and **intravenous**.

Oral Anticoagulants

Routinely used oral anticoagulants are vitamin K antagonists, glycosaminoglycans, inhibitors of factor Xa and inhibitors of thrombin.

Vitamin K Antagonists

The commonly used vitamin K antagonist is **warfarin**. This is a coumarin derivative.

1. Warfarin is an acronym for WARF, i.e. Wisconsin Alumini Research Foundation that first synthesized it in 1942 (Coumarin of WARF, named as warfarin).

2. The four ***vitamin K-dependent coagulation factors*** are II, VII, IX and X. They undergo ***post-translational γ-carboxylation*** of approximately 10 glutamic acid residues in the N-terminal Gla- domain (the domain where γ-carboxylation of clotting proteins takes place is called the ***Gla-domain***).
3. The γ-carboxylation of these cofactors is necessary to enable them to bind calcium and to localize enzymatic processes to a phospholipid surface like membrane of activated platelet.
4. When γ-carboxylation is reduced by 1 to 6 glutamic acid residues, coagulation activity of factors II, VII, IX and X is impaired significantly.

Mechanism of action of warfarin: Warfarin inhibits γ-carboxylation of about 3 to 10 glutamic acid residues, especially of factor II (prothrombin). Warfarin achieves this by ***inhibiting the reductase enzymes that cause formation of vitamin KH_2*** (Fig. 21.3).

- Vitamin KH_2 is required for γ-carboxylation of vitamin K-dependent coagulation factors.
- During the process of γ-carboxylation, vitamin KH_2 is converted to vitamin K-epoxide by *vitamin K epoxide reductase*, vitamin K-epoxide is converted back to vitamin KH_2 by *vitamin K reductase*.
- Both these enzymes are inhibited by coumarin derivatives such as warfarin.

Protein C and protein S (the inhibitors of blood coagulation) also undergo γ-carboxylation and vitamin K antagonists prevent their activity by inhibiting the process.

Dicoumarol is another commonly used vitamin K antagonist.

Glycosaminoglycans

Oral heparin sulfate and **iduronyl-glycosaminoglycan** are used as anticoagulants.

Inhibitors of Factor Xa

Formation of Xa is the key step in blood coagulation. Therefore, **selective inhibitor of Xa** is a ***potent antithrombotic agent*** without affecting bleeding time as demonstrated in animal models. However, its use in human is under trial.

Inhibitors of Thrombin

Many low-molecular weight selective inhibitors of thrombin have been recently identified and are under clinical trials.

Intravenous or Subcutaneous Anticoagulants

Most commonly used intravenous anticoagulants are heparin and hirudin.

Heparin

Heparin is a glycosaminoglycan consisting of chains of alternating residues of D-glucosamine and iduronic acid. Due to its variation in chain lengths, heparin is available as ***LMW-heparin and HMW-heparin***, molecular weight

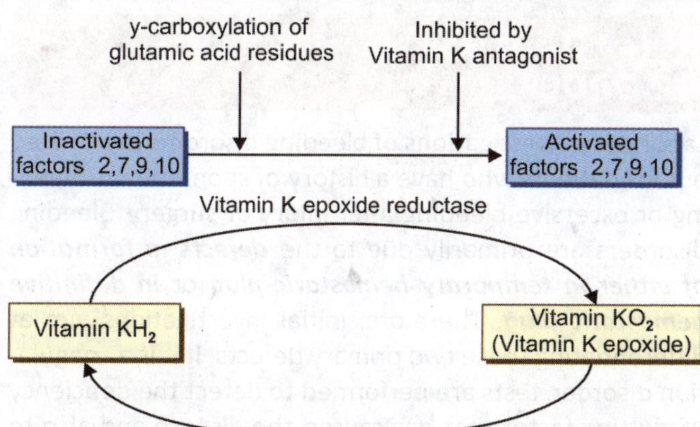

Fig. 21.3: Mechanism of action of Vitamin K antagonist in the prevention of blood coagulation. Factors 2, 7, 9 and 10 are Vitamin K-dependent clotting factors. Vitamin K antagonists inhibit both Vitamin K epoxide reductase and Vitamin K reductase that are essential for Vitamin KO_2 and Vitamin KH_2 formations. Vitamin KH_2 is required for γ-carboxylation of these clotting factors that activate them.

ranging between 5,000 to 30,000. Its anticoagulant activity is due to its **facilitation of the effects of antithrombin III** (AT-III).

1. The pentasaccharide component of heparin has high affinity binding to AT-III.
2. AT-III inactivates thrombin, Xa and IXa. However, heparin inhibition of thrombin is different from inhibition of Xa and IXa.

HMW heparin: HMW heparin molecules ***inhibit thrombin*** by forming a ternary complex in which it binds with both thrombin and AT-III, and *facilitates the thrombin inhibition by AT-III*. But for inhibition of Xa, AT-III/heparin complex does not require heparin to bind directly to factor Xa or IXa in a ternary complex.

LMW heparin: LMW heparin molecules are unable to bind thrombin and AT-III simultaneously. Therefore, they can not augment the inhibition of thrombin by AT-III. However, they retain the ability to ***inhibit factor Xa and IXa***. LMW heparin is as effective as unfractionated heparin for the **treatment of venous thromboembolism** or **acute coronary syndrome**. It is given subcutaneously and is cost-effective in comparison to IV heparin.

Hirudin

Hirudin is a polypeptide containing 65 amino acids. It is produced by the salivary glands of *Hirudo medicinalis*, a medicinal leech.

1. It is a **naturally occurring most specific inhibitor of thrombin**.
2. It is also produced by recombinant DNA technology. It directly inactivates thrombin by binding to the active site and main fibrinopeptide binding region of thrombin.
3. It has been tried in the treatment of acute coronary syndrome, patients undergoing coronary angioplasty and deep vein thrombosis.
4. It is mainly used as anticoagulant in patients who develop heparin-induced thrombocytopenia.

INVESTIGATIONS OF BLEEDING DISORDERS

Laboratory investigations of bleeding disorders are carried out for patients who have a history of spontaneous bleeding or excessive bleeding after injury or surgery. Bleeding disorders are primarily due to the ***defects in formation of either in temporary hemostatic plug*** or ***in definitive hemostatic plug***. Therefore, initial investigations aim at differentiating these two primary defects. If it is a coagulation disorder, tests are performed to detect the deficiency of clotting factor that has caused the disease and also to assess whether the ***defect is in intrinsic or extrinsic system***.

Assessment of Defects in Temporary Hemostatic Plug

1. Bleeding time
2. Capillary fragility test
3. Platelet aggregation test
4. Platelet adhesiveness test

Bleeding Time (BT)

The normal BT by **Duke method** is 1 to 5 minutes and by **Ivy method** is 5 to 11 minutes. BT assesses platelet number and functions.

Capillary Fragility Test

This test measures the ability of the capillaries to withstand increased stress. **Petechiae** appear in the fore arm of the subject when the blood pressure cuff in the arm is inflated to a maximum pressure of 100 mm Hg for about 5 minutes.

1. Normally, **zero to 10 petechiae appears**.
2. **More than 10** petechiae indicate ***capillary weakness, thrombocytopenia or both***.

Platelet Aggregation Test

An aggregating agent is added to a suspension of platelets in plasma and the response is measured turbidometrically as a change in the transmission of light by the instruments called ***aggregometers***. Measurement of platelet aggregation is an essential part of the investigation of any patient with suspected platelet dysfunction in a modern laboratory.

Pletelet Adhesiveness Test

This test measures the ability of platelets to adhere to glass surface. When anticoagulated blood is passed through a plastic tube containing glass beads at a constant rate, some platelets will adhere to the glass beads.

1. The percentage difference of the platelet count done prior to and after passage through the glass bead column is calculated.
2. The normal range is 75 % to 95 % of platelet retention.
3. The platelet adhesiveness test is nonspecific. It is abnormal in several platelet functional disorders.

Assessment of Defects in Definitive Hemostatic Plug

1. Clotting time
2. Prothrombin time
3. Prothrombin consumption test
4. Partial thromboplastin time
5. Activated partial thromboplastin time
6. Thrombin time
7. Plasma recalcification time
8. Clot retraction time

Clotting Time (CT)

Determination of CT is routinely performed before any surgical procedure. It is usually performed by two methods: **capillary tube method**, and **Lee-White (venipuncture) method**.

1. **The capillary method** is used routinely in clinical laboratories. The normal range of CT by capillary glass tube method ranges from ***2 to 8 minutes***. CT is prolonged in diseases in which there is deficiency of clotting factors.
2. If the CT is prolonged more than 10 minutes, the patient should be subjected to more detailed investigations for the identification of the missing coagulation factors.
3. The normal range of CT by **Lee-White method** ranges from 5 to 12 minutes.

Prothrombin Consumption Test

This test is performed to **determine the quantity of prothrombin** remaining in the serum after clot is formed. Normally, prothrombin is used if it is converted to thrombin. Increased serum prothrombin results from a ***quantitative or qualitative platelet deficiency***.

Prothrombin Time (PT)

PT detects the **integrity of stage 2 clotting process**. In this, preparation of rabbit brain emulsion (which contains tissue thromboplastin) is added to plasma in the presence of calcium. This, in the presence of factor VII, triggers stage 2 of the coagulation mechanism, and the clotting time is recorded after the addition of calcified thromboplastin to the plasma.

1. Normal PT is 12 to 16 seconds. Prolonged PT suggests the possibility of ***deficiency of factor II, V, VII, and X***.
2. In stage 2, prothrombin is converted to thrombin which triggers the transformation of fibrinogen to fibrin. Thus, abnormal prothrombin time suggests **defect in stage 2**.

Partial Thromboplastin Time (PTT)

PTT detects the **integrity of stage 1 clotting process**. The platelet substitute in the form of partial thromboplastin is prepared from rabbit brain as chloroform extract. The extract is mixed with test plasma containing excess of calcium, which leads to clot formation.

1. Normal PTT is 60 to 80 seconds. PTT is prolonged when there is a ***deficiency of one or more clotting factors XII, XI, IX, VIII, X, V, II, and I***.
2. Abnormal PTT indicates **stage 1 defect** and missing of one or more of these intrinsic factors.

Activated Partial Thromboplastin Time (APTT)

APTT is a more reliable test than PTT in evaluating the coagulation disorders. Its use in conjunction with PT provides a simple method for **differentiating between stage 1 intrinsic defects and deficiency of other factors**. The platelet substitute, in the form of partial thromboplastin, is prepared from rabbit brain. This is incubated with a contacting agent (kaolin) to provide optimal activation of the intrinsic coagulation factors. The clotting time is determined after the addition of an excess of calcium.

1. Normal APTT is **35 to 40 seconds**.
2. APTT is prolonged in ***deficiencies of factor XII, XI, X, IX, and VIII***.
3. APTT is mainly estimated in hemophilias that involve deficiencies of factor VIII, IX or XI.

Thrombin Time (TT)

TT assesses the **integrity of stage 3 of blood coagulation**. Thrombin (commercially available) is added to the plasma along with calcium and clotting time is determined.

1. Normal value of TT is **15 to 20 seconds**.
2. Thrombin time detects the ***effectiveness of the final stage of coagulation*** in which fibrinogen is converted to fibrin.
3. A prolonged TT is considered to be due to either a **decrease in fibrinogen concentration** or the presence of **dysfunctional fibrinogen**.

Plasma Recalcification Time (PRT)

PRT assesses **efficiency of intrinsic system of coagulation**. When excess of calcium is added to the citrated plasma, clotting occurs. As platelet factor 3 acts as a cofactor for coagulation, clotting occurs in less time in platelet rich plasma than in platelet poor plasma.

1. Normal value of PRT of platelet rich plasma is **100 to 150 seconds** and of platelet poor plasma is **135 to 240 seconds**.
2. PRT is a screening test to detect the deficiencies of the factors of the intrinsic pathway, especially **XII, XI, IX, VIII, X, V, and II** (all coagulation factors except VII and XIII).

Clot Retraction Time

It assesses the clot stability and platelet functions (for detailsof clot retraction time, refer to previous chapter).

ABNORMALITIES OF COAGULATION

Hemorrhagic disorders are broadly classified into inherited and acquired defects.

1. **Acquired defects are more common than inherited defects** and *platelet defects are more common than the coagulation defects*.
2. Deficiencies of factor VIII (hemophilia) and factor IX (Christmas disease) are more common inherited coagulation defects.
3. The **common acquired defects** are thrombocytopenia, vitamin K deficiency, disseminated intravascular coagulation and liver failure resulting in clotting defects.

Hemophilia A

Etiology

Hemophilia A, also known as **classic hemophilia**, is a bleeding disorder that occurs due to **deficiency of factor VIII**. It is an **X-linked recessive** hereditary disease. Though it is less common than von Willebrand disease, it is more common than other inherited defects of coagulation. **Women are carriers** and generally do not suffer from the disease as they are protected by the second X-chromosome which is usually normal.

Clinical Features

The disease manifests with the ***bleeding tendency*** which appears in infancy, but in mild cases, may appear in adult life.

1. *Soft tissue hematomas* and *hemarthroses* (bleeding into joints) leading to severe *crippling hemarthropathy* are highly characteristic of the disease.
2. In severe cases, spontaneous hemarthropathy from infancy is the common feature.
3. In mild to moderate cases, continuation of hemorrhage secondary to trauma or surgery is the feature.
4. Bleeding usually persists from days to weeks inspite of formation of clots.
5. Bleeding may also occur spontaneously into tissues, and cavities of the body.

Diagnosis

Patients have ***prolonged activated partial thromboplastin time*** (APTT). Prothrombin time and bleading time are normal. **Assay of factor VIII in plasma is diagnostic**. Functional factor VIII coagulant activity can also be measured.

Treatment

The treatment consists of **transfusion of fresh blood** (as on storage factor VIII is rapidly lost), or transfusion of **factor**

VIII-concentrate. Many plasma products are available for raising factor VIII to hemostatic level. **Fresh-frozen plasma and cryoprecipitate** both contain factor VIII. Attempt should be made to avoid aspirin, nonsteroidal anti-inflammatory drugs and other drugs that interfere with platelet aggregation.

Christmas Disease (Hemophilia B)

Etiology

Christmas disease or hemophilia-B occurs due to **deficiency of factor-IX** (antihemophilic factor-B or Christmas factor). This is a sex-linked recessive hemorrhagic disease.

Features

The disease is clinically indistinguishable from hemophilia A. Bleeding episodes are clinically identical to those in hemophilia A. Therefore, this is also called ***hemophilia-B***. Hematoma, hemarthroses and crippling hemarthropathy occur.

Diagnosis

In most cases, PT is normal and partial thromboplastin time **(PTT) is prolonged**. Specific assay of factor IX coagulant activity confirms diagnosis.

Treatment

The specific treatment of hemophilia B is the **replacement of factor IX**.

Scientist contributed

In 1947, **Dr Alfredo Pavlovsky**, a doctor in Buenos Aires, Argentina, distinguished **two types of hemophilia** in his lab—***A*** and ***B***. He reported that the blood from some hemophiliac patients corrected the abnormal clotting time in others. In 1952 this was called ***Christmas disease***, after the family in which it was discovered

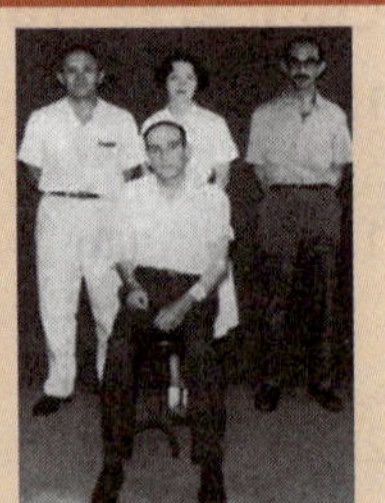

Alfredi Pavlovsky

von Willebrand Disease

Etiology

von Willebrand disease (vWD) is the **most common inherited bleeding disorder** in humans that occurs due to **deficiency of von Willebrand factor** (vWF). In 1926, ***Eric von Willebrand*** described this bleeding disorder in both genders of 24 persons of a 66 members of family from Åland Island.

1. vWF plays a central role in hemostasis as it serves as a **carrier for factor VIII** and is essential for **adhesion of platelets** to the injured vessel wall.
2. Therefore, deficiency of vWF leads to **defects in the formation of both temporary and definitive hemostatic plugs.**

Variants

There are different variants of vWD: **Type 1, type 2A, type 2B, type 2M, type 2N** and **type 3**.

1. **Type 1** is the most common variant, which occurs due to decrease in 20–50% in quantity of vWF.
2. **Type 2** variants are mainly qualitative abnormalities of vWF.
3. **Type 3** is the most severe form in which vWF is grossly decreased.

Factor VIII activity is decreased in type 1, decreased or normal in type 2, and markedly decreased in type 3.

Clinical Features

Mucocutaneous bleeding is the ***most commonest presentation in type 1***. Epistaxis, easy bruising, hematoma, menorrhagia and GI bleeding are common. In type 3, patients suffer from severe bleeding and present with hemarthroses and muscle hematomas like hemophilia A. Type 2 presents with moderate symptoms.

Diagnosis

As vWF is primarily responsible for platelet adhesion, **prolongation of bleeding time** is a standard screening test for vWD. However, *clotting time is prolonged or normal* depending on the degree of deficiency of factor VIII. Quantitative and functional **assays of plasma vWF** are diagnostic.

Treatment

Desmopressin (DDAVP), an analogue of ADH increases factor VIII activity, vWF-Ag concentration and ristocetin cofactor activity. Therefore, DDAVP is very useful in type 1 and 2 diseases. However, **vWF replacement** therapy is required in type 3 disease.

Disseminated Intravascular Coagulation (DIC)

Definition and Etiology

DIC is a clinicopathological syndrome in which there is **widespread intravascular coagulation** that occurs due to procoagulants that are introduced into or produced by blood circulation.

1. The procoagulant activity overcomes the natural anticoagulant mechanisms. This is also called ***consumption coagulopathy*** or ***defibrination syndrome.***
2. This is a hemorrhagic disorder in which diffused intravascular coagulation results in defects of hemostasis.
3. In this disease, **coagulation factors and platelets are overutilized**. This results in bleeding.
4. The most common procoagulant stimulus is the ***tissue factor (tissue thromboplastin) exposure to the blood***, that activates extrinsic pathway of coagulation (Fig. 21.4).

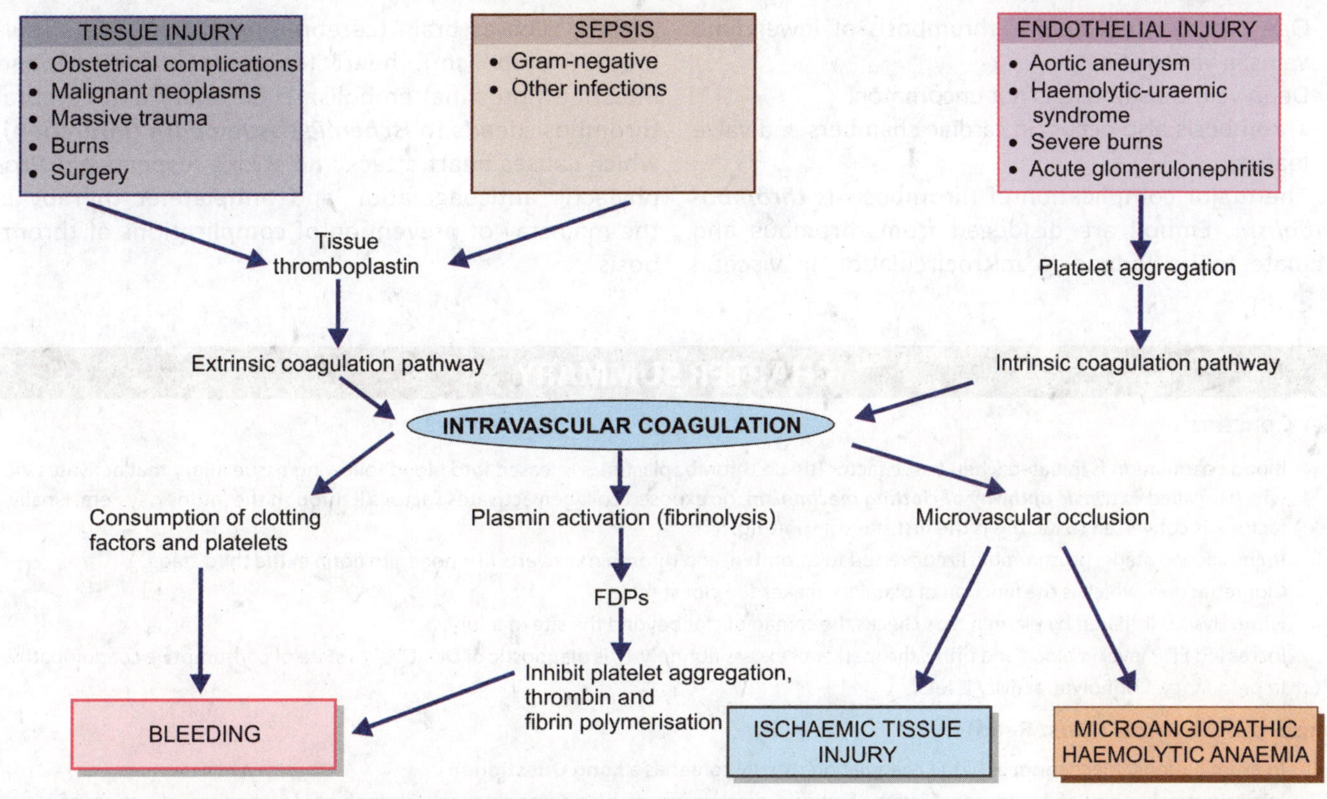

Fig. 21.4: Pathophysiology of disseminated intravascular coagulation.

5. **Activation of plasmin** causes excess fibrinolysis, resulting in increased levels of fibrin degradation product (FDP)

Common causes of DIC are:

1. Septic abortions
2. Amniotic fluid embolism
3. Gram-negative septicemia
4. Fungemia
5. Severe trauma
6. Severe eclampsia
7. Burns (burn sepsis)
8. Snake bite (Russell viper)
9. Sometimes in hemolytic transfusion reactions.

Manifestations

The clinical manifestations of DIC include two important features:

1. **Multiorgan dysfunctions** caused by widespread micro-embolism
2. **Bleeding** caused by consumption of platelets, fibrinogen, factor V and factor VIII.

Therefore, this is also called ***consumption coagulopathy***. There is also activation of secondary fibrinolysis (hence, called ***defibrination syndrome***).

Diagnosis

Laboratory features include thrombocytopenia, hypofibrinogenemia, increased d-dimer and fibrin degradation product (FDP) and prolonged PTT, PT and thrombin time (TT). Diagnosis is usually done by **demonstrating FDP in urine** and **decreased concentration of coagulation factors** and fibrin monomers in blood.

Treatment

Treatment is based on early diagnosis, elimination of the precipitating factors, and replacing coagulation factors and platelets. Blood component therapy is needed for those who bleed excessively.

Thrombosis

Thrombus is an intravascular clot. Normally, a balance is maintained between the processes of coagulation and anticoagulation and therefore thrombus is not formed. However, in pathological situations, intravascular clotting occurs. Three factors (**Virchow's triad**) predispose to the formation of thrombosis. These are:

1. **Endothelial injury:** Injury to vascular endothelium occurs in chronic and sustained hypertension, ulcerated atherosclerosis, arterial diseases etc. Injured site becomes the site for platelet adhesion and aggregation and intravascular clot formation.
2. **Sluggishness of blood flow:** Stasis of blood promotes thrombosis (as described above).
3. **Hpercoagulability of blood:** Increased activity of procoagulants such as fibrinogen, prothrombin and other coagulants leads to thrombosis.

Platelet aggregation at the site of injury initiates the process of thrombosis. Venous thrombosis is more common than arterial thrombosis.

1. One common example is thrombosis of lower limb veins in varicosities.
2. Deep vein thrombosis is not uncommon.
3. Thrombosis also occurs in cardiac chambers and valve leaflets.

The major complication of thrombosis is ***thromboembolism***. Emboli are dislodged from thrombus and circulate to be lodged in microcirculation in visceral organs, such as brain (cerebral embolism), lungs (pulmonary embolism), heart (coronary embolism) and intestine (intestinal embolism). Coronary and cerebral thrombosis leads to ***ischemic tissue death (infarction)***, which causes heart attack and stroke respectively. Prophylactic anticoagulation and antiplatelet therapy is the mainstay of prevention of complications of thrombosis.

CHAPTER SUMMARY

Key Concepts

1. Blood coagulation is initiated when tissue factor (tissue thromboplastin) is released into blood following tissue injury that activates VII, which is called ***extrinsic pathway of clotting mechanism***, or, exposed collagen activates Factor XII through the intrinsic system. Finally, factor X is converted to Xa. This is the first stage in clotting.
2. In the second stage, prothrombin is converted to thrombin, and thrombin converts fibrinogen to fibrin in the third stage.
3. Clot retraction, which is the function of platelets, makes the clot stable.
4. Fibrinolysis is initiated by plasmin that checks the spread of clot beyond the site of injury.
5. Increased FDP level in blood and urine, the marker of excess fibrinolysis, is diagnostic of DIC. DIC is a state of consumptive coagulopathy.
6. In pregnancy, fibrinolytic activity is less.

Important to Know (Must Read)

1. In examinations, 'Mechanism of blood coagulation' usually comes as a **Long Question**.
2. Intrinsic mechanism of blood coagulation, Extrinsic mechanism of blood coagulation, Fibrinolysis, Mechanism of action of Vit K antagonists, Anticoagulant, Tests for detecting defects in temporary hemostatic plug, Tests for detecting defects in definitive hemostatic plug, Hemophilia, DIC, and Thrombosis usually come as **Short Questions** in exams.
3. In **Viva**, examiners may ask... name the clotting factors, stages of blood clotting, steps of intrinsic and extrinsic pathways of clotting, clot retraction and its importance, mechanism of fibrinolysis, mechanism of action of Vitamin K antagonist, anticoagulants and their mechanisms, tests to detect defects in extrinsic and intrinsic mechanisms of clotting, and causes, features and treatment of common coagulation disorders.
4. Anticoagulants are frequently asked for as they are commonly used in clinical as well as laboratory practices.

SECTION–3

Nerve and Muscle

PART A: NERVE

22. Structure and Functions of Neurons
23. Nerve Potentials
24. Properties, Classification and Applied Aspects of Nerve Fibers

PART B: NEUROMUSCULAR JUNCTION

25. Neuromuscular Transmission

PART C: MUSCLES

26. Structure of Skeletal Muscle: Physiological Aspects
27. Mechanism of Skeletal Muscle Contraction
28. Skeletal Muscle: Properties, Fiber Types and Applied Aspects
29. Smooth Muscle and Cardiac Muscle

"The great are strongest when they stand alone.
A God-given might of being in their force,
A ray from self's solitude of light the guide;
The soul that can live alone with itself meets God."

Sri Aurobindo (in 'SAVITRI')

CHAPTER 22

Structure and Functions of Neurons

Learning Objectives

On completion of study of this chapter, the student **WILL** be able to:

1. Draw the labeled diagram of a neuron.
2. Give the structure and functions of different parts of the neuron.
3. Understand the functions of Schwann cells and the process of myelinogenesis.
4. Appreciate the concept and purposes of axonal transport.
5. Classify neurons and give examples for each.
6. List the neurotrophins and give their functions.

A neuron is the structural and functional unit of the nervous system. Its primary function is to receive the various stimuli and transmit the signals to other neurons and tissues. The neuron is an excitable cell where message transmission occurs in the form of action potentials. There are about 10^{11} neurons present in the human central nervous system (CNS). There are also supporting cells called glial cells, which are 10 to 30 times more in number than the neural cells.

Scientists contributed

Camillo Golgi
(1843–1926)

SR y Cajal
(1852–1934)

The **Nobel Prize in Physiology or Medicine, 1906,** was awarded jointly to Italian neurophysiologist and neuroanatomist, Prof. **Camillo Golgi** and neurophysiologist and neuroanatomist of Spain, Prof. **Santiago Ramón y Cajal** *"in recognition of their work on the structure of the neuron and the nervous system".*

STRUCTURE OF A NEURON

A neuron has three parts: a cell body, dendrites, and an axon that ends at axon terminal (Fig. 22.1).

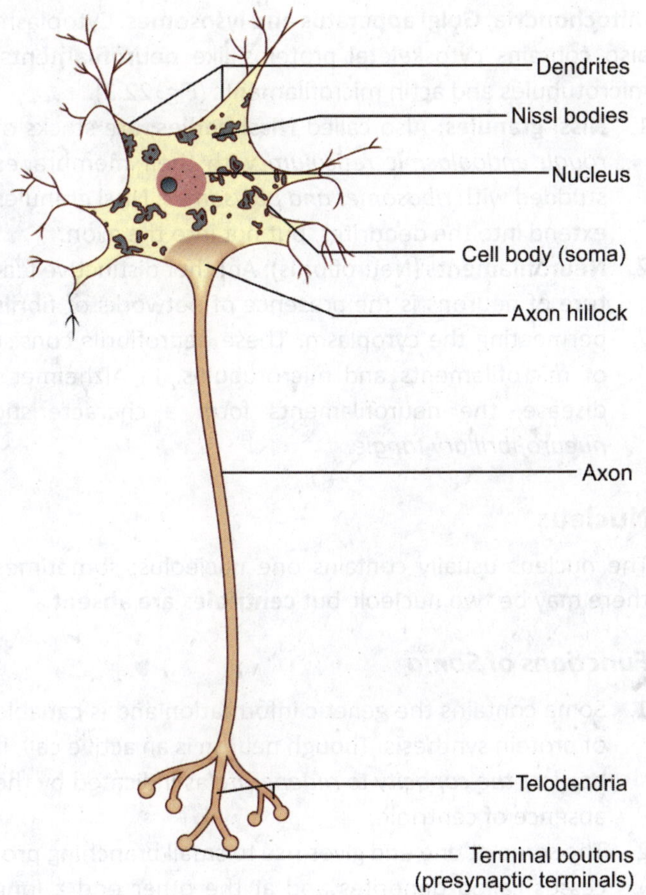

Fig. 22.1: Structure of a neuron.

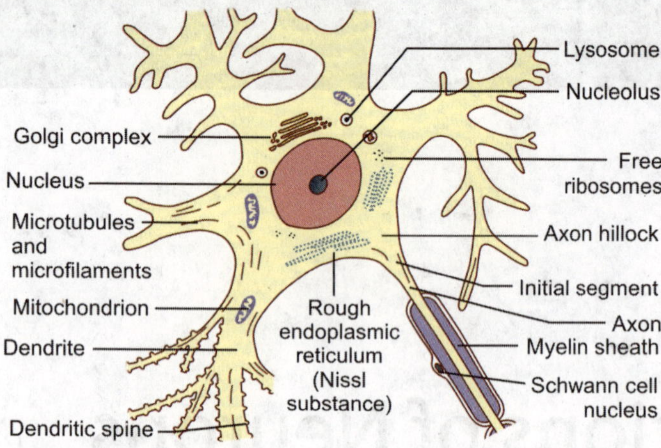

Fig. 22.2: Detailed structure of the proximal part of neuron, highlighting the cell body region.

Table 22.1: Differences between axons and dendrites.

Axons	Dendrites
1. Axon is a single long thin process of nerve cell which terminates away from the nerve cell body	Dendrites are multiple, short, thick and tapering processes of the nerve cell which terminate near the nerve cell
2. Axon rarely branches at the right angle (axon collaterals) but ends by dividing into many fine processes called axon terminals	Dendrites are highly branched. Their branching pattern forms a dendritic tree
3. Free of Nissl granules	Nissl granules are present in dendrites.
4. The nerve impulse travel away from the cell body	Nerve impulse travels toward the cell body

Cell Body

Cell body, also known as soma or **perikaryon** is the center of the neuron. It contains the **nucleus** and **cytoplasm** containing ***cell organelles***. The plasma membrane of the soma is a bilayered lipid protein membrane, called *plasmalemma.*

Cell Organelles

Cell organelles are mainly numerous **Nissl granules**, many **mitochondria, Golgi apparatus and lysosomes**. Cytoplasm also contains cytoskeletal proteins like **neurofilaments**, microtubules and actin microfilaments (Fig. 22.2).

1. **Nissl granules:** Also called **Nissl bodies**, are stacks of *rough endoplasmic reticulum* with their membranes studded with *ribosomes and polysomes*. Nissl granules extend into the dendrites, but not into the axon.
2. **Neurofilaments** (Neurofibrils): Another distinctive feature of neurons is the presence of networks of fibrils permeating the cytoplasm. These neurofibrils consist of microfilaments and microtubules. In Alzheimer's disease, the neurofilaments form a characteristic *nueurofibrillary tangle*.

Nucleus

The nucleus usually contains one nucleolus; sometimes there may be two nucleoli, but **centrioles are absent**.

Functions of Soma

1. Soma contains the genetic information and is capable of protein synthesis. Though neuron is an active cell, it has *lost the capacity to regenerate* as indicated by the absence of centriole.
2. The soma at one end gives rise to small branching processes called dendrites and at the other end a long process called axon.

Dendrites

The numerous short extensions from the cell body are called dendrites.

1. They increase the cell surface area many folds. Dendrites have **dendritic spines**, that help in increasing the surface area for receiving information.
2. In neurons of cerebral and cerebellar cortex, small knobby projections called **dendritic spines** further increase the surface area.
3. Dendrites receive the incoming signals from other cells and transmit it to the cell body.
4. At some areas of the brain, they *can cause protein synthesis*, also generate and conduct the action potentials.
5. On an average, there are about 10,000 dendrites per neuron present in the CNS.

Axon

Axon or the axis cylinder of the neuron forms the nerve fiber. It is a long tubular process that extends away from the cell body to transmit output signals to target organs. Dendrites transmit impulses toward cell body, whereas axons carry impulses away from cell body (Table 22.1).

1. The cytoplasm is known as **axoplasm** that contains mitochondria, Golgi apparatus, and cytoskeletal proteins.
2. The axon arises from a thickened, tapered area of the cell body called the **axon hillock.**
3. The initial portion of the axon is known as the **initial segment**.
4. The axon hillock continues as initial segment and this part is known as **axon hillock—initial segment portion** of the neuron.
5. The action potential is generated at the initial segment in motor neurons and at the first node of Ranvier in sensory neurons.

Axon terminal: The terminal part of axon loses myelin and divides into several branches, called **telodendria**. The endings of telodendria form bulb like enlargements

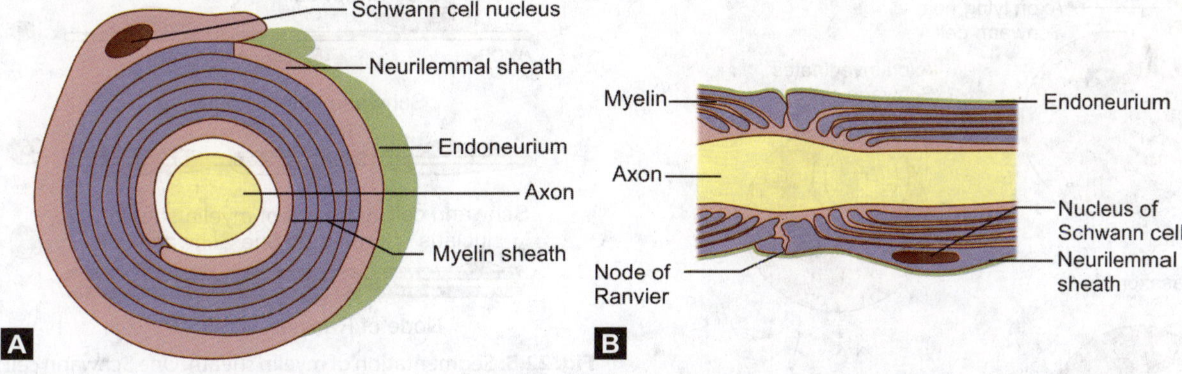

Figs. 22.3A and B: Myelin sheath, shown in transverse section (A) and longitudinal section (B) of the axon.

called terminal buttons or **synaptic knobs**. The buttons contain ***neurotransmitter vesicles***.

Types of Axon

Axons are of two types: myelinated and unmyelinated.

Myelinated Axons

In the peripheral nervous system (PNS), myelinated axons have a sheath around, called myelin sheath (Figs. 22.3A and B).

1. Myelin sheath in PNS formed by the **Schwann cells**. The large diameter somatic nerve fibers as well as the preganglionic fibers of the autonomic nervous system are myelinated.
2. In the CNS of mammals, myelination is carried out by **oligodendrocytes**. Each oligodendrocyte projects several processes that wrap around many axons.

Role of Schwann Cell in Myelination

The double layers of the membrane of a single Schwann cell wrap several times (about 100 times) over 1 mm length of the axon forming a covering of 8–10 µm thickness (Figs. 22.3A and B).

1. The adjacent layers stick to each other tightly with the help of a protein called **protein zero** (P_0) present in the Schwann cell membrane.
2. The extracellular portion of P_0 in one layer locks to the extracellular portion of P_0 in the apposing layer resulting in compaction of myelin.
3. ***Mutation of P_0 cause defective myelination*** and decreased conduction as occurs in various peripheral neuropathies.
4. The nucleus of the Schwann cell lies beneath the plasma membrane in the outermost layer (Fig. 22.3A). Thus, the myelin sheath extending along the length of an axon is formed by many Schwann cells, which are present at regular intervals along the course of the axon.
5. The gaps between the Schwann cells are called the ***nodes of Ranvier*** (Fig. 22.3B), where the plasma membrane is exposed to the ECF. Each node is 0.5–1.0 µm in length and the internodal distance is 1–2 mm.
6. In multiple sclerosis, an autoimmune disease, patchy destruction of myelin occurs causing decreased conduction velocity in both motor and sensory neurons.

Myelinogenesis

Myelin sheath when present is seen outside the axolemma. The cells providing this sheath for axons in the peripheral nervous system are called Schwann cells and in CNS are oligodendrocytes. The nature of this sheath is best understood by considering the mode of its formation.

1. An axon lying near a Schwann cell invaginates into the cytoplasm of Schwann cell. In this process the axon comes to be suspended by a fold of the cell membrane of the Schwann cell. This fold is called **mesaxon** (Fig. 22.4).
2. In some situations the mesaxon becomes greatly elongated and comes to be spirally wound around the axon, which is thus surrounded by several layers of cell membrane. Lipids are deposited between adjacent layers of the membrane. These layers of the mesaxon, along with the lipids, form the myelin sheath.
3. Outside the myelin sheath a thin layer of Schwann cell cytoplasm persists to form an additional sheath that is called **neurilemma** (also called the neurilemma sheath or Schwann cell sheath).
4. An axon is related to a large number of Schwann cells over its length. Each Schwann cell provides the myelin sheath for a **short segment of the axon**. At the junction of any two such segments there is a short gap in the myelin sheath. These gaps are called the **nodes of Ranvier** (Fig. 22.5).
5. The nodes of Ranvier have great physiological importance. When an impulse travels down a nerve fiber it does not proceed uniformly along the length of the axis cylinder, but jumps from one node to the next. This is called saltatory conduction (in unmyelinated neurons the impulse travels along the axolemma). Such conduction is much slower than saltatory conduction and consumes more energy.
6. The segment of myelin sheath between two nodes of Ranvier is called **internode**.

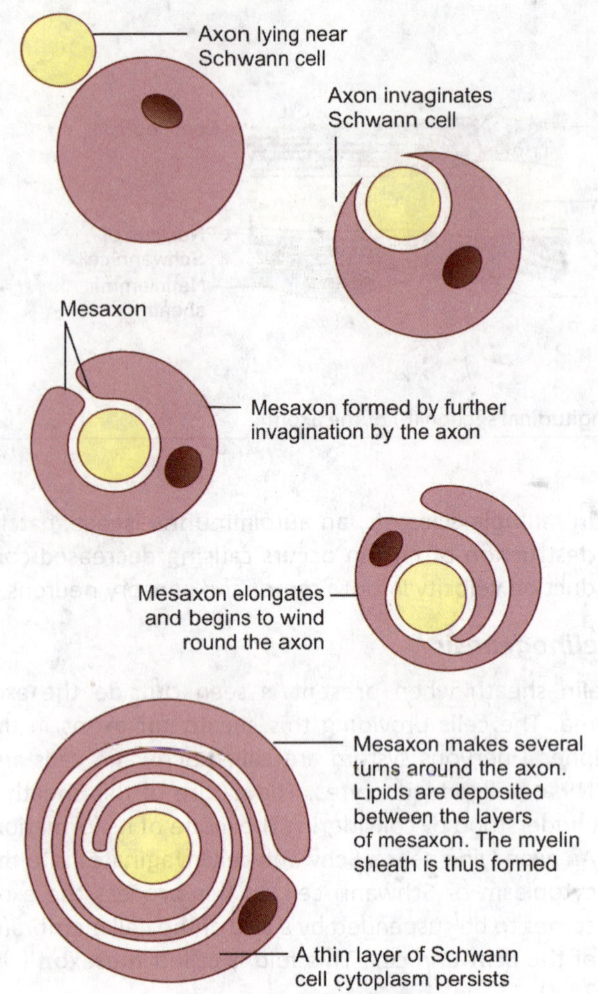

Fig. 22.4: Stages of formation of myelin sheath by Schwann cell.

Composition of Myelin Sheath

Myelin contains **protein, lipids,** and water. The main lipids present include ***cholesterol, phospholipid, and glycosphingolipids***. Other lipids are present in smaller amount.

Important Note

Myelin sheath defects: Myelin sheath can be seriously impaired and there can be abnormal collections of lipids, in disorder of lipid metabolism. Various proteins have been identified in myelin sheath and abnormality in them can be the basis of some neuropathy.

Objectives of Myelination

Myelination serves following four purposes.

1. It increases the speed of conduction.
2. It reduces energy expenditure by the cell.
3. It provides a protective covering to the axon.
4. It is responsible for the color of the white matter of the brain and spinal cord.

Timing of Myelination during Development

Myelination of different types of nerve fibers takes place at different times.

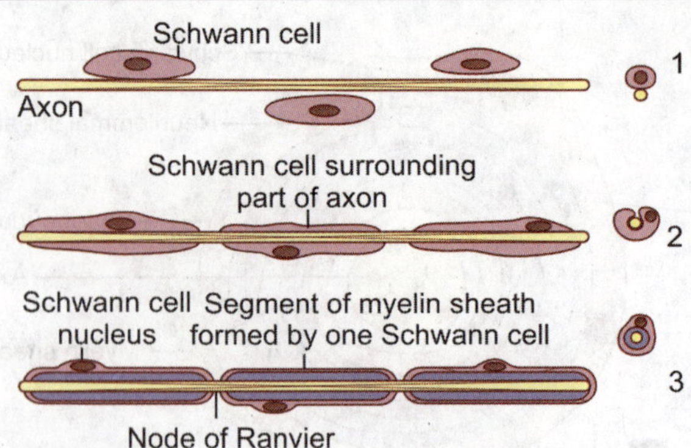

Fig. 22.5: Segmentation of myelin sheath. One Schwann cell forms a small segment. Gap between the segment is called node of Ranvier.

1. The sensory fibers of the dorsal column system first get myelinated, which occurs at 4th–5th month of intrauterine life.
2. The corticospinal tract fibers start myelinating at two months of age and the process gets completed at about 2nd year of life, when the child has learned to walk (Application Box 22.1).

Application Box 22.1

Axonal Growth: During development of a neuron, axonal growth depends on the interaction between the growing axon and the surrounding tissue environment. At the growing end is present a **growth cone**, which is motile and contains actin. The direction of axonal growth is determined by cell adhesion molecules, influenced by trophic factors secreted from target cells and guided by glial cells.

Unmyelinated Axons

Unmyelinated axons do not have myelin sheath.

1. The Schwann cells are present near these axons, but their mesaxons do not completely spiral around them (Fig. 22.6).
2. Another difference is that several such axons may invaginate into the cytoplasm of a single Schwann cell.
3. Somatic nerve fibers of very small diameter, postganglionic sympathetic neurons of the autonomic nervous system, dorsal root fibers and most of the fibers in invertebrates are unmyelinated.
4. The speed of conduction of impulse is slower in unmyelinated nerve fibers (Table 22.2).

Scientist contributed

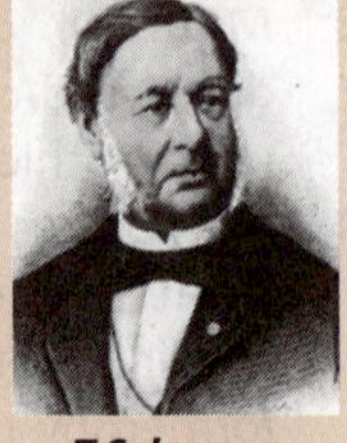

T Schwann (1810–1882)

Theodor Schwann advanced the concept of cellular organization of living beings, described the structure of neurilemma (covering of the nerve) and showed the necessity of air for embryonal growth. His intense study on digestion was important, in which he discovered pepsin and its action, and highlighted the importance of bile in digestion. His discovery of yeast and its role in purification and fermentation was an important revelation. He is popularly remembered for his discovery of myelin sheath and myelinogenesis (**Schwann cells** that form the covering of myelinated neurons) of axons; hence these cells are known as Schwann cells.

Source: Uber das W. des Verdauungs processes. *Arch Anat Physiol Med* 1836; 90–138.

Axoplasmic Transport

Transfer of substances between cell body and axon terminal is called axoplasmic transport.

1. Various proteins, organelles and other cellular substances required for the development, growth, and maintenance of the neuron are transported mainly along the length of the axon.
2. Axoplasmic transport can be ***abolished by*** application of colchicine, dinitrophenol, azide, cyanide, and prolonged anoxia.
3. **Colchicine disrupts the movement of microtubules**; others block the process of oxidative phosphorylation.

Types of Axoplasmic Transport

In the axoplasm, transport process can occur in both directions by different transport mechanisms. Accordingly, they are called anterograde, retrograde, and transneuronal transports.

Anterograde Transport

The transport of materials ***from the cell body toward the axon*** terminals is known as anterograde transport. For example, various neurotransmitters synthesized in the cell body are packaged in vesicles and get secreted at the nerve endings through axoplasmic microtubules. Anterograde transport process is mapped by [^{3}H]-leucin. The rate of transport process may be fast or slow.

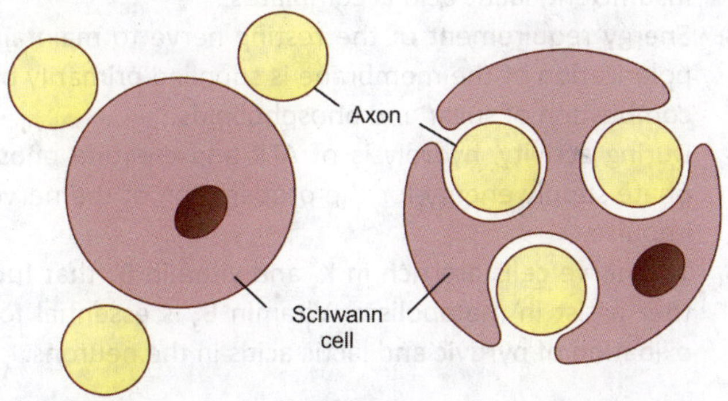

Fig. 22.6: Relation of unmyelinated fibers with Schwann cells. Mesaxons do not totally spiral around the axon.

Fast axoplasmic transport: Fast axoplasmic transport occurs at the speed of about 400 mm/day, which is accomplished by *kinesin*, a microtubule associated protein that transports many organelles, vesicles and membrane glycoproteins.

Slow axoplasmic transport: Slow axoplasmic transport occurs at the rate of about 0.5–2 mm/day. Various structural proteins like actin, neurofilaments and microtubules get transported by slow transport. It has an important role in supplying the required materials for the regeneration of axons following nerve injury.

Retrograde Transport

Transport of substances ***from the axon terminals to the cell body*** is known as retrograde transport. It occurs at a speed of about 200 mm/day, brought about by ***dynein***, another microtubule associated protein. This mechanism keeps the soma informed about the synaptic environment. Retrograde transport is ***mapped by horse-radish peroxidase***.

The examples of retrograde transport are:

1. **Transport of viruses:** The chickenpox virus, known as varicella zoster that causes herpes simplex reaches cell body from nerve terminals in the skin by retrograde transport. The virus may remain in a dormant state in nerve root for many years before causing herpes zoster afterwards.
2. **Transport of toxins:** Tetanus toxin at motor neuron ending is transported to the cell body by this retrograde process.
3. **Transfer of nerve growth factor:** Nerve growth factor is taken up by presynaptic terminal and transferred to soma by retrograde transport.
4. **Reuptake of synaptic transmitters:** Neurotransmitters like norepinephrine (NE) released at the nerve terminals are rapidly removed from the synaptic cleft by reuptake

Table 22.2: Differences between myelinated and unmyelinated nerves.

Myelinated nerves	Unmyelinated nerves
1. Have axons of large diameter.	Have axons of small diameter.
2. Axons surrounded by concentric layers of Schwann cell plasma membrane.	Axons surrounded by cytoplasm of Schwann cells.
3. Nerve impulse jumps from one node to the other node, which is called saltatory conduction.	Nerve impulse travels uniformly along the axolema.
4. Density of voltage gated Na^+ channels are more (about 350 to 500/μm^2 at initial segment, and 2,000 to 12,000/μm^2 in node of Ranvier).	Na^+ channels are less in axons (about 110 /μm^2).
5. Saltatory conduction seen in myelinated nerves is fast and consumes less energy.	Conduction seen in unmyelinated nerves is slow and consumes more energy.
6. Examples: All preganglionic fibers in ANS. In PNS, fibers more than 1 μm in diameter.	All post-ganglionic fibers in ANS. In PNS, fibers less than 1 μm in diameter.

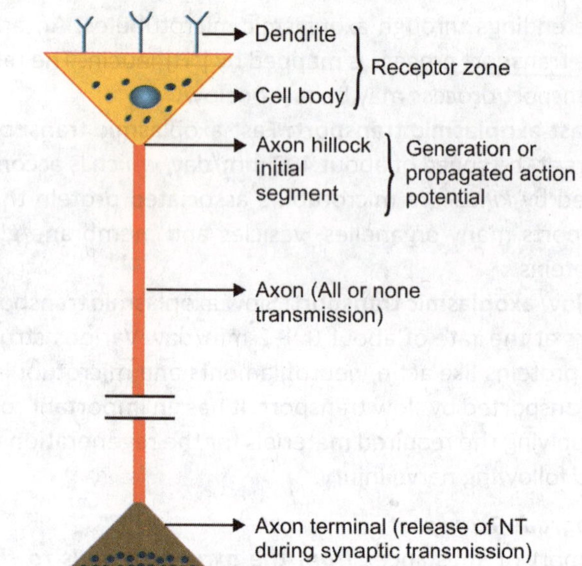

Fig. 22.7: Functions of different parts of the neuron.

into the presynaptic neuron. In the presynaptic terminal, NE is repackaged into vesicles or deaminated by mitochondrial monoamine oxidase. This reuptake is an active retrograde transport process. Some of the vesicles may be transported back to the cell body and this may provide a feedback signal to the cell body for further synthesis of transmitters. Choline is also taken up by the axon terminal and reused for new Ach synthesis.

Transneuronal Transport

Trophic substances like nerve growth factors are transported **across the synapse** to the presynaptic membrane of another neuron. This is called transneuronal transport. This helps in maintenance of the synaptic contacts.

FUNCTIONS OF NEURONS

The cell body and dendrites serve as the receptor zone to receive the information, axon hillock and initial segment for generation of action potential, axon for transmission of nerve impulse, axon terminal for discharge of neurotransmitters (Fig. 22.7).

Cell body: It maintains the functional and anatomical integrity of the axon. The proteins associated with synaptic transmitters are synthesized in Nissl granules of the cell body and are transported to axon terminal by axoplasmic flow.

Dendrites: They form the receptor zone of the neuron, i.e. they receive impulses and transmit the impulses toward the cell body. In this region, non-conducted local potential changes generated by synaptic connections are integrated.

Axon: The ***initial segment*** is the site where propagated action potentials are generated. The axonal process transmits propagated impulses from the cell body to the axon terminal.

Synaptic knobs: This is the nerve ending where arrival of action potentials results in the release of synaptic transmitter.

Important Note

Concentration of voltage gated Na^+ channels: Na^+ channels are highly concentrated in the nodes of Ranvier and the initial segment in myelinated nerve fibers.

METABOLISM AND GROWTH OF NEURONS

Metabolism

Neurons are metabolically active cells as mitochondria are present in adequate numbers. Neurons are always active as the membrane potentials and neuronal cytosolic activities are continuous phenomena. About 70% of total energy required is used to maintain polarization of the membrane by the action of Na^+-K^+ pump. During the peak activity, the metabolic rate of nerve doubles compared to skeletal muscle cell metabolism.

Special features of neuronal metabolism are:

1. The excitability, conductivity and recovery process from the activities can happen in a nerve for a considerable period in the absence of oxygen.
2. Chemical changes in the nerve are similar to that in muscles, i.e. pyruvic acid is formed and if O_2 supply is insufficient, lactic acid accumulates.
3. Energy requirement of the resting nerve to maintain polarization of the membrane is supplied primarily by combustion of sugar and phospholipids.
4. During activity, hydrolysis of ATP and creatine phosphate supply energy for the propagation of the nerve impulse.
5. The nerve cells are rich in K^+ and vitamin B_1 that further assist in metabolism. Vitamin B_1 is essential for oxidation of pyruvic and lactic acids in the neurons.

Growth of Neurons

Various factors affecting neuronal development, growth and survival have been isolated and studied. These can be broadly arranged into two groups:

1. **Neurotrophins**
2. **Other growth factors:** Other factors affecting neural development such as ciliary neurotrophic factor (CNTF), glial cell line-derived neurotrophic factor (GDNF), leukemia inhibitory factor (LIF), fibroblast growth factor (FGF), platelet-derived growth factor (PDGF), transforming growth factor (TGF), insulin like growth factor (IGF-I), etc.

Neurotrophins

Neurotrophins are trophic proteins to the neurons, as they promote nerve growth and survival. They are produced by the nerves, muscles, glands, and astrocytes.

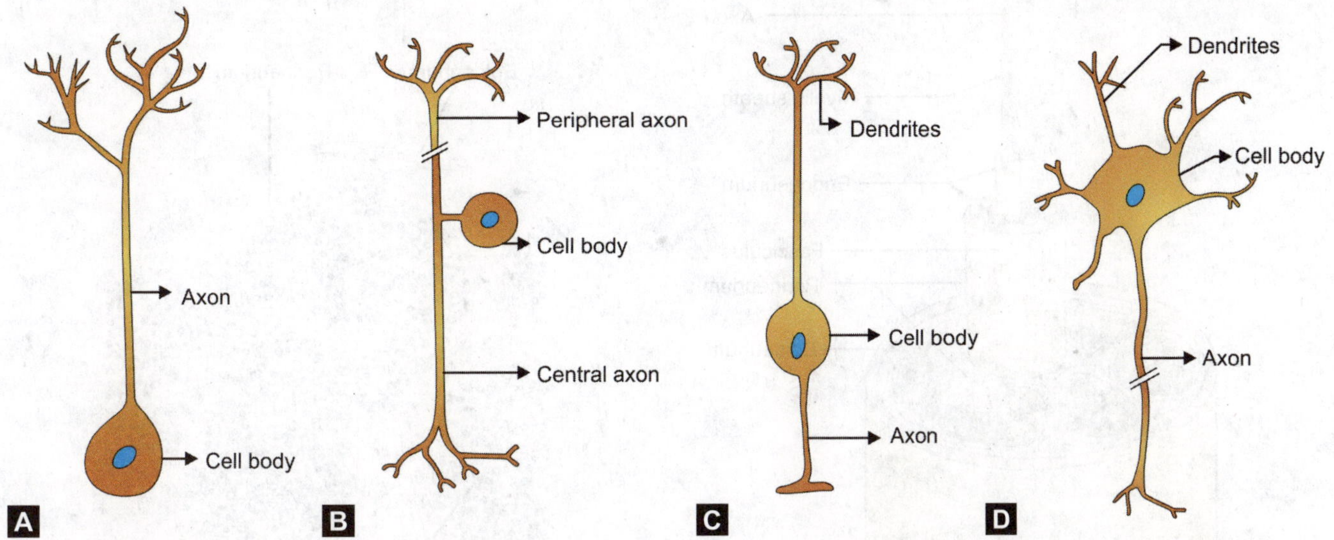

Figs. 22.8A to D: Types of neurons based on arrangement of axon. (A) Unipolar neuron; (B) Pseudo-unipolar neuron; (C) Bipolar neuron; (D) Multipolar neuron.

Known neurotrophins are:

1. Nerve growth factor (NGF),
2. Brain-derived neurotrophic factor (BDNF),
3. Neurotrophin-3 (NT-3), and
4. Neurotrophin-4/5

Nerve Growth Factors

Nerve growth factor (NGF) is the first neurotrophin to be identified. It promotes the growth of sympathetic nerves and some sensory nerves. NGF is made up of 2α, 2β, and 2γ subunits.

1. The α subunits have trypsin-like activity.
2. The β subunits are similar to insulin and have nerve growth-promoting activity.
3. The γ subunits are serine proteases.

NGF decreases apoptosis of neurons by acting through tyrosine kinase A receptor.

Brain-derived Neurotrophic Factor (BDNF)

BDNF promotes growth of peripheral sensory nerves. It acts through tyrosine kinase A.

Neurotrophin 3

The neurotrophin-3 (NT-3) promotes growth of cutaneous mechanoreceptors. It acts through tyrosine kinase A, B, and C.

Neurotrophins 4 and 5

They act through tyrosine kinase B. Exact function is not known.

TYPES OF NEURONS

Neurons are classified according to the number of processes, length of axon, functions of neurons, and patterns of dendrites.

According to the Arrangement of Axon

According to the arrangement and number of processes, the neurons are classified into unipolar, pseudounipolar, bipolar, and multipolar neurons (Figs. 22.8A to D).

Unipolar Neurons

They have a **single process** (Fig. 22.8A). They are usually found in invertebrates. In vertebrates, they are found in ANS.

Pseudounipolar Neurons

In pseudounipolar neurons, axon after originating from soma **splits into central and peripheral processes** (Fig. 22.8B). The example is dorsal root ganglion cell (primary sensory neurons with cell bodies in dorsal root ganglion).

Bipolar Neurons

In these neurons, **two processes arise from the cell body** (Fig. 22.8C). The example is the bipolar cell of retina.

Multipolar Neurons

In multipolar neurons, **many processes arise from the soma** (Fig. 22.8D). The example is a spinal motor neuron.

According to the Length of Axon

According to the length of the axon, neurons are classified into two categories: Golgi type 1 and type 2.

Golgi Type 1

Axons of Golgi type 1 neurons ***are long***. Cortical motor neurons (pyramidal cells that give rise to corticospinal tract) are the examples.

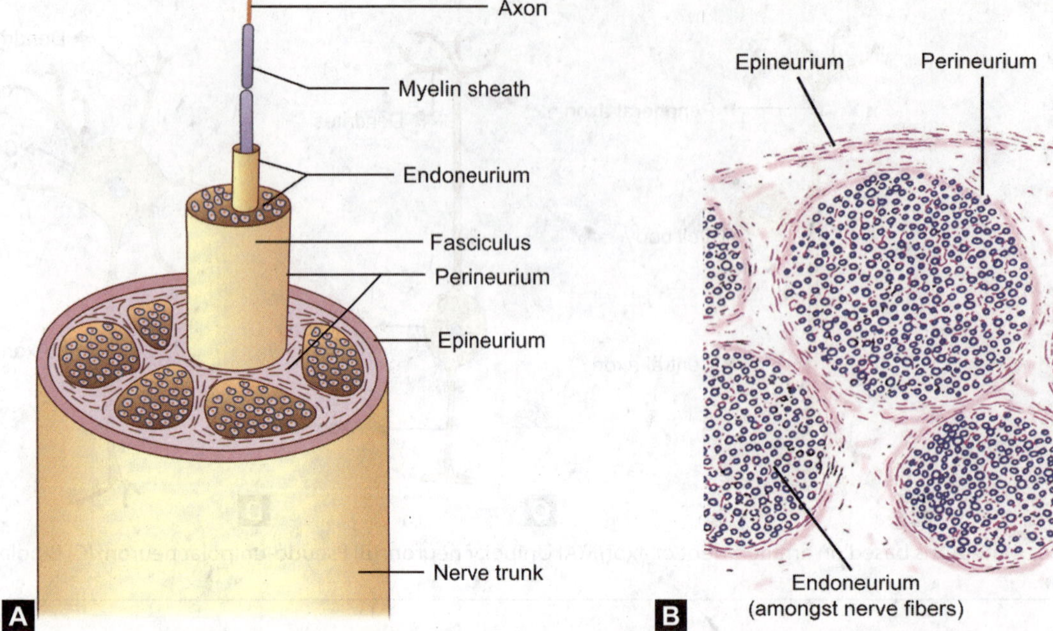

Figs. 22.9A and B: Placement of nerve fiber and axon in nerve trunk. (A) Longitudinal section; (B) Transverse section.

Golgi Type 2

These are the neurons ***with short axons***. Dendrites of these neurons terminate near the soma. The example is cortical inhibitory neurons and Golgi cells in cerebellar cortex.

According to Function

According to functions, neurons can be divided into sensory and motor neurons.

Sensory Neurons

These are the neurons that carry impulses from the receptors to the central nervous systems. These are called **afferent neurons** *(afferent fibers)*.

Motor Neurons

These are the neurons that carry impulses from the central nervous system to the target organs. These are called **efferent neurons** *(efferent fibers)*.

According to Dendritic Pattern

According to dendritic pattern, two types of neurons are present: pyramidal cells and stellate cells.

Pyramidal Cells

Dendrites of these cells spread like pyramids. The example is hippocampal pyramidal neurons.

Stellate Cells

Radial shaped spread of dendrites occurs in these cells. The examples are cortical stellate cells.

ARRANGEMENT OF NEURONS AND NEROGLIA

Arrangement of Neurons in Nerve Fibers

Basic Structure of Peripheral Nerves

The neuronal structures are present in endoneurium, perineurium, and epineurium (Figs. 22.9A and B).

Endoneurium

In the peripheral nerves each nerve fiber with its Schwann cell and basal lamina is surrounded by a layer of connective tissue called **endoneurium**.

1. The endoneurium contains collagen, fibroblast, Schwann cells, endothelial cells and macrophages.
2. Many nerve fibers together form ***bundles or fasciculi***.
3. Endoneurium holds adjoining nerve fibers together and facilitates their aggregation to form fasciculi.

Perineurium

Each fasciculus is surrounded by thicker layer of connective tissue called **perineurium**.

1. The perineurium is made up of layers of flattened cells separated by layers of collagen fibers.
2. The perineurium probably controls diffusion of substances in and out of axons.
3. A very thin nerve may consist of **single fasciculus**, but usually a nerve is made of ***several fasciculi***.

Epineurium

The fasciculi are held together by a fairly dense layer of connective tissue that surrounds the entire nerve and is called the epineurium.

Flowchart 22.1: Types of neuroglia in the nervous system (PNS and CNS).

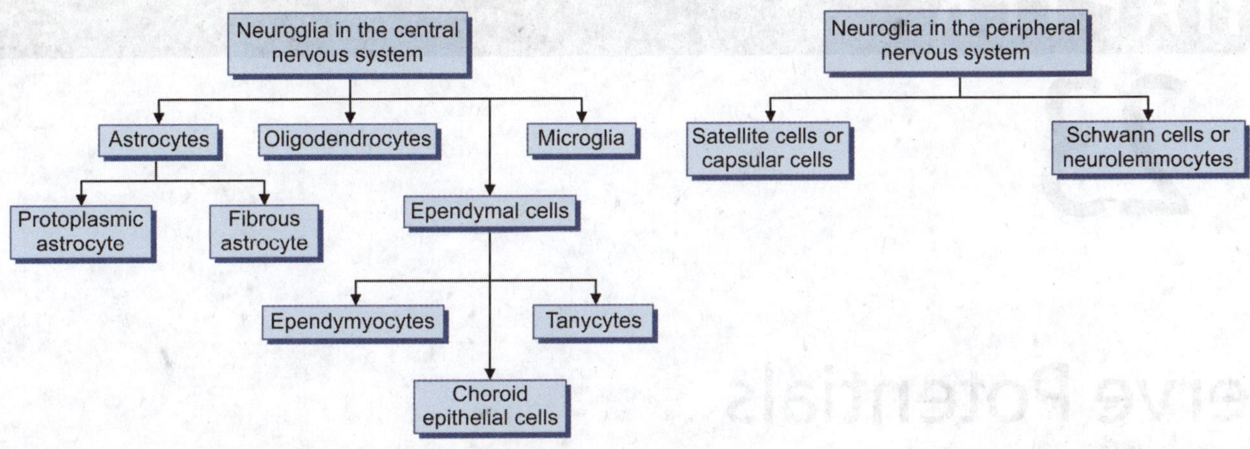

(PNS: Peripheral neurons system; CNS: Central neurons system).

Important Note

Clinical Correlation of Neuronal Structures:

- The epineurium contains nerve fibers. Loss of this fat in bedridden patients can lead to pressure on nerve fibers and paralysis.
- Blood vessels to a nerve travel through the connective tissue that surrounds it. Severe reduction in blood supply can lead to ischemic neuritis and pain.

Neuroglia

In addition to neurons, the nervous system contains several types of supporting cells called neuroglia (Flowchart 22.1). As neuroglia are present mostly in CNS, their structure and functions are discussed in first chapter of Neurophysiology, in Section XI.

CHAPTER SUMMARY

Key Concepts

1. Neuron is the structural and functional unit of the nervous system.
2. Neurons are divided into myelinated and unmyelinated, based on the presence or absence of myelin sheath. Myelination improves the speed of conduction.
3. Myelination of axon in PNS occurs by Schwann cells and in CNS by oligodendroglia.
4. The cell body and dendrites serve as the receptor zone to receive the information from other neurons. Axon hillock and initial segment are the sites of generation of action potential. Axon is meant for transmission of nerve impulse. Axon terminal is for discharge of neurotransmitters into the synapse.
5. Neurotrophins are the main nerve growth factors.

Important to Know (Must Read)

1. In examinations, usually **Long Questions** are not asked from this chapter.
2. Structure of neuron, Mechanism of myelination, Axoplasmic transport, Types of neurons, and Neurotrophins are usually **Short Questions** in exams.
3. In **Viva**, examiners may ask…… different parts of neurons and their functions, how the myelination occurs and what are the functions of myelination, functions of Schwann cells, types of axoplasmic transport, types of neurons, special features of metabolism of neurons, axoplasmic transport, types of neurons with examples for each, and different neurotrophins.

CHAPTER 23

Nerve Potentials

Learning Objectives

On completion of study of this chapter, the student **MUST** be able to:

1. Appreciate the distribution and working of ion channels on the neuronal membrane.
2. Understand the importance of electrotonic potentials.
3. Define rheobase, chronaxie and utilization time and draw the strength-duration curve.
4. Draw a labeled schematic diagram of nerve action potential (AP) and describe the ionic basis of each phase of AP.
5. Define refractory periods (ARP and RRP) of nerve AP and explain their importance.
6. Explain the mechanism of propagation of action potential along the axon and understand the importance of saltatory conduction.
7. List the differences between graded potential and action potential.

The student **MAY** also be able to:

1. Describe the mechanism and genesis of electrotonic potentials.
2. Describe the mechanism of strength-duration curve.
3. Explain the application of nerve potential in various aspect of neuromuscular physiology.

ELECTROPHYSIOLOGICAL ASPECTS

For nerve impulses to be transmitted from neuron to neuron, the action potential must be generated and propagated along the nerve cell membrane. All these events depend on the activities of ion channels present on the membrane of the neurons.

Neuronal Ion Channels

Like any other cell membrane, neuronal membrane possesses numerous ion channels like Na^+, K^+, Ca^{++}, Cl^-, etc. They are broadly categorized into **three types**:

i. Nongated or leaky channels
ii. Gated (voltage-gated, ligand-gated and mechanical-gated) channels.
iii. ATP-driven pumps:
   1. The nongated or leaky channels of Na^+, K^+, Cl^- are present throughout the neuronal membrane.
   2. The **voltage-gated Na^+ channels** are *concentrated at the nodes of Ranvier*.
   3. The **voltage-gated Ca^{++} channels** are mainly present at the axon terminals, where they play important role in the secretion of neurotransmitters.
   4. The **mechanical-gated Na^+ channels** are involved in the genesis of receptor potential in the somatic sensory nerve endings.
   5. **Ligand-gated ion channels** are present predominantly on dendritic spines, dendrites and cell body of the neuron. They are important for receiving information from other neurons at synaptic sites, in the form of released neurotransmitters.

Distribution of Na^+ Channels

In myelinated neurons, the number of Na^+ channels per square micrometer of membrane in different segments of the neuron is as follows:

1. At cell body: 50–75
2. At axon hillock-initial segment: 350–500
3. On the surface of the myelin: 25
4. At the nodes of Ranvier: 2000–12,000
5. At the axon terminals: 20–75

Thus, the channels are concentrated in areas where the action potential is first initiated (initial segment) and in regions where it is regenerated (nodes of Ranvier) during its propagation.

In unmyelinated neurons, about 110 Na^+ channels are present per square micrometer of the axonal membrane. Abnormalities of channels are called channelopathies (Clinical Box 23.1).

Clinical Box 23.1

Channelopathies: The diseases caused due to the structural or functional changes in the ion channels are known as channelopathies. Those affecting neurons include episodic and spinocerebellar ataxias, some forms of epilepsy and familial hemiplegic migraine.

Recording of Nerve Responses

To study the various activities and properties of a nerve, intracellular and extracellular recording methods are adopted. For both recordings, electrical stimulus is usually used as it is convenient to apply the stimulus and accurately measure the strength of the stimulus.

Intracellular Recording

Usually, an isolated single giant axon taken from invertebrates such as cuttlefish (sepia) or squid (Loligo) is used for experimental set-up. As their fiber diameter is large (about 500 µm) it allows vertical penetration of **microelectrode** (diameter of 100 µm). The tip of the recording electrode is placed inside the axon, and the reference electrode is kept on the surface of the axon. A steady negative potential of –70 mV is recorded by the cathode ray oscilloscope (CRO) in the resting set-up. Then on application of a stimulus, the **monophasic response** obtained, is observed.

Extracellular Recording

In this type of recording, both the recording and reference electrodes are placed on the external surface of the isolated nerve fiber or on the skin surface of the intact animals or human beings. When the set-up is arranged, at rest, no potential is recorded by the CRO. Since both the electrodes are placed in same environment, both pick up the same voltage and there is no potential difference. On stimulation, a **biphasic response** is observed.

Scientists contributed

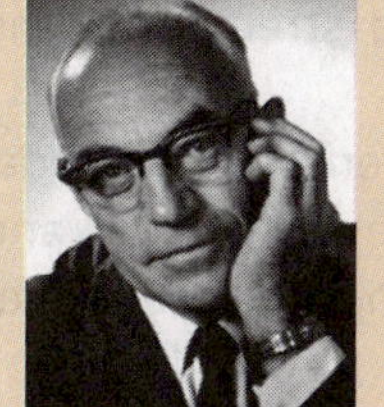

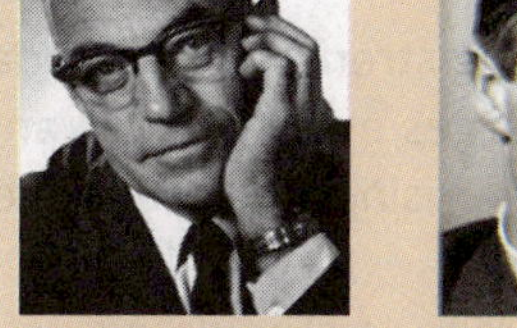

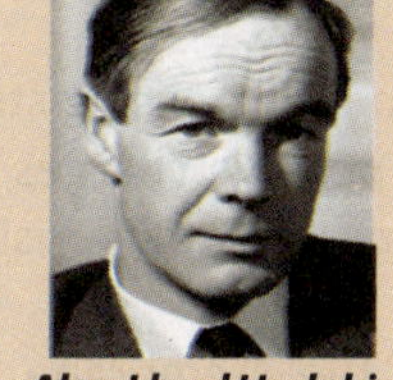

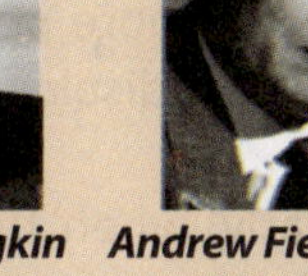

Sir John Carew Eccles (1903–1997) *Alan Lloyd Hodgkin* (1914–1998) *Andrew Fielding Huxley* (1917–2012)

The **Nobel Prize in Physiology or Medicine 1963** was awarded jointly to **Sir John Carew Eccles, Alan Lloyd Hodgkin** and **Andrew Fielding Huxley** "for their discoveries concerning the ionic mechanisms involved in excitation and inhibition in the peripheral and central portions of the nerve cell membrane". They worked extensively in the field of neurophysiology related to nerve impulse transmission.

The **Nobel Prize in Physiology or Medicine 1936** was awarded jointly to neurophysiologist from UK Sir **Henry Hallett Dale** and neurophysiologist from USA Prof. **Otto Loewi** *"for their discoveries relating to chemical transmission of nerve impulses"*. Their pioneering works were mainly in the field of transmission of nerve impulses in ANS (sympathetic and parasympathetic systems).

Terms Used for Membrane Potentials

Certain terms are used to explain the change in membrane potential relative to the resting membrane potential (RMP):

1. When there is a voltage difference between the inside and outside of the membrane, the membrane is said to be **polarized**.
2. When a stimulus allows influx of positive charges or efflux of negative charges, it decreases the membrane potential (i.e. the membrane potential approaches towards zero) and the stimulus is called a **depolarizing stimulus**. Thus, the membrane is said to be **depolarized** when the membrane potential becomes positive or less negative in relation to RMP.
3. After the depolarization phase, return of the potential towards the resting value is known as **repolarization**.
4. Similarly, as the interior of the cell becomes more negative in relation to RMP, due to influx of negative charges or removal of positive charges, the membrane is said to be **hyperpolarized**. In this state, the membrane potential is more negative in relation to RMP.

GENESIS OF NERVE POTENTIALS

The ability of the cells to generate action potential in their membrane is known as **excitability**. Nerve is a highly excitable tissue, which can be stimulated by electrical, chemical and mechanical forms of energy. When a stimulus is applied, it induces ions to flow across the membrane and alters the ionic balance on both sides of the membrane, producing a **voltage change**. With application of a stronger stimulus, much larger disturbance in ionic balance occurs. However, the **ionic balance is promptly restored by 2 factors (repolarizing forces)**:

1. Diffusion of ions across the cell membrane
2. Increased activity of Na^+-K^+ ATPase.

The voltage changes across the membrane generate electrical signals, which on recording show a wave like pattern. The transient and small voltage changes spread along the length of the nerve fiber and die out after some time. When the stimulus is strong enough, the response does not die out fast, rather, it travels along the whole length of the axon, being regenerated at regular intervals. This phenomenon is possible because the neuronal membrane is a biological membrane studded with different ion channels, whose activation time is modifiable with change in external environment.

In the neuron, processing of information takes place chiefly in the cell body and to some extent in the dendrites.

The message transmission occurs by means of generation and propagation of the electrical signals in the axon from one end to the other. These generated signals can be of **two types**:

1. Electrotonic or graded potentials
2. Action potentials.

Graded potentials spread the signal over short distances, whereas **action potentials** transmit the message throughout the length of the plasma membrane. Another type of response is seen in neuronal membrane that is called **local response**.

Electrotonic or Graded Potentials

Definition

Electrotonic potentials are local, nonpropagated potentials of small magnitude, in response to a depolarizing or hyperpolarizing stimulus of lesser strength.

Types

Electrotonic potentials are two types: catelectrotonic and anelectrotonic.

Catelectrotonic potential: When a membrane is electrically stimulated, the cathodal end of the stimulator evokes a depolarizing response called catelectrotonic potential.

Anelectrotonic potential: The hyperpolarizing potential produced due to stimulation at the anodal end is known as anelectrotonic potential (Fig. 23.1).

Concept

In the resting state, negatively charged ions are lined along the interior of the membrane and positively charged ions are lined along the exterior of the membrane:

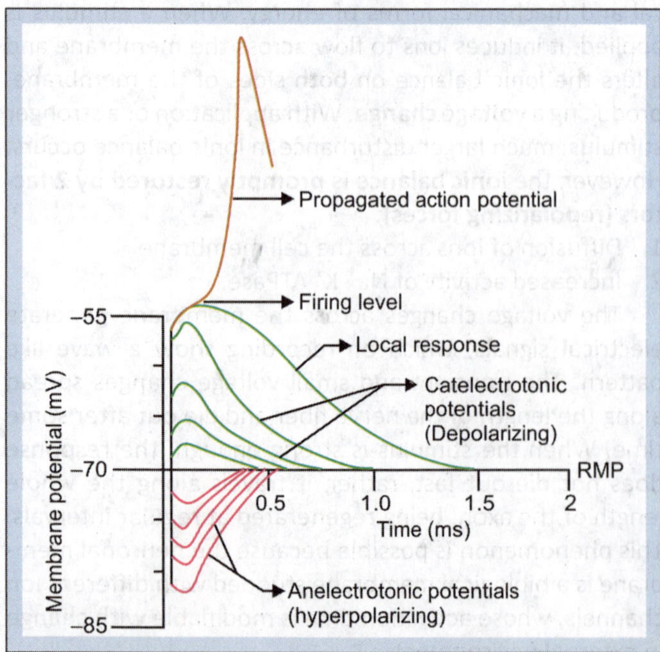

Fig. 23.1: Electrotonic potential and local response. (RMP: Resting membrane potential).

1. With the application of a cathodal stimulus of smaller strength to a small area of the membrane, few Na^+ ions enter through the leaky sodium channels into the cell.
2. At that instant, at the site of stimulus, the inside of the membrane becomes positive compared to the previous resting state.
3. With application of greater strength of stimulus, more positive charges enter into the cell and the voltage change is larger.
4. The repolarizing forces try to neutralize the disturbance in RMP, created by the Na^+ entry. **K^+ tends to come out** of the cell and **Cl^- enters** through the leaky channels to maintain the electrical neutrality. Also, Na^+ moves away by diffusion from the site of stimulus. Moreover, activity of the Na^+-K^+ ATPase is increased **pumping 3 Na^+ out and 2 K^+ in**. All these lead to the gradual return of the membrane potential towards the resting value.

In the neuron, graded potentials are recorded from the membranes of dendrites and cell body.

Properties of Graded Potential

1. **Graded in nature:** The term **graded potential** comes from the fact that the potential change increases in a stepwise manner with application of increasing strength of stimulus, i.e. **the magnitude of potential change is proportionate to the stimulus strength**.
2. **Decremental conduction:** Graded potentials decay progressively with time and distance, which is known as decremental conduction:
   i. When recorded near the site of stimulus, the amplitude of the potential is larger and recorded at a farther place, it is smaller. The potentials die out within a distance of 3 mm from the site of stimulus.
   ii. If recorded immediately after the application of the stimulus, the amplitude is larger and with delay in recording, the amplitude is smaller.
3. **Depolarizing or hyperpolarizing nature:** If the change in potential is plotted in the y-axis and time in the x-axis, the graph will be like a wave (Fig. 23.1), which primarily depends on the type and strength of the stimuli:
   i. With application of increasing strength of cathodal stimulus, more positive charges enter the cell and the graph displays gradually rising **upward waveforms**.
   ii. Similarly, when the membrane is stimulated with anodal end, due to entry of negative charges or removal of positive charges, the membrane potential becomes more negative; the graph displays a **downward waveform**.

   Therefore, according to the type of stimulus, graded potentials can occur in either a depolarizing or a hyperpolarizing direction.

4. **Summation:** if a second stimulus is applied before the potential produced by the first stimulus has disappeared, both the potential changes are added together producing a larger and/or prolonged wave in the recording. This happens due to the arrival of more Na^+ ions at the site of stimulus before neutralization of all Na^+ influx caused by the first stimulus. Similarly the anelectrotonic potentials exhibit the property of summation.

Forms of Graded Potentials

Wherever a cell responds to a stimulus, graded potentials are produced along its membrane:

1. According to the type and location of the membrane from where they are recorded, they are described as **end-plate potential**, recorded from skeletal muscle membrane at neuromuscular junctions.
2. **Receptor potential**, recorded from sensory nerve endings.
3. **Synaptic potential**, recorded from membrane of postsynaptic neurons at neuro-neuronal junctions.
4. **Pacemaker potential**, recorded from pacemaker cells in the heart, intestine, etc. and so on.

Local Response

As the axon is stimulated with slowly increasing strength of stimuli, the amplitude of the electrotonic potential gradually rises. When the membrane potential is decreased by 7 mV, the **pattern of graded potential is altered**. The response becomes greater than what is expected for that strength of stimulus. This **enhanced response** is known as **local response**:

1. Similar to the graded potential, the local response gradually dies out with increasing distance.
2. Local response is seen only with a depolarizing stimulus of lower strength, and not with a hyperpolarizing one.

Ionic Basis of Local Response

As the applied cathodal stimulus is progressively raised from zero the **influx of Na^+ ions through the leaky sodium channels** increases proportionately. Consequently, the membrane potential gradually **decreases from –70 to –63 mV.** At –63 mV, the few **voltage-gated sodium channels start opening**, which allows entry of some more Na^+ ions. The **extra Na^+ ions** entering into the cytoplasm are added to the existing Na^+ influx, resulting in a heightened response called local response. This is observed within a potential change from –63 to –55 mV.

Types of Stimuli

Threshold, Subthreshold and Suprathreshold Stimuli

At membrane potential of –55 mV, the neuron starts generating action potentials:

1. This is termed as *firing* or *discharge* of the neuron and the membrane potential at –55 mV is known as the **firing level** or *threshold*.
2. The stimulus that brings the membrane potential to –55 mV is known as threshold stimulus. **Threshold stimulus** is defined as the lowest strength of stimulus that elicits an action potential.
3. The stimuli less in strength than the threshold are known as **subthreshold stimuli** and the stimuli higher in strength than the threshold are known as **suprathreshold stimuli.**

Strength-Duration Relationship

Strength and duration are two important aspects of a stimulus. Both of them have a complimentary role in determining the excitability of a tissue. These two parameters are inversely related to each other. The relationship between the strength and duration of stimuli depicted in graph form is known as **strength-duration curve** (Fig. 23.2):

1. To excite a tissue, the lowest amplitude of current required is termed as **rheobase.**
2. The minimum time for which the rheobase must be applied to elicit an action potential is known as **utilization time**. A stimulus weaker than rheobase does not excite the tissue and a stimulus stronger than rheobase requires less time (less than utilization time) to elicit a response.
3. **Chronaxie** is the time required for a stimulus of double the rheobase strength to produce an action potential.
4. Usually chronaxie gives us a better idea about the excitability of a tissue. The lesser the chronaxie, the greater is the excitability.
5. Nerves have a shorter chronaxie compared to muscles.

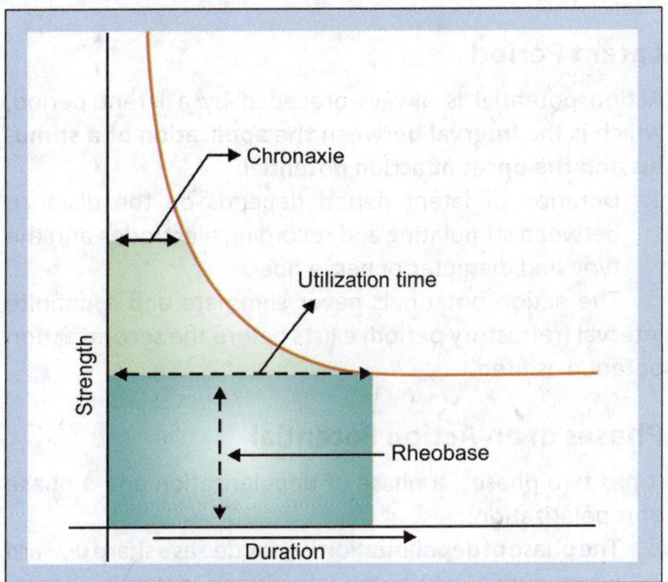

Fig. 23.2: Strength-duration curve.

Accommodation

If the intensity of a stimulus is slowly raised to the threshold value, the tissue fails to produce an action potential because it adapts to the stimulus. This phenomenon is known as accommodation:

1. During the slow depolarization, some of the voltage-gated Na^+ channels start opening at a membrane potential of –63 mV. But, they soon get inactivated before another set of channel opens; because, the membrane takes longer time to arrive at the next level of potential.
2. Thus, the sufficient number of activated sodium channels required to fire an action potential is never accomplished. Like this, the membrane may attain the normal threshold level or even surpass that level, but action potential is not produced.
3. Besides, the potassium channels that open in response to the depolarization drain off the positive charges.

Action Potential

Definition

Action potential is defined as a transient change in membrane potential of about 100 mV, which is conducted along the axon in an all-or-none fashion.

It has following featues:

1. It is characterized by a gradual depolarization to threshold, and a rapid ascent in the membrane potential followed by a phase of repolarization.
2. It travels along the axon with the same shape and amplitude being regenerated at regular intervals.
3. It is also known as an **impulse** or **spike potential**.

Duration and Amplitude

The duration of a single nerve action potential is about 1 msec, during which the membrane potential sharply rises from –70 to +35 mV, and then returns to its resting value.

Latent Period

Action potential is always preceded by a latent period, which is the **interval between the application of a stimulus and the onset of action potential**:

1. Duration of latent period depends on the distance between stimulating and recording electrodes and the type and diameter of nerve fiber.

The action potentials never summate and a definite interval (refractory period) exists before the second action potential is fired.

Phases of an Action Potential

It has two phases, a phase of depolarization and a phase of repolarization:

i. **The phase of depolarization** is recorded as a sharp upward wave during which the membrane potential approaches zero and then attains a positive value. It consists of slow depolarization to threshold, rapid rising phase, overshoot and peak. During overshoot, the membrane potential crosses the zero or isopotential level and then at peak, it reaches a maximum potential of +35 mV.

ii. **The phase of repolarization** is recorded as downstroke during which the membrane potential returns to the resting level. It includes a rapid falling phase and slower terminal part called **after-depolarization.**

The phase of repolarization is followed by an **after-hyperpolarization** phase during which the membrane potential undershoots (becomes more negative) and then returns back to the resting level (Fig. 23.3).

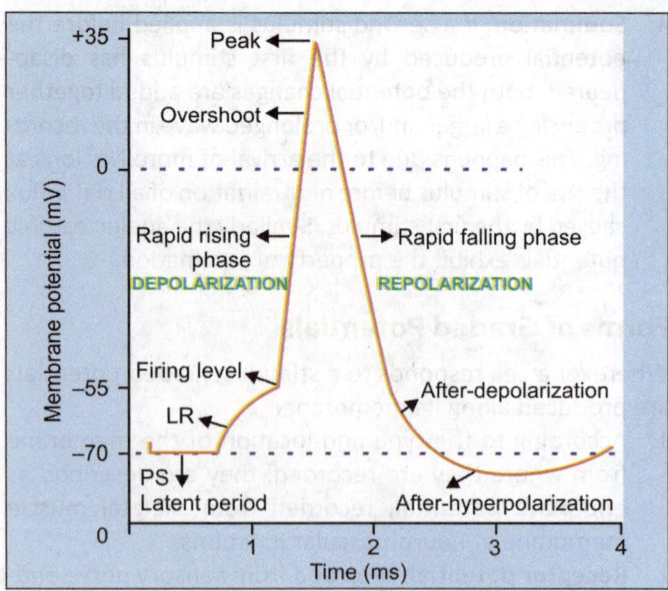

Fig. 23.3: Phases of action potential recorded from a neuron. Note, depolarization phase, overshoot and peak; and repolarization phase consists of rapid falling phase and after-depolarization. (LR: Local response; PS: Point of stimulation).

Ionic Bases of Action Potential

The depolarization and repolarization phase of the action potential are due to sequential changes in membrane permeability to sodium and potassium leading to large fluxes of these ions across the membrane, along their gradients. **Depolarization is due to influx of sodium** and **repolarization is due to efflux of potassium**. The voltage-gated Na^+ and K^+ channels contribute to the different phases of the action potential.

Depolarization

Depolarization is due to **opening of voltage-gated Na^+ channels,** causing massive *influx of sodium ions*:

1. When a threshold or suprathreshold stimulus is applied, the influx of Na^+ through leaky channels and later through opening of few voltage-gated Na^+ channels decreases the membrane potential from –70 mV to –55 mV (threshold level).

2. At this **threshold potential**, there occurs *simultaneous opening of a large number of the voltage-gated Na^+ channels*, increasing the membrane permeability to sodium ions several hundredfold. This leads to **massive influx of sodium ions** producing a swift, large and steep depolarization, changing the membrane potential to +35 mV (a change in membrane potential by 105 mV starting from the resting value of –70 mV to +35 mV).

The initial change in membrane potential by +15 mV (–70 mV to –55 mV) is essential for instantaneous activation of a large number of voltage-gated Na^+ channels. At threshold level, the number of Na^+ channels that have already opened, cause concomitant opening of almost all the Na^+ channels in the stimulated part of the membrane (**positive feedback control**) (Application Box 23.1). The activation gate of Na^+ channels opens that brings them to the activated state (for details, see below). Therefore, this process of simultaneous activation of huge number of Na^+ channels is called **auto-activation**, which occurs very rapidly.

Application Box 23.1

Hodgkin's cycle: The opening of few Na^+ channels leading to further opening of other Na^+ channels is called Hodgkin's cycle. This is an example of positive feedback control in which a stimulus triggering an event further facilitates the process (Refer to Fig. 3.3, Chapter 3).

The concentration gradient as well as electrical gradient favors the entry of sodium ions across the membrane. In fact, there occurs reversal of membrane potential with the inside becoming positive than outside as the membrane potential crosses the isopotential value of 0 mV and finally attains a peak potential of +35 mV.

Membrane Potential Remains Below Na^+ Equilibrium Potential

During depolarization, the membrane potential approaches but does not reach the equilibrium potential for sodium, which is +60 mV as derived from Nernst equation, because of the **following three factors.**

At the peak of the action potential:

1. Sodium influx abruptly ceases due to the closure of the *inactivation gates* of the Na^+ channels. The Na^+ channels open very fast, remain open for a very brief period, and they close very fast. The process of speedy closure is called **rapid autodeactivation.**
2. The voltage-gated potassium channels being fully open, allow the exit of positively charged K^+ ions.
3. The electrical gradient for Na^+ is reversed subsequent to the overshoot, i.e. after crossing RMP of 0 mV, inside of the cell membrane becomes positive and it hinders the positively charged Na^+ to enter the positive interior, slowing down further sodium entry.

During an action potential, approximately 20,000 Na^+ ions enter into the cell. The repolarizing forces try to restore the resting membrane potential, but the depolarization is large enough to overcome the opposing forces and produce an action potential.

Repolarization

Repolarization is due to **opening of voltage-gated K^+ channels, causing efflux of** K^+. Actually, these K^+ channels are sensitive to the same depolarization that opens the voltage-gated Na^+ channels but they open more slowly:

1. At the peak of the action potential, the voltage-gated Na^+ channels enter a closed state whereas the voltage-gated K^+ channels are fully open.
2. The membrane permeability to potassium ions increases several times causing increased potassium efflux. The K^+ concentration is much higher inside the cell and at the peak of the action potential, outside of the membrane is negative in comparison to inside, which is positive (+35 mV).
3. These two factors favour the electrochemical gradient for potassium efflux.
4. Thus, the *rapid falling phase of repolarization* is brought about by **decline in sodium influx together with increase in potassium efflux**.
5. The termination of action potential due to activation of voltage-gated potassium channels is a negative feedback process.

Following the phase of rapid fall, once the membrane potential drops close to the isopotential level and moves towards RMP, the inside of the membrane becomes negative that limits the efflux of potassium. Thus, *after-depolarization phase* is due to the slower exit of potassium ions that considerably decreases the rate of repolarization and makes the repolarization curve oblique (less steep).

Voltage-gated Na^+ and K^+ Channels

The Na^+ channel has two gates, an **activation gate** and an **inactivation gate**:

1. When the membrane is at rest, the inactivation gate is open and the activation gate is closed. This is the **resting state of the channel** in which Na^+ influx cannot occur. The K^+ channel has only one gate that remains closed during the resting state (Fig. 23.4A).
2. As the membrane is depolarized to the firing level, the activation gate of Na^+ channel opens. This is the **activated state of the Na^+ channels** in which, both the gates are open permitting massive influx of Na^+ that brings the membrane potential to +35 mV (Fig.23.4B).
3. The gate of the K^+ channel start opening at the same time as the activation gate of Na^+ channel, but K^+ gates open slowly.
4. At the peak of the action potential, the inactivation gate of Na^+ channel closes. This is the **inactivated state of the Na^+ channels**, in which Na^+ influx stops. Also, the activation gate of Na^+ channel is about to close (Fig. 23.4C).
5. At this time, the gates of K^+ channel are fully open allowing K^+ efflux and causing rapid repolarization (Fig. 23.4D).
6. In the later part of repolarization, the activation gate of Na^+ channel is closed and the inactivation gate starts opening slowly. This is the **closed state of the Na^+ channels (Fig. 23.4E)**.

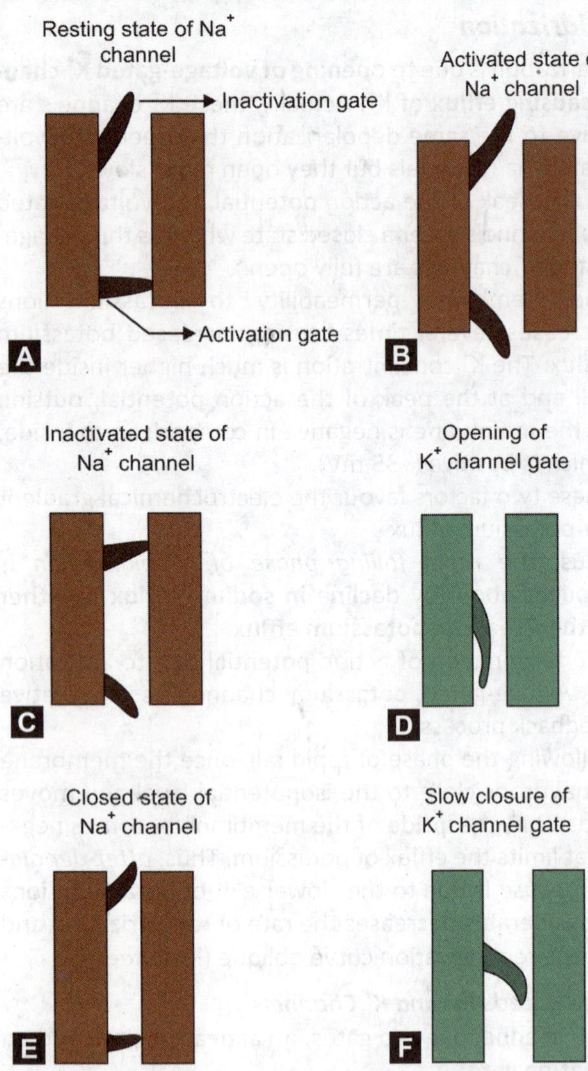

Figs. 23.4A to F: States of Na^+ and K^+ channels during depolarization and repolarization of action potential. (A) In the resting state, inactivation gate of Na^+ channels remains open, but activation gate remains closed; (B) During depolarization (activated state of Na^+ channels), both inactivation and activation gates of Na^+ channels remain open allowing massive influx of sodium; (C) At the peak of action potential (inactivated state of Na^+ channels), inactivation gate closes and activation gate is about to close, causing cessation of Na^+ influx; (D) At the same time (peak of action potential), gate of K^+ channel remains fully open allowing K^+ efflux to occur; (E) During later part of repolarization (closed state of Na^+ channels), inactivation gate of Na^+ channels starts opening when activation gates are completely closed; (F) At the same time (during later part of repolarization), gate of K^+ channel slowly starts closing, causing gradual cessation of K^+ efflux.

7. By now, the K^+ channel gates have started to close but they take a longer time to shut down completely (Fig. 23.4F).
8. Then the channels proceed to the resting state, where, the inactivation gate of Na^+ channel is fully open; the activation gates of Na^+ channels and the K^+ channel gates are fully closed causing no ion movement across the channels.

After-Hyperpolarization

1. Following after-depolarization, the membrane reaches the resting potential (RMP). At this level, though most of the voltage-gated K^+ channels are closed, some of them still remain open allowing continued efflux of K^+.
2. As a result, the membrane potential becomes more negative than the RMP, giving rise to the prolonged and slow undershoot, which is called as phase of after-hyperpolarization.
3. Finally, the K^+ channels completely close, restoring the membrane potential back to the resting level.

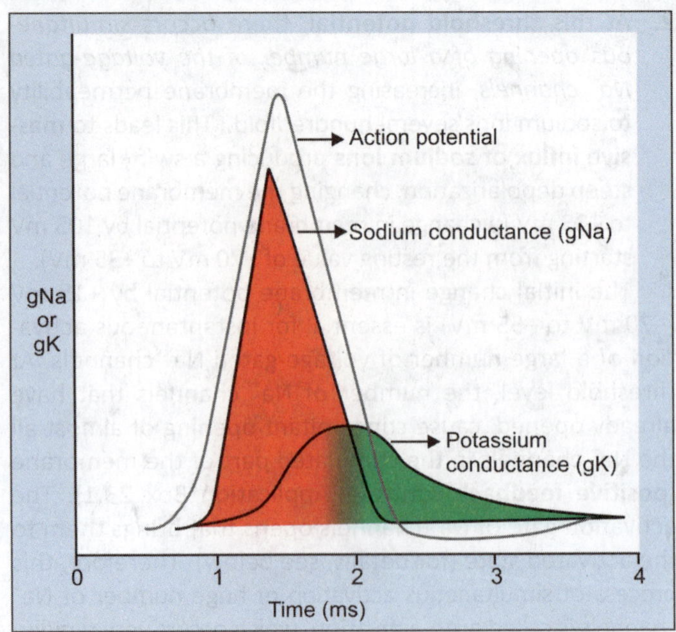

Fig. 23.5: Conductance of sodium and potassium across the membrane during action potential.

Ionic Conductance during Action Potential

Conductance of an ion means the ease with which the ion passes through the plasma membrane. It indicates the **permeability of the membrane to the ion**. Conductance is reciprocal of resistance, offered by the membrane as well as the potential gradient across the membrane hindering the passage of the ion through the membrane:

1. The **Na^+ conductance** rises gradually from the RMP to the firing level, and then it fast increases reaching a peak. At the peak of the action potential, it declines rapidly and comes to the base line.
2. The **K^+ conductance** rises after the rise in Na^+ conductance. Initially, the conductance increases at a much slower rate during the phase of depolarization. Just after the peak of the action potential, the conductance increases to its maximum during the rapid falling phase of repolarization. After that, the K^+ conductance decreases but takes a long time to reach the base line (Fig. 23.5).

Ionic Activity after Action Potential

At the end of an action potential, the ionic composition on both sides of the membrane is altered. This leaves more sodium and less potassium inside the cell:

1. The ionic composition is restored by **increased activity of the Na^+-K^+ ATPase.**
2. The number of ions that take part in generation of a single action potential is very little compared to the total number of ions in the cell (1 of every one million Na^+ go into the cell and about the same number of K^+ come out of the cell during an action potential). This produces a negligible change in the intracellular ionic concentration.
3. However, if this imbalance was not taken care of, in the long run, following repeated generation of action potentials, it would be difficult to generate action potentials further, because slowly the concentration gradients of sodium and potassium across the membrane will cease to exist.

Effects of Extracellular Ionic Changes

1. When the **extracellular Na^+ concentration is decreased**, the amplitude of the action potentials becomes smaller than usual because the concentration gradient for Na^+ that drives sodium into the cell is reduced.
2. When the **extracellular Na^+ concentration is increased**, the amplitude of the action potentials may increase.
3. When the **extracellular K^+ concentration is decreased**, the membrane potential becomes more negative as the resting K^+ efflux is increased favoured by the increased concentration gradient across the membrane.
4. When the **extracellular K^+ concentration is increased**, the membrane potential come closer to the firing level and the membrane becomes more excitable.
5. When the **extracellular Ca^{++} concentration is decreased**, the electrical potential difference across the membrane is decreased, as the inside becomes less negative compared to outside. The RMP come closer to the firing level, so that, the magnitude of depolarization needed to reach the firing level is less. Hence, decrease in extracellular Ca^{++} concentration increases the excitability of the tissue, as observed in hypocalcemic tetany, occurring in hypoparathyroidism.
6. If the **extracellular Ca^{++} concentration is increased**, the RMP goes away from the firing level due to increased potential difference across the membrane. Consequently, the magnitude of depolarization needed to reach the firing level is more, decreasing the tissue excitability.

Ion Channel Blockers

Na^+ Channel Blockers

The drugs like lidocaine, procaine 'etc., and neurotoxins like tetrodotoxin, saxitoxin' etc., block the voltage-gated Na^+ channels and hinder the generation of action potentials.

Local Anesthetics

Lidocaine and procaine are used clinically as local anesthetics during various surgical procedures. When injected into the affected tissue or sprayed over an area, the ionizable hydrophobic drug molecules diffuse readily through the plasma membrane and block the Na^+ channels and decrease the transmission of pain and other sensations. Axons with a smaller diameter are more sensitive to the local anesthetics than the large diameter fibers.

Membrane Toxins

The neurotoxins like **tetrodotoxin** (TTX) is found in ovaries of puffer fish and in tissues of salamanders, and **saxitoxin** (STX) is accumulated in the tissues of shellfish. Both are lethal paralytic toxins and eating a small quantity of tissue containing the toxins can lead to death. These animals have survived by developing resistance against the toxins' i.e. they have TTX-resistant or STX-resistant sodium channels.

K^+ Channel Blockers

The voltage-gated K^+ channel blockers are **tetraethylammonium** (TEA) and **4-aminopyridine** (4-AP). These chemicals along with TTX are used extensively by scientists in electrophysiological research, like study of voltage-clamp techniques.

Na^+– K^+ ATPase Blocker

Drugs like **digitalis and dinitrophenol** block the Na^+–K^+ ATPase pump.

All-or-None Law

Definition

All or none states that the action potential occurs with a constant amplitude and shape irrespective of magnitude of the stimulus. A **subthreshold stimulus** fails to excite the tissue. Only a stimulus of **threshold magnitude** elicits an action potential. If **suprathreshold stimuli** are applied, the action potentials resulting from them have the same amplitude, duration and form as those produced by threshold stimuli, provided the experimental conditions like electrical potentials on both sides of the membrane, concentration of ions in ICF and ECF, temperature' *etc.* remain same (Fig. 23.6).

Mechanism

The activation gates of voltage-gated Na^+ channels open as soon as 15 mV of depolarization is achieved. Following that, any extra degree of depolarization is of no further use, as the membrane automatically achieves another +90 mV of depolarization (–55 to +35 mV):

1. Thus, *after the threshold level is achieved,* the amount of **sodium influx becomes independent of the stimulus factor.**
2. The number of voltage-gated Na^+ channels over the axonal membrane of unmyelinated axons as well as at the nodes of Ranvier in myelinated axons remain fairly constant.

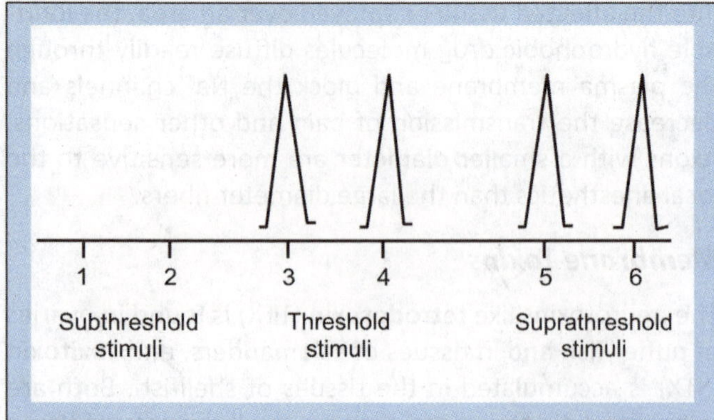

Fig. 23.6: All or none law for action potential. Note, sub-threshold stimuli (1 and 2) do not evoke formation of action potential, whereas, threshold (3and 4) and supra-threshold (5 and 6) stimuli evoke similar action potentials.

3. Once the action potential is formed, it appears with its maximum size and shape, otherwise it does not form at all.
4. Therefore, the action potential follows the all-or-none law; i.e. the action potential occurs with a constant amplitude and shape whether the stimulus is of threshold or suprathreshold magnitude.

Refractory Periods

During the action potential, the stimulated area of the membrane happens to be unresponsive to a second stimulus in most part, and later it requires a stronger stimulus to get excited again. The **length of time during which the membrane is unresponsive to a second stimulus** no matter how strong is the stimulus, is known as refractory period. The periods of total and relative refractoriness are known as absolute and relative refractory periods respectively.

Absolute Refractory Period

Definition and Duration

Absolute refractory period (ARP) is defined as the period in the action potential during which, application of a second stimulus of any strength and duration does not produce another action potential. The ARP corresponds to the period from the time the firing level is reached until repolarization is about one-third complete (Fig. 23.7).

Mechanism

At the peak of the action potential, the inactivation gates of the voltage-gated sodium channels close and they remain in that inactivated state for some time before returning to the resting state. These sodium channels can reopen in response to a second stimulus, only after attaining the resting state. Hence, even if a stronger stimulus is applied during this interval, it will not produce a second action potential, and the membrane is said to be in its absolute refractory period.

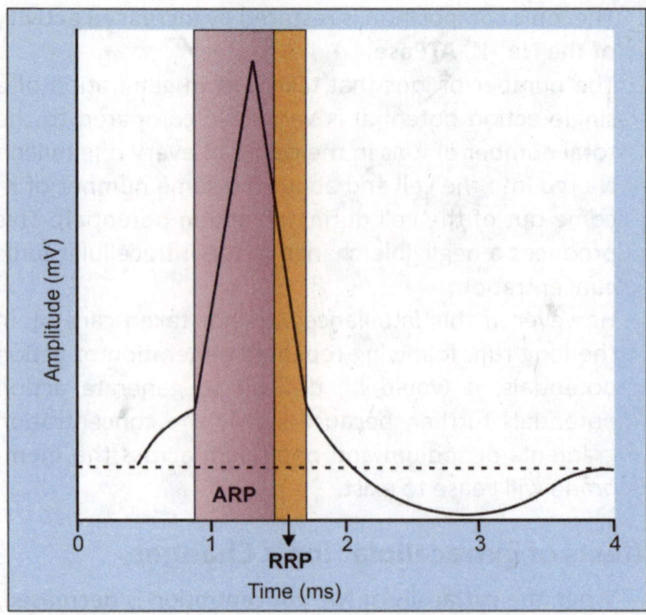

Fig. 23.7: Refractory periods of nerve action potential. (ARP: Absolute refractory period; RRP: Relative refractory period).

Physiological Importance

The absolute refractory period limits the number of action potentials that the nerve can fire in a given period of time. ARP serves **two important functions:**

1. ARP determines the **rate of discharge of nerve fiber.** In our body, nerves fire at a rate of 10 to 1000 impulses per second. Generally, **large diameter nerve fibers** have an ARP of about 0.4 msec, with a firing rate of 2500 impulses per second, whereas **small diameter fibers** have an ARP of about 4 msec, with a firing rate of 250 impulses per second.
2. The ARP is also responsible for the **one-way conduction of action potentials** (this will be discussed under the propagation of action potential).

Relative Refractory Period

Definition and Duration

Relative refractory period (RRP) is defined as the period following ARP during which, application of a suprathreshold stimulus can elicit a second action potential. The RRP **starts from the end of ARP to the** start of after-depolarization.

Mechanism

The following factors contribute to RRP:

1. All the sodium channels present at the site of stimulus do not achieve the open state or inactivated state or resting state, exactly at the same time. Few of them open when the membrane potential is –63 mV, causing local response. By the time of relative refractory period, some of the channels have returned to their initial resting state. These channels in resting state can open their activation gate and allow the influx of Na^+.
2. A suprathreshold stimulus can spread to larger area over the membrane and open extra voltage-gated sodium channel.

Thus, only a suprathreshold stimulus and not any threshold stimulus can open up sufficient number of sodium channels to elicit an action potential during the RRP.

The **excitability of the membrane** keeps on changing in different phases of the action potential. Usually, the time the membrane potential is closer to the firing level, the membrane is more excitable; and the excitability of the membrane decreases, when its potential is away from the firing level. During the ARP, it is least excitable.

Initiation and Propagation of Action Potential

Initiation of Action Potential

The production of action potentials requires the presence of large number of voltage-gated ion channels that are present mostly on the axons. Therefore, it is the axon, not the cell body or the dendrites that generate and conduct the action potentials:

1. The action potential is first initiated in the specialized areas in the axon called the **first node of Ranvier in sensory neurons** and **initial segment-axon hillock area in motor neurons.**
2. These areas are known as **trigger zones** that have a very high concentration of voltage-gated sodium and potassium channels.
3. The synaptic potential generated at the dendrites and, or the cell body is integrated by the cell body and transmitted to the axon hillock.
4. If this potential is sufficient to depolarize the membrane of the axon hillock to firing level, the membrane easily fires an action potential.

Propagation of Action Potential

Once formed, the action potential is regenerated at regular intervals to be transmitted from the initial segment of the axon to the axon terminal. This is known as the propagation of action potential. In myelinated axon, the speed and mode of propagation of action potential is different from that in unmyelinated axon.

The *speed of conduction of the impulse* depends on **two factors**:

1. **Myelination:** Conduction velocity is more in myelinated axon and is proportionate to the degree of myelination.
2. **Diameter of the axon:** Conduction velocity is proportionate to the diameter of the fiber. Fibers with larger diameter have faster rate of conduction. The large diameter fibers have less cytoplasmic resistance. So, the flow of ions across the membrane is easier.

In Unmyelinated Axon

At the site of genesis of an action potential, large influx of positive charges into the membrane occurs, which is known as **current sink**. The positive charges diffuse away from the site of accumulation. The adjacent membrane, which is in its resting state, has a potential of –70 mV:

1. This potential difference allows the positive charges to flow toward the adjacent negative area. Consequently, *the potential of the adjacent membrane decreases and reaches the threshold* value, as the fraction of Na^+ ions that move to the nearby negative area are sufficient enough to bring the **adjacent membrane to the firing level.** This results in opening of the voltage gated Na^+ channels present in that area, firing an action potential.
2. Similarly, from the site of second action potential, positive charges flow to the adjacent resting membrane and decrease its potential to the threshold level. This activates the voltage gated Na^+ channels present in that part of the membrane resulting **in another action potential.**
3. In this manner, each point of the membrane gets depolarized to the firing level and produces an action potential.
4. As the depolarization and repolarization phases of the ensuing action potentials go on, there is a sequential opening and closing of sodium and potassium channels along the axonal membrane (Fig. 23.8).
5. The action potential does not move by itself but helps to generate a new action potential in the membrane ahead of it. As the number of voltage gated Na^+ and K^+ channels are distributed uniformly along the axon, the action potential arriving at the end of the axon is almost identical in appearance to the initial one. Thus, due to the **local current flow** produced following an action potential, there occurs serial depolarization of the adjacent membrane to the firing level and action potential travels, being successively regenerated along the membrane in an all-or-none manner.
6. At the same time, the exterior of the membrane which becomes negative due to current sink attracts flow of positive charges from the adjacent regions toward the site of application of stimulus. Thus, on both sides of the site of action potential, a **circular pattern of current flow** occurs across the membrane; i.e. inside the membrane, positive charges flow away from the site of action potential, whereas outside the membrane, positive charges flow towards the site of action potential. This circular pattern of current flow tries to restore the resting potential of the membrane where the action potential was previously generated.

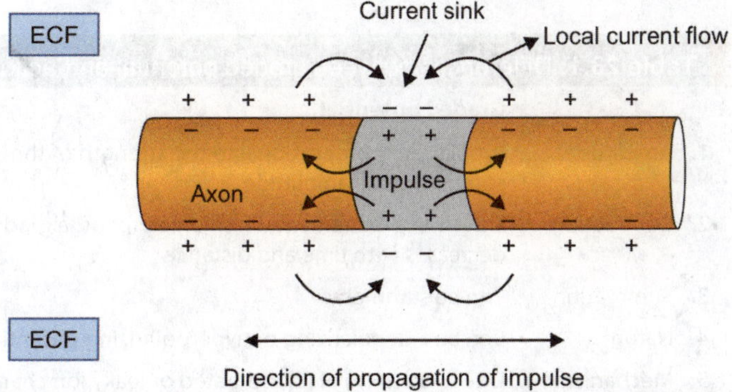

Fig. 23.8: Propagation of action potential in unmyelinated axon.

In Myelinated Axon (Saltatory Conduction)

There are few voltage gated Na^+ channels on the surface of the myelin:

1. **Myelin acts as an insulator** and does not allow free flow of ions across the membrane. Therefore, as the positive charges flow from the site of action potential to the adjacent area, large Na^+ influx (as occurs during an action potential) does not occur in the myelinated portion of the membrane, though it may attend the threshold potential of –55 mV. Also, in the myelin sheath, the concentration of positive charges does not decrease fast because of less 'leakage'. This helps the charges to spread farther along the axon.
2. The local current (the positive charges) travels like a graded potential and dies away 37% of its maximal strength over a distance of about 3 mm.
3. As the internodal distance is 1–2 mm, the local current definitely arrives at the adjacent node of Ranvier and decreases its membrane potential. Most importantly, the **voltage gated Na^+ channels are present in large numbers** *at the nodes of Ranvier*. Therefore, as soon as the nodal membrane gets depolarized to threshold level, an action potential is quickly fired.
4. Thus, in the myelinated axon, the **action potential is generated at each node of Ranvier** (Fig. 23.9).
5. Because the action potential rapidly proceeds from one node to the next and pause at each node to get regenerated, the mode of propagation of action potential in myelinated axon is known as **saltatory conduction** (Latin word *'saltare'* means to jump).

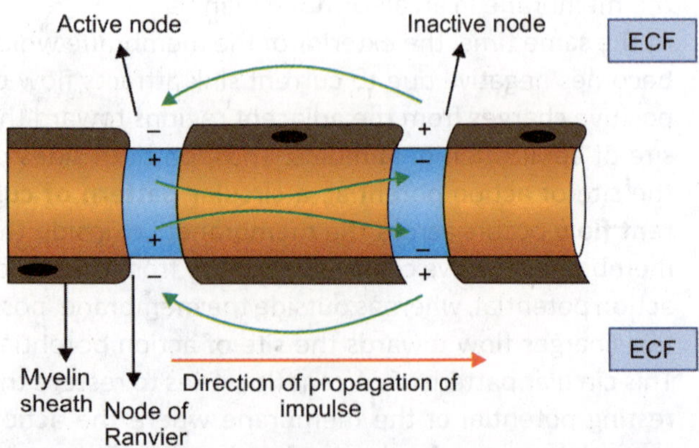

Fig. 23.9: Propagation of action potential in myelinated axon.

Advantages in Myelinated Axon

In myelinated axon, the velocity of conduction is faster. Besides, myelination also helps to conserves energy. Since the ionic flux occurs only at the nodes of Ranvier, the total membrane area across which ionic balance has to be restored is much less compared to the unmyelinated axon. Therefore, in unmyelinated axons, voltage-gated channels open throughout the axonal length causing activation of larger number of Na^+-K^+ ATPase and higher expenditure of energy.

Direction of Propagation of Action Potential

In the motor neuron, the action potential is conducted from axon hillock toward axon terminal. In the sensory neuron, it propagates from the first node of Ranvier toward CNS. This is called **anterograde conduction** of impulse:

1. The axon contains a large number of voltage gated Na^+ channels that promotes in quick generation of an action potential in the axonal membrane next to the trigger zone.
2. The action potential **does not travel from the axon back toward the trigger zone.** This is because; following depolarization, the area on the membrane where action potential was produced becomes refractory.
3. Therefore, though local currents from the site of next action potential tend to bring the membrane toward threshold value, the membrane does not fire an action potential, as the sodium channels remain inactivated.
4. Hence, the action potential can be conducted **only in the direction away from the site of previous action potential.**
5. The action potential can spread from the point of stimulus in both directions along the axon, if it is initiated between trigger zone and axon terminal.

Differences between Graded Potential and Action Potential

From the above discussions, we note that many differences exist between graded potentials and action potentials. The major differences are listed in Table 23.1.

Table 23.1: Differences between graded potential and action potential.

	Graded potential	Action potential
1. Amplitude	Amplitude is proportional to the strength of the stimulus; small amplitude	Once threshold potential is reached, amplitude remains same irrespective of the strength of the stimulus; large amplitude
2. Conduction	Travels in a decremental fashion; amplitude gradually decreases with time and distance	Conducted in an all-or-none manner; appears with the same amplitude and shape all along the axon
3. Summation	Can be summated	Cannot be summated
4. Nature	Can be a depolarizing or hyperpolarizing potential	Always a large depolarizing potential
5. Mechanism	Due to opening of ligand-gated or leaky ion channels	Due to opening of voltage-gated ion channels
6. Properties	Does not have a threshold or refractory period	Has a threshold and refractory period

CHAPTER SUMMARY

Key Concepts

1. Electrotonic potentials are local, non-propagated potentials of small magnitude, in response to a depolarizing or hyperpolarizing stimulus of lesser strength.
2. **Threshold stimulus** is the lowest strength of stimulus that elicits an action potential. This brings the membrane potential to –55 mV. The stimuli less in strength than the threshold are known as **subthreshold stimuli** and the stimuli higher in strength than the threshold are known as **suprathreshold stimuli**.
3. **Chronaxie** is the time required for a stimulus of double the rheobase strength to produce an action potential. Chronaxie indicates excitability of a tissue. Lesser the chronaxie, greater is the excitability.
4. In an action potential, **depolarization is due to influx of sodium** and **repolarization is due to efflux of potassium**.
5. Absolute refractory period (ARP) is defined as the period in the action potential during which, application of a second stimulus of any strength and duration does not produce another action potential. ARP is the period from the firing level to the one-third of repolarization.
6. The speed of conduction of impulse in myelinated neuron is much faster due to presence of large number of Na^+ channels at nodes of Ranvier that makes the conduction saltatory in nature.

Important to Know (Must Read)

1. In examinations, usually **Long Questions** are not asked from this chapter.
2. Electrotonic potentials, Local response, Strength-duration curve, Labeled diagram and ionic basis of action potential, All or none law, Refractory period, Propagation of action potential along the axon, and Saltatory conduction, are usual **Short Questions** in exams.
3. In **Viva**, examiners may ask........ definition and importance of electrotonic potentials, meaning and ionic basis of local response, definition and importance of rheobase, chronaxie and utilization time, different phases and ionic basis of action potential, latent period, definition of firing level, threshold, subthreshold and suprathreshold stimuli, All or none law, definition of absolute and relative refractory period, their mechanisms and importance, how is action potential propagated in unmyelinated and myelinated axons, saltatory conduction, and differences between graded potential and action potential.

CHAPTER 24

Properties, Classification and Applied Aspects of Nerve Fibers

LEARNING OBJECTIVES

On completion of study of this chapter, the student **MUST** be able to:

1. List the properties of nerve fibers.
2. Classify nerve fibers and mention their functions.
3. Describe the degenerative (Wallerian degeneration) and regenerative changes following nerve injury.

The student **MAY** also be able to:

1. Describe the properties of nerve fibers.
2. Classify nerve fibers and mention their functions.
3. Explain the changes in nerve fibers following injury.

PROPERTIES OF NERVE FIBERS

Important properties of the nerve fibers are as follows:

1. Excitability
2. Conductivity
3. Unfatigability
4. Refractory period
5. All-or-none law
6. Summation
7. Accommodation

Refractory period and 'All-or-none law' of nerve fibers have already been described in the previous chapter.

Excitability

Excitability is the property by virtue of which cells or tissues respond to changes in the external or internal environments. It is due to the disturbances in the ionic equilibrium across the receptive zone of cell membrane. The nerve fibers are highly excitable tissues. They respond to various forms of stimuli—mechanical, thermal, chemical or electrical. In experiment set-up, 'electrical' stimulus is usually employed, because its strength and frequency can be accurately controlled, nerves respond well to chemical and thermal stimuli. The production of a wave of depolarization, and (excitation or activation) impulse demonstrates that a nerve has been excited.

Factors Affecting Excitability

1. Strength and duration of the stimulus
2. Effect of extracellular Ca^{++}
   i. Decrease in ECF Ca^{++} increases excitability of neuron by decreasing the amount of depolarization necessary to initiate the changes in the Na^+ and K^+ permeability that produces the action potential.
   ii. Increase in ECF Ca^{++} stabilizes the membrane by decreasing excitability. Ca^{++} entry contributes to depolarization.

Conductivity

On stimulation, action potential is generated in the nerve fiber, which is propagated along its entire length to the axon terminal (described in detail in the previous chapter).

Orthodromic and Antidromic Conduction

An axon can conduct in either direction. If the stimulus is applied in the middle junction of axon, the action potential initiated in the middle of it can travel in both directions, due to set-up of electronic depolarization on either side of the initial current sink.

1. Impulses normally pass from synaptic junction to the axon terminal, which is called ***orhtodromic conduction***.
2. Conduction in the opposite direction is called ***antidromic conduction***, seen in sensory nerve supplying the blood vessels. *Axon reflex* is an example of antidromic conduction.

Summation

Application of a subthreshold stimulus does not evoke an action potential. However, if subthreshold stimuli are applied in rapid succession, they are summated and they produce an action potential. This property is called ***summation***.

Accommodation

Application of continuous stimuli may decrease the excitability of the nerve fiber, a phenomenon called ***accommodation***. More than nerve fiber, it is nerve endings that adapts. This decreases the transmission of impulse across the neurons.

1. If a nerve is submitted to the passage of constant strength of current, the site of stimulation shows decrease in excitability. The accommodation consists of a rise in threshold of the membrane during stimulation
2. A similar feature observed at at nerve endings is called ***adaptation***.
3. Thus, nerve fiber accommodates while the nerve endings adapt.

Unfatigability

Nerve fibers cannot be fatigued, even when they are stimulated continuously. This is because the nerve fibers primarily conduct impulses (propagation of action potential) that do not involve expenditure of energy (ATP).

CLASSIFICATION OF NERVE FIBERS

Based on function, nerves are classified as motor, sensory and secretomotor, and based on myelination, they are classified as myelinated and unmyelinated. Likewise, though there are many classifications of nerve fibers, the most appreciated and popular classification is of **Erlanger and Gasser**, which is based mainly on their diameter and conduction velocity.

Scientists contributed

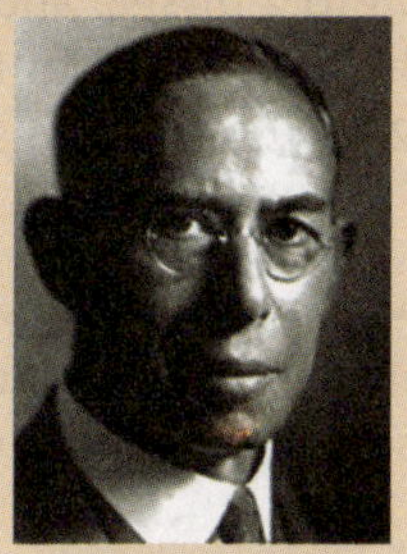

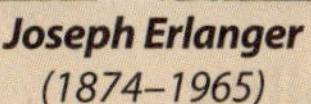

Joseph Erlanger
(1874–1965)

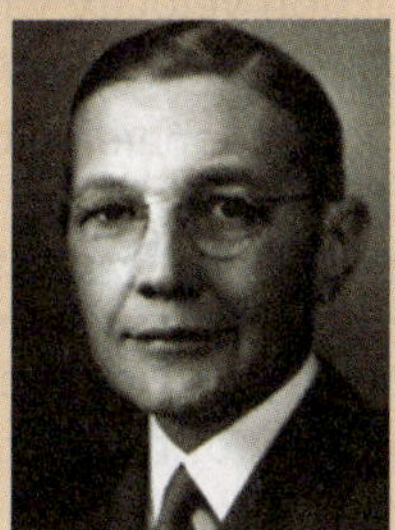

Herbert S. Gasser
(1888–1963)

The **Nobel Prize in Physiology or Medicine for the year 1944** was awarded jointly to two neurophysiologists from USA, **Joseph Erlanger** and **Herbert Spencer Gasser,** *"for their discoveries relating to the highly differentiated functions of single nerve fibers".* They worked extensively on nerve fiber types and the classification of nerve fibers is named after them **'Erlanger-Gasser classification'**).

Erlanger-Gasser Classification

This is the most popular classification of nerve fibers, based on their diameter and conduction velocities. Broadly fibers are classified into three categories: A, B and C.

Type A Nerve Fibers

These are the fastest conducting fibers with conduction velocity ranging from 70 to 120 m/sec. The fiber diameter varies from 12 to 20 µm. Type A fibers are further subdivided into α, β, γ and δ fibers (Table 24.1).

1. **Aα fibers** supply extrafusal fibers in skeletal muscles and also carry proprioception.
2. **Aβ fibers** carry touch pressure sensation and act as motor fibers.
3. **Aγ fibers** supply intrafusal fibers in muscle spindles.
4. **Aδ fibers** are mainly fast conducting nociceptive fibers.

Type B Nerve Fibers

These are preganglionic autonomic afferent and efferent fibers. They have a diameter of less than 3 µm and conduction velocity ranging from 3 to 15 m/sec.

Type C Nerve Fibers

These are unmyelinated fibers. They are subdivided into two broad categories: ***dorsal root fibers*** that carry various

Table 24.1: Classification of nerve fibers.

Fiber types	Fiber diameter (µm)	Conduction velocity (m/s)	Function
Aα	12–20	70–120	Somatic motor and proprioception
Aβ	5–12	30–70	Touch-pressure
Aγ	3–6	15–30	Motor to muscle spindle
Aδ	2–5	12–30	Pain, cold and touch
B	< 3	3–15	Autonomic preganglionic fibers
C-dorsal root fiber	0.4–1.2	0.5–2	Somatic sensations
C-sympathetic fiber	0.3–1.3	0.7–2.3	Postganglionic sympathetic fibers

sensations and have diameter of 0.4 to 1.2 μm and their conduction velocity varies from 0.5 to 2 m/sec, and ***post-ganglionic sympathetic fibers*** with diameter 0.3 to 1.3 μm and conduction velocity of 0.7 to 2.3 m/s (Table 24.1).

Numerical Classification

Sensory nerve fibers are typed into Ia, Ib, II, III and IV. A comparison of the numerical classification and the earlier classification is shown in Table 24.2.

Classification by Susceptibility to Various Agents (Hypoxia, Pressure and Local Anesthetics)

Hypoxia: Type B fibers are most susceptible to hypoxia. Type C is the least susceptible.

Pressure: Type A fibers are most susceptible to pressure and type C is the least. This is because of fiber diameters.

Local anesthetics: Type C fibers are most susceptible to local anesthetics and type A is least susceptible.

APPLIED ASPECTS

Demyelinating Diseases

Multiple Sclerosis

In multiple sclerosis, **patchy loss of axonal myelin** occurs at several areas in the nervous system, resulting in decreased conduction velocity along the fiber.

1. The pathways commonly affected are pyramidal tracts, cerebellar tracts, medial longitudinal fasciculus, optic nerve and posterior columns.
2. The symptoms vary depending on the site of affection. The usual symptoms are **sensory abnormalities** (decreased or abnormal sensations or pain), **muscle weakness**, fatigue, spasticity, optic neuritis, diplopia and ataxia (poor coordination).

Demyelinating Form of GBS

In demyelinating form of Guillain-Barre syndrome, loss of myelin causes abnormal conductions.

Table 24.2: Numerical classification of sensory fibers.

Types	Origin	Fiber types
Ia	Primary spindle afferent from annulospiral ending	Aα
Ib	From Golgi tendon organ	Aα
II	Secondary spindle afferent from flower spray endings Also from touch and pressure receptors	Aβ
III	Mainly from pain and cold receptors	Aδ
IV	Mainly from pain and temperature	C fibers in dorsal root

Nerve Injury

When a nerve is sectioned, the distal part of the nerve separated from the cell body degenerates. This is called ***Wallerian degeneration***. The proximal portion of the axon still attached to the cell body and then develops a growth cone and grows distally toward the distal portion; the changes associated are known as ***regenerative changes***. The soma gets informed about the injury by absence of substances transported retrogradely from the axon terminals.

Scientist contributed

Augustus Volney Waller showed the relation of nerve fibers to nerve cells, by describing peripheral degeneration of nerve fibers after sectioning the main trunk of the nerve, the central stump remaining alive. He experimented neural degeneration changes by making sections of glossopharyngeal and hypoglossal nerves of frog. He is widely known for his description of changes in neurons following injury, which is popularly known as ***Wallerian degeneration***.

Source: Phil. Tr. Royal Society of London 1850; 140: 423-429.

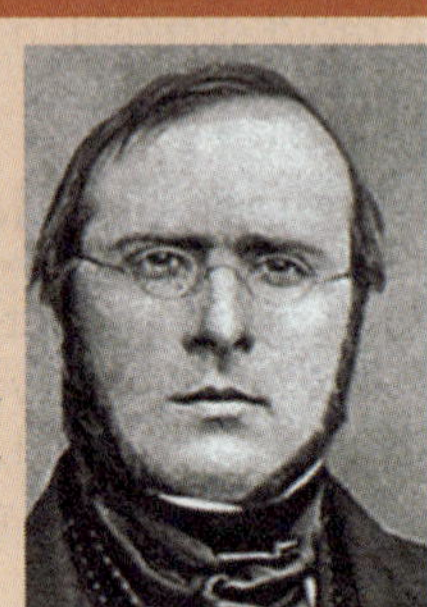

AV Waller
(1816–1870)

Grading of Nerve Injury

Based on severity, nerve injury is typed into **five degrees**:

1. **First-degree injury** is transient loss of function that occurs due to a mild pressure on the nerve. The temporary loss of function is mainly caused by local ischemia following obstruction to the blood flow. Nerve fibers completely recover within few hours to few weeks.
2. **Second-degree injury** includes nerve damage with intact endoneural tube. This occurs due to prolonged pressure on the nerve. The regeneration is delayed but complete as endoneural tube is intact.
3. **Third-degree injury** is the severe damage to the nerve fiber that interrupts endoneural tube.
4. **Fourth-degree injury** refers to a severe damage to the nerve associated with disorganization of nerve fasciculi.
5. **Fifth-degree injury** is the complete transection of the nerve. The degenerative changes occur early.

Degenerative Changes (Wallerian Degeneration)

The degenerative changes occurring in the distal segment of the axon are called ***Wallerian degeneration,*** named after its discoverer August Waller. The changes are as follows (Figs. 24.1A to D):

1. **Transmission of impulse:** Shortly after the injury, synaptic transmission occurring at the axon terminal stops within hours.
2. **Axonal changes:** *The axon swells and the terminals retract from the postsynaptic target*. Gradually, over a period of several weeks, the **axon and all its terminals degenerate**. If the axon is myelinated, round

fatty enlargements form all over the myelin sheath that looks like a series of beads (Fig. 24.1B). The myelin sheath breaks down but the *myelinating cells remain viable* (Schwann cell in the PNS and oligodendrocyte in the CNS). The debris created by the disintegration of the axon and its myelin is devoured by macrophages and Schwann cells in the PNS and microglia in the CNS. The phagocytic process is rapid in the PNS than in the CNS.

3. **Effect of stimulation:** On stimulation, the distal axon can conduct an action potential upto 3 days; this ability is impaired from 3rd to 5th day, and action potential cannot be initiated after the 5th day.
4. **Changes in soma and the stump:** Following injury, degenerative changes are seen in the soma and, to some extent in the proximal stump. These changes are known as ***retrograde degeneration***. The changes are:
   i. Cell body swells and become rounded.
   ii. The nucleus also swells and moves to an eccentric position (Fig. 24.1B).
   iii. Endoplasmic reticulum instead of being closer to the nucleus reassembles around the periphery of the cell body.
   iv. The ribosomes appear disorganized.
   v. The Nissl granules gradually disintegrate and are stained weakly with basic dyes; this is known as ***chromatolysis*** (Fig. 24.1C).

Regenerative Changes

The soma tries to repair the axon by synthesizing new structural proteins that fills up and distends the cisterns of the rough endoplasmic reticulum. This is known as ***axonal reaction***. Chromatolysis is reversible, if the neuron survives and re-establishes its contact with the appropriate target.

Axonal Changes

The proximal end of the axon develops **many sprouts** (Fig. 24.1C).

1. The sprouts elongate by formation of a **growth cone** at their growing ends (Fig. 24.1D).
2. The Schwann cells that had survived the degeneration *multiply* and *form rows* along the pathway previously taken by the disintegrated distal axon.
3. Out of the many sprouting branches, one branch finds the way through the Schwann cells and finally *reinnervates the original target structure*.
4. The regeneration rate of the growing axon is about 1–4 mm/day.
5. The Schwann cells then lay down their bilayered membrane to form the myelin sheath around the newly formed axon.

Somatic Changes

The soma regains its size. The number of Nissl granules slowly reappears. Other organelles also reappear. The cell loses excess fluid and regains its normal size. The nucleus occupies the central position (Fig. 24.1E).

Changes in Target Structure

Following degeneration of the nerve, the neurotransmitter release at axonal terminal decreases.

1. Decreased neurochemical at the synaptic cleft leads to **upregulation of the receptors** in the target structure.

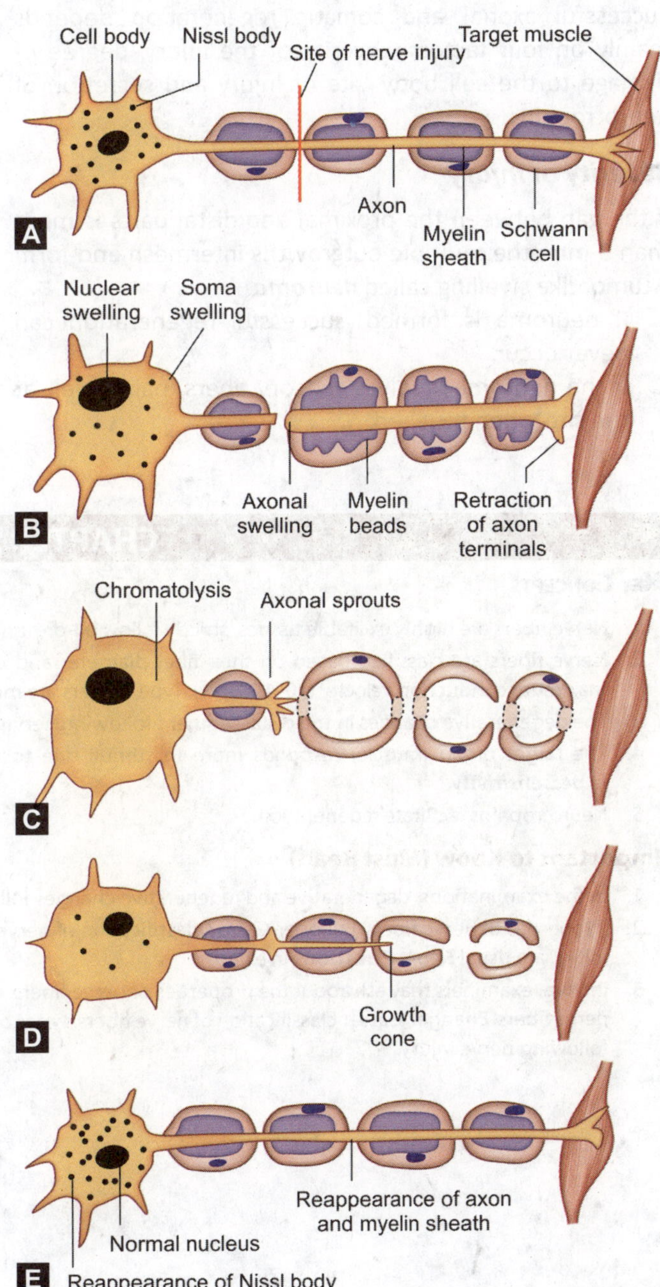

Figs. 24.1A to E: Changes in neuron following nerve injury. (A) Normal neuron indicating the site of axon section; (B) Immediate change depicting swelling of soma, swelling of nucleus, which is eccentrically placed, swelling of axon distal to the section; (C) Continuation of degenerative changes depicting chromatolysis, disappearance of organelles in soma cytoplasm, disintegration of axon and some degeneration of myelin sheath, and beginning of regeneration in the form of sprouting from proximal stump of axon; (D) Regenerative changes with reduction in soma swelling, appearance of few Nissl bodies, development of growth cone and initiation of myelination; (E) Normalization of the soma and axon with re-establishment of axon contact with the target muscle.

2. Therefore, when a neurotransmitter is released following regeneration, the response of the target tissue to the neurotransmitter is increased. This is called ***denervation hypersensitivity*** (for details, refer to next chapter).

Factors Influencing Regeneration

Successful axonal and somatic regeneration depends mainly on four factors: severity of the injury, degree of damage to the cell body, site of injury and secretion of neurotrophins.

Severity of Injury

If the gap between the proximal and distal parts is more than 3 mm, the multiple outgrowths intermesh and form a tumor like swelling called ***neuroma***.

1. If neuroma is formed, successful regeneration can never occur.
2. If the neuroma involves sensory fibers, pain is felt at the site when touched.

Condition of Soma

If the axonal damage is close to the cell body, a lager part of the neuronal membrane and cytoplasm is lost. In such situations, the neuron often dies instead of regenerating.

Location of Injury

In the CNS, a single oligodendroglia sends out many processes to myelinate several (around 15) axons. Therefore, even though the axonal sprouting occurs, the oligodendroglia cannot form a path along which the sprouts can grow. Besides, glial scars formed by astrocytes pose obstruction in the pathway of the growth cone. Hence, axons in the CNS regenerate less successfully than axons in the PNS.

Neurotrophins

When specific neurotrophins are administered to the site of injury, the growth of the regenerating sprout is enhanced and enmeshing of the branches does not occur.

CHAPTER SUMMARY

Key Concepts

1. Nerve fibers are highly excitable tissues, strictly follow all-or-none law, and they do not exhibit fatigability.
2. Nerve fibers are classified based on their fiber diameter and conduction velocity. A fiber has maximum diameter (12–20 µm) and maximum conduction velocity (70–120 m/s). Type C fibers are most susceptible to local anesthetics.
3. The degenerative changes in the distal segment following nerve injury are called ***Wallerian degeneration***.
4. The target organ (muscle) responds more to stimuli due to upregulation of receptors. This phenomenon in called ***denervation hypersensitivity***.
5. Neurotrophins facilitate regeneration.

Important to Know (Must Read)

1. In the examinations, 'degenerative and regenerative changes following nerve injury' may sometimes come as a **Long Question**.
2. 'Properties of nerve fibers, Erlanger-Gasser classification of nerve fibers, Wallerian degeneration, Regenerative changes following nerve injury' are usual **Short Questions** in exams.
3. In **Viva**, examiners may ask about the properties of nerve fibers, definition of refractory period, All-or-none law, types of classification of nerve fibers, Erlanger-Gasser classification of nerve fibers, types of nerve fibers, features of Wallerian degeneration, regenerative changes following nerve injury.

CHAPTER

25

Neuromuscular Transmission

Learning Objectives

On completion of study of this chapter, the student **MUST** be able to:

1. Draw the schematic diagram of neuromuscular junction (NMJ).
2. Describe the events of neuromuscular transmission at presynaptic, synaptic and postsynaptic parts of NMJ.
3. Classify neuromuscular blockers and give their mechanism of action.
4. Name the common disorders of NMJ and give their physiological basis.
5. Understand the mechanism of denervation hypersensitivity.

The student **MAY** also be able to:

1. Explain the physiological basis of etiology, features and treatment of myasthenia gravis and Lambert-Eaton syndrome.

The junction between a motor neuron and a muscle fiber is known as the neuromuscular junction (NMJ). This is also called **myoneural junction** or **motor end plate**, through which action potential from the neuron is transmitted to the muscle fiber. At this junction, the neuronal membrane and the sarcolemma remain apposed to each other, but do not touch.

1. The nerve endings release vesicles containing **acetylcholine** (ACh) that diffuse across the gap and initiates action potential in the muscle fiber.
2. The NMJ is the most extensively studied and best understood synaptic connection in the nervous system where *chemical synaptic transmission was first studied*.
3. It is readily visible under the light microscope, has a relatively simple mechanism and easily accessible to experimentation. Therefore, it is an ideal site for *studying the basic features of chemical transmission*.

STRUCTURE OF NEUROMUSCULAR JUNCTION

The anatomy of neuromuscular junction may be broadly divided into three parts: Presynaptic, synaptic and postsynaptic portions.

Presynaptic Portion (Axon Terminal)

The neurons innervating skeletal muscle fibers are known **as motor neurons** that have their cell bodies in anterior horn of the spinal cord or in the brainstem. Their axons are myelinated and are the *largest-diameter axons in the body*.

The **features of presynaptic portion** of NMJ are:

1. As the axon of motor neuron approaches the muscle fiber, it **loses its myelin sheath** and divides extensively into **several fine branches** of about 2 μm in diameter, called **axon terminals**.
2. The terminals are covered by Schwann cells, known as **teloglia** (glial cells at terminals).
3. Each terminal forms a junction with a single skeletal muscle fiber, midway along its length. Thus, each muscle fiber is supplied by one motor neuron terminal. The motor neuron, including its axon and axon terminals and the muscle fibers supplied by it are called a **motor unit**.
4. Each terminal is expanded at its end to form a knobby structure, called **synaptic knob (terminal button)**, which contains plenty of mitochondria and neurotransmitter vesicles (Fig. 25.1). The terminal button lies in the groove (**synaptic trough**) in the surface of the muscle fiber, but outside the muscle cell membrane. Presence of large number of mitochondria indicates higher metabolic activity at terminal region.

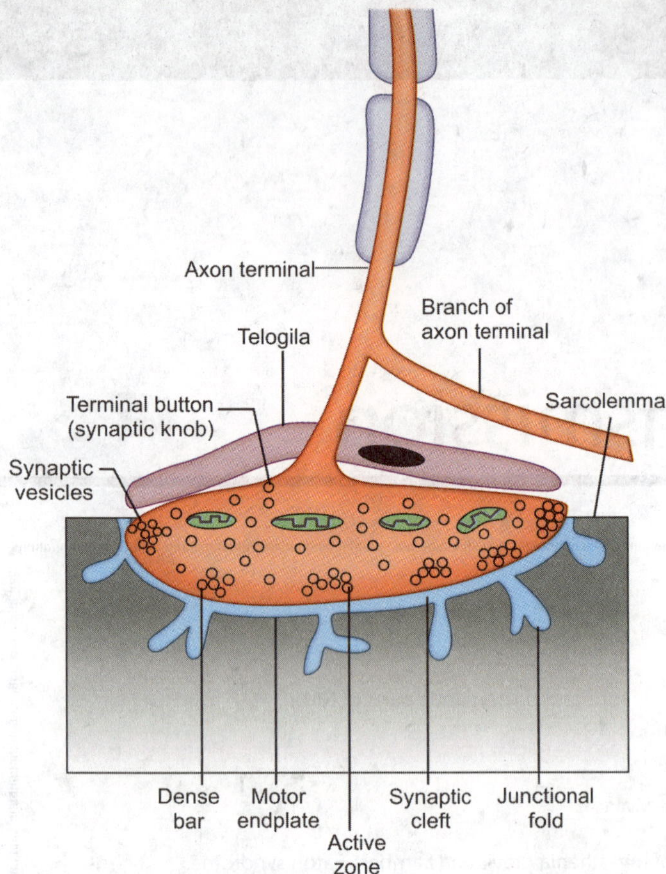

Fig. 25.1: Structure of neuromuscular junction. Note that acetylcholine vesicles are clear vesicles that are clustered at active zones in the terminal buttons opposite to junctional folds. Junctional folds are invagination of motor end plate into the muscle cell that contains more acetylcholine receptors and increase surface area for generation of electrical activities.

5. The vesicles are clustered around specific points called **active zones**. The membrane at the active zones is modified to form **dense bar** that contains numerous **voltage-gated Ca^{++} channels.** These channels mediate ACh release.

Synaptic Cleft

This is the gap between the terminal button and the muscle fiber, which is about 40–100 nm wide.

1. The muscle fiber is covered by a layer of amorphous connective tissue called the **basement membrane** or **basal lamina**, consisting of collagen, glycoproteins and other extracellular matrix proteins.
2. The basement membrane in the cleft contains the enzyme **acetylcholine-esterase** (AChE), which is anchored to the collagen fibrils and is secreted into the basement membrane by the presynaptic terminal and the muscle fiber.
3. AChE rapidly hydrolyzes ACh into acetate and choline. The basal lamina helps organize the presynaptic buttons with the postsynaptic junctional folds.

Postsynaptic Portion (End Plate Membrane)

The postsynaptic portion of the neuromuscular junction is known as the end-plate membrane (**motor end plate**). This is the part of the sarcolemma that lies directly under the terminal button (Fig. 25.1).

1. The area of the end plate membrane increases many times as it is thrown into several folds called **junctional folds.**
2. The endplate membrane contains numerous **ACh receptors** (AchR), which are concentrated at the crests of the junctional folds. It also contains voltage-gated Na^+ channels.

ACh Receptors at NMJ

ACh receptors (AChR) at NMJ are **nicotinic type**. An average end plate contains about 15–40 million AChR, which accounts for about **10,000 AchR per square micrometer** of end-plate membrane.

1. The AChR protein is a **chemically gated ion channel** that undergoes a configurational change and opens when two molecules of Ach bind to it.
2. The channel is **blocked by α-bungarotoxin**.
3. Because of its larger pore diameter (0.8 nm), AChR is permeable to both Na^+ and K^+. But, as the electrochemical gradient is favorable for Na^+ entry, more sodium moves in than potassium coming out resulting in **net Na^+ influx**.
4. AchR allows the **passage of only cations** because the anions are repelled by the fixed negative charges present in it.

MECHANISMS OF NEUROMUSCULAR TRANSMISSION

Neuromuscular transmission (NMT) is the transmission of impulse from the motor neuron to the skeletal muscle fibers supplied by the neuron. Mechanisms involved in NMT are broadly divided into **three parts**: presynaptic events, synaptic-cleft events and postsynaptic events.

Presynaptic Events

The purpose of presynaptic mechanism is to release acetylcholine into the synaptic cleft. This occurs in following steps:

1. Arrival of an action potential at the axon terminal **depolarizes the membrane** of the terminal buttons.
2. This causes activation and **opening of the voltage-gated calcium channels**, which leads to **calcium influx**.
3. Increased cytoplasmic calcium concentration increases movement of microtubules and microfilaments that leads to **migration of neurotransmitter vesicles** to the inner surface of the presynaptic membrane.

4. The vesicles **fuse with the membrane** and discharge their contents into the synaptic cleft by **exocytosis**. Various membrane proteins present in the vesicular membrane as well as in the neuronal membrane are involved in the fusion process. Effective interaction between **synaptobrevin**, a vesicular membrane protein with **syntaxin**, a neuronal membrane protein occurs in the presence of SNAP-25, α/γ SNAP, NSF and many other associated proteins.

Quantal Release

Depolarization of the terminal button causes synchronous releases of about 60–200 vesicles from different parts of the presynaptic membrane. All the vesicles are roughly of the same size. Each vesicle contains around 4000–10,000 Ach molecules.

1. The vesicle or the multimolecular **packet of ACh** is known as **quanta**, and, the process of release is known as **quantal release** of neurotransmitter.
2. With each action potential, the presynaptic terminal discharges about the same amount of neurotransmitter, collectively known as a "quantum of neurotransmitter" or "**quantal content**", which is synonymous with "number of vesicles released".

Scientists contributed

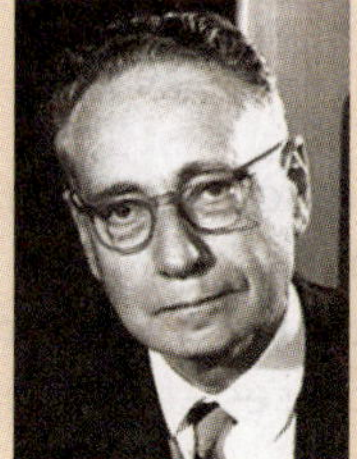

Bernard Katz
_(1911–2003)_

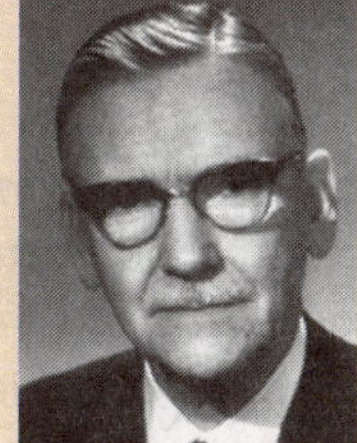

Ulf von Euler
_(1905–1983)_

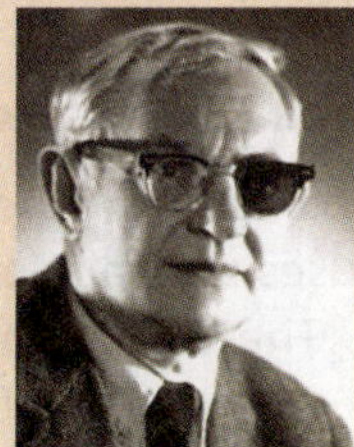

Julius Axelrod
_(1912–2004)_

The **Nobel Prize in Physiology or Medicine 1970** was awarded jointly to **Sir Bernard Katz, Ulf von Euler and Julius Axelrod** *"for their discoveries concerning the humoral transmitters in the nerve terminals and the mechanism for their storage, release and inactivation"*. They contributed to the understanding of synaptic transmission, especially they explained the mechanism of presynaptic events.

Events at the Synaptic Cleft

The released Ach molecules diffuse across the synaptic cleft and **bind to the receptors present at the post-synaptic membrane**.

1. On their way to the end plate membrane, some Ach molecules are **hydrolyzed by AChE**, and some **diffuse out of the synaptic cleft**.
2. However, the amounts that arrive at the end plate region and get bound to AchR, is **sufficient enough** to produce an action potential in the muscle fiber.

Events at the End Plate

The major purpose of postsynaptic mechanism is to **generate action potential in sarcolemma** adjacent to end plate. This occurs in following steps (Flowchart 25.1):

Flowchart 25.1: Major events of neuromuscular transmission.

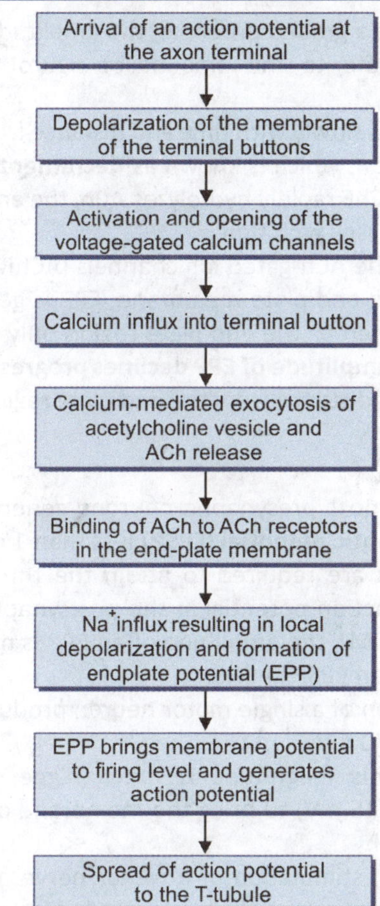

1. The binding of ACh to AChR in the end-plate membrane allows Na^+ influx, producing a rapid local depolarization of the motor end plate known as **end plate potential (EPP)**.
2. EPP decreases the membrane potential to the firing level and opens the voltage-gated Na^+ channels resulting in an **action potential** at the membrane adjacent to the end plate region. The voltage-gated Na^+ channels are present all over the sarcolemma.
3. The action potential propagates along the sarcolemma and T-tubule network, activating the contractile machinery. As the motor end-plate is present at the middle of a muscle fiber, action potential **propagates in both directions**.
4. The binding of ACh to AChR is **loose and reversible**. Soon ACh diffuses away and gets **rapidly hydrolyzed by AChE to acetate and choline**.
5. The action of ACh is terminated leading to **closure of ion channels, cessation of end plate potential** and consequently action potential. The membrane potential of the end plate **returns to the resting state**.
6. The acetate diffuses away into the extracellular fluid and choline is taken up by the presynaptic terminal to be reused for the synthesis of new ACh.

All these events at the neuromuscular junction occur in a **few milliseconds** and can be repeated several times per second without fatigue.

End Plate Potential (EPP)

The EPP is like a graded potential, the amplitude of which is proportionate to the amount of neurotransmitters released.

1. EPP decays slowly with time and distance from the end plate region, which is known as **decremental conduction**. As AChE rapidly hydrolyzes ACh, the amplitude of EPP decreases with time.
2. Because the ACh-gated ion channels (AChR) are localized to the end plate membrane, EPP is generated at and confined to the end plate region only and therefore, the **amplitude of EPP declines progressively** with increasing distance from the end plate region.

EPP vs EPSP

In the CNS, most presynaptic neurons generate **excitatory postsynaptic potential (EPSP)** less than 1 mV, so that several EPSPs are required to attain the threshold and generate an action potential in the postsynaptic neuron. Whereas, in NMJ, the amplitude of an EPP is much larger compared to an EPSP in CNS.

1. Stimulation of a single motor neuron produces an EPP of about 70 mV.
2. EPP of this magnitude is much bigger than that required (15 mV) to bring the membrane potential to firing level.
3. Therefore, stimulation of a motor nerve always produces action potential in each muscle fiber supplied by it; i.e. all the muscle fibers in a motor unit contract in response to discharge of its motor neuron. In skeletal muscle, the **EPP is always a depolarizing potential.**
4. The **EPP rises quickly** resulting in an action potential as soon as the end plate membrane attains threshold level. During intracellular voltage recording, the magnitude of EPP gets flanked by the rising phase of action potential (Application Box 25.1).

The EPP was first recorded in **1950 by Paul Fatt and Bernard Katz** by application of curare to the end plate membrane that blocked the Ach receptors, thereby decreased the amplitude of EPP below threshold level.

Application Box 25.1

Safety factor of EPP: A stimulated motor neuron produces an EPP of about 70 mV. Under normal circumstances, the amount of neurotransmitters released is enough to activate about 10 times the number of receptors required to produce an EPP that can bring the membrane potential to firing level. Due to this 10-fold safety factor, stimulation of a motor neuron never fails to excite an action potential in the muscle fibers of its motor unit. This reserve helps to elicit muscle contraction even in different pathological situations like (i) decrease in number or function of AchR receptors, (ii) decline in the quantity of Ach released, and (iii) abnormal voltage-gated Na^+ channels in the end plate region.

Miniature End Plate Potential

When the motor nerve is at rest, spontaneously occurring potentials of minute amplitude (0.1 to 4 mV) are recorded from the postsynaptic membrane. These potentials are known as **miniature end plate potential** (MEPP).

1. They occur several times a second and have all the properties of an EPP.
2. MEPP occurs due to release of the contents of a single Ach vesicle by exocytosis (**a quantal event**) that opens around 2000 Ach channels in a very small area of the end plate membrane.

BLOCKADE OF NEUROMUSCULAR TRANSMISSION

The neuromuscular transmission is disrupted at different steps by drugs, chemicals, toxins and trauma. Failure to generate required EPP leads to paralysis of the skeletal muscles. The paralysis of the respiratory muscles endangers the life of the patient and has to be taken care of immediately. The drugs causing muscle relaxation are used during surgery and in some hyperactive states. The blockade can occur at presynaptic or postsynaptic level.

Presynaptic Blockade

Interruption of events taking place at the presynaptic axon terminal leads to impaired calcium influx causing decreased vesicle release.

Botulinum Toxins

The bacterium *Clostridium botulinum* releases a toxin that causes a paralytic disease called **botulism.**

1. The botulinum toxin is one of the most potent natural toxins, a minute amount of which causes serious illness.
2. The **lethal dose** for an adult human is around 2 to 3 µg.
3. Botulinum toxin B, D, F and G **inactivate synaptobrevin,** a vesicle membrane protein that is required for the binding and fusion of ACh vesicles with the plasma membrane of the axon terminal.
4. Botulinum toxin A and B **act on SNAP-25** and toxin C **breaks down syntaxin.**
5. Thus, the botulinum toxin inhibits the release of acetylcholine from the axon terminals resulting in cessation of muscle contraction (flaccid paralysis) (Clinical Box 25.1).

Clinical Box 25.1

Clinical Uses of Botulinum Toxin: The paralytic effect of botulinum toxin is utilized for **therapeutic and cosmetic purposes**. Local injections of highly diluted toxin (*botox treatment*) produce muscle relaxation at the desired site. It is injected into the lower esophageal sphincter to treat **achalasia cardia**; into extraocular muscles to decrease their overactivity, which is used in the management of **strabismus** and **blepharospasm**; into facial muscles to reduce aging-related skin wrinkle and is used in cases of **cervical dystonia**. However, it can also be a **lethal bioterrorism agent** by dispersing it as an aerosol or by contaminating the food supply.

Hemicholinium

The drug inhibits choline uptake by the presynaptic terminal resulting in depletion of ACh. Consequently, the EPP decreases and action potential cannot be formed.

Postsynaptic Blockade

A variety of agents can act on the postsynaptic membrane interfering with generation of EPP by different mechanisms. They may be classified into competitive blockers and depolarizing blockers.

Competitive Blockers

Competitive blockers are blockers that block the receptors on postsynaptic membrane. Curare and gallamine are examples of competitive blockers of AChR. These substances diffuse to the end plate membrane and compete with ACh for AChR. Their attachment with AchR does not lead to opening of ion channels, as they do not have the biological activity of ACh. Moreover, they do not get hydrolyzed by AChE. So, the Ach binding sites in the receptors remain occupied permanently. In these conditions, motor nerve releases ACh, but ACh fails to bind to its receptor resulting in absence of EPP and lack of muscle contraction.

Curare

Curare is a plant product used as a South American arrowhead poison for hunting. The animal hit by such arrow suffers from **paralysis in all skeletal muscles** including the respiratory muscles. Consequently, the animal dies of asphyxiation.

Gallamine

Gallamine is given before surgery to **relax the skeletal muscles.**

1. It reduces the required dose of general anesthetic as well as bleeding and other complications.
2. As the respiratory muscles are also relaxed, patients are supported with artificial ventilation.

Depolarizing Blockers

Drugs like **succinylcholine** and **carbamylcholine** have the biological activity of ACh, but they are not hydrolyzed by AChE. Therefore, their action is long lasting. When they bind to AChR, the **ion channels remain open** in the end plate. The maintained depolarization keeps the **voltage-gated Na^+ channels in an inactivated state** and **blocks subsequent action potentials.** There are other drugs that produce the blockade by inactivating AChE reversibly or irreversibly.

Reversible AChE Inhibitors

These agents compete with ACh to bind to AChE, thereby, **prevent the hydrolysis of ACh** by AChE. The accumulated ACh at the synaptic cleft binds to AchR, leading to a **depolarizing block.**

1. This is of use in diseases like myasthenia gravis, where excess ACh is a requirement in the face of decreased AChR.
2. **Neostigmine** and **physostigmine** (eserine) are examples of reversible AChE inhibitors. Their attachment with AchE decreases, when the concentration of the drug falls and so the block is removed after some time.
3. This block can be overcome by application of curare that attaches to AChR and reduces the effect of excess ACh on the end plate membrane.

Irreversible AChE Inhibitors

The **organophosphorous compounds** (pesticides like parathion, malathion and baygon) and **nerve gases** used in chemical warfare like disopropylfluro-phosphate (DFP) and sarin, **bind to AChE very tightly.** This binding is irreversible.

1. Lack of hydrolysis of ACh produces **sustained depolarization** of the end plate resulting in no further contractions in response to subsequent nerve stimulation.
2. Poisoning with these agents lead to skeletal muscle paralysis and death from asphyxiation.
3. Nerve gases also cause accumulation of ACh at the cardiac pacemaker cells. Therefore, in cases of nerve gas exposure, **atropine** (a muscarinic receptor antagonist) **is given as antidote.**

NEUROMUSCULAR DYSFUNCTIONS

Myasthenia Gravis

It is a neuromuscular disorder of **autoimmune nature,** characterized by weakness and fatigability of skeletal muscles that gradually worsens as the muscles are used.

Etiology

Myasthenia gravis results from a **decrease in the number of AChR** present on the motor end plate due to production of **circulating autoantibodies** against these receptors (Figs. 25.2A and B). Moreover, the **postsynaptic folds are flattened**, or simplified. Due to these changes, though **ACh is released normally**, the magnitude of the end plate potential falls below the threshold for initiating a muscle action potential.

The anti-AChR antibodies have following **three major functions**:

i. They compete with Ach to bind to AChR, producing receptor blockade.
ii. They induce endocytosis of AChR.
iii. They damage the postsynaptic membrane.

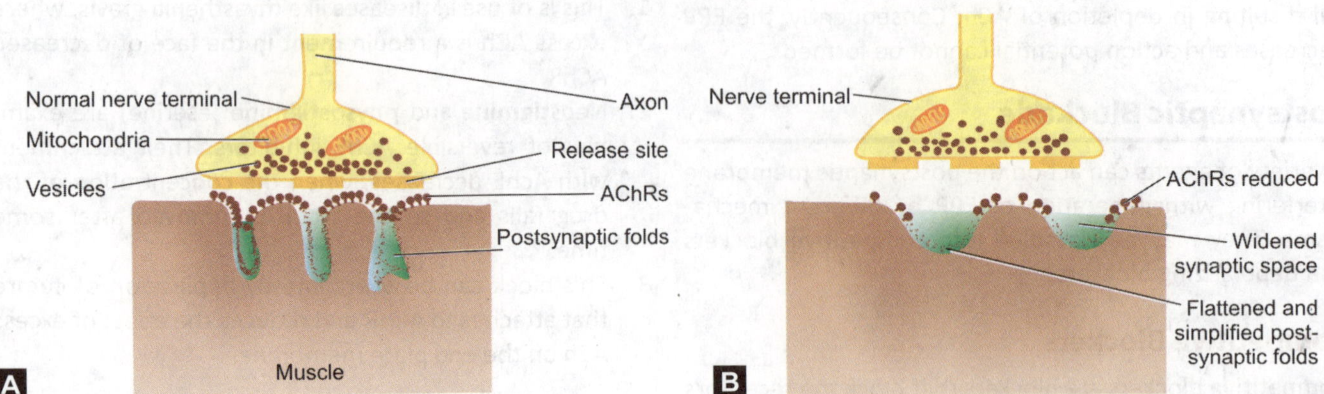

Figs. 25.2A and B: Neuromuscular transmission in normal (A), and in myasthenia gravis (B). In myasthenia gravis, number of AChR is reduced, postsynaptic folds are flattened and simplified, and synaptic space is widened.

Features

1. **Fatigue:** Normally, on repeated stimulation of the motor nerve, the amount of ACh released per action potential gradually decreases (**presynaptic rundown**). But the amount is enough to generate an EPP well above the threshold level. In myasthenic patients, due to the postsynaptic changes along with the presynaptic rundown, after a few motor nerve impulses, the successive contractile responses become feebler, causing **fatigue**. So there is **decremental response to repetitive nerve stimulation** on EMG recording from the affected muscle.
2. **Women are affected more** than men in a ratio of 3:2.
3. The **muscle weakness** increases during prolonged use of the muscle and improves after rest or sleep. Thus, the patient feels better in the morning, but **symptoms aggravate toward evening** or after exertion.
3. The **extraocular muscles and eyelids are often involved** early in the course of the diseases. Therefore, **diplopia and ptosis** (drooping of eyelids) are early symptoms (Fig. 25.3).
4. Proximal limb muscles are commonly affected. In severe cases, respiratory muscle paralysis leads to death.

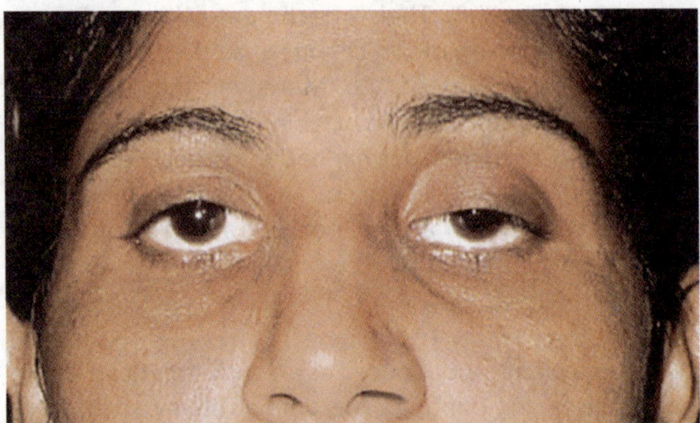

Fig. 25.3: Ptosis (as seen in myasthenia gravis). The left eye is more affected than the right eye of this female.
Courtesy: Figure 15.33A, Comprehensive Ophthalmology, 6th edition, 2015, by A. K. Khurana; Jaypee Brothers Medical Publishers (P) Ltd.

Physiological Basis of Treatment

Current modalities of treatment are as follows.

1. **Administration of AChE inhibitors:** Examples of these drugs are **pyridostigmine and neostigmine**. They increase the concentration of ACh at the neuromuscular junction.
2. **Thymectomy:** Recently it has been observed that immune responses mediated by **T cells** are part of the pathophysiologic mechanisms. Thymectomy is therefore helpful. It blunts down the immune response and improves the condition.
3. **Immunosuppression:** Immunosuppressive drugs glucocorticoids and azathioprine are useful. They inhibit the immunological mechanisms.
4. **Plasmapheresis:** Plasmapheresis removes AChR antibodies from plasma.

Lambert-Eaton Myasthenic Syndrome

It is a presynaptic disorder of the neuromuscular junction due to production of **autoantibodies against voltage-gated Ca^{++} channels**. The decreased Ca^{++} influx in the presynaptic axon terminals results in impaired ACh release from the nerve endings. The muscular weakness is primarily seen in the limb muscles. Patients show **incremental response to repetitive nerve stimulation** as Ca^{++} level raises with each action potential. Thus, with prolonged contractions, muscle strength increases.

NERVE ENDINGS IN SMOOTH AND CARDIAC MUSCLES

The smooth and cardiac muscle cells are innervated by autonomic nervous system. There are no well-defined end plate regions or precise synaptic terminals.

1. Especially in smooth muscles, the neurotransmitter vesicles are present in dilated areas of the axon all along its length. These dilated portions (swellings) are known as **varicosities** (Fig. 25.4).
2. On stimulation of the neuron, the neurotransmitters are released and then diffused to the adjacent muscle fibers, initiating action potentials in many fibers simultaneously.

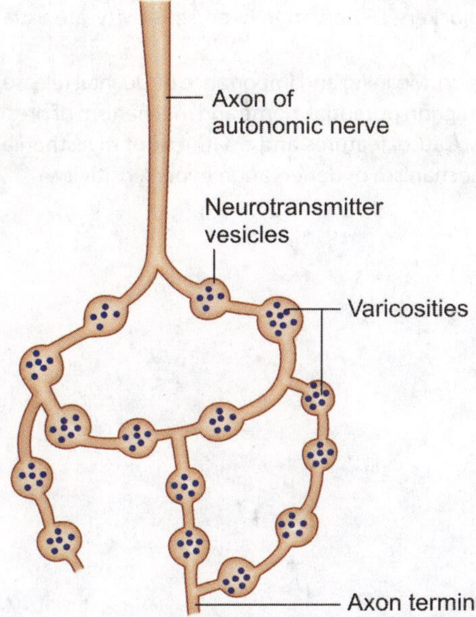

Fig. 25.4: Termination of autonomic neurons on smooth muscles. Note axon does not end in a typical neuromuscular junction, rather the axon has numerous dilations (varicosities) at the axon terminal. These varicosities contain neurotransmitters.

3. In a noradrenergic nerve, there can be as many as 20,000 varicosities per neuron. This type of synaptic arrangement is called **synapse en passant**.
4. The depolarizing potentials produced in the smooth muscle cells are known as **excitatory junction potentials** (EJPs).
5. EJPs are like graded potentials and can be summated. The hyperpolarizing potentials produced in the smooth muscle cells are known as **inhibitory junction potentials** (IJPs).

DENERVATION HYPERSENSITIVITY

When a neuron is cut and the distal axon degenerates, the target tissue innervated by its synaptic terminals becomes more reactive to the neurotransmitter secreted at the nerve endings. This **phenomenon of increased responsiveness** is known as **denervation hypersensitivity**. This is *seen in both skeletal and smooth muscles*. Due to degeneration of the nerve endings, the chemical is no more released from the terminals. The tissue reacts to the neurotransmitter present in the circulation, where concentration of the chemical is lower than at the synaptic endings.

The hypersensitivity occurs due to **three reasons**:

1. **Increased number of receptors** at the postsynaptic membrane (**up-regulation**). Both number and distribution of receptors increase. For example, after degeneration of the motor nerve, the AChR appears all over the sarcolemma (Fig. 25.5B), whereas normally it is confined to the end plate region only (Fig. 25.5A).
2. **Increased responsiveness** (sensitivity) of receptors to the chemical.
3. In case of noradrenergic neurons, the reuptake of neurotransmitter molecules by the presynaptic terminals is decreased resulting in **higher plasma noradrenaline concentration.**

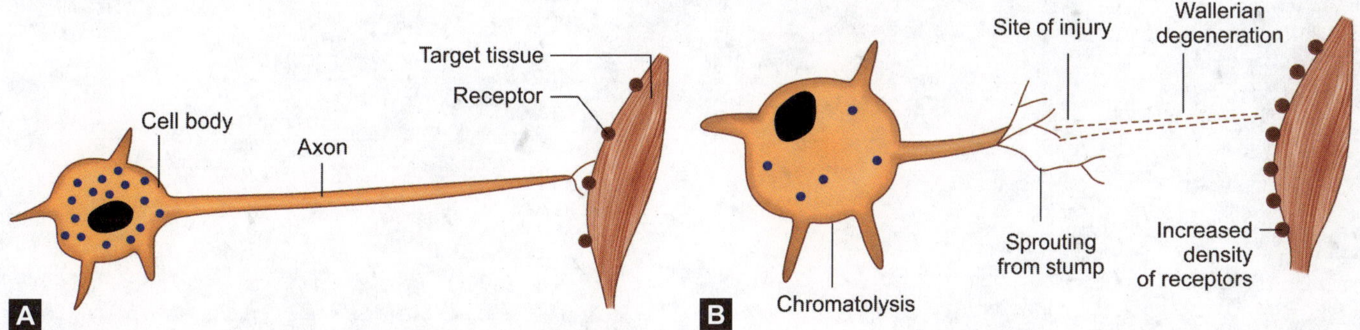

Figs. 25.5A and B: Denervation hypersensitivity following nerve injury. Note the increased density of receptors in the target tissue that increases responsiveness of the tissue to the neurotransmitter.

CHAPTER SUMMARY

Key Concepts

1. Arrival of an action potential at the axon terminal causes opening of the voltage-gated calcium channels, and causes calcium influx. Calcium mediated exocytosis of neurotransmitter vesicles is facilitated by membrane proteins synaptobrevin and syntaxin
2. Binding of Ach to AChR causes Na^+ influx that leads to genesis of end plate potential (EPP).
3. EPP at threshold causes activation of voltage-gated Na^+ cannels causing influx that causes genesis of muscle fiber action potential.
4. Botulinum toxin causes presynaptic blockade and curare causes postsynaptic blockade (competitive blockade of AChR) of neuromuscular transmission.
5. Myasthenia gravis results from a decrease in the number of AChR present on the motor end plate due to production of circulating autoantibodies against these receptors.
6. When the distal axon degenerates, the target tissue innervated by its synaptic terminals becomes more reactive to the neurotransmitter secreted at the nerve endings, which is known as denervation hypersensitivity. This is due to increased number of receptors as well as sensitivity of receptors to chemicals.

Important to Know (Must Read)

1. In examinations, 'Structure of NMJ and Neuromuscular transmission' usually come as a **Long Question**.
2. Mechanism of neuromuscular transmission, end-plate potential, Neuromuscular blockers, Denervation hypersensitivity, are usual **Short Questions** in exams.
3. In **Viva**, examiners may ask...... Structure of NMJ, Steps of neuromuscular transmission, Meaning and importance of Quantal release, role of syntaxin and synaptobrevin, Features of end-plate potential, and how it differs from action potential, Name and mechanism of presynaptic blocker, Name and mechanism of post-synaptic blocker, Neuromuscular blockers, Cause, features and treatment of myasthenia gravis, Special feature of autonomic innervation in smooth muscle, and Definition and mechanism of denervation hypersensitivity.

CHAPTER 26

Structure of Skeletal Muscle: Physiological Aspects

Learning Objectives

On completion of study of this chapter, the student **MUST** be able to:

1. Understand the organization of muscle fibers and fibrils in skeletal muscle.
2. Name the contractile proteins in the skeletal muscle and give their functions.
3. Draw the labeled diagram of sarcomere.
4. Draw the picture of sarcotubular system (STS) and give function of each component of STS.

The student **MAY** also be able to:

1. Describe the details muscle proteins.
2. Describe the role of STS in muscle contraction and relaxation.

For muscle contraction, muscles use chemical energy to generate force. All muscles transduce a chemical or electrical command into a mechanical response. The trigger for muscle contraction is the rise in free cytosolic Ca^{++} concentration. However, on the basis of structure, metabolism, control mechanisms and contractile properties like rate and duration of contraction, fatigability and the ability to regulate contractile strength, muscles can be classified into three types:

1. Skeletal muscle
2. Smooth muscle
3. Cardiac muscle.

Skeletal muscle, as the name implies, is attached to the skeleton (bones). Its contraction supports and moves the skeleton (through joint movements). The contraction in skeletal muscle is mostly under voluntary control and is initiated by discharge of the motor neuron supplying it. Skeletal muscle is capable of rapid force development and shortening. It can maintain contractile force for relatively longer periods.

STRUCTURE OF SKELETAL MUSCLE

A typical skeletal muscle contains many **muscle bundles or fascicles**. Each fascicle consists of large number of muscle fibers arranged parallel to each other (Figs. 26.1A and B). Connective tissue layers in the muscle bundles are epimysium, perimysium and endomysium (Fig. 26.2).

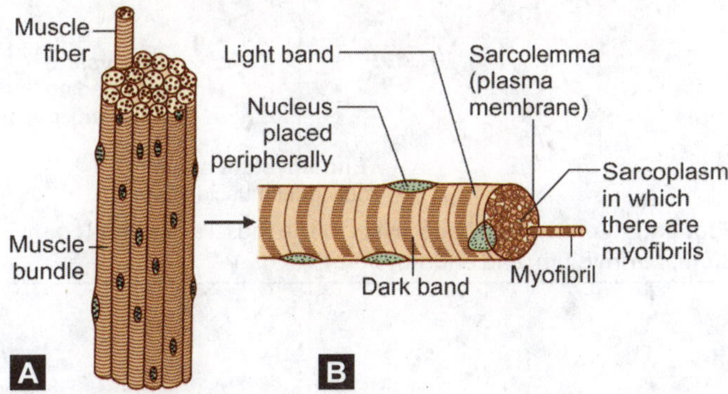

Figs. 26.1A and B: Structure of skeletal muscles. (A): Muscle bundle; (B) Muscle fiber.

1. The connective tissue layer around the muscle is called **epimysium**.
2. The layer covering each fascicle is known as **perimysium**.
3. The layer surrounding each muscle fiber is termed as **endomysium**.

The blood vessels and nerves supplying the muscle fibers are present within the perimysium. All the three layers are made up of **collagen and elastin** that helps to transmit the force from the muscles to the bones. Muscles are usually attached to bones by collagen fibers known as tendons.

Myocyte

The structural unit of muscle is muscle fiber that is a single skeletal muscle cell (myocyte). The cell membrane of myocyte is known as ***sarcolemma*** and the cytoplasm as ***sarcoplasm*** (Fig. 26.1B).

1. The muscle fibers are long, cylindrical, ***multinucleated cells***, extending the entire length of the muscle, and attach to tendons at both ends.
2. They are 10–100 µm in diameter and may extend up to 20 cm in length.
3. In embryonic fibers, the nuclei are centrally placed; but following differentiation after birth, they lie beneath the sarcolemma, hence peripherally placed (Fig. 26.3A).

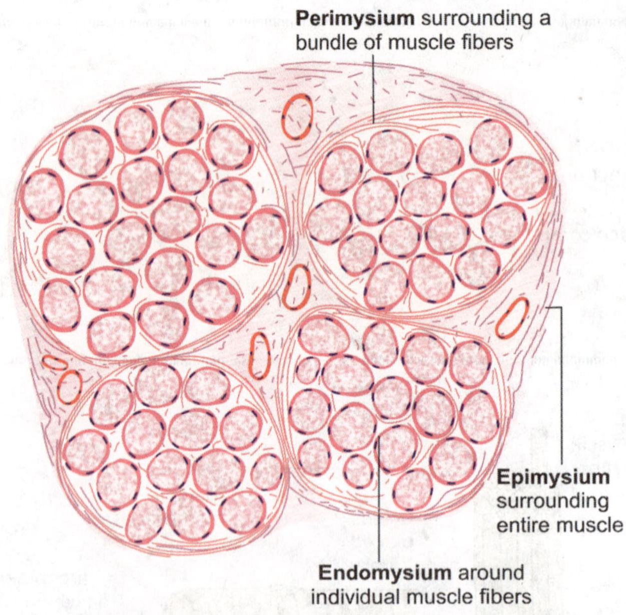

Fig. 26.2: Connective tissue layers in the muscle bundles (epimysium, perimysium, and endomysium).

The **important functions of sarcolemma** are:

1. It **transmits the wave of depolarization** originating at the motor end plate over the entire cell surface to initiate contraction.
2. Besides shielding the muscle fiber, the sarcolemma contributes to the parallel **elastic resistance,** i.e. the resistance to stretch offered by all the connective tissue layers.
3. It has *no gap junctions or tight junctions*, thereby promotes **electrical separation** between fibers.

Myofibrils and Organelles

Characteristically, the sarcoplasm is filled with myofibrils that extend along the axis of the cell and are connected to the tendons at both ends of the muscle fiber.

1. Each myofibril is 1 µm in diameter and consists of cylindrical bundles of two types of **myofilaments** that are referred to as thick and thin filaments.
2. The sarcoplasm contains the usual cytoplasmic organelles including mitochondria (sarcosomes), sarcoplasmic reticulum, and Golgi apparatus.

Development of Myocytes

The muscle fibers are formed during fetal development by the fusion of a number of undifferentiated, mono-nucleated cells, known as **myoblasts.**

1. At the time of birth, the **differentiation of skeletal muscle fibers is complete**. These differentiated fibers continue to increase in size during growth from infancy to adulthood, but ***no new fibers are formed*** from myoblasts.
2. After birth, following destruction of skeletal muscle due to any cause, the existing muscle fibers do not divide to replace the damaged fibers. Instead, *new fibers are formed by differentiation* of **satellite cells** that are located in the adjoining myocytes.

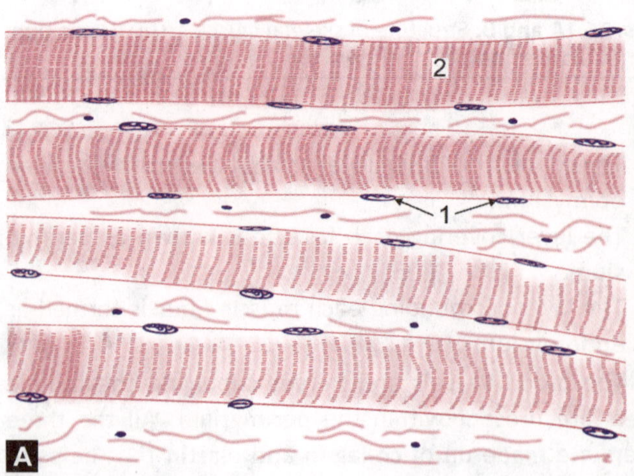

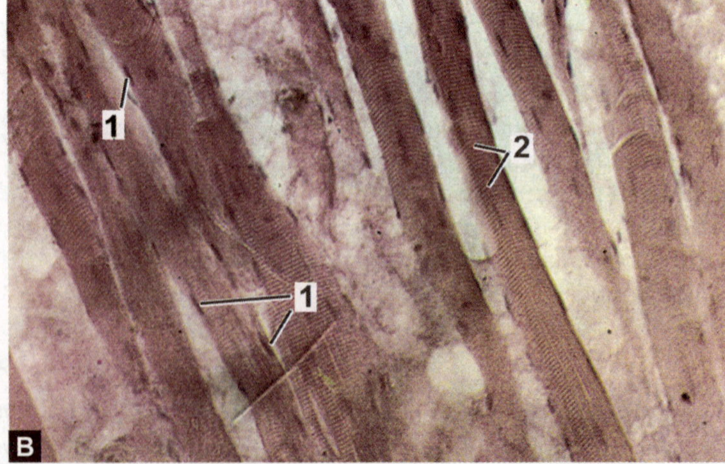

Figs. 26.3A and B: Longitudinal section through skeletal muscle showing multinucleate myocytes (A) and photomicrograph showing transverse striations (B). 1. Peripherally placed nuclei; 2. Transverse striations.

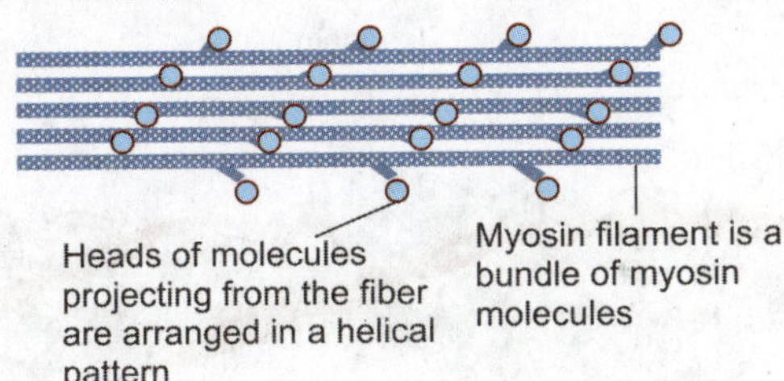

Fig. 26.4: Structure of myosin filament. Note, heads of myosin molecules project out and arranged in a helical manner.

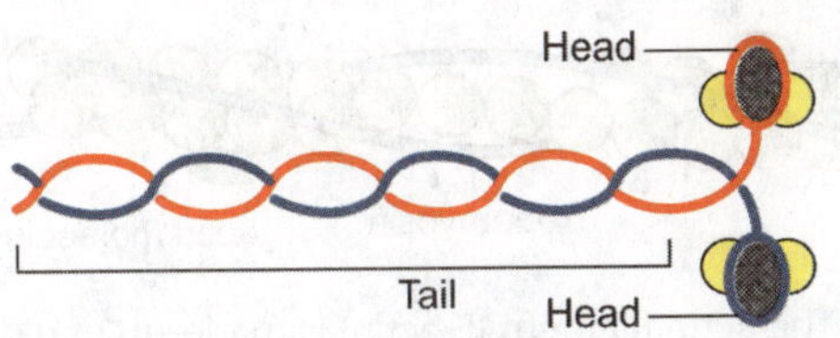

Fig. 26.5: Structure of myosin molecule. Note, the joining region between head and tail is called the hinge.

3. Though the satellite cells are capable of forming a large number of new muscle fibers, that may not be adequate enough to restore a severely damaged muscle to its full strength. In such situations, *hypertrophy* (increase in cell size) *of the remaining muscle fibers usually compensates for the loss.*
4. Recently, it has been demonstrated that a transcription factor called **myogenin** stimulates fibroblasts to become muscle cells.

Striations: The most striking feature of skeletal muscle is the **presence of striations** due to alternate light and dark bands throughout the length of the fiber as seen through a light microscope (Fig. 26.3B).

1. The dark band is also called **A band** because it is *anisotropic to polarized light.*
2. The light band is known as **I band** because it is *isotropic to polarized light* (refer to Fig. 26.1B).

Each myofibril is made up of units called **sarcomere** that contains different muscle proteins (*see* below).

Muscle Proteins

There are **three types of proteins** in skeletal muscle:

1. **Contractile proteins:** myosin and actin
2. **Regulatory proteins:** troponin and tropomyosin
3. **Attachment proteins:** titin, nebulin, alpha actinin, desmin, myomesin, and dystrophin

Contractile Proteins

There are two contractile proteins in skeletal muscle: **myosin and actin**.

Myosin

There are thick and thin filaments in muscle. The **thick filaments are polymers of myosin II** (MW 480,000). Myosin filament is a bundle of myosin molecules. The head of myosin molecules projects from the filaments that are arranged in a helical manner (Fig. 26.4). The filament is composed of following units:

1. Two intertwined heavy chains,
2. Two regulatory light chains, and
3. Two alkali (essential) light chains.

The myosin II has **three regions**: two globular heads, neck (hinge region) and a long tail (Fig. 26.5).

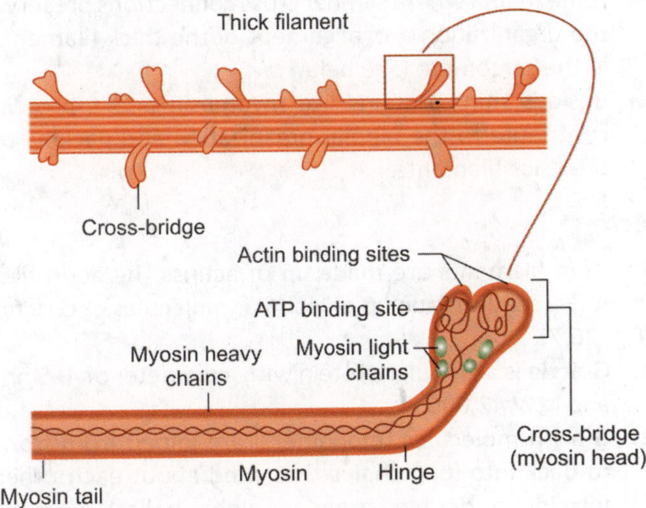

Fig. 26.6: Structure of myosin II molecule.

Myosin Head

Each head is made up of amino terminal portions of one heavy chain forming a complex with two light chains, one regulatory and one alkali.

1. The myosin head contains **two binding sites**, one for actin and one for ATP (Fig. 26.6).
2. The **ATP binding site** functions as an ATPase (hydrolyzes ATP).
3. The carboxy terminals of the heavy chains coil around each other in an alpha-helical configuration forming a long rod-like tail.
4. The **alkali light chain** stabilizes the myosin head and the **regulatory light chain** regulates its ATPase activity.

Myosin Tail

The tail of each myosin molecule lies along the axis of the thick filament, and the two globular heads extend out to the sides, forming the **cross-bridges**.

Myosin Hinge

In the hinge region, the tail joins the globular head.

Arrangement of myosin molecules: The myosin molecules aggregate with a definite directional arrangement, such that their **tail-ends are directed toward the center** of the thick filaments creating a bare region in the middle consisting of myosin tails only, while the **globular heads point away from both sides** of the tail.

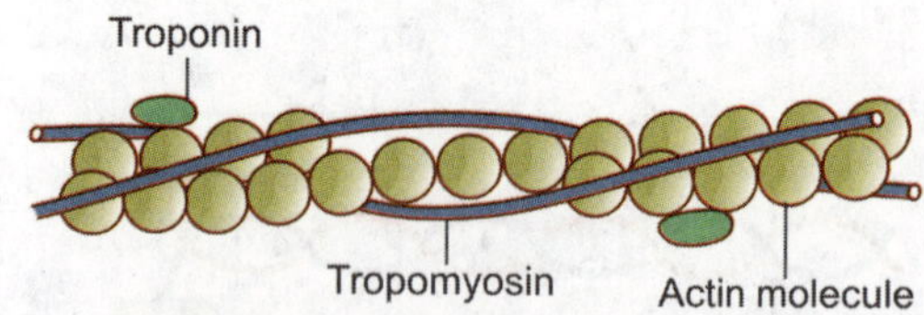

Fig. 26.7: The actin filament (F-actin) is made-up of globular molecules of G-actin.

1. The site of the reversal of polarity of myosin molecules is the **M line** where slender cross connections preserve the organization and alignment of the thick filaments in the sarcomere (*See* below).
2. Besides titin, proteins like myomesin and C-protein contribute to the bipolar organization and packing of the thick filaments.

Actin

The thin filaments are made up of actins. The actin filament (F-actin) is made up of globular molecules of G-actin (Fig. 26.7).

1. **G-actin** is a globular protein with a diameter of 4–5 nm and MW 42,000.
2. G-actin molecules (monomers) are joined from front to back into long chains that wind about each other forming a double stranded alpha helical filament known as **F-actin** (or filamentous actin) that forms the backbone of the thin filament.
3. The cytoskeletal protein **nebulin** extends along the length of the F-actin and plays a role in the regulation of the length of the thin filament.
4. Each actin monomer contains ***binding sites*** for myosin, tropomyosin, troponin I, and other actin monomers.
5. As the F-actin undergoes a half-turn every seven G-actin monomers, a groove is formed down the length of the helix where lies the long, filamentous protein *tropomyosin*.
6. Each thin filament contains 300–400 actin molecules and 40–60 tropomyosin molecules.

Regulatory Proteins

Regulatory proteins are **tropomyosin and troponin.**

Tropomyosin

Tropomyosin is a rod-shaped molecule (MW 70,000) composed of **two strands of polypeptides** intertwined in an alpha helical configuration with a ***length approximately equal to seven actin monomers***. It is located in the groove between two chains of actin (Fig. 26.8).

1. The tropomyosin molecules are connected to one another serially that extends over the entire actin filament covering myosin-binding sites on the actin monomers.
2. The function of tropomyosin is to *interfere with the binding of myosin head to actin*.

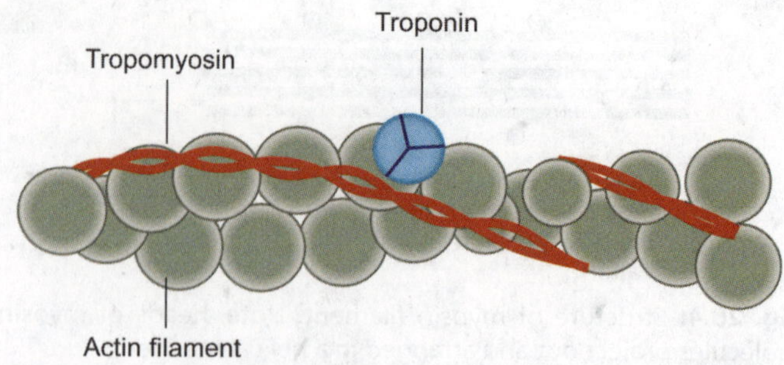

Fig. 26.8: Structure of tropomyosin and troponin. Note the double helical structure of tropomyosin and three component (I, T, C) of troponin.

Troponin

Troponin is a complex of three proteins: Troponin T, Troponin I, and Troponin C (Fig. 26.8)

Troponin T

Troponin T has molecular weight 30,000. It binds the troponin complex to tropomyosin.

Troponin I

Troponin I (MW 22,000) binds the troponin complex to actin. It is called I, because it inhibits the binding of actin to myosin by blocking the myosin binding site on actin.

Troponin C

Troponin C (MW 18,000) binds to calcium.

Note:

Interaction of troponin with tropomyosin: Each troponin complex interacts with one tropomyosin molecule, which in turn interacts with seven actin monomers. The troponin complex also interacts directly with the actin filaments. Troponin is known as the regulatory protein in the contraction of skeletal muscle.

Attachment Proteins

Titin

It is a large, elastic, filamentous, cytoskeletal protein, which extends from the Z line to the M line. It provides framework for the thick filaments by connecting the Z line to the M line. It *prevents overextension of the thick filaments* and maintains the central location of the A band.

Nebulin

This is a large, filamentous protein that extends along the length of the thin filaments. It is believed to play a role in *stabilizing the length of the actin filaments* during muscle development.

Alpha Actinin

Alpha actinin anchors the thin filaments to the Z line.

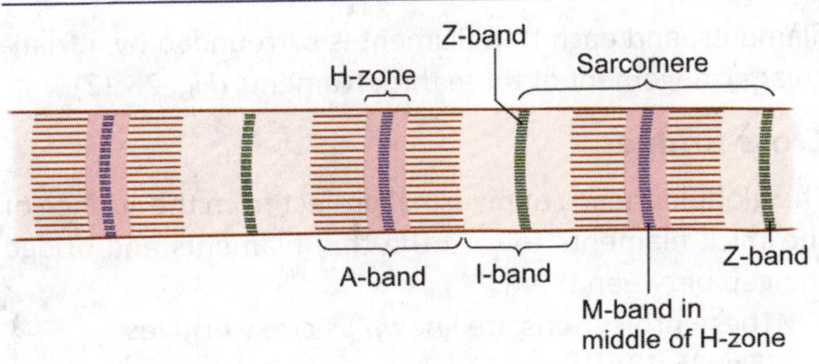

Fig. 26.9: Arrangement of sarcomere in a myofibril. Note, light band is I band and dark band is A band.

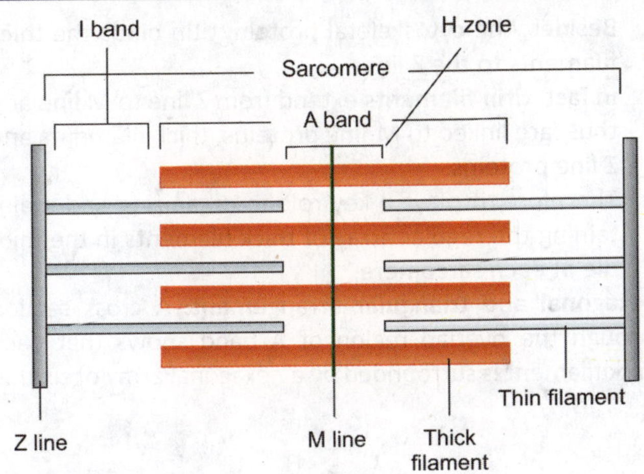

Fig. 26.10: Structure of sarcomere.

Desmin

Desmin is present in the intermediate filament of cytoskeleton of myocyte. It connects the Z line to the sarcolemma. It also connects myofibrils to each other.

Dystrophin

It is a large rod like protein that anchors the thin filaments to the membrane spanning protein **beta-dystroglycan**, which in turn is connected to the extracellular matrix protein **laminin** through alpha-dystroglycan.

1. Dystrophin helps in *transfer of force from the contractile system to extracellular regions* through the transmembrane proteins.
2. These proteins are disrupted in the group of genetic diseases called **muscular dystrophy**.
3. Absence of these proteins or their mutations leads to muscle degeneration, weakness and even death.

Myomesin

It is present in the region of M disc. It binds the tail end of myosin filament to the disc.

Sarcomere

Sarcomere (in Greek; *sarco* means muscle, and *mer* means part) is the structural and functional unit of myofibril. A single myofibril may be composed of hundreds or thousands of sarcomeres that are joined end-to-end. In each myofibril, thick and thin filaments are arranged in a repeating pattern in the form of sarcomere (Fig. 26.9).

1. Sarcomere is **defined** *as the portion of the muscle fibril between two successive Z lines.*
2. The ***average length*** of a sarcomere is **2 µm**.

Structure

Electron micrographic studies reveal the detailed structure of sarcomere (Fig. 26.10).

Z Line

The Z line or **Z disc** is a network of interconnecting proteins. It is oriented perpendicular to the axis of the muscle fiber. The thin filaments are anchored to the two sides of each Z line by **alpha actinin**.

Thin Filament

Each thin filament is **1 µm long and 7 nm in diameter**.

1. It is composed of the contractile proteins actin, tropomyosin, and troponin in a ratio of 7:1:1.
2. From the Z line, the thin filaments project in parallel arrays toward the center of the sarcomere where they overlap a portion of the thick filaments.
3. Thus, each sarcomere contains **two sets of thin filaments**, one at each end. The Z disc not only binds the thin filaments of a single myofibril together, but connections between the Z discs also anchor each myofibril to its neighbors.

Thick Filament and A Band

The parallel array of thick filaments located in the middle of each sarcomere produces **A band**.

1. The thick filament is **1.6 µm long and 10 nm in diameter**.
2. It consists of the protein myosin (*see* above).

I Band

I band lies between the ends of A bands of two adjacent sarcomeres and includes those portions of the thin filaments that do not overlap the thick filaments. The Z line bisects I band.

1. During muscle contraction, the length of the sarcomere (the distance between two Z lines) decreases. This results in shortening of I band but, length of A band remains unchanged (Fig. 26.11).
2. Thus, **sarcomeric length is decided by the length of I band.**

H Band

H band (H zone) is a narrow, light band in the center of A band. This is the portion of A band showing no overlap (represented by thick filaments only) as can be seen in a relaxed muscle.

M Line

A transverse M line runs through the middle of H band. The M line contains proteins that bind the parallel array of thick filaments.

1. Besides, the cytoskeletal protein, titin binds the thick filaments to the Z lines.
2. In fact, **titin filaments** extend from Z line to M line and thus, are linked to M-line proteins, thick filaments and Z line proteins.
3. Therefore, it plays a key role in organizing and maintaining the regular array of thick filaments in the middle of each sarcomere.

Hexagonal and triangular arrangement: A cross section through the overlap region of A band shows that each thick filament is surrounded by a hexagonal array of six thin filaments, and each thin filament is surrounded by a triangular arrangement of three thick filaments (Fig. 26.12).

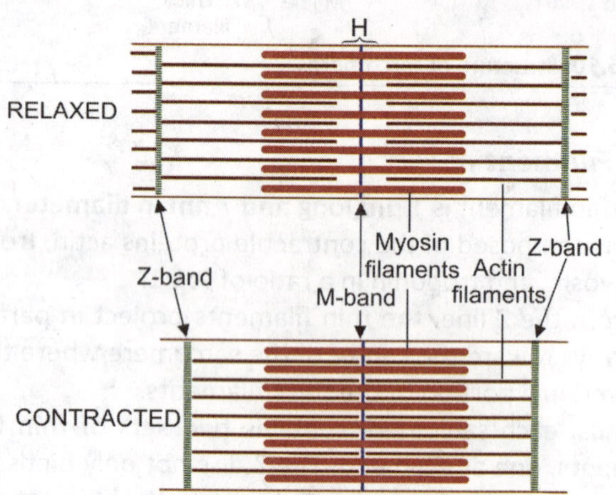

Fig. 26.11: State of sarcomere in muscle contraction. Note, the length of I band decreases (without change in A band) during contraction that decreases in sarcomeric length.

Cross-Bridges

The globular heads of myosin II project from the surface of the thick filaments toward the thin filaments and bridge the gap between them.

1. These projections are known as **cross-bridges** (Fig. 26.13).
2. During muscle contraction, they attach to the thin filaments and pull them.

Sarcotubular System

Inside a muscle fiber, fibrils are surrounded by membranous structures known as sarcotubular system. The relationship of sarcotubular system with the I and A bands of sarcomere in a myofibrils is shown in Figure 26.14.

Structure

It consists of sarcoplasmic reticulum and T (transverse) tubules (Fig. 26.15).

T-tubules

The T-tubules, also called **sarcotubules** are tubular extensions of the sarcolemma, about 0.03 µm in diameter.

1. They penetrate to the center of the muscle fiber and surround the individual myofibrils at the junctions of A and I band.

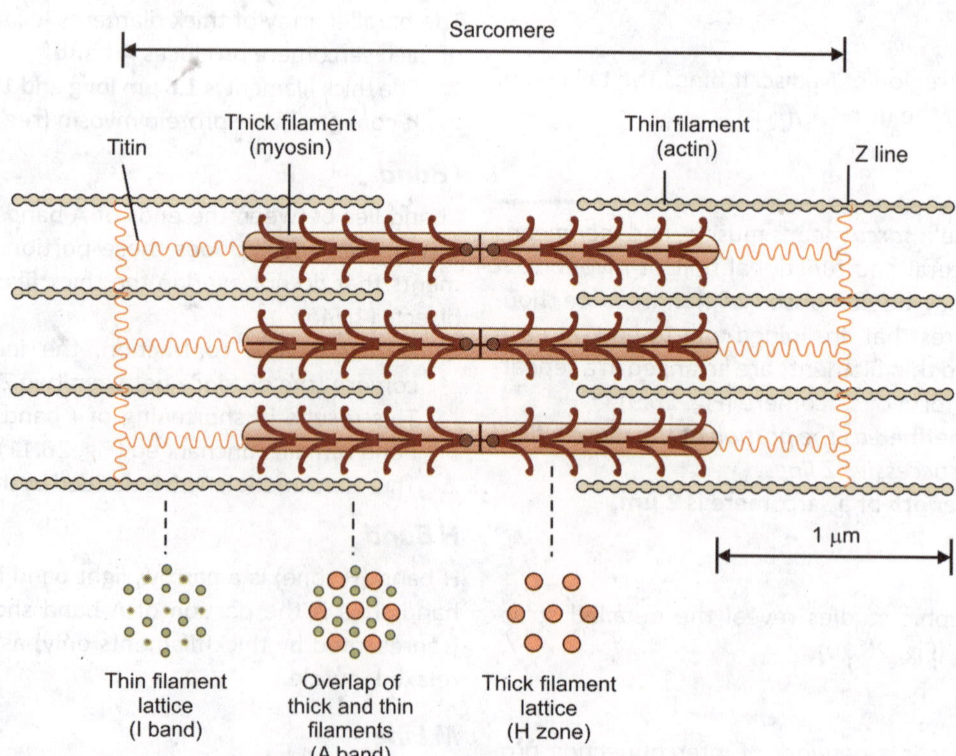

Fig. 26.12: Hexagonal and triangular arrangement of thin and thick filaments. A cross section through the overlap region of A band shows that each thick filament is surrounded by a hexagonal array of six thin filaments, and each thin filament is surrounded by a triangular arrangement of three thick filaments.

2. The lumen of the T tubule contains extracellular fluid, which is a continuation of the ECF surrounding the muscle fibers.
3. Once initiated, an ***action potential is rapidly conducted*** along the sarcolemma over the surface of the muscle fiber as well as into the interior of the muscle cell by the way of the T-tubules so that deep lying myofibrils are fast activated.

Sarcoplasmic Reticulum

The sarcoplasmic reticulum (SR) in skeletal muscle corresponds to the endoplasmic reticulum found in other cells.

1. It forms an elaborate **membranous network** having extensive anastomosis around each myofibril and runs parallel to the myofilaments.
2. The slender tubules, about 0.04 µm in diameter, have an elongated portion in the middle and dilated region at both ends known as lateral sacs or **terminal cisternae**.
3. The cisternae lie in close contact with the T-tubules **at the A-I junction**.
4. The combination of the T-tubule membrane and its two neighboring cisternae is called a **triad**, which plays a vital role in linking membrane action potentials to muscle contraction (details see below). In cardiac muscle, it forms a diad due to the presence of one cistern.

Receptors and Channel Proteins in STS

The T-tubules are separated from the terminal cisternae by a narrow space of about 12–14 nm that contains areas of densities known as *feet*. The **junctional feet** involve two integral membrane proteins, one in the T-tubule membrane, and the other in the membrane of the terminal cistern.

1. The T-tubule protein is a modified *voltage-sensitive calcium channel* known as the **dihydropyridine (DHP) receptor**. It is so named because it is blocked by the drug dihydropyridine.
2. The DHP receptors are **L-type calcium channels** and they are clustered in groups of four called *tetrads*.
3. Primarily the receptor acts as a ***voltage sensor*** *rather than a calcium channel*.
4. The portion of the terminal cisternae membrane that faces the T-tubules contains proteins known as the **ryanodine receptors**. They are so called because they bind to the plant alkaloid ryanodine. They mainly act **as *calcium release channels***.
5. There is also **calcium ATPases** present on the membrane of SR that pumps calcium back into the SR.

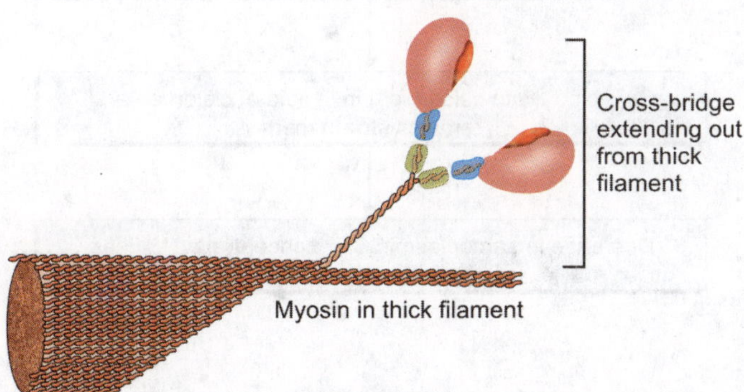

Fig. 26.13: The structure and position of cross bridge.

Functions

Role of STS in Muscle Contraction and Relaxation

Sarcotubular system (STS) plays a vital role in muscle contraction as it links T-tubular action potentials (excitation) with calcium release from the SR that activates the contractile machinery (**contraction**). When calcium is pumped back into the SR, decline in cytoplasmic calcium level leads to muscle **relaxation**. Thus, STS is crucial in both contraction and relaxation process by mediating ***calcium release*** and ***calcium uptake***.

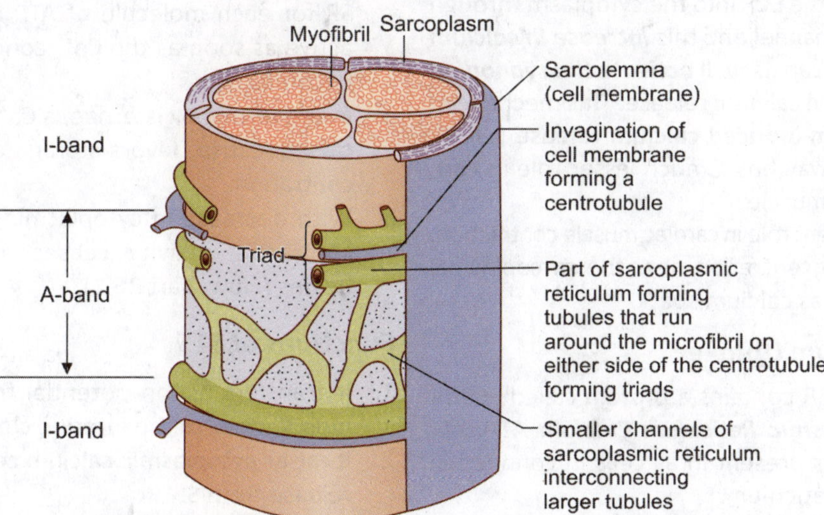

Fig. 26.14: Arrangement of sarcotubular system in the myofibril. Note the relationship of sarcoplasmic reticulum and T tubules with I and A bands of sarcomere, in a myofibrils.

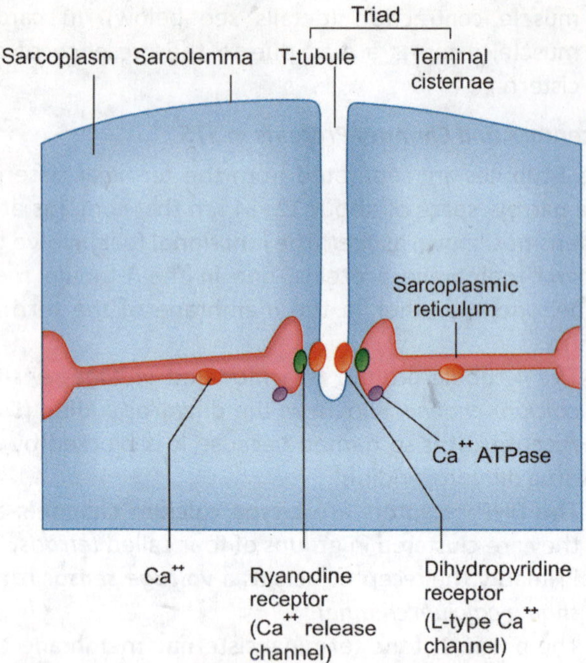

Fig. 26.15: Structure of sarcotubular system.

Mechanism of Calcium Release

Following depolarization at the motor end plate, action potentials propagate along the sarcolemma and down the T-tubule membrane.

1. Depolarization of the triad region of the T-tubules induces *conformational changes* in each of the four DHP receptor proteins, which leads to a ***conformational change in the ryanodine receptor*** resulting in **opening of the ryanodine receptor channel**.
2. Calcium is thus released from the terminal cisternae of the SR into the cytoplasm, **activating cross-bridge cycling**.
3. The entire process, starting from depolarization of the T-tubule membrane to the initiation of the cross-bridge cycling is termed *excitation-contraction coupling*.
4. Further, conformational change in DHP receptor allows calcium entry from the ECF into the cytoplasm through the DHP receptor channel and this ***increase in calcium level*** inside the cell can as well ***activate the ryanodine receptors*** resulting in calcium release. This mechanism is known as **calcium-induced calcium release** (CICR). However, this pathway has a much lesser role in contraction of skeletal muscle.
5. CICR plays an important role in cardiac muscle contraction.
6. Increase in Ca^{2+} concentration near the sarcoplasmic reticulum is known as calcium spark.

Mechanism of Calcium Uptake

The membrane of the SR contains a **protein** called SERCA (***Sarcoplasmic Endoplasmic Reticulum Calcium ATPase***). This is so named as it is present in all cells in connection with the endoplasmic reticulum.

1. The protein is a **Ca^{2+} ATPase** that pumps free calcium ions from the sarcoplasm to the SR, from where the calcium ions are moved to their storage sites in the terminal cisternae.
2. The pump relocates two molecules of Ca^{2+} into the SR for each molecule of ATP hydrolyzed. It becomes active as soon as the Ca^{2+} concentration in cytoplasm becomes high.
3. In the terminal cisternae, a Ca^{2+} binding protein called **calsequestrin**, favors storage of calcium at high concentration.
4. With decrease in cytoplasmic calcium concentration, contractile activity ceases and relaxation process begins (Flowchart 26.1).

Flowchart 26.1: Role of sarcoplasmic reticulum in muscle contraction and relaxation.

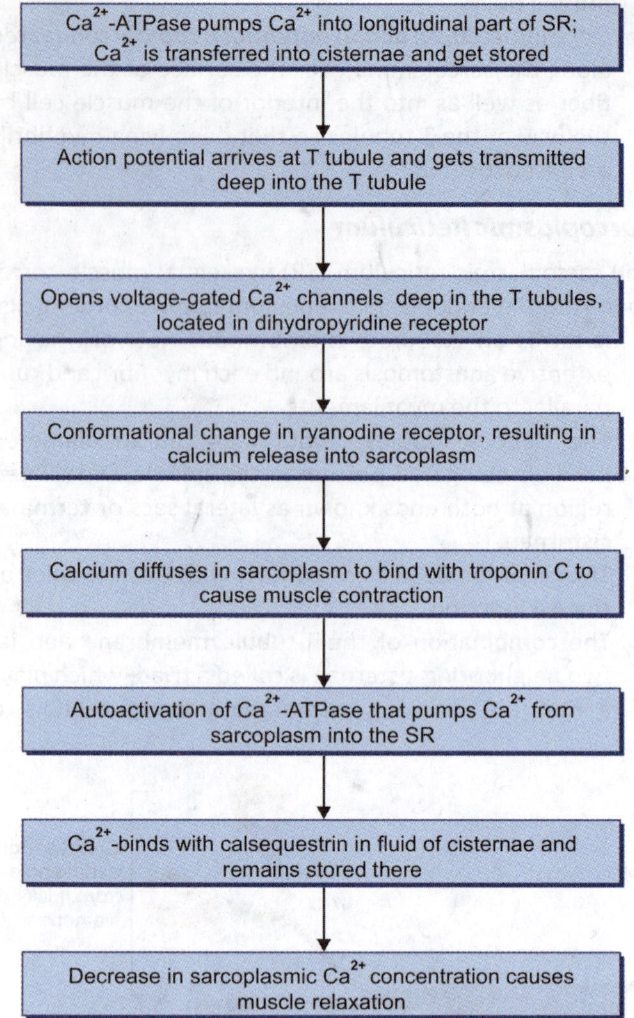

Functions of STS

1. It transfers action potential from the surface of the muscle fiber to the interior, closer to the myofibrils.
2. It raises cytoplasmic calcium concentration by calcium release from SR.
3. It ensures muscle relaxation by calcium reuptake by SR
4. The cisternae of SR act as storage sites for calcium.

CHAPTER SUMMARY

Key Concepts

1. Sarcomere, the functional unit of muscle fibril, is the distance between two Z lines.
2. During muscle contraction, the length of the sarcomere decreases, due to shortening of I band, but the length of A band remains unchanged.
3. The globular heads of myosin project from the thick filaments toward the thin filaments and bridge the gap between them. Hence, this head region is called cross-bridges. During muscle contraction, cross bridge attach to the thin filaments and pull them.
4. T tubule of sarcotubular system that invaginates into the myofibril transmits action potential to the contractile machinery. Release of calcium from cistern causes muscle contraction and active pumping of calcium back into the cistern causes muscle relaxation.

Important to Know (Must Read)

1. In examinations, usually **Long Questions** are not asked from this chapter.
2. Muscle proteins, Sarcomere, Sarcotubular system, Role of sarcotubular system in muscle contraction, are usual **Short Questions** in exams.
3. In **Viva**, examiners usually ask… Type of muscle proteins, Structure and function of each muscle protein, what is cross bridge, What are the regulatory proteins and their functions, What are the attachment proteins and their functions, Definition and structure of sarcomere, What are the I and A bands and what are their significance, Components of sarcotubular system and function of each component, Name the receptors and channel proteins in sarcotubular system, and what are their functions, and, How sarcotubular system participates in muscle contraction and relaxation.
4. Types of muscle proteins, sarcomere and sarcotubular system are usually asked.

CHAPTER

27

Mechanism of Skeletal Muscle Contraction

Learning Objectives

On completion of study of this chapter, the student **MUST** be able to:

1. Describe the mechanism of excitation-contraction coupling in skeletal.
2. Understand the process of cross-bridge cycle.
3. Appreciate the relationship between the action potential and contractile response.
4. List the types of muscle contraction and the differences between them.

The student **MAY** also be able to:

1. Describe the detailed mechanism of cross-bridge cycle.

The action potential from sarcolemma spreads to the interior of muscle fiber through T tubules and results in calcium release from cisternae. This increases sarcoplasmic calcium concentration. The muscle response to the action potential (through increased calcium) is the **excitation**, and the mechanical response is the **contraction** of the muscle. Calcium diffuses to troponin C and induces muscle contraction through a series of well controlled steps. Therefore, this phenomenon of pairing of electrical event with the mechanical event is called **excitation-contraction coupling**.

EXCITATION-CONTRACTION COUPLING

Increase in sarcoplasmic calcium concentration in response to arrival of action potential from sarcolemma leads to muscle contraction. The process is called excitation-contraction coupling.

1. The term contraction means attachment of myosin heads to actin and activation of the cross bridge cycles so that force is generated within to shorten the muscle fibers.
2. However, it may not always lead to shortening as occurs in isometric contraction. While lifting a heavy object, shortening occurs, but holding the object at a constant position, activates the cross bridge cycles without apparent shortening.

Sliding-Filament Theory of Muscle Contraction: In 1957, **AF Huxley** proposed the sliding filament theory of muscle contraction based on the changes observed in the lengths and widths of various bands and zones of the sarcomere. Shortening of a muscle fiber occurs due to **sliding of thin filaments over thick filaments** toward the center of the sarcomere (described below in "molecular mechanisms of muscle contraction"). It was observed that the **length of A band does not change** during contraction, but **the H zone and I band decrease in width** and the Z lines move closer together.

Scientists contributed

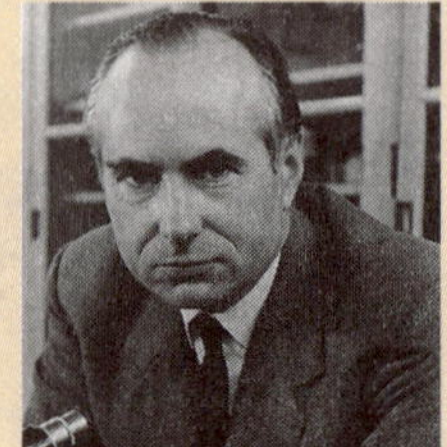

Sir AF Huxley (1917–2012)

Sir Andrew Fielding Huxley was a Nobel Prize-winning **English physiologist and biophysicist**. He discovered the basis for propagation of nerve impulses (called an action potential) earned the **Nobel Prize in Physiology or Medicine in 1963**. He developed *interference microscopy* suitable for studying muscle fibers. In 1952, German physiologist **Rolf Niedergerke** joined him, and in 1954 together they discovered the mechanism of muscle contraction, popularly called the "Sliding filament theory", which established the foundation of understanding of muscle mechanics. He contributed enormously to the understanding of nerve impulses and muscle contraction. He was conferred a ***Knight Bachelor by Queen Elizabeth II*** in 1974, and was appointed to the ***Order of Merit in 1983***. He was a ***fellow of Trinity College***, Cambridge, until his death.

Molecular Mechanisms of Muscle Contraction

The molecular mechanism of muscle contraction is based on the principle that the **sliding motion of the filaments** occurs as a result of a ***cyclic interaction between the myosin cross bridges and the actin filaments***, in the presence of calcium and ATP.

1. This is known as the **cross bridge theory** or the **ratchet theory** as the strokes are similar to the action of a ratchet.
2. The force generation and shortening are produced at the cross bridge sites where the chemical energy stored in the muscle is converted into mechanical energy.

Role of Troponin, Tropomyosin and Calcium

Calcium ions provide the most important chemical link in the regulation of muscle protein interactions during the course of excitation-contraction coupling.

1. **In resting skeletal muscle**, cytoplasmic calcium ion concentration is low, which is about 10^{-7} M in the region of the myofilaments. Troponin I is attached to myosin binding site on actin and partially covers the myosin binding site. Rest of myosin binding site is covered by tropomyosin filament.
2. Thus, in normal condition, **troponin I and tropomyosin inhibits myosin-actin interaction.**
3. Troponin T is attached to tropomyosin.
4. Each tropomyosin molecule is held in this blocking position by troponin that is bound to both tropomyosin and actin.
5. Thus, the troponin-tropomyosin complex behaves as a ***relaxing protein*** that prevents undesirable contraction.

Troponin–Tropomyosin Interaction

Following propagation of action potential along the sarcolemma and down the T tubules, calcium is released from the SR and **calcium concentration rises to 10^{-4} M** in the sarcoplasm, which accounts for about 1,000-fold rise of the ion.

1. Calcium binds to troponin C and induces a conformational change in the troponin molecule.
2. This result in ***shifting of troponin I from the actin filament***, allowing tropomyosin to move deeper into the actin groove, **unmasking the myosin binding sites** (Figs. 27.1A and B). Moreover, the conformational change alters the position of troponin T that drags tropomyosin away from the myosin-binding sites.
3. The exposure of the binding sites allows myosin heads to interact with actin and engage in **cross-bridge cycling.**
4. Thus, the troponin-tropomyosin complex ***regulates the contraction of skeletal muscle***.
5. As the regulation of the contractile process by calcium is implemented through the actin filaments, it is also called **actin-linked regulation.**

Role of Calcium

An increase in cytoplasmic Ca^{2+} concentration triggers the contractile process by removing the inhibition on cross bridge cycling. On the contrary, decrease in cytoplasmic Ca^{2+} concentration leads to detachment of calcium from troponin that reverses the process and turns off contractile activity.

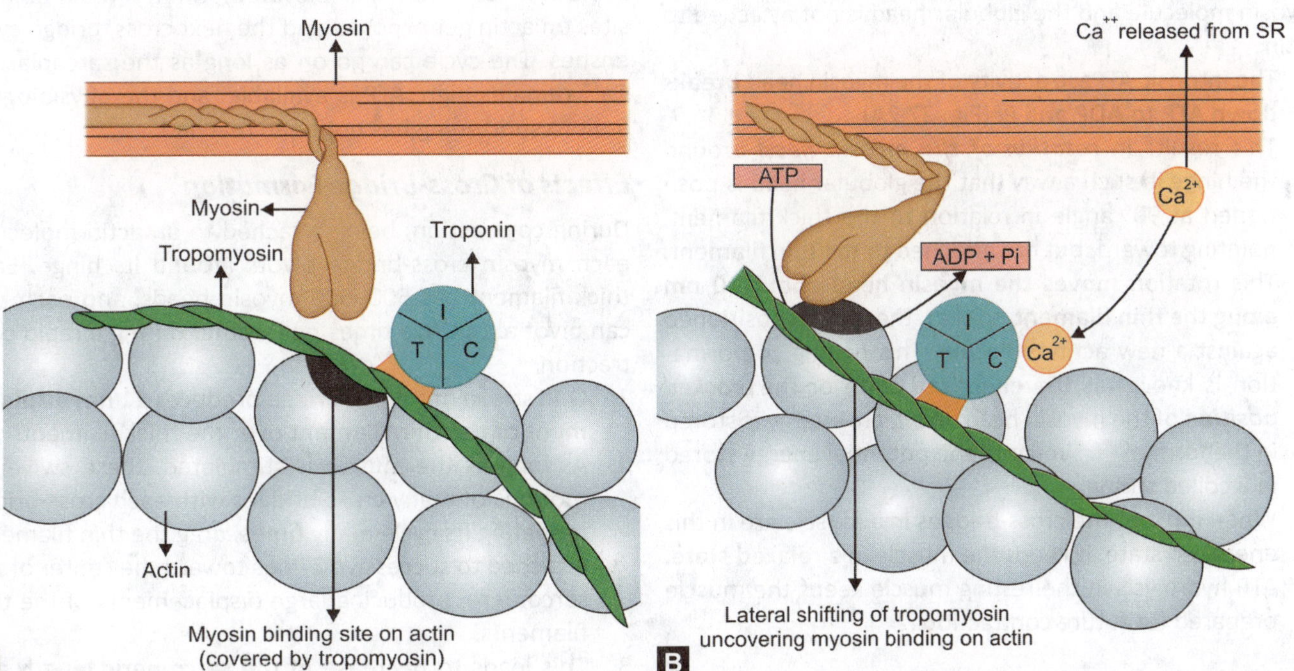

Figs. 27.1A and B: Role of troponin-tropomyosin interaction in muscle contraction. Binding of calcium with troponin C induces conformational change in the troponin molecule, which shifts troponin I from the actin filament, and simultaneously troponin T that drags tropomyosin away from the myosin-binding site on actin. Exposure of this binding site allows myosin heads to interact with actin and engage in cross-bridge cycling. Note, ATP is converted to ADP during this interaction.

1. **In skeletal muscle**, increase in cytosolic calcium in response to a single action potential is usually sufficient to saturate all troponin-binding sites on actin filaments.
   - At a calcium concentration of 10^{-4} M, there is full force development and the *contractile system is fully saturated*.
   - With further increase in concentration, there is only small increase in the force.
2. Whereas, **in cardiac and smooth muscle**, the amount of calcium regulates the degree of actin-myosin interaction as the *contractile system is only partially saturated* under normal conditions.

Cross-Bridge Cycle

The sequence of events that occur during the interaction between the myosin cross-bridges and the actin molecules is termed as a cross-bridge cycle.

1. During each cycle, cross bridge (myosin head) attaches to thin filament causing displacement of thick filament over thin filament followed by detachment of myosin head in a repetitive fashion.
2. ATP is required during the cycle; for the movement of the cross bridge as well as for its detachment.
3. However, all the cross-bridges do not go through the same phase at any instant during a cycle. This helps in a smooth and sustained contraction.

Events in the Resting Muscle

When the muscle is at rest, the cytoplasmic ATP gets attached to its specific binding site in the head of the myosin molecule and the globular head is not attached to actin.

1. The intrinsic ATPase activity of the myosin head **breaks down ATP to ADP and Pi** (Fig. 27.2A).
2. This results in ***rotation of the myosin head*** around the hinge in such a way that the globular head is positioned at 90° angle in relation to the thick filament, pointing toward, but not attached to the thin filament.
3. This rotation **moves the myosin head about 10 nm along the thin filament**, so that, the head is positioned against a new actin molecule. This resting conformation is known as the **energized state** or the ***'cocked position*** of the myosin head' in which, energy is stored in the form of Pi, similar to the potential energy stored in a coiled spring.
4. When most of the cross-bridges in a muscle are in this energized state, it keeps the muscle in a **relaxed state.** ATP hydrolysis in the resting muscle keeps the muscle prepared for future contraction.

Events in the Stimulated Muscle

When action potential arrives at the T-tubules, calcium is released from the SR and the myosin-binding sites on actin are exposed.

1. The ***myosin-ADP-Pi complex has higher affinity for actin***, which is called as the charged or energized myosin head. The charged myosin head binds to actin forming the actomyosin complex, also called **cross-bridge formation** (Fig. 27.2B).
2. The binding of myosin head to actin has **two effects**:
   - First, Pi is released from myosin head producing the **power stroke,** i.e. a conformational change in which the myosin head bends on the hinge at an angle of about 45 degrees pulling the actin filament about 11 nm toward the center of the sarcomere (Fig. 27.2C).
   - Second, the binding causes the **dissociation of ADP** from the myosin head leaving the actomyosin complex in a **rigid state**. That means the myosin head stay attached to the actin molecule in the same position and at a 45° angle with respect to the thick and thin filaments.
3. For detachment to occur, a new molecule of ATP must bind to the myosin head and initiate next cycle. Usually, the sarcoplasmic ATP concentration in normal physiological conditions is always adequate to produce the necessary detachment of cross-bridges. So, the ADP-free actomyosin complex (***attached state***) quickly binds to ATP.
4. This decreases the affinity of myosin for actin resulting in detachment of cross-bridges from the thin filaments, called as **detached state** (Fig. 27.2D). Soon after, ATP hydrolysis occurs and the myosin head attains the energized state.

If the stimulus for contraction persists, i.e. the sarcoplasmic Ca^{2+} remains elevated, then myosin-binding sites on actin get exposed and the next cross, bridge cycle ensues. The cycle can go on as long as the sarcoplasmic Ca^{2+} remains high, ATP is available, and the physiological limit to shortening has not been reached.

Effects of Cross-Bridge Formation

During contraction, being attached to an actin molecule, each myosin cross-bridge pivots around its hinge. Each thick filament has 500–600 myosin heads, and each one can pivot about five times per second during a rapid contraction.

1. One stroke of a cross-bridge produces **11 nm displacement of the thin filament** over the thick filament.
2. As long as the muscle is stimulated, these swiveling motions of many cross-bridges with each cross-bridge repeating its cycle many times, drag the thin filaments attached to successive Z lines toward the center of the sarcomere, producing large displacements of the thin filaments.
3. This leads to **decrease in the sarcomeric length** and ultimately muscle shortening.
4. **When shortening does not occur** as in isometric contraction, the repetitive binding and pull on the actin generate tension.

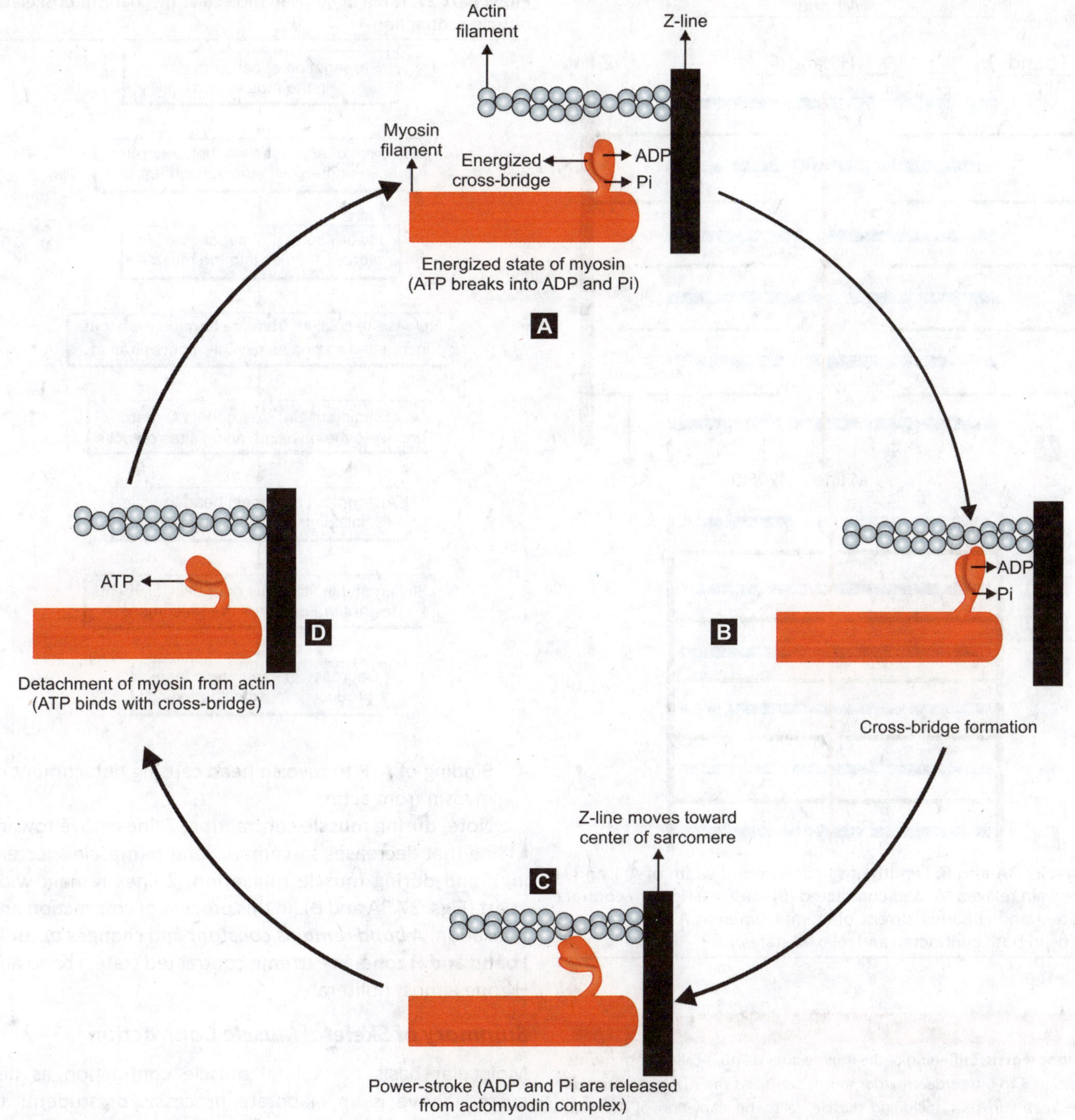

Figs. 27.2A to D: Cross-bridge cycle. (A) Resting state (cross-bridge is energized by braking down of ATP to ADP and Pi that provides energy; (B) Myosin head-ADP-Pi complex develops more affinity for actin and bind with actin to form actomyosin complex; (C) Myosin Head pulls actin filament that moves Z line toward center of sarcomere (power-stroke), and actomyosin complex is free of ADP and Pi; (D) ATP binds with myosin head and detaches it from actin filament (detached state).

Role of ATP in Cross-Bridge Formation

ATP is required for the **detachment of myosin head from the thin filaments.**

1. If most of the cross-bridges in a muscle remain in the detached state, it would produce relaxation in the muscle.
2. *Not all the cross bridges remain in the detached state* even in a completely relaxed muscle; some of them bind to actin and generate tension that **contributes to the tone of the muscle.**
3. If cellular ATP stores are depleted, as happens after death, the cross-bridges cannot detach and it is called a **rigor cross bridge**, the cycle stops there and the filaments remain in the attached state. This produces stiffening in the muscle, known as ***rigor mortis*** (Clinical Box 27.1).

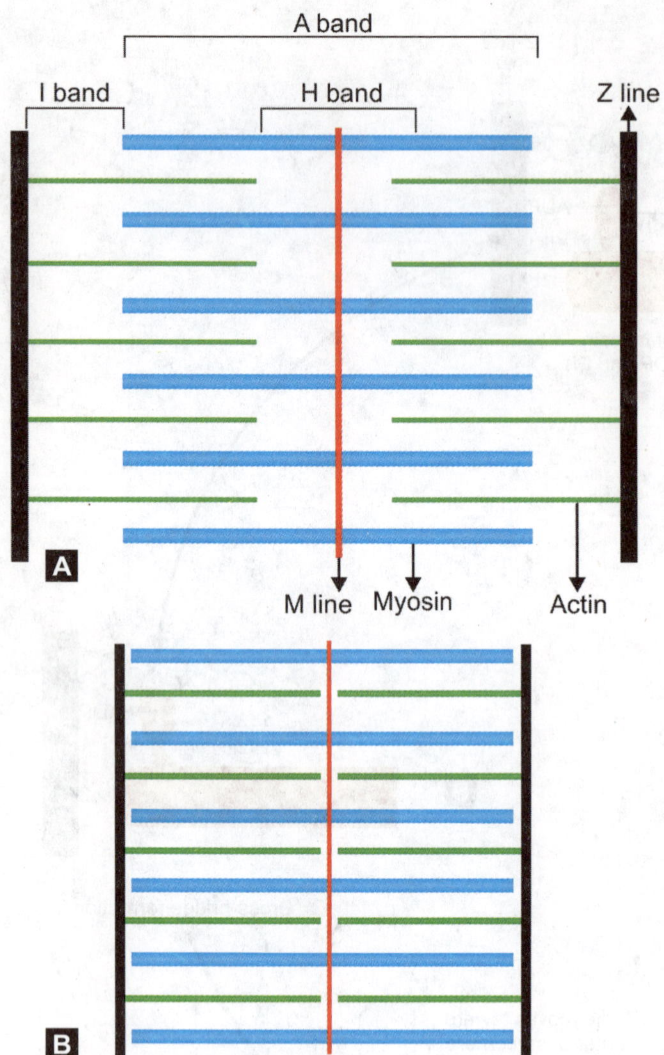

Figs. 27.3A and B: Length of sarcomeric and width of A, I, and H bands in relaxed (A) and contracted (B) muscles. Note, in contract state, I and H bands almost obliterate, whereas A band remains same in both contracted and relaxed states.

Clinical Box 27.1

Rigor mortis: Stiffening of the muscle after death is called rigor mortis. Within 3 to 6 h of death, rigor mortis sets in as the ATP concentration decreases in cells, including muscle cells. The depletion of ATP fails to detach the cross-bridge. Therefore, muscle remains in a state of contraction or rigidity. The rigidity of rigor mortis completes in about 12 h and disappears about 40 to 60 h after death due to disintegration and putrefaction of muscle fibers. Due to rigor mortis, body remains in same position for a longer time. Thus, rigor mortis not only speaks about the time of death, but also the nature of death, which helps in medicolegal investigations in case of mysterious deaths.

The process of cross-bridge cycle can be **summarized in four steps** (Figs. 27.2A to D, as depicted above):

1. ATP hydrolysis in the myosin head leading to energized state of the myosin.
2. Cross-bridge formation in the presence of increased calcium.
3. Release of Pi and ADP from myosin head producing power stroke.

Flowchart 27.1: Major steps in molecular mechanism of skeletal muscle contraction.

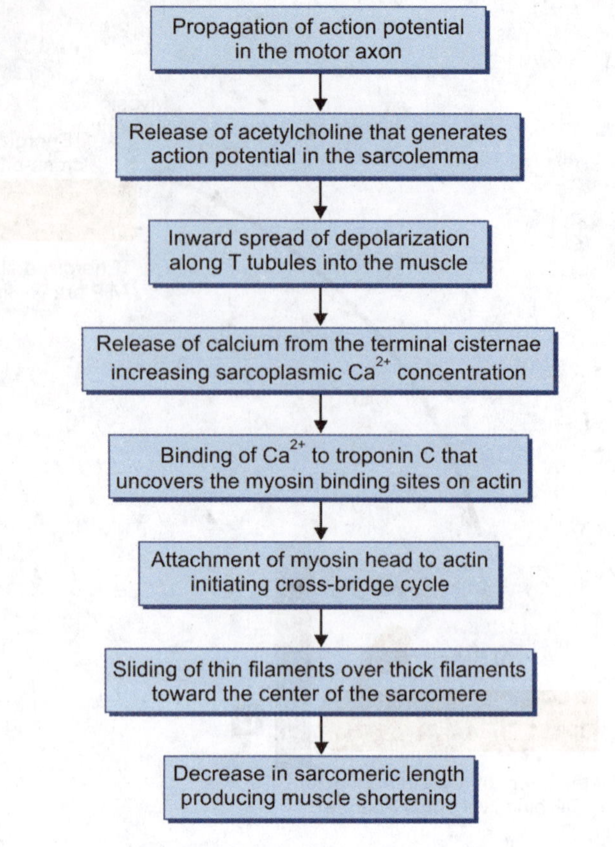

4. Binding of ATP to myosin head causing detachment of myosin from actin.

    Note, **during muscle contraction**, Z lines move toward M line that decreases sarcomeric length (muscle shortening), and **during muscle relaxation**, Z lines remain wide apart (Figs. 27.3A and B). In this process of contraction and relaxation, ***A band remains constant*** and **changes occur in I band and H zone**. In extreme contracted state, I band and H zone almost obliterate.

Summary of Skeletal Muscle Contraction

Molecular basis of skeletal muscle contraction as discussed above is an elaborate process. For students to quickly revise, understand and memorize quickly, it is summarized in Flowchart 27.1.

Mechanism of Muscle Relaxation

Like muscle contraction, relaxation is also an ***active process***.

1. The ***Ca^{++} ATPase*** present on the membrane of SR pumps Ca^{2+} from the sarcoplasm into the SR (for details read the mechanism of calcium uptake by Sarco-Tubular System (in previous chapter).
2. If no further action potential arrives at the myoneural junction, the activity of ***Ca^{++}ATPase*** decreases calcium concentration in the vicinity of the myofilaments to a very low level.
3. Consequently, ***very few calcium ions are available*** to bind with troponin.

Flowchart 27.2: Major events in skeletal muscle relaxation.

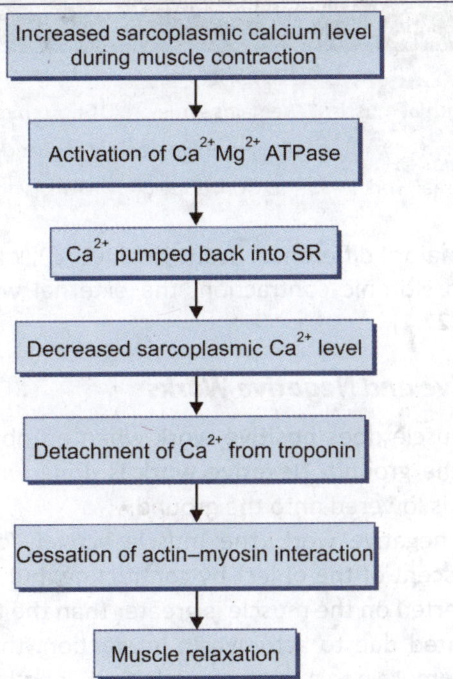

4. This leads to ***cessation of interaction*** between actin and myosin.
5. The contractile activity stops and relaxation process begins (Flowchart 27.2).

Thus, contraction as well as relaxation in skeletal muscle requires energy in the form of ATP.

Action Potential and Contractile Response

Action Potential

The **resting membrane potential** of skeletal muscle is **–90 mV**. The action potential is generated at the end plate region and spreads at a speed of 5 m/sec along the sarcolemma and down the T tubules activating the myofilaments.

1. The **duration** of the action potential is **2–4 ms** and **absolute refractory period is 1–3 ms.**
2. The **depolarization phase** of the action potential is due to ***sodium influx*** and **repolarization** is a manifestation of ***potassium efflux***.
3. The action potential does not directly activate the contractile proteins but instead produces a state of increased cytosolic calcium concentration, which activates the contractile apparatus long after the electrical activity in the membrane has ceased (Fig. 27.4A).

Contractile Response

In response to the motor nerve discharge, the thick and thin filaments slide past each other producing shortening of the activated fibers. This contractile response (twitch contraction) can be recorded in a graphical form (Fig. 27.4B).

1. A **twitch** is defined as the mechanical response of single muscle fiber to an action potential consisting of a phase of contraction followed by a relaxation phase.

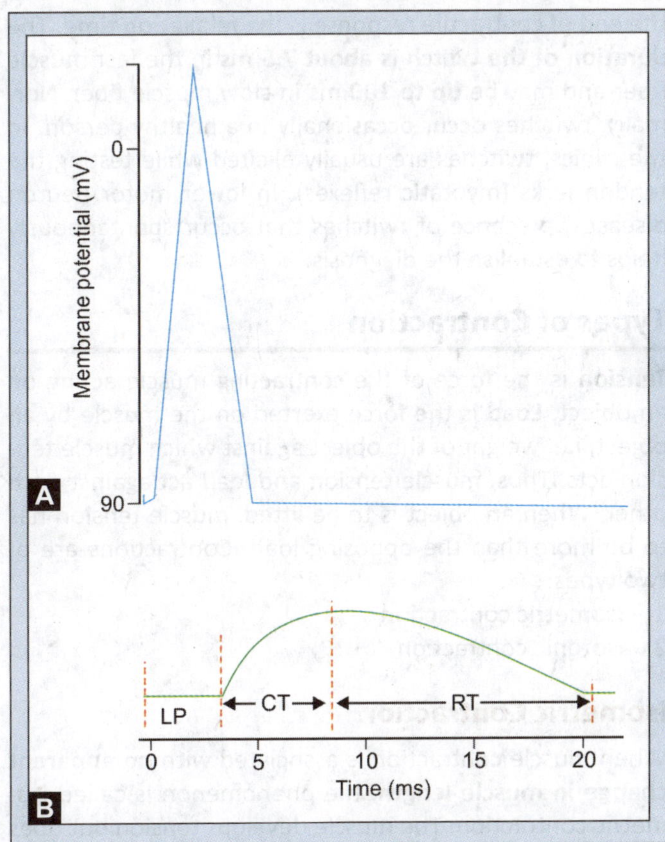

Figs. 27.4A and B: Comparison of electrical and mechanical responses of skeletal muscle. (A) Action potential recorded from skeletal muscle fiber; (B) Simultaneous recoding of contractile response on same time scale. (LP: Latent period; CT: Contraction time; RT: Relaxation time).

2. When the action potential and the twitch contraction are plotted on the same time scale, the contractile response begins about 2 ms after the onset of the action potential. This delay is known as the **latent period**, during which the excitation-contraction coupling takes place.

In nerve-muscle preparation, where a motor nerve is stimulated to obtain a contraction, the latent period occurs due to the time taken for:

1. Conduction of impulse along the axon from the point of stimulus.
2. Secretion of Ach, its diffusion through the synaptic cleft and generation of end plate potential.
3. Origin and spread of action potential along the sarcolemma and T tubules
4. Activation of the contractile mechanism.
5. Overcoming the viscous resistance of the muscle.
6. Overcoming the inertia of the writing lever (if the twitch is being recorded).

Calcium released during a twitch can fully activate the contractile machinery, but the relaxation process starts soon after. So, the magnitude of peak tension developed is relatively low. The duration from the start of the contractile response to the attainment of peak tension is the **contraction time** and from the point of peak tension to the end of contractile response is the **relaxation time**. The **duration of the twitch is about 7.5 ms** in the fast muscle fiber and may be **up to 100 ms** in slow muscle fiber. Normally, twitches occur occasionally in a healthy person. In the clinics, twitches are usually elicited while testing the tendon jerks (myotatic reflexes). In lower motor neuron diseases, presence of twitches that occur spontaneously helps to establish the diagnosis.

Types of Contraction

Tension is the force of the contracting muscle acting on an object. **Load** is the force exerted on the muscle by an object, i.e. weight of the object against which muscle tension acts. Thus, muscle tension and load act against each other. When an object is to be lifted, muscle tension has to be more than the opposing load. Contractions are of two types:

1. Isometric contraction
2. Isotonic contraction

Isometric Contraction

When muscle contraction is associated with **no apparent change in muscle length**, the phenomenon is called isometric contraction. The muscle develops tension but does not shorten or lengthen; for example, when somebody is trying to lift a heavy object.

1. During this type of contraction, the cross bridges bind with the actin molecules and attempt to pull them but cannot drag the thin filaments because the load is greater than the tension exerted by the muscle fiber. This exerts a force on the thin filament, the **isometric tension**.
2. If isometric contraction is continued, cycling cross bridges again and again bind to the same actin molecule.
3. According to the law of physics, if displacement is zero (position of the object does not change), the work done (force × displacement) is also nil, though force is generated and energy is spent. Thus, in isometric contraction **no external work is done**.
4. Isometric tension can be recorded with the help of an isometric lever when the muscle is stimulated to contract with its two ends held at fixed points.

Isotonic Contraction

When muscle contraction is associated with **no apparent change in muscle tone**, the phenomenon is called isotonic contraction.

1. The shortening of the muscle fiber occurs due to sliding of thin over thick filaments. Examples of such muscle contractions are walking, running, lifting an object, etc.
2. Isotonic contraction is also known as ***concentric contraction***.

Table 27.1: Differences between isometric and isotonic contractions.

	Isometric	Isotonic
1. Length of muscle	Remains same	Shortening occurs
2. Tension	Tension increases	No change
3. External work	No work done	Work is done

The major difference from isometric contraction is that in isotonic contraction, the external work is done (Table 27.1).

Positive and Negative Works

The muscle does **positive work** when an object is lifted from the ground. **Negative work** is done when a heavy object is lowered onto the ground.

1. In negative work, the muscle actively opposes the descent of the object by contracting, but, as the load exerted on the muscle is greater than the tension generated due to actomyosin interaction, the load pulls the muscle to a longer length. Such lengthening of the muscle is called **lengthening contraction** or **eccentric contraction**, for example, the extensors of the knee lengthen when somebody sits on the ground.
2. This is not an active process produced by cross bridge activation, rather a passive phenomenon, where external load stretches the muscle.

When stimulated, a muscle fiber always tends to shorten, unless an external lengthening force is present. While recording for isotonic contraction, one end of the muscle is fixed and the other kept free, so that on stimulation, the muscle shortens by contraction producing a constant force.

Processes in Isometric and Isotonic Contractions

When an object is to be lifted, initially tension increases in the muscle till it becomes equal to the downward pulling force (due to the weight of the object) without any change in muscle length, i.e. the fibers undergo isometric contraction.

1. Once the tension in the muscle is greater than the opposing load, shortening contraction of the muscle lifts the object and brings it to the new position; here the fibers undergo isotonic contraction.
2. Now, if the object is to be held in space in the new position, the fibers undergo isometric contraction, the tension generated being just equal and opposite to the load of the object.
3. Pushing against a wall is an example of isometric contraction if the elbow does not bend during the act, i.e. the distance between shoulder and hand remains unchanged.

CHAPTER SUMMARY

Key Concepts

1. Muscle contraction is an active process in which ATP is utilized, and muscle relaxation is also an active process.
2. Sliding filament theory of muscle contraction is based on cross-bridge formation, in which myosin head pulls the thin filament on thick filament.
3. During each cross bridge cycle, cross bridge (myosin head) attaches to thin filament causing displacement of thick filament over thin filament followed by detachment of myosin head in a repetitive fashion.
4. ATP is required during the cycle for the movement of the cross bridge as well as for its detachment.
5. In skeletal muscle, the contractile response (that lasts for about 15 ms) begins almost toward the end of electrical response (that lasts for about 4 ms). Therefore, skeletal muscle can be tetanized.

Important to Know (Must Read)

1. In examinations, "Describe the molecular basis of muscle contraction" is a very common **Long Question**. Cross bridge cycle may sometime come as long question.
2. Excitation-contraction coupling, Molecular basis of muscle contraction, Cross bridge cycle, Relationship between electrical and mechanical response in skeletal muscle, Types of muscle contraction, are usual **Short Questions** in exams.
3. In **Viva**, examiners usually ask… What is the meaning of Excitation-contraction coupling, Who described Sliding-Filament Theory, What is the meaning of Sliding-Filament Theory, Steps in molecular basis of muscle contraction, Mechanism of calcium release from cisterns, Mechanism of cross-bridge cycle, Role of troponins and tropomyosin, Steps of muscle relaxation, Relationship between electrical and mechanical response in skeletal muscle and its importance, and Types of muscle contraction.
4. Mechanism of skeletal muscle contraction is invariably asked in both theory and oral exams.

CHAPTER 28

Skeletal Muscle: Properties, Fiber Types and Applied Aspects

LEARNING OBJECTIVES

On completion of study of this chapter, the student **MUST** be able to:
1. List the properties of skeletal muscle.
2. Understand the link of muscle properties to function.
3. Name the energy sources in skeletal muscle.
4. Explain the mechanism of oxygen debt.
5. Define the motor unit and understand the concept of size principle.
6. Define different types of muscle heat and understand their importance.
7. Name the type of muscle fibers and basic differences between them.
8. Correlate the application of knowledge of function with dysfunctions.

The student **MAY** also be able to:
1. Describe each property of skeletal muscle.
2. Understand the mechanism of muscle fatigue and rigor mortis.

PROPERTIES OF SKELETAL MUSCLE

Important Properties

Important properties of skeletal muscles (in addition to the properties, like contractility, excitability, fatigability, etc.) are:
1. Summation of contraction
2. Staircase phenomenon
3. Tetanization
4. Post-tetanic potentiation
5. Length-tension relationship
6. Load-velocity relationship

Summation of Contraction

It states that isometric tension developed in a single fiber or a muscle depends on the frequency of the stimulus applied to it.
1. The action potential of the skeletal muscle is brief (1–4 ms) compared to its contraction time. The absolute refractory period (which includes the depolarization phase and part of the repolarization phase) of the action potential is over by the time contraction starts.
2. Thus, during the contraction period, if the motor neuron is stimulated repeatedly, it will generate several action potentials in the muscle fiber. The **contractile elements have no refractory period**; they do not follow-all-or none law and contraction can continue till Ca^{++} and ATP are available.

If a second twitch is produced when the contraction phase of the first twitch is still continuing, the phase of contraction of the second twitch is added to the phase of contraction of the first twitch, resulting in a **summated contractile response** (Figs. 28.1A to C).
1. The Ca^{++} released due to the second action potential is added to the Ca^{++} released due to the first action potential, producing a higher sarcoplasmic Ca^{++} concentration that results in a *bigger contractile response*. Therefore, the tension generated during summated response is greater than that of a single twitch. The tension increases further as the stimulus interval shortens (Fig. 28.1C).
2. Thus, repeated stimulation of the muscle before relaxation has occurred produces a phenomenon known as **summation of contractions**.

Staircase Phenomenon

If a skeletal muscle is stimulated rapidly (but below the tetanizing frequency) with a maximal stimulus, there is a progressive increase in the force of contraction for the

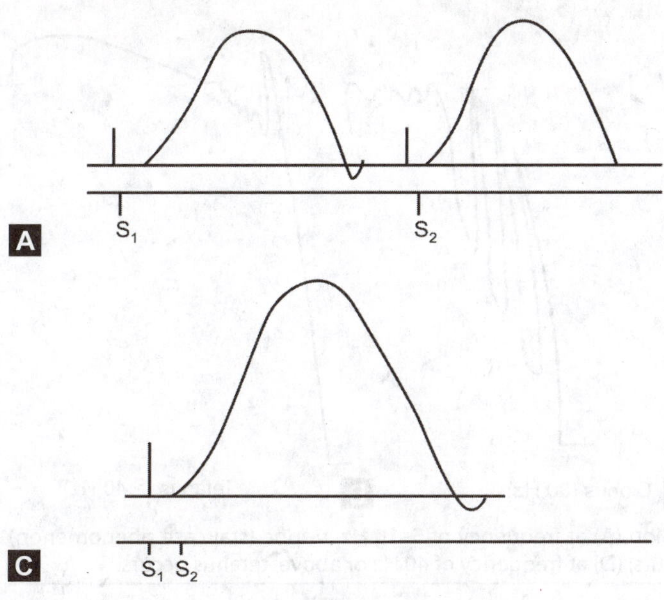

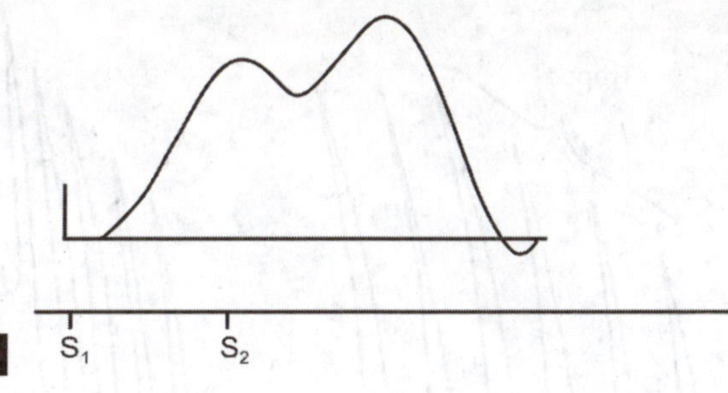

Figs. 28.1A to C: Summation of contraction. (A) Second stimulus (S_2) was applied after the contractile response of first stimulus (S_1) was over; (B) S_2 was applied in the contraction phase of S_1; (C) S_2 was applied close to the latent period of S_1. Note that the second stimulus applied before relaxation period of first response leads to summation of contraction and increases in magnitude of contraction.

first few contractions, until a maximum uniform tension per contraction is reached. This is the staircase phenomenon or **treppe** (in German). Treppe is also seen in cardiac muscle. In 1871, **Bowditch** first described Treppe in the frog's heart.

1. During repeated and rapid stimulation, if a second contraction occurs during the relaxation phase of the first one, the amplitude of the second twitch happens to be higher than the first one (Figs. 28.2A to D).
2. This is because when the muscle has not completely relaxed, the cytoplasmic calcium concentration remains elevated as all the calcium released due to the first stimulus has not been pumped back into the sarcoplasmic reticulum.
3. This leftover calcium is added to the calcium released during the second contraction and results in greater amplitude. Also, the heat produced during preceding contraction decreases sarcoplasmic viscosity and facilitates the enzymatic activity that increases the height of succeeding contractions.
4. In this manner, if subsequent contractions occur before the relaxation phase of the previous one is over, first few twitches gradually increase in amplitude.
5. This is known as staircase phenomenon as the graph is in an ascending order, like a staircase. The amplitude does not increase after a few contractions as the calcium level becomes saturated.

Scientist contributed

There is an autoregulation method by which myocardial tension increases with an increase in heart rate, which is known as the **Treppe phenomenon**, Treppe effect or staircase effect. The treppe phenomenon was first observed by **Henry Pickering Bowditch** in 1871, in cardiac muscle. Later, it was described in skeletal muscle. This is also called **Bowditch effect.**

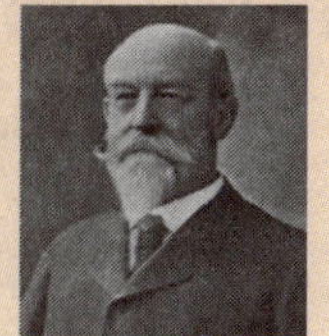

HP Bowditch
(1840–1911)

Tetanization

If the muscle is stimulated repeatedly at a very high frequency, continuous activation of the contractile mechanism occurs without any relaxation, resulting in a sustained contraction known as tetanus *(tetanic contraction)*.

1. In *complete/fused tetanus*, there is no relaxation between the contraction phases.
2. In clonus or *incomplete* or *unfused tetanus*, there are periods of incomplete relaxation between the maintained contractions (Figs. 28.2C and D).
3. While the frequency of the action potentials progressively increases to tetanizing frequency, the tension generated in the muscle gradually rises and summated until a maximal **tetanic tension** is reached. Beyond this, tension does not increase further with increase in frequency of the action potentials.

The **critical frequency** (CF) at which summation of contractions occur differs from muscle to muscle since it depends on the twitch duration of a fiber.

$$CF = \frac{1}{\text{Twitch duration (in sec)}}$$

For example, a fiber has twitch duration of 10 ms or 0.01s. The CF for this fiber will be 1/0.01s = 100/s.

When a muscle is stimulated with a frequency more than CF, summation of contractions occurs. Stimulation of the muscle with less than CF produces distinct contractions with intermittent relaxations. A fast muscle needs a larger CF and a slow muscle needs a smaller CF to summate the contractions. The tension generated during a complete tetanus is usually about four times that of a single twitch.

1. Following a single action potential, enough Ca^{++} is released to expose all the myosin-binding sites on actin molecules. But, the attachment of activated myosin heads to these sites takes time. Also, the Ca^{++} concentration starts decreasing as the pumping back of Ca^{++} into the sarcoplasmic reticulum commences immediately.

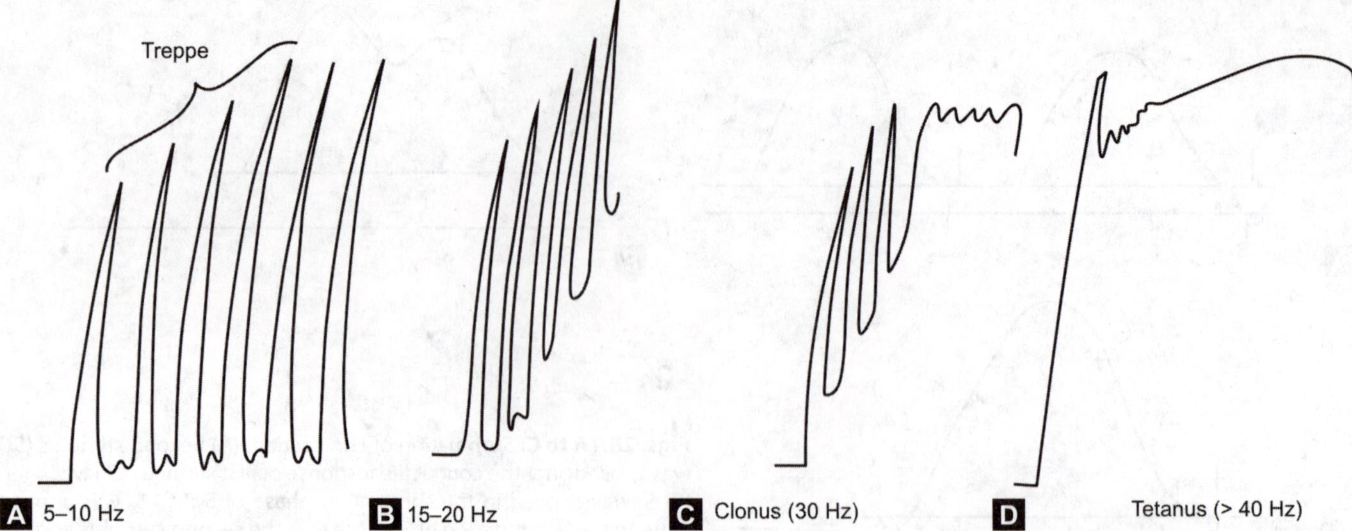

Figs. 28.2A to D: Effect of frequency on muscle contraction and tension (A) at frequency of 5–10 Hz, treppe (staircase phenomenon) occurs; (B and C) at frequency of 15–30 Hz, clonus (partial tetanus) occurs; (D) at frequency of 40 Hz or above, tetanus occurs.

2. Therefore, all the cross-bridges are not engaged and the *tension-generating mechanism is not saturated.*
3. In a tetanic contraction, more and more Ca^{++} is released with each successive action potential, exhausting the pumping-back mechanism.
4. Thus, the cytosolic calcium remains at a constantly high level so that all the myosin-binding sites on the thin filaments are available.
5. Therefore, the *tension generated during tetanic contraction is very high*. Such contraction occurs in a disease called tetanus caused by the clostridium tetani.

Post-Tetanic Potentiation

When a single stimulus is applied to a muscle immediately after the tetanic contraction is over, the amplitude of contraction is higher than that of a single twitch. This phenomenon is known as *post-tetanic potentiation*.

1. Following tetanic contraction, the released Ca^{++} takes some time to be pumped back into the sarcoplasmic reticulum.
2. This left-over Ca^{++} is added to the Ca^{++} released by the next stimulus resulting in a higher cytosolic Ca^{++} level and, therefore, a bigger contraction.

Length-Tension Relationship

Isometric tension developed in a muscle depends on the initial length of the muscle. For the isometric tension to be recorded in an experimental set-up, the ends of the muscle are attached to two fixing points so that changing the distance between the fixing points can alter the length of the muscle.

1. When the muscle fiber is stretched, the tension registered by it is known as the **passive tension**, which is due to the elongation of the elastic titin filaments, not due to activation of the contractile elements.

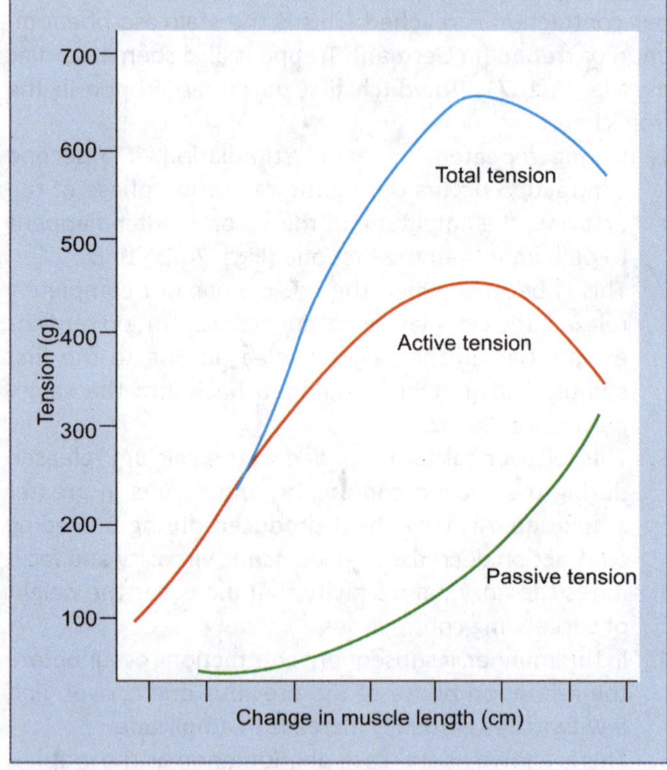

Fig. 28.3: Length-tension relationship in skeletal muscle.

2. If this stretched muscle is stimulated, the tension developed by it is known as the **total tension**.
3. At any length, the amount of tension actually generated by the cross-bridge movements is known as the **active tension**, which is the difference between the two values, that is the total tension minus passive tension.

The length-tension relationship graph (Fig. 28.3) shows that within physiological limit, the tension in the muscle increases, as the length is gradually increased.

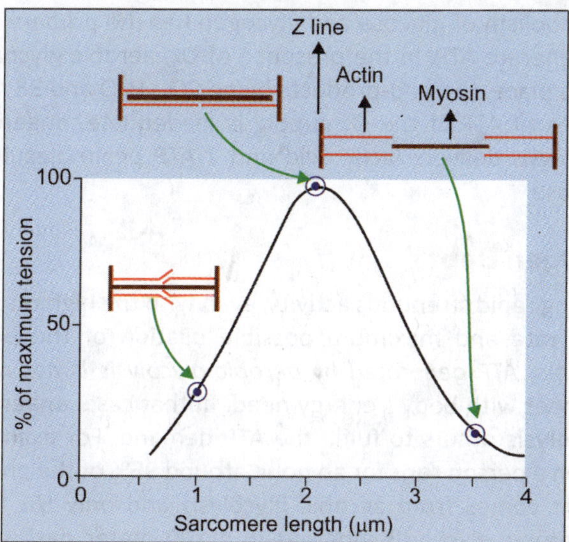

Fig. 28.4: Active tension developed at different sarcomere length. Note that the interaction between actin and myosin is maximum at the peak of active tension, which corresponds to the resting muscle length.

1. The length of the muscle prior to contraction is called the **initial length**.
2. The length of the muscle at which it develops maximal isometric active tension is known as the optimal length or **resting length**, beyond which the tension generated on stimulation decreases until the muscle fibers are torn by the stretch.
3. It has been found that when the skeletal muscles in the body are relaxed, if the tendon is cut from its bony attachment, the muscle *shortens about 20%*. This indicates that the skeletal muscles are under a certain degree of stretch in the resting state.
4. Experiments have shown that this degree of stretch of resting muscles generates maximum tension on stimulation. Therefore, the term 'resting' length is used to describe the muscle length at which maximum response is produced when it is stimulated.

Length-Tension Relationship in a Sarcomere: The length-tension relationship in skeletal muscle has been explained by the sliding filament mechanism of muscle contraction described earlier. According to this mechanism, during contraction, the amount of tension generated depends on the total number of cross-linkages formed due to interaction between actin and myosin molecules.

1. **At resting length**, there is utmost overlap between actin and myosin filaments that can lead to maximum tension development.
2. As the muscle is stretched beyond this length, overlap between thick and thin filaments decreases progressively and the active tension developed declines proportionately, such that, when there is no overlap, the tension generated becomes nil (Fig. 28.4).
3. On the contrary, when the length becomes less than the resting length, overlap decreases and the tension declines.

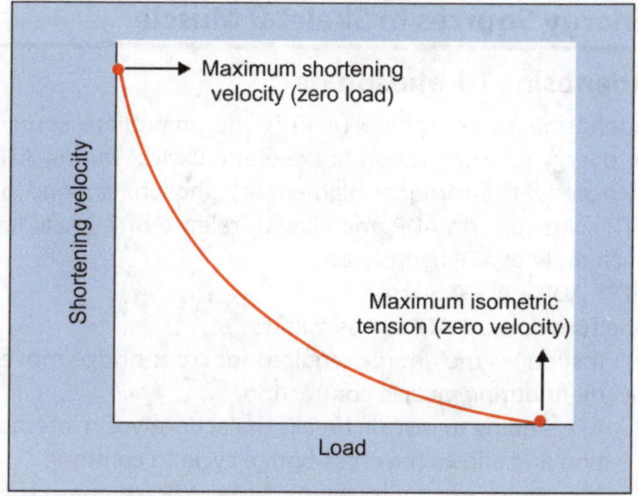

Fig. 28.5: Load-velocity relationship.

4. With extreme reduction in length, the thin filaments overlap each other in the center of the sarcomere so that the binding sites on actin are in the bare area of the thick filaments, producing minimal tension. The optimal sarcomeric length in frog muscle is 2.0–2.2 μm.

Load-Velocity Relationship

When a muscle contracts against a load (isotonic contraction), the velocity of fiber-shortening is inversely proportional to the degree of load. When there is no load, the muscle contracts with maximum velocity and the velocity decreases with increasing load on the muscle (Fig. 28.5).

1. When the load becomes equal to the maximal isometric tension the muscle can develop, the shortening velocity is zero. If the load increases further, the muscle lengthens (**lengthening contraction**).
2. This load-velocity relationship is a common experience in our day-to-day life. As we know, light objects can be lifted faster than heavy objects.
3. The rate of cross-bridge cycling in a muscle, which *depends on its ATPase activity, determines the shortening velocity of that muscle*. In general, a light load offers less resistance to the sliding of the filaments so that thin filaments move quickly over thick filaments allowing few cross-bridges to form at a time, producing less tension and faster contraction.
4. On the contrary, increasing the load on a cross-bridge slows its forward movement during a power stroke and reduces the ATP hydrolysis; the slower contraction allows more time for actomyosin interaction and greater tension development.

Now, if we correlate both the length-tension and load-velocity relationships in a skeletal muscle, we can derive that for any given load, the shortening velocity is maximal when the muscle is at its resting length. When a muscle is stretched by a load prior to start of contraction, the condition is known as free-loaded (pre-loaded); and when the load is applied to the muscle after it starts contracting, the condition is called after-loaded.

Energy Sources in Skeletal Muscle

Adenosine Tri-phosphate

Adenosine Tri-phosphate (ATP) is the immediate source of energy for contraction in skeletal muscles. During ATP hydrolysis, the terminal high-energy phosphate bond of ATP splits to form ADP and Pi, with release of 7.3 kcal for each mole of ATP hydrolyzed.

ATP® ADP + Pi + 7.3 kcal

The functions of ATP are as follows:

1. It supplies the energy required for cross-bridge movement during muscle contraction.
2. ATP binding to myosin breaks the actin-myosin interaction and allows the cross-bridge cycle to continue.
3. It provides energy to the Ca^{++}-Mg^{+} ATPase pump that transports Ca^{++} back into the SR and initiates relaxation.
4. The Na^{+}-K^{+} pump in the sarcolemma utilizes the energy derived from ATP hydrolysis to maintain the membrane excitability (RMP).

In resting muscle, less ATP molecules are present in the sarcoplasm. Once contraction is initiated, ATP store can sustain contraction for fraction of a second. For contractions to continue, muscle requires an enormous supply of ATP, which has to be generated immediately. ATP is regenerated by the addition of one phosphate group to ADP by **three pathways**:

1. Phosphorylation of ADP by creatine phosphate
2. Oxidative phosphorylation of ADP in the mitochondria
3. Phosphorylation of ADP by the breakdown of glucose to CO_2 and H_2O.

Creatine Phosphate

Creatine phosphate (CP) is also called phosphorylcreatine. Phosphorylation of ADP by creatine phosphate is a very rapid, nonoxidative process, which provides ATP by transfer of a phosphate group from CP to ADP, catalyzed by the enzyme creatine kinase (CK).

$$CP + ADP \xrightarrow{CK} C + ATP$$

The concentration of CP is about five times that of ATP in the resting muscle. The above reaction is stimulated by a fall in ATP and a rise in ADP concentration. The amount of ATP that can be formed is limited by the initial concentration of CP in the sarcoplasm. The ATP supplied by this mechanism sustains contractions for a few seconds. During recovery period, the concentration of CP is restored back to the normal level by addition of ATP formed by glycolysis to creatine (C). Also some mitochondrial ATP transfers its phosphate group to creatine.

$$C + ATP \xrightarrow{CK} CP + ADP$$

As the levels of ATP and CP fall, other mechanisms are activated to provide ATP to the contracting muscle. At rest and during light exercise, muscle utilizes free fatty acids as its energy source. During moderate to heavy exercise, metabolism of glucose and glycogen has the primary role to generate ATP. In the presence of O_2, aerobic glycolysis takes place, the end-products being CO_2, H_2O and 38 molecules of ATP. If the O_2 supply is inadequate, anaerobic glycolysis delivers lactic acid and 2 ATP per molecule of glucose.

Oxygen Debt

During rapid strenuous activity, even with the high respiratory rate and maximum possible dilation of the blood vessels, *ATP generated by aerobic glycolysis is not rapid* to meet with body's energy need. In that case, **anaerobic glycolysis** occurs to fulfill the ATP demand. For example, when a person runs for an hour, around 95% of the energy spent comes from aerobic glycolysis and only 5% from anaerobic glycolysis whereas in a 100 meter dash completed in 10 seconds, 85% of the energy is derived from anaerobic glycolysis.

After the exercise is over, body has to accomplish the following functions:

1. Convert the surplus lactate into pyruvate
2. Replenish the ATP and CP stores in the muscle
3. To replaced the O_2 that came from myoglobin.

For all the above functions, O_2 is required. Therefore, even after the termination of the exercise, the respiratory rate remains high for some time according to the severity of the exercise. The **amount of extra oxygen taken up by the body above the basal O_2 consumption** following exercise is known as oxygen debt (Application Box 28.1).

Application Box 28.1

Effects of training: Trained athletes can increase muscle oxygen consumption greatly than the nonathletes. They can also effectively utilize free-fatty acids. Thus, they sustain exercise without loss of glycogen and accumulation of lactate. Hence, oxygen debt in them is much smaller even for severe exercise. They also practice more carbohydrate meal several days before the final competition to increase their muscle glycogen store.

Muscle Fatigue

When a skeletal muscle is repeatedly stimulated, the tension developed by the muscle gradually decreases, even though the stimulation continues. The *decrease in muscle tension as a result of previous contractile activity is known as muscle fatigue*. There is decline in the amplitude of contraction as well as the shortening velocity, and the relaxation period is prolonged. Fatigue can be of early or late onset and the rate of its progress can be fast or slow.

In general, the factors affecting skeletal muscle fatigue are:

1. The types of fibers present in the muscle
2. The intensity and duration of the exercise
3. Availability of nutrients like oxygen and glucose
4. Accumulation of metabolites like lactic acid, H^{+}, K^{+} and substance P
5. Previous regular training of the similar type of activity
6. CNS factor

Out of all these, the CNS factor plays an important role in delaying the muscle fatigue in human beings. As we know, **motivation and encouragement** significantly prolong the duration of exercise. They lead to secretion of certain neurotransmitters by an unknown mechanism that reduces the sensory inputs from the exercising muscle as well as the whole body, reaching the level of consciousness. One probable mechanism is that they activate the **endorphin system**. The degree and source of encouragement also affect fatigue significantly. A muscle that fatigues early also recovers early and the one that takes longer time also recovers late.

Rigor Mortis

During the cross-bridge cycle, binding of ATP to the myosin head breaks the actin-myosin interaction and brings in relaxation of the muscle. If cellular energy stores are depleted, as happens after death, **cross-bridge detachment cannot** occur due to lack of ATP. Therefore, the *myosin heads remain in the attached state*. Following death, the **cytoplasmic calcium concentration remains elevated** because of the following reasons:

1. Calcium is not pumped back into the sarcoplasmic reticulum in the absence of ATP.
2. Ca^{2+} diffuses from ECF into the cytoplasm. This is because after death, the muscle membrane becomes inactive, which cannot maintain the high gradient of Ca^{++} between ECF and ICF, as occurs in life.
3. The inactive membrane of the SR cannot hold back Ca^{++}, which diffuses out of SR to the sarcoplasm.

The raised cytoplasmic calcium concentration initiates contraction by exposing the myosin heads on actin and permitting **formation of cross-bridges that do not detach** due to lack of ATP. This leads to stiffness in the muscle, which is known as **rigor mortis**. It starts about 3 to 4 h after death and gets completed in about 12 h after death. The stiffness disappears 48 to 60 h after death due to disintegration of muscle proteins.

Heat Production in Muscles

During muscle contraction, most of the energy is spent in the form of heat, part of the energy is used to do the work and a small portion is used to build up the ATP stores. The *mechanical efficiency* of a muscle is expressed as the percentage of total energy spent for the work done. **In isometric contraction**, work done is zero; so the mechanical efficiency is 0%, whereas **in isotonic contraction**, the efficiency lies between 20 and 25%, and can be as much as 50%. The amount of heat generated can be measured accurately with the help of sensitive thermocouples.

The heat generated is of the following types:

a. **Resting heat:** When the muscle is at rest, the heat generated due to basal metabolism is known as resting heat.
b. **Initial heat:** Initial heat is the heat liberated during muscle contraction in excess of resting heat. It can be further divided into two parts:
   i. **Activation heat,** which is produced after the muscle is stimulated and before the contraction starts.
   ii. **Shortening heat,** which is released during contraction leading to shortening and is proportionate to the degree of shortening.
c. **Relaxation heat:** When a previously shortened muscle returns to its original length, the heat generated is known as relaxation heat.
d. **Recovery heat:** This is the heat produced by the metabolic processes to restore the muscle to its resting state, in excess of resting heat. The recovery heat is liberated for a prolonged period and is equal in magnitude to the initial heat.

Scientists contributed

Archibald Vivian Hill
(1886–1977)

Otto Fritz Meyerhof
(1884–1951)

The **Nobel Prize in Physiology or Medicine 1922** was divided equally between muscle physiologist from UK **Archibald Vivian Hill** 'for his discovery relating to the production of **heat in the muscle**' and American muscle physiologist **Otto Fritz Meyerhof** 'for his discovery of the fixed relationship between the consumption of oxygen and the metabolism of lactic acid in the muscle'.

Fiber Types in Skeletal Muscle

Based on the speed of contraction and the process of deriving energy from the body metabolism, skeletal muscle fibers can be classified into two categories: type I and type II (Table 28.1).

Table 28.1: Differences between type I and II muscle fibers.

	Type I	Type II
1. Other names	Slow; red; oxidative	Fast; white; glycolytic
2. Contraction velocity	Slow	Fast
3. Myosin ATPase	Low	High
4. Ca^{2+}-pumping capacity of SR	Low	High
5. Rate of fatigue	Slow	Fast
6. Fiber diameter	Moderate	Large
7. Size of motor unit	Small	Large
8. Glycogen content	Low	High
9. Glycolytic capacity	Low	High
10. Oxidative capacity	High	Low
11. Mitochondria	Numerous	Less
12. Myoglobin content	High	Low
13. Capillaries	Many	Few
14. Primary source of ATP production	Oxidative phosphorylation	Glycolysis

Type I Muscle Fibers

Muscles consisting mainly of type I fibers have **many capillaries and high myoglobin** content that imparts them the **red color**. This ensures an increased blood flow to supply more oxygen.

1. As there are plenty of mitochondria and the oxygen binding protein myoglobin, they synthesize ATP by oxidative phosphorylation and are named as **oxidative fibers**.
2. Due to their low myosin ATPase activity, they break down ATP slowly; thus, the rate of cross-bridge cycling is less causing a decreased contraction velocity and so they are known as the **slow fibers**.
3. They are more *resistant to fatigue*; that means they can remain contracted for longer time, thereby help maintain posture.
4. Therefore, type I fibers in back and proximal limb muscles are known as postural muscles.

Type II Muscle Fibers

Muscles containing mainly type II fibers have a greater contraction velocity and are mainly **white muscles**. They carry out fine, precise movements. The examples are intrinsic muscles of the hand and extraocular muscles of the eye.

Motor Units

Definition

A motor unit consists of a single motor neuron, its axonal branches and all the muscle fibers supplied by them (Fig. 28.6).

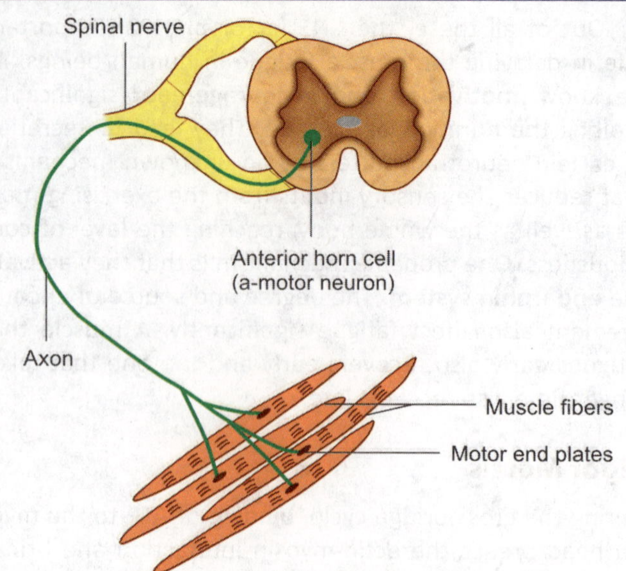

Fig. 28.6: Structure of a motor unit. Note the number of muscle fibers innervated by a single motor neuron is the motor unit.

Size of a Motor Unit

The cell bodies of motor neurons are present in the anterior horn of the spinal cord. A single motor neuron branches out and innervates many muscle fibers. When a motor neuron discharges, contraction is produced in all the muscle fibers supplied by it.

1. The size of a motor unit can be large or small depending on the number of muscle fibers innervated by it.
2. In the intrinsic muscles of the hand, one motor neuron innervates less than ten muscle fibers so, stimulation of a motor unit produces a small rise in tension.
3. The back muscles have hundreds or even thousands of muscle fibers per motor unit, where activation of a single motor unit causes a large increase in tension.

Recruitment of Motor Units

At the resting state of the muscle, hardly any motor unit is activated. When a single motor neuron discharges, there is some rise in tension in the muscles of the concerned limb. If a greater total tension has to be attained, additional motor neurons fire and there is increase in the number of active motor units. *The process of activating more number of motor units is called recruitment of motor units*.

1. In hand muscles, gradual activation of motor units produces a stepwise increase in muscle tension because, with activation of each new unit, a small amount of tension is added. As the tension goes up in a graded manner, it can precisely be regulated. Therefore, the **muscles carrying out skilled movements have smaller motor units**, for which finer regulation of muscle tension is of primary importance.
2. In contrast, in back muscles, with recruitment of additional motor units, each time a huge amount of tension is added. Therefore, the back muscles are useful in maintenance of posture, as there is need to develop a greater tension to resist the downward pull of the gravity (Application Box 28.2).

> **Application Box 28.2**
>
> **Asynchronous discharge of motor units prevents fatigue:** The motor units discharge asynchronously. When some of the motor units are active, other units are silent. Afterward, the active units go to rest and the silent units become active. At any instant of time, the inputs from different units are summated and this results in a smooth contraction of the muscle. This also helps the muscle to work for longer time without being fatigued.

Size Principle

All the muscle fibers in a motor unit are of the same type, i.e. the muscle fibers innervated by a spinal motor neuron are either oxidative or glycolytic in nature. Based on this, the motor units can be designated as oxidative or slow and glycolytic or fast motor units. Usually the large diameter, fast-conducting motor neurons innervate the muscle fibers of the fast motor units and the small diameter, slow conducting motor neurons innervate muscle fibers of the slow motor units. This is called the size principle. As the strength of contraction gradually increases, the small motor units are recruited initially, followed by the recruitment of large motor units. Thus, during the activity of mild to moderate intensity, the less fatigable, oxidative fibers mostly take part in the contractile activity, whereas the glycolytic fibers are recruited during more intense contraction. In general, *a muscle has both types of motor units* (Application Box 28.3).

Application Box 28.3

Nature of exercise determines type of muscle fibers: The proportion of fast and slow motor units determines the overall strength, fatigability or contraction velocity of a muscle. There are both types of motor units in a muscle. Regular practice of isometric exercise increases the amount of slow fibers and practice of isotonic exercise increases the percentage of fast fibers.

Whole-Muscle Contraction

During any voluntary activity, muscles contract or relax around a joint to facilitate or inhibit movement in a particular direction. A **whole muscle** (for e.g. biceps or triceps) consists of many muscle fibers that are organized into several motor units. The central nervous system exerts a precise control over the voluntary movements by matching the force required by the act with the **tension** developed in the active muscles. Depending on the *type and degree of activity*, tension develops in the muscles in a smooth and graded fashion. The CNS achieves this by **recruitment of more motor units** and increasing the **frequency of discharge** of the motor units. The motor units discharge **asynchronously** and this results in a *smooth and sustained contraction* **preventing early fatigue** of the muscle.

The total tension developed in a muscle depends on the number of active fibers at any instant during contraction, which is decided by the following factors:

1. The total number of active motor units
2. The number of fibers present in each motor unit
3. The type of fibers present in each motor unit (based on the initial length of the fiber, its diameter and fatigability).

Muscle Strength

The strength of a muscle is measured by the maximum load it is capable of lifting. There are muscles of different lengths and shapes. Therefore, in order to compare the relative strengths of muscles, the maximum load it can lift in kilograms is divided by the cross-sectional area in square centimeters. The strength of human skeletal muscles is about **3–4 kg/cm^2**, a value typical of all mammals. In the same age group, males have a higher value than females, the ratio being 1:0.65. The male hormone testosterone contributes to better development and growth of skeletal muscles. So, the differences are apparent in the postpubertal life. Genetic build plays a role. Also, regular and systematic training enhances muscle power.

Applied Aspects

Muscular Dystrophy

Muscular dystrophy (MD) includes a variety of degenerative muscle diseases that are due to mutations in the genes coding for the various components of the dystrophin-glycoprotein complex.

Duchenne Muscular Dystrophy

The commonest of muscular dystrophy is Duchenne muscular dystrophy (DMD), also called pseudohypertrophic MD, an *X-linked recessive disease* that affects mostly male children.

1. DMD is characterized by progressive muscular weakness that becomes apparent by age 4, and enlargement of affected muscles (muscle hypertrophy), especially of the calf muscles, and pelvifemoral muscles. Cardiomegaly is common.
2. Enlargement occurs due to gradual degeneration and necrosis of muscle fibers that are replaced by more fibrous and fatty tissue.
3. Typically, the child uses his hands to climb up, while getting up from the floor. By age 12, most sufferers are no longer ambulatory and death occurs by age 30.
4. The pathology is mainly due to absence of dystrophin in the muscles, caused by mutations of the dystrophin gene.
5. Dystrophin gene is a large gene, located in the p21 region of the X chromosome and has a high mutation rate.

Baker's Muscular Dystrophy

Baker's muscular dystrophy (BMD) is a less severe and rare form MD. It is similar in presentation to DMD, but patients often survive into adulthood.

1. In BMD patients, dystrophin is reduced in amount or present in an abnormal form. Research is underway to identify and stimulate the production of dystrophin-related proteins that may help to correct the symptoms of BMD.
2. A gene expressing a truncated form of dystrophin, called utrophin, has been inserted into mice using transgenic methods and has improved the myopathy.
3. In several forms of MD, laminin 2, a protein associated with the basal lamina of muscle cells and concerned

with mechanical connections between the exterior of muscle cells and the extracellular matrix, is absent along with dystrophin.

Myopathies

Mutations in the gene coding for the protein **desmin** cause skeletal and cardiac myopathies.

Metabolic Myopathies

Metabolic myopathies occur due to mutations in the genes coding for various enzymes involved in the metabolism of carbohydrates, proteins and fats. In these patients, muscle breakdown occurs due to accumulation of toxic metabolites.

Inflammatory Myopathy

Poliomyelitis is an inflammatory myopathy in which weakness of proximal limb muscles is an early feature. It is due to destruction of motor neurons present in the anterior horn of spinal cord by the poliovirus, resulting in paralysis of skeletal muscles. Death may occur due to respiratory failure.

Myotonia

These are conditions where muscle relaxation is prolonged after voluntary contraction. They are due to abnormal genes on chromosomes 7, 17 or 19 that lead to malfunction of Na^+ or Cl^- channels.

Focal Dystonias

Dystonia means faulty contraction. Usually the abnormal contraction is limited to a small and specific region of muscles, so it is called focal dystonia.

1. These are neuromuscular disorders characterized by involuntary and repetitive or sustained skeletal muscle contractions that cause twisting, turning or squeezing movements in a body part.
2. They often result in abnormal postures, considerable pain and also physical impairment.
3. The common dystonias are spasmodic torticollis and cervical dystonia that usually affect neck and shoulder muscles, blepharospasm that affects eyelid muscles, strabismus and nystagmus that affect extraocular muscles, writer's cramp that affect finger muscles, spasmodic dysphonia that affect muscles of speech apparatus including vocal cord and hemifacial spasm that affect facial muscles.
4. Injection of botulinum toxin into the affected muscles has shown promising results in the treatment of these disorders.

Muscle Sprain

Muscle sprain often occurs during sports activity or physical labor due to overstretching or forced extension of an active muscle.

1. Very often the myotendinous junction is injured or, at times, there is separation of the fibers.
2. Ultrastructural damage to the contractile elements especially at the Z lines may occur. Pain, soreness, weakness, and swelling are the usual symptoms.
3. Treatment includes ice packs, rest and immobility. Drugs to relieve pain may be prescribed and surgery is performed to correct the damage if needed.

Muscle Cramp

This is a painful condition due to involuntary tetanic contraction of skeletal muscle.

1. It is caused by *generation of nerve action potentials at a very high rate*.
2. This abnormal activity of nerve occurs in conditions like electrolyte imbalances in the extracellular fluid surrounding both the muscle and nerve fibers due to overexercise or persistent dehydration.

CHAPTER SUMMARY

Key Concepts

1. Skeletal muscle exhibits properties, such as summation of contraction, treppe, tetanization and typical lenth-tension and load-velocity relationship that are suited for its functions.
2. Major energy sources in skeletal muscles are ATP, and creatine phosphate.
3. After the termination of the exercise, the respiratory rate remains high for some time to meet the amount of extra oxygen taken up by the body above the basal O_2 consumption during exercise. It is known as *oxygen debt*. Oxygen debt is much less in athletes compared to nonathletes, even in severe exercise.
4. A motor unit consists of a single motor neuron, its axonal branches and all the muscle fibers supplied by them. At rest, hardly any motor unit is activated. For more muscle tension to be attained, additional motor neurons should fire and there should be increase in the number of active motor units. The process of activating more number of motor units is called recruitment of motor units.

Important to Know (Must Read)

1. In examinations, 'properties of skeletal muscle' may be asked as a **Long Question**.
2. Treppe, Length-tension relationship, Load-velocity relationship, Oxygen debt, and Heat produced in muscle come as usual in **Short Questions** in exams.
3. In **Viva**, examiners usually ask: Name the properties of skeletal muscle, What is staircase phenomenon, Define treppe and speak about it mechanism and importance, What is the difference between tetanization and tetany, What are the critical frequency for tetanization, What is post-tetanic potentiation, Define initial length and resting length, What is passive tension, active tension and total tension, What is Length-tension relationship and Load-velocity relationship, Define oxygen debt, what is its mechanism and its importance, What are the types of heat produced in a muscle, How muscle fatigue can be delayed, What is rigor mortis and what is its mechanism, What are the types of muscle fibers and what are the differences between them, Define motor unit, What is motor unit recruitment, What is size principle, Name common muscle dystrophies and myopathies, What is the defect in Duchenne muscle dystrophy and what are the features in this problem.
4. Oxygen debt, length-tension relationship and motor units are invariably asked in both theory and oral exams.

CHAPTER 29

Smooth Muscle and Cardiac Muscle

Learning Objectives

On completion of study of this chapter, the student **MUST** be able to:

1. Classify smooth muscle, and mention the differences between them.
2. List the properties of smooth muscle.
3. Describe the mechanism of smooth muscle contraction.
4. List the special features of cardiac muscle.
5. List the differences between skeletal, smooth, and cardiac muscle.

The student **MAY** also be able to:

1. Describe the properties of smooth muscle and cardiac muscle.
2. Explain the differences between skeletal, cardiac, and smooth muscles.

SMOOTH MUSCLES

Smooth muscles are mainly present in the visceral organs and blood vessels. The distinctive features in smooth muscles and major differences from skeletal and cardiac muscles are:

1. They are characterized by absence of regular pattern of cross-striations as found in skeletal and cardiac muscles, hence the name *smooth muscles*.
2. The nerve supply to smooth muscles is through the branches of autonomic nervous system.
3. Another striking difference is that the length tension relationship is not linear as in skeletal and cardiac muscle.
4. Smooth muscles can remain contracted for relatively longer periods without expenditure of much energy, a property that endows them with a better metabolic economy.

Types of Smooth Muscles

In some organs, groups of smooth muscle fibers behave as ***syncytium***, like that of cardiac muscles and in few other organs they follow the functional properties of skeletal muscles. Based on this, they are classified into two types: **single-unit** smooth muscles, and **multiunit** smooth muscles.

Single-unit Smooth Muscle

The muscle fibers in single-unit smooth muscles are connected to each other by **gap junctions**.

1. The action potential generated at one place spreads rapidly to all the fibers of that unit. Therefore, contraction occurs simultaneously in all the fibers. Due to this ***synchronous electrical and mechanical activity***, the fibers behave as a **syncytium** or a single unit.
2. Single-unit smooth muscles are far more abundant. They form the **walls of hollow viscera** such as the gastrointestinal tract, from the esophagus to the rectum, including the gallbladder and ducts of digestive glands; the ureters and urinary bladder; the uterus and small diameter blood vessels.
3. As they are present in many visceral organs, they are also called **visceral smooth muscles**.

Multiunit Smooth Muscle

Multiunit smooth muscles **do not have gap junctions**; therefore, they do not act as a syncytium.

1. They *resemble skeletal muscles functionally* as they are largely under neural control, though not under voluntary control.
2. They are abundantly innervated by the fibers of the autonomic nervous system.

3. The intrinsic muscles of the eye (ciliary body and iris), muscle in the large airways to the lungs, precapillary sphincters, and piloerector muscles are examples of multiunit smooth muscles.

Functional Organization

Though the structure of smooth muscles remains apparently same in various body parts, they accomplish different tasks at different body locations. For example, they regulate movement of fluids in the blood vessels, cause propulsive movements at different parts of GIT, expel the contents of the hollow organs like uterus, etc. To suit these varieties of functional needs, arrangements of smooth muscles differ in body parts.

Chiefly, arrangement of fibers is of **three types**:

1. **Circular:** Circular pattern of arrangement is seen in the ***blood vessels and in the airways*** of the lungs where contraction of the muscles narrows the diameter of the passage and reduces the flow. In sphincters, the contraction can totally block the passage and stop the flow.
2. **Circular and longitudinal:** Circular and longitudinal organization is found in ***GI tract***, where an inner thick circular muscle layer and an outer thin longitudinal muscle layer regulate the many types of movements of intestine and promote the mixing and forward movement of the digested food.
3. **Circular, longitudinal and oblique:** Circular, longitudinal and oblique arrangement is typically found in the ***uterus and urinary bladder***. When the increased contents of these viscera stretch these muscles, they contract and decrease the volume by expelling the contents.

Structure

Unlike skeletal muscle fibers that cannot multiply once differentiation is complete around birth, the smooth muscles are ***capable of dividing throughout the life*** of the individual. The special features of smooth muscles are as follows:

1. The cells are quite ***small in size*** compared to the whole tissue. The small size of cells is an advantage for smooth muscle for precisely controlling visceral functions.

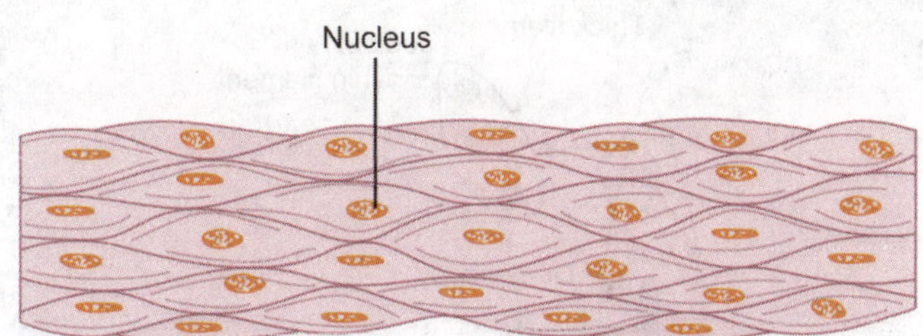

Fig. 29.1: Smooth muscle. Note the spindle shaped cells.

2. Each smooth muscle fiber is a spindle-shaped cell, **100–300 μm long and 5–10 μm in diameter** at the middle (Fig. 29.1).
3. Smooth muscle cells contain a single elongated nucleus at the center and few mitochondria. The cell ***derives energy mainly from glycolytic pathway***.
4. The ***sarcoplasmic reticulum is well developed*** only in some types of smooth muscles; in others it is rudimentary.
5. Myofilaments are organized differently.
6. There are ***no sarcomeres*** and ***striations are not visible*** (Figs. 29.2A and B).
7. There is ***lack of an organized T tubular system***.
8. The cell membrane shows invaginations called **caveolae** that increase the surface area.

Myofilaments

The cytoplasm contains three types of myofilaments: ***thick, thin, and intermediate***. In addition to the filaments, the cytoplasm contains a calcium-binding protein called **calmodulin**, which is structurally related to troponin.

Thick Filaments

The thick filaments are about 2.2 μm long and composed of myosin molecules that are not arranged in a regular pattern around the axis of the filament as in the skeletal muscle. They are interspersed among the thin filaments (Fig. 29.3) and are much fewer than in skeletal or cardiac muscle.

Intermediate Filaments and Dense Bodies

The diameter of intermediate filaments is about 10 nm, which is present between the thick and thin filaments. Intermediate filaments provide cytoskeletal support and have negligible roles in contractile activity.

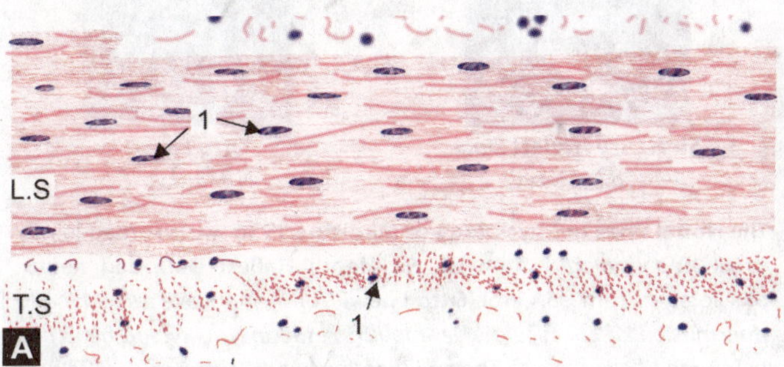

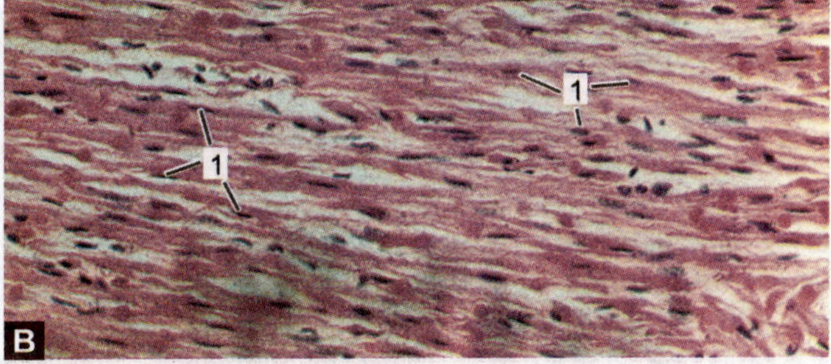

Figs. 29.2A and B: Ultrastructure (A) and photomicrograph (B) of smooth muscle. No. 1 indicates oval centrally placed nucleus. Note, there is no striations and sarcomere.

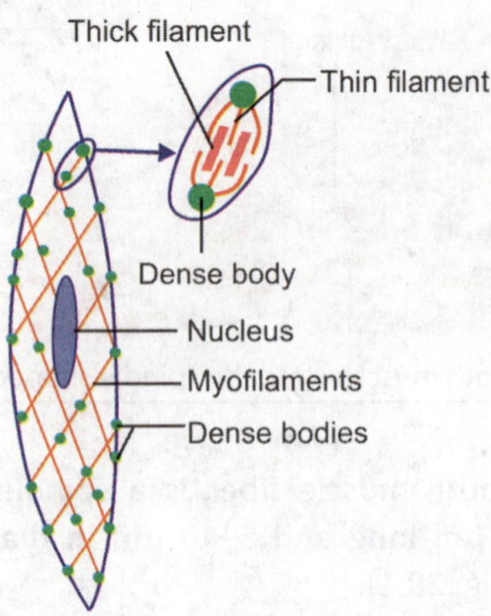

Fig. 29.3: Arrangement of myofilaments in smooth muscles.

1. Small, electron-dense, dark areas called **dense bodies** are present throughout the cytoplasm, as well as attached to the cell membrane.
2. Those associated with the cell membrane are often called membrane-associated dense bodies or patches, or **focal adhesions**. Dense bodies are functionally analogous to the Z lines in skeletal muscle fibers.

Thin Filaments

In smooth muscles, thin filaments are composed of actin and tropomyosin molecules but ***troponin protein complex is absent***.

Organization of Filaments

The relationship between the thick and thin filaments is poor and they are less well organized.

1. In cross sections through the overlap region of the filaments, the geometric pattern as found in striated muscles are not seen.
2. Because of the absence of a highly organized arrangement of contractile apparatus, the ***length tension relationship in the smooth muscles is very much flexible***.
3. The thick and thin filaments are *obliquely oriented* to the long axis of the cell. The actin filaments anchor to the dense bodies by means of the protein ***α-actinin***.
4. During the sliding-filament mechanism, the gap between the actin filaments reduces and the shortening force is transmitted through the dense bodies to the plasma membrane producing contraction of the muscle fiber.

Organization of Muscle Fibers

The smooth muscle fibers are ***organized in sheets*** and the cells are connected to adjacent cells by short strands of connective tissue. In addition, collagen and elastin fibers are embedded in a reticular connective tissue that traverses through the whole organ, connecting and holding the cells together.

1. Most importantly, the cells are linked to each other by ***gap junctions***, by which many cells are activated at a time by single action potential.
2. With the help of the stroma and the gap junctions, the mechanical as well as ***electrical activities of the cells are coupled***, so that contraction occurs in an integrated and coordinated fashion.

Innervations of Smooth Muscles

Smooth muscles exhibit a spontaneous, slow wave rhythm. Neural stimulation only modulates (increases or decreases) this basic pattern. Branches of the autonomic nervous system innervate the smooth muscles, most of which are supplied by **sympathetic** as well as **parasympathetic fibers**:

1. In response to a nerve action potential, neurotransmitters are secreted from the numerous varicosities present along the axon, and then diffuse to the adjacent tissues.
2. Since the release of neurotransmitters is not confined to the axon terminals, highly ***specialized neuromuscular junctions are absent*** in smooth muscles.
3. Unlike the skeletal muscle, the receptors for neurotransmitters are not gathered at the neuromuscular junctions, they are scattered along the postsynaptic membrane.

Electrical Properties

Unlike the skeletal muscle where the stimulus arrives in the form of an all-or-none action potential, in smooth muscles the contraction may or may not be preceded by an action potential. The smooth muscles react to a variety of stimuli, which may be **neural** (sympathetic or parasympathetic); **hormonal** (circulating catecholamines, serotonin, histamine, angiotensin, vasopressin, oxytocin, estrogen, and progesterone); **chemical** (hypoxia, hypercapnia, and H^+); cold; and stretch. The transmission of nerve impulse in sympathetic and parasympathetic nerves supplying visceral muscles and properties of visceral muscle were studied in detail by Dale.

Scientists contributed

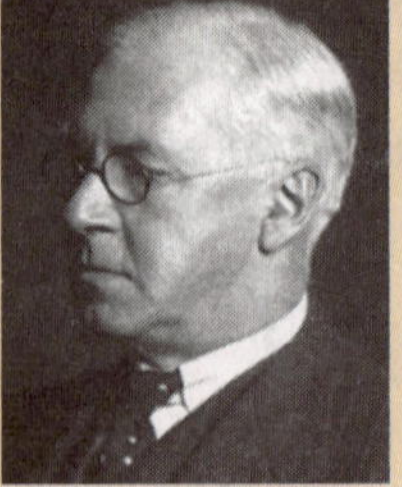

Sir Henry Hallett Dale
(1875–1968)

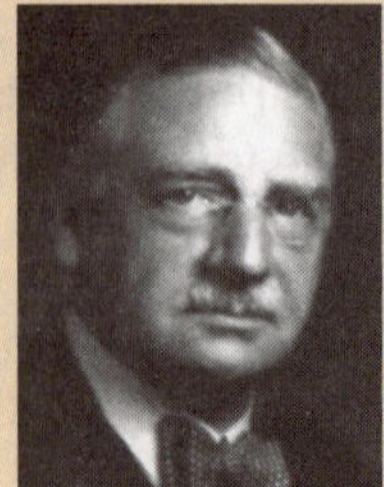

Otto Loewi
(1873–1961)

The **Nobel Prize in Physiology or Medicine 1936** was awarded jointly to neurophysiologist from UK **Sir Henry Hallett Dale** and neurophysiologist from USA Prof. **Otto Loewi** *"for their discoveries relating to transmission of chemical nerve impulses, especially in sympathetic and parasympathetic nerves"*. Their pioneering works were in the field of transmission of nerve impulses, especially its chemical basis. Dale had also studied the details of smooth muscle functions

Characteristic Electrical Activities

1. When the stimulus is excitatory, the membrane potential decreases and it increases in response to an inhibitory stimulus.
2. The membrane potential of visceral smooth muscles is variable (no fixed resting potential), ranging from –30 mV to –70 mV with an average of –50 mV.
3. The visceral smooth muscle shows spontaneous oscillations in a wave like pattern. Some of the oscillations lead to action potentials that may occur in the rising or falling phase of the wave.
4. The multiunit smooth muscles do not discharge spontaneously; they also do not respond to stretch.
5. Most of the visceral smooth muscles generate action potentials inherently; any stimulus acting on it only alters the rate and pattern of action potentials formed.
6. The **shapes of action potentials** vary widely, which may be a spike, or action potential with a prolonged plateau, or multiple spikes, superimposed on the membrane potential (Fig. 29.4). Other forms of spikes or action potentials of smooth muscle have been described in GI system).
7. In some cells, in response to stimuli like hormones or mechanical stretch, the membrane potential shows a graded change that may culminate into an action potential.

Action Potential

The action potentials are generally of low amplitude, which is about 60 mV, and the duration is around 100 ms. ***The depolarization phase*** is caused by influx of calcium from ECF due to the opening of voltage-gated Ca^{++} channels. Compared to the striated muscles, the ***upstroke of actions potential is prolonged*** in smooth muscles, because the Ca^{++} channels take more time to open than the Na^{+} channels. ***The repolarization phase*** occurs due to closure of Ca^{++} channels, which occurs slowly. Opening of voltage-gated K^{+} channels contributes toward the later part of repolarization. Action potentials are generally observed in visceral smooth muscles. Some smooth muscle cells contract without any change in membrane potential.

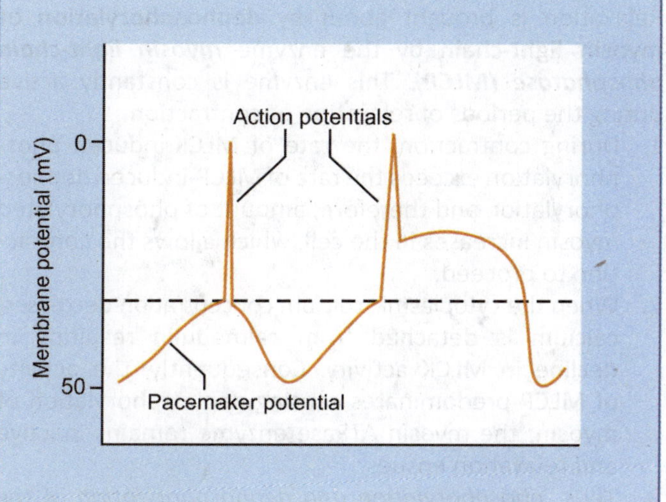

Fig. 29.4: Electrical activities (pacemaker potential and action potential) in smooth muscle.

Junctional Potential

Generally, action potentials are not observed in multiunit smooth muscles. Instead, in response to neurotransmitters like Ach, local depolarization called junctional potential is recorded that spreads electrotonically along the muscle fiber and decreases the membrane potential causing calcium influx through the opening of voltage-gated Ca^{++} channels, leading to contraction.

Pacemaker Potential

In addition to action potentials, pacemaker potentials are recorded in visceral smooth muscle. However, unlike cardiac muscle, the pacemaker activity is not generated at a fixed location; rather it shifts from place to place. In visceral smooth muscles like intestine, pacemaker activities occur at several sites at the same time and then they travel for a short distance in the muscle.

Mechanism of Contraction

Role of Calcium

As in other muscle types, changes in sarcoplasmic calcium ion concentration plays a major role in smooth muscle contraction.

1. The strength of the stimulus (the degree of stretch or the amount of neurotransmitter/hormone reaching the cell membrane) acting on the smooth muscle fiber can be graded. Accordingly, the change in cytosolic calcium concentration may be minute, more or very high, producing different degrees of contraction.
2. The cytosolic calcium concentration is increased mainly by **entry of calcium from the interstitial fluid** (calcium influx) or to some extent by its *release from cytoplasmic calcium stores* (calcium release).
3. However, the concentration of calcium in cytosol ***decreases due to binding of calcium to calmodulin,*** pumping back of calcium to the SR and calcium efflux.

Calcium Influx

Calcium influx occurs through voltage-gated Ca^{++} channels, ligand-gated Ca^{++} channels and a few leaky channels. The ECF calcium concentration is about 12,000 times higher than that of the cytoplasm (1,200,000 nmol/L versus 100 nmol/L). This high inwardly directed gradient favors calcium entry into the smooth muscle as soon as calcium channels open.

Calcium Release

Calcium release from the SR takes place by two mechanisms.

1. IP_3-mediated pathway activated by second messengers.
2. *Calcium-induced calcium release (CICR)* mechanism (as described above) in which, some amount of calcium influx stimulates further calcium release from the SR.

Binding of Calcium to Calmodulin

Binding of calcium to calmodulin starts when cytoplasmic calcium concentration is above 10^{-7} M and is completed at 10^{-4} M.

Pumping Back of Calcium to the SR

Pumping back of calcium to SR is mediated via a Ca^{++} ATPase present on the membrane of SR.

Calcium Efflux

Calcium efflux to the ECF occurs by **Na^{+}-Ca^{++} antiport**, a process of secondary active transport and by ***Ca^{++}-ATPase***, both the mechanisms being present on the cell membrane.

In smooth muscles, tension is generated in the same manner as in skeletal muscles, by the attachment of energized cross-bridges to actin, followed by detachment from and reattachment to actin.

Molecular Basis of Contraction

As described above, calcium concentration increases in the cell mainly by influx from ECF, and partly by release from SR. The following step-wise processes take place sequentially to culminate in muscle contraction.

1. Rise in cytosolic calcium mainly due to calcium influx from ECF.
2. Calcium binds to calmodulin following which *activation of* **myosin light-chain kinase** (MLCK) occurs. **Calmodulin** is a small protein associated with MLCK, which is a *Ca^{++}-calmodulin dependent protein kinase*. When calmodulin binds with four calcium ions, the calcium-calmodulin complex activates MLCK.
3. Activated MLCK brings about **phosphorylation of myosin head** and ***stimulates myosin ATPase activity***. MLCK utilizes one molecule of ATP and causes phosphorylation of the *regulatory light chains* of myosin, on serine at position 19. This ***phosphorylation process is critical for the activation of myosin ATPase***.
4. Increased myosin ATPase activity and myosin-actin interaction initiates the cross-bridge cycle and shortening occurs due to the sliding-filament mechanism. The myosin ATPase enzyme is activated in the phosphorylated myosin head causing hydrolysis of one ATP molecule. The energized myosin head (***Myosin-ADP-Pi complex***) binds with actin producing the power stroke and pulls the thin filament toward the center of the thick filament. ADP and Pi are released during this process.
5. The ***cross-bridge detaches*** from actin when another ATP molecule attaches to myosin reducing its affinity for actin. Then, the myosin ATPase enzyme hydrolyses ATP resulting in the attachment of myosin head with actin.
6. Thus, the **cross-bridge cycle continues**, provided that the myosin head remains phosphorylated.
7. The cross-bridge cycle continues as long as the required cytoplasmic calcium concentration is maintained, because ***phosphorylation depends on cytosolic calcium level*** (Flowchart 29.1).

Flowchart 29.1: Major events of smooth muscle contraction and relaxation.

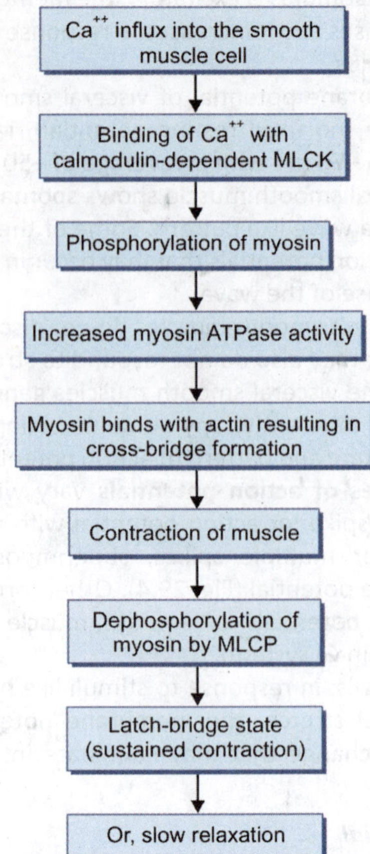

(MLCK: Myosin light-chain kinase; MLCP: Myosin light-chain phosphatase).

In skeletal muscles, contraction proceeds with activation of thin filament proteins (**actin-linked regulation**), whereas in smooth muscles, the process of contraction is myosin based (**myosin-linked regulation**).

Mechanism of Relaxation

Relaxation is brought about by **dephosphorylation of myosin light-chain** by the enzyme ***myosin light-chain phosphatase (MLCP)***. This enzyme is constantly active during the periods of relaxation or contraction.

1. During contraction, the rate of MLCK-induced phosphorylation exceeds the rate of MLCP-induced dephosphorylation and therefore, amount of phosphorylated myosin increases in the cell, which allows the contraction to proceed.
2. When the cytoplasmic calcium concentration decreases, calcium is detached from calmodulin resulting in decline in MLCK activity. Consequently, the activity of MLCP predominates causing dephosphorylation of myosin; the myosin ATPase enzyme remains inactive and relaxation ensues.
3. Thus, *phosphorylation and dephosphorylation of the myosin light-chain is regulated by respective rise and fall of cytosolic calcium concentration*.

Phasic and Tonic Contractions: Unlike the skeletal muscles that demonstrate either twitch or tetanic contraction waves on stimulation, the smooth muscles exhibit phasic or tonic type of contraction.

Phasic Contraction

In phasic type, the degree of phosphorylation, the rate of cross-bridge cycle and the cytoplasmic calcium concentration return to the resting value following the phase of contraction.

Tonic Contraction

During tonic contraction, the above-mentioned parameters do not return to the resting value, rather they remain elevated above the baseline. However, their activity remains less than their peak activity, producing a sustained tension in the muscle at a lower level of MLCK phosphorylation that occurs with less expenditure of energy. This is possible due to the operation of *latch-bridge mechanism*.

Latch-Bridge Mechanism

Muscle in this state is known as the ***latch-state***, in which dephosphorylation of attached cross-bridges occurs in an environment of elevated cytosolic calcium level.

1. When MLCP-induced dephosphorylation of myosin light-chain takes place, it does not bring about dissociation of myosin from actin until the cytoplasmic calcium concentration falls below a critical level.
2. This attached cross-bridges following dephosphorylation are known as the ***latch-bridges***. In this process the rate of cross-bridge cycle is decreased due to slower rate of detachment of cross-bridges. That means the cross-bridges spend more time in an attached state.
3. Therefore, the ATP utilization is less, which enables the visceral smooth muscles to have sustained contractions with less expenditure of energy.
4. The force of this sustained contraction can be graded over a wide range because the cytosolic calcium concentration can be finely regulated over a wide range. From the latch-state, the relaxation of the muscle occurs when the cytoplasmic calcium concentration falls below 10^{-7} M.

Properties of Smooth Muscle

The properties of visceral smooth muscles may be divided into 3 categories (Table 29.1):

The electrical properties of smooth muscles are described above. Few other important properties are discussed below.

Contractile Response

In response to a stimulus, the visceral smooth muscles show a **prolonged contraction** that has a slow initiation and the relaxation also takes longer time. The **latent period is 100–200 msec**; the **contraction period can be 200–500 msec** or even more; likewise, the relaxation period extends into few hundred milliseconds.

Table 29.1: Properties of smooth muscle.

A. Morphological properties
1. Lack of striations
2. Absence of troponin
3. Absence of T-tubules
4. Absence of well-developed neuromuscular junctions
B. Electrical properties
5. Presence of gap junctions (syncytial property)
6. Excitability
7. Variable RMP and shifting pacemakers
8. Variable action potentials
C. Mechanical properties
9. Tonus
10. Plasticity
11. Slow and prolonged contractile response
12. Length–tension relationship
13. Force–velocity relationship
14. Muscle hypertrophy

Muscle Tone

Visceral smooth muscles are continuously in a state of spontaneous irregular contraction known as **tonus**, which occurs due to generation of ***basic slow wave rhythm***. In blood vessels, especially the arterioles, this muscle tone helps to maintain the blood pressure without much expenditure of energy. The multiunit smooth muscles do not exhibit the inherent muscle tone.

Length–Tension Relationship

Unlike the skeletal and cardiac muscles, where the tension changes proportionately to the change in length, the length–tension relationship is variable in smooth muscles.

1. When a smooth muscle is stretched, it initially shortens and exerts tension. However, if the stretch is maintained, gradually the tension decreases and if the stretch is increased, the tension may not rise proportionately or at a particular length, the tension may increase considerably. Thus the relationship is ***highly inconsistent***.
2. The adaptability of the smooth muscle to the new length with less increase in tension is known as **plasticity**, which is based on the latch-bridge phenomenon.
3. In blood vessels, this feature is also known as ***stress relaxation*** that helps to maintain BP within the normal range in spite of sudden rise in pressure.
4. In hollow viscera like stomach, large volume of food and fluid can be accommodated without an undue increase in internal pressure, called ***receptive relaxation***.

Force–Velocity Relationship

Compared to the skeletal muscles, smooth muscles have a low myosin ATPase activity, less number of cross-bridges and a slower rate of cross-bridge cycling. These factors contribute to a slower contraction velocity. Moreover, a **variety of force-velocity graphs** can be obtained in response to different stimuli, which can alter the plasma

Ca^{++} in a graded manner. Thus, the degree of phosphorylation of the cross-bridges changes over a wide range.

Smooth Muscle Hypertrophy

Growth and proliferation of vascular smooth muscles are stimulated by a variety of growth factors. This is typically seen during pregnancy and in hypertension.

In pregnancy: Toward term, *estrogen* stimulates the ***hypertrophy (increase in cell size)*** and ***hyperplasia (increase in cell number) of myometrium*** as well as the growth of the connective tissue mass. There is increase in the amount of contractile proteins and the number of gap junctions that helps for an effective and coordinated contraction. ***Stretch of the uterine*** wall by the growing fetus also induces expansion of the myometrium.

In hypertension: When blood pressure is chronically elevated, the ***pressure load*** acts as a stimulus and the walls of the blood vessels undergo hypertrophy and hyperplasia. In addition, if there is sympathetic hyperactivity, increased ***catecholamines*** also stimulate the vessel wall proliferation by trophic effect. Angiotensin II stimulates, whereas glucocorticoids inhibit growth of vascular smooth muscles. Some other factors like arachidonic acid derivatives, adenosine, serotonin and heparin like substances also affect smooth muscle hypertrophy.

Other examples: When a hollow viscus like small intestine gets obstructed, the prolonged elevation of the intraluminal pressure stimulates hypertrophy of its muscle layer. Another example is hypertrophy of urinary bladder in men due to enlargement of the prostate gland.

Neural and Hormonal Influences

Autonomic Control

The autonomic nervous system influences the intrinsic rhythmic or pacemaker activity of the visceral smooth muscles. The effect of **sympathetic or parasympathetic** stimulation depends on the type of receptor involved and the mechanisms of the second messenger(s) released subsequently.

Parasympathetic control: Parasympathetic stimulation is ***excitatory***. It releases acetylcholine. In intestine, *acetylcholine is stimulatory*.

1. It decreases the membrane potential, which makes the tissue more excitable.
2. It also increases the frequency of action potentials. As a result, there is increase in the number of rhythmic contractions as well as the duration of tonic contractions.
3. Ach acts by ***increasing the cytoplasmic*** Ca^{++} through phospholipase C and IP3.

Sympathetic control: Sympathetic stimulation is ***inhibitory***. It releases catecholamines. The effects of catecholamines on intestine are just opposite to that of Ach. Catecholamines increase the membrane potential and decrease the frequency of spikes producing *relaxation of the muscle*. ***Norepinephrine*** (NE) acts through both α and β receptors.

Action through α receptors: Acting via α receptors, NE increases calcium efflux from the cell. This leads to decline in cytoplasmic Ca^{++} and relaxation of the muscle.

Action through β receptors: Acting via β receptors, NE ***stimulates adenylyl cyclase*** that increases formation of cAMP, which activates the enzyme cAMP-dependent protein kinase. This protein kinase as well as cAMP ***increase calcium uptake by the sarcoplasmic reticulum***. This results in ***fall in cytoplasmic concentration of*** Ca^{++}. Thus relaxation occurs. In addition, the cAMP-dependent protein kinase decreases the activity of MLCK. Therefore, the cross-bridge formation is reduced that also produces relaxation.

The multiunit smooth muscles do not exhibit the inherent muscle tone. In response to the stimulation of the autonomic nervous system, their contraction is regulated in a precise, graded fashion.

Hormonal Control

Nitric oxide (NO): In response to the shearing stress caused by flow of blood, NO is released from the endothelial cells lining the arteries. It diffuses to the vascular smooth muscle fibers and binds to the receptors present on the sarcolemma. The NO-receptor complex stimulates ***guanylyl cyclase*** and ***forms cGMP***, which activates cGMP-dependent protein kinase. This protein kinase produces relaxation by increasing calcium reuptake by SR, opening of Ca^{++}activated K^{+} channels and decreasing IP3-induced Ca^{++}release by inhibiting phospholipases C.

Other hormones: ***Angiotensin II*** acting via AT II receptors, ***vasopressin*** and ***endothelin*** stimulate contraction of smooth muscles by releasing IP3. ***Adenosine*** causes relaxation by increasing the level of cAMP.

CARDIAC MUSCLE

Muscles present in heart are **cardiac muscles**. Though they are structurally close to skeletal muscle they demonstrate many properties of smooth muscles. The details of structure, properties and functions of cardiac muscles are given in "Heart" section of CVS. Here, salient features are given to differentiate it from skeletal muscles and smooth muscles (Table 29.2).

General features of cardiac muscles are:

1. Cardiac muscle is an involuntary, but striated muscle. The imuscle cell is 100 μm long and 15 μm wide.
2. The fibers are branched and attached with each other closely.
3. Intercalated discs are present at the point of contact of two muscle fibers.
4. Numerous gap junctions are present in the intercalated disc that make cardiac tissue a functional syncytium. There are two such separate syncytia in the heart. The

Table 29.2: Differences between skeletal, cardiac, and smooth muscles.

	Skeletal muscle	Cardiac muscle	Smooth muscle
A. Morphological properties			
1. Distribution	Fixed to bones, form body muscle	Heart only, not attached to bone	(A) Single (visceral) unit smooth muscle in hollowed viscera, e.g.: intestine, bronchi, uterus, ureters. (B) Multi unit smooth muscle in capillary muscle. Iris in eye, pilometer muscle of skin; muscle in blood vessels
2. Striations	It has well-developed striations, therefore, also called striated muscle	Also show cross	Lack cross striations, therefore also called "plain" muscles
3. Size and shape	Cylindrical, 1–40 mm long, 50-100 μm diameter; multinucleated cells	Short, cylindrical, 100 μm long, and 15 μm diameter; single nucleus; forms a branching network	Spindle (Elongated), single nucleus, variable sizes
4. Sarcoplasmic reticulum	Well developed	Well developed more than in the skeletal muscle	Poorly developed
5. Syncytial structure	Non-syncytial	It is functionally syncytial in character	Functionally syncytial in character
6. Sarcotubular system	Present; T system at A-I junction; terminal cistern prominent.	Present with poorly developed terminal cistern. T system prominent and present at Z lines	Present, but not so characteristic
7. Nerve supply	By somatic nerves and by special nerve endings	Via two branches of ANS with ganglia and free nerve terminals	Same as in the cardiac muscle
8. Control and rhythmicity	Voluntary control, no rhythmicity	It contracts rhythmically and spontaneously in the absence of external innervation, by pacemaker drive	Rhythmicity: two types (i) regular and (ii) irregularly discharging pacemaker
9. Blood supply and oxygen consumption	840 mL/min (3–4 mL 100 gm/min) with moderate oxygen consumption	Abundant, 250 mL/min (80 mL/100 gm/min) with high O_2 consumption	350 mL/min (1.4 mL per 100 gm/min) with less O_2 consumption
B. Electrical properties			
10. RMP	–90 mV	–90 mV	–50 mV (Range between –30 mV and –50 mV), Fluctuating
11. Action potential (AP)	Rapid depolarization Spike duration is 2–4 ms Total amplitude120 mV, Conduction velocity 5 mts/sec	Rapid depolarization, 15 to 20 mV produces, AP duration 250 ms, Amplitude 100 Mv, variable speed of conduction	Variable (rapid rise and fall in action potential). Total duration 50 msec. Total amplitude up to 60 mV, variable speed of conduction
C. Mechanical properties			
12. Mechanical events	Contraction starts 2 msec after the start of depolarization, before repolarization ends. Can summate the contractile response, Tetanization occurs	More than half of mechanical contraction is over, during absolute Tetanization not seen	Muscle starts to contract approximately 200 msec after the start of the spike (150 msec after the spike is over). Peak contraction is reached approximately 500 msec after the spike. Tetanus is seen
13. Duration of muscle twitch	Varies with types of muscle fibers; 7.5 msec in fast muscles, 100 msec in slow muscles	One and half times the total duration of action potential	Approximately 1,000 msec
14. Excitation contraction coupling	Rapid process, time from initial depolarization to initiation of contraction is 10 msec	More rapid process time (< 10 msec)	Very slow process
15. All or none law	Applicable, true for single muscle fiber	Applicable, true for whole of the atria or ventricles	Applicable, true for single muscle fibre
16. Length tension relationship	Maximum active tension is developed at the optimal length	Same as in skeletal muscle	Shows property of plasticity
17. Phenomenon of fatigue	Occurs	Not seen	Possible but difficult to demonstrate
D. Metabolic properties			
18. Energy	Under basal state 20% by fats. >60% from carbohydrates; 20% by proteins	65% by fats, 25% by carbohydrates; and 10% by ketones bodies and amino acids.	Low, mainly provided by the utilization carbohydrates and fats

atrial and ventricular syncytia, connected with each other by A-V bundle.

5. Each syncytium obeys all or none law.
6. The cardiac muscle fibers are highly vascular, i.e. surrounded by a very rich capillary network.
7. They show well developed sarcoplasmic reticulum with plenty of cytoplasm, mitochondria and rich in glycogen.

Differences between skeletal, cardiac, and smooth muscles are summarized (Table 29.2).

CHAPTER SUMMARY

Key Concepts

1. Though smooth muscles do not have organized sarcomeres, they have myofilaments for muscle contraction.
2. Membrane potential fluctuates between –30 mV and –70 mV.
3. Cytosolic calcium concentration plays a great role in muscle contraction. Calcium from sarcoplasmic reticulum mainly determines to cytosolic level of calcium, though calcium influx by voltage-gated and ligand-gated channels contribute.
4. Phosphorylation of myosin and latch-bridge mechanism, are special characteristics.
5. There is no definitive length-tension relationship. Plasticity is the main feature.
6. Control of smooth muscle is by autonomic nerves (sympathetic inhibitory and parasympathetic excitatory), and hormones.

Important to Know (Must Read)

1. In examinations, "Mechanism of smooth muscle contraction, and properties of smooth muscle" may come as a **Long Question**.
2. Special morphological features of smooth muscle, Electrical properties of smooth muscle, Mechanism of smooth muscle contraction, Role of calcium in smooth muscle contraction, Latch bridge mechanism, Properties of smooth muscle, Plasticity, Regulation of smooth muscle activity, and Differences between skeletal muscle, cardiac muscle and smooth muscle, come as **Short Questions** in exams.
3. In **Viva**, examiners usually ask... list the special features of smooth muscle, How membrane potential and action potential differ in skeletal muscle and smooth muscle, Steps of smooth muscle contraction, How calcium-calmodulin complex influences smooth muscle contraction, What are phosphorylation and phosphorylation processes, What is Latch-bridge mechanism, What is plasticity, Properties of smooth muscle, Regulation of smooth muscle activity, and List the differences between skeletal muscle, cardiac muscle, and smooth muscle.

SECTION–4

Autonomic Nervous System

30. Functional Organization of Autonomic Nervous System
31. Sympathetic System
32. Parasympathetic System
33. Control of Autonomic Functions and Applied Aspects
34. Antonomic Function Tests
35. Heart Rate Variability

"A soul shall wake in the Inconscient's house:
The mind shall be God-vision's tabernacle,
The body intuition's instrument,
And life a channel for God's visible power."

Sri Aurobindo (in 'SAVITRI')

CHAPTER 30

Functional Organization of Autonomic Nervous System

Learning Objectives

On completion of study of this chapter, the student **MUST** be able to:

1. Understand the importance of autonomic nervous system (ANS) in regulation of body functions.
2. Differentiate functional specialization of sympathetic and parasympathetic divisions of ANS.
3. Appreciate the differences in central connections and reflex arc of somatic nervous system and ANS.
4. Understand the differences in pre- and post-ganglionic fibers of sympathetic and parasympathetic divisions of ANS.
5. Name the common neurotransmitters in ANS and their receptors.
6. Comprehend the general organization of ANS at different levels of the neuraxis.

The student **MAY** also be able to:

1. Describe the details of organization of neurons of ANS.
2. Describe the details of neurotransmitters of ANS.

The term 'autonomic' is derived from the words *auto* means 'self' and *nomos* means 'control'. Emotional responses of the body and responses to environment occur without conscious knowledge of the individual. These responses are therefore, called autonomic responses that are executed by the autonomic part of the nervous system. The ANS controls functions of the involuntary organs of the body that include heart and blood vessels, exocrine and endocrine glands, and all visceral organs. Thus, ANS controls all major functions of the body such as circulation, respiration, digestion, excretion and reproduction. Circulating hormones and locally produced chemicals assist in mediating these autonomic functions.

The **functions of ANS** can be broadly categorized into ***five parts***:

1. Maintenance of homeostatic conditions of the body.
2. Regulation of visceral activities.
3. Smoothening body's responses to environmental changes.
4. Coordination of body's responses to exercise and stress.
5. Assisting the endocrine system to regulate reproductive functions.

Scientists contributed

WH Gaskell and JN Langley laid the foundation for study of Physiology of ANS.

Walter Holbrook Gaskell was the first scientist who thoroughly investigated the innervation of the cardiovascular system and viscera. He **discovered the cardioaccelerator nerve** and laid the foundation for an understanding of autonomic nervous system.

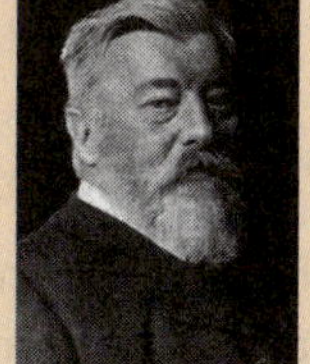

WH Gaskell
(1847–1914)

Sources:

1. On the rhythm of the heart of the frog. *Phil Tr Roy Soc Lond* 1882; 173: 993-1033.
2. *The Involuntary Nervous System*. London: Longman Publication, 1916.

John Newport Langley analyzed the functional significance of autonomic nervous system (ANS) in vertebrates. He was the first scientist to **classify ANS into the sympathetic and parasympathetic divisions**, indicating their anatomical, physiological and pharmacological relations and characteristics.

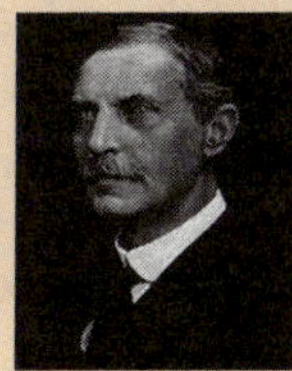

JN Langley
(1852–1925)

Source: Heffer W. *The Autonomic Nervous System*. Cambridge Publication: Cambridge, 1921.

FUNCTIONAL OVERVIEW

Divisions of Autonomic Nervous System

Autonomic nervous system is traditionally divided into two subdivisions: **sympathetic** and **parasympathetic**, based on their anatomic, functional and neurochemical properties. Enteric nervous system is considered to be the ***third division*** of ANS.

Sympathetic System

When the body requires support to meet emergency conditions and stressful situations, sympathetic system provides the desirable assistance. For its sympathy to help the body to face and overcome such critical situations in life, this division of ANS is called sympathetic system. Sympathetic system also helps to control normal functions of the body such as regulation of blood pressure, respiration, metabolism, etc. The importance of sympathetic system is realized in its dysfunctions. For example, a person with sympathetic imbalance will not be able to stand up from sitting or supine posture and will not be able to maintain the standing posture. Thus, sympathetic system is a friend of the body not only in emergency needs but also in its routine deeds.

1. The cell bodies of sympathetic system are located in the thoracic and abdominal segments of the spinal cord and sympathetic ganglia are present as a chain close to the vertebral column.
2. This system is also termed as the **thoracolumbar division of the ANS** for the location of the ganglia and cell bodies of neurons at thoracic and lumbar segments of spinal cord (Fig. 30.1).

Parasympathetic System

The component of ANS that works by the side of the sympathetic system is the parasympathetic division of ANS. It has a reciprocal influence on organ functions to that of sympathetic influence. In fact, it checks the overactivity of sympathetic system and smoothens the autonomic responses.

1. The cell bodies are found in the brainstem cranial nerve nuclei (*cranial component*), and in the most caudal part of the spinal cord (*spinal or sacral component*).
2. Hence, it is also termed as **craniosacral division *of ANS*** (Fig. 30.1).

Enteric Nervous System

The enteric nervous system (ENS) is the local neural network in GI system which has strong anatomical and physiological link with ANS. Therefore, ENS is considered as the **'Third division of ANS'**. It is concerned with the regulation of gastrointestinal function.

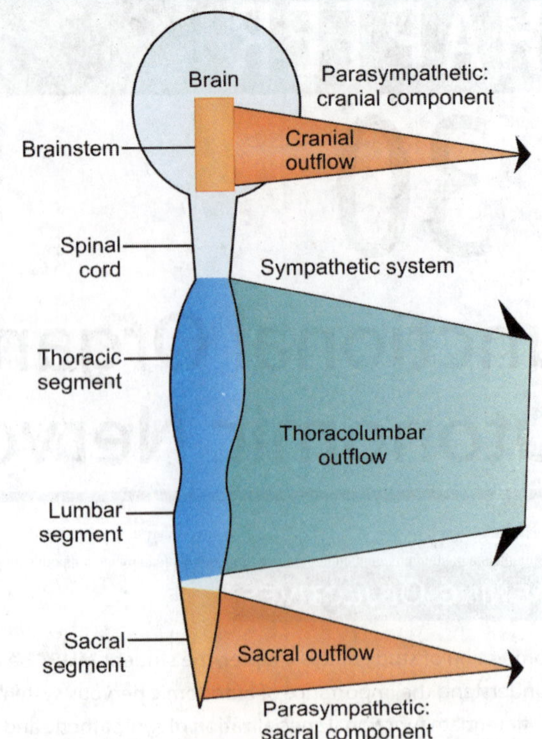

Fig. 30.1: General view of sympathetic (thoracolumbar outflow) and parasympathetic (craniosacral outflow) systems.

FUNCTIONAL SPECIALIZATION

The neurochemical differences between two divisions of sympathetic system led to the description of the *sympathetic system as adrenergic* for adrenaline (or noradrenaline) like actions resulting from sympathetic activation; and the *parasympathetic system as cholinergic* for acetylcholine like actions from parasympathetic activation. Some of the important functional characteristics of sympathetic and parasympathetic divisions are as follows:

1. The sympathetic division is primarily meant for **utilization of metabolic resources and emergency responses** of the body, whereas the parasympathetic division helps in **restoration and build-up of the body's reserves** and the ***elimination of waste products***.
2. Almost all the organs are supplied by both sympathetic and parasympathetic nerves and usually they are **activated in a reciprocal fashion**. Therefore, when the discharge rate in one division is increased, the rate in the other division is decreased. For example, when sympathetic activation occurs during exercise to increase heart rate, simultaneous decrease vagal activity also contributes to achieve the target increase in heart rate.
3. In some organs, sympathetic and parasympathetic systems work ***synergistically***. For example, to enhance gastrointestinal secretions, when parasympathetic stimulation increases volume and enzyme content, simultaneous sympathetic activation contributes to increased mucus content of the secretory product.

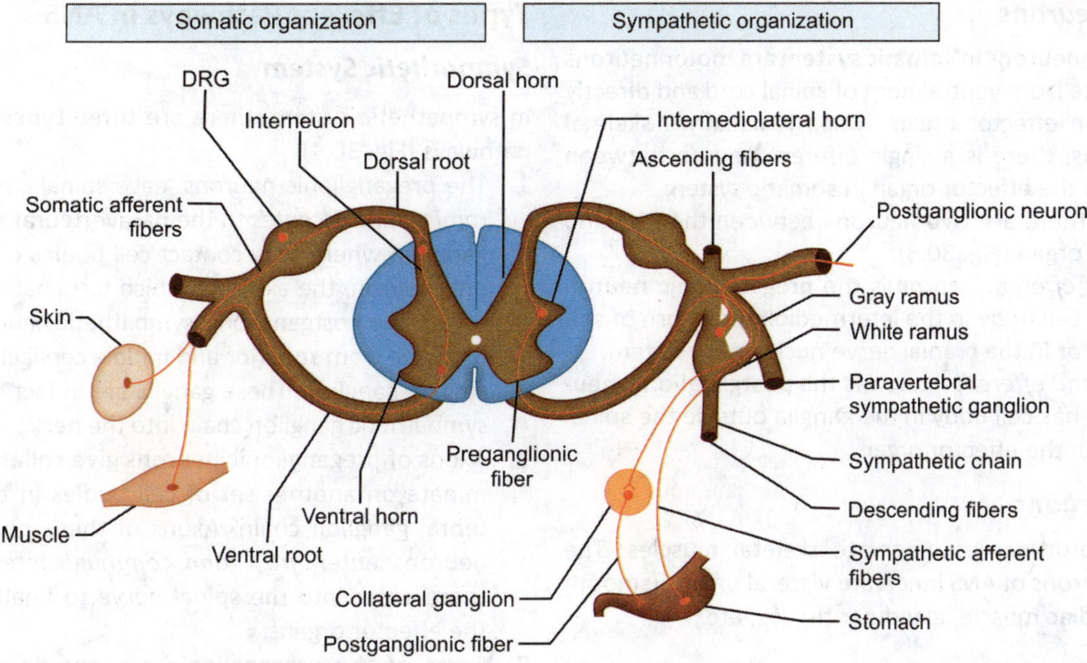

Fig. 30.2: Differences between segmental organization of somatic nervous system and sympathetic component of ANS.

4. Also, few structures such as blood vessels and skin receive only sympathetic innervation and therefore, their functions are regulated by alteration in the rate of sympathetic discharge to these structures.

Somatic vs Autonomic Nervous System

The nervous system contacts all organs and tissues of the body via the sensory system (afferent innervation), motor system (efferent innervation) and the ANS.

Central Connections

For efferent innervation of somatic system (i.e. the motor pathway), axons originate from cell body of neurons in the motor cortex and terminate directly or indirectly on motor neurons in the ventral horn of the spinal cord or in the brainstem motor nuclei, and usually the second order neuron (or sometimes the third order neuron) innervates the skeletal muscle. Similarly, **in ANS**, efferent pathway consists of ***two or three-neuron tract*** with one or two synapses interposed between the center and the effector cells.

1. The cell bodies of autonomic motor neurons are located in the intermediolateral horn of spinal cord or in the specific brainstem cranial nerve nuclei.
2. The efferent fiber emerges from CNS as the **preganglionic axon** and then synapses with the cell bodies of neurons located in a peripheral ganglion. The neuron from the ganglion then projects as **postganglionic axon** to the effector cells (usually a visceral organ).

Reflex Arc

The somatic nervous system collects information from the external environment, whereas the ANS collects information usually from inside the body, i.e. the changes in visceral structures (Fig. 30.2).

Receptors

Receptors are located in the body surface or in the musculoskeletal system in somatic system. In ANS, the receptors are present in the visceral structures.

Afferent Pathway

The **afferent neurons of somatic system** enter spinal cord via dorsal root with their cell bodies in the dorsal root ganglion and terminate on interneurons in deeper layers of dorsal horn or on motor neurons in the ventral horn. The **afferent neurons of ANS** enter spinal cord in a similar fashion, but they terminate on autonomic efferent neurons having their cell bodies in intermediolateral horn (ILH) of spinal cord.

Central Neurons

Central component **in somatic system** consists of the cell body of a motor neuron in the ventral horn of the spinal cord on which the afferent neuron directly terminates monosynaptically. The afferent neuron may also contact motor neuron through interneurons via disynaptic or polysynaptic connections.

In ANS, the cell bodies of central neurons are located in intermediolateral horn of spinal cord on which the afferent neuron directly terminates.

Efferent Neurons

The efferent neurons **in somatic system** are motor neurons that originate from ventral horn of spinal cord and directly terminate on effector organ, which is usually a skeletal muscle. Thus, there is a single efferent neuron between the CNS and the effector organ in somatic system.

In **ANS,** there are **two neurons** between the CNS and the effector organ (Fig. 30.3).

1. *The first efferent neuron* is the **preganglionic neuron** that has cell body in the intermediolateral horn of spinal cord or in the cranial nerve nuclei in brainstem.
2. *The second efferent neuron* is the **postganglionic neuron** that has cell body in the ganglia outside the spinal cord or in the effector organ.

Effector Organs

Somatic motor nerves innervate skeletal muscles. The efferent neurons of ANS innervate visceral organs (smooth muscle, cardiac muscle, glandular tissues, etc.).

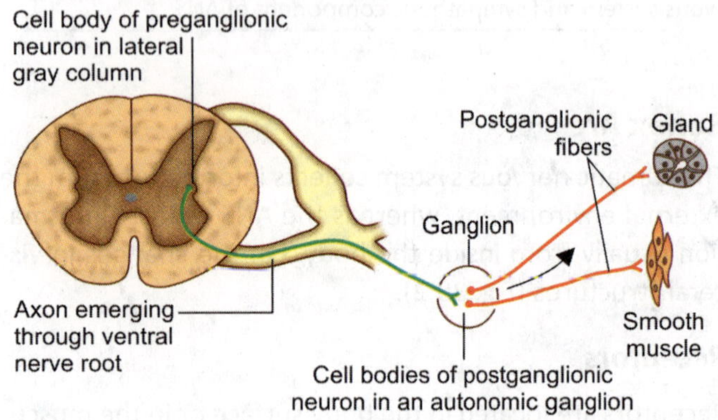

Fig. 30.3: Typical arrangement of efferent neurons in ANS.

Types of Efferent Pathways in ANS

Sympathetic System

In sympathetic system, there are **three types** of efferent pathways (Fig. 30.4):

1. The preganglionic neurons leave spinal cord via *white rami communicantes* to the **paravertebral sympathetic ganglion** where they contact cell bodies of postganglionic neuron, the axons of which terminate on effector organ. The postganglionic sympathetic neurons to head originate from superior and middle cervical ganglia and stellate ganglion. These ganglia are in fact extension of sympathetic ganglion chain into the neck.
2. Axons of preganglionic neurons **give collaterals** to terminate on another set of cell bodies in the paravertebral ganglion chain. Axons of these postganglionic neurons enter *gray rami communicantes* and from there enter into the spinal nerve to finally innervate the effector organs.
3. Some of the preganglionic neurons do not relay in paravertebral ganglion chain, rather they come out directly of the ganglion chain to terminate on the cell bodies of postganglionic neurons located in **collateral ganglion** that are present close to the effector organ. In this efferent pathway of sympathetic system, the preganglionic fibers are longer than the postganglionic fibers. Thus, the postganglionic neurons in this system form **short noradrenergic neurons.**

Parasympathetic System

In parasympathetic system, the preganglionic neurons of cranial part originate from cell bodies in the cranial nerve

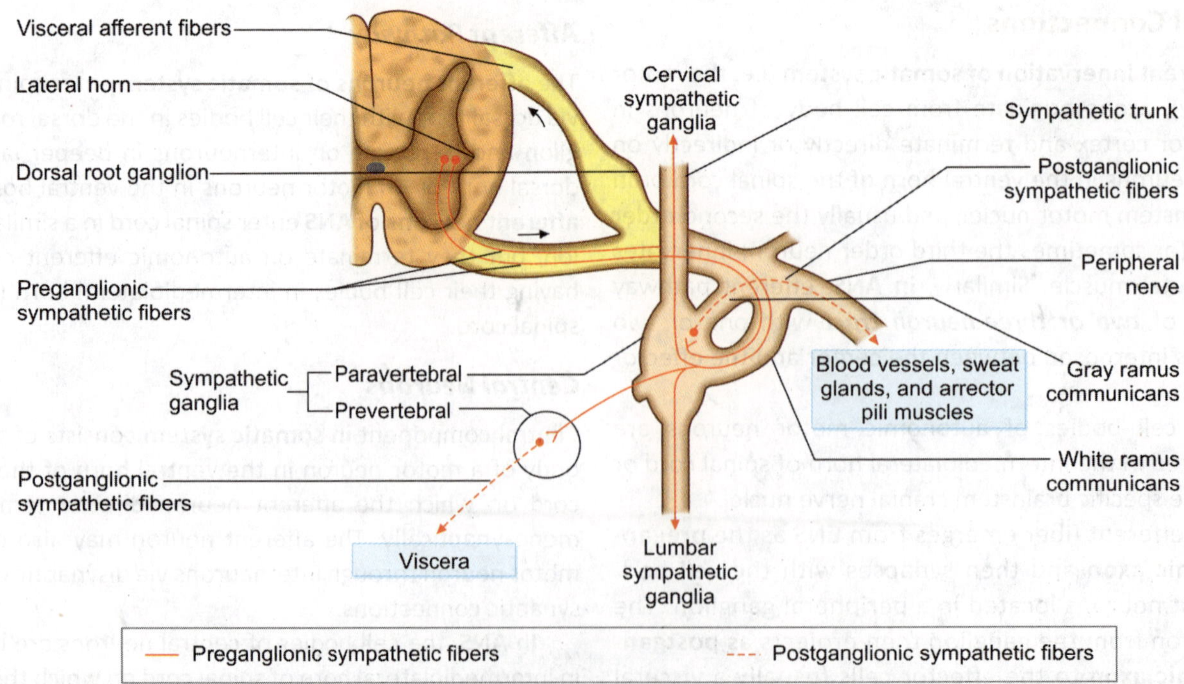

Fig. 30.4: Gray and white rami connecting a spinal nerve to sympathetic trunk.

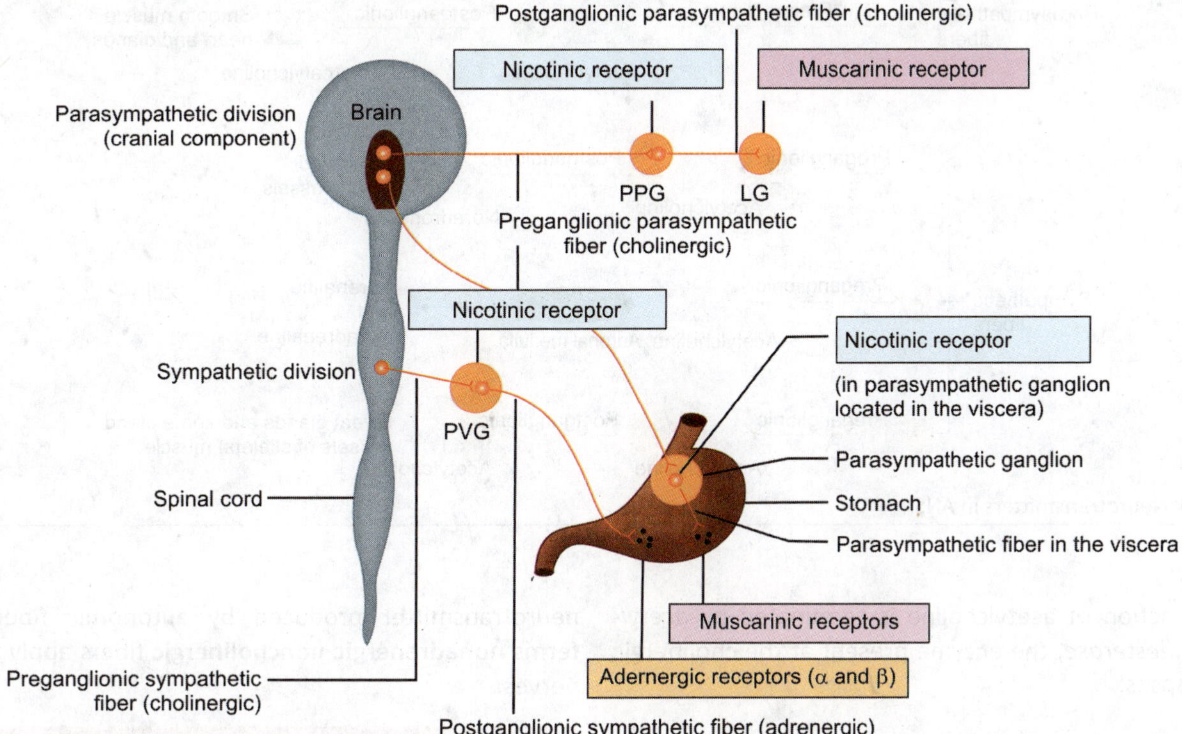

Fig. 30.5: Distribution of (pre- and post-ganglionic) fibers and receptors in both the divisions of ANS. (PVG: Paravertebral ganglia; PPG: Pterygopalatine ganglion; LG: Lacrimal gland).

nuclei (III, VII, IX and X) in the brainstem and terminate in the **postganglionic neuron located very close to or in the visceral organ**. The preganglionic neurons of sacral part follow a similar route except that the fibers originate from cell bodies in the intermediolateral horn of spinal cord and traverse in spinal nerve.

In general, **in sympathetic system**, the preganglionic fibers are smaller than the postganglionic fibers (Application Box 30.1), whereas **in parasympathetic system**, the preganglionic fibers are much longer than the postganglionic fibers (Fig. 30.5).

Application Box 30.1

Intrinsic cardiac adrenergic cells: Evidences of recent research studies indicate that few postganglionic sympathetic neurons are embedded in the cardiac tissue like that of postganglionic neurons of parasympathetic systems that are usually located in the visceral organs. These neurons form intrinsic cardiac adrenergic cells (ICAC). Secretion from ICAC accounts for about 15% of adrenaline and noradrenaline content of the heart. It is believed that during fetal and early childhood, catecholamine content of ICAC plays an essential role in development of the heart.

Neurotransmitters in ANS

In the somatic nervous system, the efferent fibers terminate on motor end plate usually with one axon terminal to one skeletal muscle fiber. The neurotransmitter is acetylcholine.

1. In ANS, postganglionic axons terminate in **varicosities**, the swellings enriched in synaptic vesicles that release the transmitter into the extracellular space surrounding the effector cells.
2. The electrical activity for discharge of autonomic fibers originates in some of the effector cells and then propagates to cells of rest of the tissue via gap junctions.
3. The neurotransmitters in ANS are acetylcholine, noradrenaline and others (Fig. 30.6).

Acetylcholine

Acetylcholine is the neurotransmitter at the following nerve terminals (**cholinergic fibers**) in ANS:

1. Preganglionic nerve terminals of both the sympathetic and the parasympathetic divisions.
2. All parasympathetic postganglionic neurons.
3. Postganglionic sympathetic neurons to sweat glands and blood vessels in skeletal muscle.

The synapse at preganglionic nerve terminals utilizes **nicotinic receptors** similar to that found at neuromuscular junction. The synapse between the postganglionic neuron and the target tissues utilizes **muscarinic receptors**. The receptor classification is based on the response of the synapses to the alkaloids nicotine and muscarine at respective type of synapse.

1. The nicotinic receptor is blocked by *hexamethonium* in autonomic ganglion, in contrast to blockade by *curare* at neuromuscular junction. The nicotinic cholinergic receptor is of **direct ligand-gated type** as it contains ion channel in it.
2. The muscarinic receptor is blocked by *atropine*. The muscarinic receptor is of **indirect ligand-gated type** as it uses a G protein to mediate effector functions.

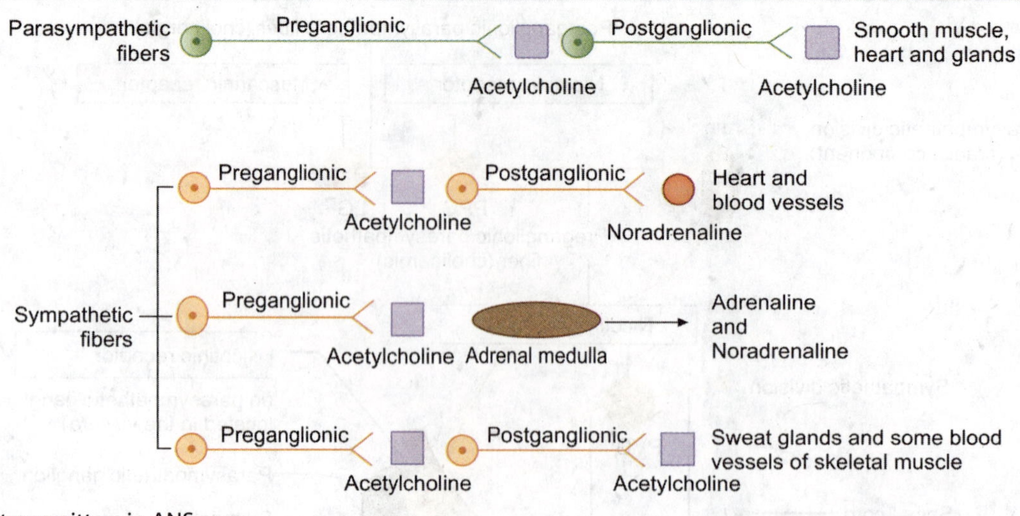

Fig. 30.6: Neurotransmitters in ANS.

The action of acetylcholine is terminated by *acetylcholinesterase*, the enzyme present at the cholinergic synapses.

Norepinephrine

Noradrenaline (NA) or norepinephrine is the neurotransmitter at postganglionic sympathetic nerve terminals (**adrenergic fibers**). NA released from adrenergic synapses utilize adrenergic receptors that can also be activated by adrenaline or epinephrine released from adrenal medulla. Therefore, these receptors are designated as adrenergic.

1. **Adrenergic receptors** are broadly classified into two types: α and β. **The α receptors** respond more to NA and less to epinephrine, and least to isoproterenol, the synthetic catecholamine.
2. **The β receptors** respond best to isoproterenol and epinephrine and less to NA. Propranolol is the antagonist for β receptors. Each class of receptors is further classified as α_1 or α_2, and β_1, β_2 or β_3 (for details, refer 'Adrenal Medulla' in 'Endocrine Physiology').
3. The adrenergic receptors are of the **indirect ligand-gated type** as they utilize G protein for their effects. The α_1 **receptors** activate phospholipase C. The α_2 **receptors** inhibit adenylyl cyclase, whereas β ***receptors*** stimulate it.

Other Neurotransmitters

In ANS, especially in the intrinsic plexuses of the gut many amines, amino acids and active peptides are widely distributed as **co-neurotransmitters**. For example, *neuropeptide Y* is co-released by vasoconstrictor nerve, *vasoactive intestinal polypeptide* (VIP) and *calcitonin-gene-related peptide* (CGRP) are released along with cholinergic nerve terminals. *Nitric oxide* is another neurotransmitter produced by autonomic fibers. The terms **nonadrenergic noncholinergic** fibers apply to such nerves.

GENERAL ORGANIZATION OF ANS

Organization of ANS occurs at five different levels: cortical organization, hypothalamic organization, brainstem organization, spinal organization and peripheral organization.

Cortical Organization

Cortical areas controlling functions of ANS are mainly **limbic areas and prefrontal cortex**.

1. The sympathetic responses to emotion originate in the limbic and prefrontal cortical areas.
2. These areas *activate sympathetic system* by stimulating hypothalamic and brainstem areas that have influence on the system.

Hypothalamic Organization

Hypothalamus considerably influences autonomic functions. Hypothalamus via hypothalamo-pituitary axis controls secretions of major endocrine glands.

1. Hypothalamus receives collaterals from ascending pathways, especially from spinothalamic tracts that transmit pain impulses.
2. Thus, **hypothalamus integrates** somatosensory, endocrine and autonomic responses that are essential components of homeostatic mechanisms during stressful situations like major surgical procedures, exposures to extreme weathers, trauma and hemorrhage.
3. For its profound influence on autonomic responses, Sherrington had correctly pointed out that hypothalamus is the **head-ganglion** of sympathetic nervous system.

Table 30.1: Location of cell bodies of ganglia in autonomic nervous system.

Location	Sympathetic	Parasympathetic
Neck	Superior, middle and inferior cervical	In the wall of the cervical viscera
Thorax	Paravertebral	Cardiac and pulmonary plexus
Abdomen	Paravertebral and plexus along the abdominal aorta (e.g: coeliac plexus)	In the wall of the viscera (myenteric and submucosa)
Pelvis	Paravertebral and plexus along the internal iliac artery (hypogastric plexuses)	In the wall of the viscera (myenteric, submucosal and viscera)

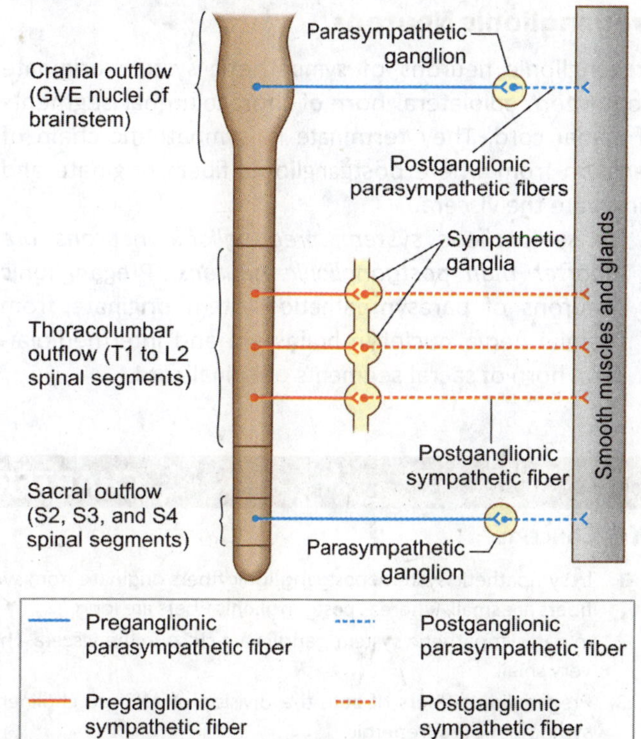

Fig. 30.7: Location of ganglia, pre- and post-ganglionic fibers in sympathetic and parasympathetic systems of ANS.

Brainstem Organization

Brainstem areas contain major nuclei of ANS. These are broadly classified into two categories: parasympathetic nuclei and sympathetic nuclei.

Parasympathetic Nuclei

The **cranial outflow** of parasympathetic system originates from **cranial nerve nuclei** that are located in the brainstem.

1. The cranial nerves that carry parasympathetic fibers are oculomotor (III cranial nerve), facial (VII cranial nerve), glossopharyngeal (IX cranial nerve) and vagus (X cranial nerve).
2. ***Nucleus tractus solitarius*** (NTS) in the medulla receives general visceral sensation via IX and X cranial nerves. It is also closely connected with reticular formation containing cardio-respiratory centers. Therefore, NTS mediates respiratory and cardiovascular responses to autonomic activation. Special visceral sensations in VII, IX and X cranial nerves reach NTS.
3. ***Edinger-Westphal nucleus*** in the midbrain is the nucleus of III cranial nerve.
4. ***Salivary nucleus*** is located in pons and ***dorsal motor nucleus of vagus*** in medulla.

Sympathetic Nuclei

Sympathetic fibers originate from ***vasomotor center*** in the medulla and project to the intermediolateral horn of spinal cord via bulbospinal pathway.

1. Nucleus gigantocellularis and parvocellularis in the reticular formation on stimulation depress activity of vasomotor center.
2. Stimulation of NTS inhibits sympathetic outflow and stimulates vagal activity.

Spinal Organization

Cell bodies of autonomic efferent neurons are located in the intermediolateral column of the spinal cord.

Sympathetic Outflow

Sympathetic fibers originate from thoracic and lumbar segments (T_1 to L_3) of spinal cord. Hence, sympathetic system is called **thoracolumbar outflow** of ANS.

Parasympathetic Outflow

Spinal component of parasympathetic system originates from sacral segments (S_2 to S_4) of spinal cord. For its cranial and sacral origin, parasympathetic system is called **craniosacral outflow** of ANS.

Peripheral Organization

Ganglia

Autonomic fibers from CNS reach visceral organs in the cranial nerves and somatic nerves. They are distributed to target organs via various ganglions (Table 30.1). The ganglia of sympathetic system are close to spinal cord and the ganglia of parasympathetic system are close to the organs (Fig. 30.7). There are two sets of neurons in the efferent pathway: preganglionic and postganglionic neurons.

Preganglionic Neurons

Preganglionic neurons of sympathetic system originate from intermediolateral horn of thoracolumbar segments of spinal cord. They terminate in sympathetic chain of ganglion from where postganglionic fibers originate and innervate the viscera.

1. *In sympathetic system, preganglionic neurons are shorter than postganglionic neurons.* Preganglionic neurons of parasympathetic system originate from cranial nerve nuclei in brainstem and intermediolateral horn of sacral segments of spinal cord.
2. *In parasympathetic system, preganglionic neurons are much longer than postganglionic neurons, as the ganglion is located either near the viscera or in the viscera.*

Postganglionic Neurons

1. In sympathetic system, postganglionic fibers originate from **sympathetic chain of ganglia** and terminate in the viscera.
2. In parasympathetic system, postganglionic fibers are located close to or in the effector organs. Hence, postganglionic parasympathetic fibers are very small.

CHAPTER SUMMARY

Key Concepts

1. In sympathetic system, postganglionic fibers originate from sympathetic chain of ganglia close to spinal cord. Therefore, preganglionic fibers are small, whereas postganglionic fibers are long.
2. In parasympathetic system, ganglia are close to the viscera. Therefore, preganglionic fibers are long, whereas postganglionic fibers are very small.
3. Preganglionic fibers of both the division of ANS are cholinergic. Postganglionic parasympathetic is cholinergic, and postganglionic sympathetic is adrenergic.

Important to Know (Must Read)

1. In examinations, usually there will be no **Long Question** from this chapter.
2. Difference between spinal organization of somatic system and sympathetic system, Neurotransmitters of ANS, General organization of ANS, may come as **Short Questions** in exams.
3. In **Viva**, examiners usually ask... What the components of ANS, General organization of ANS, General functions of sympathetic and parasympathetic systems, Say the differences between spinal organization of somatic system and ANS Organization of pre-ganglionic and postganglionic fibers of sympathetic and parasympathetic systems, Location of ganglia in sympathetic and parasympathetic systems, List the neurotransmitters of sympathetic and parasympathetic systems.

CHAPTER 31

Sympathetic System

LEARNING OBJECTIVES

On completion of study of this chapter, the student **MUST** be able to:

1. Understand the importance of sympathetic system in regulation of body functions.
2. Appreciate the anatomical and functional specializations of sympathetic divisions of autonomous nervous system (ANS).
3. Trace the course of pre- and postganglionic neurons of sympathetic system.
4. Name the sympathetic ganglia and give the segmental distribution of sympathetic fibers to various visceral organs.
5. Understand the importance of basal sympathetic tone.
6. List the widespread responses to sympathetic stimulation.
7. Give the effects of sympathetic stimulation to various organs and name the receptors that mediate these effects.
8. Comprehend the features, mechanism and importance of fight-or-flight responses.
9. List the differences between sympathetic and parasympathetic systems.

The student **MAY** also be able to:

1. Describe the detailed widespread responses to sympathetic stimulation.
2. Describe the effects of sympathetic stimulation to various organs.
3. Explain the basis of fight-or-flight responses.

Sympathetic system is the system of **energy utilization**. At the time of activity, urgency, anxiety, emotion, excitement and combating stressful situations, sympathetic system is activated to provide energy to the body. Excessive and chronic stimulation of this system leads to leanness, degeneration ad decay, and underutilization of it leads to lethargy and adiposity.

FUNCTIONAL ANATOMY

Sympathetic Neurons

Preganglionic Neurons

Cell bodies of preganglionic neurons of the sympathetic division are located in the intermediolateral horn of the thoracic (T_1 to T_{12}) and upper lumbar (L_1 to L_3) segments of spinal cord. Hence, sympathetic division is known as **thoracolumbar outflow** of ANS. The preganglionic neurons come out of the spinal cord via ventral roots. After the merger of dorsal and ventral roots, spinal nerve emerges. Sympathetic preganglionic axons leave the spinal nerve via

Scientists contributed

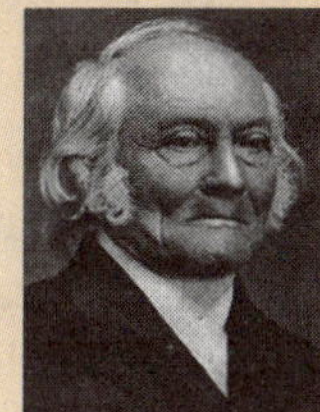

Ernst Heinrich Weber
(1795–1878)

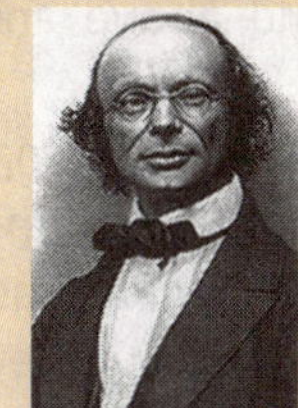

Wilhelm Eduard Weber
(1804–1891)

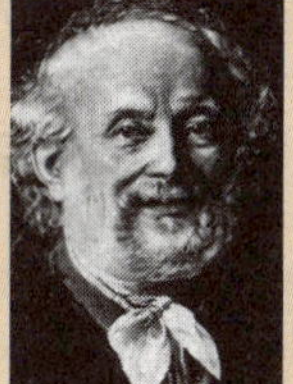

Eduard Friedrich Wilhelm Weber
(1806–1871)

In 19th century, three Weber brothers (Ernst Heinrich Weber, Wilhelm Eduard Weber, and Eduard Friedrich Wilhelm Weber) had contributed greatly to Physiology, especially in the field of **autonomous nervous system** (ANS). Ernst Heinrich first made a **comparative study of sympathetic nerves**. With his younger brother, Eduard Friedrich measured the speed of pulse wave and correctly explained the nature of arterial pulse. Eduard Friedrich studied the hearing mechanism. Wilhelm and Eduard completed the full study of locomotion and demonstrated that vagal stimulation stops heart.

Source: Anatomical comparata nervi sympathici. Leipzig. CH Reclam: 1871.

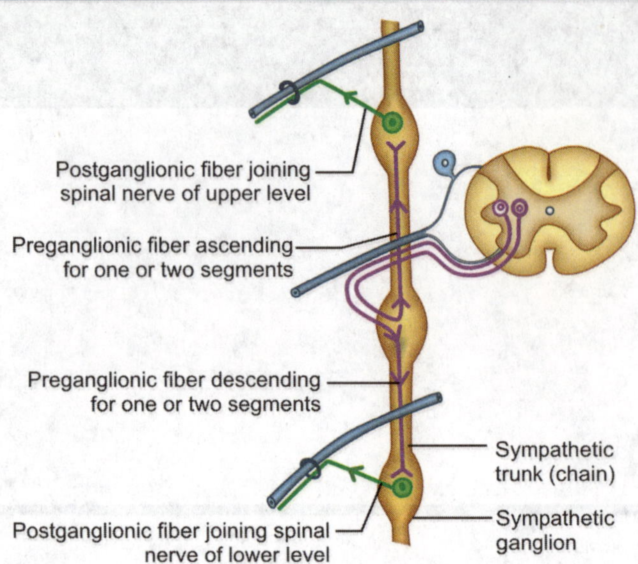

Fig. 31.1: Termination of preganglionic neuron in spinal cord. Note that the preganglionic axons (in addition to synapse with postganglionic neurons in the paravertebral ganglion at the same level) ascend or descend to the several spinal segments and then synapse with the postganglionic neuron.
Courtesy: Figure 18.7, Human Neuroanatomy by Samar Deb, 1st edition, 2014; Jaypee Brothers Medical Publishers (P) Ltd.

the white rami communicantes and enter the paravertebral sympathetic ganglia, which is an interconnected chain located on both sides of the vertebral column.

Preganglionic fibers have any of the following destinations (refer to Fig. 30.4, Chapter 30):

1. Preganglionic fibers emerging from spinal cord **synapse with cell bodies of postganglionic neuron located in the paravertebral sympathetic ganglion** at the same spinal cord level. The postganglionic sympathetic axons then travel in the cervical and lumbosacral spinal nerves. However, few fibers of sympathetic ganglion chain extend above and below the spinal level.
2. The chain of sympathetic ganglia extends above and below the thoracolumbar spinal levels, in which branches of preganglionic fibers ascend to the cervical levels or descend to the sacral level. Thus, preganglionic axons may synapse with postganglionic neurons in the paravertebral ganglion at the same level, or **ascend up or descend down** to the several spinal segments and then synapse with the postganglionic neuron (Fig. 31.1).
   - **Preganglionic axons that ascend to cervical level** arise from T_1 to T_5 and form three major ganglia: superior, middle and inferior cervical ganglia.
   - **Preganglionic axons descend below L_3**, form two additional lumbar and at least four sacral ganglia. Preganglionic fibers ***synapse with postganglionic neurons in these sympathetic ganglia*** **that are present beyond the thoracolumbar segments** of spinal cord.
3. The preganglionic axons may pass through the paravertebral ganglia *en route* without synapsing there to **terminate in a prevertebral ganglion (collateral ganglion)**, which is located close to the organ.

Postganglionic Neurons

Postganglionic neurons **for somatic structures** such as sweat glands, piloerector muscles, cutaneous blood vessels and blood vessels of skeletal muscles leave the paravertebral ganglion in the gray rami communicantes and reenter the spinal nerve to supply the target tissues.

Postganglionic neurons **to head, heart and lungs** originate in the cervical or upper thoracic paravertebral ganglia and proceed to the organs as *separate nerves*, for example the cardiac nerve to the heart, or as *perivascular plexuses* of axons that accompany arteries.

Sympathetic Ganglia

Sympathetic ganglia are of **three types**: paravertebral, prevertebral, and terminal.

Paravertebral Ganglia

There are two paravertebral chains of ganglia on either side of the spinal cord. Each chain has 22 or 23 ganglia (Fig. 31.2).

Cervical Ganglia

There are **three cervical ganglia**: superior, middle, and inferior.

1. The **superior cervical ganglion** provides sympathetic fibers that innervate the structures in the head. These sympathetic fibers travel in the perivascular plexus along the carotid arteries and innervate radial muscle of the iris that causes dilation of the pupil, supply Muller's muscle that assists in elevating the eyelid, and innervate lacrimal and salivary glands. Therefore, diseases involving this pathway produce prominent ophthalmic signs.
2. The **middle and inferior cervical ganglia** innervate structures in the chest, including the trachea, esophagus, heart and lungs. Often, inferior cervical ganglion and first cervical ganglion fuse to form **stellate ganglion.**

Thoracic Ganglia

There are about 12 thoracic ganglia. Fibers from these ganglia supply mainly thoracic structures. Preganglionic fibers from T_1 and T_2 supply structures in head and neck, from T_3 and T_4 supply thoracic viscera, from T_5 to T_9 supply structures in upper limb, and from T_6 to T_{12} supply upper abdominal viscera (Table 31.1).

Lumbar and Sacral Ganglia

There are three lumbar ganglia for three lumbar segments. However, there are **two additional lumbar** and at

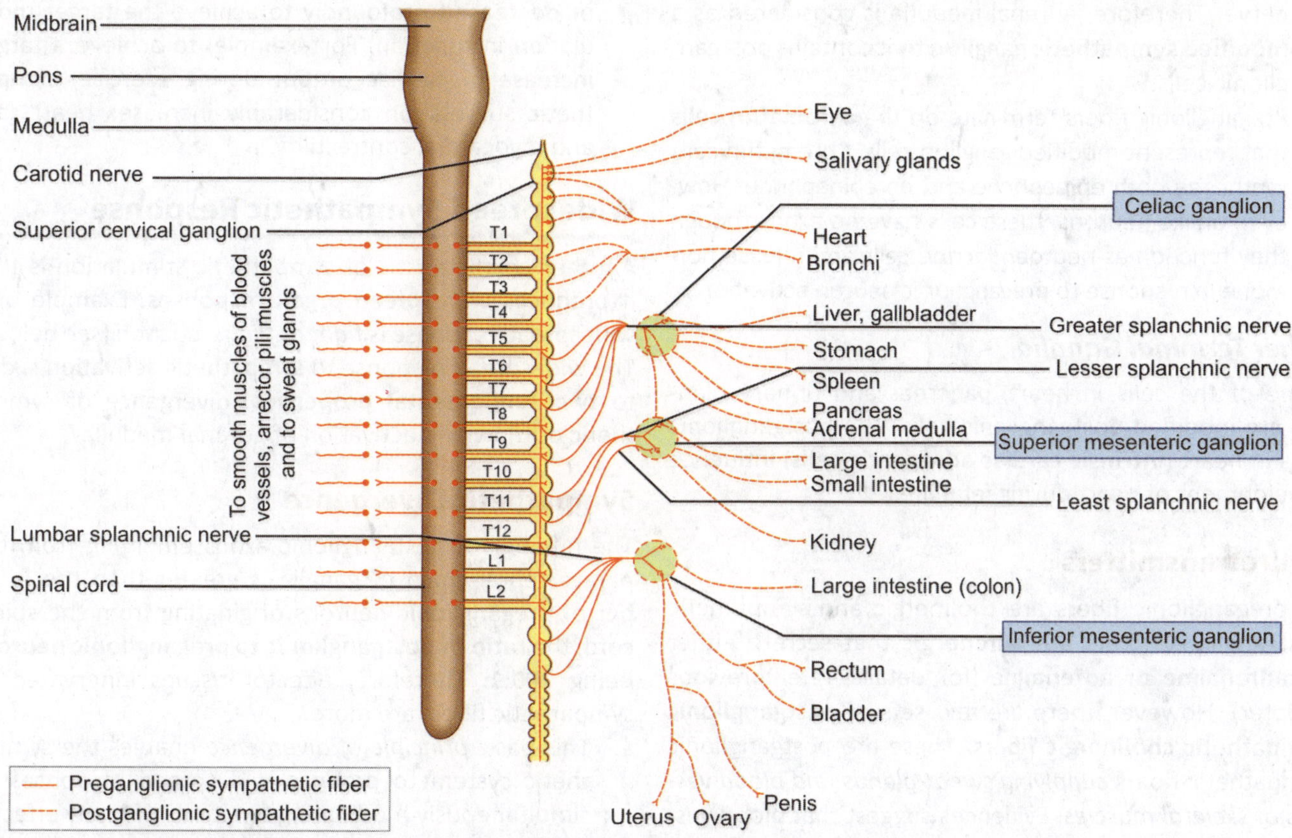

Fig. 31.2: Sympathetic nervous system. Note the thoracolumbar outflow of fibers.

Table 31.1: Segmental distribution of sympathetic fibers.

Preganglionic neurons from spinal segments	Structures innervated by postganglionic fibers
T_1 and T_2	Dilator pupillae, Muller's muscle, blood vessels, and sweat glands of head and neck.
T_3 and T_4	Heart, esophagus, trachea, bronchi, and lungs.
T_5 to T_9	Blood vessels and sweat glands of upper limbs.
T_6 to T_{12}	GI tract, liver, urinary tract, adrenal medulla, and spleen.
T_{10} to L_2	Blood vessels and sweat glands of lower limbs.
L_1 and L_3	Bladder, uterus, fallopian tube, testes, vas deferens, seminal vesicle, and prostate.

least **four sacral ganglia** that are present below the lumbar segments. Preganglionic fibers from T_{10} to L_2 supply structures in lower limbs, and from L_1 and L_2 supply lower abdominal viscera (Table 31.1).

Prevertebral Ganglia

Postsynaptic neurons for the abdominal and pelvic visceral organs arise from the prevertebral ganglia. They are also called **collateral ganglia**. There are three major prevertebral ganglia: celiac, superior mesenteric, and inferior mesenteric (Fig. 31.2). They are so named as they overlie the celiac, superior mesenteric and inferior mesenteric arteries at their origin from the aorta respectively.

1. **Celiac ganglion:** The preganglionic axons for celiac ganglion originate in the T_5 to T_{12} spinal levels and provide innervation to the stomach, small intestine, liver, pancreas, gallbladder, spleen and kidneys.
2. **Superior mesenteric ganglion:** The preganglionic fibers for superior mesenteric ganglion originate primarily in T_{10} to T_{12} and innervate the small and large intestines.
3. **Inferior mesenteric ganglion:** The preganglionic fibers for inferior mesenteric ganglion originate from L_1 to L_3 and innervate the lower part of colon, rectum, urinary bladder, and reproductive organs.

Terminal Ganglia

These are located in the organ innervated by sympathetic fibers. Examples are adrenal medulla, heart, pancreas, and urinary bladder.

Adrenal Medulla

Adrenal medulla is a neuroendocrine structure. It forms the inner core of the adrenal gland.

1. Cells of the adrenal medulla are innervated by *preganglionic sympathetic fibers* originating in the lower thoracic spinal segments that travel in lesser splanchnic

nerve. Therefore, adrenal medulla is considered as a **modified sympathetic ganglion** that contains postganglionic cells.

2. Preganglionic fibers terminate on the **chromaffin cells** that represent modified ganglion cells. Chromaffin cells synthesize both epinephrine and norepinephrine. However, unlike neurons, these cells have no axons though they function as neuroendocrine cells and release hormone in response to preganglionic neuron activation.

Other Terminal Ganglia

Some of the cells in heart, pancreas and urinary bladder are modified postganglionic cells. The postganglionic cells in heart (**intrinsic cardiac adrenergic cells**) influence development of heart during fetal life.

Neurotransmitters

All preganglionic fibers are cholinergic and sympathetic postganglionic fibers are **adrenergic** that secrete either **noradrenaline or adrenaline** (for details, refer previous chapter). However, there are few sets of **postganglionic sympathetic cholinergic fibers**. These are postganglionic sympathetic fibers *supplying sweat glands and blood vessels of skeletal muscles*. Evidences suggest that blood vessels of heart, lungs, kidney and uterus also receive some cholinergic innervation.

Scientists contributed

The **Nobel Prize in Physiology or Medicine 1936** was awarded jointly to neurophysiologist from UK **Sir Henry Hallett Dale** and neurophysiologist from USA **Prof. Otto Loewi** *"for their discoveries relating to chemical transmission of nerve impulses".* Their pioneering works were in the field of neurotransmission in ANS. HH Dale had studied the details of neurotransmitters of sympathetic nervous system and sympathetic visceral responses.

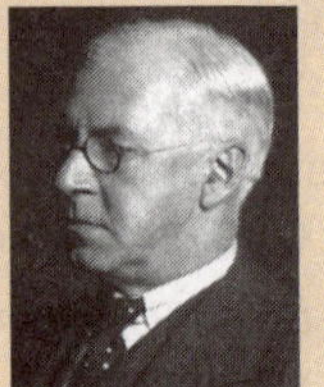

Sir Henry Hallett Dale *(1875–1968)*

SYMPATHETIC RESPONSES

Sympathetic activities are broadly two types: basal level activity at rest and widespread responses following activation.

Basal Sympathetic Activity

The sympathetic fibers impart a basal influence on many organs they innervate. This basal rate of discharge is called **basal sympathetic tone**.

1. Usually, functions of many viscera can be altered by **changing the basal level of sympathetic discharge** to the organs. Many such changes occur during normal physiological activities. For example, change in heart rate and blood pressure in response to change in posture.
2. But, if situations warrant for greater changes, **basal firing rate in sympathetic nerves can be increased or decreased** profoundly to achieve the target modulation in function. For example, to achieve a target increase in cardiac output during exercise, sympathetic stimulation considerably increases heart rate and myocardial contractility.

Widespread Sympathetic Response

Another characteristic of sympathetic stimulation is that it produces **widespread organ responses**. Example of a widespread response is *fight or flight reaction* (*see* below). The widespread response to sympathetic activation is due to **two fundamental properties**: divergence of sympathetic outflow and activation of adrenal medulla.

Sympathetic Divergence

The number of postganglionic axons emerging from the paravertebral chain of ganglia is greater than the number of preganglionic neurons originating from the spinal cord, the **ratio of postganglionic to preganglionic neurons being 100:1**. Therefore, effector tissues innervated by sympathetic fibers are more.

1. This basic *principle of divergence* enables the sympathetic system to produce widespread responses by simultaneously modulating functions of many effector organs.
2. The divergence is due to branching of the preganglionic sympathetic axons in the paravertebral chain of ganglia that makes synaptic connections with multiple postganglionic neurons both above and below their original level of emergence from the spinal cord.

Role of Adrenal Medulla

The adrenal medulla mediates many sympathetic responses. In addition to its **anatomical divergence of postganglionic neurons**, sympathetic system activates hormonal mechanism to achieve its widespread responses. These are mediated by **catecholamine** secreted from adrenal medulla.

1. The adrenal medulla is a *neuroendocrine gland*, which is basically a **modified sympathetic ganglion.**
2. The **chromaffin cells** of the adrenal medulla secrete both epinephrine and norepinephrine in a ratio of about 8:1 and store them in their secretory vesicles.
3. They release hormone directly into the bloodstream in response to activation by sympathetic preganglionic fibers. Catecholamines released from adrenal medulla by sympathetic stimulation modulate many organ functions and therefore, further promote sympathetic effects.
4. Thus, adrenomedullary secretion by sympathetic activation forms the **physiological basis of divergence** for widespread sympathetic responses.

Circulating **epinephrine plays a greater role** than norepinephrine in physiologically mediating widespread responses for ***three reasons***:

1. From adrenal medulla, ***epinephrine secretion is considerably more*** than norepinephrine.
2. Norepinephrine secretion is limited only to the axon terminals of sympathetic fibers, and therefore its effects are restricted only to the postsynaptic receptors in the target tissues, whereas ***circulating epinephrine reaches almost all tissues*** of the body.
3. Epinephrine ***potentiates sympathetic effects*** with greater efficacy than norepinephrine as it is more effective in stimulating both α and β-adrenergic receptors (though in general, epinephrine is a better β receptor agonist and norepinephrine is a better α receptor agonist).

EFFECTS OF SYMPATHETIC STIMULATION

Effects of sympathetic stimulation are summarized in Table 31.2. Effects are mediated by release of **noradrenaline** from sympathetic nerve endings and **adrenaline** from adrenal medulla.

Effects via Adrenergic Receptors

Catecholamines elicit their effects by acting on adrenergic receptors. Adrenergic receptors are broadly divided into two types: α and β. The α **receptor** has two subtypes: α_1 and α_2; and β **receptor** has three subtypes: β_1, β_2, and β_3. Generally, β receptors are more sensitive to adrenaline and α receptors to noradrenaline.

Effects of α Receptor Stimulation

Effects of α_1 Stimulation: The α_1 receptors are present in vascular smooth muscles of cutaneous and splanchnic circulation, sphincters of bladder and GI tract and radial muscles of iris. Stimulation of these receptors causes contraction or constriction of the structures in which they are present. They are equally sensitive to adrenaline and noradrenaline. The effects are mediated by formation of **intracellular IP_3**.

Effects of α_2 Stimulation: α_2 receptors are present in presynaptic nerve endings, wall of GI tract, platelets and adipocytes. Stimulation of these receptors often causes relaxation or inhibition of the structure. The effects are mediated by **decreased formation of intracellular cAMP**.

Effects of β Receptor Stimulation

Effects of β_1 Stimulation: β_1 receptors are present in SA node, AV node and ventricular muscle. Stimulation of these receptors causes excitation of these structures. They are more sensitive to adrenaline than noradrenaline. The effects are mediated by increased formation of ***intracellular cAMP***.

Effects of β_2 Stimulation: β_2 receptors are present in blood vessels of skeletal muscles, bronchial smooth muscles

Table 31.2: Effects of sympathetic and parasympathetic stimulation.

Effector organ	Sympathetic	Parasympathetic
Eye		
Dilator pupillae	Contraction (α_1) (dilation of pupil)	–
Sphincter pupillae	–	Contraction (constriction of pupil)
Ciliary muscle	Relaxation (β_2)	Contraction
Muller's muscle	Contraction (α_1)	–
Glands		
Lacrimal gland	–	↑ secretion
Nasal glands	↓ secretion (α_1)	↑ secretion
Salivary glands		
Secretion	Amylase secretion	↑ secretion
Blood vessel	Constriction (α_1, α_2)	Dilation
Heart		
SA node	↑ heart rate (β_1, β_2)	↓ heart rate
AV node	↑ conductivity (β_1, β_2)	↓ conductivity
Conduction paths	↑ conductivity (β_1, β_2)	↓ conductivity
Atria	↑ contractility (β_1, β_2)	↓ contractility
Ventricles	↑ contractility (β_1, β_2)	↓ contractility
Blood vessels		
Cutaneous	Constriction (α_1)	No supply
Skeletal muscle	Dilation (β_2)	No supply
	Constriction (α)	
Visceral	Constriction (α_1)	No supply
Coronary	Dilation (β_2) Constriction (α_1, α_2)	Dilation
Cerebral	Constriction (α_1)	Dilation
Pulmonary	Constriction (α_1) Dilation (β_2)	Dilation
Renal	Constriction (α_1, α_2) Dilation (β_1, β_2)	No supply
Systemic veins	Constriction (α_1, α_2) Dilation (β_2)	No supply
Lungs		
Bronchioles	Dilation (β_2)	Constriction
Glands	↑ secretion (β_2)	
	↓ secretion (α_1)	
Skin		
Sweat glands	Less secretion	More secretion
Pilomotor muscle	Contraction (α_1)	No supply
GI tract		
Motility and tone	Decrease (α_1, β_1, β_2)	Increase
Sphincter	Contraction (α_1)	Relaxation
Secretion	Inhibition (α_2)	Stimulation
Gallbladder	Relaxation (β_2)	Contraction
Liver	Glycogenolysis and gluconeogenesis(α_1, β_2)	–

Contd...

Contd...

Effector organ	Sympathetic	Parasympathetic
Pancreas		
Islets	↓ secretion (α_2) ↑ secretion (β_2)	↑ secretion
Acini	↓ secretion	↑ secretion
Adrenal medulla	↑ secretion of Epinephrine and NE	–
Urinary system		
Detrusor muscle	Relaxation (β_2)	Contraction
Trigone-Sphincter	Contraction (α_1)	Relaxation
Ureter	Contraction (α_1)	Relaxation
Other structures		
Male sex organ	Ejaculation (α_1)	Erection
Uterus	Contraction (α_1) Relaxation (β_2)	Variable
Adipose tissue	Lipolysis (α_1, β_1, β_3)	None
Pineal gland	↑ melatonin secretion (β)	None
JG cells	↑ renin secretion (β_1)	None

and wall of GI tract. Stimulation of these receptors causes relaxation of these structures. They are more sensitive to adrenaline than noradrenaline. The effects are mediated by change in the level of ***intracellular cAMP***.

Effects of β_3 Stimulation: β_3 receptors are present in adipose tissues. Stimulation of these receptors causes lipolysis. The effect is mediated by increase in the level of ***intracellular cAMP***.

Fight-or-Flight Response

The fight-or-flight response is a typical widespread response of sympathetic activation. This occurs in critical situations of life when one has to either fight the situation or flee from the situation. Though many components of response are due to direct effects of sympathetic stimulation, secretion of catecholamine from adrenal medulla contributes considerably. The effects are as follows:

1. **Sympathetic stimulation of CVS** *increases blood pressure* due to increased cardiac output and vasoconstriction. Also, *redistribution of the blood flow* occurs to skeletal muscles and heart from splanchnic and cutaneous territories so that ***performance enhances***.
2. In lungs, **increased exchange of blood gases** occurs due to *stimulation of the respiratory rate and dilation of bronchiolar tree*. This **increases supply of oxygen** to the tissues.
3. Sympathetic stimulation to salivary gland **decreases salivary secretion**. However, *secretion of mucus increases proportionately*, permitting lubrication of the mouth despite increased ventilation and reduced salivation.
4. **Supply of metabolic substrates increases**, which is an essential component of effective stress reaction. The demand for increased supply of substrates like glucose and fatty acids is met by the actions of circulating epinephrine on hepatocytes and adipocytes. **Glycogenolysis** increases plasma glucose concentration and **lipolysis** promotes plasma free fatty acid level.
5. **Sympathetic stimulation to sweat glands** causes *secretion of a watery fluid*, and *evaporation of body heat*. **Cutaneous vasoconstriction** with concurrent sweat gland activation causes *cold, clammy skin* of a frightened individual.
6. **Activation of piloerector muscles** of hair follicles causes hair-standing-on the skin. The hair erection helps in *preservation of body temperature* or gives a *ferocious appearance* to threaten the enemy.
7. **Pupillary dilation** *enhances visual acuity* and perception to make the individual environmentally maximal alert.
8. **Stimulation of brainstem reticular system** makes the individual maximally alert and mentally conscious to take appropriate decisions in quick successions.
9. Activity of **bowel and bladder** *temporarily ceases* due to constriction of sphincters.

CHAPTER SUMMARY

Key Concepts

1. In sympathetic system (thoracolumbar outflow), preganglionic fibers in the paravertebral chain can ascend up or descend down to terminate in the postganglionic neurons of many segments in spinal cord, which can activate many visceral structures.
2. Sympathetic activation results in widespread sympathetic response that occurs due to divergence (more postganglionic fibers than preganglionic fibers), and secretion of catecholamines from adrenal medulla.
3. Generally, β receptors are more sensitive to adrenaline and α receptors to noradrenaline.

Important to Know (Must Read)

1. In examinations, usually there will be no **Long Question** from this chapter.
2. Sympathetic ganglia, Sympathetic neurons, Sympathetic neurotransmitters, Effects of sympathetic stimulation, Fight-or-flight response, may come as **Short Questions** in exams.
3. In **Viva**, examiners usually ask... Organization of sympathetic system, How preganglionic fibers come out of spinal cord, Sympathetic pre- and postganglionic neurons, Name the sympathetic ganglia, Specialities of sympathetic responses, Effects of sympathetic stimulation, Sympathetic neurotransmitters, Receptors for sympathetic neurotransmitters, Details of effects of sympathetic stimulation on each organ, What is Fight-or-flight response, and its features.

CHAPTER 32

Parasympathetic System

Learning Objectives

On completion of study of this chapter, the student **MUST** be able to:

1. Understand the importance of parasympathetic system in regulation of body functions.
2. Appreciate the anatomical and functional specializations of parasympathetic division of ANS.
3. Trace the course of pre- and post-ganglionic neurons of parasympathetic system.
4. Name the parasympathetic ganglia and give their distribution to various visceral organs.
5. Understand the importance of basal parasympathetic tone.
6. Narrate the responses of parasympathetic stimulation.
7. Give the effects of parasympathetic stimulation to various organs and name the receptors that mediate these effects.

The student **MAY** also be able to:

1. Describe the effects of parasympathetic activation.

The parasympathetic system is the system of **energy restoration**. This system works when the body is at rest. It helps in generating and restoring the energy and recovering the body from energy loss. Thus, this helps in repair and renovation of the body systems. In general, parasympathetic activity is synonymous with the vagal activity, as vagus nerve controls most of the visceral functions.

Structural Organization

The parasympathetic system is the **craniosacral outflow** of autonomic nervous system.

1. The **cranial component** emanates from the brainstem, and the **sacral component** originates from intermediolateral gray column of sacral segments of spinal cord.
2. In contrast to the stimulation of sympathetic system that causes widespread responses, parasympathetic activation causes localized responses (Table 32.1). The divergence of parasympathetic outflow is minimal. The **divergence ratio** of the presynaptic output to postsynaptic output is about 1:15, in contrast to 1:100 in sympathetic system.
3. There is no circulating hormonal mechanism to aid to the divergence of parasympathetic activation. Hence, stimulation of parasympathetic nerve to an organ-system results in a limited activation of the concerned structures. For example, vagal stimulation to heart slows the heart rate without significantly altering the vagal influence on stomach.

Parasympathetic ganglia are located either close to the organ or embedded in the organ. Therefore, preganglionic neurons are much longer than postganglionic neurons. The differences between sympathetic and parasympathetic systems are summarized in Table 32.1.

Cranial Component

Cell bodies of preganglionic neurons of cranial component of parasympathetic system are located in the brainstem. Hence, this component is also called **brainstem parasympathetic division**. Brainstem parasympathetic neurons innervate structures in the head, neck, thorax and abdomen. Parasympathetic axons from brainstem travel in **III, VII, IX, and X cranial nerves** (Fig. 32.1). Nuclei of these cranial nerves are present in the midbrain in tectum, pons and medulla. Therefore, these nuclei serve as the centers for the integration of autonomic reflexes for the organ systems they innervate.

Table 32.1: Differences between sympathetic and parasympathetic systems.

	Sympathetic system	Parasympathetic system
A. General Features		
Origin	Thoracolumbar outflow (cell bodies of preganglionic fibers are located in IML horn of thoracic and lumbar segments of spinal cord).	Craniosacral outflow (cell bodies of preganglionic fibers are located in brainstem cranial nerve nuclei and sacral segments of spinal cord).
Preganglionic fibers	Short and cholinergic, along with ventral nerve roots of thoracolumbar nerves	Long and cholinergic, along with cranial nerves III, VII, IX, X and ventral nerve roots of sacral nerves
Ganglia	Located close to spinal cord, forms chain of paravertebral ganglia.	Located close to the target organ or in the organ
Postganglionic fibers	Long, unmyelinated and adrenergic, along spinal nerves, blood vessels and visceral branches of paravertebral chain	Short, myelinated and cholinergic, through branches of trigeminal in head region; and direct ganglionated branches
Ratio of pre to postganglionic fibers	1:100	1:1 to 1:15
Organs innervated	Almost all organs of the body	Mainly visceral organs
Responses	Widespread	Localized
Impact on body energy	Utilizes energy	Restores energy
Highest modulators	Limbic region	Limbic region
Hypothalamus	Caudal	Rostral
Brainstem control	Reticular formation	Reticular formation
Supraspinal fibers	Hypothalamus fibers	Dorsal longitudinal fasciculate and hypothalamospinal fibers
Preganglionic neurons (connector neurons)	Intermediolateral grey column of T_1 to T_{12}	General visceral efferent nuclei and intermediolateral grey column of cranial nerves III, VII, IX, X and S_2 to S_4.
Myelination of preganglionic fibers	Myelinated (white ramus communicans)	Myelinated
Length of preganglionic fibers	Relatively short	Relatively long
Preganglionic neuron terminal (and receptor) /neurotransmitter	Acetylcholine (nicotinic receptor)	Acetylcholine (nicotinic receptor)
Ganglia of relay effector neuron	Paravertebral and plexus along the abdominal aorta and internal iliac artery	Ciliary, pterygopalati submandibular, otic, cardiopulmonary plexus and in the wall of the viscera
Ratio of preganglionic fibers to neurons of ganglia	One is many (therefore mass discharge)	One is to a few (therefore localized effect
Myelination of postganglionic fiber	Unmyelinated	Unmyelinated
Length of postganglionic fiber	Relatively long	Relatively short
Postganglionic neuron terminal (and receptor) /neurotransmitter	Noradrenaline (α and β adrenergic receptor) and acetylcholine (muscarinic receptor to sweat gland and some blood vessels to skeletal muscle)	Acetylcholine (muscarinic receptor)
Effect	Response as in 'fright-flight-fight' response	Responsible for homeostasis
Metabolism	Catabolic	Anabolic
B. Effects of organ stimulation		
Eye	Dilatation of pupils and contraction of orbitalis and smooth muscles of tarsals	Constriction of pupils and ciliary muscle for accommodation
Lacrimal gland	-------	Secretion
Salivary glands	Thick, viscous secretion	Profuse, watery secretion
Heart	Increases heart rate, increases contractility	Deceases heart rate, decreases Contractility
Lung	Bronchial smooth muscle relaxation	Bronchial smooth muscle relaxation
Gastrointestinal tract	Decreases motility, contraction of sphincters and inhibition of secretion	Increases motility, relaxation of sphincters and stimulation of secretion
Urinary bladder	Relaxation of detrusor and contraction of involuntary sphincter vesicae	Contraction of detrusor and relaxation of involuntary sphincter vesicae
Male sex organs	Ejaculation	Erection
Skin	Contraction of erector pili and secretion of sweat glands	-----------
Blood vessels	Vasoconstriction, dilation in some vessels	

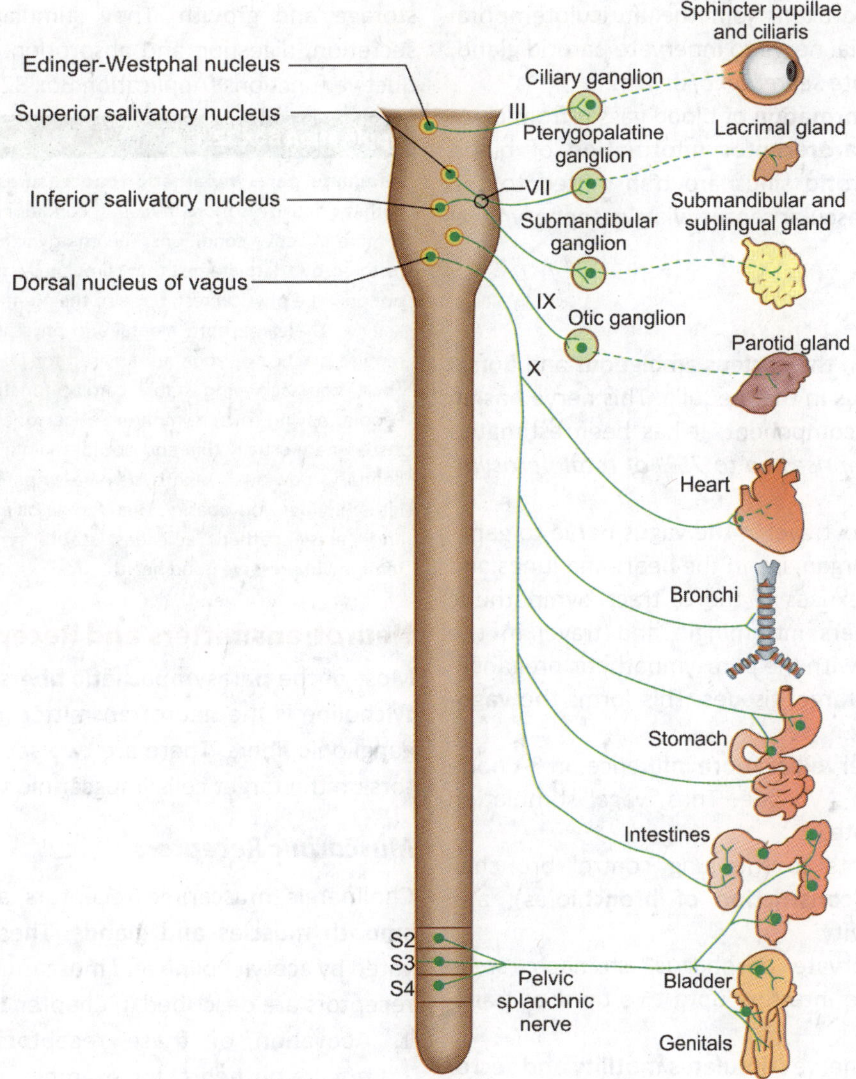

Fig. 32.1: Parasympathetic nervous system. Note the craniosacral outflow.

Cranial Nerve III

Cranial nerve III is the **oculomotor nerve** that originates from tectum of the midbrain. The cell bodies are located in the **Edinger-Westphal nucleus.**

1. The preganglionic axons travel in the III cranial nerve to terminate on the cell bodies of postganglionic neuron in **ciliary ganglion**, which is located inside the orbit of the eye.
2. The postganglionic axons enter eyeball near the optic nerve and innervate sphincter muscle of the iris (*sphincter pupillae*) that control the diameter of the pupil, the *ciliary muscle* that focuses the lens for accommodation for near vision, and the *choroidal blood vessels*.
3. The postganglionic fibers project mainly to the iris muscles. About 90% of fibers innervate ciliary muscle, 3 to 5% innervate sphincter pupillae and rest of the fibers terminates on blood vessels of choroid. Optic nerve projects to tectum and provides input for ocular reflexes.

Cranial Nerve VII

The preganglionic fibers in facial nerve emerge from the **superior salivary nuclei** in the rostral medulla and then pass from the facial nerve into the greater superficial petrosal nerve to synapse in the **pterygopalatine ganglion.**

1. The postganglionic fibers innervate the *lacrimal gland and the glands of nasal and palatal mucosa*. Another set of preganglionic fibers in the facial nerve travel via the chorda tympani nerve to synapse in the **submandibular ganglion.**
2. These postganglionic fibers from submandibular ganglion innervate *submandibular and sublingual glands*. Stimulation of this nerve **increases saliva production.**

Cranial Nerve IX

The preganglionic axons of the glossopharyngeal nerve originate form the **inferior salivary nuclei** in the medulla. The fibers take a tortuous course through the lesser petrosal nerve to terminate in **otic ganglion.**

1. The postganglionic axons join the auriculotemporal branch of 5th cranial nerve to innervate parotid gland, where they *facilitate secretion of saliva.*
2. **Chemosensory information** of blood gasses from carotid bodies and **baroreceptor information** of blood pressure from carotid sinus are transmitted to the medullary cardiovascular centers via glossopharyngeal afferents.

Cranial Nerve X

Vagus nerve arises from the **nucleus ambiguous** and **dorsal motor nucleus of vagus** in the medulla. This nerve has an extensive autonomic component. It has been estimated that *vagal output comprises up to 75% of total parasympathetic activity*.

1. Preganglionic fibers travel in the vagus nerve to ganglia located in the organ, i.e. in the heart and lungs and in the intrinsic plexuses of the GI tract. Sympathetic postganglionic fibers intermingle and travel in the same nerve trunk with the parasympathetic preganglionic fibers to the target tissues. This forms the **vago-sympathetic trunk**.
2. The **right vagus nerve** has more influence on SA node and left vagus on AV node. Thus, vagal stimulation **slows the heart rate**.
3. The vagal efferents to the lung control bronchial smooth muscle (**constriction of bronchioles**), and secretory cell activity.
4. Vagal fibers innervate esophagus, stomach, small intestine and large intestine upto two-third of transverse colon.
5. On GI tract, vagus nerve **stimulates motility and secretory functions.** Acetylcholine and VIP are the transmitters of the postganglionic neurons.
6. There are vagal innervations of kidneys, liver, spleen and pancreas.

Sacral Component

Sacral parasympathetic neurons innervate structures in the pelvis.

1. **Preganglionic fibers** originate in the intermediolateral gray column of the sacral segments S_2, S_3, and S_4 of spinal cord.
2. The preganglionic fibers terminate in ganglia in or near the viscera that include descending colon, sigmoid colon, rectum, internal anal sphincter, urinary bladder and the reproductive organs.

PARASYMPATHETIC FUNCTIONS

Parasympathetic system **restores body's energy reserve.** Favorable conditions in both external and internal environments herald parasympathetic activation. Except on cardiovascular system, most parasympathetic effects are stimulatory, especially for the processes that facilitate energy storage and growth. They stimulate intestinal motility, secretion, digestion and absorption. They promote reproductive functions (Application Box 32.1).

Application Box 32.1

Adequate parasympathetic tone ensures good health: Parasympathetic activity is more in resting conditions and sympathetic activity is more in active conditions. The energy lost during activities must be restored by adequate rest that stimulates parasympathetic system. It is not only the physical rest, but also the mental rest that promotes vagal activity. Therefore, both mental and physical relaxations as occurs by regular practice of yoga are advised for improving health in general, apart from achieving stable cardiac functions and blood pressure. People having hypersympathetic personality (always anxious and restless) are usually thin and do not maintain good health, and in the contrary, individuals with hyperparasympathetic personality (lazy and lethargic) develop obesity. Therefore, a balanced state of sympathetic and parasympathetic activities (**stable sympathovagal balance**) is required to preserve good health.

Neurotransmitters and Receptors

Most of the **parasympathetic fibers are cholinergic.** Acetylcholine is the neurotransmitter in both pre- and postganglionic fibers. There are two sets of cholinergic receptors on the target cells: muscarinic and nicotinic.

Muscarinic Receptors

Cholinergic muscarinic receptors are present in **heart, smooth muscles and glands**. These receptors are activated by acetylcholine and muscarine (Types of muscarinic receptors are described in Chapter 116).

1. Activation of these receptors produce *inhibitory effects on heart*, for example, decreased heart rate, and *excitatory effects on smooth muscle and glands*, for example, increased GI motility and secretion etc.
2. Effects are mediated by **decreased cAMP formation** in the cytosol of cardiac cells and **direct opening of K^+ channels** in nodal tissues of heart.
3. In smooth muscles and glandular tissues, effects are mediated by **intracellular IP_3 and Ca^{++}**. Muscarinic receptors are **blocked by atropine**.

Nicotinic Receptors

Cholinergic nicotinic receptors are present in **autonomic ganglia** (both sympathetic and parasympathetic), **neuromuscular junctions** and **adrenal medulla**. These receptors are activated by acetylcholine and nicotine.

1. Activation of these receptors produces *excitatory effects* on target tissue. Effects are mediated by **direct binding of acetylcholine to α subunits** of the receptors.
2. Receptors also contain Na^+ and K^+ channels.
3. Nicotinic effects are **blocked by ganglion blockers** such as hexamethonium that prevent action of acetylcholine in the ganglia and at neuromuscular junction by curare drugs.

CHAPTER SUMMARY

Key Concepts

1. In parasympathetic system (craniosacral outflow), preganglionic fibers are very long as ganglions are located close to the organs.
2. Parasympathetic activation is considered to be similar with vagal activation, as 75% of parasympathetic functions are mediated by vagus nerve.
3. Greater vagal tone is essential for good health.

Important to Know (Must Read)

1. In examinations, usually there will be no **Long Question** from this chapter.
2. Parasympathetic ganglia, Parasympathetic cranial nerves, Parasympathetic neurotransmitters and receptors, Effects of parasympathetic stimulation, Parasympathetic functions, Vagal tone, may come as **Short Questions** in exams.
3. In **Viva**, examiners may ask… Name parasympathetic ganglia, Name parasympathetic cranial nerves, Parasympathetic neurotransmitters and receptors, Effects of parasympathetic stimulation on different organs, especially on CVS, Parasympathetic functions, Importance of vagal tone, and the differences between sympathetic and parasympathetic systems.

CHAPTER 33

Control of Autonomic Functions and Applied Aspects

Learning Objectives

On completion of study of this chapter, the student **MUST** be able to:

1. List the control mechanisms of autonomic functions.
2. Understand the importance of regulation of autonomic functions.
3. Classify autonomic disorders .
4. Name the features of common autonomic disorders.

The student **MAY** also be able to:

1. Describe the regulation of autonomic functions.

CONTROL OF AUTONOMIC FUNCTIONS

Visceral organs are innervated by sympathetic and parasympathetic divisions of autonomic nervous system (ANS). Effects of stimulation of sympathetic and parasympathetic systems are usually opposite. But due to robust regulatory mechanisms, the process that activates one division of ANS usually inhibits and moderates the function of the other. Therefore, sympathetic and parasympathetic divisions are also reciprocal to each other. Consequently, under normal circumstances excessive stimulation or activation of both the systems, which might have deleterious effects, is avoided. Autonomic functions are regulated by various reflexes and supraspinal mechanisms.

Reflex Regulation

Previously, ANS was regarded as an efferent system, and the sensory neurons (afferents) that innervate autonomic structures were not considered as part of ANS. However, afferent fibers also constitute an important component of autonomic system and ***sensory input from visceral structures is part of autonomic organization***.

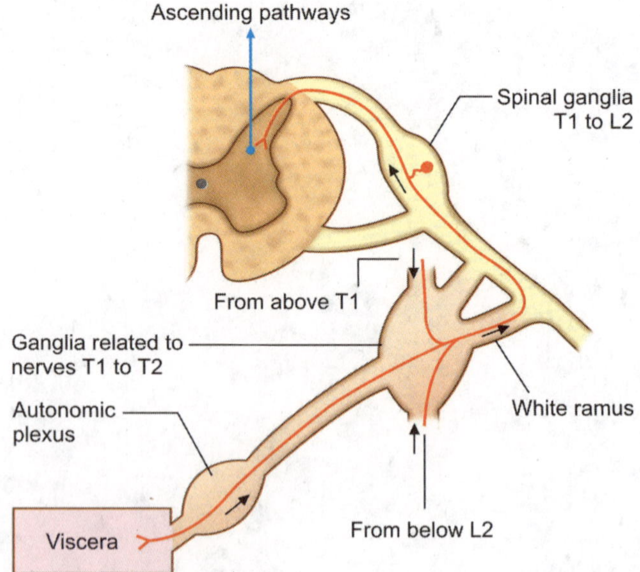

Fig. 33.1: Afferent autonomic pathways from visceral structures involving sympathetic nerves.

1. The sensory innervation to the visceral organs including blood vessels and cutaneous structures forms the **afferent limb** of autonomic reflexes. The information from visceral organs reach the spinal cord through afferent fibers and, from there, the second order of neurons convey information to the higher centers via **ascending pathways** (Fig. 33.1).
2. Sensory information in the afferent pathways may not always reach higher center for finer integration and

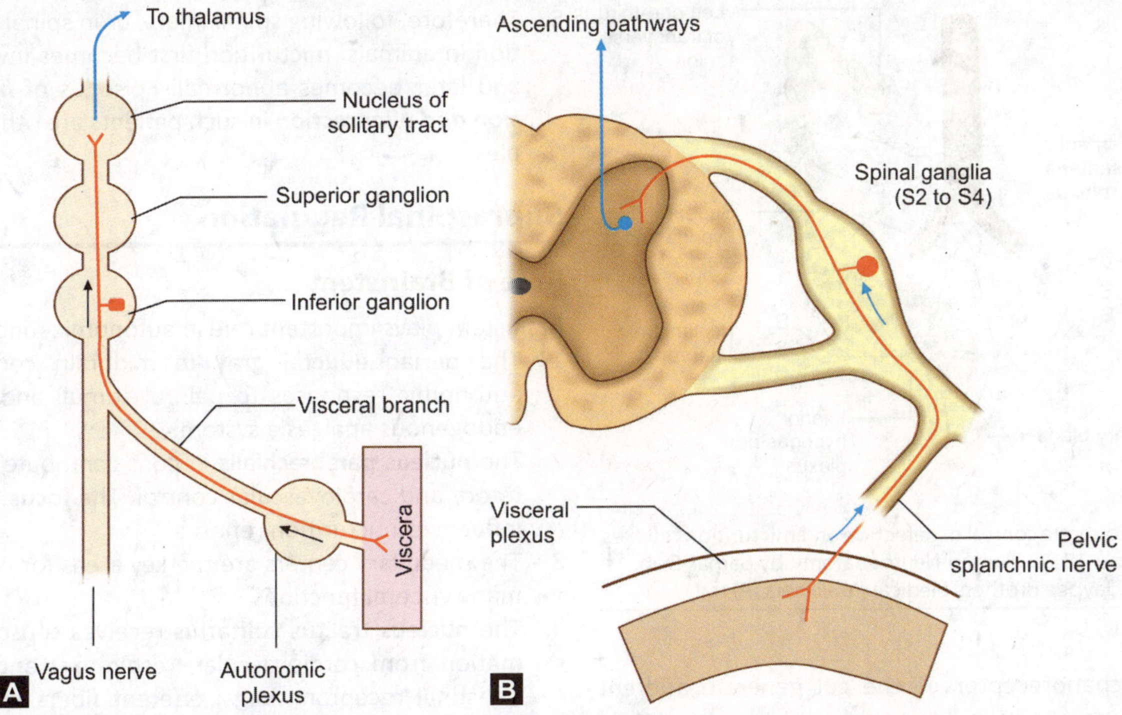

Figs. 33.2A and B: Arrangement of (A) afferent autonomic neurons related to the vagus; and (B) pelvic splanchnic nerves.

conscious perception, but definitely reaches **different levels of autonomic neuraxis** up to the level of subcortical structures, especially the thalamus (Figs. 33.2A and B).

3. Thus, ANS integrates a ***hierarchy of reflexes*** to control organ functions. According to their level of integration, the autonomic reflexes are subjected to control by various part of CNS.

Local Reflexes

A sensory neuron (afferent autonomic fiber) has many terminal branches peripherally.

1. As a result, sensory action potential that propagates ***orthodromically*** in one of the afferent branch to CNS may also enter a branch of the same axon and then conduct ***antidromically*** to **release neurotransmitters at the sensory terminals** that end on other structure.
2. The process results in spreading initial reaction produced by the stimulus.
3. For example, when the branch of a sensory neuron innervates blood vessels, the response is the spread of reddening of skin as a result of arteriolar dilation (refer to the **'Axon Reflex'** in 'Cutaneous circulation' in CVS), or if sensory neuron innervates sweat glands, the response will be local sweating as a result of sweat gland activation. This process is called **'Local axon reflex'**.
4. Persistent activation of such reflexes in nociceptive afferents following trauma can produce dramatic features.

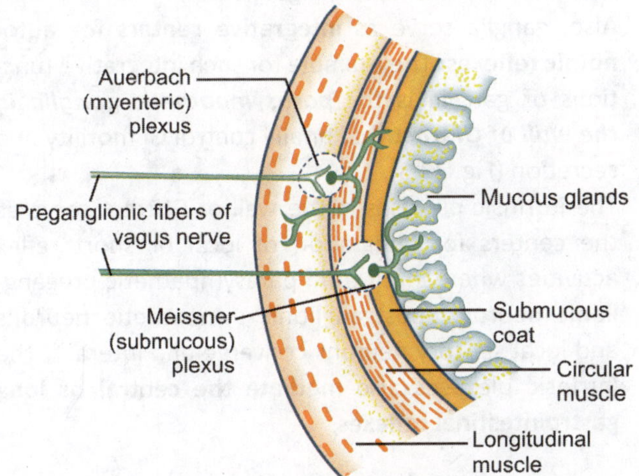

Fig. 33.3: Parasympathetic plexuses in GI tract control secretion and motility.
Courtesy: Figure 18.19, Human Neuroanatomy by Samar Deb, 1st edition, 2014; Jaypee Brothers Medical Publishers (P) Ltd.

Role of Autonomic Ganglia

Ganglia in ANS serves as relay stations for preganglionic and postganglionic neurons. Recent evidences suggest that **synaptic activity in the ganglia may influence final efferent output.**

1. Inputs arriving from many preganglionic neurons alter the activity in ganglia, which in turn alter the visceral activity. The best example is the regulation of GI functions by ***ganglia of GI tract*** *(Fig. 33.3)*. Chemoreceptors

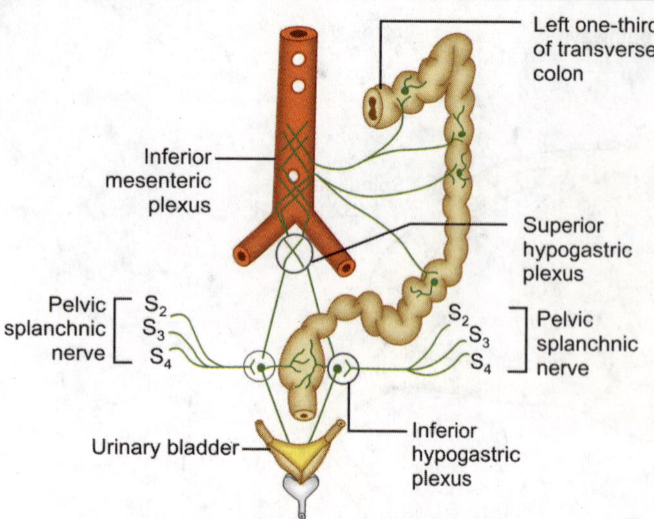

Fig. 33.4: Autonomic control of defection and micturition reflexes. *Courtesy*: Figure 18.20, Human Neuroanatomy by Samar Deb, 1st edition, 2014; Jaypee Brothers Medical Publishers (P) Ltd.

and mechanoreceptors in the gut generate afferent action potentials that pass to the spinal cord and then from there to the *celiac and mesenteric ganglia*. The output from these ganglia *changes the GI motility and secretion required during digestion*.

2. Also, ganglia serve as **integrative centers for autonomic reflexes**. The example for such integrative functions of ganglia is the ***parasympathetic ganglia in the wall of GI tract*** that finally control GI motility and secretion (Fig. 33.3).
3. The intrinsic plexuses in the wall of GI tract serve as the centers for integration of local or short reflex activities where input from parasympathetic preganglionic neurons, postganglionic sympathetic neurons and local sensory neurons converge and interact. The intrinsic plexuses also **mediate the central or long gastrointestinal reflexes**.

Spinal Autonomic Reflexes

Many autonomic reflexes are integrated in the spinal cord. The examples are micturition, defecation and sexual reflexes. These reflexes are coordinated by centers in the lumbar and sacral spinal cord.

1. **Micturition reflex** causes emptying of urinary bladder, **defecation reflex** causes emptying of rectum, and **sexual responses** in male cause erection and ejaculation and in female produce vaginal lubrication (Fig. 33.4).
2. Sensory input from the wall of the bladder and bowel inform the degree of distension of these hollow viscera.
3. Coordination between sympathetic and parasympathetic systems is required for many of these responses.
4. **Higher centers usually inhibit spinal cord reflex centers.**
5. Therefore, following spinal injury, or in spinal preparation in animals, micturition first becomes involuntary and later becomes abnormal. Episodes of ***hypertension and piloerection*** in such patients are other examples.

Supraspinal Regulation

Role of Brainstem

Brainstem plays important role in autonomic functions.

1. The **periaqueductal gray** in midbrain coordinates autonomic responses to painful stimuli and induces endogenous analgesia system.
2. The **nucleus parabrachialis** in pons contribute to respiratory and cardiovascular control. The **locus ceruleus** influences micturition reflexes.
3. The medullary centers are the key areas for control of many visceral functions.
4. The **nucleus tractus solitarius** receives sensory information from cardiovascular, respiratory and gastrointestinal receptors. Vagal efferent fibers arise from this area in the medulla.
5. The **vasomotor center** in the ventrolateral medulla is the key center for sympathetic output as it directly controls preganglionic sympathetic neurons in the spinal cord.

Major autonomic reflexes integrated in the brainstem include:

1. Pupillary light reflex
2. Accommodation reflex
3. Reflex salivation
4. Reflex lacrimation
5. Deglutition reflex
6. Vomiting reflex
7. Reflexes for regulation of heart rate and blood pressure
8. Reflexes for regulation of respiration.

Role of Hypothalamus and Cortex

Hypothalamus and cortex provide the highest levels of autonomic control.

1. The periventricular hypothalamus, and medial and lateral hypothalamic areas control homeostatic functions such as thermoregulation, appetite behaviors etc.
2. Stimulation of ***lateral and posterior hypothalamus*** causes sympathetic activation, and stimulation of ***posterior hypothalamus*** causes parasympathetic activation.
3. **Hypothalamus** controls ***circadian rhythms*** that influence many autonomic functions.
4. Hypothalamus also contributes to the *regulation of blood pressure and blood volume*.
5. For its major role in autonomic functions, hypothalamus was designated (by Charles Sherrington) in the past as **'head ganglion of the ANS'**.

6. Hypothalamus, due to its close proximity and reciprocal interaction with limbic system, is influenced by limbic activities. Therefore, autonomic functions are easily affected by limbic functions and dysfunctions.
7. The **prefrontal cortex** is involved in the regulation of autonomic function.
8. The **amygdala** coordinates the autonomic components of emotional responses.
9. Cortex, limbic structures, brainstem and their spinal connections for control of autonomic functions are collectively referred to as **central network for autonomic control**.

AUTONOMIC DYSFUNCTIONS

Following are the two fundamental types of lesion of autonomic nervous system
1. Diseases
2. Injury

Autonomic Diseases

Autonomic disorders are broadly termed as **autonomic failures**. Autonomic failures are of two types: primary and secondary.

Primary Autonomic Failure

Primary autonomic failure is **idiopathic autonomic dysfunction** that invariably manifests as ***orthostatic hypotension***.

Secondary Autonomic Failure

Secondary autonomic failure occurs in various diseases.
1. Commonly seen in **diabetes**, amyloidosis, beriberi, syringomyelia, tabes dorsalis and subacute combined degeneration of spinal cord.
2. It also occurs in patients receiving **sympatholytic drugs** of those who have undergone **surgical sympathectomy**.
3. Autonomic imbalance also occurs in patients with **prolonged bed rest**.

Features of Autonomic Dysfunctions

Autonomic dysfunctions manifest as multiple organ dysfunctions as autonomic nerves innervate many visceral organs.

Commonly affected are cardiovascular, gastrointestinal, renal and reproductive organs.

Cardiovascular features: Usual manifestation is ***orthostatic hypotension***. **Tachycardia** may also be seen.

Gastrointestinal features: Either ***constipation or diarrhea*** can occur. Dysphagia is not uncommon. Dryness of mouth occurs frequently.

Renal features: Increased ***frequency of micturition*** is the usual feature. Nocturia and incontinence may occur.

Reproductive features: ***Erectile dysfunction*** is common in male. ***Premature ejaculation*** is also common. In females, decreased vaginal lubrication during sexual act is common.

Sudomotor features: ***Anhydrosis*** is common. Heat intolerance and hyperhydrosis may occur.

Neurological symptoms: Weakness, lethargy and giddiness.

Treatment

Treatment should start immediately for the cause of the disease, if it is of secondary variety of autonomic failure. Treatment otherwise is mostly symptomatic depending on the nature of the failure.

Diseases affecting Sympathetic System

Horner's Syndrome

This is a syndrome (described by Johan Horner) of autonomic dysfunction, characterized mainly by:
1. Presence of **ptosis** (drooping of the upper eyelid)
2. **Miosis** (constriction of pupil)
3. **Facial anhydrosis** (lack of sweating on the affected side of face and neck).

Etiology

Horner's syndrome is a condition of **oculo-sympathetic paralysis**. Horner's syndrome commonly occurs in ***malignancy of cervical lymph nodes*** that presses on cervical sympathetic chain, and ***Pancoast tumor of lungs***.

Pathophysiology

Clinical manifestations of this syndrome occur due to **interruption of sympathetic nerve supply to the head and neck**.
1. Venter (connector neurons) for the sympathetic outflow to head and neck lies in lateral horn cells of first thoracic segment of spinal gray matter. Proximally, it gets supraspinal control through reticulospinal tract descending from brainstem reticular formation.
2. Preganglionic sympathetic fibres for head and neck arising from 1st thoracic segment ascend through cervical part of sympathetic chain.
3. After relay in cervical sympathetic ganglia, postganglionic fibres are distributed to head and neck through following branches:
   - Lateral branches: Gray rami to join cervical spinal nerve to arterial wall and sweat gland.
   - Medial splanchnic branches.
   - Internal carotid branch: It runs along internal carotid artery to enter inside the cranium. Apart from vascular branches, fibers along ophthalmic artery, entering the orbit supply dilatorpupillae and part of levator palpebrae superioris.

A patient may suffer from Horner syndrome **due to lesion of anyone of following three levels** of sympathetic pathway for head and neck.

1. First neuron lesion:	Affecting reticulospinal tract	Due to degeneration of diseases like Multiple myeloma, Syringomyelia
2. Second neuron lesion:	Affecting first thoracic segment of spinal gray matter	
3. Third neuron lesion:	Affecting cervicothoracic (stellate) ganglion	Due to Penetrating injury at root of neck Traction by cervical rib

Physiological Basis of Clinical Features

Ptosis occurs due to paralysis of Muller's muscle, and **miosis** occurs due to paralysis of dilator pupillae. **Anhydrosis** is due to decreased sympathetic activity.

1. **Miosis:** Constriction of pupil due to unopposed action of sphincter pupillae for non-functioning dilator pupillae.
2. **Ptosis:** Partial dropping of upper eyelid due to paralysis of levator palpebrae superioris.
3. **Anhidrosis:** Dryness of one half of the face with head and neck due to impaired secretion of sweat gland.
4. **Flushing or blanching of same half of face** due to loss of vasoconstrictor effect on skin.

Scientist contributed

Horner's syndrome, a disorder of the sympathetic nervous system, was named after **Johann Friedrich Horner,** a 19th century Swiss ophthalmologist following his description of the condition in 1869. His name is also associated with "***Horner's muscle***", the lacrimal portion of the orbicularis oculi muscle that is sometimes referred to as the tensor tarsi muscle. With *Alexios Trantas* (1867–1960), the "***Horner-Trantas spots***" are named, being defined as small whitish-yellow chalky concretions of the conjunctiva around the corneal limbus.

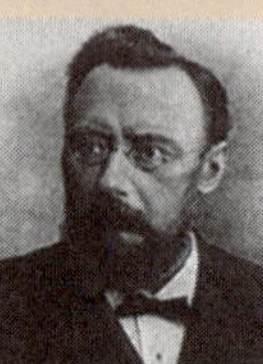

JF Horner
(1831–1886)

Raynaud Disease

It is a vasospastic disease due to **hyperactivity of vasoconstrictor sympathetic fibres** affecting digital arteries of fingers. It is a bilateral disorder which is precipitated by exposure to cold and smoking. In case of smokers, nicotine aggravates vasospasm. Clinical manifestations are pain, pallor and cyanosis due to impaired vascular supply. Fingertips show black discoloration with formation of dry gangrene.

Buerger Disease

It is arterial occlusive disease of lower limb. Ischemia of muscle of leg causes pain due to muscular cramps intermittently. That is why the disorder is named as intermittent claudication.

Diseases affecting Parasympathetic System

1. **Argyll Robertson pupil:** It is a disorder in a patient of neurosyphilis due to lesion of pretectal nucleus of midbrain which is one of the cell stations in light reflex pathway. The disease is characterized by narrow pupil with no reaction to light due to interruption of light reflex pathway which is as follows:

   Retina—optic nerve—optic chiasma—optic tract—lateral geniculate body — superior brachium — pretectal nucleus — Edinger—Westphal nucleus occulomotor nerve — ciliary ganglion — short ciliary nerve — sphincter pupillae.

   In case of Argyll Robertson pupil, accomodation reflex is not disrupted as it is not passing through pretectal nucleus and its pathway id as follows.

   Retina — optic nerve — optic chiasma — optic tract — lateral geniculate body — optic radiation — primary visual cortex — superior — longitudinal fasciculus frontal eye lid — corticonuclear tract — occulomotor nucleus —(somatic as well as visceral efferent) — occulomotor nerve to supply medial rectus, sphincter pupillae and ciliaris for accommodation.

   A simple formula mentioned below may be helpful to remember manifestation of Argyll Robertson pupil.

   Argyll Robertson pupil { ARP (Accommodation reflex present)
   PRA (Pupillary reflex absent)

2. **Adie tonic pupil:** This is a syndrome characterized by following clinical presentations.
   i. Diminished or absent light reflex due to disorder of function sphincter pupillae.
   ii. Slow or delayed dilation of pupil in the dark.
   iii. Slow or delayed accommodation to near vision because of ciliary muscle which is responsible for increase of curvature of lens.

   All the above features are supposed to be due to suppression of parasympathetic ocular function.
3. **Frey syndrome:** It is a clinical condition that is found to occur following healing of a penetrating wound of face over parotid gland. During healing process, injured nerves of this area of face communicate with one another, as done by auriculotemporal nerve supplying parasympathetic postganglionic secretomotor fibers to parotid gland with great auricular nerve supplying sweat glands of this area of face. So stimulation of salivary secretion during mastication of food causes sweating of area of face supplied by great auricular nerve.
4. **Hirschsprung disease:** This disease is also called **'megalocolon'**. It is a congenital disease characterized by failure of development of Auerbach (myenteric) plexus with absence of postganglionic parasympathetic neurons in the wall of distal part of colon. So, this part of colon does not show peristaltic activity,

for which part of the colon proximal to it presents huge dilation with stagnant fecal matter.

Injuries to Autonomic Nervous System

Injury to Parasympathetic System

It may be cranial or spinal. Causes of damage to the cranial component of parasympathetic system are head injury. Head injury may cause impairment of function of following components of parasympathetic system.

Occulomotor Nerve Injury

It is affected when head injury is associated with herniation of uncus of temporal lobe. Visceral afferent fibers of the nerve supply of sphincter papillae and ciliary muscles. So, damage of the nerve causes **loss of light reflex with dilation of pupil** due to non-functioning of sphincter papillae. **Accommodation reflex is also affected** due to non-functioning of ciliary muscle along with medial rectus and sphincter papillae.

Facial Nerve Injury

Facial nerve containing visceral efferent fibers with other functional components may be affected in fracture of base of skull affecting internal auditory meatus of petrous part of temporal lobe. Lesion of preganglionic secretomotor fibers to the lacrimal gland causes **impaired lacrimation**. Salivary secretion is not fully impaired, as parotid gland remains functioning, because it is supplied by visceral efferent fibers through glossopharyngeal nerve.

Spinal Injury

Spinal injury affecting the parasympathetic system alone with sympathetic system leads to disorders of bladder, bowel and sexual function.

Injury to Sympathetic System

It is the sympathetic trunk which is injured opposite the level of cervicothoracic (stellate) ganglion at the root of neck.

1. This injury may occur due to stab or gunshot wound.
2. It may also occur due to traction by cervical rib. Beside injury, metastatic lesion at the root of neck may affect stellate ganglion.

Clinical condition arising from this lesion is known as **Horner syndrome** which is described earlier.

CHAPTER SUMMARY

Key Concepts

1. All visceral functions are controlled by both sympathetic and parasympathetic divisions of ANS. Though sympathetic and parasympathetic systems have opposite effects, they are reciprocal to each other.
2. Regulation of sympathetic and parasympathetic systems occurs at spinal cord, brainstem, hypothalamic, limbic and cortical levels.
3. As hypothalamus is the head ganglion of ANS, hypothalamic control is important. Nevertheless, all medullary visceral centers influence autonomic functions that could in turn be controlled by limbic-hypothalamic projections.
4. Autonomic functions are disturbed by metabolic diseases such as diabetes.

Important to Know (Must Read)

1. In examinations, Control of autonomic functions may sometimes come as a **Long Question**.
2. Control of autonomic functions, supraspinal control of autonomic functions, autonomic dysfunction, Horner syndrome, orthostatic hypotension may come as **Short Questions** in exams.
3. In **Viva**, examiners my ask... Name levels of control of autonomic functions, Name autonomic reflexes, Name supraspinal control mechanisms of autonomic functions, Classify autonomic dysfunction, Causes and features of Horner syndrome, Causes and features of Argyll Robertson pupil and Adie's pupil, Causes and features of orthostatic hypotension.

CHAPTER 34

Autonomic Function Tests

Learning Objectives

On completion of study of this chapter, the student **MUST** be able to:

1. Classify autonomic function tests (AFTs).
2. Appreciate the application of AFTs in clinical physiology.
3. List the AFTs for assessment of sympathetic and of parasympathetic functions.

The student **MAY** also be able to:

1. Describe the physiological basis, method and merits and demeris of AFTs.

Sympathetic and parasympathetic systems control all visceral functions. Neurons of sympathetic and parasympathetic systems are affected in metabolic diseases. Therefore, autonomic dysfunctions are common in metabolic diseases such as diabetes, obesity, hypertension, hyperlipidemia, hyper and hypothyroidism, etc. India is the epicenter of diabetes, hypertension and heart diseases. Therefore, assessment of sympathetic and parasympathetic functions by conventional ***autonomic function tests*** (AFTs) is now part of routine clinical management.

CLASSIFICATION OF AFTs

Autonomic function tests (AFTs) are performed to confirm the clinical diagnosis of autonomic dysfunctions and to assess the degree of sympathetic and parasympathetic involvement in the process of dysfunction.

AFTs are classified as:

A. Tests for cardiovascular autonomic functions
   1. Heart rate and Blood pressure (BP) response to standing
   2. Heart rate and BP response to passive tilting
   3. Assessing baroreceptor sensitivity (BRS)
   4. Heart rate response to deep breathing
   5. Valsalva ratio
   6. BP response to hand grip
   7. Cold pressure test
   8. Nor-epinephrine spillage technique
   9. Standing to lying ratio
   10. Spectral analysis of heart rate variability (HRV)

B. Tests for sudomotor functions
   1. Sympathetic skin response
   2. Thermoregulatory sweat test (TST)
   3. Quantitative sudomotor axon reflex test (QSART)

C. Vasomotor test
   1. Laser Doppler Velocimetry for skin blood flow measurement
   2. Cold pressor test

C. Tests for pupillary functions
   1. Cocaine test
   2. Adrenaline test

D. Tests for bladder functions
   1. Test for sphincter-detrusor dysynergia
   2. Cystometrogram

E. Other methods
   1. Muscle sympathetic nerve activity (MSNA)

Tests for Cardiovascular Autonomic Functions

Heart Rate Response to Standing

Changing the posture from supine to standing, heart rate increases immediately by about 10 to 20 beats per minute.

1. On standing, the heart rate increases until it reaches a maximum at about the 15th beat, after which it slows down to a stable state at about 30th beat.
2. The ratio of R-R intervals corresponding to the 30th and 15th heart beat is called **the 30:15 ratio**.

3. The 30:15 ratio is a *measure of parasympathetic function*.
4. However, relative bradycardia at 30th beat depends also on the sympathetic reactivity.
5. The normal 30:15 ratio is 1.15–1.12 at 21 to 30 years and 1.12 to 1.10 at 31 to 40 years of age.
6. This ratio decreases with age. Ratio less than 1.04 is considered abnormal.

Blood Pressure Response to Standing

The changes in blood pressure on standing are studied to assess the *integrity of the sympathetic system*.

1. Immediately on standing, blood pressure falls, which activates baroreceptor reflex and blood pressure returns to normal within 15 seconds.
2. When there is sustained fall in systolic pressure more than 20 mm Hg or diastolic fall more than 10 mm Hg within three minutes of standing, ***orthostatic hypotension*** is said to be present.

Assessing Baroreceptor Reflex Sensitivity (BRS)

Baroreceptor reflex sensitivity is a newer method of assessing autonomic reactivity to various stimuli, such as orthostatic challenge and injection of chemicals and drugs that change the blood pressure.

1. This is assessed by continuous blood pressure variability (BPV) measurement. Sensitivity of baroreceptors to change in dynamic component (fluctuations) of blood pressure is an important marker of sympathetic and parasympathetic systems. Thus, it is a reflection of integration of both the components.
2. BRS is expressed as ms/mm Hg.
3. BRS less than 20 ms/mm Hg reflect poor cardiovascular (CV) health, and BRS less than 15 ms/mm Hg is an indicator of increased CV risk.
4. BRS 25 ms/mm Hg or more indicates enhanced autonomic tone and improved CV health.

Norepinephrine (NE) Spillage Technique

Norepinephrine level in plasma is measured in supine position and after 5 minutes of standing. The difference in level of NE represents alteration in sympathetic-hormonal reactivity.

Heart Rate Response to Tilting

Heart rate response to **head up tilt** (HUT) is a useful tool in the diagnosis of autonomic dysfunctions. It is more accurate because the active change of position is avoided by passively tilting the subject on a tilt-table. Moreover, variation in time taken by individuals to stand and the manner in which they stand from supine position is avoided in this method.

1. On changing from recumbent to operate position on a tilt table to 60 to 80 degrees HUT, pooling of about 30% venous blood occurs in the peripheral vascular compartment, especially in lower limbs.
2. This decreases cardiac filling pressure and stroke volume by about 40%.
3. Heart rate rises immediately due to withdrawal of parasympathetic activity and afterward due to increased sympathetic activity.

Standing to Lying Ratio (SLR)

Heart rate (RR interval) response to lying down from standing posture is assessed by continuous recoding of ECG.

1. Following lying from standing position, increase in venous return produces reflex bradycardia.
2. Longest RR interval in standing to shortest RR interval in lying down is calculated as SLR.
3. Value of SLR below 1 is considered as abnormal.

Heart Rate Response to Deep Breathing

The variation of heart rate with respiration is known as *sinus arrhythmia*. Inspiration increases and expiration decreases heart rate.

1. This is primarily mediated via parasympathetic innervation of heart. Pulmonary stretch receptor, and cardiac mechanoreceptors and baroreceptors contribute to sinus arrhythmia.
2. The difference between the maximum and minimum heart rate during a deep breathing is called **deep breathing difference** (DBD).
3. DBD is more than 15 beats per minute in normal individual. It **assesses the parasympathetic activity**. DBD decreases with age.
4. It is one of the ***best parasympathetic reactivity test***.
   Normal values of DBD at different age group are:
   10 to 40 years : > 18 beats per minute
   41 to 50 years : > 16 beats per minute
   51 to 60 years : > 12 beats per minute
   61 to 70 years : > 8 beats per minute

Usually, subject is asked to inhale deeply for five seconds and then exhale for five seconds for six cycles. The ratio of longest RR interval in expiration to shortest RR interval in inspiration is calculated for each, which is called expiration-inspiration ratio (E/I ratio). The average E/I ratio of six cycles in a normal young individual is about 1:20.

The E/I ratio decreases with age (Table 34.1).

Normally, instead of DBD expressed in terms of beats per minute, **E:I ratio** is usually considered for assessing parasympathetic reactivity to deep breathing.

DBD is abnormal in **multisystem atrophy, progressive autonomic failure, diabetes mellitus, autonomic neuropathy and CNS depression.**

Valsalva Ratio

The Valsalva ratio is a measure of parasympathetic and sympathetic function.

1. In **Valsalva maneuver** (named after scientist **AM Valsalva**, who described it), parasympathetic is the afferent and the efferent, and sympathetic is the part

Table 34.1: Normal values of E:I ratio.

Age (years)	E:I ratio
16 to 20	: > 1.23
21 to 25	: > 1.20
26 to 30	: > 1.18
31 to 35	: > 1.16
36 to 40	: > 1.14
41 to 45	: > 1.12
46 to 50	: > 1.11
51 to 55	: > 1.09
56 to 60	: > 1.08
61 to 65	: > 1.07
66 to 70	: > 1.06

of the efferent pathway. Therefore, Valsalva ratio assesses more of **parasympathetic (cardiovagal)** than sympathetic functions.

2. The procedure is performed by closing both nostrils and then blowing into a tube connected to sphygmomanometer. By putting strain, blowing pressure is maintained at 40 mm Hg for 15 seconds.

Valsalva Maneuver

Valsalva maneuver has four phases:

Phase I: Phase I consists of the onset of strain. In this phase, there is transient increase in blood pressure that lasts for a few seconds. This occurs due to increased intrathoracic pressure and mechanical compression of the great vessels. However, heart rate does not change much.

Phase II: This is the phase of straining. In the early part of this phase, venous return decreases, which in turn decreases cardiac output and blood pressure. This change persists for 4 seconds. In the later part of this phase, blood pressure returns towards normal, which occurs due to increased peripheral resistance as a result of sympathetic vasoconstriction. However, heart rate increases steadily throughout this phase due to vagal withdrawal (in the early phase) and sympathetic activation (in the later phase).

Phase III: This phase occurs following the release of strain during which there is transient decrease in blood pressure lasting for a few seconds. This is caused by mechanical displacement of blood to pulmonary vascular bed, which was under increased intrathoracic pressure. There is little change in heart rate.

Phase IV: This is the phase that occurs with further release of strain. The blood pressure slowly increases and heart rate proportionately decreases. It occurs following 15 to 20 seconds after release of strain and lasts for about 1 minute or more. The cardiovascular changes occur due to increase in venous return, stroke volume and cardiac out put.

Table 34.2: Normal values of Valsalva ratio at different age.

Age (years)	Valsalva ratio
10 to 40	: > 1.5
41 to 50	: > 1.45
51 to 60	: > 1.40
61 to 70	: > 1.35

Valsalva ratio is the ratio of minimal heart rate in phase IV to maximum heart rate in phase II as depicted in terms of RR interval.

$$\text{Valsalva ratio} = \frac{\text{Longest R-R interval during phase IV}}{\text{Shortest R-R interval during phase II}}$$

Clinical Correlation

Valsalva ratio more than 1.45 is considered to be normal.

1. Ratio 1.2–1.45 is considered borderline, and ratio less than 1.2 is regarded abnormal.
2. The normal ratio is different at different age groups (Table 34.2).
3. Valsalva ratio is also affected by gender, posture of subject in which recording is done, expiratory pressure, duration of strain and level of yoga practice of the subject.

Changes in Valsalva ratio occur due to changes in cardiac vagal efferent and sympathetic vasomotor activity, which are stimulated by carotid sinus and aortic arch baroreceptors and other intrathoracic stretch receptors. *Failure of heart rate to increase during strain suggests a* ***sympathetic dysfunction*** and *failure of heart rate to slow down after the strain suggests* ***parasympathetic dysfunction***. If the cardiovascular response to Valsalva maneuver is abnormal but that to cold pressure test (see blow) is normal, the lesion is supposed to be present in the baroreceptors or their afferent nerves. Such types of abnormalities occur commonly in diabetes, other neuropathies, multisystem atrophy and autonomic failure.

Scientist contributed

Antonio Mario Valsalva (1667-1723), an early Italian anatomist and physiologist who had his research focused on the anatomy of the ears and ear functions. He coined the term Eustachian tube and he described the aortic sinuses of Valsalva in his writings, published posthum ously in 1740. His name is associated with the Valsalva antrum of the ear and the **Valsalva maneuver**, which is used as a test of circulatory function, i.e. alteration in HR and BP by this maneuver. Anatomical structures bearing his name are ***Valsalva's muscle*** and ***taeniae Valsalvae***.

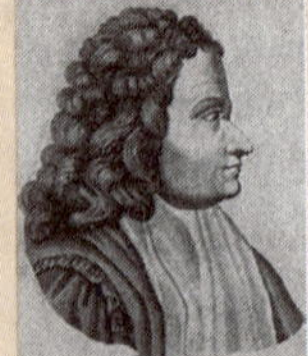

AM Valsalva (1667–1723)

BP Response to Sustained Hand Grip

In hand-grip test is an isometric exercise in which the subject is asked to maintain hand grip against resistance.

1. Resistance usually offered by using a hand grip dynamometer at a 30% of maximum voluntary contraction for 5 min. BP and heart (HR) are recorded before and after the hand grip.

2. In hand-grip test, heart rate and blood pressure increase.
3. These cardiovascular responses to isometric exercise are mediated partly by central motor command and partly by mechanical changes or both, in response to contraction of the muscles that activate small fibers in the afferent limb of the reflex arch.
4. The normal response is **rise in diastolic pressure more than 15 mm Hg** and rise in heart rate by about 30%.
5. The blood pressure rise is due to *increased sympathetic activity* and heart rate rise is due to *decreased parasympathetic activity*.
6. The responses to hand grip test are usually not dependent on age.
7. Isometric handgrip test is one of the ***best sympathetic reactivity tests***.

Cold Pressure Test

This test is performed by submerging the upper limb of the subject in ice cold water at 4°C for 30 to 60 sec. and BP is recorded before and after the procedure. The submersion of hand in cold water increases systolic pressure by about 20 mm Hg and diastolic pressure by 10 mm Hg.

1. The afferent limb of the reflex pathway is somatic fibers whereas the efferent pathway is the sympathetic fibers.
2. Thus, it assesses sympathetic activity.
3. Cold pressor test is one of the ***best sympathetic reactivity tests***.

Tests for Sudomotor Functions

Sympathetic Skin Response

Sympathetic skin response (SSR) helps in studying the functions of **peripheral sympathetic cholinergic (sudomotor) fibers** by evaluating the changes in resistance of skin in response to electrical stimuli.

1. SSR is age dependent and is present in both hands and feet till the age of 60.
2. Composition of surface electrodes, stimulus frequency, skin temperature, and mental state of the subject affect the parameters of SSR.
3. The latency and amplitude of SSR are measured.
4. The amplitude of SSR in hand is 1.6 mV and in feet is 2.1 mV. SSR is helpful in diagnosing multisystem atrophy, progressive autonomic failure, diabetes, uremic patients and alcoholic neuropathy.

Thermoregulatory Sweat Test (TST)

Assessment of sweating response to heat also assesses sudomotor functions.

1. The subject's body temperature is raised to by 1°C by exposing to heat of the electric heater.
2. Sweating response is studied by demarcating the area of sweating with the help of iodide starch or quinizarin powder that changes the color of the moist skin.
3. Absence of sweating in TST indicates sympathetic pre- and post-ganglionic lesions.

Quantitative Sudomotor Axon Reflex Test

Quantitative sudomotor axon reflex test **(QSART)** is a measure of regional autonomic function by Ach-induced sweating.

1. In this test, Ach is injected intradermally and the sweat production rate is assessed.
2. Reduced or absence of sweating indicates post-ganglionic lesion of sudomotor fibers (sympathetic fibers concerned with sweating).

Tests for Pupillary Functions

Pupillary function tests assess the function of sympathetic nerve supplying iris. Two tests usually performed are: cocaine test and adrenaline test.

Cocaine Test

Dilation of pupil is observed following instillation of 4% cocaine on both eyes. Cocaine prevents reuptake of norepinephrine at adrenergic nerve endings. Therefore, pupils dilate in response to cocaine, but, Horner's pupils do not.

Adrenaline Test

Instillation of 1:100 or 1% noradrenaline on eyes dilate Horner's pupil more than normal pupil. This is due to the mechanism of denervation hypersensitivity of Horner's pupil.

Tests for Bladder Function

Cystometrogram (CMG) is performed to detect autonomic dysfunctions of urinary bladder. CMG reveals decreased ability of bladder to accommodate urine. Absence of accommodation to filling indicates autonomic dysfunction. Also, contraction of bladder muscle is poor in response to the act of micturition (evacuation).

Spectral Analysis of HRV

Recently, spectral analysis of heart rate variability (HRV) has evolved as a sensitive tool for assessing integrity of sympathetic and parasympathetic functions and for determining the **sympathovagal balance**. (Details are given in the next chapter)

AFTs to Assess Sympathetic and Parasympathetic Functions

A. AFTs for assessment of sympathetic functions:

1. BP response to standing/tilt
2. Cold pressor test
3. Isometric hand grip
4. Galvanic/sympathetic skin response
5. Thermoregulatory sweat test
6. Tachycardia ratio
7. Valsalva ratio
8. NE spillage test
9. LF and LFnu of HRV

B. AFTs for assessment of parasympathetic functions:

1. Resting heart rate: Basal heart rate is a good index of parasympathetic functions as **heart rate in resting conditions is a measure of vagal tone.** Resting HR more 75 indicates poor vagal tone and is presently considered as a CV risk.
2. 30:15 ratio
3. E:I ratio
4. Valsalva ratio
5. Bradycardia ratio
6. Baroreceptor sensitivity
7. Standing to lying ratio
8. HF and HFnu of HRV

Concept of Reactivity and Activity Tests and CAFTs

Reactivity Tests

Tests that are based on stimuli or disturbances such as change in position (standing, lying, dipping finger in cold water, hand grip against resistance, Valsalva maneuver etc.) are called **reactivity tests.** Accordingly, they are grouped as ***sympathetic and parasympathetic reactivity tests.***

Activity Tests

Tests that are performed without disturbing the subject (subject at rest usually lying on couch in a comfortable room for 15 to 20 min) are called **activity tests.**

1. Recording of Resting HR and BP, and HRV analysis are examples.
2. Accordingly, they are grouped as *sympathetic and parasympathetic activity tests.*
3. **Resting heart rate is parasympathetic test and resting BP is sympathetic test.**

CAFTs

CAFTs refer to **conventional autonomic function tests.** HR and BP response to standing, HR response to deep breathing, isometric hand grip, cold pressor test and Valsalva maneuver are CAFTs.

CHAPTER SUMMARY

Key Concepts

1. AFTs are noninvasive and conventional tests for assessing autonomic functions.
2. Resting heart rate is the commonest and simplest parasympathetic function test, and DBD (E/I ratio) is the best parasympathetic reactivity test.
3. Isometric hand grip and Cold pressor test are the best sympathetic reactivity tests.

Important to Know (Must Read)

1. In examinations, 'Classification, procedure, merits and demerits of AFTs', 'Classification, procedure, merits and demerits of sympathetic tests' and 'Classification, procedure, merits and demerits of parasympathetic tests' may come as **Long Questions**.
2. Parasympathetic function tests, Sympathetic function tests, HR and BP response to standing, HR and BP response to tilting, HR and BP response to lying, Deep breathing difference, E/I ratio, 30:15 ratio, Valsalva ratio, QSART, SSR, Cold Pressor Test, may come as **Short Questions** in exams.
3. In **Viva,** examiners may ask... Classify AFTs, List parasympathetic function tests, List sympathetic function tests, Importance of HR and BP response to standing, Importance of HR and BP response to tilting, Importance of HR and BP response to lying, Importance of deep breathing difference, Importance of E/I ratio, 30:15 ratio, Importance of Valsalva ratio, Importance of QSART, Importance of SSR, Importance of Cold Pressor Test, What is the best sympathetic function test, What is the best parasympathetic function test, What are Reactivity tests, What are Activity tests, What are CAFTs.

CHAPTER

35

Heart Rate Variability

Learning Objectives

On completion of study of this chapter, the student **MUST** be able to:

1. Define and explain the term heart rate variability (HRV).
2. List different spectral components (time domain and frequency domain) of HRV.
3. Mention physiological significance of each HRV component.
4. Understand the principle of short-term HRV measurement.
5. Comprehend the concept of sympathovagal balance and understand the importance of HRV recording in assessing sympathovagal balance.
6. Explain the importance of HRV analysis and its clinical utility in health and diseases.

The student **MAY** also be able to:

1. Describe different methods of measurement of HRV indices.
2. Explain the technical aspects of HRV components.
3. Describe the clinical application of HRV in in health and disease.

PHYSIOLOGICAL ASPECTS

Heart rate variability (HRV) is the **cardiac beat-to-beat variation** (variation in cardiac cycle length), a physiological phenomenon that occurs mainly due to variation in cardiac activity during the respiratory cycle (***respiratory sinus arrhythmia***) at rest, though the circadian rhythm, environmental factors and exercise also contribute to it. Resting heart rates can vary; some have rates of 100 beats/min while others beat at only 60 beats/min for no obvious reason.

1. The rate of the heart and its **beat-to-beat variations** are dependent on the rate of discharge of the primary pacemaker, the SA node, which is influenced by autonomic activities that are controlled in a complex way by a variety of reflexes, central irradiations and cortical factors.
2. As SA nodal discharge is largely controlled by **parasympathetic (vagal) influence**, and ***sinus arrhythmia is primarily due to alteration in vagal tone*** in inspiration and expiration, **HRV is mainly influenced by vagal activity**, though both the divisions of ANS influence it.
3. Recently, HRV has been proposed as the most sensitive indicator of autonomic function, especially for the assessment of **sympathovagal balance**, the balance between the sympathetic and parasympathetic activity of the individual at any given time.
4. The state of sympathovagal balance is used for the prediction of **many cardiovascular (CV) dysfunctions** and other dysfunctions affecting cardiovascular function, its main use is in the CV risk stratification. However, the use of HRV analysis is limited in the diagnosis and management of CV and other diseases.

Technical Terms

Heart rate variability can be quantified in **time and frequency domains.**

1. **Time domain measures** include the usual tools of assessment of variations, as done in statistics. Time domain is easier to assess but finer aspects of variations are not appreciated. Shortly, the ***overall magnitude of HRV is assessed*** well but the individual contribution of various factors is not elucidated.
2. On the other hand, the variations in the instantaneous heart rate can be **assessed spectrally**. That is, an **RR tachogram** is plotted using the ***RR intervals in the five-minute lead II ECG.***

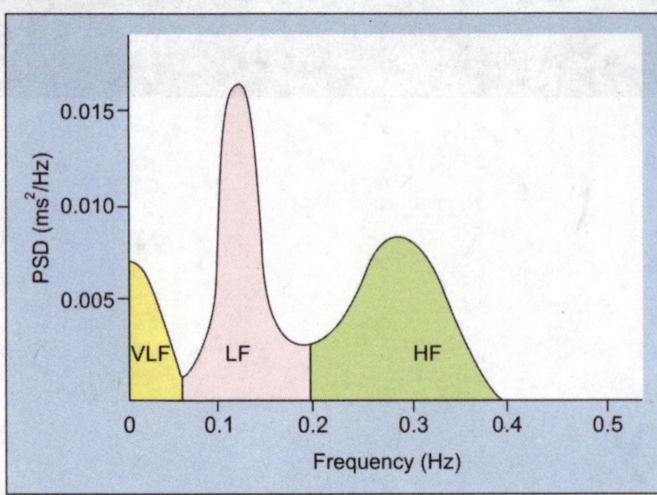

Fig. 35.1: Distribution of VLF, LF and HF in HRV power spectrum. Note, in this picture, the TP was 920 ms^2, of which VLF was 70 ms^2, LF was 500 ms^2 and HF was 350 ms^2.

3. The RR tachogram is considered as a non-periodic signal which is transformed to its frequency spectrum using **fast-Fourier transformation algorithm** or ***autoregressive modeling***.
4. The biggest advantage of this complex mathematical transformation is that the distribution of magnitude of variations in **different frequency bands** corresponds to the activity of different physiological systems. The entire frequency spectrum 0 to 0.4 Hz is divided as follows:

HRV Components

The power spectrum of HRV in mammals usually reveals three spectral components. These components are (Fig. 35.1):

1. A high frequency band (HF) 0.15–0.4 Hz
2. A low-frequency band (LF) 0.04–0.15 Hz
3. A very low-frequency band (VLF) 0–0.04 Hz

HF Component

HF component is caused by **vagal tone** during the respiratory cycle.

1. The **inspiratory inhibition of vagal activity** is evoked centrally in the cardiovascular center and explains why heart rate fluctuates with the respiratory frequency.
2. In addition, **peripheral reflexes** arising from thoracic stretch receptors also contribute to this so-called respiratory sinus arrhythmia (RSA).
3. As RSA is clearly **abolished by atropine or vagotomy,** the power of the ***HF component has been used as an index of the vagal drive***.

LF Component

LF component of HRV is usually characterized by an oscillatory pattern with a period of 10 seconds.

1. This rhythm originates from self-oscillation in the **vasomotor part** (*sympathetic component*) of the baroreflex loop as a result of negative feedback and it is commonly associated with synchronous fluctuations in blood pressure, the so-called Mayer waves.
2. Thus, LF component mainly represents **sympathetic power**. However, ***parasympathetic drive*** also contributes to it.

VLF Component

VLF component accounts for all other heart rate changes, including those associated with thermoregulation and humoral (especially, **rennin-angiotensin mechanism**) and local factors.

Power Spectrum Analysis of HRV

Power spectrum of HRV is analyzed by two methods: Fast-Fourier transform and autoregressive modeling.

Fast Fourier Transform

Any electrophysiological signal can be described as a sum of sine waves and this decomposition is called the Fast Fourier Transform (FFT). An efficient algorithm to carry out this transformation is the FFT, which, with some improvements and modifications, is still in use in many applications, such as voice analysis or vibration studies.

1. The analysis of short-term HRV (SHRV) is another one of these applications.
2. FFT algorithms impose some constraints on the signal to analyze because an evenly sampled, infinite and stationary time series is required.

Autoregressive Modeling

An alternative method to the FFT is the autoregressive (AR) identification algorithm combined with power spectral estimation for the assessment of SHRV. This method fits the data to a prior defined model and estimates the parameters of the model. The power spectrum implied by the model is then computed.

1. FFT or AR modeling methods share a common goal: the estimation of the power spectrum of a signal.
2. FFT-based methods are also called **nonparametric methods** because the time domain prior to spectral analysis is greatly simplified.

Physiological basis: The FFT and autoregressive algorithms are the most commonly used tools to study the SHRV.

1. The final step in SHRV analysis includes the application of power spectrum estimation methods to ***characterize the frequency components*** associated with vagal and/or sympathetic outflow.
2. AR methods are parametric because they require prior information of the system under study. Thus, it was suggested that FFT-based methods are still the ***best***

choice for the assessment of SHRV in comparative studies, where no previous knowledge of the system is available.
3. In addition, FFT algorithms are readily available in many different languages, even in commercial statistical packages.
4. Once the basic spectral content of the system is known and an initial model of the signal can be formulated, ***AR algorithms should be a better choice*** because they provide better frequency resolution and avoid the problems of spectral leakage.
5. The electrocardiogram (ECG) is the most appropriate signal to study SHRV because it offers the most ***accurate representation of the electrical cardiac events***.
6. In particular, the QRS complex of the ECG sharply defines the ***onset of ventricular electrical depolarization*** and is the closest approach to ***time the occurrence of pacemaker potentials***, which, in turn, are modulated by the autonomic outflow.

HRV Indices

Analysis of HRV has two parts: time-domain and frequency-domain.
1. HRV assessed by calculation of indices is based on statistical operations on R-R intervals (**time domain analysis**) or by spectral analysis of an array of R-R intervals (**frequency domain analysis**).
2. Both methods require accurate timing of R waves.
3. The analysis can be performed on short electrocardiogram (ECG) segments (lasting from 0.5 to 5 minutes) or on 24-hour ECG recordings.
4. The analysis of 5 min ECG recording is called **short-term HRV** and of 24-hour ECG recording is called **long-term HRV**.

Time Domain Analysis

Two types of heart rate variability indices are distinguished in time domain analysis. Beat-to-beat or **short-term variability** (STV) indices represent fast changes in heart rate. **Long-term variability** (LTV) indices are slower fluctuations (fewer than 6 per minute). Both types of indices are calculated from the ***R-R intervals occurring in a chosen time window*** (usually between 0.5 and 5 minutes).
1. An example of a simple STV index is the **standard deviation** (SD) of beat-to-beat R-R interval differences within the time window.
2. Examples of LTV indices are the SD of all the R-R intervals, or the difference between the maximum and minimum R-R interval length, within the window.
3. With calculated heart rate variability indices, respiratory sinus arrhythmia contributes to STV, and baroreflex- and thermoregulation-related heart rate variabilities contributes to LTV.

Frequency Domain Analysis

Ever since spectral analysis was introduced as a method to study heart rate variability, an increasing number of investigators have preferred this method to time domain analysis for the calculation of heart rate variability indices.
1. The **main advantage** of spectral analysis of signals is the possibility to study their ***frequency-specific oscillations***.
2. Thus, not only the amount of variability but also the oscillation frequency (number of heart rate fluctuations per second) can be obtained.
3. Spectral analysis involves decomposing the series of sequential R-R intervals into a sum of sinusoidal functions of different amplitudes and frequencies by the Fourier transform algorithm.
4. The result can be displayed (power spectrum) with the magnitude of variability as a function of frequency. Thus, the power spectrum reflects the amplitude of the heart rate fluctuations present at different oscillation frequencies.

Measurement of HRV Indices

Time Domain Methods

The variations in heart rate may be evaluated by a number of methods. Perhaps the simplest to perform are the time domain measures.
1. In these methods, either the heart rate at any point in time or the intervals between successive normal complexes are determined.
2. In a continuous ECG record, each QRS complex is detected, and the so-called **normal-to-normal (NN) intervals**, i.e. all intervals between adjacent QRS complexes resulting from sinus node depolarization or in the instantaneous heart rate are determined.
3. Simple time domain variables that can be calculated include the **mean NN interval**, the **mean heart rate**, the **difference between the longest and shortest NN interval**, the difference between **night and day heart rate** and so forth.

Statistical Methods

From a series of instantaneous heart rates or cycle intervals, particularly those recorded ***over longer periods***, traditionally **24 hours**, more complex statistical time domain measures can be calculated.
1. These may be divided into **two classes**: (a) Those derived from direct measurements of the NN intervals or instantaneous heart rate, and (b) those derived from the differences between NN intervals.
2. These variables may be derived from analysis of the total ECG recording or may be calculated using smaller segments of the recording period.
3. The most commonly used measures derived from interval differences include **RMSSD**, the square root of

Table 35.1: Selected time-domain measures of HRV.

Variable	Units	Description
SDNN	ms	Standard deviation of all NN intervals
SDANN	ms	Standard deviation of the averages of NN intervals in all 5 min segments of the entire recording
RMSSD	ms	The square root of the mean of the sum of the squares of the differences between adjacent NN intervals
SDNN index	ms	Mean of the standard deviations of all NN intervals for all 5 min segments of the entire recording
SDSD	ms	Standard deviation of differences between adjacent NN intervals
NN50 count		Number of pairs of adjacent NN interval differing by more than 50 ms in the entire recording
pNN50	%	NN50 count divided by the total number of all NN intervals

the mean squared differences of successive NN intervals; **NN50**, the number of interval differences of successive NN intervals greater than 50 ms; and **pNN50**; the proportion derived by dividing NN50 by the total number of NN intervals (Table 35.1).

4. All of these measurements of the short-term variation estimate high-frequency variations in heart rate and, thus, are highly correlated.

Geometrical Methods

A series of NN intervals also can be converted into a geometric pattern, such as the **sample density distribution of NN interval durations**, sample density distribution of ***difference between adjacent NN intervals***, **Lorenz plot** of NN or RR intervals and so forth.

1. A simple formula is used that judges the variability on the basis of the geometric and/or graphics properties of the resulting pattern.
2. The **HRV triangular index** measurement is the integral of the density distribution (that is, the number of all NN intervals) divided by the maximum of the density distribution.
3. The **major advantage** of the geometric methods lies in their relative insensitivity to the analytical quality of the series of NN intervals.
4. The **major disadvantage** of the geometric methods is the need for a reasonable number of NN intervals to construct the geometric pattern.

The methods expressing overall HRV and its long-and short-term components cannot replace each other. The selection of method used should correspond to the aim of each particular study.

Frequency Domain Methods

Various spectral methods for the analysis of the tachogram have been applied since the late 1960s.

1. **Power spectral density** (PSD) analysis provides the basic information of how power (variance) distributes as a function of frequency.
2. Independent of the method used, only an estimate of the true PSD of the signal can be obtained by proper mathematical algorithms.

Nonparametric and Parametric Methods

Methods for the calculation of PSD may be generally classified as nonparametric and parametric. In most instances, both methods provide comparable results.

The advantages of nonparametric methods are:

1. The simplicity of the algorithm used [fast Fourier transform (FFT)] in most of the cases.
2. The high processing speed.

The advantages of parametric methods are:

1. Smoother spectral components that can be distinguished independent of preselected frequency bands.
2. Easy post processing of the spectrum with an automatic calculation of low- and high-frequency power components with easy identification of the central frequency of each components.
3. An accurate estimation of PSD even on a small number of samples on which the signal is supposed to remain stationary.

The basic **disadvantage of parametric methods** is the need for verification of the suitability of the chosen model and of its complexity (that is, the order of the model).

Spectral Components of Frequency Domain

Short-term Recordings

Three main spectral components are distinguished in a spectrum calculated from short term recordings of 2 to 5 minutes: VLF, LF and HF components (Table 35.2). The distribution of the power and the central frequency of LF and HF are not fixed but may vary in relation to changes in autonomic modulations of heart period. The physiological explanation of the VLF component is much less defined and the existence of a specific process attributable to these changes might even be questioned. The non-harmonic component, which does not have coherent properties and is affected by algorithms of baseline or trend removal, is commonly accepted as a major constituent of VLF. Thus VLF assessed from short-term recordings (≤ 5 minutes) is a dubious measure and should be avoided when the PSD of short-term ECG is interpreted.

1. The measurement of VLF, LF and HF power components is usually made in absolute values of power (milliseconds squared).
2. LF and HF may also be measured in **normalized units**, which represent the relative value of each power component in proportion to the total power minus the VLF component.

3. The representation of LF and HF in normalized units (**LFnu and HFnu**) emphasizes the controlled and balanced behavior of the two branches of the autonomic nervous system. Moreover, the normalization tends to ***minimize the effect of the changes in total power*** on the values of LF and HF components.
4. Nevertheless, normalized units **should always be quoted with absolute values of LF and HF power** in order to describe completely the distribution of power in spectral components.
5. LF-HF ratio provides a better indicator of spectral powers.

Long-term Recordings

Spectral analysis also may be used to analyze the sequence of NN intervals of the entire 24-hour period. The result then includes an **ultra-low frequency** (ULF) component, in addition to VLF, LF and HF components. The slope of the 24-hour spectrum also can be assessed on a log-log scale by linear fitting the spectral values. Frequency domain measures are summarized below.

Table 35.2: Selected frequency domain measures of HRV

Variable	Units	Description analysis of short-term recordings (5 mins)	Frequency range
Total power (5 min)	ms^2	The variance of NN intervals over the temporal segment.	Approximately ≤ 0.4 Hz
VLF	ms^2	Power in very low-frequency range	0–0.04 Hz
LF	ms^2	Power in low frequency range	0.04 – 0.15 Hz
LF norm	nu	LF power in normalized units LF/(Total Power – VLF) x 100	
HF	ms^2	Power in high frequency range	0.15-0.4 Hz
HF norm	nu	HF power in normalized units HF/(Total Power – VLF) x 100	
LF/HF		Ratio LF (ms^2)/HF (ms^2)	

(TP: total power; nu: normalized unit)

Technical Aspects

The basic principle is that beat-to-beat variation in SA nodal discharge as recorded by ECG is computed and analyzed by the software for determination of spectral indices of HRV.

Brief methodology: There are two types of HRV recordings: the short-term 5 min HRV recording and day-night long-term HRV recording. Though long-term HRV recording is the ideal one, **short-term HRV recording** is usually performed for research and clinical investigations. We shall briefly describe the procedure of short-term recording as depicted in the **Task Force Report on HRV**.

1. The subject is asked to lie down comfortably in supine position in the laboratory, and ECG electrodes are connected for Lead II ECG recording.
2. After 5 minutes of supine rest, ECG signals are acquired at a rate of 1000 samples/second during supine rest using data acquisition system, such as BIOPAC MP 100 (BIOPAC Inc., USA) (minimum 250 Hz sampling rate). The raw ECG signal and the RR intervals are acquired on a moving time base.
3. Data from BIOPAC are transferred to a windows-based PC loaded with software for HRV analysis, such as Acknowledge software version 3.8.2. Ectopics and artifacts are removed from the recorded ECG.
4. **RR tachogram** is extracted from the edited 256 sec ECG using the R wave detector in the Acknowledge software and saved in ASC-II format, which is later used offline for short-term HRV analysis (RR tachogram should have minimum 288 RR intervals) (Fig. 35.2).
5. HRV analysis is performed by using the HRV analysis software version 1.1 (Bio-signal Analysis group, Finland).

Calculation of Time Domain Indices

In a continuous ECG record, each QRS complex is detected, and the so-called normal to-normal (NN) intervals (i.e. all intervals between adjacent QRS complexes resulting from sinus node depolarizations) or instantaneous heart rate is

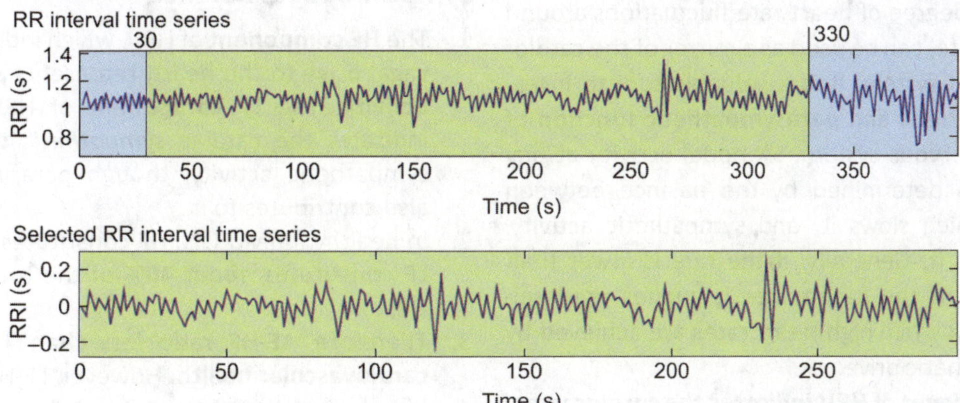

Fig. 35.2: RR tachogram obtained from continuous ECG recordings for HRV analysis. Note, 300 RR intervals (30 to 330) were selected from RR interval time series (upper RR tracing), and selected RR intervals (lower RR tracing)

determined. Simple time domain variables that are calculated include:

1. The mean RR
2. Standard deviation of normal-to-normal interval (SDNN)
3. Square root of the mean squared differences of successive normal-to-normal intervals (RMSSD) of HRV.
4. NN50
5. pNN50

Calculation of Frequency Domain Indices

Frequency domain variables that are usually calculated include **total power** (TP), **low frequency** (LF) component, LF component expressed as ***normalized unit*** (LFnu), **high frequency** (HF) component, HF component expressed as ***normalized unit*** (HFnu) and **LF/HF ratio** (Table 35.2).

Normalizing spectral powers are calculated by the formula as follows:

1. LF nu = LF x 100 (TP – VLF)
2. HF nu = HF x 100 (TP – VLF)
3. LF/ HF ratio = Ratio of LF to HF spectral powers

IMPORTANCE OF HRV ANALYSIS

Physiological Significance

HRV analysis is used to precisely assess the **efficiency of vagal control** of the individual, as it reflects the heart rate variability that occurs mainly due to **sinus arrhythmia**.

1. Due to inspiratory inhibition of the vagal tone, the heart rate shows fluctuations with a frequency similar to the respiratory rate.
2. The inspiratory inhibition is evoked primarily by central irradiation of impulses from the medullary respiratory to the cardiovascular center.
3. Respiratory sinus arrhythmia can be abolished by atropine or vagotomy as it is parasympathetically mediated.

HRV Analysis for Assessment of Sympathovagal Balance

HRV, that is, the degree of heart rate fluctuations around the mean heart rate, can be used as a mirror of the cardiorespiratory control system. It is a valuable tool to investigate the **sympathetic and parasympathetic function** of the autonomic nervous system. SA nodal activity at any particular time is determined by the balance between vagal activity, which slows it, and sympathetic activity, which accelerates it. Generally, if the rate is lower than the intrinsic rate of the pacemaker, it implies predominant vagal activity, while high heart rates are achieved by increased sympathetic drive.

1. The ***HF component of HRV indicates the cardiac vagal drive*** of the individual. Increased HF power (or more specifically, increased HFnu) represents increased vagal drive and decreased HF power (decreased HF nu) represents decreased vagal drive to the heart.
2. The ***LF component of HRV mainly indicates the cardiac sympathetic drive*** of the individual. Increased LF power (or more specifically, increased LFnu) represents increased sympathetic drive while decreased LF power (decreased LFnu) represents decreased sympathetic drive.
3. The **sympathovagal balance** is assessed by the LF–HF ratio. Increased LF–HF ratio reflects increased sympathetic activity, while decreased LF–HF ratio indicates increased parasympathetic and decreased sympathetic activity.

Physiological basis: The relationship between vagal stimulation frequency and the resulting change in heart rate is hyperbolic, with changes in frequency at low heart rates having a much greater effect that does not directly control the heart rate, but which regulates the interval between successive beats.

1. The ***effect of vagal stimulation is rapid***. Vagal stimulation releases the neurotransmitter acetylcholine, which inhibits the pacemaker potentials.
2. ***Sympathetic responses*** differ from vagal effects in that they *develop much more slowly*. Hence, responses with longer latency are likely to be mainly sympathetic.
3. ***Peripheral vascular resistance*** exhibits intrinsic oscillations with a low frequency. These oscillations can be influenced by thermal skin stimulation and are thought to arise from *thermoregulatory peripheral blood flow* adjustments.
4. The fluctuations in peripheral vascular resistance are accompanied by fluctuations with the same frequency in blood pressure and heart rate and are *mediated by the sympathetic nervous system*.
5. Hence, analysis of HRV also indicates the tone of sympathetic outflow and, therefore, reflects the individual's state of sympathetic function and susceptibility to sympathetic dysfunction.

Importance of LF-HF Ratio and Sympathovagal Balance

1. The **HF component** of HRV, which indicates the cardiac vagal drive to the heart, represents ***parasympathetic activity***. The **LF component** of HRV, which mainly indicates the cardiac ***sympathetic drive***, represents sympathetic activity, though parasympathetic drive also contributes to it.
2. In healthy individuals, **HF constitutes about 60%, and LF constitutes about 40%** of the total power (TP) of HRV.
3. Therefore, **LF-HF ratio less than 1 indicates good cardiovascular health**. However, LF-HF ratio in normal population varies **from 0.5 to 1.5**.
4. The sympathovagal balance is assessed by the LF-HF ratio.

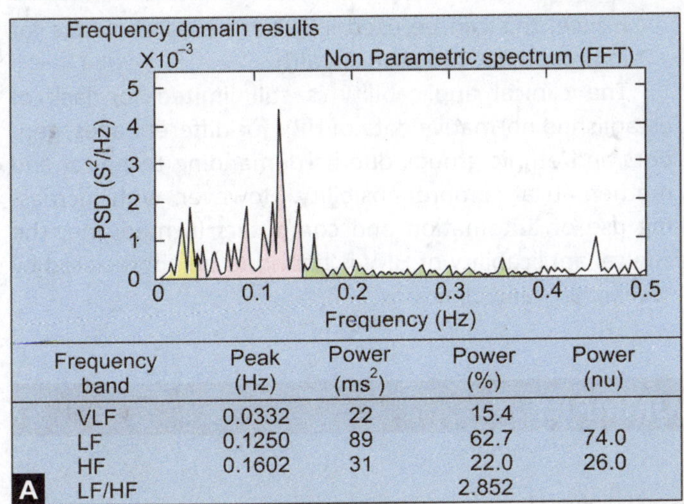

Frequency band	Peak (Hz)	Power (ms^2)	Power (%)	Power (nu)
VLF	0.0332	22	15.4	
LF	0.1250	89	62.7	74.0
HF	0.1602	31	22.0	26.0
LF/HF			2.852	

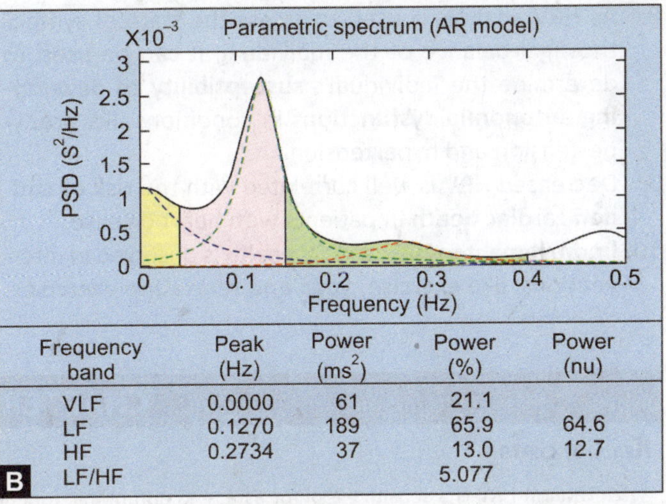

Frequency band	Peak (Hz)	Power (ms^2)	Power (%)	Power (nu)
VLF	0.0000	61	21.1	
LF	0.1270	189	65.9	64.6
HF	0.2734	37	13.0	12.7
LF/HF			5.077	

Figs. 35.3A and B: Frequency domain indices of HRV analysis of a subject having increased sympathetic activity. Refer to Fig. 35.1 for PSD of VLF, LF and HF of HRV. Note, as depicted in parametric spectrum, LF Power (ms^2) is significantly increased (189 ms^2) compared to HF Power, which is grossly reduced (37 ms^2) and LF-HF ratio is increased to 5.077. Also, total power is only 287 (VLF 61 + LF189 + HF 37).

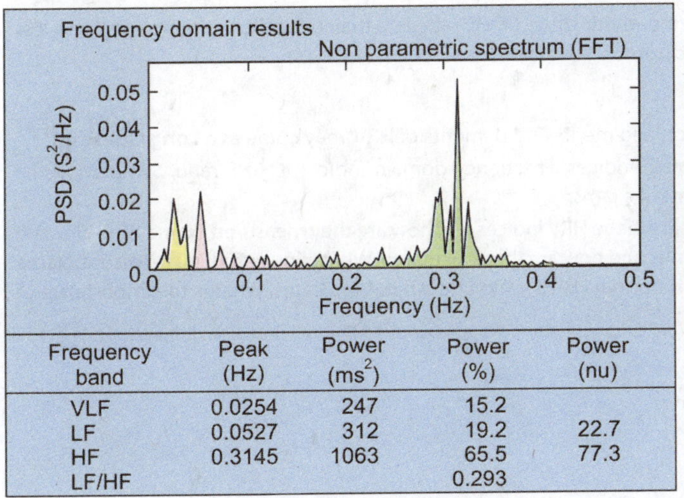

Frequency band	Peak (Hz)	Power (ms^2)	Power (%)	Power (nu)
VLF	0.0254	247	15.2	
LF	0.0527	312	19.2	22.7
HF	0.3145	1063	65.5	77.3
LF/HF			0.293	

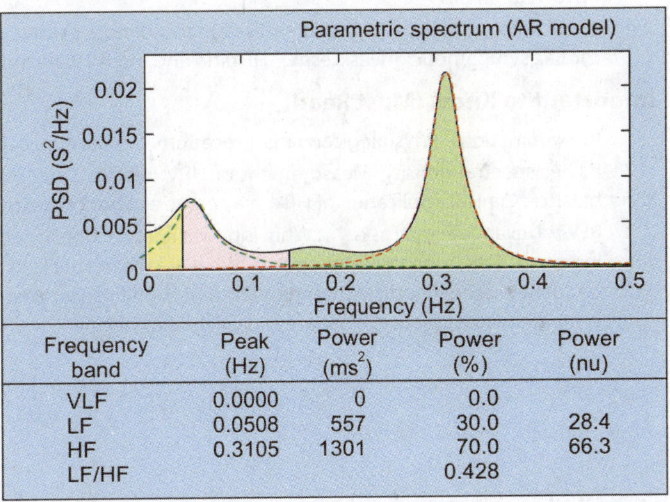

Frequency band	Peak (Hz)	Power (ms^2)	Power (%)	Power (nu)
VLF	0.0000	0	0.0	
LF	0.0508	557	30.0	28.4
HF	0.3105	1301	70.0	66.3
LF/HF			0.428	

Fig. 35.4: Frequency domain indices of HRV analysis of a subject having more parasympathetic activity. Refer to Fig. 35.1 for PSD of VLF, LF and HF of HRV. Note, as depicted in parametric spectrum, HF Power (ms^2) is significantly increased (1301 ms^2) compared to LF Power, which is much less (557 ms^2) and LF-HF ratio is increased to 0.428. Also, total power is 1858 (VLF 0 + LF 557 + HF 1305), which is quite high and reflects increased HRV, the indicator of good CV health.

5. **Increased LF-HF ratio** reflects **increased sympathetic activity** (Figs. 35.3A and B) that is invariably associated with decreased TP.
6. Decreased LF-HF ratio indicates increased parasympathetic and decreased sympathetic activity that is invariably associated with increased TP (Fig. 35.4).

Clinical Application

Though there is considerable discussion regarding the physiology of HRV, it is well correlated and studied in many physiological and pathological conditions:

1. Total power (TP) of HRV indicates the **magnitude of heart rate variability**.
2. **Decreased TP** (decreased overall cardiac vagal modulation) has been implicated with future adverse ***cardiovascular (CV) morbidities*** and ***mortalities***.
3. **Decreased HRV** (decreased total power of HRV) is observed in many cardiovascular disease conditions and generally indicated **poor prognosis** in these conditions.
4. Much before the onset of clinical symptoms of the cardiovascular disease, alterations are observed in HRV, indicating that HRV could be used as **sensitive tool in the prediction of CV risks**. However, more research is required to establish the predictive value of HRV in CV dysfunctions.
5. Presently, HRV is used as a **prognostic tool in conditions like postmyocardial infarction** and cardiac transplantation.
6. The most important application of HRV analysis is the surveillance of postinfarction and diabetic patients.
7. HRV gives information about the sympathetic-parasympathetic autonomic drives, and used as tool for assessment of **autonomic imbalance**.

8. As HRV analysis is used to assess the state of sympathovagal balance of the individual, it can be used to determine the individual's **susceptibility to developing autonomic dysfunctions** in conditions like prehypertension and hypertension.
9. Decreased HRV is well correlated with the **risk of sudden cardiac death** in patients with heart disease.
10. **Improvement in HRV** and CV health is observed in interventions, like **exercise, yoga and relaxation exercises**.

Hence, this can be used in future research works for improvement of holistic health.

The clinical applicability is still limited for lack of established normative data of HRV for different ages, genders and ethnic groups due its demanding technical and mathematical comprehensibility. However, with increasing use of automation and computers in medicine, the clinical applicability of HRV is bound to be appreciated by researchers and clinicians.

CHAPTER SUMMARY

Key Concepts

1. Though HRV is a sensitive tool for assessing autonomic functions and dysfunctions, due to lack of wide range of normative data, its application in clinical medicine is limited.
2. HRV has less diagnostic application, though it is widely used in assessing prognosis of the diseases and in prediction of CV risks for morbidity and mortality.
3. TP of HRV depicts overall vagal modulation of heart. HF and HFnu indicate cardiac vagal drive, and LF and LFnu indicate sympathetic drive in general.
4. LF-HF ratio more than 1.5 indicates less vagal and more cardiac sympathetic drive, LF-HF ratio less than 0.5 indicates more vagal and less cardiac sympathetic drives. Less LF-HF ratio and more TP are indicators of good CV health.

Important to Know (Must Read)

1. In examinations, 'Physiological basis, procedure, clinical application and merits and demerits of HRV' may come as a **Long Question**.
2. Power spectral density, Measurement of HRV indices, Time-domain indices, Frequency-domain indices, LH-HF ratio, Sympathovagal balance, Clinical application of HRV, may come as **Short Questions** in exams.
3. In **Viva,** examiner may ask...... What is power spectral density, What are the HRV indices and how are they measured, Name Time-domain indices and mention their significance, What are the normalized units and how are they calculated, What LFnu and HFnu represent, Name frequency-domain indices and mention their significance, What is normal LH-HF ratio and what it indicates, What is the importance of sympathovagal balance, What are clinical utilities of HRV.

SECTION–5

Gastrointestinal System

PART A: INTRODUCTION TO GI SYSTEM

36. Functional Organization of GI System and Principles of GI Regulations
37. Gastrointestinal Hormones

PART B: GI SECRETIONS

38. Principles of GI Secretion and Secretion of Saliva
39. Gastric Secretion
40. Pancreatic Secretion
41. Physiology of Liver, Liver Function Tests and Pathophysiology of Jaundice
42. Biliary Secretion
43. Intestinal Secretion
44. Secretion of Large Intestine

PART C: GI MOTILITY

45. Introduction to GI Motility
46. Chewing and Deglutition
47. Esophageal Motility
48. Gastric Motility
49. Small Intestinal Motility
50. Motility of Large Intestine

PART D: DIGESTION AND ABSORPTION

51. Principles of Digestion and Absorption

"Where ignorance is, there suffering too must come.
...Your grief is a cry of darkness to the Light above;
Pain was the first-born of the Inconscience
Which was the body's dumb original base"

Sri Aurobindo (in 'SAVITRI')

CHAPTER 36

Functional Organization of GI System and Principles of GI Regulations

Learning Objectives

On completion of study of this chapter, the student **MUST** be able to:

1. Appreciate the importance of GI physiology in learning medicine.
2. List the functions of GI tract and correlate the functional anatomy with functions of GI tract.
3. Name the layers of wall of GI tract, and give their functional importance.
4. Understand the difference in sympathetic and parasympathetic stimulation on GI functions.
5. Appreciate the organization of enteric nervous system.
6. Learn the principles of GI regulations.

The student **MAY** also be able to:

1. Describe the innervation of GI tract
2. Describe the principle of GI regulations

Gastrointestinal (GI) system is a fundamental design of the nature to provide nutrition to the individual by ingestion. The food particles that enter GI tract as larger molecules like polysaccharides, proteins and fats must be broken down into smaller absorbable molecules in the lumen of stomach and intestine to cross the GI epithelium and enter blood. Though, a person can survive on parenteral (usually, intravenous) nutrition, this restricts the mobility of the individual and requires assistance for connecting intravenous infusion. Therefore, parenteral nutrition is advocated temporarily in patients who cannot eat, or in whom oral feeding is prohibited due to some other cause. It is also difficult to provide all nutritional ingredients for a longer duration through parenteral route. Therefore, gastrointestinal dysfunctions invariably lead to malnutrition.

1. When food enters GI system, starting from the mouth cavity, exocrine secretions (**GI secretions**) pour into the tract.
2. GI secretions (mainly salivary, gastric, pancreatic, biliary and intestinal) contain enzymes that split various food materials into their absorbable form. This is called **digestion of food.**
3. For adequate enzymatic digestion to take place, food should be thoroughly grinded and then mixed with GI secretions.
4. The process of grinding and mixing is initiated when food is present in oral cavity. Contraction of smooth muscle in the wall of the gastrointestinal tract produces various movement of the tract. This is called **GI motility**.
5. Chewing, and gastric and intestinal motilities help in grinding food particles and facilitate their mixing with the digestive juices.
6. GI motility also exposes chyme (digested food) to the epithelial surface of the intestine for their transfer into general circulation. This is called **absorption of food**.
7. GI motility is essential for propulsion of food in aboral direction.

Keeping the sequence of GI activities in mind, while describing GI physiology, we shall first discuss GI secretions, followed by GI motility and finally, the digestion and absorption of food.

Scientist contributed

RENÉ ANTONIE FERCHAULT DE REAUMUR, the French entomologist explored the comparative physiology in insects and birds. He studied the digestive process in birds and ***isolated gastric juice***. He demonstrated the ***solvent action of gastric juice on food***. His pioneering works in comparative physiology included regeneration in crustacean, electric organs of torpedo, star-fish movement, marine phosphorescence, formation of silk from silkworms and digestion in birds.

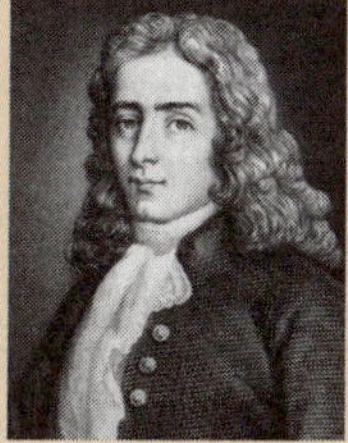

RAF De Reaumur
(1683–1757)

Sources: Sur les diverses reproductions que se font dan les ecrevisses. *Med Acad Roy Sci* 1712; 224–245.

FUNCTIONAL ORGANIZATION

Functions of GI Tract

Gastrointestinal system, in addition to its principal functions of digestion and absorption of nutrients, carry out many other functions of the body. The GI functions may be listed as follows:

1. **Digestion and absorption of food:** The primary functions of GI system are to digest food materials and absorb essential nutrients of digestive products into the bloodstream.
2. **Excretion of waste materials:** Digestive tract excretes waste materials in the form of feces. Fecal matter includes mainly the excretory products of digestion and undigested food particles.
3. **Fluid and electrolyte balance:** On average, an adult consumes ***1 kg of food and 1.5 liters of water*** per day. An additional amount ***of 7 liters of fluid is secreted*** into GI tract in the form of secretions from various exocrine glands. Thus, intestine is presented with ***about 8.5 liters of fluid per day***. About 99% of this fluid and 90% of solids are absorbed in small and large intestines along with absorption of various electrolytes, so that only about 100 ml of liquid and 100 g of solids are excreted in feces per day. Decreased absorption of this water content results in dehydration. *Diarrhea occurs when capacity of intestine to absorb fluid is decreased or secretion of fluid is increased.*
4. **Immunity:** The GI tract is approximately a 15 feet long tube, which is open at both the ends. Therefore, anatomically it is continuous with the external environment. Consequently, it provides a fine channel for organisms from external world to pass through it. However, the **gut associated lymphoid tissues** (GALTs) protect the body from pathogenic organisms. GALTs are of two types: **Peyer's patches** (aggregates of lymphoid tissue in the submucosa) and **diffuse population of immune cells** (discussed below). GALTs prevent entry of organisms from gut into the body. **Acidic secretion of stomach** also prevents entry of organisms through oral route.
5. **Intestinal bacterial flora:** Many nonpathogenic bacteria inhabit intestine. They form the normal **bacterial flora of intestine.** This normal flora is essential for **many intestinal functions** like epithelial cell permeability to electrolytes and water, synthesis and absorption of vitamins, stimulation of enzymatic activity, peristalsis and mucus secretion. Decreased flora impairs intestinal functions and increased flora increases the susceptibility to diarrhea and steatorrhea. These bacteria also **detoxify many toxins** present in the chyme and prevent their absorption into the bloodstream.

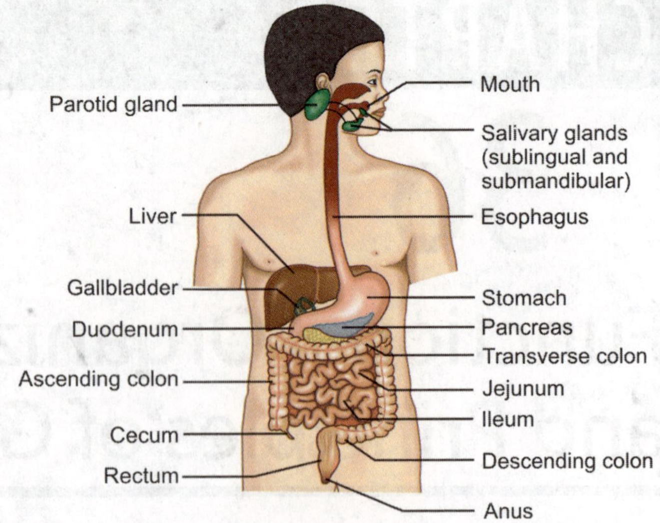

Fig. 36.1: Parts of GI system.

Parts of GI System

Gastrointestinal system consists of gastrointestinal tract (GIT) and its associated glandular structures that produce exocrine secretions essential for digestion and absorption of various nutrients. The parts of GIT include **mouth, pharynx, esophagus, stomach, small intestine** (duodenum, jejunum, and ileum), **colon** (ascending, transverse, descending and sigmoid colons), **rectum, and anus** (Fig. 36.1). The major **associated glandular structures** are salivary glands, liver, exocrine pancreas and intestinal glands.

1. GI tract begins with the **mouth** (oral cavity). Digestion of food starts in mouth with chewing. ***Salivary glands*** open into the oral cavity and pour their secretion (saliva) into it. Salivary amylase helps in partial digestion of complex sugars (polysaccharides).
2. Oral cavity opens into **pharynx** which in turn is continuous with the esophagus.
3. **Esophagus** transmits food from oropharynx into stomach.
4. **Stomach** is a bag like structure that stores and grinds food, and mixes food with gastric juice. HCl and pepsin secreted in stomach help in partial digestion of proteins and stomach converts food into chyme. Chyme from stomach enters intestine through pyloric sphincter by controlled gastric emptying.
5. **Small intestine** is a 9 feet tube that extends from pyloric sphincter to the ileocecal valve. It consists of ***three parts***: duodenum, jejunum and ileum.
6. **Biliary and pancreatic secretions** are poured into duodenum.
7. Intestinal glands secrete *succus entericus*.
8. **Pancreatic and intestinal secretions** are rich in various enzymes that cause digestion of carbohydrates, fat and proteins.
9. Absorption of most of the nutrients takes place in jejunum and ileum.

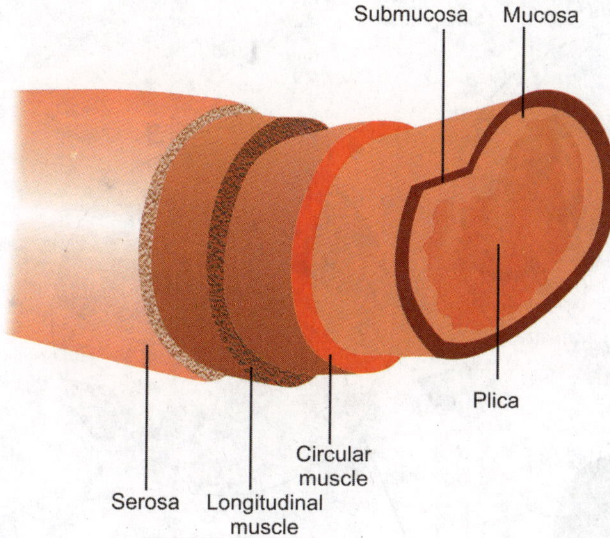

Fig. 36.2: Layers of wall of the gut.

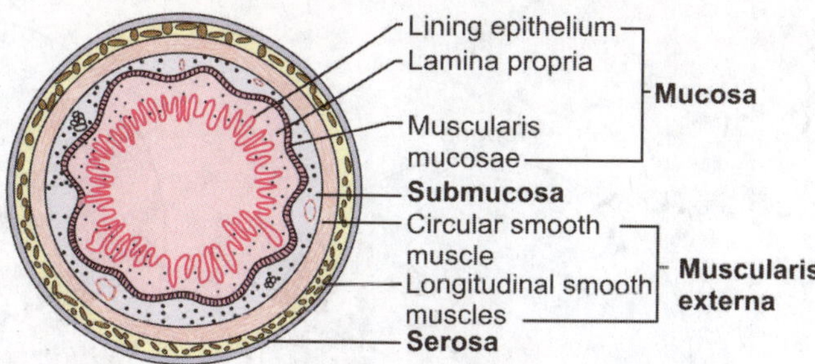

Fig. 36.3: Details of the layers of the gut.

10. Small intestinal motility propels food into large intestine through ileocecal sphincter.
11. **Large intestine** absorbs water and electrolyte and temporarily stores the concentrated and undigested material, which then enters the rectum.
12. **Rectum**, the final segment of large intestine stores fecal matter and contracts when distended. *Defecation reflex* relaxes the anal sphincters and expels feces from rectum to outside through **anal canal**.

Structure of the Wall of GI Tract

The basic nature of arrangement of tissues in the wall of GI tract starting from esophagus to the rectum is similar. In general, there are four layers from interior to exterior: mucosa, submucosa, muscle layer, and serosa (Fig. 36.2).

Mucosa

The innermost layer of GI tract is the mucosa, which has an epithelium, lamina propria and muscularis mucosa (Fig. 36.3).

Epithelium

A single layer of epithelial cells line the mucosa. The cells are tightly bound to each other at their edges by **tight junctions**.

1. The epithelium is mainly a *stratified squamous epithelium*.
2. In stomach and intestine, the mucosa is lined by simple columnar epithelium that facilitates secretion and absorption.
3. At places, the epithelium contains endocrine cells (**enterochromaffin cells**) that secrete local hormones.

Lamina Propria

Just below the epithelium is the lamina propria consisting of mainly **loose connective tissue** that contains *collagen and elastin fibers*.

1. This sub-layer is rich in blood vessels, lymph nodes and lymphatic ducts, nerve fibers, and capillaries. This layer supports the epithelium and also binds epithelium to the muscularis mucosa.
2. The **lymphatic tissues** present in this layer form the *local immune system* and prevent the entry of pathogens that try to penetrate mucous membrane to enter into the body.

Muscularis Mucosa

This is the innermost layer of the intestinal smooth muscle present in the mucosa. The muscle fibers are arranged in **two layers**: an inner circular and outer longitudinal layer.

1. Contraction of muscularis mucosa in the stomach and intestine throws the mucous membrane into folds and ridges.
2. In the intestine, these mucosal folds called **plica** *increase the surface area for absorption* (Fig. 36.4).
3. Contraction of muscularis mucosa in small intestine produces ***local movements*** that facilitate the process of digestion and absorption.

Submucosa

Next to the mucosa is the submucosa. It consists mainly of loose connective tissue and is highly vascular.

1. The submucosal layer contains a network of nerve fibers known as *submucosal plexus* or **plexus of Meissner**.
2. Autonomic nerve fibers supplying muscles and blood vessels of GI tract closely interact with Meissner's plexus.
3. In some regions, especially in intestine, submucosa contains **lymphatic tissue**.

Muscular Layer

This is called **muscularis externa**. It consists of **two layers** of smooth muscles: the ***inner circular*** and the ***outer longitudinal*** layers.

1. A nerve plexus is located between the muscle layers, called as *myenteric plexus* or **plexus of Auerbach**.
2. Auerbach's plexus contains fibers from both divisions of ANS.
3. Muscularis externa primarily **controls the motility of GI tract** that mixes and circulates the gastrointestinal contents and propels them along the lumen of the tract.

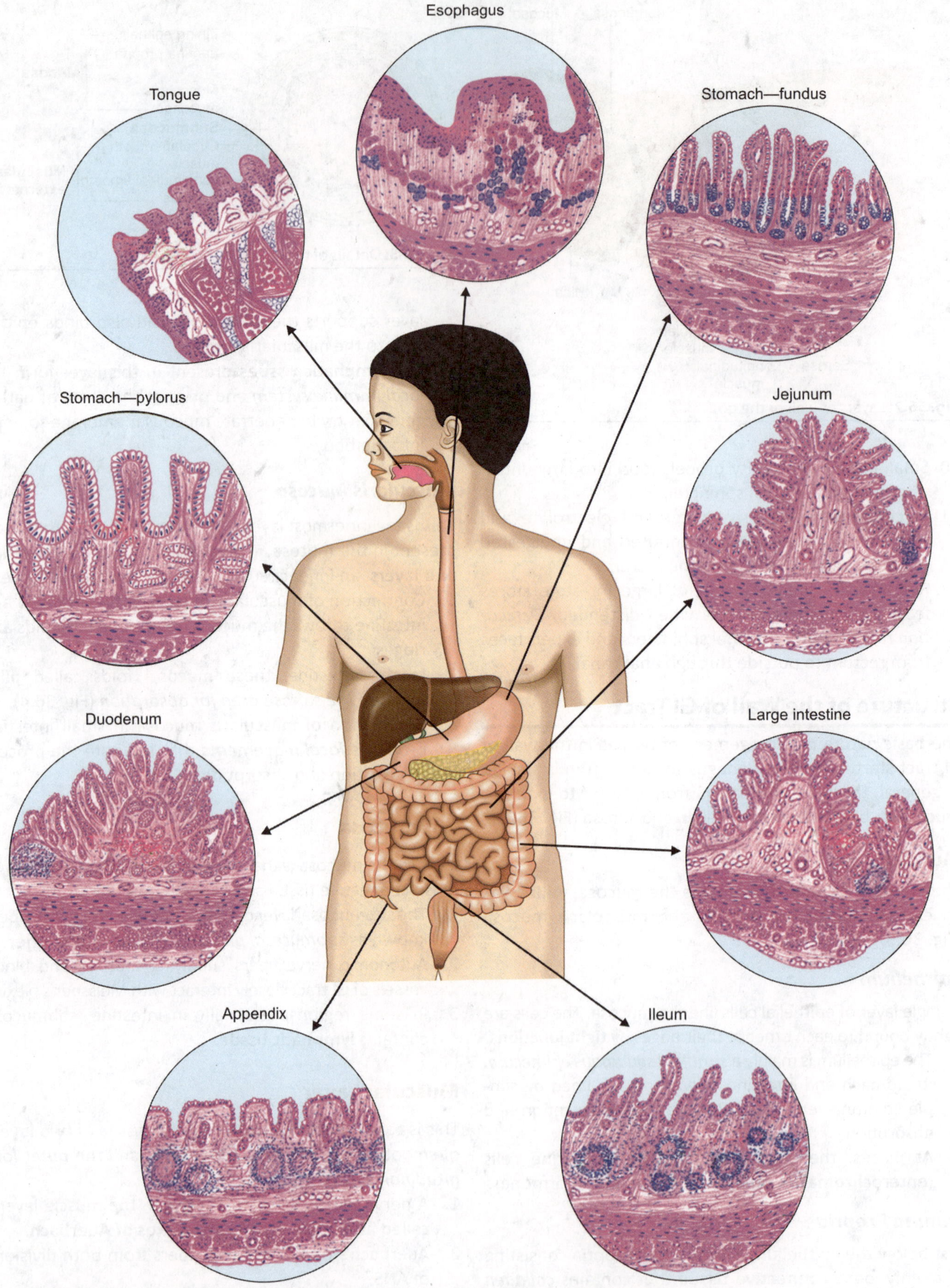

Fig. 36.4: Differences in the layers of the wall in different parts of GIT. Note that mucosa is simple columnar in stomach and intestine. In jejunum, the muscularis mucosa is folded to form plica that increases the surface area for absorption.
Courtesy: Figure 13.1, Basic Histology, by V Subhadra Devi, 1st edition, 2016; Jaypee Brothers Medical Publishers (P) Ltd.

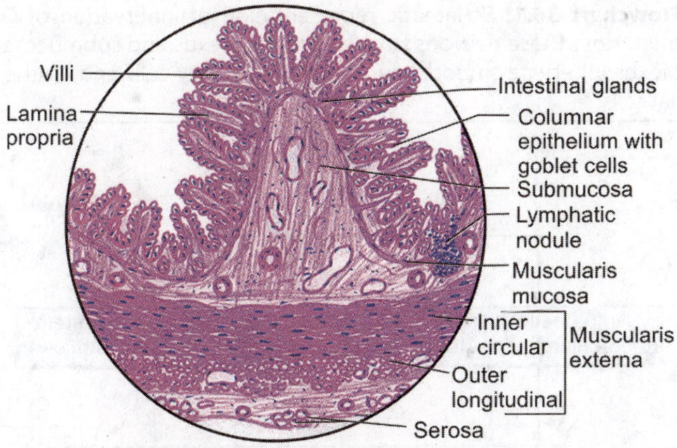

Fig. 36.5: Modifications of mucosal layer in the intestine. Note, there are numerous microvilli on the villi.
Courtesy: Figure 13.23A, Basic Histology, by V Subhadra Devi, 1st edition, 2016; Jaypee Brothers Medical Publishers (P) Ltd.

Serosa

This is the outermost layer of the GIT. It consists mainly of a *thin layer of connective tissue* covered with a layer of **squamous mesothelial cells**. It provides **external protection** to the GIT.

Intestinal Modifications

Villi

In small intestine, from the luminal surface, finger like projections extend into the lumen. These are called villi. Surface of each villus is covered with an epithelial cell layer.

1. Small projections arise from the surface of these epithelial cells, known as **microvilli** (Fig. 36.5).
2. Microvilli are collectively called as **brush border**.
3. Folded mucosa, villi and microvilli increase the surface area of the intestinal luminal epithelium by **600 fold**.
4. The **total luminal surface area** of human intestine is about 300 m^2, which is about the *area of a tennis court*.
5. Intestinal epithelial cells are **continuously replaced** by new cells. About *17 billions of epithelial cells are replaced* every day and the entire intestinal epithelium is replaced almost every five days.
6. Center of each villus is occupied by lymphatics called **lacteals**, and capillaries, venules and nerve fibers.

Peyer's Patches

These are the **aggregates of lymphoid tissue** in the mucosal-submucosal regions of the intestinal wall.

1. They serve *local immune functions* in the intestine. They prevent organisms to enter blood stream from the intestinal lumen.
2. They also *secrete mediators of inflammation* (cytokines) that alter motility. These cytokines play role in genesis of inflammatory bowel disease and Crohn's disease.

Innervation of GI Tract

Gastrointestinal tract is innervated by sympathetic and parasympathetic fibers. Also, it has its own neural circuits (*enteric nervous system*).

Sympathetic Innervation

Stimulation of sympathetic fibers to GI tract is **generally inhibitory**. Sympathetic innervation is via **noradrenergic fibers** having their cell bodies in the prevertebral and paravertebral chain of ganglia. The postganglionic fibers mainly originate from **celiac, superior and inferior mesenteric ganglia** (Refer to Fig. 31.2; Chapter 31).

Usually, sympathetic fibers do not directly innervate the target GI tissues. Instead, they terminate on neurons of intrinsic nerve plexuses that in turn contact the target structures (Fig. 36.6). However, the vasoconstrictor fibers directly innervate blood vessels of GI tract.

Sympathetic stimulation results in:

1. Inhibition of motor activity resulting in relaxation of GI smooth muscles.
2. Stimulation or contraction of sphincters.
3. Inhibition of GI secretions.

Parasympathetic Innervation

Parasympathetic innervation is **mainly via vagus nerve**, which innervates GI tract from oral cavity upto transverse colon. Remaining parts (descending and sigmoid colons, rectum, and anal canal) receive parasympathetic fibers from **pelvic nerves** (*see* Fig. 32.1; Chapter 32).

1. Parasympathetic fibers are **cholinergic** and generally **excitatory**.
2. They terminate mainly on the intrinsic nerve plexuses.
3. *Parasympathetic stimulation leads* to increased motility and exocrine secretions of GI tract.

Enteric Nervous System

Enteric nervous system (ENS) is the intrinsic nervous system of the GI tract.

1. This includes **myenteric and submucosal nerve plexuses** in the GI tract (Fig. 36.6). These two plexuses are the network of nerve fibers and ganglion cells.
2. The neurons of these plexuses are **small interneurons** that connect afferent neurons and efferent neurons to smooth muscles, secretory cells and epithelial cells (Flowchart 36.1), and they form the *anatomical basis of local GI reflexes*. Therefore, the reflex arc for local GI reflexes is located within the GI tract. Hence, ENS is capable of coordinating GI activity in the absence of external innervation.
3. The neurons of ENS closely interact with the autonomic nervous system. The sympathetic and parasympathetic fibers project to the neurons of the myenteric and submucosal plexuses, and control GI activities via these neurons.

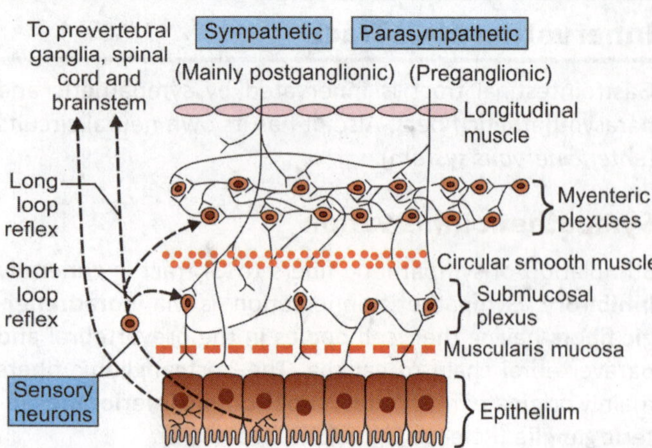

Fig. 36.6: Innervation of GIT by sympathetic and parasympathetic neurons of the enteric nervous system. Note the arrangement of neurons in the myenteric plexus and submucosal plexus.
Courtesy: Figure 5.2, Physiology Preparatory Manual for Undergraduates, by Sanoop KS et al., 1st edition, 2012; Jaypee Brothers Medical Publishers (P) Ltd.

4. Therefore, ENS is also known as **third division of ANS**. However, it should be remembered that *regulation of GI functions by ENS is independent of autonomic control*.

ENS as the Mini-brain of gut: ENS consists approximately of 100 millions of neurons, the number of neurons that are roughly present in spinal cord or in entire ANS. These neurons are clustered exclusively in the gut.

1. They have sensory neurons, interneurons and motor neurons. Therefore, ENS is loosely called the '***mini brain***' for the gut.
2. The ENS afferent neurons monitor changes in luminal activity like distension, alteration in osmolality, pH etc. and activate gut interneurons.
3. The interneurons signal the changes in ENS motor fibers that alter the activities of effector tissues like smooth muscle cells, glandular cells, epithelial cells and vascular cells.

Neurotransmitters in the ENS: Many neurotransmitters in the ENS have been recently identified.

1. **Acetylcholine** (ACh) is the primary neurotransmitter in preganglionic and postganglionic neurons that regulate secretory and motor activities of GI tract.
2. **VIP, serotonin, enkephalins, substance P, norepinephrine, GABA, ATP, NO and CO** have also been described as neurotransmitters in ENS, and these chemicals play important role in regulation of GI functions.

GI Sphincters

Sphincters are **specialized circular muscles** that are present at the *beginning or at the end of a gut structure*. Sphincters regulate antegrade (forward) movement of food and prevent retrograde (reverse) expulsion of the same. There are **six sphincters** in GI tract:

1. Upper esophageal sphincter
2. Lower esophageal sphincter

Flowchart 36.1: Schematic representation of innervation of GI tract. Note these neurons from myenteric plexus and submucosal plexus innervate smooth muscle cells, secretory cells and epithelial cells.

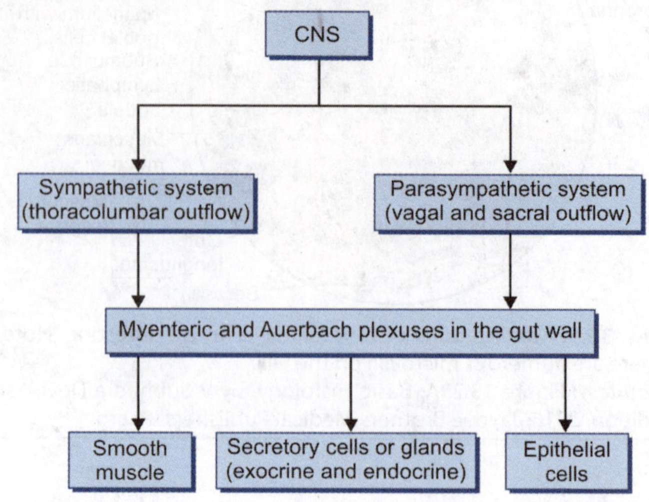

3. Pyloric sphincter
4. Ileocecal sphincter
5. Internal anal sphincter
6. External anal sphincter

There is another sphincter located in the wall of the duodenum called **Sphincter of Oddi** that regulates secretion of bile and pancreatic juice into the intestine.

GI Immune System

An extensive immune mechanism is developed in GI system, which is called **gastrointestinal immune system**. This system includes:

1. **Mesenteric lymph nodes**
2. **Peyer's patches** (aggregation of lymphatic tissues in the submucosa)
3. **Phagocytic cells and immunocytes** present in the mucosa and submucosa throughout the GI tract (For details, refer to Chapter 18).

Immunological Cells in GI System

The **immunological cells** in GI system constitute about **50% of the total immunocytes in the body**.

1. Immunocytes in GI tract are **B and T cells, epithelial lymphocytes, plasma cells**, mast cells and macrophages.
2. These cells *secrete chemicals* that mediate immunological and inflammatory responses in GI tract.
3. They *secrete antibodies* locally in response to antigens that enter through GI tract.
4. *Other chemicals* secreted by immunocytes are **leukotrienes, cytokines, prostaglandins and histamine**. These chemicals not only mediate immunological responses, but also influence activities of smooth muscles of GI tract.

Flowchart 36.2: Short and Long reflexes in the regulation of GI functions.

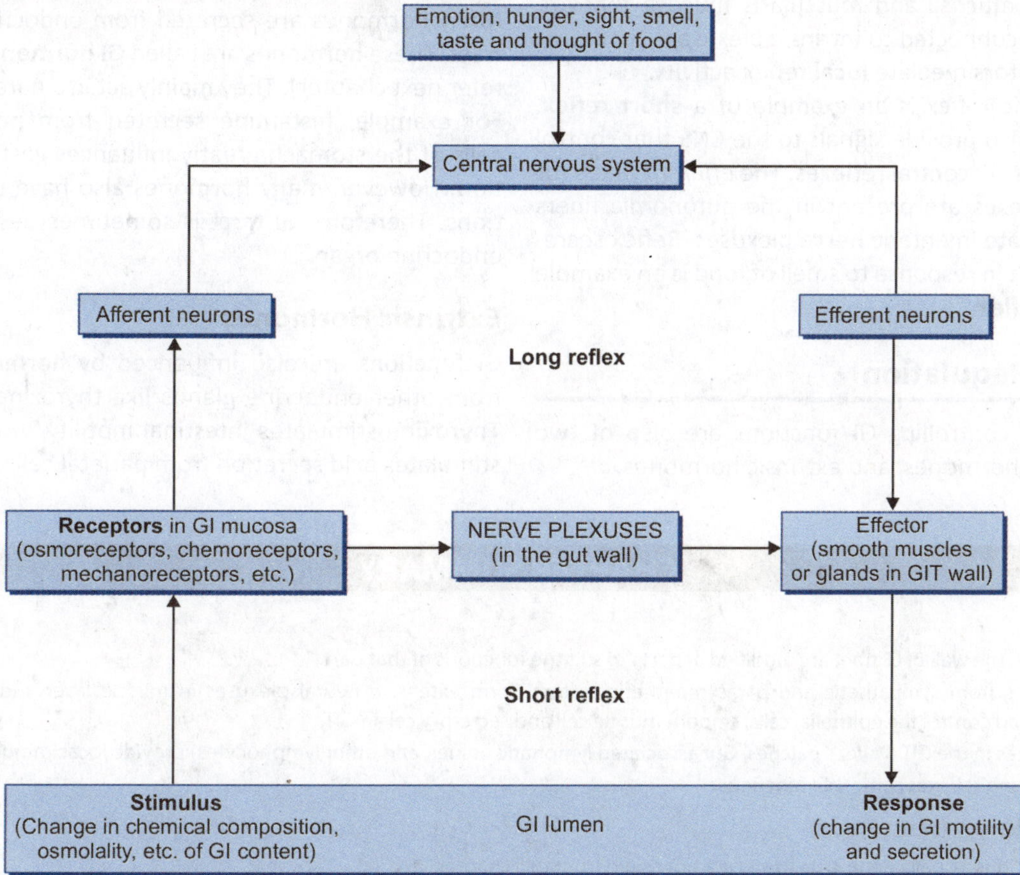

5. GI immune system plays an important role in the ***pathogenesis of inflammatory bowel diseases*** like ulcerative colitis.

PRINCIPLES OF GI REGULATIONS

The functions of GI tract are regulated mainly by neural and hormonal influences. Interestingly, the hormonal and neural control systems of GI functions are mostly intrinsic to GI tract.

Neural Regulation

The digestive system is regulated by the nerves arising locally in the GI tract (**intrinsic neural control**) and the nerves innervating the gut (**extrinsic neural control**). The GI reflexes modify activities of GI system depending on the state of digestion and absorption taking place in the tract.

Intrinsic Neural Regulation

The intrinsic nerves of the GI system form the **enteric nervous system**, sometimes called as *third component of ANS.*

1. The nerves are arranged in the submucosal layer as *Meissner's plexus* and in the muscle layer as *Auerbach's plexus.*
2. These nerve plexuses control local secretion and movement of GI tract.
3. The Meissner's plexus performs sensory functions and Auerbach's plexus performs motor functions.
4. The intrinsic neurons mediate **local or short reflexes**.
5. The intrinsic nerve plexuses are connected and controlled by extrinsic nerves.

Extrinsic Neural Regulation

Extrinsic nerves regulating GI functions belong to sympathetic and parasympathetic systems.

1. In general, the **sympathetic system to the GI tract is inhibitory** and the **parasympathetic system is stimulatory**.
2. The autonomic innervations also control GI functions by altering the activity of neurons in the enteric nervous system.
3. Extrinsic nerves **mediate long reflexes**.

Reflex Control

There are **two types of neural reflexes** that operate in GI system: **short or local reflexes** and **long or central reflexes** (Flowchart 36.2).

1. Afferent pathway in the GIT forms *afferent limb* for both local and central reflexes.

2. There are many chemoreceptors and mechanoreceptors in the mucosa and muscularis mucosa that are extensively connected to intrinsic plexuses. Actions of these receptors mediate **local reflex** activity.
3. Enterogastric reflex is an example of a **short reflex**. Receptors also provide signals to the CNS that control GI functions via **central reflexes**. The *efferent fibers* for central reflexes are present in the autonomic fibers that terminate in enteric nerve plexuses. Reflex secretion of saliva in response to smell of food is an example of a **long reflex**.

Hormonal Regulation

The hormones controlling GI functions are also of two types: intrinsic hormones, and extrinsic hormones.

Intrinsic Hormones

Many hormones are secreted from endocrine cells of GI tract. These hormones are called **GI hormones** (for details, refer next chapter). They mainly act in a paracrine fashion. For example, histamine secreted from neuroendocrine cells of the stomach greatly influences gastric acid secretion. However, many hormones also have systemic functions. Therefore, GI tract is sometimes designated as an endocrine organ.

Extrinsic Hormones

GI functions are also influenced by hormones secreted from other endocrine glands like thyroxine and cortisol. **Thyroxine** stimulates intestinal motility, whereas **cortisol** stimulates acid secretion from parietal cells of stomach.

CHAPTER SUMMARY

Key Concepts

1. The layers in the wall of GI tract are modified at parts to suit the functions of that part.
2. Interneurons from sympathetic and parasympathetic system (form extensive neural plexuses in muscle layer and mucosal layer) innervate and control the epithelial cells, smooth muscle cell and secretory cell in GIT.
3. Immunocytes in the GIT (Peyer's patches, Gut associated lymphatic tissues, and other lymphocytes) provide local immunity.
4. Short and long reflexes control GI functions.

Important to Know (Must Read)

1. In examinations, usually **Long Questions** are not asked from this chapter.
2. Layers of GIT, Innervation of GIT, Immune system of GIT, Enteric nervous system, and Reflex control of GI functions, may come as **Short Questions** in exams.
3. In **Viva**, examiner may ask... What are the parts of GIT and what are their main functions, What the layers of GIT and what are their functions, What is the system of innervation of GIT, What are the effects of stimulation of sympathetic and parasympathetic system to GIT, Name the immune mechanisms in GIT, How is enteric nervous system formed and how it works, What are neurotransmitters secreted by GI neurons, What are short and long reflexes and how they work.
4. If a student fails to answer the part of GIT, their organization and functions, it becomes difficult for examiner to give pass mark.

CHAPTER 37

Gastrointestinal Hormones

Learning Objectives

On completion of study of this chapter, the student **MUST** be able to:

1. Classify GI hormones.
2. Give the structure, source, and functions of GI hormones.
3. Understand the role of GI hormones in the regulation of GI functions.
4. Appreciate the dysfunctions produced by alteration in secretion of GI hormones.

The student **MAY** also be able to:

1. Describe the details of GI hormones.
2. Explain the role of GI hormones in GI functions and dysfunctions.

The hormones secreted from the endocrine cells of the GI tract are collectively known as gastrointestinal hormones (GI hormones). Endocrine cells are scattered throughout epithelium of GI tract, especially in stomach and small intestine. The apical surface of epithelial endocrine cells is continuously exposed to chemical changes in the luminal contents of the gut, which directly stimulates the release of hormones from these cells.

1. Endocrine cells that secrete GI hormones are called **enteroendocrine cells**.
2. Cells that secrete serotonin are called **enterochromaffin cells**, and cells that secrete amines and polypeptides are called **APUD cells** (amine precursor uptake and decarboxylation).
3. APUD cells are also found in other organs like lungs. They are also called **neuroendocrine cells**. *Carcinoid tumors* originate from these neuroendocrine cells.

Families of GI Hormones: GI hormones are broadly divided into ***three categories***:

1. ***Gastrin family*** that includes cholecystokinin and gastrin.
2. ***Secretin family*** that includes GIP, glucagon, secretin, and VIP.
3. ***Other polypeptides.***

GI HORMONES OF GASTRIN FAMILY

Gastrin

Source

Gastrin is produced by **G cells** in the stomach that are located mainly in the antral region.

1. G cells are conical cells with apex projecting toward the lumen. Apical surface of G cells contains numerous microvilli. Microvilli of G cells contain receptors for chemicals that mediate gastrin release.
2. **Gastrin producing cells are also present in** hypothalamus, anterior pituitary, medulla, and fetal pancreas.
3. Gastrin as a neurotransmitter is also secreted from ***vagus and sciatic nerve***.

Structure

Gastrin is a polypeptide hormone. Gastrin has marked heterogeneity; but its physiological significance is not clearly known.

1. Gastrin exhibits both **macroheterogeneity** (gastrins having different polypeptide lengths) and **microheterogeneity** (gastrins having different molecular structures).

2. Though different types of gastrins have been described, **three types of gastrin** are physiologically important. Depending on the number of amino acids they possess, they are named as **G 34, G 17, and G 14.** Other types of gastrins are **C-tetrapeptide** (carboxyl terminal tetrapeptide, which is also called *minigastrin*), and gastrin containing 45 amino acids (*megagastrin*).
3. However, **G 17 is the principal gastrin *secreted from the stomach*** and is the major stimulator of gastric acid secretion.
4. Though C-tetrapeptide executes all the actions of G-17, it has only 10% of its physiological strength.

Metabolism

Gastrin secreted from G cells enters general circulation. In blood, half-life of gastrin is less. Half-life of G 14 and G 17 is 2–5 min and of G 34 is about 15 min. Gastrin is inactivated in the intestine and degraded in the kidney.

Functions

1. Primary function of gastrin is the **stimulation of gastric acid and pepsin secretion**. In fact, gastrin is the most potent natural stimulator of HCl secretion from parietal cells of stomach. Therefore, hypergastrinemia causes peptic ulcer.
2. Gastrin **stimulates growth of gastric mucosa** and mucosa of intestine. This is called **trophic action** of gastrin.
3. It stimulates gastric motility.
4. It causes contraction of muscles at the gastroesophageal junction (lower esophageal sphincter). Therefore, it *prevents reflux esophagitis*.
5. It stimulates exocrine pancreatic secretion.
6. It also **stimulates insulin secretion**.
7. It stimulates mass movement of large intestine.
8. It causes colonic contraction that initiates gastrocolic reflex after a meal. Therefore, usually defecation is activated after a meal.
9. It stimulates histamine secretion from ECL (enterochromaffin like cells) in GI mucosa.

Mechanism of Action

The primary function of gastrin is to stimulate acid secretion from parietal cells of the stomach. Gastrin acts on **gastrin** or **CCK receptors** on parietal cells and *increases intracellular calcium* concentration via second messenger, IP3. Increased cytosolic calcium ***activates protein kinase*** that *stimulates* H^+*–*K^+ *ATPase* to promote acid secretion.

Control of Gastrin Secretion

1. **Stimuli that increase gastrin secretion:** Gastric distention, products of protein digestion (peptides and amino acids) in the stomach, increased vagal discharge via GRP (**non-cholinergic**), epinephrine and calcium (Flowchart 37.1). Hypergastrinemia occurs in **ZE syndrome** (Clinical Box 37.1). Gastrin secretion is also elevated in **pernicious anemia**, in which acid secretion in the stomach is less as parietal cells are damaged. This causes feedback release of gastrin from G cells.
2. **Stimuli that decrease gastrin release:** Acid in the stomach, somatostatin, secretin, GIP, VIP, calcitonin, and glucagon. Acid in the antrum inhibits gastric secretion by **negative feedback mechanism**, which is partly by direct action of acid on G cells and partly by release of somatostatin.

Flowchart 37.1: Regulation of gastrin secretion. Minus (–) sign indicates inhibition.

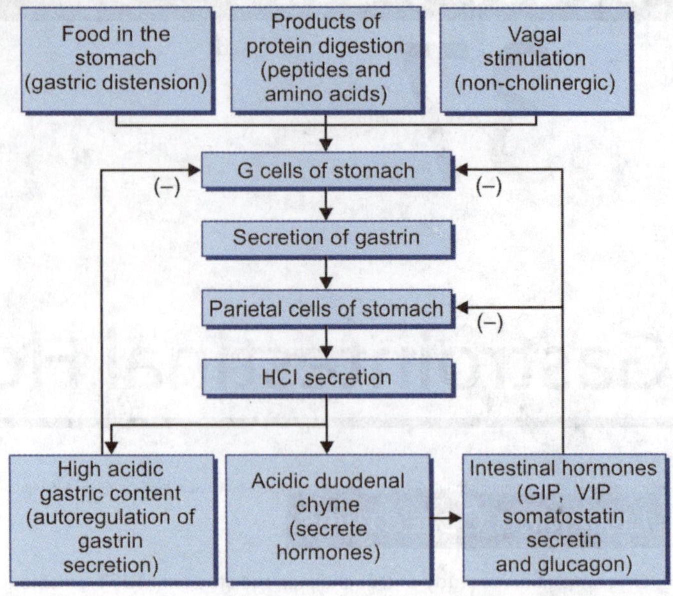

Clinical Box 37.1

Gastrinoma: Gastrinoma is a neuroendocrine tumor (NET) that produces gastrin. Though gastrin is not secreted from pancreas after birth, tumor of pancreatic islet (non-α-non-β cell tumor) secretes gastrin. Gastrin secreting tumor causes severe and chronic hypergastrinemia that causes peptic ulcer disease, which is often refractory and severe. This is called **Zollinger-Ellison syndrome**. The disease is characterized by abdominal pain, diarrhea and gastroesophageal reflux.

Cholecystokinin

Source

Secreted from I cells in the **mucosa of upper small intestine**. CCK is present as neurotransmitter in cerebral cortex, in somatic nerves and in nerves of distal ileum and colon.

Structure

Cholecystokinin (CCK) is a polypeptide hormone. There are different forms of CCK depending on the number of amino acids present, like **CCK 58, CCK 39, CCK 33, CCK 12, CCK 8, and CCK 4** (carboxyl terminal tetrapeptide). CCK secreted from duodenum and jejunum are usually CCK 12 and CCK 8. CCK in the enteric and pancreatic nerves is mainly CCK 4. The forms of CCK in brain are primarily CCK 58 and 8. **Half-life** of CCK is about 5 minutes.

Functions

1. CCK causes **contraction of gallbladder**. Therefore, CCK increases bile release into the intestine following a meal.
2. It stimulates pancreatic secretion rich in enzymes. Therefore, CCK is also called **cholecystokinin-pancreozymin** (CCK-PZ).
3. It also **augments the action of secretin** to produce alkaline pancreatic secretion.
4. It **inhibits gastric acid secretion**.
5. It **inhibits gastric motility**, thereby delays gastric emptying.
6. Causes **relaxation of sphincter of Oddi** that allows both bile and pancreatic juice to enter duodenum.
7. Stimulates growth of pancreas.
8. Increases secretion of enterokinase.
9. Enhances motility of small intestine.
10. Stimulates colonic movements.
11. Augments contraction of pyloric sphincter. Therefore, prevents reflux of duodenal contents into the stomach.
12. Stimulates glucagon secretion.
13. In brain, it acts as an anorexigenic neurotransmitter. It inhibits food intake.
14. It also produces analgesia and anxiety.

Mechanism of Action

There are **two CCK receptors**: CCK A and CCK B. **CCK A receptors** are mainly located in the peripheral structures like gallbladder, pancreas, GI tract etc., whereas, **CCK B receptors** are present in central structures like brain areas. CCK acting on both receptors activates membrane phospholipase–C and stimulates production of intracellular IP_3 and DAG.

Regulation of Secretion

Factors that increase CCK secretion:

1. Contact of intestinal mucosa with products of digestion especially fatty acids, peptides, and amino acids.
2. *Bile and pancreatic juice*: Bile and pancreatic juice facilitate digestion of protein and fat. Therefore, they provide **positive feedback** for CCK secretion (Flowchart 37.2).

Flowchart 37.2: Regulation of cholecystokinin secretion.

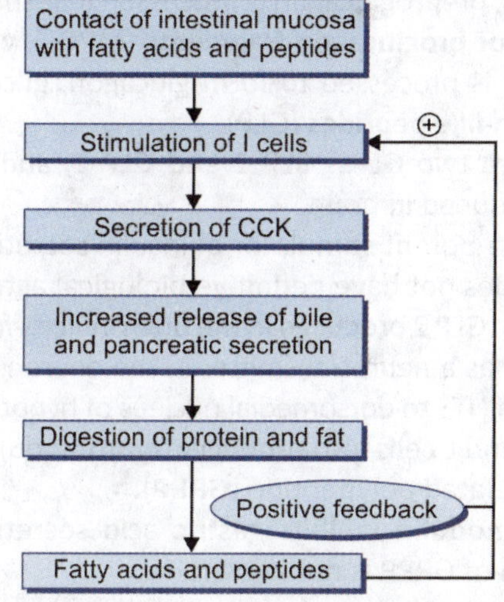

GI HORMONES OF SECRETIN FAMILY

Secretin

Secretin has an important place in the history of endocrine physiology, as it was the **first hormone to be discovered** (Bayliss and Starling; 1902).

Source

Secretin is secreted from **S cells** located in the mucosa of upper part of small intestine.

Structure

Secretin is a polypeptide hormone containing 27 amino acids.

Functions

1. Secretin **increases secretion of pancreatic juice rich in bicarbonate** (watery and alkaline pancreatic secretion).
2. It also increases **alkaline bile secretion**.
3. Augments the action of CCK to produce pancreatic secretion rich in enzymes.
4. Decreases gastric acid secretion and motility.
5. Causes contraction of pyloric sphincter.

Mechanism of Action

Secretin acts on adenylate cyclase on the cell membrane and increases cytosolic formation of cAMP.

Regulation of Secretion

Secretion of secretin is increased by acidic chyme and products of protein digestion entering the upper part of intestine. Secretin stimulates watery and alkaline pancreatic secretion. When watery and alkaline pancreatic juice enters intestine, the acidic content of upper small intestine is neutralized. The increased pH of duodenal and upper jejunal content decreases secretin secretion by **feedback mechanism** (Flowchart 37.3).

Flowchart 37.3: Regulation of secretin secretion.

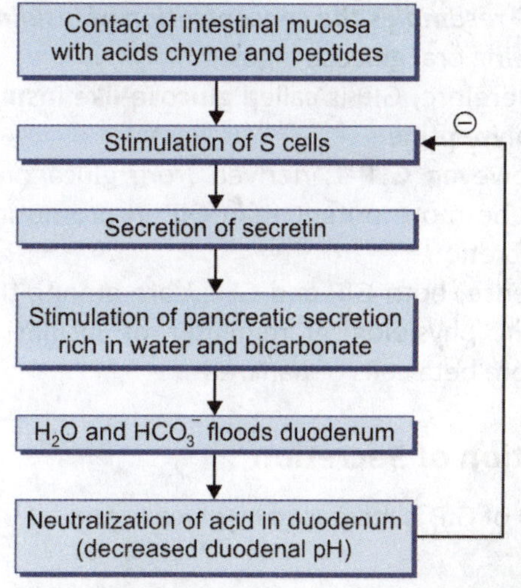

Scientists contributed

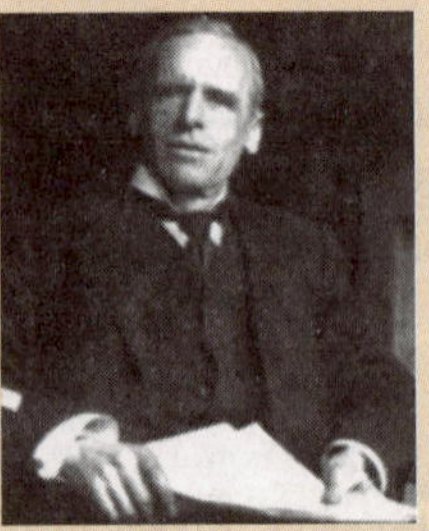
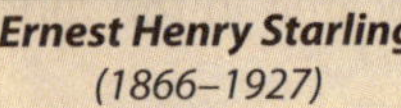

Ernest Henry Starling (1866–1927)

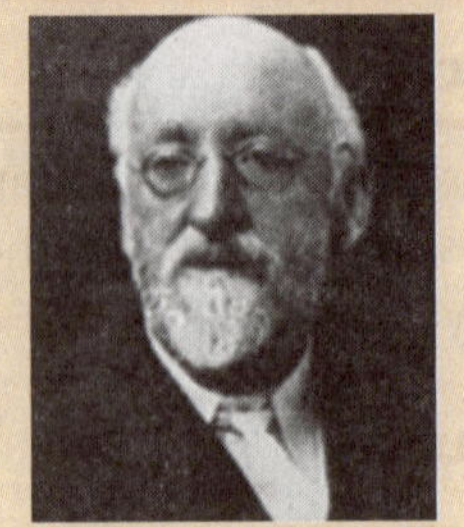

Sir William Maddock Bayliss (1860–1924)

Ernest Henry Starling (1866–1927) an English physiologist worked with his brother-in-law, **Sir William Maddock Bayliss.** Both of them had discovered the first hormone, **Secretin**. Starling is most famous for developing the *"Frank–Starling law of the heart"*, presented in 1915 and modified in 1919. In 1891, when he was 25, Starling married Florence Amelia Wooldridge, the widow of Leonard Charles Wooldridge, who had been his physiology teacher at Guy's and died at the age of 32. She was a great support to Starling as a sounding board, secretary, and manager of his affairs as well as mother of their four children. To be noted, **Bayliss was born on 2nd May and Starling died on 2nd May.**

GIP

Structure

Glucose-dependent insulinotropic polypeptide (GIP) is a polypeptide hormone containing 42 amino acids. This is also called **gastric inhibitory peptide** (GIP).

Source

GIP is produced by **K cells** present in the mucosa of duodenum and jejunum.

Functions

1. It **inhibits gastric secretion and motility**.
2. It **stimulates insulin secretion**. For this function, GIP is considered as an *important physiological regulator of insulin secretion*. Though other hormones like gastrin, CCK, secretin and glucagon also stimulate insulin secretion, plasma insulin ***level of insulin in response to GIP resembles the concentration of insulin*** attained following oral glucose ingestion.
   - Therefore, GIP is called **glucose-like insulinotropic polypeptide**.
   - However, **GLP-1**, derived from glucagon appears to be more potent than GIP in promoting insulin secretion.
   - Hence, both GIP and GLP-1 are among the important physiological regulator of insulin secretion from beta cells of pancreas.

Regulation of Secretion

Secretion of GIP is increased by glucose and fat in the duodenum.

VIP

Structure

VIP is a polypeptide containing 28 amino acids. It is formed from prepro-VIP that contains both VIP and PHM-27, a closely related peptide.

Source

VIP is secreted from mucosal cells of entire GIT, starting from stomach to colon. However, the secretion is more in the colon. It is found in the nerves of GIT, other autonomic nerves, blood and also in brain. Its half-life is 2 minutes.

Functions

1. It markedly **increases intestinal secretion rich in electrolytes and water**. Therefore, in excess it produces watery diarrhea.
2. It causes **vasodilation**. Therefore, it ***decreases blood pressure***.
3. It decreases GI motility. It causes **relaxation of intestinal smooth muscle including sphincters.**
4. It potentiates the action of acetylcholine on salivary glands.
5. It inhibits gastric acid secretion.

Clinical Significance

The tumor of VIP secreting cells is called **VIPoma**. Profuse watery ***diarrhea and hypotension*** are major features of VIPoma.

Glucagon

This is structurally similar with glucagon secreted from A cells of pancreas. In GIT, it is secreted from A cells in the stomach and L cells in intestine, where it is known as **enteroglucagon**. This produces hyperglycemia.

Glucagon-like Polypeptides

Glucagon is mainly produced from *A cells in pancreas* and *L cells in intestine*.

1. In A cells, preproglucagon is processed to form glucagon and **major proglucagon fragments** (MPGF), whereas in L cells it is processed to form glucagon, **glicentin** and **glucagon-like peptides** (GLP).
2. There are two GLPs: **GLP 1 and GLP 2,** and both are also produced in brain.
3. **GLP 1** is a potent stimulator of insulin secretion.
4. **GLP 2** does not have definitive biological activity.
5. However, GLP 2 produced in the brain inhibits food intake and acts as a neurotransmitter in the neurons that project from NTS to dorsomedial nucleus of hypothalamus.
6. Both A and L cells also produce oxyntomodulin and glicentin related polypeptide (**GRPP**).
7. **Oxyntomodulin** inhibits gastric acid secretion. Exact function of GRPP is not known.

MISCELLANEOUS FAMILY

Motilin

Structure and Source

This is a polypeptide hormone containing 22 amino acids. It is secreted from **enterochromaffin cells** and **Mo cells** present in the mucosa of all parts of GIT, except esophagus and rectum. It acts on G-protein coupled receptors on enteric neurons.

Functions

1. It causes contraction of intestinal smooth muscle and therefore, **increases GI motility**, especially *in the interdigestive phase*.
2. It is a **major regulator of migrating motor complex** (MMC), that regulates GI motility between meals.
3. Secretion of motilin is decreased following ingestion of a meal and its concentration remains low until the digestion and absorption of that meal is complete. Then the concentration increases and activates MMC that sweeps and cleans the intestine. Thus, it **prepares the intestine for next meal**.

Applied Physiology

Erythromycin can be used in patients having hypomotility of GI tract, as this antibiotic and its derivative bind to motilin receptors and facilitate intestinal motility.

Other Hormones

Neurotensin

This is a polypeptide hormone containing 13 amino acids. It is produced by neurons and mucosal cells of intestinal epithelium, mainly in ileum. **It inhibits GI motility** but increases ileal blood flow.

GRP

Gastrin releasing polypeptide (GRP) is a polypeptide containing 27 amino acids.

1. It is secreted from non-cholinergic vagal fibers.
2. It mediates gastrin release via **non-cholinergic vagal stimulation**.
3. The 10 amino acid residues at the carboxyl terminal of GRP is almost similar to the **bombesin** of amphibians.

Somatostatin

This is a polypeptide containing either 14 (***SS 14***) or 28 (***SS 28***) amino acids.

1. Somatostatin is secreted from GIT (starting from stomach to colon), hypothalamus and D cells of pancreas.
2. It *inhibits gastrin secretion*.
3. It also inhibits secretion of VIP, GIP, secretin, and motilin.
4. It is an inhibitory neurotransmitter in many parts of brain, especially in hypothalamus and pituitary.

Guanylin

Structure and Source

This is a polypeptide hormone containing 15 amino acids. It is secreted from the cells of intestinal mucosa. In human, it is produced by **Paneth cells** (endocrine cells located in the crypts of Lieberkuhn of small intestine).

Mechanism of Action

It acts by stimulating the **activity of guanylyl cyclase** (hence called guanylin) which increases the concentration of cGMP. The cGMP in turn **increases activity of chloride channels** and increases **chloride secretion** into the intestine.

Functions

Guanylin **increases secretion of chloride ions** into the intestinal lumen and therefore **regulates fluid movement** across intestinal tract. Guanylin receptors are present in kidney, liver and female reproductive tract. In these organs, guanylin appears to control fluid movement and particularly integrates the actions of intestine and kidneys.

Applied Physiology

Enterotoxins of some ***strains of E. coli*** that cause diarrhea have structural similarity with guanylin. They ***activate guanylin receptors*** in intestine and produce fluid secretion into the intestinal lumen.

TRH

This is structurally similar to the hypothalamic TRH. But, as it does not enter circulation, it does not produce any effect on thyroid. However, it is involved in the regulation of secretory immunity of intestine.

ACTH

Structurally, it is **similar to the ACTH** of anterior-pituitary. The function of intestinal ACTH is not clearly known.

Ghrelin

It is a 28 amino acid polypeptide secreted mainly from stomach. It has more systemic effects than local actions. It is a **strong orexigenic** agent that increases food intake by acting on arcuate nucleus of hypothalamus. It stimulates secretion of growth hormone from anterior pituitary.

Peptide YY

It is a polypeptide hormone secreted from small intestine and colon. It **inhibits gastric secretion and motility**.

Hence, it is proposed to be an **effective gastric inhibitory peptide**. Its secretion is stimulated by presence of fat in jejunum. Though, structurally it resembles neuropeptide Y that stimulates food intake, peptide YY inhibits feeding.

Substance P

Substance P is secreted from endocrine cells and neurons of entire GIT starting from stomach to colon. It **increases intestinal motility**. Its role in modulation of pain is discussed in "Physiology of Pain" in Sensory System.

CHAPTER SUMMARY

Key Concepts

1. Though of GI hormones have local effects, and they are called local hormones, many of them have systemic effects.
2. In addition to influence on GI secretion and motility, they affect food intake, metabolic functions, insulin and glucagon secretion, cardiovascular function and many brain functions.

Important to Know (Must Read)

1. In examinations, "Classify GI hormones and describe their functions" may come as a **Long Question**.
2. GI hormones of Gastrin family, GI hormones of secretin family, Gastrin, Cholecystokinin, Secretin, VIP, GIP, Enteroglucagon, Guanylin, Motilin, may come as **Short Questions** in exams.
3. In **Viva**, examiner may ask… Classification of GI hormones, structure and functions of any GI hormone, Applied aspect of any GI hormone.
4. GI hormones are usually asked in oral examination.

CHAPTER 38

Principles of GI Secretion and Secretion of Saliva

LEARNING OBJECTIVES

On completion of study of this chapter, the student **MUST** be able to:

1. Name the phases of GI secretion and give their physiological importance.
2. List the general functions of GI secretions.
3. Name salivary glands, and give the composition and function of saliva.
4. Outline the mechanism and control of salivary secretion.
5. Understand the dysfunctions that occur due to abnormalities of salivary secretion.

The student **MAY** also be able to:

1. Describe the regulation of salivary secretion.
2. Explain the physiological basis of salivary dysfunctions.

Secretions from exocrine glands associated with GI tract are called GI secretions. The major GI secretions include secretion from:

1. Salivary glands (***salivary secretion***)
2. Gastric glands (***gastric secretion***)
3. Exocrine pancreas (***pancreatic secretion***)
4. Liver (***bile secretion***)
5. Intestinal glands (***intestinal secretion***).

The major objectives of GI secretions are to facilitate digestion of food in the gut lumen, promote absorption of nutrients from the GI tract, and to assist in passage of luminal contents in aboral direction.

PRINCIPLES OF GI SECRETION

Phases of GI Secretions

Most of the GI secretions occur in **three phases**: cephalic, gastric, and intestinal. These phases are classified based on stimulus location.

Cephalic Phase

When stimuli activate the **brain mechanisms** (*cephalic* means "head") to alter GI secretions, the phase is called cephalic phase.

1. **Sight, smell, and thought** of food initiates cephalic phase of secretion. **Taste of food** (food in mouth) and chewing of food that increase GI secretions are also stimuli for cephalic phase.
2. Various **emotional states** also activate cephalic phase of secretions.
3. The **efferent pathway is the vagus nerve** that activates neurons in the ENS, which in turn influence gastric secretion and motility.

Physiological Importance of Cephalic Phase

Cephalic phase is important for **salivary, gastric, pancreatic, and bile secretions.**

1. It accounts for about **90% of volume of salivary secretion**. It contributes to about **40% of gastric and pancreatic secretions**. This simply indicates that GI tract *prepares for digestion* even before food enters into stomach and intestine.
2. In fact, sufficient GI secretions ***accumulate in advance*** in this phase so that the process of digestion starts as soon as food arrives in the gut, especially in the intestine.
3. Therefore, *it is desirable to spend some time in taking soup and starters before taking a major meal.*

Gastric Phase

Gastric phase starts **when food enters stomach**. Stimuli that influence GI secretions when food is present in the stomach are:

1. Distension of stomach
2. Chemical composition (especially, amino acids, and peptides) of food in the stomach
3. pH of the gastric content
4. Gastrin secreted from G cells.

Physiological Importance of Gastric Phase

Distension of stomach is the major mechanical event of gastric phase.

1. **Gastric distension** is the primary regulator of satiety.
2. It also greatly ***influences digestion*** of food by controlling GI secretions.
3. Gastric distension along with acidic chyme in the stomach and gastrin secreted from stomach, **activate short and long GI reflexes** to influence gastric, pancreatic, biliary, and intestinal secretions.
4. These secretions control the processes of digestion and absorption.

Intestinal Phase

Intestinal phase is initiated when **chyme enters duodenum**.

1. Products of digestion (fatty acids, peptides, etc.), presence of acidic chyme, intestinal distension and osmolality of intestinal contents are important stimuli in the intestinal phase of GI secretions.
2. They activate various **intestinal reflexes** to alter GI secretions.
3. **CCK, secretin, GIP, VIP,** and many other hormones are secreted during this phase.

Physiological Importance of Intestinal Phase

Chyme in the intestine requires enzymes for digestion of food particles in which the first step is to **hydrolyze macromolecules into their smaller absorbable forms**. This is achieved mainly by pancreatic and intestinal secretions.

1. Acidic chyme in duodenum stimulates secretion of CCK and secretin from upper part of small intestine that profoundly influence pancreatic and bile secretions.
2. Through reflex mechanisms, food in intestine inhibits gastric secretion and motility.

Principles of Regulation

Regulation of GI secretions occurs mainly by **neural and hormonal factors**. However, mechanisms specifically controlling these regulations *depend on the phase* of GI secretion.

1. For example, **cephalic phase is predominantly regulated by neural mechanisms,** whereas **gastric and intestinal phases are regulated by both hormonal and neural mechanisms.**
2. Accordingly, tests detecting the integrity of GI secretions are different for different phases.

General Functions of GI Secretion

1. **Digestion:** Enzymes in GI secretion are key elements for digestion of food particles in the GI tract. Broadly, these enzymes are amylases that digest carbohydrates, peptidases that digest proteins and lipases that digest lipids.
2. **Protection from infections:** Chemicals present in GI secretions protect the body from infections. For examples, lysozyme in secretions is antibacterial, IgA in saliva provides local immunity and HCl in gastric secretion kills all types of organisms.
3. **Mixing:** The aqueous part of secretions help in mixing of food with chemicals and enzymes in the secretions. This is essential for thorough exposure of food particles with chemicals for proper digestion of each ingredient in the food.
4. **Lubrication:** Mucus secretions facilitates passage of bolus of food or chyme along the GI tract in aboral direction. This especially helps in propulsion of food.
5. **Protection of mucosa:** The mucus and alkaline pH of secretions protect mucosal epithelium of gut from the harmful effects of HCl, bile acids, and toxins in the food.
6. **Absorption:** GI secretions present digested food materials to the epithelium of GI tract for absorption. Many food particles are dissolved and carried in GI secretions to the absorptive surface of the GI tract for absorption into blood and lymph.
7. **Appetite regulation:** Chemicals in GI secretions stimulate appetite. For example, bile acids and HCl are appetizers in physiological concentration. Therefore, patients with achlorohydria (gastric atrophy) and bile deficiency (liver disease) develop anorexia. However, in high concentration these chemicals may also inhibit appetite.

SALIVARY SECRETION

The secretion from the salivary glands is called salivary secretion. It is secreted from a heterogeneous group of salivary glands located in and around the mouth cavity. Salivary secretion is distinctive for its exclusive neural regulation.

Scientists contributed

Niels Stensen (1638–1686) was a prominent Danish scientist who laid the foundations of paleontology, geology, and crystallography. Though he is known eponymously for the discovery of the duct of the parotid gland (**Stensen's duct**) and ***study of salivary secretion***, he researched more on the anatomy of the brain, and did seminal investigation on ***methods in neuroscience***. His scientific letter on a hydrocephalic calf represents an early pathophysiological ***investigation on hydrocephalus***.

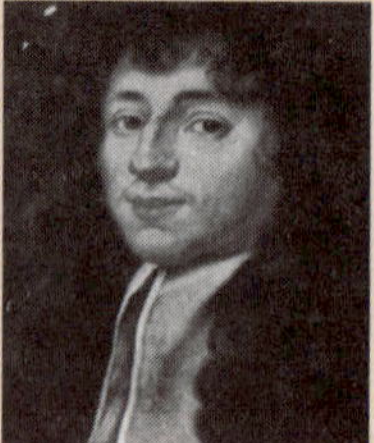

Niels Stensen
(1638–1686)

Source: Perrini P, Lanzino G, Parenti GF. Niels Stensen (1638-1686): scientist, neuroanatomist, and saint. Neurosurgery. 2010 Jul;67(1):3-9; doi: 10.1227/01.

Thomas Wharton (1614–1673), a great physician from Cambridge, received fellowship of Royal College of Physicians for his extensive studies on **salivary and pancreatic secretions.** Wharton described the glands more accurately relying on his dissection and experiment. He was the discoverer of the duct of the sub-mandibulary gland for the conveyance of the saliva into the mouth, which bears his name (**Wharton's duct**). He made a special study of the minute anatomy of the pancreas.

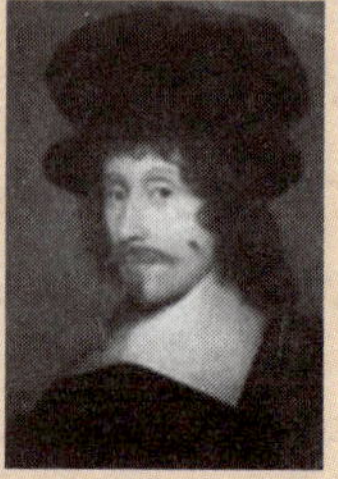

Thomas Wharton
(1614–1673)

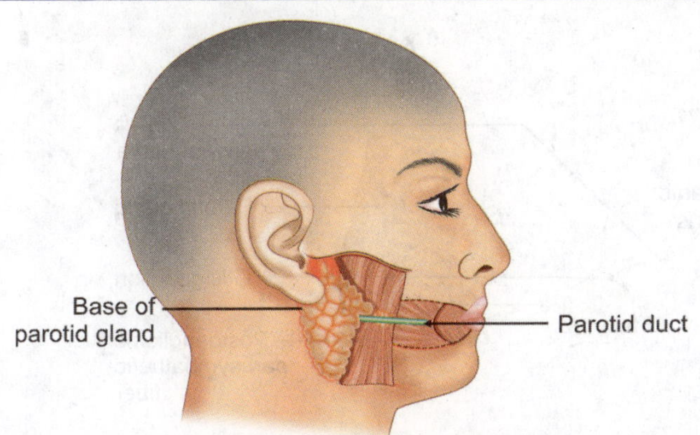

Fig. 38.1: Location of parotid gland and the parotid duct.
Courtesy: Figure 63.1, Clinical Anatomy, by Neeta Kulkarni, Vol. 2, 3rd edition, 2016; Jaypee Brothers Medical Publishers (P) Ltd.

Salivary Glands

Types

There are **major and minor salivary glands**.

1. **Major salivary glands** are three pairs: parotid, sublingual and submandibular glands.
2. There are many **minor salivary glands** located in the mucosa of oral cavity, at the pharyngeal outlet, in the palates and in buccal pouches.

Based on nature of secretion: Salivary glands may be **serous** that exclusively release watery secretions, **mucous** that secrete viscous secretion mainly containing mucus and **mixed** that secrete moderately viscous secretions.

Parotid Glands

Parotid glands are the largest salivary glands.

1. They are **entirely serous glands**. Serous cells are usually arranged in the form of rounded acini.
2. The parotid secretion is rich in water and electrolytes, and lacks mucins.
3. They pour their secretion into the mouth cavity by means of parotid duct (***duct of Stensen***), which opens into the oral cavity at the level of second molar tooth (Fig. 38.1).

Sublingual Glands

These glands are situated below the tongue in the floor of the mouth.

1. Secretions from these glands drain directly into the mouth by means of sublingual ducts (***ducts of Rivinus***).
2. There are about 10 sublingual ducts. Sublingual glands are **predominantly mucous glands**.
3. They secrete thick viscous saliva.

Submandibular Glands

Submandibular, also called *submaxillary glands* are situated below the inner ramus of mandible on both sides.

1. They pour their secretion into the mouth cavity by means of submandibular ducts (***ducts of Wharton***).
2. These glands are **mixed type** (both serous and mucous).

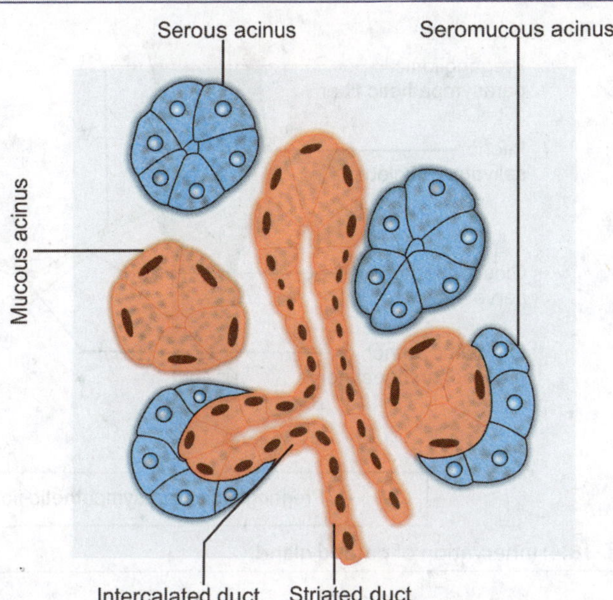

Fig. 38.2: Structure of a salivon (with types of acini in salivary glands). Note the location of intercalated and striated ducts in the gland.

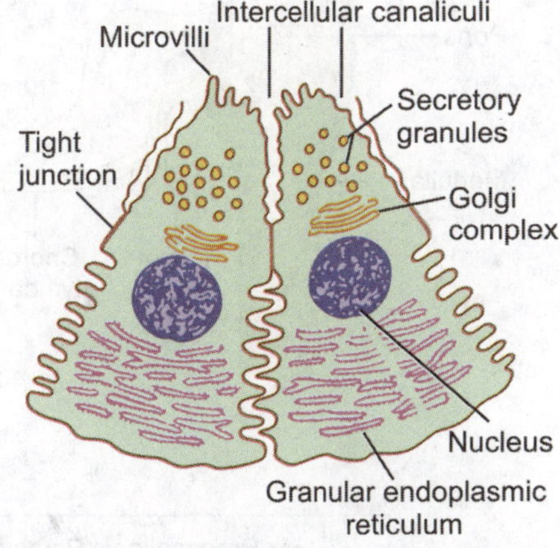

Fig. 38.3: Features of serous cells in a salivary gland.

Histology of Salivary Glands

Salivary gland consists of base units called **salivon**. Each salivon consists of acinus, intercalated duct and striated duct (Fig. 38.2).

Acinus

Acinus is a sac like structure containing many **pyramidal cells**. Myoepithelial cells are present at places surrounding the pyramidal cells.

1. **Serous cells** of acinus contain many endoplasmic reticulum and zymogen granules, and secrete digestive enzyme, whereas **mucous cells** contain mucin droplets and secrete mucin (Fig. 38.3).
2. The secretion in the acinus is called **primary secretion**. Electrolyte composition of primary secretion is similar to that of plasma.

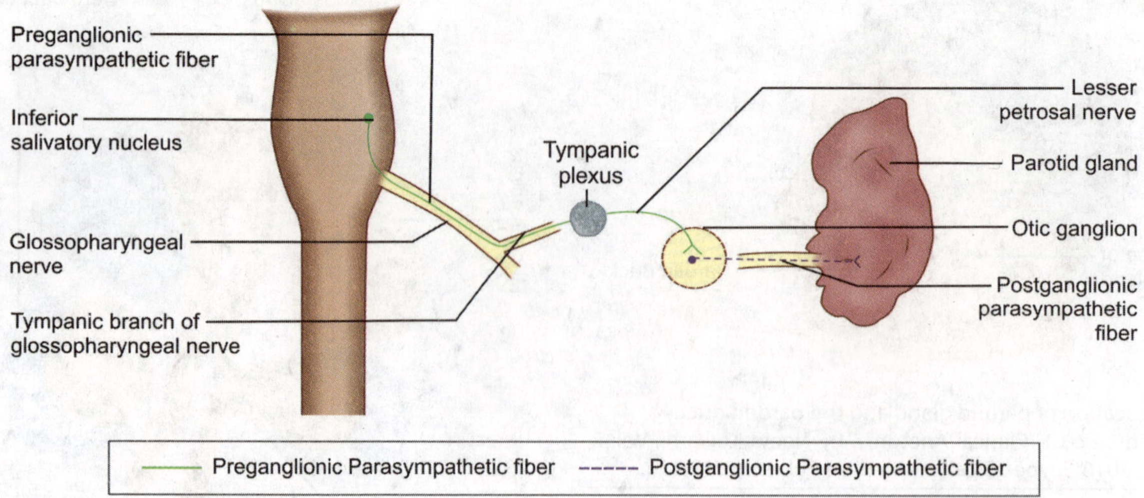

Fig. 38.4: Innervation of parotid gland.

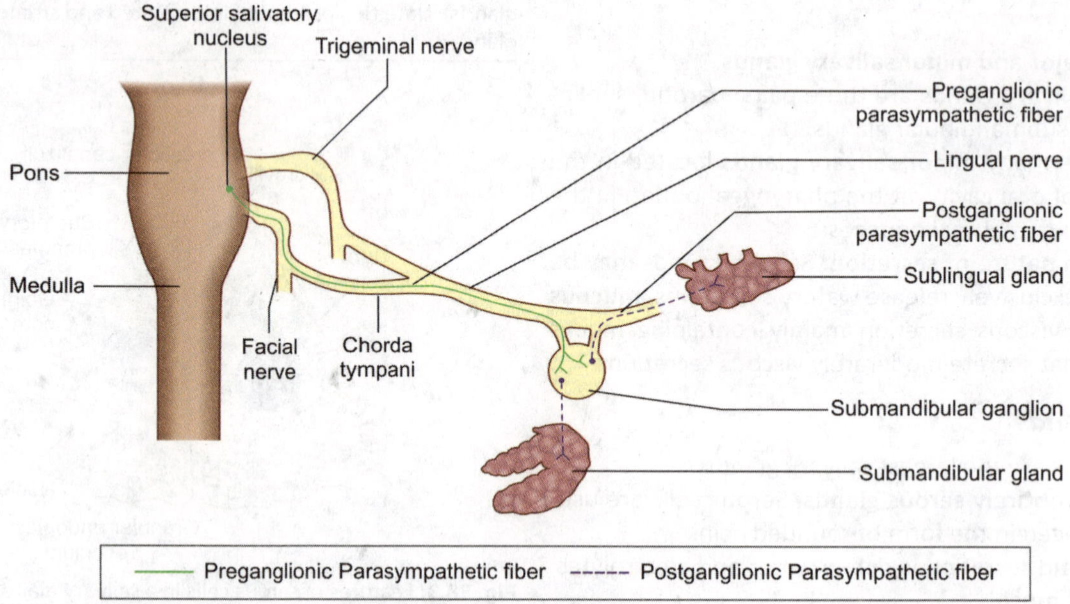

Fig. 38.5: Innervation of submandibular and sublingual glands.

Intercalated and Striated Ducts

These ducts are lined by cuboidal cells. Secretion from these duct epithelial cells modifies the ionic composition of secretion from acinus and determines the final composition of saliva. Secretion coming out of duct is called **modified or final secretion.**

Innervation of Salivary Glands

Salivary glands are innervated by both the divisions of autonomic nervous system. In normal situation, parasympathetic innervation is the major neural factor for salivary secretion.

Parasympathetic Innervation

The centers for parasympathetic fibers are located in medulla.

1. Preganglionic fibers for parotid gland are present in 9th cranial nerve that originate in **inferior salivary nucleus** and terminate in **otic ganglion** from where postganglionic fibers originate and innervate the gland (Fig. 38.4).
2. Fibers for **submandibular and sublingual glands** are present in the 7th cranial nerve that originate from ***superior salivary nucleus*** and terminate in ***submandibular ganglion*** from where postganglionic fibers come out and supply the glands (Fig. 38.5).
3. In general, **parasympathetic stimulation is excitatory**.

Sympathetic Innervation

Sympathetic fibers originate from upper cervical segments and terminate in **superior cervical ganglion**. Postganglionic fibers leave the ganglion and innervate acini, duct and blood vessels. In general, **sympathetic stimulation is inhibitory**.

Salivary Blood Flow

Salivary glands have a high rate of metabolism and a high blood flow. Blood flow and metabolism are *proportionate to the rate of saliva formation*.

1. The **rate of salivary secretion** in human is about ***50 mL/min/100 g*** of salivary tissue.
2. Blood flow to salivary glands is about 10 times the blood flow to that of active skeletal muscles.
3. **Stimulation of parasympathetic nerve** to salivary gland ***increases blood flow*** by about 10 times by causing vasodilation, which occurs due to secretion of ***VIP, bradykinin, and acetylcholine*** at nerve terminals.
4. **Sympathetic stimulation** *decreases blood flow*.

Salivary Secretion

Rate of Secretion

About **1.5 liters** (1,000–1,800 mL) of saliva is secreted every day. Normally, we never realize the amount of saliva secreted as it is a continuous and slow process. Salivary secretion even continues in minimum amount during sleep. However, an **orexigenic stimulus**, especially sight, smell or thought of food causes immediate and profuse salivation. We realize the importance of salivation when the secretion becomes less and mouth becomes dry. Salivary secretion **increases in response to feeding**.

Composition of Saliva

Saliva contains mainly water (99.5%) and some solids (0.5%). Solids are organic and inorganic.

Organic Solids

Organic solids are mainly **enzymes** such as ptyalin, lysozyme, lactoperoxidase, carbonic anhydrase, lingual lipase, RNAase, and DNAase. ***Other organic solids*** include kallikrein, blood group substances, secretory immunoglobulin (IgA), and nerve growth factor.

Inorganic Solids

Cations like sodium, calcium, potassium, and magnesium ions, and **anions** like chloride, bicarbonate, phosphate, sulfate, and bromide ions constitute the inorganic solids.

Tonicity of Saliva

In human beings, **saliva is always hypotonic to plasma**. The concentration of sodium and chloride ions in saliva is less than that of plasma. The tonicity of saliva depends on the rate at which saliva is produced. Greater the rate of secretion, higher is the tonicity. The tonicity of saliva is about 70% of that of plasma.

The pH and K^+ Content of Saliva

The pH of saliva is alkaline (about 8).

1. The pH of the original secretion in the salivary gland is slightly acidic. But as saliva flows down the salivary ducts, it becomes alkaline because of secretion of bicarbonate from the duct epithelium.
2. The decrease in flow rate in duct increases bicarbonate concentration as time to add more bicarbonate increases, and therefore, this increases pH.
3. However, if the **increase in flow is due to parasympathetic stimulation**, secretion of bicarbonate from duct cells is more that increases salivary content of bicarbonate.
4. Therefore, invariably with increased flow rate, bicarbonate content becomes high.
5. The concentration of **K^+ in saliva is always greater than that in plasma**, but with increase in flow rate, K^+ concentration decreases.

Functions of Saliva

Saliva performs many important digestive and non-digestive functions.

1. Saliva contains **ptyalin**. This is an enzyme called *salivary amylase*, which causes **splitting of starch**. Salivary amylase reduces starch to oligosaccharide molecules. However, digestion of starch is not impaired in the absence of salivary amylase (if pancreas is intact). Action of salivary amylase is maximum at pH 6.8. But, digestion by ptyalin takes place in the stomach, as food remains for a short duration in mouth. In the stomach, digestion occurs at the center of food bolus which is still alkaline, until the food is thoroughly mixed with the acidic gastric secretion of the stomach.
2. Saliva has many **protective functions**. Saliva keeps the mouth clean and therefore **prevents oral infection**. Saliva contains **lysozyme**, which is anti-bacterial. **IgA** in saliva provides local immunity and **lactoferrin** in saliva is bacteriostatic.
3. Saliva keeps the mouth cavity and tongue moist, which **facilitates speech**. The importance of this function of saliva is realized when mouth becomes dry due to decreased salivary secretion that impairs speech. Dryness of mouth is usually felt before appearing for an interview, especially for learners.
4. Saliva increases the **taste of food**. Taste is perceived by the taste buds present in the tongue. For taste of food to be well appreciated, food particles should better be present in solution. Saliva dissolves the food and makes the solution of food.
5. Saliva helps in **mastication and swallowing**. This is due to lubricant property of saliva. The mucin in saliva lubricates food. In the absence of saliva, deglutition becomes impossible, especially for dry foods.
6. Saliva contains bicarbonate which **buffers gastric acid** to some extent in the stomach, and therefore reduces heart burn.
7. Proline rich protein in saliva **protects enamel** of the teeth and thus provides them strength. Proline also binds with tannin & reduces its toxicity.
8. Saliva **prevents injury to buccal mucosa** by diluting the hot and irritant food materials.

9. In animals, salivation (panting) is an important process of dissipation of heat and therefore, has contribution in **temperature regulation**.
10. Saliva ***excretes certain heavy metals, thiocyanate and morphine*** from the body.

Mechanism of Secretion

Salivary secretion occurs in **two stages**: secretion in the acinus and secretion in the duct.

Secretion in Acinus of Gland

In the gland acini, the secretion is called **primary secretion** in which ***amylase concentration is more***.

1. The enzyme is produced and stored in the zymogen granules.
2. On stimulation, granules are exocytosed and the enzyme is released.
3. The electrolytes secreted from the epithelial cells of the end pieces are Na^+, K^+, HCO_3^-, and Cl^-.
4. The **fluid of primary secretion is almost isotonic** to that of plasma.

Secretion in Ducts

The composition of secretion in the ducts when the fluid passes through the intercalated and striated ducts, is modified. This is called **modified** or **final secretion**.

1. This is because Na^+ and Cl^- are extracted from the fluid and K^+ and HCO_3^- are added to the fluid.
2. The ducts do not change the volume of saliva but only modify the composition of the primary secretion (Fig. 38.6).

Stimuli for Salivary Secretion

Saliva is continuously secreted. However, a large number of stimuli increase the secretion. The important stimuli are **anticipation, thought, sight and smell of food, discussion on food, and presence of food** in the mouth cavity. **Chewing** is also an important stimulus for salivary secretion.

Control of Salivary Secretion

Salivary secretion is controlled exclusively by the neural mechanisms. Both sympathetic and parasympathetic stimuli influence salivary secretion.

Neural Control

Parasympathetic Stimulation

Parasympathetic stimulation occurs by sight, smell, and taste of food.

1. **Chewing** of food is a potent stimulus for salivary secretion. These factors act through **salivary nucleus** in the medulla (Flowchart 38.1).

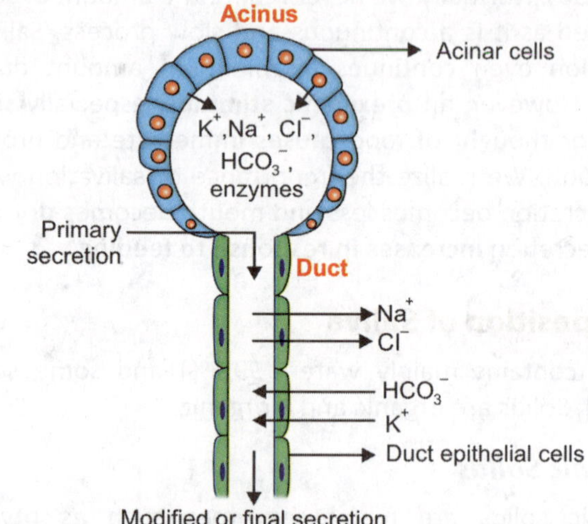

Fig. 38.6 : Mechanism of salivary secretion. Note the processes that determine ionic compositions of primary and modified secretions.

Flowchart 38.1 : Mechanism of increased salivary secretion by parasympathetic stimulation.

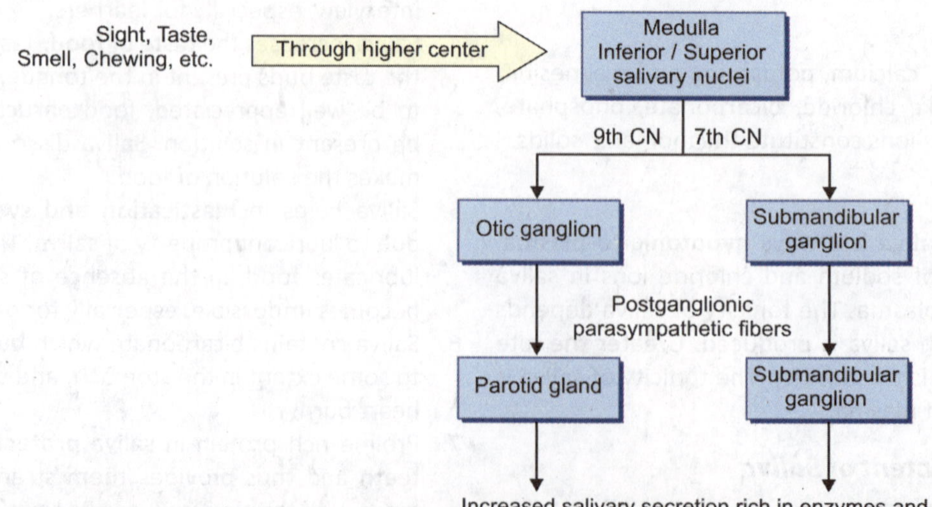

(CN: Cranial nerve).

2. Parasympathetic activation **increases salivary secretion rich in enzymes, and mucin.**
3. It increases secretion by causing *vasodilation* (via bradykinin, VIP, and acetylcholine), and *stimulation of glandular tissue*.

Sympathetic Stimulation

Stimulation of sympathetic fibers (sympathetic fibers to salivary gland originate from superior cervical ganglion) temporarily increases secretion but finally decreases it.

1. The *transient increase* is due to contraction of myoepithelial cells of the glandular tissue.
2. However, sympathetic stimulation causes *vasoconstriction* that decreases saliva formation and makes the secretion thick.

Reflex Secretion

Saliva is secreted reflexly by contact of food with the mouth cavity. This reflex secretion is **unconditioned** as this is present since birth (does not need learning). However, salivary secretion due to smell or thought of food is a **condition reflex** as these are learnt by social and environmental factors. Conditioned salivary secretion was described by Pavlov.

Salivary secretion exclusively occurs in the **cephalic phase** (sight, smell and thought of food, presence of food in mouth, chewing food, etc.). Secretion is almost nil in gastric and intestinal phase of digestion of food. Hormonal regulation of saliva is negligible.

Applied Physiology

Xerostomia

This is a condition in which there is consistent decreased secretion of saliva. This causes dryness of mouth, and predisposes to oral infections. Xerostomia (dryness of mouth) is a common in acute stressful situation that happens due to sympathetic stimulation

Sialorrhea

In this condition, salivary secretion is increased persistently.

Sialolithiasis

This is the condition in **which stone is formed in the ducts** of salivary gland.

Infections

Viral infection of parotid gland is seen commonly in children (mumps).

CHAPTER SUMMARY

Key Concepts

1. Though salivary secretion does not help much in digestion, it is very essential for chewing, deglutition, speech and oral and dental hygiene.
2. Parasympathetic stimulates and sympathetic inhibits salivary secretion.
3. Xerostomia (dryness of mouth) is a common condition in acute stressful situations that happens due to sympathetic stimulation.

Important to Know (Must Read)

1. In examinations, "Composition, mechanism and regulation of salivary secretion" may sometimes come as a **Long Question**.
2. Phases of GI secretions, Salivary secretion, Composition and function of salivary secretion, Mechanism of salivary secretion, Regulation of salivary secretion may be asked as **short questions**.
3. In **Viva**, examiner may ask... What are the Phases of GI secretions and how are they generally controlled, Amount of salivary secretion/day, Name of salivary glands, Histologic types of salivary glands, Innervation of salivary glands by parasympathetic and sympathetic fibers, Composition and function of salivary secretion, Function of each constituent of saliva, Mechanism of salivary secretion, What are the differences between primary and secondary salivary secretion, Regulation of salivary secretion, What are the effects of parasympathetic and sympathetic stimulation, What is Xerostomia, silaorrhea and sialolithiasis.
4. Composition and functions of saliva are usually asked in oral examination. A student is expected to answer this; otherwise it may be difficult for him to pass.

CHAPTER 39

Gastric Secretion

Learning Objectives

On completion of study of this chapter, the student **MUST** be able to:

1. List the functions of stomach.
2. Give the structure of gastric glands.
3. Understand the difference in the structure of resting and activated parietal cell.
4. Give the composition and functions of gastric juice.
5. Describe the mechanism of HCl secretion.
6. Describe regulation of gastric secretion in different phases.
7. Name gastric function tests and their normal values.
8. Understands the physiological basis of etiology of peptic ulcer.

The student **MAY** also be:

1. Describe the physiological basis and application of gastric function tests.
2. Appreciate the physiological basis of treatment of peptic ulcer.

Stomach is an important part of GI system. Though the major function of stomach is the storage of food, it regulates controlled emptying of food into the duodenum and prepares the chyme for digestion and absorption in the small intestine. Chyme results from grinding of food into smaller particles and mixing of food with gastric secretion.

FUNCTIONS AND FUNCTIONAL ANATOMY OF STOMACH

Functions of Stomach

1. **Temporary storage of food:** The primary function of stomach is the temporary storage of food. It serves as a **reservoir for food** so that ingestion of a large meal at a time becomes possible.
2. **Grinding and mixing of food**: Stomach causes grinding and mixing of food. It churns the food and breaks larger food particles (macromolecules) into smaller molecules. It also mixes food with gastric juice. The content of stomach after proper mixing with gastric juice is called **chyme**.
3. **Controlled emptying of food:** Stomach performs its ***own controlled emptying (gastric emptying)***. It allows food to enter into duodenum and jejunum at a lesser but controlled rate so that load on the upper part of the small intestine is not more than the amount that it can handle. This allows intestine to digest and absorb nutrients slowly, steadily and adequately.
4. **Secretion of hydrochloric acid:** Stomach secretes hydrochloric acid (HCl), which is essential for digestion of food. Though the exact nature of digestion by HCl is not clearly known, hypochlorohydria decreases the process of digestion and impairs appetite.
5. HCl in the stomach **converts ferric form of iron into ferrous form**. Iron is absorbed from gut only in the ferrous form. Therefore, ***HCl deficiency in the stomach results in iron deficiency anemia***.
6. **Kills the microorganism**: Gastric HCl kills the bacteria and other ingested microorganisms. Therefore, entry of microbes into body through GI system is prevented in the stomach.
7. **Activates pepsinogen to pepsin:** HCl activates pepsinogen to pepsin, an *endopeptidase*. Pepsin cleaves protein molecules to form smaller peptides. The optimal pH

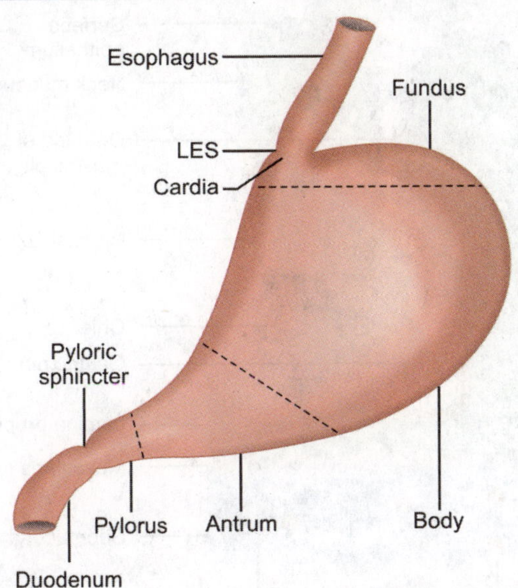

Fig. 39.1: Parts of the stomach. (LES: Lower esophageal sphincter).

Fig. 39.2: Interior of the stomach (in empty condition). Note the presence of gastric rugae.
Courtesy: Figure 50.5, Clinical Anatomy, by Neeta Kulkarni, Vol. 2, 3rd edition, 2016; Jaypee Brothers Medical Publishers (P) Ltd.

for endopeptidase activity is 1.8 to 3.5. Thus, HCl not only activates pepsin, but also ***provides acidic environment*** for action of pepsin.

8. **Secretes intrinsic factor:** Stomach secretes intrinsic factor (IF) which is essential for **reabsorption of vitamin B_{12}** (the extrinsic factor) in the terminal ileum. Vitamin B_{12} binds with intrinsic factor to from IF-B_{12} complex, which is taken up by **cubilin**, a lipoprotein present in the terminal part of ileum and then absorbed by endocytosis. Therefore, gastrectomy or chronic gastric atrophy results in **megaloblastic anemia** (Clinical Box 39.1).
9. Stomach helps in **absorption of water and lipid soluble substances**, such as alcohol and few drugs.

Clinical Box 39.1

Dimorphic anemia: When red cell morphologies in an anemia have both microcytic and macrocytic features, the type of anemia is called dimorphic anemia. Anemia following gastrectomy or chronic gastric atrophy results in such type of anemia, as HCl deficiency causes microcytic hypochromic anemia due to iron deficiency and intrinsic factor deficiency causes megaloblastic anemia due to B_{12} deficiency.

Functional Anatomy

Anatomically, stomach is divided into **three major parts**: fundus, body and antrum (Fig. 39.1). Esophagus opens into stomach through *gastro-esophageal junction* that contains ***lower esophageal sphincter*** (LES). The initial portion of the stomach close to gastroesophageal junction is called ***cardia***. The proximal part of stomach is called **fundus**, the middle and major part of stomach is the **body or corpus**, and the distal portion of the stomach is the **antrum**. Antrum opens into the duodenum through pylorus which contains pyloric sphincter:

1. The capacity of the stomach depends on age, gender and eating habit. On average, it is about 1.5 liter in adults, though it varies from 1 to 4 liters.
2. The **mucous membrane of stomach** is thick and thrown into large folds, called **gastric rugae**. These rugae are more prominent in empty stomach (Fig. 39.2).
3. The mucosal epithelium is formed by ***simple columnar epithelial cells*** that secrete mucous and alkaline fluid.
4. These mucous and alkaline fluids protect gastric epithelium from acidic content and mechanical injury. The mucosal surface of stomach is studded with **gastric pits** (faveola) into which gastric glands empty (Fig. 39.3).
5. The gastric glands are situated deep in the mucosal infoldings that open into the pits.

Gastric Glands

The mucosal lining of the stomach is a glandular mucosa that contains surface mucous cells in the gastric pit and glands deep in the mucosal infoldings. There are three types of gastric glands:

1. **The cardiac glands**: Located below the lower esophageal sphincter and contain mainly mucous secreting cells. They secrete mucous and bicarbonate ions.
2. **The oxyntic glands:** Located in the fundus and body of the stomach and contain mainly the oxyntic cells.
3. **Pyloric glands:** Present in the pyloric-antral region and consist mainly of mucous neck cells that secrete mucous and G cells that secrete gastrin.

Oxyntic Gland

The acid secreting oxyntic gland is typically a tubular and straight gland (Fig. 39.4). It consists of neck, body and base. The cells in the neck are mainly mucous secreting cell. The **oxyntic cells** are present mainly in the body of the gland. Chief or **peptic cells** are present at the base.

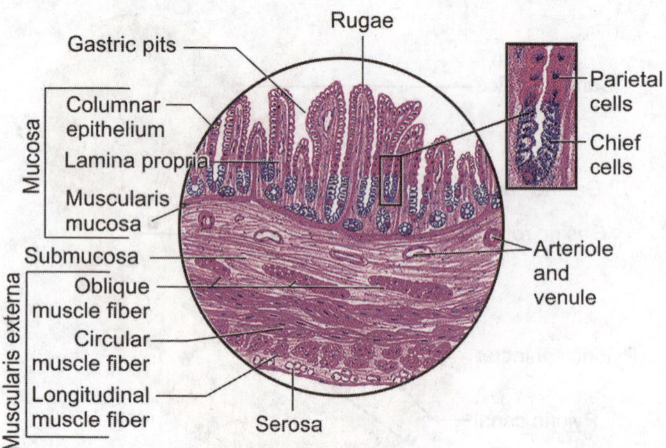

Fig. 39.3: Layers of stomach wall in the body of stomach. The epithelium of the mucosa is simple columnar epithelium. Note the location of gastric pit, into which the gastric glands open. Structure of a gastric gland containing chief cell and parietal cell is depicted in the inset.
Courtesy: Figure 13.17A, Basic Histology, by V Subhadra Devi, 1st edition, 2016; Jaypee Brothers Medical Publishers (P) Ltd.

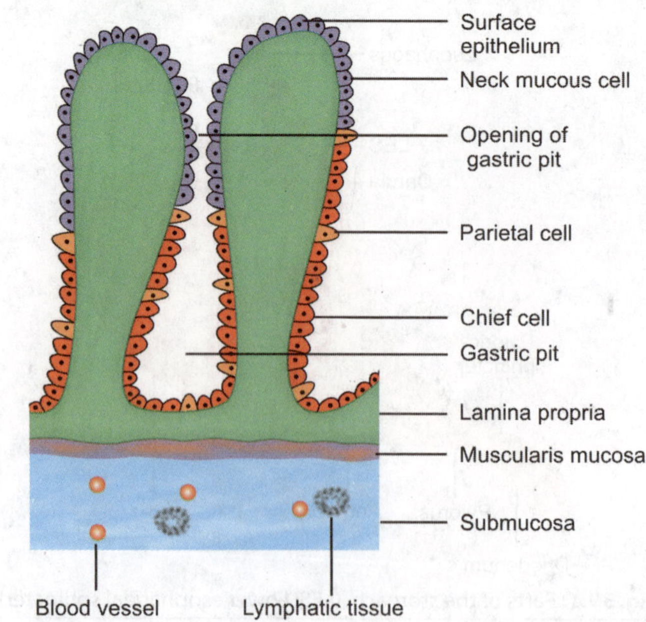

Fig. 39.4: Parts of a gastric oxyntic gland.

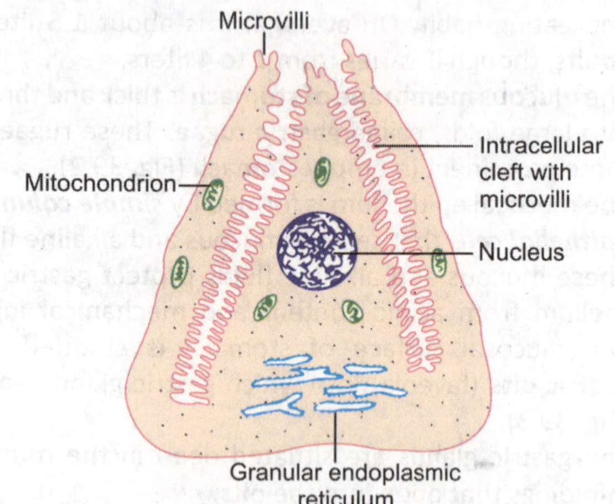

Fig. 39.5: Structure of a parietal cell in the resting state. Note the intracellular cleft contains tubules and vesicles.

Different cell types in the oxyntic glands are:

1. **Mucous cells:** They are present in the neck region of the gland. The mucous and bicarbonate ions secreted by them protect the stomach epithelium from acidic gastric secretion.
2. **Oxyntic or Parietal cells:** Oxyntic cells are present mainly in the body part of the gland. They secrete hydrochloric acid and intrinsic factor.
3. **Chief or peptic cells:** Chief cells are present towards the base of the gland. They secrete pepsinogen.
4. **Endocrine cells:** The endocrine cells are also called *enterochromaffin cells*. The major endocrine cells in oxyntic glands are **enterochromaffin-like cells (ECL)** or **mast-like cells** that secrete histamine. There are also other endocrine cells that secrete somatostatin, VIP, glucagon, and enkephalin. **G cells** are present in antral region that secrete gastrin. Antrum also contains **D cells** that secrete somatostatin.

Structure of Oxyntic Cells

Oxyntic cells or parietal cells are present in the body and neck of the oxyntic glands. They secrete hydrochloric acid and intrinsic factor:

1. They have extensive **tubulovesicular system** and **open canalicular system**.
2. The apex of the parietal cells faces towards the lumen of the gastric glands. The canaliculi extend from apical surface into the cell. The tubules and vesicles open into the canaliculi.
3. **In resting cells**, tubules and vesicles are present abundantly (Fig. 39.5) and microvilli are rudimentary. The membrane of these tubulovesicular structures contains **H^+-K^+ ATPase**.
4. **On activation**, the tubulovesicular membranes fuse with the cell membrane and microvilli that project into the canaliculi (Fig. 39.6), so that the *area of cell membrane in contact with gastric lumen is greatly increased*.
5. Fusion of tubules and vesicle with microvillar or canalicular membrane ensures ***increased H^+-K^+ ATPase activity of the membrane*** in the active state.

Nerve Supply of Stomach

Stomach is supplied by both divisions of ANS:

1. Parasympathetic innervation is by vagus nerve.
2. **Vagal stimulation facilitates** and **sympathetic stimulation inhibits** gastric secretion and motility.

Gastric Juice

Composition of Gastric Juice

The amount of gastric secretion per day varies from 1 to 2.5 liters. The gastric juice is **highly acidic**; having **pH** 0.7–4. It has following constituents:

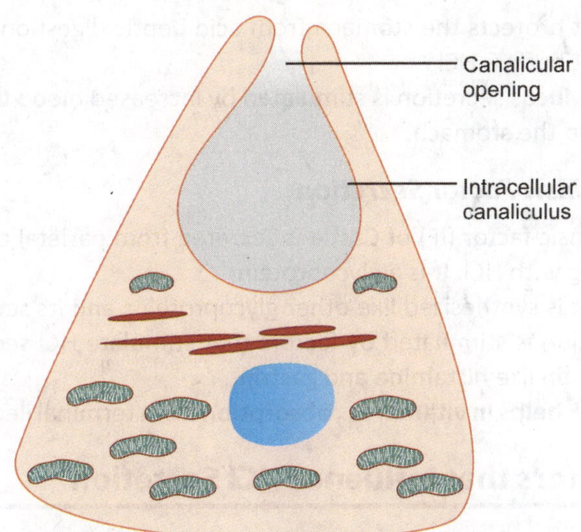

Fig. 39.6: Structure of a parietal cell in the activated state. Note that tubules and vesicles are inserted to the membrane of canaliculus.

1. Water (99.5%)
2. Solids (0.5%)

   Solids contain inorganic and organic substances.

   Inorganic constituents: Anions are Cl^-, PO_4^{3-}, SO_4^{2-}, and HCO_3^-; and cations are H^+, Na^+, K^+, Ca^{2+}, and Mg^{2+}.

   Organic constituents: Pepsinogen, intrinsic factor, mucin, rennin, gastric lipase, gelatinase, carbonic anhydrase, and lysozyme.

Functions of Constituents

Normal concentration of HCl is 40–60 mEq/L. The maximum concentration can increase upto 150 mEq/L:

1. *Pepsinogen* is secreted from the peptic cells. There are **two types of pepsinogens**:
   - **Type-I pepsinogen** is found in chief cells in fundus and body.
   - **Type-II pepsinogen** is found in the chief cells throughout the stomach.
2. Pepsinogen is **converted into pepsin** by HCl. Pepsin is a proteolytic enzyme that breaks down protein molecules into peptones. Pepsin acts best at pH of 2–4.
3. The **mucin** secreted by mucous cells is of ***two types***: the ***insoluble mucin***, and the ***soluble mucin***. Mucin forms a protective layer on the gastric epithelium. It retains bicarbonate and has alkaline pH. Thus, it protects the stomach from acid peptic digestion, as it buffers HCl.
4. **Intrinsic factor helps in vitamin B_{12} absorption** from terminal ileum.

GASTRIC SECRETION

Mechanism of HCl Secretion

HCl is secreted from **parietal cells** that are located in the fundus and body of the stomach. H^+ secretion is possible in stomach due to the presence of numerous **H^+–K^+ ATPases** in apical membrane of the parietal cells:

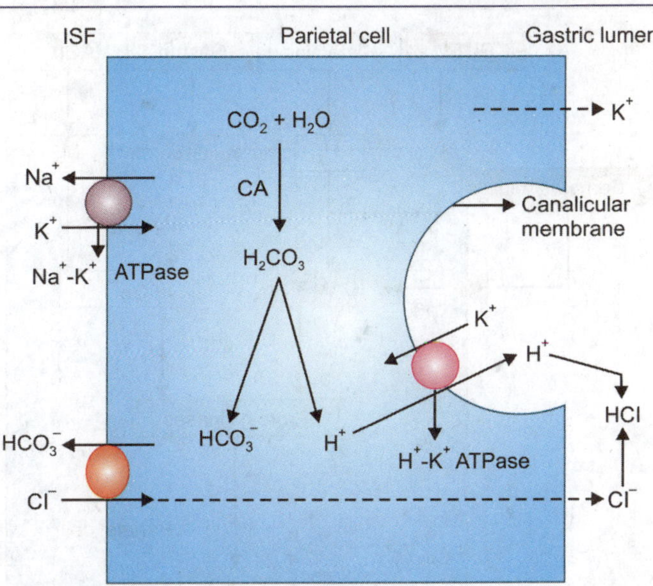

Fig. 39.7: Mechanism of HCl secretion from gastric parietal cell. (CA: Carbonic anhydrase). The dashed lines for K^+ and Cl^- depict their passive diffusion into the gastric lumen. Note the presence of H^+–K^+ ATPase on the canalicular membrane that pumps K^+ into the cell for H^+ into the gastric lumen. (ISF: Interstitial fluid).

1. H^+–K^+ pump actively pumps H^+ (against its concentration gradient) out of the cell into the gastric lumen. In exchange for H^+, the K^+ enters the cell (Fig. 39.7). As this is an active transport, energy is provided for the process by hydrolysis of ATP.
2. In the cytosol of parietal cell, H^+ is derived from the ***break down of carbonic acid*** (H_2CO_3). H_2CO_3 is formed by combination of CO_2 and H_2O in a reaction catalyzed by **carbonic anhydrase.** This step can be blocked by *acetazolamide*, the carbonic anhydrase inhibitor.
3. CO_2 utilized for formation of H_2CO_3 is derived from intracellular metabolisms and plasma.
4. HCO_3^- formed by break down of H_2CO_3 is exchanged for Cl^- on the basolateral membrane of the cell by **HCO_3^--Cl^- exchanger.**
5. The Cl^- that enters parietal cell is transported into the gastric lumen.
6. In the lumen, Cl^- combines with H^+ to form HCl.
7. The **HCO_3^- enters blood stream** from the interstitial fluid.

Thus, *for each H^+ secreted into the gastric lumen, one HCO_3^- is reabsorbed into the plasma*. Therefore, with ***increase in the rate of HCl secretion, HCO_3^- level increases in the blood.*** Consequently, following a meal that stimulates gastric acid secretion, pH of blood increases. As blood becomes alkaline, the urine becomes alkaline. This is called **post-prandial alkaline tide.**

K^+ that enters the oxyntic cell by H^+-K^+ ATPase is transported back into the gastric lumen, which is ***reutilized*** for further H^+secretion (recycling of K^+). K^+ entering the

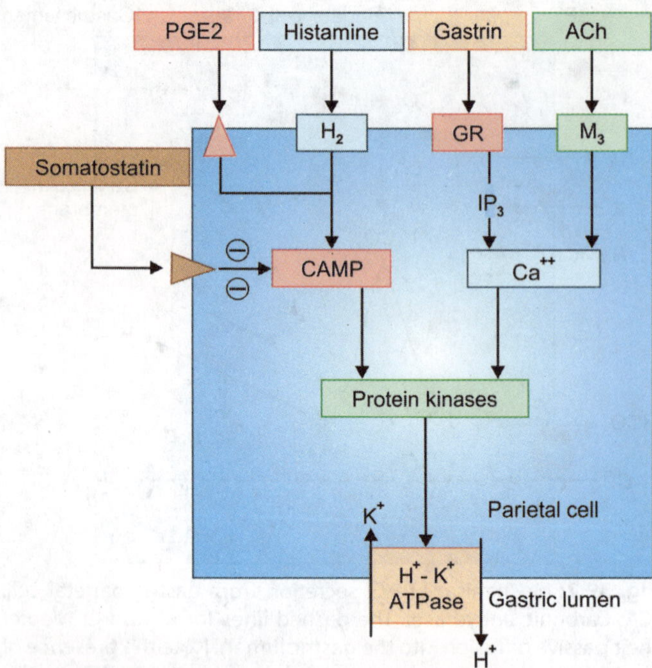

Fig. 39.8: Mechanism of actions of hormones on parietal cell. (GR: Gastrin receptor; M_3: Muscarinic type 3 receptor; H_2: Histamine type 2 receptor; ACh: Acetylcholine; PGE_2: Prostaglandin E_2). Note, finally calcium and cAMP acts as second messengers for hormones that activate H^+-K^+ ATPase to pump H^+ into the gastric lumen. Minus sign indicates inhibition.

cell from basolateral membrane is also secreted into the lumen. Thus, adequate $K^+$is available in the lumen for effective H^+-K^+ pump activity.

Secretion of Other Constituents

Pepsinogen Secretion

Pepsinogen is secreted from chief cells. It is synthesized in the cell like other proteins and stored in the zymogen granules:

1. There are two types of pepsinogens: **type-I pepsinogen**, found in chief cells in fundus and body and **type-II pepsinogen** found in the chief cells throughout the stomach.
2. Pepsinogen is converted into pepsin by HCl.
3. Pepsin is a strong proteolytic enzyme.
4. Pepsinogen secretion is stimulated by gastrin and histamine.

Mucus Secretion

Mucus is secreted by mucus secreting cells that are plentily available in the neck region of gastric glands:

1. The **mucin** secreted by mucous cells is of two types: the ***insoluble mucin***, which is secreted by mucus secreting cells of entire gastric mucosa and the ***soluble mucin***, secreted from mainly cardiac and pyloric mucosal cells.
2. Mucin forms a protective layer on the gastric epithelium. It retains bicarbonate and has alkaline pH. Thus, it protects the stomach from acid peptic digestion, as it buffers HCl.
3. Mucus secretion is stimulated by increased blood flow to the stomach.

Intrinsic Factor Secretion

Intrinsic factor (IF) of Castle is secreted from parietal cells along with HCl. It is a glycoprotein:

1. It is synthesized like other glycoproteins and its secretion is stimulated by factors that stimulate HCl secretion like histamine and gastrin.
2. IF **helps in vitamin B_{12} absorption** from terminal ileum.

Factors that Influence HCl Secretion

Factors that Stimulate Gastric Acid Secretion

Factors that increase HCl secretion from the parietal cells of stomach mainly act through locally altering the concentration of three hormones: **acetylcholine, gastrin and histamine**. In the parietal cells, there are specific receptors for these hormones and other hormones. Hormones bind with the receptors and change the intracellular second messenger concentration that finally stimulate HCl secretion (Fig. 39.9).

Acetylcholine

Acetylcholine is an effective stimulator of gastric acid secretion. It is released at the nerve endings of **vagal cholinergic fibers** that innervate parietal cells:

1. Acetylcholine acts on the **M_3 cholinergic receptors** on the parietal cells and **increases intracellular Ca^{++}**.
2. It acts directly on the parietal cell to increase HCl secretion and acts indirectly by secreting histamine and gastrin from ECL cells and G cells respectively that in turn stimulate parietal cells.

Gastrin

Gastrin is the *most potent stimulus for HCl secretion*:

1. Gastrin acts on *gastrin receptors* on the parietal cells and increases HCl secretion by **increasing intracellular Ca^{++}** (Fig. 39.8).
2. Gastrin is secreted from G cells that are present in the antral mucosa of the stomach.
3. Vagal fibers innervate G cells and vagal stimulation increases gastrin release. However, vagal fibers that mediate gastrin release are **non-cholinergic** (Fig. 39.9) as the neurotransmitter is GRP (**gastrin releasing peptide**).
4. Gastrin also stimulates histamine release from ECL cells that in turn increases secretion of HCl from parietal cells. Gastrin secretion from stomach is increased by gastric distension, noncholinergic vagal stimulation, protein rich food, and catecholamines. **Pentagastrin** is used for assessing gastric acid output (Application Box 39.1).

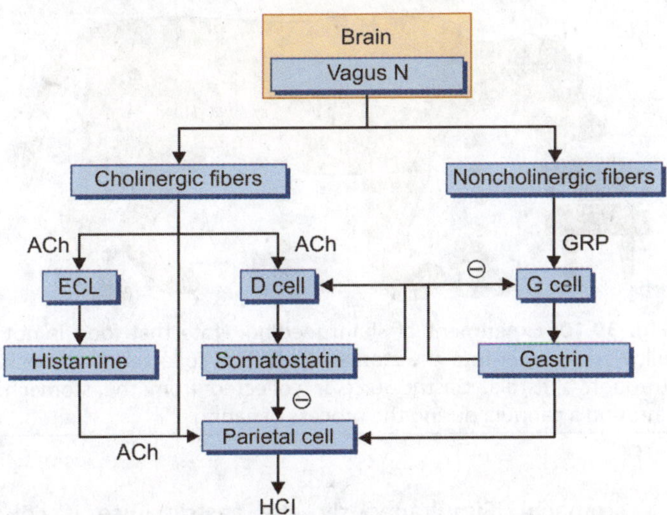

Fig. 39.9: Regulation of gastric secretion by vagus nerve. (ECL: Enterochromaffin cell; GRP: Gastrin releasing peptide; ACh: Acetylcholine; Minus sign indicates inhibition).

Application Box 39.1

Pentagastrin test; and Gastrectomy: As gastrin is the most potent stimulator of HCl secretion, exogenously administered synthetic gastrin (pentagastrin) assesses the degree of acid output from parietal cell mass of the stomach. This forms the physiological basis of pentagastrin test. As G cells are present in antral part of stomach and gastrin is the strong stimulus for parietal cells, **antrectomy** (partial antral gastrectomy) is performed for surgical treatment for protracted peptic ulcer. It is useful in patients with protracted peptic ulcer.

Histamine

Histamine is a powerful stimulator of HCl secretion from stomach:

1. It acts on H_2 receptors on the parietal cells and **increases intracellular cyclic AMP** as second messenger. Cyclic AMP stimulates protein kinase, which increases the activity of H^+-K^+ ATPase and HCl secretion.
2. Histamine is secreted from enterochromaffin-like (ECL) cells.
3. Histamine release is stimulated by both acetylcholine and gastrin.
4. Thus, histamine is considered as a major mediator of HCl secretion. Therefore, patients with peptic ulcer are usually first treated with histamine type-2 receptor antagonists.

Mechanical and Chemical Factors

Accumulation of food in the stomach increases acid secretion. This mainly occurs due to **mechanical distension that stretches G cells** and stimulates gastrin release. Also, **products of protein digestion** (peptides and amino acids) increase gastrin secretion, and **hot and spicy foods** facilitate HCl secretion from the stomach (Table 39.1).

Table 39.1: Stimuli that alter gastric acid secretion.

A. Factors that increase HCl secretion
Luminal factors 1. Distension of stomach 2. Products of protein digestion
Hormonal (locally acting) factors 1. Acetylcholine 2. Gastrin 3. Histamine
Neural factors – Vagal stimulation (cholinergic and noncholinergic)
Blood borne – Epinephrine
B. Factors that decrease HCl secretion
Luminal factors – Increased acid content (highly acidic chyme)
Hormonal (locally acting) factors – Somatostatin
Blood-borne factors – Secretin, GIP, glucagon

Factors that Inhibit Gastric Acid Secretion

Increased acid output, somatostatin and acidic content of duodenum decrease gastric acid secretion.

pH of Gastric Luminal Content

Decreased pH of gastric content is an important and natural inhibitor of HCl secretion:

1. When secretion of acid is high enough to decrease pH of gastric content to below 2, secretion of HCl is inhibited by negative feedback mechanism. Hence, this is called as **autoregulation of acid secretion.**
2. The highly acidic gastric pH does not inhibit parietal cell directly; rather inhibition of acid secretion is **mediated by gastrin and somatostatin.**
3. The highly acidic chyme directly inhibits gastrin secretion from G cells, and stimulates somatostatin secretion from D cells of stomach.
4. Somatostatin inhibits secretion of gastrin from G cells that decreases acid secretion.

Somatostatin

Somatostatin is secreted from the D cells of the gastric mucosa:

1. Decreased pH of gastric content (pH less than 2) increases the secretion of somatostatin, which inhibits gastrin release.
2. As gastrin is the most potent stimulator of acid secretion, decreased gastrin release decreases HCl secretion from the stomach.

Chyme in the Duodenum

When acidic chyme enters duodenum, **secretin** is secreted from upper intestinal mucosa:

1. **Secretin inhibits gastric secretion** and motility, and gastrin release from G cells.
2. Products of carbohydrate and lipid digestion in the duodenum, and hyperosmolality of duodenal content inhibit acid secretion by increasing the release of an **enterogastrone** called GIP (***gastric inhibitory peptide***).
3. There are other enterogastrones also that inhibit gastric secretion.

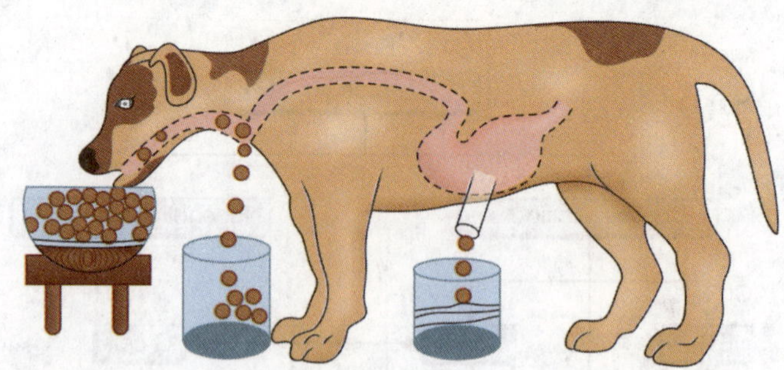

Fig. 39.10: Experiment of sham feeding. Note that food is not allowed to enter into the stomach, which is collected from neck through a fistula. Gastric juice is collected from the stomach through a cannula during the process of eating.

Regulation of Gastric Secretion

Gastric secretion is regulated by neural and humoral mechanisms. The mechanism of regulation depends on the phase of gastric acid secretion. The **neural mechanisms** are autonomic influences, short and long GI reflexes, and central influences mediated by vagus nerve. The **hormonal mechanisms** regulating gastric secretion are discussed above.

Gastric secretion occurs in **three phases** (cephalic, gastric and intestinal) and the mechanisms regulating secretion are different for each phase of secretion.

Cephalic Phase

The cephalic phase of gastric secretion is elicited by smell, sight, thought, taste and chewing of food. This is called cephalic phase as impulses to increase acid secretion originate mainly in the brain:

1. The sensory stimuli activate dorsal motor nucleus of vagus in the medulla. Therefore, cephalic phase of gastric secretion is **entirely mediated by vagus nerve** and the fibers are both **cholinergic and noncholinergic** (*see* Fig. 39.9).
2. The vagal fibers that directly contact parietal cells are cholinergic and fibers that contact G cells are **noncholinergic (neurotransmitter is GRP)**.
3. As noncholinergic effects are stronger than cholinergic effects, *atropine can not effectively prevent vagally mediated acid secretion*. Therefore, atropine is not prescribed in the management of peptic ulcer.

The gastric juice secreted in the cephalic phase occurs before food reaches the stomach. Therefore, this is also called **pregastric phase**. This phase accounts for 40–50% of total gastric secretion (Application Box 39.2).

Experimental Design to Study Cephalic Phase

The usual experimental design to assess the integrity of the cephalic phase is the **sham feeding**. In this procedure, a dog is taken as the experimental animal:

1. A fistula is made in the esophagus of the dog; so that when animal eats the food comes out of the neck ***through the fistula*** (food is not allowed to reach stomach). Simultaneously, the gastric juice is collected from the stomach by *placing a cannula into it* (Fig. 39.10). Gastric juice obtained during the cephalic phase is analyzed for volume and composition.
2. Then, **bilateral vagotomy** is performed and the gastric juice is collected following vagotomy for analysis.
3. **Vagotomy abolishes gastric secretion during cephalic phase,** which proves that this phase is primarily vagally mediated.

Application Box 39.2

Appetite juice: The gastric juice secreted during cephalic phase stimulates the appetite, and therefore, this is called *appetite juice*, as it occurs in anticipation of food. Usually in parties and special dinners, enough time is spent initially in taking soup and appetizers before actual dinner is served. This is meant to stimulate appetite for food and to collect enough gastric juice in stomach before food enters the stomach, so that digestion becomes easier.

Gastric Phase

The gastric phase of gastric secretion starts when food enters the stomach:

1. The primary stimulus for secretion in this phase is the **distension of the stomach.**
2. Also, products of digestion like peptides and amino acids produced by pepsin action that breaks proteins stimulate gastric secretion.
3. The distension of the stomach elicits acid secretion by both local as well as central reflexes (Fig. 39.11). **The central reflex** is mediated by vagus nerve (*vagovagal reflex*), and is both cholinergic and noncholinergic. **The local reflex** releases acetylcholine that directly stimulates parietal cell. Distension of stomach *per se* also increases gastrin release from the antral G cells that in turn increases HCl secretion.
4. Amino acid and peptides stimulate G cells to release gastrin.
5. Therefore, mechanisms of acid secretion in the gastric phase are **mechanical, neural, and chemical.**
6. Gastric phase accounts for 50–60% of gastric secretion.

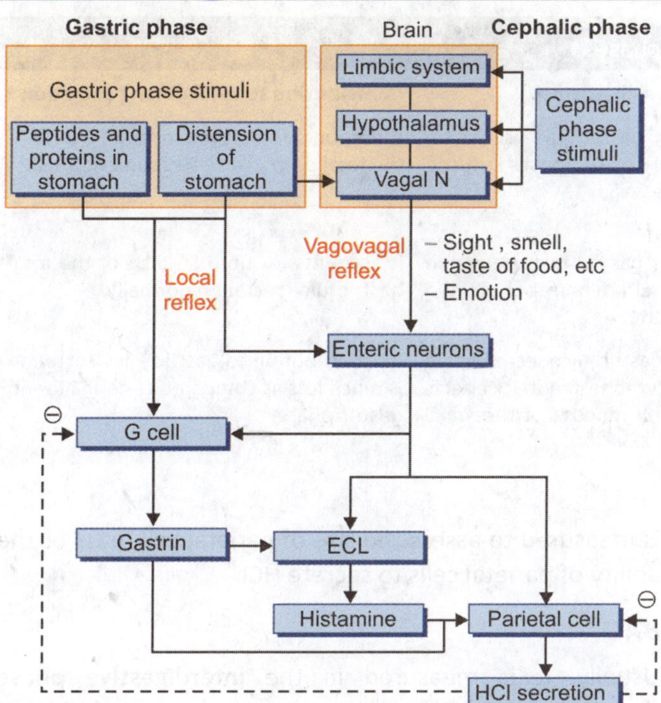

Fig. 39.11: Regulation of HCl secretion in cephalic and gastric phases of gastric secretion. (ECL: Enterochromaffin cell). Dotted lines depict HCl inhibition of G cell to reduce gastrin release and direct inhibition of parietal cell by HCl is indicated by minus signs.

HCl secretion in this phase is decreased by the acidic pH of the chyme bathing in the gastric mucosa. When pH of gastric content becomes less than 2, HCl secretion is effectively reduced. This is called **autoregulation of gastric acid secretion** (discussed above). HCl *inhibits both G cells and parietal cells*.

Experimental Designs to Study Gastric Phase

Gastric phase of gastric secretion is studied by making five different types of pouches: **Pavlov pouch, Heidenhain pouch, Bickel pouch, Farrell pouch and Ivy pouch**. However, the pouch experiment to study gastric secretion is not performed nowadays. This is mainly of academic and historical importance.

1. **Pavlov pouch** is a small pouch separated from the main body of the stomach by a double layer of mucous membrane. This gastric pouch of mucous membrane has intact nerve and blood supply. Therefore, it helps to study both neural and chemical factors of gastric acid secretion.
2. **Heidenhain pouch** is a denervated pouch, which helps to study the influence of neural factors on gastric secretion.

Scientist contributed

Rudolf Peter Heinrich Heidenhain (1834–1897) pioneered in the study of salivary and gastric secretions. He developed experimental designs to study secretion of salivary and gastric juices. The pouch made in experimental animals to study gastric secretion is named as **Heidenhain's pouch**. He also studied the functions of secretory and trophic nerves of glands and promoted the intracellular theory of secretory phenomena.

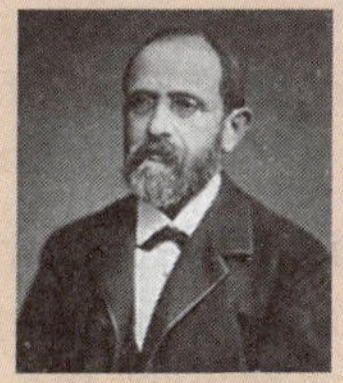

RPH Heidenhain
(1834–1897)

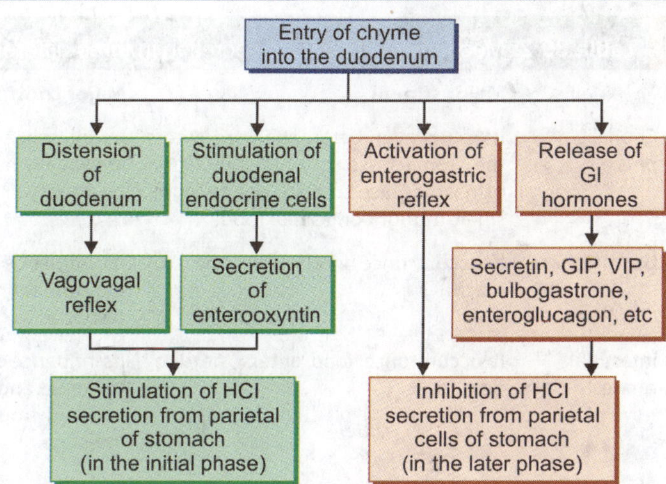

Fig. 39.12: Regulation of HCl secretion in the intestinal phase of gastric secretion. Though initially in the intestinal phase gastric secretion is stimulated, inhibition occurs in the later part of the phase.

Intestinal Phase

When chyme enters the intestine, intestinal phase of gastric secretion starts. This is also called **postgastric phase**. Initial part of intestinal phase is stimulatory to gastric secretion, but later part is inhibitory.

Stimulation of Secretion

1. Distension of duodenum increases gastric acid secretion by activating **vagovagal reflex**.
2. The chemical composition of chyme, especially the products of protein digestion like amino acids and peptide ***stimulate G and other endocrine cells in the duodenum*** and upper jejunum to secrete ***enterooxyntin***, which in turn stimulates gastric acid secretion (Fig. 39.12).

Inhibition of Secretion

1. Acidic chyme in the duodenum (decreased pH of duodenal content) inhibits gastric secretion via **enterogastric reflex**.
2. Acid also stimulates release of ***secretin***, which inhibits gastrin secretion from G cells. Secretin also decreases the response of parietal cells to gastrin and histamine.
3. Acid in the duodenum and hyperosmolality of duodenal content also secrete a hormone called ***bulbogastrone*** that inhibits acid secretion from parietal cells of the stomach.
4. Products of fat digestion especially fatty acids and triglycerides stimulate secretion of ***GIP and CCK*** from upper part of small intestine. These hormones ***inhibit secretion of acid*** from parietal cells.

Thus, the net effect of intestinal phase is the inhibition of gastric secretion. Hence, intestinal phase accounts for about **10% of gastric secretion**.

The differences between cephalic, gastric and intestinal phase of gastric secretion are summarized in Table 39.2.

Table 39.2: Mechanisms of gastric secretion in three different phases.

	Major stimuli	Major control mechanisms	Contribution to total gastric secretion
Cephalic phase	It occurs even before the food enters the stomach, i.e. psychic stimulation of gastric juice in response to sight, smell, thought or taste of food.	Its influence on gastric juice secretion are vagally mediated responses induced by activity in the CNS.	It accounts for approximately 30-50% of the total gastric juice secretion normally.
Gastric phase	It occurs once food enters the stomach.	Its influence on gastric juice secretion are primarily local reflex responses and response to gastrin.	It accounts for upto 50-60% of the total gastric juice secretion normally.
Intestinal phase	It occurs once food enters the duodenum.	Its influence on gastric juice secretion are the reflex and hormonal feedback effects initiated from the mucosa of the small intestine.	Its contribution to gastric juice secretion is much less as compared to cephalic and gastric phase.

GASTRIC FUNCTION TESTS

To diagnose various diseases of stomach, the laboratory tests measuring gastric secretion, serum gastrin, etc carries much importance. Therefore, gastric function tests (GFTs) are performed to diagnose various gastric and duodenal anomalies and to monitor the effectiveness of the therapy. It includes:

1. Examination of gastric contents
2. Test for gastric acid secretion
3. Tests for pepsin, mucous, intrinsic factor
4. Tests for gastrin
5. Visualization of the interior of stomach
6. Tests for gastric motility and electrical activities (gastrography)
7. Obtaining biopsy from the suspected tissue.

Classification

Gastric content is examined for the normal and abnormal constituents. The following parameters are looked for in the gastric content sample: Volume of acid (acid output), pH, colour, acidity (total and free), and presence of blood, mucous and food particles.

Examination of gastric contents can be divided into ***three types*** according to the time of examination:

1. **At rest:** Gastric juice is collected after the patient awakes in the morning, but still lying on the bed.
2. **After a meal in the post absorptive phase:** A specific diet is provided, which has a fixed composition (also known as ***fractional test meal analysis***) followed by that gastric content is collected for analysis.
3. **After a specific stimulus:** A specific stimulus for induction of acid secretion is applied following which the gastric content is withdrawn. Mainly the maximum amount of acid output is checked in these type of tests.

Measurement of Acid Output

Two types of acid outputs are assessed: **basal acid output** (BAO), and **maximal acid output** (MAO). Acid output is measured to assess the size of parietal cell mass or the ability of parietal cells to secrete HCl.

BAO

Usually, it is measured in the **interdigestive phase** (between two meals, when stomach is supposed to be at rest). The gastric juice is collected for about 60 minutes through a Ryle's tube introduced into patient's empty stomach following an overnight fast and complete sleep.

Normal value: Usually, it is 10–40 mEq/L or 0.5–2 mEq/hour.

Significance: Increased BAO indicates high gastrin activity as occurs in Zollinger-Ellison syndrome. A pH more than 2.5 for the acid, rules out this syndrome.

MAO

This is the ***maximum quantity of acid that can be secreted*** by the stomach. Usually, estimation of MAO is performed by a ***stimulation test*** in which a stimulant is injected to increase acid secretion. The chemical is injected and gastric juice is collected by Ryle's tube. Usual tests performed are given below.

Normal value: The MAO is usually 12–60 mEq/hour.

Special Test to Detect Acid Output

Histamine Test

Historically, histamine was the first standard stimulant used for gastric acid secretion test. 0.01 mg/kg bodyweight of histamine phosphate is injected subcutaneously with simultaneous administration of antihistaminic agent to prevent the untoward side effects. Then the acid output is measured, every 10 minutes for 1 hour. Upto 10 ml of gastric content is aspirated and analyzed. It is helpful in the diagnosis of pernicious anemia, subacute combined degeneration of spinal cord and assessing the maximum acid output following duodenal surgery.

Histalog (Betazole) Test

Histalog, is a better replacement for histamine as it does not require the simultaneous administration of antihistaminic agent due to its fewer side effects. 1-15 mg/kg of histalog is injected subcutaneously and similar protocol as in histamine test is followed.

Pentagastrin (Peptavlon) Test

Pentagastrin is injected subcutaneously at a dose of 6 µg/kg and acid output is measured. Being a synthetic analogue of gastrin, it is a potent stimulus for acid secretion.

Insulin Test (Hollander test)

This test is based on the fact that in a state of hypoglycemia, produced by insulin, in turn causes **vagal stimulation.** The direct vagal action on parietal cells, leads to acid secretion. Therefore, insulin can be used for measuring acid output. 15 IU of soluble insulin is injected intravenously and gastric content is collected every 15 minutes interval for two and half hours. Usually, insulin test is performed **to assess the completeness of vagotomy**. No increase in acid production should occur if the vagal resection is complete.

Fractional Test Meal Analysis

Patient is allowed to take a meal that has a particular composition, following which small fractions (10 ml) of gastric content is removed through Ryle's tube every 15 min to estimate the acid secretion for about 3 hours (in 13 samples). This test indicates the **acid secretion capacity in the post-absorptive phase**. It is useful in the detection of hyperchlorhydria, hypochlorhydria and achlorohydria.

Tubeless Gastric Analysis

To decrease the discomfort by Ryles tube, this is an alternative. However, it may not be always accurate:

1. **Diagnex blue** which contains a cation exchange resin with an indicator Azure A is given orally to the patient.
2. The acid present in stomach releases the indicator by virtue of its low pH.
3. The released indicator gets absorbed by intestine and gets excreted subsequently via urine. The intensity of its color is compared with standards to check for the concentration of gastric acid.
4. This test can also be repeated after giving stimulant of gastric secretion.
5. It is *contraindicated* in renal disorders, malabsorption, etc.

The Significance of BAO and MAO

In gastric ulcer, the values of BAO and MAO are usually normal or slightly below normal.

Higher values are found in:

i. Duodenal ulcer
ii. Zollinger-Ellison syndrome (gastrinoma)
iii. Anastomotic ulcer

Higher values are found:

i. Pernicious anemia (atrophic gastritis)
ii. Gastric malignamcy (Achlorhydria in the presence of gastric ulcer is highly suggestive of gastric malignancy)

Tests for other Gastric Secretory Products

Test for Pepsin

Pepsin inhibitors are used for analysis of pepsin derived from pepsinogen for research purposes. The level of pepsin is low in atrophic gastritis.

Test for Mucous

Protein content of gastric mucous is measured, normal value being 1.8 mg/ml. The level is increased in chronic hypertrophic gastritis (Menetrier disease).

Test for Intrinsic factor

Intrinsic factor (IF) is essential for vitamin B_{12} absorption from the small intestine. In its absence, the absorption of vitamin B_{12} is impaired as occurs in chronic atrophic gastritis and gastric atrophy. Schilling test is used for evaluation of patients with suspected pernicious anemia but can also be used as diagnostic test for pancvreatic efficiency resulting in impaired absorption of vitamin B_{12} since gastric R binder protein is not cleared from intrinsic factor due to reduced pancreatic proteolytic activity.

Test for Gastrin

Gastrin is secreted by G cells present in the antropyloric and proximal duodenal mucosa. The circulating gastrin level is normally 0-200 pg/mL. it can be tested by following methods:

1. **Serum gastrin level:** Radioimmunoassay (RIA) is the commonly used method for gastrin measurement. Normal fasting level of gastrin is 20-150 pg/mL. its levels are higher in:
   i. Atrophic gastritis (with low gastric acid secretion)
   ii. Zollinger-Ellison syndrome or gastrinoma (with high gastric acid secretion)
   iii. Following surgery of the stomach
2. **Gastrin provocative tests:** These tests are used to differentiate between hypergastrinaemia and gastric acid hypersecretion as follows:
   i. Secretin test: an intravenous injection of secretin (1 U/kg body weight) is given. If the serum level rises by more than 50% of basal value in 5-15 minutes, it is diagnostic of Zollinger-Ellison syndrome (gastrinoma). This rise does not occur in other conditions.
   ii. Calcium infusion test: Intravenous infusion of calcium (5 mg/kg per hour) is given for 3 hours. Rise in serum gastrin levels by more than 50% of basal value is diagnostic of Zollinger-Ellison syndrome (gastrinoma).

Other Tests

Barium-Meal X-Ray

A barium-mixed food is swallowed by the subject following which X-rays of upper GI tract are obtained. This gives

Table 39.3: Tests for gastric analysis.

A. Tests for gastric secretions
1. Tests for gastric secretions i. Histamine stimulation ii. Histalog stimulation iii. Pentagastrin (peptavlon) stimulation iv. Insulin test (Hollander test) v. Tubeless analysis
2. Tests for pepsin
3. Tests for mucous and its protein content
4. Tests for intrinsic factor
B. Tests for gastrin
1. Serum gastrin
2. Gastrin provocative tests i. Secretin test ii. Calcium infusion test

the details of the contour of the lower esophagus, stomach and upper small intestine. The **location and size of the ulcer and tumor** can be delineated.

Endoscopy (Gastroscopy)

A fiber-optic gastroscope is introduced into the stomach to study the details of the ulcer or other pathologies. The advantages are:

1. It gives an opportunity to visualize the lumen of the stomach, so that the ulcer details can be seen.
2. A **biopsy of the ulcer** can be taken to study the type of ulcer (to exclude malignancy).
3. The tissue is also cultured to study the organism (***to confirm H. pylori infection***).
4. The gastroscope can be introduced into the duodenum and biliary tract to study further details.
5. **Urease test** is performed from the biopsy sample for *H. pylori* confirmation.

The major tests for analysis of gastric secretory functions are summarized in Table 39.3.

APPLIED ASPECTS

The common diseases related to gastric secretion are gastritis and peptic ulcer.

Gastritis

The term gastritis is commonly employed for any clinical condition with upper abdominal discomfort like indigestion or dyspepsia in which the specific clinical signs and radiological abnormalities are absent. The condition is of great importance due to its relationship with peptic ulcer and gastric cancer. Broadly, gastritis is of 2 types: acute and chronic. Chronic gastritis can further be of various types.

A simple classification of various types of gastritis is presented in Table 39.4.

Table 39.4: Classification of gastritis.

A. Acute gastritis
1. Acute *H. pylori* gastritis
2. Other acute infective gastritis (bacteria, virus, fungi, parasites)
B. Chronic gastritis
1. Type A (autoimmune) gastritis: Body-fundic predominant
2. Type B (*H. pylori* related) gastritis: Antral predominant
3. Type AB (mixed environmental) gastritis: Antral body predominant
4. Chemical (reflux) gastritis: Body fundic predominant: Antral body predominant
5. Miscellaneous forms of gastritis

Etiopathogenesis

A variety of etiologic agents have been implicated in the cause of acute gastritis. These are as follows:

1. Diet and personal habits:
2. Infections
3. Drugs
4. Chemical and physical agents
5. Severe stress

Chronic gastritis, if untreated leads to peptic ulcer.

Peptic Ulcers

Peptic ulcer means ulcer in the stomach (**gastric ulcer**) or duodenum (**duodenal ulcer**). Acid of the gastric juice or pepsin in the gastric secretion produces damage to the gastroduodenal mucosa in abnormal conditions. Therefore, peptic ulcer is called **acid-peptic disease.**

Pathophysiology

Peptic ulcer is caused either by decreased mucosal defense, or by hypersecretion of acid or infection.

A. Diminished Effectiveness of Mucosal Barrier

The defense barrier of the stomach is the mucous coat on the gastric epithelium. This is called **mucosal defense barrier**:

1. The mucus is secreted by mucous cells. Mucus is a viscous gel that contains mucin, phospholipid, electrolytes (mainly HCO_3^-) and water.
2. The **mucous gel layer** is about 0.2 mm thick and effectively separates the bicarbonate rich secretion of epithelial cells from the acidic content of the stomach (Fig. 39.13).
3. This allows the **pH of the epithelial cells to remain alkaline** despite acidic pH of gastric content. It protects mucosal epithelium from injury caused by acidic chyme.
4. However, when secretion of mucus is impaired, or bicarbonate production is decreased or when the mucosal coat is mechanically damaged, acid and pepsin cause ulcer formation.

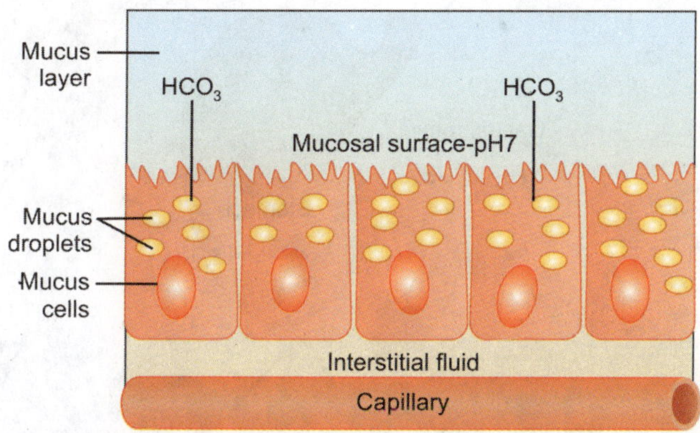

Fig. 39.13: Mucosal defense barrier by bicarbonate.

Such damage is usually produced by **use of aspirin and NSAID** (nonsteroidal anti-inflammatory drugs) that inhibit the secretion of mucus and bicarbonate. Catecholamines also inhibit mucus secretion. In ***chronic stress***, ulcer is produced (**stress ulcer**) by chronically elevated level of catecholamines in blood.

B. Hypersecretion of Acid

Gastric acid secretion increases in chronic anxiety. Peptic ulcer is common in business executives as most of them lead a life either in hurry or in worry. Intake of *more spicy food* is known to increase acid secretion. Therefore, it is generally believed that **hurry**, **worry**, and **curry** are the causes of peptic ulcer. Chronically increased secretion of acid (hyperchlorhydria) produces peptic ulcer by damaging the mucosal barrier.

Conditions that cause hyperchlorhydria are:

- Zollinger-Ellison syndrome
- Gastric outlet obstruction syndrome (as occurs in pyloric stenosis)
- Systemic mastocytosis (histamine secreted from mast cell increases HCl secretion)

Zollinger-Ellison syndrome is a non-α non-β ***gastrin secreting tumor of pancreas***.

C. Helicobacter Pylori Infection

Recently it is observed that infection by *H. pylori* is the major cause of peptic ulcer:

1. This is a ***Gram-negative bacillus*** that secretes an enzyme called **urease** that converts urea into carbon dioxide and ammonia. Ammonia buffers the acid surrounding the bacteria.
2. *H. pylori* colonizes the antral mucosa, where it causes **local inflammation** and **disrupts immune responses**. It also **inhibits somatostatin secretion** from D cells that facilitates gastrin release and consequently increased HCl secretion.
3. Therefore, serum gastrin level is moderately elevated in duodenal ulcer.
4. *H. pylori* causes gastritis initially, but later, ulcer is produced.

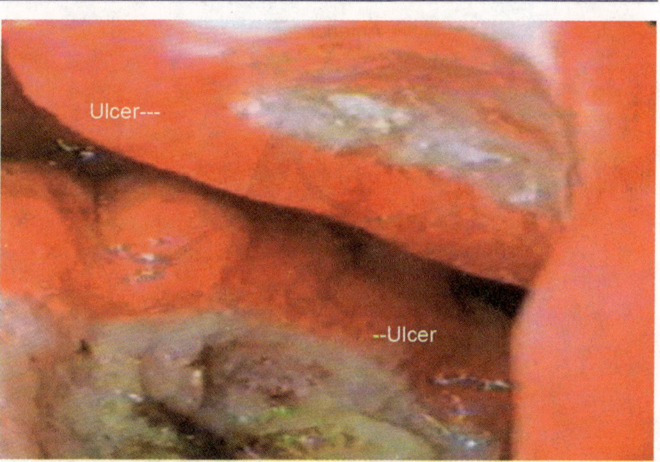

Fig. 39.14: Endoscopic view of chronic peptic ulcer (note, two ulcers in the duodenum seen through endoscope).
Courtesy: Figure 2.3, Gastrointestinal Surgery, by S Devaji Rao, 1st edition, 2009; Jaypee Brothers Medical Publishers (P) Ltd.

5. Therefore, antibiotic therapy to kill *H. pylori* is frequently successful in the treatment of peptic ulcer.

Scientists contributed

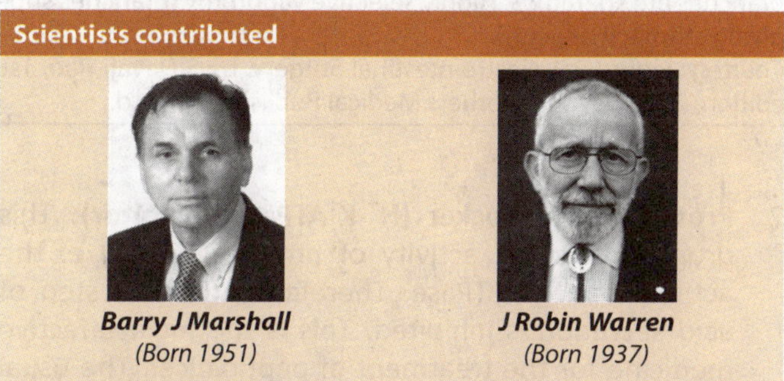

Barry J Marshall *(Born 1951)*

J Robin Warren *(Born 1937)*

The **Nobel Prize in Physiology or Medicine 2005** was awarded jointly to two Australian physicians **Barry J. Marshall** and **J. Robin Warren** *"for their discovery of the bacterium Helicobacter pylori and its role in gastritis and peptic ulcer disease"*

Features

In most of the cases ulcer is located in the duodenum (Fig. 39.14), usually above the ampulla of Vater, as in this area acidic chyme is not neutralized by alakaline pancreatic juice. The main feature of peptic ulcer is **upper abdominal pain** (*epigastric pain*). Typically, pain is experienced in empty stomach and is relieved by taking water, food or antacid. If disease is untreated, **hematemesis** (vomiting of blood) or **malena** (dark, tarry stool), **vomiting** (due to pyloric obstruction), and peritonitis due to **perforation of ulcer** into the peritoneal cavity occurs.

Treatment

Specific Treatment

The specific treatment includes use of following drugs:

1. **H_2 receptor antagonists:** Ranitidine, cimetidine, famotidine, and nizatidine are different generations of H_2 receptor blockers. These drugs block the H_2 receptor and inhibit histamine secretion. As histamine is a potent stimulator of HCl release from parietal cells, H_2 receptor blockers inhibit HCl secretion.

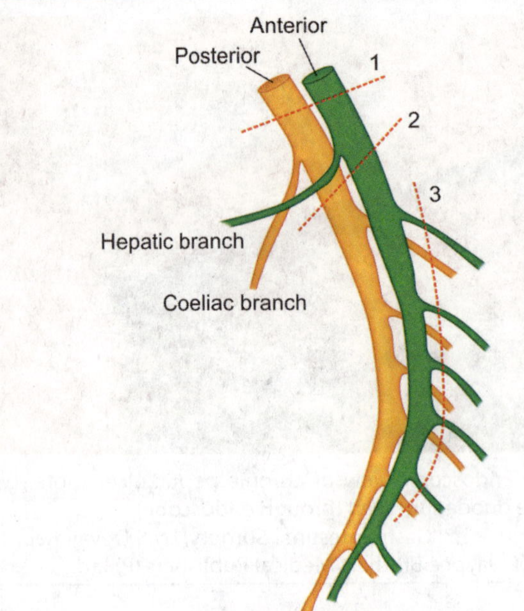

Fig. 39.15: Types of vagotomy. [1: Truncal vagotomy (main trunk of the vagus is cut); 2: Selective vagotomy (hepatic and celiac branches are spared); 3: Highly selective vagotomy (branches supplying stomach are cut)].
Courtesy: Figure 2.2, Gastrointestinal Surgery, by S Devaji Rao, 1st edition, 2009; Jaypee Brothers Medical Publishers (P) Ltd.

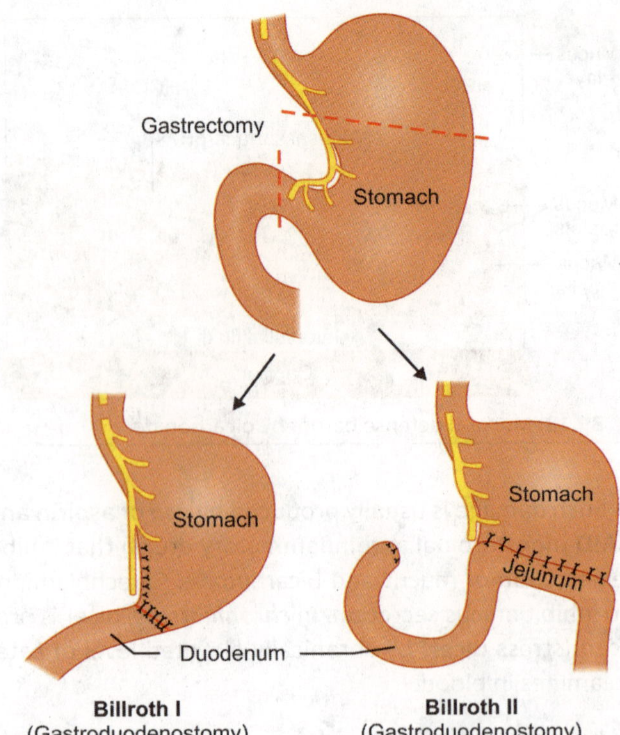

Fig. 39.16: The procedure of gastrectomy followed by gastroduodenostomy (Billroth I surgery) or gastrojejunostomy (Billroth II surgery). Note the portion of stomach (as shown within the two dotted lines) removed in gastrectomy Surgery for peptic ulcer.
Courtesy: Figure 4.9, Gastrointestinal Surgery, by S Devaji Rao, 1st edition, 2009; Jaypee Brothers Medical Publishers (P) Ltd.

2. **Proton-pump blocker (H^+-K^+ATPase inhibitor):** This drug inhibits the activity of proton-pump, i. e. the activity of H^+-K^+ATPase. Therefore, the final step of acid secretion is inhibited. This is the most effective medicine for the treatment of peptic ulcer. The usual proton-pump blocker used is omeprazole.
3. **Sucralfate:** This is a sucrose octasulfate. It provides a protective layer on the ulcer. Therefore, it promotes ulcer healing.
4. **Muscarinic blockers:** Atropine and pirenzepine are used to block the M_1 and M_3 receptors. Therefore, acetylcholine does not act on parietal cells. However, as the ***noncholinergic vagal innervation dominates over the cholinergic innervation*** for acid secretion, **atropine does not produce encouraging results.** Therefore, muscarinic blockers are not used in peptic ulcer treatment.
5. **Gastrin blockers:** As gastrin is the most potent stimulator of acid secretion, effort has been made to discover gastrin antagonists. However, a successful gastrin blocker has not yet been discovered. Proglumide, a gastrin blocker is used recently for the purpose.
6. **Antibiotics:** Recently, high dose of antibiotics such as amoxicillin to kill *H. pylori* has provided promising result.

Nonspecific Measures

Antacids

Antacids give immediate and temporary relief from pain. As the disease is mostly due to stress, measures to reduce the stress level are very helpful.

Yoga Therapy and Other Measures

Yoga therapy like practice of relaxation techniques, adequate **sleep** and rest, regulation of **diet**, and withdrawal of **drugs** like aspirin and NSAID improve the condition. **Use of cold milk** and **avoidance of spicy food & alcohol** also help in curing the disease.

Surgical Treatment

Sometimes inspite of effective use of medicines, the disease is not cured. In such patients, surgery is advocated. The usual surgical procedures performed are:

1. **Vagotomy:** There are different types of vagotomy such as **truncal vagotomy** (cutting the trunk of vagus nerves in abdomen just below the diaphragm), **selective vagotomy** (cutting the vagus nerve that supplies only stomach), and **highly selective vagotomy** (cutting the vagus nerve that preferentially innervate the parietal cell) (Fig. 39.15). Usually, the *parietal cell vagotomy is preferred* as other two types are associated with complications.
2. **Gastrectomy:** Partial gastrectomy **removes the antral portion of stomach**, as this part contains G cells. Antrum is the pump of the stomach that propels food into duodenum. Therefore, *antrectomy results in stasis of food*. To avoid such complication, usually gastroduodenostomy or **gastrojejunostomy** (the ***drainage procedures***) is performed with gastrectomy (Fig. 39.16). Gastrojejunostomy is also performed with truncal vagotomy.

CHAPTER SUMMARY

Key Concepts

1. Though the primary function of stomach is temporary storage, grinding and mixing of food and controlled emptying of chyme into the intestine, gastric acid secretion is useful for acid-peptic digestion of food, providing IF for Vitamin B_{12} absorption and killing microorganisms in food in stomach.
2. Gastric distension, spicy food, emotion and stress are important stimulant for gastric secretion. Mental relaxation, healthy food, Yoga and adequate sleep are important to have control over secretion of gastric acid.
3. *H. Pylori* is an important causative factor for gastritis and peptic ulcer.
4. Though endoscopy is the surest method for diagnosis of gastritis and peptic ulcer, estimation of gastrin level is useful in the management.

Important to Know (Must Read)

1. In examinations, 'Mechanism and regulation of gastric secretion' comes as a **Long Question**.
2. Phases of gastric secretion, Composition and functions of gastric secretion, Mechanism of gastric secretion, Regulation of gastric secretion, Gastric function tests, can come as **Short Questions**.
3. In **Viva**, examiner may ask....... Structure and functions of stomach, Amount of gastric secretion/day, Names of gastric glands, Innervation of stomach, Composition and function of gastric secretion, Function of each constituent of gastric secretion, Mechanism of gastric secretion, What are the Phases of gastric secretions and how are they regulated, What are the stimuli for different phases of gastric secretion, How different phases of gastric secretion can be studied, What are the gastric pouches and how they differ from each other, What are the effects of parasympathetic and sympathetic stimulation on gastric secretion, What is appetite juice, Classify gastric function tests, Procedure and normal values of important gastric function tests, Causes of gastritis and peptic ulcer, Who got Nobel prize for discovery of *H. pylori*, What is the role of *H. pylori* in peptic ulcer.
4. Functions of stomach, and Composition and functions of gastric juice are usually asked in viva. Mechanism of HCl secretion, and Regulation of different phases of gastric secretion are usually asked in theory exam. A student is expected to answer these questions; otherwise it may be difficult for him to pass.

CHAPTER 40

Pancreatic Secretion

Learning Objectives

On completion of study of this chapter, the student **MUST** be able to:

1. Understand the importance of exocrine pancreas in digestion and absorption of food.
2. Give the composition and functions of pancreatic juice.
3. Describe the mechanism of pancreatic secretion.
4. Explain regulation in different phases of pancreatic secretion.
5. Understand the physiological basis of pancreatic function tests.

The student **MAY** also be able to:

1. Describe pancreatic function tests.
2. Learn the physiological basis of pancreatic abnormalities.

FUNCTIONAL ANATOMY

The **exocrine pancreas** plays a major role in digestion and absorption of all essential nutrients from the GI tract. The exocrine pancreas constitutes about 80% of the total mass of the pancreas (12% by ducts and blood vessels, and 2% by endocrine tissues). This is a unique organ in the body having both major endocrine and exocrine tissues in it. The **endocrine pancreas** is involved in energy metabolism, deficiency of which results in diabetes mellitus, exocrine pancreatic deficiency results in severe indigestion, malabsorption and malnutrition.

Structure of Exocrine Pancreas

Pancreas forms the major part of the stomach bed. The head of pancreas fits into the "C" curvature of the duodenum. Pancreatic duct combines with common bile duct to form hepatopancreatic duct (form hepatopancreatic ampulla *or ampulla of Vater)* that opens into second part of duodenum as major duodenal papilla via sphincter of Oddi (Fig. 40.1A). Often, an accessory pancreatic duct opens separately into duodenum as minor duodenal papilla (Fig. 40.1B).

Histology and Secretory Apparatus

Histologically, exocrine pancreas *resembles salivary glands*. The exocrine tissue of pancreas consists of **lobules** that contain multiple **acini** (Fig. 40.2).

1. **Acini** are sac-like dilatations composed of single layer of pyramidal (acinar) cells. Acinar cells contain multiple endoplasmic reticulum, Golgi apparatus and zymogen granules that are located in the apical region of the acinar cells (Fig. 40.3).
2. A few **centroacinar cells** line the lumen of the acinus.
3. Acini open to **intercalated duct** which in turn empty into **intralobular duct**.
4. Intralobular duct drains into extralobular duct that finally open to the main collecting duct, the *duct of Wirsung*.
5. Sometimes an accessory pancreatic duct, the *duct of Santorini*, drains separately from the head of the pancreas into the duodenum.
6. Collecting ducts combine to form **pancreatic duct** that drains into the common bile duct and form hepatopancreatic duct with an ampulla (Ampulla of Vater), which opens to the second part of duodenum through the ***sphincter of Oddi***.
7. The acini secrete enzymes of the pancreatic juice.

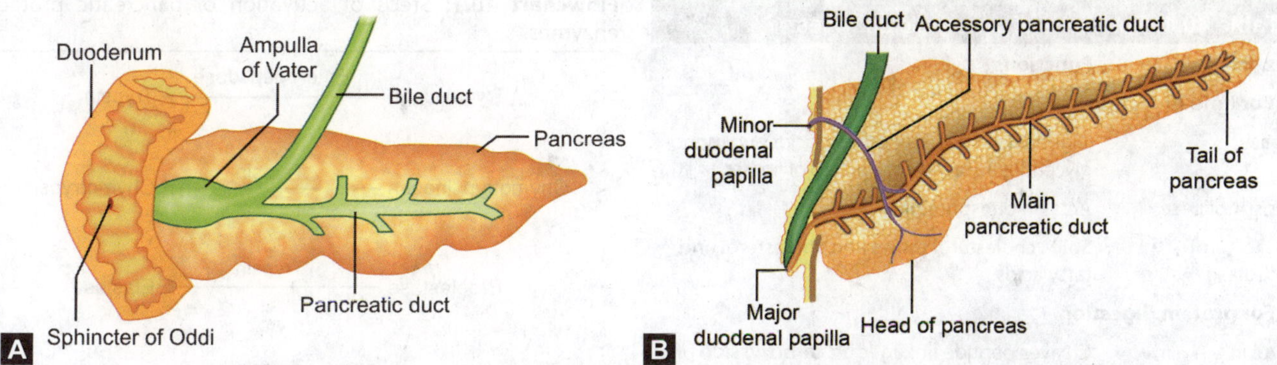

Figs. 40.1A and B: (A) Position of pancreas in the C curvature of duodenum, showing the pancreatic duct and hepatic duct opening into duodenum through sphincter of Oddi via ampulla of Vater. (B) Structure of pancreas showing the opening major and accessory duodenal papilla draining from major and accessory pancreatic ducts respectively.

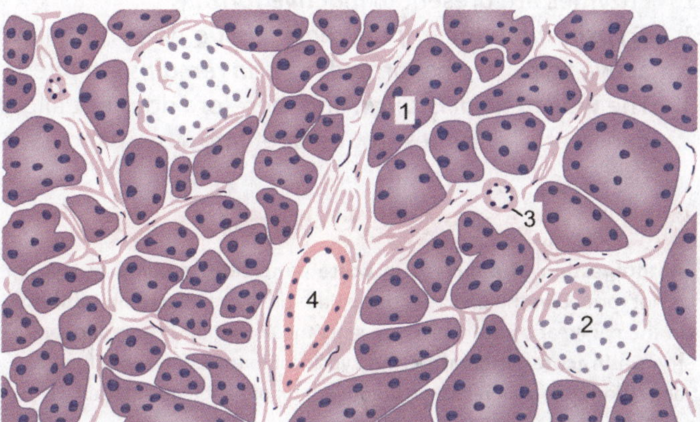

Fig. 40.2: Histology of pancreas. 1: Serous acini inside lobules; 2: Islets of Langerhans; 3: Intralobular duct; 4: Interlobular duct.

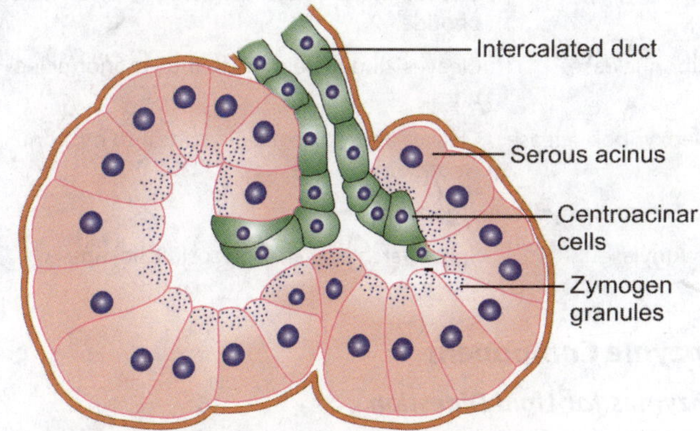

Fig. 40.3: Structure of pancreatic acinus and ducts.

8. The aqueous component of pancreatic juice is produced by epithelial cells that line the pancreatic ducts.

Scientist contributed

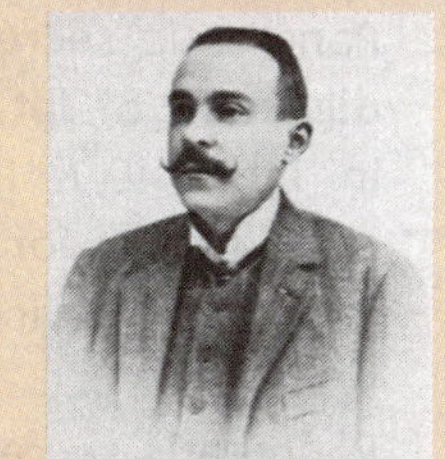

Ruggero FAGV Oddi *(1864–1913)*

Ruggero Ferdinando Antonio Giuseppe Vincenzo Oddi (1864–1913) was an Italian physiologist, studied medicine at Perugia, Bologna and Florence, and in 1894 was appointed as Head of the Physiology Institute at the University of Genoa. While still a student, Oddi described a small group of circular and longitudinal muscle fibers that wrapped around the end of the bile and pancreatic ducts, and he demonstrated the physiology of these muscles. This structure was later named as the eponymous "**sphincter of Oddi**". Though this sphincter was initially identified by English physician ***Francis Glisson,*** it was Oddi who was first to characterize its physiological properties. Inflammation of the junction of the duodenum and common bile duct at the sphincter of Oddi is referred to as "Odditis".

Nerve supply

Pancreas is supplied by both parasympathetic (vagal fibers) and sympathetic fibers.

Vagal Fibers

These fibers innervate both the acinar cells (exocrine tissue) and islet cells (endocrine tissue). Stimulation of parasympathetic fibers **increases exocrine pancreatic secretion**.

Sympathetic Fibers

The postganglionic sympathetic fibers from celiac and superior mesenteric plexuses innervate pancreatic blood vessel and tissue. Stimulation of sympathetic fibers **inhibits pancreatic secretion**.

PANCREATIC SECRETION

Composition and Functions

Composition

The pancreatic secretion has aqueous component (98%) and enzyme component (2%).

Aqueous Component

This contains mainly water and ions. The **cations** are Na^+, K^+, Ca^{++}, Mg^{++}, and Zn^{++}, and the **anions** are HCO_3^-, Cl^-, PO_4^{3-}, and SO_4^{3-}.

Table 40.1: Functions of pancreatic enzymes.

Enzymes	Functions
A. For lipid digestion	
Lipase	Digests neutral lipids into fatty acids and monoglycerides. Facilitates the action of lipase.
Phospholipase	Acts on phospholipids.
Cholesterol hydrolase	Splits cholesterol esters into cholesterol and fatty acids.
B. For protein digestion	
Trypsin	Cleaves peptide linkages on carboxyl side of basic amino acids.
Chymotrypsin	Cleaves peptide linkages on carboxyl side of aromatic amino acids.
Elastase	Cleaves peptide linkages on carboxyl side of aliphatic amino acids.
Carboxypeptidase	Cleaves amino acids from carboxyl end of the peptide.
Ribonuclease	Cleaves ribonucleic acids into mononucleotides.
Deoxyribonuclease	Cleaves deoxyribonucleic acids into mononucleotides
C. For carbohydrate digestion	
Amylase	Splits starch at α–1, 4-glycosidic linkage

Enzyme Component

Enzymes for Lipid Digestion

Enzymes for lipid digestion are **pancreatic lipase** (triacylglycerol hydrolase, cholesterol ester hydrolase, and phospholipase A_2), **colipase** and **phospholipases**.

1. The **pancreatic lipase** digests neutral lipids into fatty acids and monoglycerides.
2. The **colipase** facilitates the action of lipase.
3. The **phospholipase** acts on phospholipids.
4. **Cholesterol hydrolase** splits cholesterol esters into cholesterol and fatty acids.

Enzymes for Protein Digestion

Enzymes for protein digestion are trypsin, chymotrypsin, carboxypeptidase, procollagenase, proelastase, and nucleases.

1. These proteolytic enzymes are **secreted in the inactive forms** like trypsinogen, chymotrypsinogen, procarboxypeptidase, procollagenases, proelastase, and pronucleases (Table 40.1).
2. The enzymes are activated in the intestine.
3. The **first step** in the process of activation is the **activation of trypsinogen to trypsin**, which is mediated by the intestinal enzyme **enteropeptidase (*enterokinase*)**.
4. Once trypsin is formed, it converts other proenzymes to their active forms (Flowchart 40.1).
5. ***Trypsin is strongly proteolytic.*** Therefore, once it is activated in the pancreas, it digests the pancreatic tissue (Clinical Box 40.1). However, normally it *remains inactivated* in pancreas.

Flowchart 40.1: Steps of activation of pancreatic proteolytic enzymes.

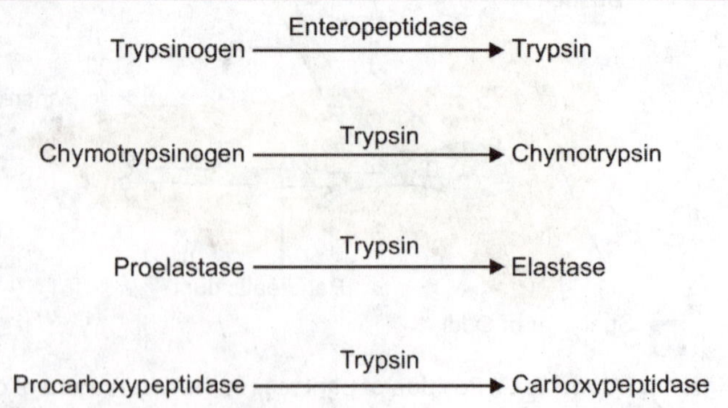

Factors that normally ***prevent autodigestion*** *of pancreas are*:

1. Enzymes are present in ***inactive form***.
2. ***Trypsin inhibitor in pancreatic tissue*** does not allow active trypsin to be formed *(trypsin remains inhibited)*.
3. The ***wall of acini is thick***, and therefore does not allow pancreatic enzymes to escape into the pancreatic tissue.

Clinical Box 40.1

Autodigestion of pancreas in acute pancreatitis: Normally, trypsin is not formed in the pancreas due to the presence of **trypsin inhibitor** in the pancreatic juice which prevents the activation of trypsinogen to trypsin. In **acute pancreatitis**, the trypsin inhibitor is deficient. Therefore, activation of trypsin results in *autodigestion* of pancreatic tissue.

Enzymes for Carbohydrate Digestion

Pancreatic amylase splits starch at α-1,4-glycosidic linkage. This is an α-amylase that acts on starch to produce maltose, α-limit dextrin, etc. It differs from salivary amylase by its **action on both boiled and unboiled starch** (*salivary amylase acts only on boiled starch*).

Functions of Pancreatic Secretion

1. Pancreatic secretion contains enzymes that help in **digestion of fat, protein and carbohydrate** as listed in Table 40.1. Pancreatic enzymes are the primary requirement for digestion and absorption. Therefore, pancreatic deficiency leads to severe malabsorption syndrome.
2. Pancreatic secretion contains bicarbonate and water that **neutralizes acidic chyme** entering intestine from stomach. It also neutralizes the effects of bile acids. Thus, it *prevents formation of duodenal ulcer* (Clinical Box 40.2).

Clinical Box 40.2

Upper part of duodenum is the commonest site for duodenal ulcer: Acidic chyme from stomach is neutralized by alkaline pancreatic juice. However, as acidic chyme in the 1st part of duodenum (part above the ampulla of Vater, the site of opening of major pancreatic duct) remains mostly unaffected by alkaline pancreatic secretion, it is the commonest site of peptic ulcer.

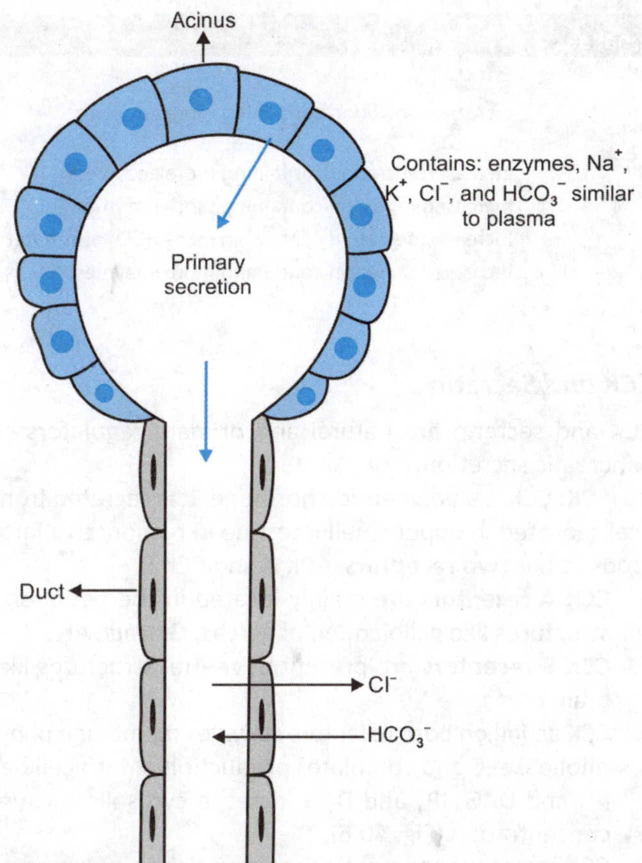

Fig. 40.4: Mechanism of pancreatic secretion. The primary secretion from acinus is modified by the exchange of ions in the duct. Note that the HCO_3^- is added by duct epithelial cells.

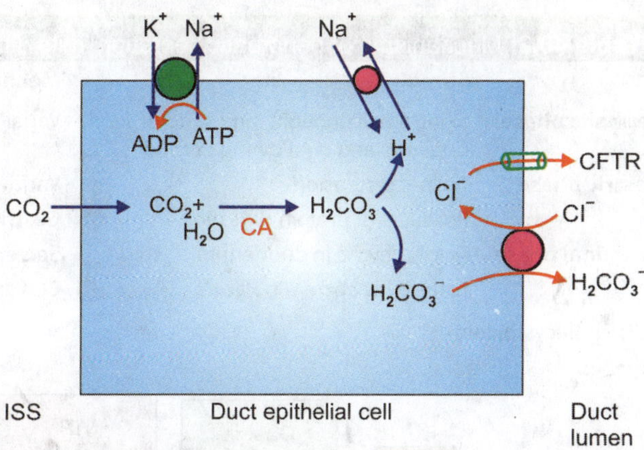

Fig. 40.5: Mechanism of bicarbonate secretion by pancreatic duct epithelial cells. (CFTR: Cystic fibrosis transmembrane regulator chloride channel; CA: Carbonic anhydrase; ISS: Interstitial tissue space).

Mechanism of Secretion

Secretion of Aqueous Component

Aqueous component of pancreatic secretion is mainly produced by the **columnar epithelial cells** that line the pancreatic ducts.

1. Pancreatic juice is **nearly isotonic with plasma** at any rate of formation and flow. The **ionic composition** includes mainly ***cations*** (Na^+ and K^+) and the ***anions*** (HCO_3^- and Cl^-). The **Na^+ and K^+ concentration** of pancreatic juice *is similar to that of plasma*. But, **HCO_3^- and Cl^- concentration** *varies according to the rate of secretion*.
   - **At lower rate of secretion**, concentration of HCO_3^- and Cl^- is about 70% of plasma.
   - **At higher rate of secretion,** their concentration is more than 100% of plasma (Fig. 40.4).
2. The aqueous component **secreted by the duct cell** is hypertonic to plasma as it contains more HCO_3^-.
3. But, when the secretion passes through the ducts, **water moves into the duct lumen** to make the pancreatic juice ***isotonic***, during which HCO_3^- is partly exchanged with Cl^- by **HCO_3^--Cl^- exchanger** present on the luminal membrane (Fig. 40.5).
   - HCO_3^- in epithelial cell is derived from carbonic acid, which is formed by CO_2 and water.
   - In duct epithelial cells, on the basolateral surface, Na^+-K^+ pump actively pumps K^+ into the cell.
   - The cytosolic H^+ is exchanged by Na^+-H^+ exchanger.
4. **In the resting state** (interdigestive phase), the secretion of aqueous component occurs ***mainly from intercalated and intralobular ducts***, but **in the stimulated state** (after eating) the secretion occurs additionally ***from extralobular ducts***, which has higher HCO_3^- concentration.

   Defect in the chloride channel causes thick exocrine secretion in the duct (Clinical Box 40.3)

Secretion of Enzyme Components

Pancreatic enzymes are **synthesized in the acinar cells** and stored in the zymogen granules. The granules are located toward the apical region of the cells. In response to appropriate stimulation, the granules are released by exocytosis into the lumen of acinus.

Clinical Box 40.3

Defect in CFTR produces viscid secretion: The Cl^- enters the acinar cells and duct epithelial cells via voltage gated Cl^- channels. The primary defect in **cystic fibrosis** is the **mutation of the gene that encodes for Cl^- channel.** Cystic fibrosis gene is located on chromosome 7, mutation of which alters the function of its product, cystic fibrosis transmembrane conductance regulator (CFTR). CFTR is localized in the apical membrane of epithelial cells in the pancreatic ducts. Alteration of CFTR results in decreased number of Cl^- channel. Therefore, Cl^- transport into duct lumen is impaired. This also impairs the transport of Na^+ and water. As a result, the secretion becomes thick causing duct obstruction which in turn causes destruction of acinar cells and duct system. This leads to ***severe pancreatic deficiency*** causing severe impairment of absorption of important nutrients. This is also accompanied by ***progressive pulmonary disease*** causing lung infection, especially in children.

Factor That Influence Secretion

Pancreatic secretion is influenced by neural and hormonal factors.

Table 40.2: Mechanisms of pancreatic secretion in its different phases.

	Stimuli	Mechanisms	Effects
Cephalic phase	Sight, smell, thought, and taste of food. Chewing and swallowing of food	Vagal stimulation	Increased secretion containing more enzymes.
Gastric phase	Gastric distension	Vagovagal reflex	Increased secretion containing more enzymes
	Products of protein digestion	Gastrin	Increased secretion containing more enzymes
Intestinal phase	Acidic chyme in duodenum	Secretin	Increased secretion containing more HCO_3^- and water
	Fatty acids and amino acids	CCK and vagovagal reflex	Increased secretion containing more enzymes.

(CCK: Cholecystokinin).

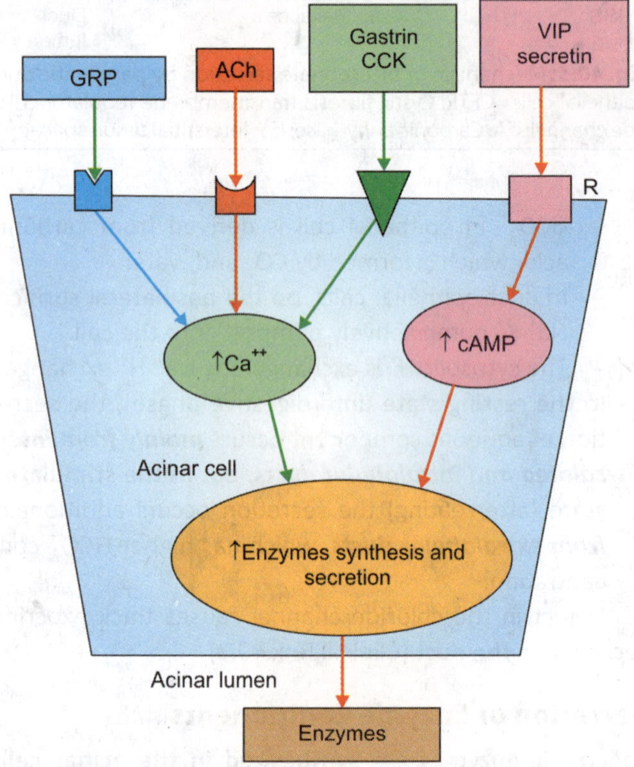

Fig. 40.6: Mechanism of different hormones acting on pancreatic acinar cells. (GRP: Gastrin releasing peptide, ACH: Acetylcholine; CCK: Cholecystokinin; VIP: Vasoactive intestinal polypeptide; R: Receptors).

1. The **hormonal factors** are mainly cholecystokinin (CCK) and secretin. **Cholecystokinin stimulates enzymatic pancreatic secretion**, whereas **secretin stimulates pancreatic secretion rich in water and bicarbonate**.
2. The **neural factors** are sympathetic and parasympathetic. *Parasympathetic stimulation increases secretion* whereas *sympathetic stimulation decreases secretion*.

However, the control mechanism varies according to the phases of secretion (described below).

Hormonal Factors

1. CCK: CCK has two receptors. (CCK A and CCK B receptors, gastrin acts through CCK B receptors)
2. Secretin
3. Gastrin: Gastrin receptors, CCK B receptors
4. GRP
5. GIP
6. VIP

CCK and Secretin

CCK and secretin are natural and primary regulators of pancreatic secretion.

CCK: CCK is a polypeptide hormone. It is secreted from I cells located in upper small intestine in response to fatty foods. It has **two receptors**: CCK A and CCK B.

1. **CCK A receptors** are mainly located in the peripheral structures like gallbladder, pancreas, GI tract, etc.
2. **CCK B receptors** are present in central structures like brain areas.
3. CCK acting on both receptors activates membrane phospholipase–C and stimulates production of intracellular IP_3 and DAG. IP_3 and DAG increase cytosolic calcium concentration (Fig. 40.6).
4. CCK increases pancreatic secretion **rich in enzymes**.

Secretin: Secretin is secreted from S cells of upper small intestine in response to acidic chyme. It acts on adenylate cyclase on the cell membrane and increases cytosolic formation of cAMP. It increases pancreatic secretion rich in bicarbonate and water. For details of CCK and secretin, refer the chapter "GI Hormones".

Neural Factors

1. Parasympathetic: stimulates secretion
2. Sympathetic: inhibits secretion

Regulation of Secretion

Phases of Pancreatic Secretion

There are ***three phases*** of pancreatic secretion: cephalic, gastric, and intestinal. Mechanisms of pancreatic secretion are different in different phases of secretion (Table 40.2).

Cephalic Phase

The cephalic phase is induced by smell, sight, thought and taste of food, and by chewing and swallowing of food.

1. Cephalic phase is mediated by **vagus nerve**. The efferent impulses originating from brain directly stimulate pancreatic secretion. The fibers mediating this response are cholinergic vagal fibers.
2. Also, **gastrin** released from the stomach in response to vagal stimulation increases pancreatic secretion.
3. The pancreatic secretion in cephalic phase is **rich in enzymes**. Cephalic phase contributes to **15–30%** of pancreatic secretion.

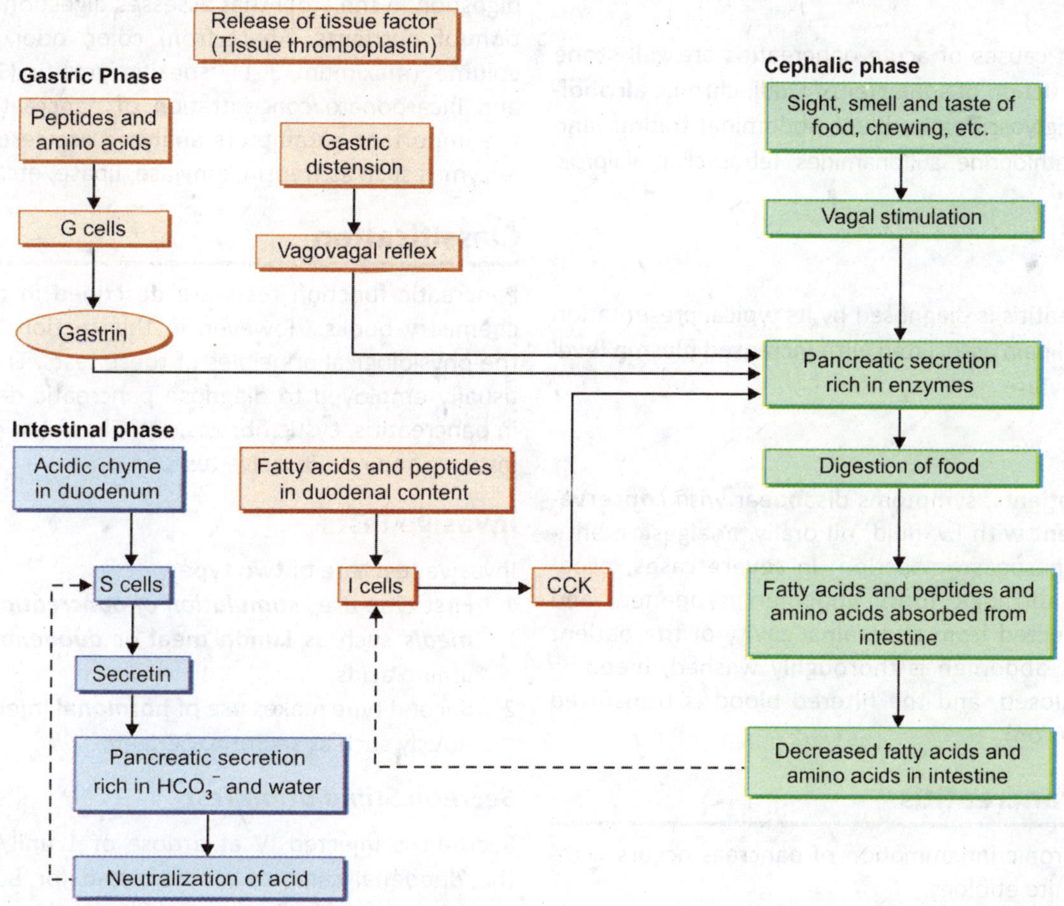

Fig. 40.7: Regulation of pancreatic secretion in cephalic, gastric, and intestinal phase. (CCK: Cholecystokinin).

Gastric Phase

When food enters the stomach, gastric phase is initiated.

1. Distension of stomach elicits **vagovagal reflex** that stimulates pancreatic secretion.
2. Presence of amino acids and peptides in the gastric content stimulate **gastrin** release from stomach that in turn stimulate pancreatic secretion (Fig. 40.7).
3. Gastric phase has ***greater effects on enzyme secretion***.
4. About **40% of pancreatic secretion** occurs in this phase.

Intestinal Phase

When chyme enters the duodenum, intestinal phase starts.

1. **Acidic chyme** increases release of **secretin** from S cells present in the mucosa of upper part of small intestine. Secretin stimulates pancreatic juice **rich in aqueous** (water and bicarbonate) component.
2. The presence of **products of protein digestion** like amino acids and peptides, and the **products of fat digestion** like fatty acids and monoglycerides in chyme evoke pancreatic secretion rich in enzymes, which is mediated by ***CCK*** secreted from I cells in intestinal mucosa (Fig. 40.7).
3. CCK potentiates the effect of secretin on ducts and secretin potentiates the effect of CCK on acinar cells.
4. The **vagovagal reflex** also mediates pancreatic secretion during gastric and intestinal phases. Intestinal phase contributes to **40–60% of pancreatic secretion**.

APPLIED PHYSIOLOGY

Acute Pancreatitis

Pathophysiology

This is a serious condition of acute abdomen that occurs due to inflammation of the pancreas.

1. The disease is characterized by **severe pain** in the epigastric or periumbilical region that often radiates to back.
2. The physiological alteration in the disease is the **activation of trypsin** inside the pancreatic tissue that causes *autodigestion of the gland*.
3. Trypsin also **activates phospholipase-A_2** which forms **lysolecithin** from fatty acid of lecithin.
4. **Lysolecithin** damages pancreatic tissue and produces necrosis of surrounding fat.
5. In severe case, hemorrhage occurs into abdominal cavity (**hemorrhagic pancreatitis**).

Etiology

The common causes of acute pancreatitis are **gall stone** causing obstruction of sphincter of Oddi, **chronic alcoholism, hypertriglyceridemia,** blunt abdominal trauma and **drugs** like azathioprine, sulfonamides, tetracycline, valproic acid, etc.

Diagnosis

Acute pancreatitis is diagnosed by its typical presentation of abdominal pain associated with **increased plasma level of serum amylase**.

Treatment

In 90% of patients, symptoms disappear with **conservative treatment** with i.v. fluid, nil orally, analgesics, antibiotics and nasogastric suction. **In severe cases**, especially in hemorrhagic form, abdomen is opened, and blood is collected from abdominal cavity of the patient and filtered, abdomen is thoroughly washed, bleeding points are closed, and the filtered blood is transfused (*autotransfusion*).

Chronic Pancreatitis

Slow and chronic inflammation of pancreas occurs without any definite etiology.

1. It may be due to improper recovery from pancreatitis or persistence of low grade acute pancreatitis.
2. Patient develops **steatorrhea** due to pancreatic lipase deficiency and **malnutrition** due to indigestion and malabsorption of various nutrients.
3. Patient *may develop diabetes mellitus* due to associated endocrine deficiency.

Cystic Fibrosis

This is an **autosomal recessive** monogenic disorder, in which the major **defect is in the Cl^- channel.**

1. The disease occurs due to **mutation in the CFTR gene** (cystic fibrosis transmembrane-conductance regulator gene), located on **chromosome 7**.
2. The disease usually starts in childhood.
3. Lung is the most common organ affected and decreased nasociliary clearance is the common pathology.
4. **Respiratory features** are chronic sinusitis, nasal obstruction, rhinorrhea and cough with expectoration of viscous-purulent sputum.
5. Common **gastrointestinal features** are intestinal obstruction and exocrine pancreatic deficiency.

PANCREATIC FUNCTION TESTS

Exocrine pancreatic function tests are based on assessment of pancreatic secretion in response to hormonal stimulation, or a meal or measurement of production of digestion in the stool that assesses digestion and absorption of nutrients. Apart from color, odor, pH (8–8.3), volume (maximum 3 L), specific gravity (1.007–1.042) and bicarbonate concentration of pancreatic secretion, the important parameters analyzed are serum and fecal enzymes such as trypsin, amylase, lipase, etc.

Classification

Pancreatic function tests are described in detail in biochemistry books. However, in this section, we describe the physiological principles of these tests. These tests are usually employed to diagnose pancreatic deficiencies as in pancreatitis, cystic fibrosis, etc. These are of two types: invasive and non-invasive tests.

Invasive Tests

Invasive tests are of **two types**.

1. First type uses ***stimulation of pancreatic secretion by meals*** such as **Lundh meal** or ***duodenal infusion*** of amino acids.
2. Second type makes use of **hormonal injection** intravenously such as secretin, CCK, etc.

Secretin Stimulation Test

Secretin is injected IV at a dose of 1 unit/kg and then the duodenal samples are collected for 80 minutes. It increases rate of formation and flow, and aqueous component of pancreatic juice.

CCK Stimulation Test

CCK increases enzymatic component of pancreatic secretion.

Meal Stimulation Test

The test meal is called Lundh meal (Lundh and Borgstrom, 1962). It consists of milk protein, corn oil, and dextrose. Following ingestion of the meal, duodenal content is aspirated for analysis.

Non-Invasive Tests

These are simpler and cheaper. Therefore, noninvasive tests are preferred to invasive tests. However, they are not as sensitive and specific as the invasive tests.

Visualization of pancreas and scanning by utrasonography, CT scan, MRI, cholangiopancreatography, etc., are usually performed before opting for biochemical pancreatic function tests. These tests are of **three types**.

1. **First type** includes estimations in stool for food particles that are not absorbed (fecal estimation of fat) and fecal enzymes (trypsin, chymotrypsin and elastase).
2. **Second type** includes estimations in blood, urine and breath for products of digested food due to action of pancreatic enzymes that are absorbed into systemic circulation.

3. **Third type** includes estimations in plasma or blood for hormones (Schilling test) and enzymes, amino acids, etc.

Fecal Estimation of Fat

Normally, about 5 g of fat is excreted per day in the feces. In pancreatic deficiency, excretion **more than 20 g of fat** is common. In severe deficiency, fat excretion may be 50 g or more.

Fecal Estimation of Nitrogen

About **7 g of nitrogen** is excreted in stool per day in a healthy individual. In pancreatic deficiency, due to decreased proteolytic enzyme activity, nitrogen excretion increases in stool.

D Xylose Absorption Test

A pentose sugar called xylose is administered (25 g, usually) and its recovery in urine is measured over next 5 hours and in blood in next 2 hours. This is a test that distinguishes between malabsorption due to pancreatic (normal absorption) and jejunal (low absorption) insufficiencies. It also helps evaluate response to therapy.

Schilling Test

It is done to assess the absorption of **vitamin B_{12}** which requires intrinsic factor. Vitamin B_{12} deficiency is seen in chronic pancreatitis because trypsin helps in binding B_{12} to intrinsic factor after which the complex is reabsorbed.

Serum Amylase Estimation

Normal level of serum amylase is **60–120 units** per liter. In acute pancreatitis, serum amylase concentration becomes very high. This differentiates pancreatitis from other conditions of acute abdomen.

Cholangiopancreatography

This is a special radiodiagnostic investigation in which the details of the contour of hepatopancreatic duct system are visualized by introducing an endoscope. The procedure is called endoscopic retrograde cholangiopancreatography (**ERCP**). This is the most accurate test for assessing pancreatic structure and function.

CHAPTER SUMMARY

Key Concepts

1. Pancreas secretes enzymes for digestion of all types of nutrients. Therefore, pancreatic deficiency leads to severe indigestion and malabsorption.
2. Pancreatic juice is alkaline. It helps in protecting the mucosa of intestine from acidic chyme that may damage the intestinal epithelium.
3. CCK stimulates pancreatic juice rich in enzymes, and secretin increases secretion of aqueous component.
4. Trypsin inhibitors prevent activation of trypsin inside pancreas. It is activated in duodenum by enterokinase. Activation of trypsin inside pancreas causes acute pancreatitis and autodigestion of pancreas, as trypsin is strong proteolytic agent.

Important to Know (Must Read)

1. In examinations, "Composition and function of pancreatic secretion, and mechanism and regulation of pancreatic secretion" may come as a **Long Question**.
2. Phases of pancreatic secretion, Composition and functions of pancreatic secretion, Mechanism of pancreatic secretion, Regulation of pancreatic secretion, Pancreatic function tests, can come as **Short Questions**.
3. In **Viva**, examiner may ask... Structure and functions of pancreatic acini, Amount of pancreatic secretion/day, Composition pancreatic juice and function of each constituent pancreatic secretion, Name pancreatic enzymes and tell their functions, Mechanism of gastric secretion, What are the Phases of pancreatic secretions and how are they regulated, What are the stimuli for different phases of pancreatic secretion, What are the effects of parasympathetic and sympathetic stimulation on pancreatic secretion, Classify pancreatic function tests, Procedure and normal values of important pancreatic function tests, Causes of acute and chronic pancreatitis, What is cystic fibrosis and which ion channel is defective in this disease.
4. Composition pancreatic juice and functions of each constituent, and Pancreatic function tests, are usually asked in viva. A student is expected to answer these questions.

CHAPTER

41

Physiology of Liver, Liver Function Tests and Pathophysiology of Jaundice

LEARNING OBJECTIVES

On completion of study of this chapter, the student **MUST** be able to:

1. List the functions of liver.
2. Understand the importance of knowing hepatic physiology in learning medicine.
3. Briefly outline functional architecture of hepatic lobule.
4. Outline the bilirubin metabolism.
5. Understand the physiological basis of classification of jaundice.
6. Appreciate the differences in laboratory findings of different types of jaundice.

The student **MAY** also be able to:

1. Describe details of bilirubin metabolism.
2. Explain the pathophysiology of jaundice.

PHYSIOLOGY OF LIVER

Liver is an essential organ of the body as it is the center of all metabolisms and crucial for many other vital functions. Therefore, liver dysfunctions result in major abnormalities of the body. In adults, liver weighs about 1.5 kg. Liver is protected by a thin but strong capsule, called *Glisson's capsule*.

Scientist contributed

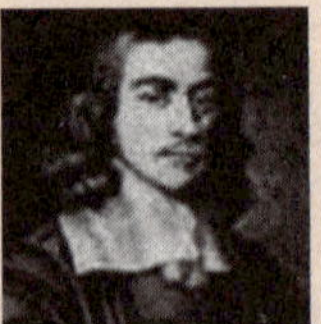
Francis Glisson
(1599–1677)

Francis Glisson (1599–1677) was a British physician, anatomist, physiologist, and writer on medical subjects. He did important work on the anatomy of the liver, and wrote on rickets. A physiology experiment he performed that helped debunk the balloonist theory of muscle contraction, as he demonstrated that when a muscle contracts under water, the water level does not rise, and thus no air or fluid could be entering the muscle. Glisson is a well-known medical eponym, the ***Glisson's capsule*** of Liver, named after him.

Functional Anatomy

The main function of the liver is the bile synthesis and secretion. The bile is secreted into hepatic ducts. The hepatic ducts join to form **common hepatic duct**. Bile is continuously formed and delivered to the gallbladder, the process known as **bile secretion** (described in detail in next chapter). In the gallbladder, the bile is stored and concentrated and delivered via the common bile duct into second part of duodenum in response to chyme entering the duodenum.

Blood Supply

Liver receives blood supply from two sources.

Portal Vein

Portal vein is formed by the union of two veins, viz. superior mesenteric vein and splenic vein. Thus portal vein supplies blood from most parts of the stomach and intestine as well as from the spleen and pancreas. Therefore, portal blood is **rich in end products of digestion, GI hormones and pancreatic hormones**. However, this blood is comparatively poor in oxygen.

Hepatic Artery

Hepatic artery contains pure arterial blood and is rich in oxygen.

Portal Circulation

The portal vein and hepatic artery break up into large number of branches.

1. Blood of these two sets of vessels get mixed up in the **sinusoids** of the liver. The hepatic cells receive oxygen and nutrients from the sinusoids.

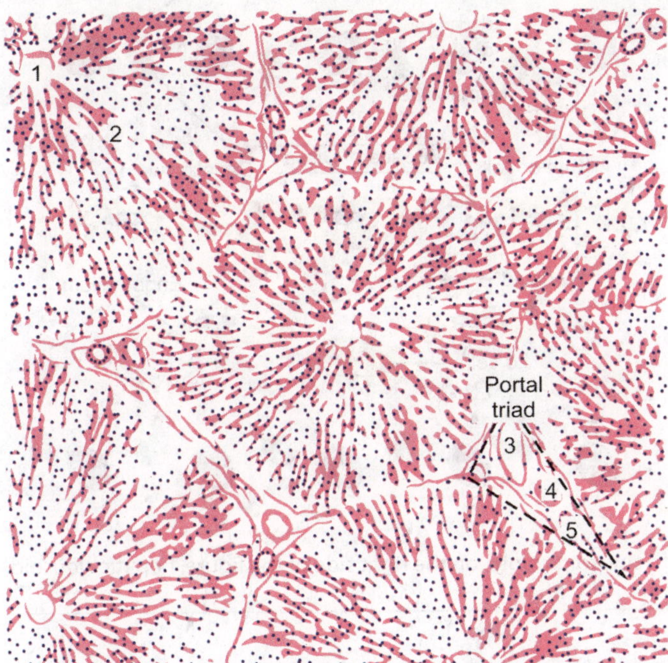

Fig. 41.1: Histology of liver showing hepatic lobules. 1: Central vein; 2: Radiating cord of hepatocytes; 3: Branch of portal vein; 4: Branch of hepatic artery; 6: Interlobular duct. Note, 3, 4, 5 form the portal triad.

2. The various substances produced by the liver, products of metabolism, the waste products and the CO_2 are discharged into the sinusoids.
3. The sinusoids drain into the central vein of the lobule.
4. Central veins from different lobules unite to form larger veins, which in turn join ultimately and drain into hepatic vein.
5. The hepatic vein opens into the inferior vena cava.

Bile Secretion by Liver Cells

The liver cells synthesize bile, which is first secreted to **small canaliculi**. The smaller canaliculi join and ultimately form two **hepatic ducts** (right and left).

Histology of Liver

Liver is formed by large number of **lobules** (Fig. 41.1). Each lobule is delineated by a connective tissue sheath.

1. The individual lobule is ***polygonal in shape*** with a central vein at the center.
2. From the central vein, plates of liver cells radiate like spokes of a bicycle wheel to the periphery of the lobule (Fig. 41.2).
3. The plates are one cell thick and are separated by liver sinusoids. Liver cells have the capacity to regenerate (Application Box 41.1).

Sinusoids and Bile Canaliculi

In a typical lobule, between the plates of hepatic cells, the **sinusoids** are present that carry blood.

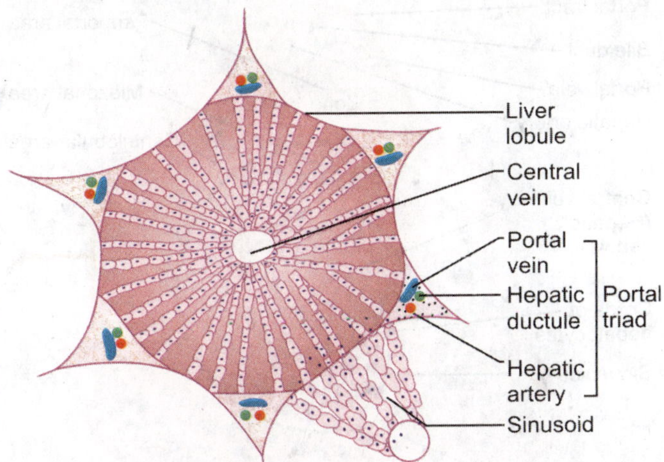

Fig. 41.2: Detailed structure of liver lobule.

1. Each sinusoid receives blood from a branch of portal vein and hepatic artery of the portal tract, and drains into the central vein.
2. Wall of the sinusoids are mostly made up of ***endothelial cells***, but at places macrophage cells, called Kupffer cells, are occasionally present.
3. The **bile canaliculi** run in between the two layers of cells (layer of cells that make the thickness of each plate) (Fig. 41.3). The liver cells (hepatocytes) synthesize the bile acids and transfer them into bile canaliculi.
4. The space that lies between sinusoid and hepatocytes is the **space of Disse** (perisinusoidal space). The space of Disse serves as a route through which hepatocytes remove certain substances from blood and discharge certain products into the blood.

Portal triad

Portal triads are typically found at the angles of liver lobules. Each portal triad consists of a branch of portal vein, a branch of hepatic artery and a bile ductule (Figs. 41.2 and 41.3).

1. The angular space that contains portal triad and its surrounding connective tissue is called **portal canal.**
2. Portal sinusoids originating from portal veins remain in close proximity with bile canaliculi that drain into interlobular bile duct (Fig. 41.4).
3. A small space between hepatocyte and portal canal is called **space of Mall**, the site of origin of lymph in liver.

Application Box 41.1

Hepatic regeneration: Despite its slow rate of cell renewal, liver has the capacity of regeneration. The loss of hepatic tissue by surgical removal, injury or effect of toxin triggers a mechanism by which hepatocytes begin to divide and grow till the normal size is attained. This property of liver tissue is used in liver transplantation, in which a small portion of transplanted liver tissue proliferates to become the normal size liver.

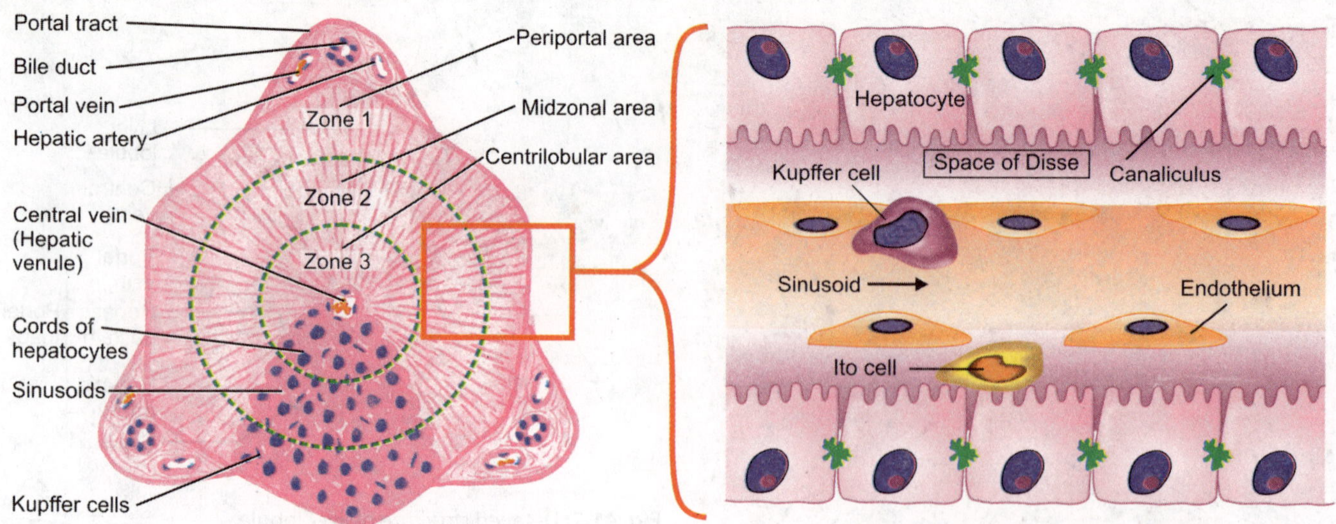

Fig. 41.3: Location of bile canaliculi in hepatocytes, and its relation with sinusoids. Note, on the right side of the figure, hepatic sinusoid, persinusoidal space and cords of hepatocytes.

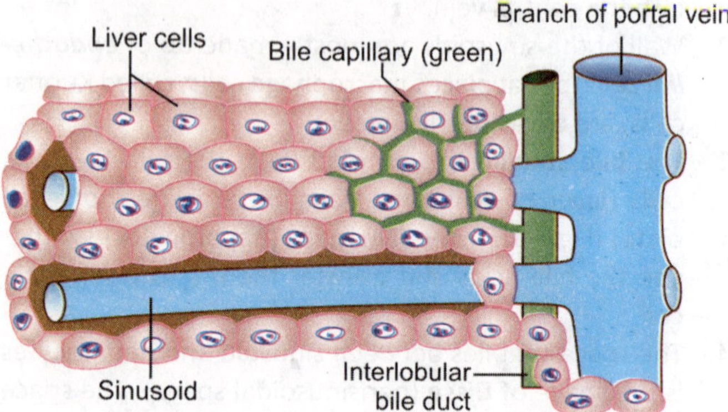

Fig. 41.4: Relation of portal sinusoids with bile capillaries.

Functions of Liver

Liver is the center for most of the metabolisms. It synthesizes many essential proteins, stores nutrients that are released into circulation at the time of starvation, and detoxifies harmful substances. It plays an essential role in maintaining blood glucose level. Therefore, liver is among the vital organs of the body.

1. **Secretory functions:** Liver forms and secretes bile into biliary tract.
2. **Metabolic functions:** Liver is involved in metabolism of major nutrients such as carbohydrate, fat, proteins, and fat soluble and water soluble vitamins. Liver plays a central role in the metabolisms of urea, iron, and alcohol.
3. **Synthetic functions:** Liver is the major organ for the synthesis of proteins that include clotting factors, acute phase proteins that mediate inflammation, hormone binding proteins, lipids, carbohydrates, vitamins and bile salts.
4. **Storage functions:** Liver stores glucose, protein, fat, and vitamins. These nutrients are released from liver and utilized during their scarcity, and are stored in liver when they are in excess.
5. **Detoxifying action:** Liver detoxifies many chemicals. Toxins released from infecting organisms are neutralized in liver.
6. **Degradation of drugs and chemicals:** Liver is the site of inactivation of many drugs. Liver degrades enzymes, hormones, cytokines, and various other chemicals.
7. **Excretory function:** Liver excretes bile pigments, cholesterol, and some metals.
8. **Immunity:** Kupffer cells of liver are part of mononuclear phagocyte system (reticuloendothelial system) that forms the nonspecific defenses of the body. These cells phagocytose and kill microorganism.
9. **Endocrine functions:** Liver converts vitamin D_3 to 25-hydroxyvitamin D_3. Liver is a major site for conversion of T_4 to T_3. Somatomedin (insulin-like growth factor) that mediates important functions of growth factor is secreted from liver. Many hormones like insulin, glucagon, growth hormone, GI hormones, etc., are degraded in liver.

LIVER FUNCTION TESTS

In view of multiplicity and complexity of the liver functions, it is obvious that no single test can establish the disturbance in liver function. Thus a battery of liver function tests is employed for accurate diagnosis, to access the severity of damage, to judge prognosis and to evaluate therapy. These tests are listed below in relation to major liver functions. A summary of various liver function tests and their significance is depicted in Table 41.1.

A. Tests for manufacture and excretion of bile
   1. Bilirubin estimation

Table 41.1: Liver function tests and their significances.

Tests	Significance
A. Tests for manufacture and excretion of bile	
1. Bilirubin estimation	
i. In serum (0.2–0.8 mg/dL)	Increased in hepatocellular, obstructive, and hemolytic disease, Gilbert disease
ii. In feces	Absent in biliary obstruction
iii. In urine	Conjugated bilirubinuria in patients of hepatitis
2. Urobilinogen	Increased in hepatocellular and hemolytic disease, absent in biliary obstruction
3. Bile acids (bile salts)	Increased in serum and detectable in urine in cholestasis
4. Bromsulphalein excretion	Helps in diagnosis of Dubin-Johnson syndrome
B. Serum enzyme assays	
1. Alkaline phosphatase (ALP) (33–96 U/L)	Increased in hepatobiliary disease (highest in biliary obstruction), bone diseases, pregnancy
2. γ-Glutamyl transpeptidase (γ-GT) (9–58 IU/L)	Rise parallels ALP but is specific for hepatobiliary diseases
3. Transaminases (aminotransferases)	
i. Aspartate transaminases (SGOT or AST)	Increased in tissue injury to liver as well as to other tissues like in myocardial infarction
ii. Alanine transaminases (SGPT or ALT)	Increase is fairly specific for liver cell injury
4. Other serum enzymes	
i. 5′ Nucleotidase	Rise parallels ALP but more specific for diseases of hepatic origin
ii. Lactate dehydrogenase	Increased in tumors involving liver
iii. Choline esterase	Decreased in hepatocellular disease, malnutrition
C. Tests for metabolic functions	
1. Amino acid and plasma protein metabolism	
i. Serum proteins (total = 6.7–8.6 g/dL; A:G ratio = 1.5 to 3.1)	Hypoalbuminemia in hepatocellular diseases; hyperglobulinemia in cirrhosis and chronic active hepatitis
i. Immunoglobulins	Nonspecific alterations in IgA, IgG, and IgM
ii. Clotting factors	Prothrombin time and partial thromboplastin time prolonged in patients with hepatocellular diseases
iii. Serum ammonia (19–60 μg/dL)	Increased in acute fulminant hepatitis, cirrhosis, hepatic encephalopathy
iv. Aminoaciduria	In fulminant hepatitis
2. Lipid and lipoprotein metabolism Blood lipids (total serum cholesterol < 200 mg/dL; triglycerides < 150 mg/dL; and lipoprotein fractions)	Increased in cholestasis, decreased in acute and chronic diffuse liver disease and in malnutrition
3. Carbohydrate metabolism Blood glucose and GTT	Decreased in hepatic necrosis
D. Immunologic tests	
1. Nonspecific immunologic reactions	
i. Smooth muscle antibody	In hepatic necrosis
ii. Mitochondrial antibody	In primary biliary cirrhosis
iii. Antinuclear Ab and LE cell test	In chronic active hepatitis
2. Antibodies to specific etiologic agents	
i. Antibodies to hepatitis B (HBsAg, HBc, HBeAg)	In hepatitis B
ii. Amoeba antibodies	Amoebic liver abscess
E. Ancillary diagnostic tests	
1. Ultrasound examination	Cholestasis of various etiologies; SOLs, US-guide-FNAC/liver biopsy
2. FNAC and/or percutaneous liver biopsy	Unknown cause of hepatocellular disease, hepatomegaly and splenomegaly; long-standing hepatitis; PUO and SOLs of the liver

i. In serum
ii. In faeces
iii. In urine

2. Urobilinogen
3. Bile acids (bile salts)
4. Bromsulphalein excretion

B. Serum enzyme assays
   1. Alkaline phosphatase
   2. γ-Glutamyl transpeptidase
   3. Transaminases (aminotransferases)
      i. Aspartate transaminases or AST
      ii. Alanine transaminases or ALT
   4. Other serum enzymes
      i. 5′ Nucleotidase
      ii. Lactate dehydrogenase
      iii. Choline esterase

C. Tests for metabolic functions
   1. Amino acid and plasma protein metabolism
      i. Serum proteins
      ii. Immunoglobulins
      iii. Clotting factors
      iv. Serum ammonia
   2. Lipid and lipoprotein metabolism
   3. Carbohydrate metabolism

D. Immunologic tests
   i. Nonspecific immunologic reactions
   ii. Antibodies to specific etiologic agents

E. Ancillary diagnostic tests
   i. Ultrasonography
   ii. FNAC and/or percutaneous liver biopsy

PATHOPHYSIOLOGY OF JAUNDICE

Jaundice is the yellowish discoloration of sclera, skin and mucous membrane due to the deposition of bilirubin. This happens when concentration of bilirubin increases in blood. Bilirubin is the product of hemoglobin breakdown. Therefore, to understand pathophysiology of jaundice, it is necessary to learn the **process of hemolysis** and hemoglobin breakdown.

Red Cell Breakdown

Red cells have an average lifespan of 120 days. The aged red cells are trapped by the macrophages of mononuclear phagocytic system (MPS) that are present in spleen, liver, lymph nodes, and bone marrow. Macrophages, especially in the spleen, after destroying red cells and hemoglobin, release their components into blood. For details of red cell destruction and bilirubin metabolism, refer to Chapter 13.

Hemoglobin Catabolism

Macrophages split hemoglobin into heme and globin.

1. **Globin** is the protein component, which is degraded into amino acids that enter the amino acid pool of the body and are reutilized whenever required.
2. **Heme** is catabolized by the *microsomal oxygenase system* to release iron, which joins the iron pool of the body.
3. Some of the heme molecules are simultaneously oxidized to **biliverdin**.
4. Then, biliverdin is reduced to **bilirubin** by the enzyme *biliverdin reductase*. Bilirubin for its lipophilic nature crosses cell membrane easily. However, for its water-insolubility, it is transported in body fluids only after conjugation in the liver or in combination with albumin.

Bilirubin Metabolism

Bilirubin released from macrophages enters the blood stream, where it forms a complex with albumin. Bilirubin bound to albumin (**albumin-bilirubin complex**) is not excreted in urine, as albumin molecule is large enough not to get filtered in renal glomeruli. Bilirubin-albumin complex is *split in the liver*, bilirubin enters liver cells and albumin stays back in the blood.

In liver cells, bilirubin undergoes **three-step metabolism**: uptake, conjugation, and excretion.

1. **Uptake:** Bilirubin after splitting from albumin-bilirubin complex is transported into the hepatocyte, where it forms a complex with a cytoplasmic protein, called **ligandin**. Formation of bilirubin-ligandin complex prevents bilirubin to return back to the blood as the complex is too big to pass through the liver cell membrane.
2. **Conjugation:** Hepatocytes conjugate bilirubin with glucuronic acid, which takes place in the endoplasmic reticulum and involves UDP-glucuronic acid and glucuronyl transferase. This forms **bilirubin glucuronide** (Fig. 41.5).
3. **Excretion:** Bilirubin glucuronide is excreted from hepatocytes into the biliary canaliculi. This is an active process, and is the ***rate-limiting step*** in the hepatic bilirubin metabolism.

Fate of Conjugated Bilirubin

Bilirubin glucuronide is excreted in bile to be discharged into the small intestine. In large intestine, bilirubin is acted upon by the bacterial flora, where glucuronic acid is split and bilirubin undergoes a series of reduction reactions to from **stercobilinogen**.

Stercobilinogen, a colorless compound ***has two fates***:

1. In the intestine, 80% of stercobilinogen is oxidized to **stercobilin**, which is excreted in stool. Stercobilin is a brownish compound that *imparts brown color to the stool.*
2. The remaining 20% stercobilinogen is absorbed into the portal circulation and re-excreted by liver into the bile, and re-enters the intestine. A part of the absorbed stercobilinogen enters the general circulation and is filtered and excreted by the kidneys. In urine, the stercobilinogen is called **urobilinogen**.
3. Conjugated bilirubin is not reabsorbable, whereas it metabolic products, urobilinogen is reabsorbed and enters enterohepatic circulation. The major differences between conjugated and unconjugated bilirubin are summarized in Table 41.2.

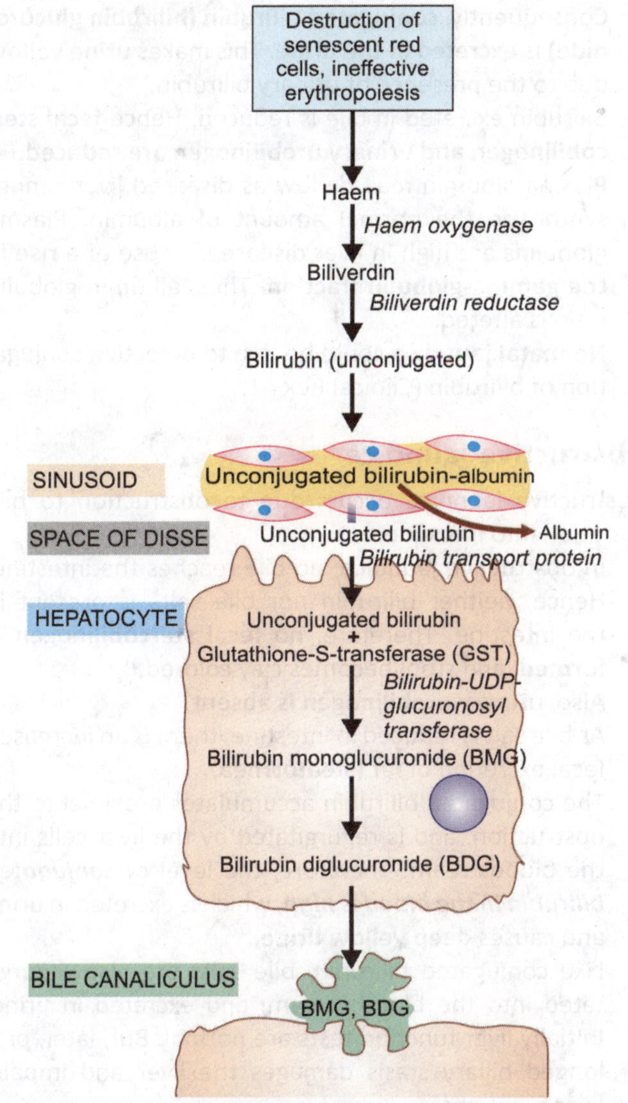

Fig. 41.5: Hepatic phase of bilirubin metabolism.

Normal Plasma Bilirubin Level: The normal concentration of bilirubin in plasma is **0.2–0.8 mg/dL**. Jaundice is detected clinically only when the bilirubin level exceeds 2 mg/dL.

Types of Jaundice

Clinically, jaundice is detected when bilirubin level is more than 2 mg/dL. Bilirubin level between 0.8 and 2 mg% is called **latent or subclinical jaundice**. Jaundice first appears in sclera (Fig. 41.6), because bilirubin has an extremely high affinity for scleral protein called **elastin**.

Physiologically, the **causes of jaundice** are divided broadly into **two categories**: increased production of bilirubin and decreased excretion of bilirubin.

Increased Production of Bilirubin

Production of bilirubin is increased in hemolysis. Therefore, the jaundice is called **hemolytic jaundice**. This is seen in hemolytic anemias (for details, refer "Pathophysiology of Anemia, Chapter 15").

Table 41.2: Differences between conjugated and unconjugated bilirubin.

Feature	Unconjugated bilirubin	Conjugated bilirubin
1. Normal serum level	More	Less (< 0.25 mg/dL)
2. Water solubility	Absent	Present
3. Affinity to lipids (alcohol solubility)	Present	Absent
4. Serum albumin binding	High	Low
5. Van den Bergh reaction	Indirect (total minus direct)	Direct
6. Renal excretion	Absent	Present
7. Bilirubin albumin covalent complex formation	Absent	Present
8. Affinity to brain tissue	Present (Kernicterus)	Absent

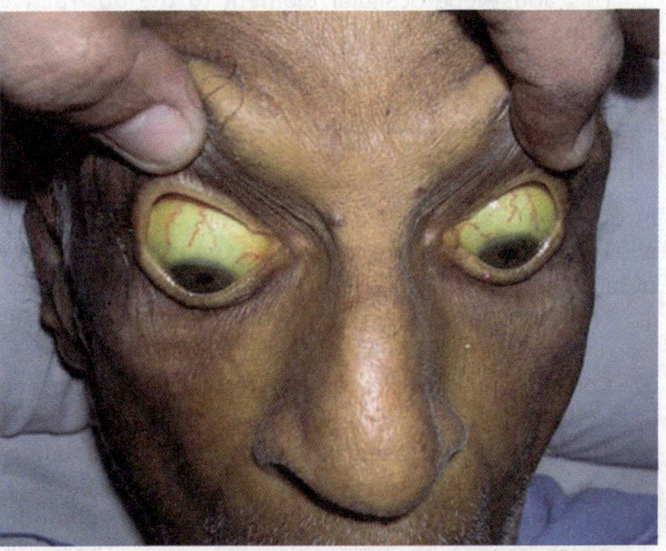

Fig. 41.6: A case of obstructive jaundice. Note the yellow discoloration of sclera.
Courtesy: Figure 12.6, Gastrointestinal surgery, by S Devaji Rao, 1st edition, 2009; Jaypee Brothers Medical Publishers (P) Ltd.

Decreased Excretion of Bilirubin

The excretion of bilirubin is impaired when liver cannot conjugate bilirubin efficiently, which is called **hepatic jaundice**, or when conjugated bilirubin cannot be excreted in bile due to biliary obstruction, which is called **obstructive jaundice**.

1. Hepatic jaundice commonly occurs in viral hepatitis and obstructive jaundice is commonly seen in gallstones (stone in the common bile duct) or stricture of bile duct. However, hepatic and obstructive jaundice overlap in their pathophysiologic processes.

Table 41.3: Differences between different types of jaundice.

	Hemolytic	**Hepatic**	**Obstructive**
Bilirubinemia	Mild	Moderate	Severe
Fecal stercobilinogen	Increased	Decreased	Absent
Urinary urobilinogen	Increased	Decreased	Absent
Urinary bilirubin	Absent	Present	Present
van den Bergh test	Indirect	Biphasic	Direct
Liver function	Normal	Impaired	May be impaired

2. In hepatic jaundice, narrowing of biliary canaliculi occurs very often resulting in **intrahepatic obstruction (stasis)**. This adds an obstructive element to the hepatic jaundice.
3. In obstructive jaundice, **biliary stasis** behind the site of obstruction causes damage to the hepatocytes. This adds hepatocellular element to the obstructive jaundice.

Laboratory Diagnosis of Jaundice

Hemolytic Jaundice

In hemolytic jaundice, **excessive production of bilirubin** allows liver to conjugate more than the normal quantity of bilirubin.

1. Therefore, more quantity of **bilirubin glucuronide** is delivered to the intestine.
2. Consequently, the amount of **stercobilinogen** formed in the intestine is increased.
3. This leads to **increased excretion of fecal stercobilinogen and urinary urobilinogen** (Table 41.3).
4. Bilirubin in plasma forms a complex with albumin, which cannot be excreted in the urine. Therefore, hemolytic jaundice is **acholuric jaundice** (absence of bilirubin in urine). Liver function tests are usually normal.

Hepatic Jaundice

In hepatic jaundice, all three steps of bilirubin metabolism **(uptake, conjugation, and excretion) are affected**. But as mentioned earlier, the ***rate-limiting step is excretion***, and therefore that may be the most affected. Therefore, not only the conjugation of bilirubin is impaired, but also some amount of conjugated bilirubin is not excreted in bile.

1. The conjugated bilirubin that accumulates in liver cells diffuses across the cell membrane into the bloodstream. Thus, in hepatic jaundice the **blood contains excess of bilirubin-albumin complex** as diseased liver may not be able to conjugate all the load of bilirubin. Also, conjugated bilirubin diffuses back into the bloodstream.
2. Consequently, **conjugated bilirubin (bilirubin glucuronide) is excreted in the urine**. This makes **urine yellow** due to the presence of urinary bilirubin.
3. Bilirubin excreted in bile is reduced. Hence **fecal stercobilinogen and urinary urobilinogen are reduced**.
4. Plasma albumin may be low as diseased liver cannot synthesize the normal amount of albumin. Plasma globulins are high in liver disease because of a **rise in the gamma-globulin fraction**. Thus, albumin-globulin ratio is altered.
5. **Neonatal jaundice** could be due to defective conjugation of bilirubin (Clinical Box 41.1).

Obstructive Jaundice

Obstructive jaundice occurs due to obstruction to bile secretion into intestine.

1. In obstructive jaundice, no bile reaches the intestine. Hence, neither bilirubin nor bile salts is present in the intestine. Therefore, **no fecal stercobilinogen is formed**, and stool becomes clay colored.
2. Also, **urinary urobilinogen is absent**.
3. As bile salt is reduced in intestine, there is an increased fecal excretion of fat (**steatorrhea**).
4. The conjugated bilirubin accumulates proximal to the obstruction, and is regurgitated by the liver cells into the bloodstream. Therefore, the level of ***conjugated bilirubin in the blood is high***, which is excreted in urine and causes **deep yellow urine**.
5. Like conjugated bilirubin, bile salts are also regurgitated into the blood stream, and excreted in urine. Initially liver function tests are normal. But, later, prolonged biliary stasis damages the liver and impairs liver functions.

van den Bergh test: Van den Bergh test detects whether *bilirubin is conjugated or not*. The test is based on the principle that excess of water soluble bilirubin-glucuronide gives a reddish-violet color when brought in contact with **diazo reagent**.

1. If the color appears immediately, the test is said to be **direct positive**.
2. If the color appears late, or only after addition of alcohol, the test is said to be **indirect positive**.
3. In hemolytic jaundice, the Van den Bergh test is **indirect positive**.
4. In obstructive jaundice, it is **direct positive**.
5. In hepatic jaundice, the test may be **biphasic**, i.e. an atypical color develops almost immediately.

Clinical Box 41.1

Physiological jaundice: This is seen in some newborns and therefore this is also known as **neonatal jaundice**. It is common in premature babies and neonates having low birth weight. The jaundice usually appears on the second or third day of life and disappears within a week. It occurs due to subnormal activity of glucuronyl transferase that impairs conjugation of bilirubin in hepatocyte. It is unlikely to be due to hemolysis.

CHAPTER SUMMARY

Key Concepts

1. Liver is the site of all metabolisms.
2. Bilirubin released from hemolysis is conjugated in liver and conjugated bilirubin is secreted in bile into intestine.
3. Excess production of bilirubin by hemolysis leads to hemolytic (Prehepatic) jaundice, diseases of liver (defect in conjugation) causes hepatic jaundice, accumulation of bilirubin due to obstruction to flow of bile causes obstructive (posthepatic) jaundice.

Important to Know (Must Read)

1. In examinations, **Long Questions** usually do not come from this chapter. However, Liver function tests may come as a question.
2. Functions of liver, Bilirubin metabolism, Pathophysiology of jaundice, Differences in laboratory diagnosis of types of jaundice, Liver function tests, can come as **Short Questions**.
3. In **Viva**, Structure of a hepatic lobule, Portal triad, Relationship between sinusoidal capillary and bile canaliculi, Functions of liver, Steps of bilirubin metabolism, How is bilirubin metabolized in liver and excreted from the body, Differences between conjugated and unconjugated bilirubin, Pathophysiology of hemolytic, hepatic, and obstructive jaundice, Common causes of hemolytic, hepatic, and obstructive jaundice, Differences in laboratory diagnosis of three types of jaundice, Classification of liver function tests (LFT), Common values and interpretation of LFT, What is physiological jaundice.
4. "Functions of liver" and "name important LFT" are very common questions in viva. A student, who fails to answer these questions satisfactorily, may get fail mark.

CHAPTER

42

Biliary Secretion

LEARNING OBJECTIVES

On completion of study of this chapter, the student **MUST** be able to:

1. Give the composition and functions of bile.
2. List the differences between hepatic and gallbladder bile.
3. Name bile salts and acids and give their functions.
4. Understand the importance of enterophepatic circulation.
5. Outline the mechanism and regulation of bile secretion.
6. Learn the physiological abnormality in gallstone formation.

The student **MAY** also be able to:

1. Describe the regulation of bile secretion.
2. Explain the mechanism of enterohepatic circulation.

HEPATOBILIARY SYSTEM

Bile is secreted from liver. Human liver secretes about **0.5 to 1 liter of bile per day**. Secretion of bile is important for digestion and absorption of fat.

Functional Anatomy

Bile is formed in the liver and is excreted through the bile ductules. The bile ductules along with the branches of portal vein and hepatic artery form the *portal triad*. The portal triad opens into the hepatic sinusoids. The sinusoids are surrounded by hepatocytes. The hepatocytes are in intimate contact with the sinusoidal blood. The **bile canaliculi** start at the space between two hepatocytes (refer to Figs. 41.3 and 41.4, Chapter 41), which opens into bile ductules. Bile ductules then form the bile duct which leads to **hepatic duct**. The right and left hepatic ducts join to form **common hepatic duct** (Fig. 42.1). The **cystic duct** from gallbladder combines with hepatic duct to form **common bile duct**. Common bile duct combines with pancreatic duct and opens to second part of duodenum through **sphincter of Oddi**.

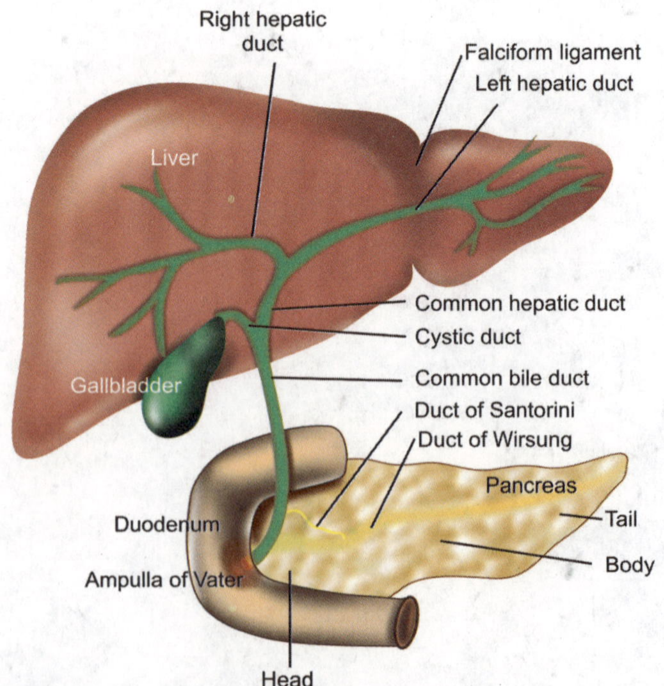

Fig. 42.1: Components of hepatobiliary system.

Composition of Bile

Bile is a greenish yellow fluid formed in the liver and stored in gallbladder. It is composed of water (98%), and solids that mainly include bile salts and pigments and different ions (Table 42.1).

Table 42.1: Composition of solids in human bile.

Bile salts
Bile pigments
Cholesterol
Inorganic salts
Fatty acids and fat
Alkaline phosphatase
Cations: Na^+, K^+, Ca^{2+}, and Mg^{2+}
Anions: HCO_3^-, Cl^-, SO_4^{2-}, and PO_4^{3-}

The color of bile is greenish yellow due to the presence of glucuronides of bile pigments. The bile pigments are bilirubin and biliverdin.

Hepatic and Gallbladder Bile

There are differences between hepatic bile (**bile formed in the liver**) and gallbladder bile (**bile stored in gallbladder**) as bile is concentrated and acidified in gallbladder (Table 42.2).

1. Water absorption is the major mechanism for concentration of bile that occurs **secondary to Na^+ absorption** (secondary active transport).
2. **Na^+-K^+ ATPase** in the basolateral membrane of epithelial cell lining transports Na^+ actively out of the cell and creates gradient for Na^+ transport into the cell.
3. Water is reabsorbed passively by **osmotic gradient** created by Na^+ movement.
4. **H^+ is exchanged with Na^+** that causes acidification of bile.

Table 42.2: Differences in hepatic and gallbladder bile.

	Hepatic bile	Gallbladder bile
1. pH	Alkaline (8–8.5)	Acidic (about 7)
2. Water content	98%	85%
3. Solids	2 g%	10–15g%
4. Bile salts and pigments	Less	More

Bile Acids and Salts

Bile Acids

There are two types of bile acids: primary and secondary.

1. The **primary bile acids** are cholic acid and chenodeoxycholic acid. The primary bile acids are ***formed in the hepatocytes*** from cholesterol.
2. **Secondary bile acids** are deoxycholic acid and lithocholic acid. The secondary bile acids are ***produced in the intestine*** where intestinal bacteria convert primary bile acids into secondary bile acids.

Bile Salts

Bile salts are **Na^+ and K^+ salts of bile acids**. Bile acids are conjugated with taurine or glycine to form **taurocholic acid** or **glycocholic acid**. These acids then combine with sodium and potassium salts to form *Na^+-taurocholate, Na^+-glycocholate, K^+-taurocholate, and K^+-glycocholate*, respectively.

Functions of Bile Salts

Bile salts are primarily responsible for absorption of fat and fat soluble nutrients. Therefore, bile deficiency causes steatorrhea. Bile salts perform following important functions.

1. **Absorption of fat:** Bile salts are essential for absorption of fat from intestine. This depends on formation of ***micelles*** by bile salts in the intestine. For their amphipathic (both hydrophilic and hydrophobic domains) property, along with lecithin and cholesterol, bile salts form cylindrical disks, called as micelles (for details, refer the chapter "Principles of Digestion and Absorption : Chapter 51". ***Lipids are transported in micelles*** from the lumen to the membrane of intestinal mucosal epithelial cells where micelle dissociates and lipids are absorbed.
2. **Emulsification of fat:** Bile salts are ***surface tension reducing agents***. Along with phospholipids and monoglycerides, they cause emulsification of fat, which is essential for digestion and absorption of fat.
3. **Source of bile acid:** Bile salts are ***converted to bile acids*** in the intestine, which are then absorbed into portal blood. Thus, bile salts are important sources of bile acids that *add to the bile acid pool of the body*.
4. **Bile secretion:** Bile salts are important ***choleretics***. They are constituent of bile and also they stimulate bile secretion.
5. **Absorption of fat-soluble vitamins:** Bile salts facilitate absorption of fat soluble vitamins (vitamins A, D, E, and K). Hence, in obstructive jaundice, features of deficiencies of fat soluble vitamins develop.
6. **Activation of pancreatic enzymes:** Bile salts activate ***pancreatic lipase***.
7. **Prevention of gallstone formation:** Bile salts along with lecithin solubilize cholesterol. Thus, they prevent formation of stones in the gallbladder.
8. **Physiological purgatives:** Bile salts act as physiological purgatives. Constipation occurs in conditions of deficiency of delivery of bile into intestine as occurs in obstructive jaundice.
9. **Stool color:** Bile salts add natural brownish color to the stool.
10. **Prevention of bacterial growth:** Bile maintains pH of intestinal content and prevents overgrowth of bacteria in intestine.

Enterohepatic Circulation

Bile acids and salts are **absorbed from the intestine and re-excreted in the bile**, and this cycle is repeated so many times, which is called enterohepatic circulation of bile acids and salts.

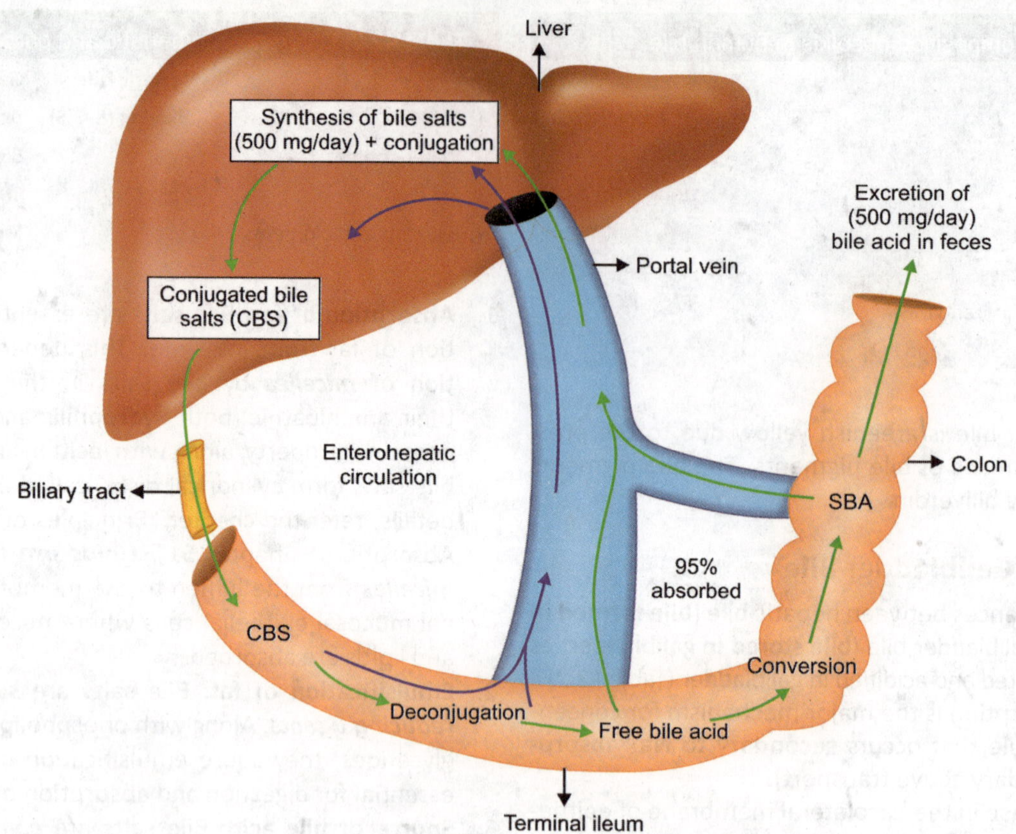

Fig. 42.2: Mechanism of enterohepatic circulation of bile salts and acids. (SBA: Secondary bile acids).

1. Bile salts are produced in liver (200 to 500 mg/day) and conjugated. **Conjugated bile salts** (CBS) through biliary tract enter intestine.
2. From intestine, they are absorbed into the portal blood to reach liver.
3. Also, in the intestine CBS is deconjugated and **unconjugated bile salt** is absorbed into portal circulation.
4. The free bile acids in terminal ileum and colon by the action of bacteria are converted into **secondary bile acids** (SBAs), i.e. deoxycholic acid and lithocholic acid.
5. SBAs are also reabsorbed into portal circulation.
6. Thus, from gut, about **95% of secreted bile salts and bile acids are transferred back to liver** via portal circulation, and only 200 to 500 mg/day of bile acids are excreted from stool.
7. From liver, again they are excreted through biliary tract into the intestine. This forms the *loop-pathway* for enterohepatic circulation (Fig. 42.2).

Enterohepatic circulation ensures **preservation and reutilization of various substances.** For example, bile salts are recirculated 4–12 times a day. The substances that undergo enterohepatic circulation include **bile salts, bile acids, bile pigments, vitamin D, vitamin B$_{12}$, thyroxine, drugs,** etc.

Importance of Enterohepatic Circulation

The primary function of enterohepatic circulation of bile acids and salts is to maintain the **total bile acid pool** of the body.

1. Total amount of bile acids (conjugated and unconjugated, and primary and secondary) in the body ranges from 2 to 4 g.
2. Bile acid is **cycled several times** a day during meals, so that a small pool of bile acid can efficiently *provide enough bile salts to facilitate adequate lipid absorption* from small intestine.
3. Though absorption of bile acids and salts from intestine occurs efficiently, some amount is lost with every cycle of passage through intestine. This accounts for loss of about ***500 mg of bile acid daily***, which is replenished by synthesis of new bile acids from cholesterol.
4. Thus, **fecal excretion of bile acid accounts for an efficient medium for loss of body cholesterol.**

Determinants of Enterohepatic Circulation

The major determinants of enterohepatic circulation of bile acids and salts are integrity of intestinal epithelium to reabsorb them and efficiency of hepatocytes to pick them up from portal blood.

Integrity of Intestinal Epithelium

Bile salts are absorbed mainly in the terminal ileum by an **efficient carrier mediated process** so that only a 5% of intestinal bile salts enter the colon. Also in the intestine, bacteria deconjugate the bile salts to bile acids, and bile acids are absorbed passively and easily as they are more lipophilic than bile salts.

1. Thus, **intestinal absorption of bile acids and salts into portal blood is an important determinant** of enterohepatic circulation of these substances.
2. Further, bacteria convert primary bile acids to secondary bile acids that are also absorbed into portal circulation. Therefore, lipid malabsorption occurs in chronic inflammatory conditions of intestine (Clinical Box 42.1).

Efficiency of Hepatic Uptake

In the portal blood, bile salts are transported bound to HDL or albumin. Once they reach liver, hepatocytes efficiently pick-up bile salts from hepatic blood, which accounts for removal of more than 80% of portal bile salts.

1. This **hepatic uptake of bile salts is an important determinant** of secretion of bile salts in the bile.
2. Thus hepatic uptake is the determinant of efficiency of enterohepatic circulation of bile salts.

Clinical Box 42.1

Enteritis and hepatitis cause lipid malabsorption: Bile salts are absorbed mainly in the distal ileum and bile salts promote lipid absorption. Therefore, inflammation of lower part of small intestine (enteritis) that inhibits absorption of bile salts in intestine results in loss of large quantity of lipid in the stool (due to malabsorption of fat). Similarly, inflammation of liver (hepatitis) impairs the uptake of bile acid and salts from portal blood that in turn decreases their secretion in the bile. This also can cause intestinal malabsorption of fat.

BILE SECRETION

Mechanism of Secretion

The secretion of bile consists of **canalicular flow** and **ductular secretion.** In the canaliculi, bile acids and Na^+-K^+ATPase contribute to bile flow. In the ducts, epithelial cells secrete HCO_3^- and Cl^- actively into the lumen.

Mechanism of Bile Acid Secretion

Bile is formed in hepatocytes. Bile acids are taken up from the sinusoidal blood by transport proteins that are present on the basolateral membrane of the hepatocytes.

1. In cytoplasm of hepatocytes, bile acids bind with *bile acid binding proteins*. This **prevents bile acids to accumulate in higher concentration** in cytoplasm. It should be noted that high concentration of free bile acids destroys the organelles of hepatocytes.
2. Bile acids are **conjugated with glycine or taurine** and then **secreted into the lumen of hepatic canaliculi by facilitated diffusion**.
3. Bile acids move into the bile down their electrochemical gradient. The concentration gradient is maintained by formation of **micelles in the bile** present in the canaliculi.

Mechanism of Water and Electrolyte Secretin

Water and electrolyte concentration of bile in the bile canaliculi is same with that of plasma.

1. The bile duct epithelial cells secrete bicarbonate rich fluid into the lumen.
2. The ions are transported in a similar way to that of pancreatic extralobular ducts.

Modification of Bile in Gallbladder

Bile is continuously synthesized and secreted from liver and is stored in the gallbladder. Gallbladder is a small sac like structure with the capacity of 30–60 mL.

Gallbladder performs ***three functions***:

1. **Storage of bile**
2. **Acidification of bile:** The hydrogen ion is secreted from gallbladder epithelial cell into the bile to make the bile acidic.
3. **Concentration of bile:** H^+ is secreted into the lumen of gallbladder in exchange for Na^+ (Na^+-H^+ exchanger). For Na^+ transport into the cell, the gradient is created by Na^+-K^+ pump located in the basolateral membrane of the epithelial cells. Water is reabsorbed from the gallbladder bile so that bile is concentrated (Fig. 42.3).

Regulation of Bile Secretion

Bile secretion is influenced by choleretics and cholagogues.

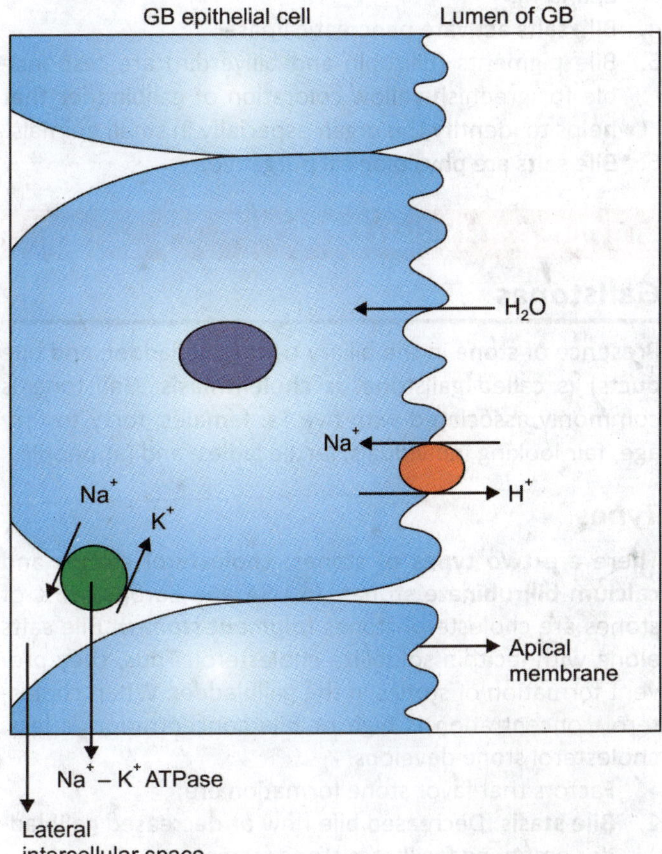

Fig. 42.3: Mechanism of water reabsorption and H secretion by epithelial cells of gallbladder (GB) that causes concentration and acidification of GB bile.

Choleretics

The substances that enhance the secretion of bile are called choleretics. The important choleretics are:

1. Bile salts
2. Secretin
3. Vagal stimulation.

Secretin increases aqueous component of bile.

Cholagogues

The substances that cause contraction of gallbladder to increase the output of bile from the structure are called cholagogues. The important cholagogues are:

1. Cholecystokinin
2. Fatty acids.

Cholecystokinin causes contraction of smooth muscles of gallbladder and empties its contents.

Functions of Bile

Functions of bile are mainly due to presence of bile salts in it.

1. Bile helps in absorption of lipids from intestine by forming micelles.
2. Bile salts in bile are important choleretics (increase bile secretion).
3. Bile promotes absorption of fat soluble vitamins (A, D, E, and K).
4. Bile salts activate pancreatic lipase.
5. Bile pigments (bilirubin and biliverdin) are responsible for greenish-yellow coloration of gallbladder that helps to identify the organ especially in small animals.
6. Bile salts are physiological purgative.

APPLIED PHYSIOLOGY

Gallstones

Presence of stone in the biliary tract (gallbladder, and bile ducts) is called gallstone or **cholelithiasis**. Gallstone is commonly associated with five Fs: females, forty to fifty age, fair looking individuals, fertile ladies, and fat people.

Types

There are **two types** of stones: **cholesterol stones** and **calcium bilirubinate stones**. In USA and Europe, 85% of stones are cholesterol stones (***pigment stones***). Bile salts along with lecithin solubilize cholesterol. Thus, they prevent formation of stones in the gallbladder. When cholesterol concentration is high or bile concentration is less, cholesterol stone develops.

Factors that favor stone formation are:

1. **Bile stasis.** Decreased bile flow or decreased gallbladder emptying facilitates stone formation.
2. **Supersaturation of bile** with cholesterol.
3. **Nucleation factor** that favors formation of stones from the supersaturated bile. Glycoproteins in gallbladder mucous form the nucleus surrounding which gallstones are formed.

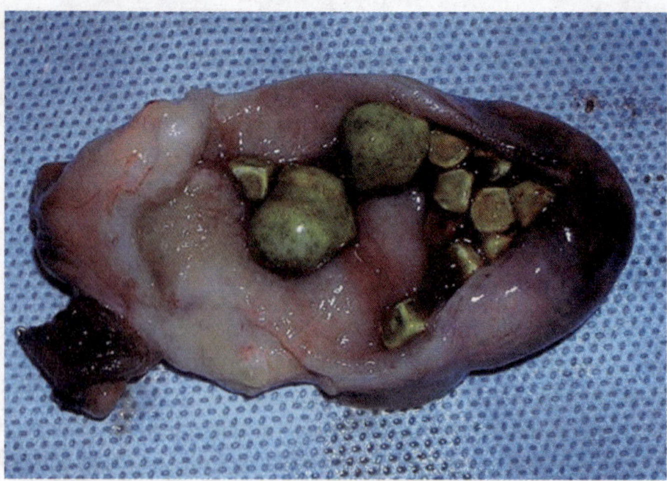

Fig. 42.4: Multiple gallstones in an edematous gallbladder having chronic cholecystitis.

Courtesy: Figure 13.2A, Gastrointestinal surgery, by S. Devaji Rao, 1st edition, 2009; Jaypee Brothers Medical Publishers (P) Ltd.

Usually cholesterol stones are big and may be one or two stones are present in gallbladder. The calcium bilirubinate stones are multiple, and more than 50 stones may be present in gallbladder of the patient (Fig. 42.4).

Features

Usually, gallstones are **silent stones**. But, when stones come out of the gallbladder and pass through the biliary ducts, **severe colicky or spasmodic acute abdominal pain** occurs.

1. Chronic gallstones may present with **acute cholecystitis**, bile stasis inducing inflammation of gallbladder.
2. The stone may induce inflammation and edema of gallbladder, resulting in chronic cholecystitis (Fig. 42.4).
3. Gallstones may also present with **obstructive jaundice**.

Diagnosis

Diagnosis is usually made by **ultrasound or cholecystography**. Plain X-ray may sometime detect stones.

Treatment

There is no effective medical treatment, though many drugs have been advocated to dissolve stone. Gallstones are treated surgically by removal of gallbladder (**cholecystectomy**).

Effects of Cholecystectomy

Gallbladder is not absolutely essential for digestive functions. The patients those who have undergone cholecystectomy, maintain normal health and usually their nutrition is not affected. Only problem they face is the **steatorrhea**, if they eat excess of fat food. Cholecystectomized patients tolerate fat foods to some extent. It decreases body fat and may be beneficial for obese people.

CHAPTER SUMMARY

Key Concepts

1. Bile is required for absorption of fat from intestine.
2. Enterohepatic circulation of bile salts and bile acids prevents loss of important metabolizes from the body and ensures their reutilization.
3. Cholecystectomy is not detrimental to health, and may be useful in the treatment of obesity.

Important to Know (Must Read)

1. In examinations, usually **Long Questions** are not asked from this chapter. However, 'Mechanism and regulation of bile secretion' may sometime come as a question.
2. Bile salts, Bile acids, Functions of bile salts, Enterohepatic circulation, Mechanism of bile secretion, Regulation of bile secretion, Choleretics and cholagogues, may come as **Short Questions**.
3. In **Viva**, examiner may ask...... Name bile salts and tell their functions, Name bile acids and tell their functions, Composition of bile and functions of bile, What is enterohepatic circulation and what is its importance, What are the common substances that undergo enterohepatic circulation, Mechanism of bile secretion, Regulation of bile secretion, Name choleretics and cholagogues, Cause, types and features of gallstones.
4. "Enterohepatic circulation" is usually asked as a short note, or in viva.

CHAPTER 43

Intestinal Secretion

Learning Objectives

On completion of study of this chapter, the student **MUST** be able to:

1. Appreciate the importance of intestinal secretion in digestion and absorption of nutrients.
2. Understand the mucosal modifications in intestinal epithelium to increase the surface area for absorption.
3. Give the composition and functions of intestinal secretion.
4. Understand the importance of intestinal flora in GI physiology.
5. Learn the physiological basis of malabsorption syndrome.

The student **MAY** be also able to:

1. Describe the details of mechanism and regulation of intestinal secretion.

FUNCTIONAL ANATOMY

Small intestine consists of duodenum, jejunum and ileum. It is the longest segment of GI tract, which is about 6.1 meters (duodenum 26 cm + jejunum-ileum 650 cm) in adults. Though duodenum is well demarcated from jejunum, there is no distinct separation between jejunum and ileum. For its length and capacity, small intestine is the most important segment of GI system for digestion and absorption of all nutrients.

1. Secretion of small intestine is called **succus entericus**.
2. It contains most enzymes for carbohydrate, protein and fat digestion.
3. Small intestine secretes about **2–3 liters** of isotonic fluid per day.

Intestinal Glands

As discussed in chapter 36, the intestinal wall has all the layers of the gut (Refer to Fig. 36.3): serosa, outer longitudinal and inner circular muscle layers, submucosa, muscularis mucosa, and mucosa (Figs. 43.1A and B). The mucosa is highly developed to contain villi and intestinal glands.

Intestinal secretion is produced by the glands in the small intestine. The intestinal glands are called **crypts of Lieberkühn**:

1. These are tubular glands present at the base of the villi. Throughout the length of small intestine, the mucous membrane is covered by **villi**. There are about **20–40 villi per square millimeter of mucosa** (Fig. 43.2).
2. Each villus is a fingerlike projection covered by a layer of columnar epithelium and contains a network of capillaries and lacteals (lymphatics).
3. The villi have numerous **microvilli** on their surface that are called **brush border.** Brush border considerably increases the surface area for absorption.
4. Some quantity of secretion is also added by **Brunner's glands** that are coiled acinotubular glands present in the duodenum in addition to crypts of Lieberkühn.
5. The intestinal mucosa is supported externally by thin layer of smooth muscle fibres, **muscularis mucosae.** The mucous membrane is thrown into folds or **plicae** which are more in the jejunum and less in the ileum, thus increasing the absorptive surface enormously.

Scientist contributed

Johann Nathanael Lieberkühn (1711–1756) was a German physician and physiologist. Initially he studied theology, then physics (mechanics) and then medicine. He served as a medical professor and medical doctor. Besides his physiological work, Lieberkühn was most known for his preparation of medical specimens—these were still presented up to the nineteenth century, especially in Moscow, as masterpieces. The **Crypts of Lieberkühn** (intestinal glands) are named after him, which he first described these in detail. He had developed microscopes for studying blood vessels that were called "Wundergläser", 'wonder-glasses' by his contemporaries.

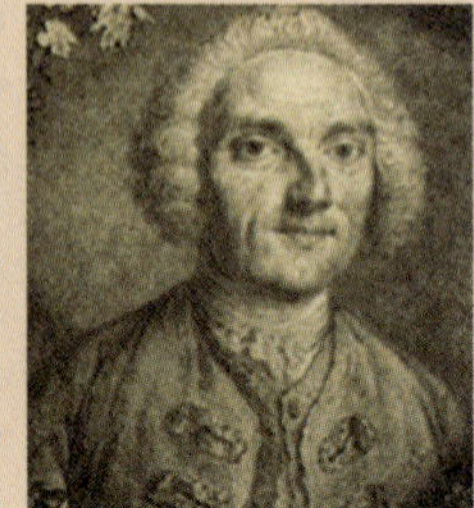

JN Lieberkühn
(1711–1756)

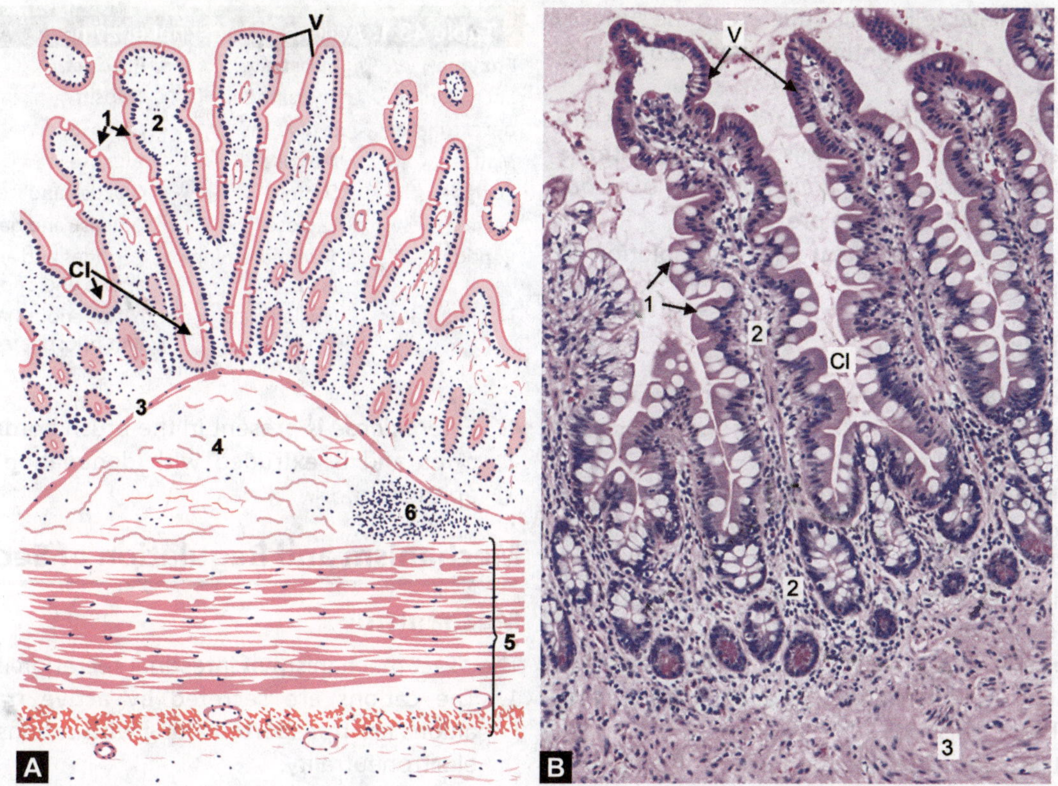

Figs. 43.1A and B: Histology of the wall of small intestine (A), and as seen in photomicrograph (B). (1: Columnar epithelial lining with goblet cells; 2: Lamina propria; 3: Muscularis mucosa; 4: Submucosa; 5: Muscularis externa; 6: Lymph nodes; V: Villi; Cl: Crypts of Leiberkuhn).

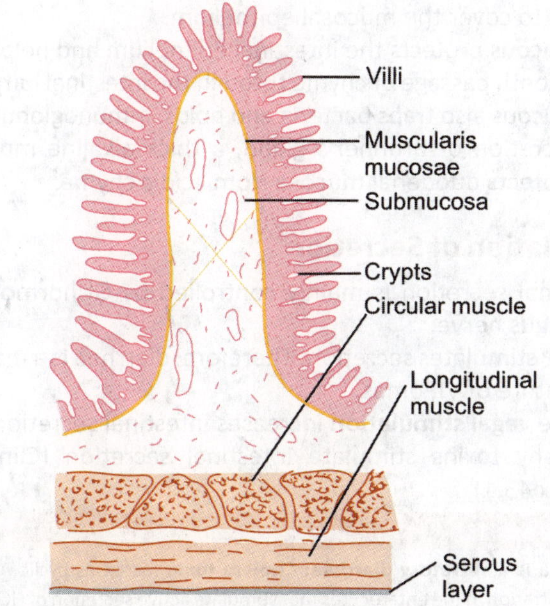

Fig. 43.2: Mucosa of jejunum showing crypts and villi.

Intestinal Mucosa

The mucosa of small intestine contains lymphatic nodules (**Peyer's patches**). There are also **enterochromaffin cells, Paneth cells and undifferentiated cells** in the intestinal mucosa (Fig. 43.3):

1. The mucous membrane of the intestine contains many valve-like folds called **valvulae conniventes**, which add to the surface area for absorption.
2. In intestine, the surface area for absorption is **increased by about 600 fold** by villi, brush border and valvulae conniventes.
3. **Paneth cells** are endocrine cells present in the crypts of Lieberkühn in their deeper part. They secrete ***defensins***, the naturally occurring antibiotics that protect developing enterocytes against infections. Paneth cells also secrete *guanylin*.
4. The **undifferentiated cells** are the progenitor cells in the mucosa present in the crypts of Lieberkühn that

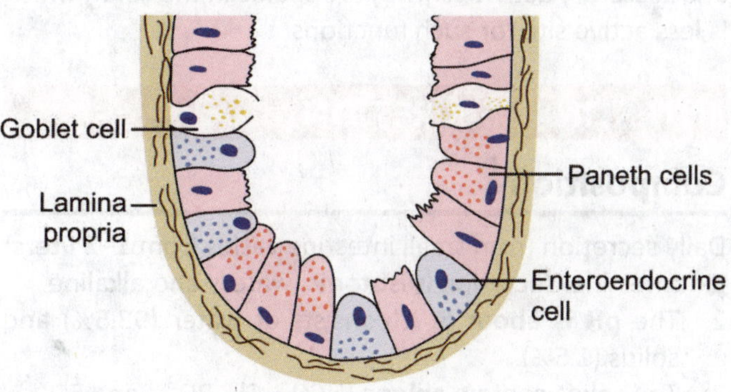

Fig. 43.3: Cells present in the intestinal glands.

form new epithelial cells, which migrate to the surface. The epithelial cells are continuously renewed by progenitor cells.

5. After the life span of about 2–5 days, enterocytes are sloughed along with mucosal cells. **Shedding of these epithelial cells** accounts for *daily excretion of about 30 g of protein* as the cells are protein-rich.
6. ***Goblet cells*** secrete mucins that form a gel solution on the surface of mucosa.

Types of Cells in Villi

The absorptive surface of intestinal mucosa is increased by the intestinal villi. Villi are finger like or leaf like projections which contain **3 types of cells**:

i. **Simple columnar cells:** They perform absorptive function due to the presence of brush border consisting of large number of villi.
ii. **Goblet cells:** These are mucous secreting cells and are interspersed between the columnar cells.
iii. **Endocrine cells:** These are scattered in the villi as well as are widely distributed throughout the gastrointestinal tract. These cells are:
   a. **Kulchitsky cells:** After the name of its discoverer
   b. **Enterochromaffin cells:** Due to their resemblance to chromaffin cells of the adrenal medulla
   c. **Argentaffin cells:** As the intracytoplasmic granules stain positively with silver salts by reduction reaction (agyrophil cells, on the other hand, require the addition of exogenous reducing substances for staining)
   d. **Endocrine cells:** As these specialized cells are considered to be part of **APUD cell system** (having common properties as amine content, Amine Precursor Uptake and Decarboxylation). APUD cells are considered to be endodermal in origin, while previously they were thought to be neural crest derivative. Other endocrine cells belonging to the APUD cell system are C-cells of the thyroid, chromaffin cells of the adrenal medulla, certain cells of the carotid body, bronchi, hypothalamus, pituitary and sympathetic ganglia.

Endocrine cells are heavily populated in the proximal small bowel as this is the most active site for absorption and secretory activities. They are sparse in the colon which is less active site for such functions.

INTESTINAL SECRETION

Composition

Daily secretion from small intestine varies from **1–2 liters**:

1. Intestinal secretion is **isotonic**, watery and alkaline.
2. The **pH is about 8**. It consists of water (98.5%) and solids (1.5%).
3. The solids contain **anions** (HCO_3^-, Cl^-, PO_4^{3-}, and SO_4^{2-}), **cations** (Na^+, K^+, Ca^{2+} and Mg^{2+}), **enzymes** (Table 43.1), and **mucous**.

Table 43.1: Actions of Intestinal enzymes.

Enzyme	Substrate	Product
Enterokinase	Trypsinogen	Trypsin
α-dextrinase	α-dextrins	Glucose
Maltase	Maltose	Glucose
Sucrase	Sucrose	Glucose and fructose
Lactase	Lactose	Glucose and galactose
Peptidases	Terminal amino acids	Peptides and amino acids at amino end of peptides
Nucleotidases	Nucleotides	Nitrogenous bases, pentoses, and phosphates

4. *Enterokinase* is present in the brush border of enterocytes and is extruded with denudation of mucosal epithelium.

Mechanism and Regulation of Secretion

Mechanism

The exact mechanism of intestinal secretion is not clear:

1. The cations are secreted by **active transport** and anions are transported along with cations to maintain electroneutrality.
2. Water follows the ions to **maintain osmotic balance**.
3. *Mucus is secreted by surface epithelial cells*, Brunner's gland and goblet cells are present in the mucosa of the intestine.
4. **Mucin** is the major component of mucous that forms a gel to cover the mucosal epithelium.
5. **Mucous** protects the intestinal epithelium and helps in smooth passage of chyme through the intestinal lumen. Mucous also traps bacteria and holds immunoglobulin.
6. Secretion of Brunner's gland, a thick alkaline mucus protects duodenal mucosa from acidic chyme.

Regulation of Secretion

Intestinal secretion is mainly controlled by GI hormones and vagus nerve:

1. **VIP** stimulates secretion. Therefore, diarrhea is a major feature of VIPomas.
2. The **vagal stimulation** increases intestinal secretion.
3. Many toxins stimulate intestinal secretion (Clinical Box 43.1).

Clinical Box 43.1

Cholera is a secretory diarrhea: Cholera toxin increases cyclic AMP concentration in the enterocytes that stimulate active secretion of HCO_3^-, and Cl^- into the lumen and produces watery diarrhea.

Experiment to Study Intestinal Secretion

In animal models, experiments are performed to study the rate and composition of intestinal secretion. In these animals, a loop of intestine is resected and both ends of the loop are connected to anterior abdominal wall in such a way that they open to outside. Thereafter, various stimuli are applied on the loop and their effects are studied. Such an intestinal loop is called **Thiry-Vella loop**.

Functions of Intestinal Secretion

1. Intestinal secretion helps in proper **mixing of chyme**. This provides suitable environment for digestion and absorption of food materials in the intestine.
2. Intestinal secretion contains enzymes for **digestion of various nutrients**.
3. Mucus of intestinal secretion **protects intestinal epithelium** from damage. It also traps and kills bacteria.
4. Mucus in the intestinal secretion contains **immunoglobulins** that play an important role in local defenses.
5. The **alkaline secretion of Brunner's gland** protects upper intestinal mucosa from damage by acidic chyme.
6. Intestinal secretion helps in **forward propulsion of chyme** in the intestine.

Absorption of Water

Normally, about 8.5 liters of fluid is added to GI tract daily. However, only about 100 ml of water is excreted in the stool. Thus, **GI tract absorbs more than 99.5% of water load** presented to it per day. 75% of water absorption takes place in the distal part of small intestine (For details, *see* next chapter).

Intestinal Bacteria

Normally, a group of bacteria are present in the intestine. They constitute normal **intestinal flora**. These microorganisms are present **mainly in the ileum** than in upper part of the intestine. This is because the acidic content of duodenum and upper jejunum do not favor growth of bacteria:

1. The organisms in the flora mainly include **E. coli, Enterobacter aerogenes and Bacteroids fragilis**.
2. There are also few other bacteria like, ***cocci and bacilli*** of various types.
3. Normally, bacteria **are lost in the stool and replaced** in the intestine by their natural growth. However, excess loss of bacterial flora in diseases like acute diarrhea results in improper digestion and absorption (Clinical Box 43.2).

Functions of Intestinal Flora

Intestinal bacteria are essential for many gut functions:

1. Normal bacterial flora is essential for **digestion and absorption of essential nutrients** including vitamins, minerals, and water.
2. They **synthesize vitamin K and B complexes**.
3. They produce chemicals that help in formation of short chain fatty acids, which help in **growth of the intestinal mucosa**.
4. Some bacteria species like Salmonella **inhibit inflammatory processes**. They do so by **inhibiting ubiquitination of $I_{K}B\alpha$**, the step that helps the transcription of factor $NF_{K}B$ to initiate inflammation. Bacteria also secrete **anti-inflammatory cytokines** like IL-10. Recently, commensal bacteria are genetically programmed to produce IL-10.
5. Some bacteria utilize substances like ascorbic acid and cyanocobalamin. Therefore, these vitamins are usually given in higher dosages.
6. Bile salts are converted to bile acids by intestinal bacteria, which are then absorbed into portal blood from intestine and colon. Thus, intestinal flora **maintains bile acid pool** of the body.
7. They **impart brown color to the stool** by forming pigments from bile pigments. Therefore, acholic (pale) stool is seen in biliary obstruction.
8. They **produce gases** that cause normal flatus. Normal flatus is required for normal distension and motility of intestine. Exaggeration or decreased flatus indicates abnormality in intestinal flora.
9. They also contribute to the **odor of the feces**. This occurs due to production of amines like **indole and skatole** by intestinal bacteria.
10. They contribute to **plasma lipid level** by interfering in absorption of LDL and cholesterol. Therefore, poorly absorbable antibiotic like neomycin that modifies bacterial flora decreases plasma cholesterol.

Though these bacteria are nonpathogenic and beneficial, their entry into systemic circulation can cause systemic sepsis as occurs in ionizing radiation that breaks the intestinal defense barrier. This results in **radiation poisoning**.

Clinical Box 43.2

Lactobacilli is used in treatment of diarrhea: Apart from antibiotics, lactobacilli are included as part of the treatment of severe acute diarrhea that causes loss of intestinal flora. Bacterial flora is not well developed in infants and is slowly established during early childhood. Therefore, **lactobacilli treatment is a must in any acute gastroenteritis in children**. Many antibiotics interfere in growth of intestinal bacteria. Hence, lactobacilli supplement is given along with higher antibiotics.

Applied Physiology

Malabsorption Syndrome

The commonest abnormality due to inappropriate intestinal secretion is malabsorption syndrome. However, malabsorption also occurs due to gastric, hepatic and pancreatic deficiencies.

1. **In malabsorption due to intestinal causes**, the digestive and absorptive functions of small intestine are impaired. The small intestine is very long (about 650 cm in adults). Therefore, unless the disease process significantly affects the adequate length of intestine, malabsorption does not develop. Similarly, only in surgical procedure that removes or bypasses more than 50% of the intestine, significant malabsorption occurs.
2. The common intestinal conditions that produce malabsorption are ***sprue*** (tropical sprue), ***celiac disease*** (gluten enteropathy), ***Chrohn's disease***, ***Whipple's disease*** and ***radiation enteritis*** (for details of malabsorption, refer the Chapter "Principles of Digestion and Absorption").
3. In these conditions, **hypoproteinemia develops early** due to deficient absorption of amino acids.

4. Absorption of carbohydrate and fat is also impaired.
5. Fat soluble vitamins (A, D, E, and K) are also not properly absorbed due to defective fat absorption. Excretion of large amount of fat (**steatorrhea**) results in bulky, pale and foul-smelling stool.

Blind Loop Syndrome

Though normal bacterial flora is essential for health, **overgrowth of bacteria is harmful**:

1. Such overgrowths occur when there is stasis of intestinal contents.
2. This condition is commonly observed in patients with **surgically created blind loops** of small intestine, which is popularly known as blind loop syndrome.
3. It causes **macrocytic anemia, malabsorption of vitamin B_{12} and steatorrhea.**
4. Steatorrhea occurs due to excessive hydrolysis of conjugated bile salts by the bacteria.

CHAPTER SUMMARY

Key Concepts

1. Intestinal secretion is very useful for digestion and absorption of nutrients from intestine, as it contain enzymes for digestion of all types of nutrients. Therefore, nature has given a vast surface area for absorption by providing microvilli and brush borders.
2. Intestinal bacteria facilitate the process of digestion and absorption and help in synthesis of few vitamins.
3. 75% of water is absorbed in distal part of small intestine. Diarrhea occurs, if the secretion of water is increased or absorption of water is decreased.

Important to Know (Must Read)

1. In examinations, usually **Long Questions** are not asked from this chapter.
2. Intestinal glands, Intestinal mucosa, Intestinal endocrine cells, Mechanism and regulation of intestinal secretion, Composition and functions of intestinal secretion, Bacterial flora of intestine, may come as **Short Questions**.
3. In **Viva**, examiner may ask...... Layers of wall of intestine, Arrangement of villi and microvilli in the mucosa, Structure of intestinal glands, Structure of intestinal mucosa, Intestinal endocrine cells and their secretions, Composition and functions of intestinal secretion, Mechanism and regulation of intestinal secretion, Experiment to study intestinal secretion, What is Thiry-Vella loop, Types of bacteria in bacterial flora of intestine, Functions of bacterial flora, Causes of malabsorption syndrome, Blind loop syndrome.

CHAPTER 44

Secretion of Large Intestine

LEARNING OBJECTIVES

On completion of study of this chapter, the student **MUST** be able to:

1. Appreciate the importance of physiology of the colon.
2. Understand the importance of colonic bacteria.
3. Learn the physiology of water absorption and secretion through GI tract.

The student **MAY** also be able to:

1. Describe the details of secretion from colon.

The secretion of large intestine is not considered so important physiologically as it does not help in digestion. The major function of large intestine is the absorption of water and electrolytes. It absorbs about 90% of its load (mainly water is absorbed) in the form of chyme presented to it from the ileum. Of about 2 liters of isotonic chyme that enters large intestine, only about 200 ml is excreted as feces.

PHYSIOLOGY OF COLON

Functional Anatomy

Large intestine consists of cecum, colon and rectum (Fig. 44.1). Colon forms the major part of the large gut:

1. Length of colon (ascending, transverse, descending and sigmoid colon) in adult is about 110 cm.
2. The **diameter of large intestine is bigger than small intestine**, which favours *slow passage of chyme* through it and also absorption of maximum quantity of water during its passage.
3. There are **no villi**, though the mucosal epithelium is folded to give villi like appearance to some extent.
4. There are many **crypts of Lieberkühn** in the mucous membrane that secrete a solution isotonic to that of plasma.
5. There are numerous ***goblet cells*** in the mucosal epithelium that secretes mucous.
6. Lamina propria contains ***intestinal glands*** and submucosa contains ***lymphatic nodules*** (Fig. 44.2).
7. No digestive enzymes are secreted in the colon.

Colonic Secretion

Composition of Secretion

Secretion of large intestine contains mainly **mucous** secreted by goblet cells. It contains **HCO_3^- and K^+** in large amount and some amount of sodium and water. The **pH is about 8.**

Mechanism of Secretion

There are **crypts** in the mucous membrane that secrete a solution **isotonic to that of plasma**.

1. There are plenty of **goblet cells** that secrete mucous. Mucous secreted from goblet cells has following functions:
   - Protects intestinal mucosa
   - Help in stool formation
   - Lubricate the intestinal mass
   - Neutralize the acid which is formed by bacteria in the large intestine.
2. Water and bicarbonate are secreted in significant amount.
3. Na^+ is reabsorbed and K^+ is secreted in large amount.
4. The **bacterial flora** of large intestine is similar to that of small intestine.

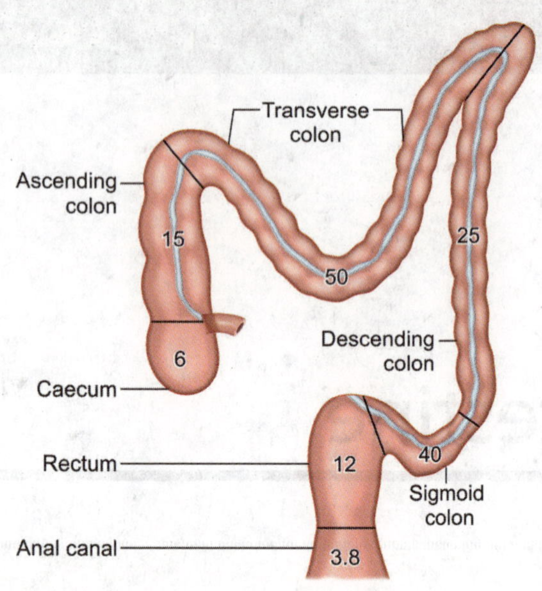

Fig. 44.1: Parts of large intestine.

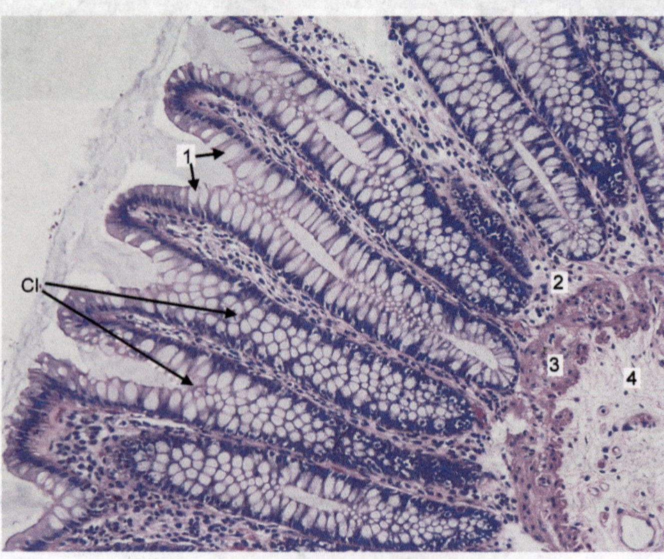

Fig. 44.2: Photomicrograph of large intestine. (1: Columnar epithelial lining with goblet cells; 2: Lamina propria; 3: Muscularis mucosa; 4: Submucosa; Cl: Crypts of Lieberkuhn).

5. About 90% water is reabsorbed from the intestinal contents:
   - Therefore, when content of large intestine passes very slowly or there is stagnation, **constipation** occurs due to absorption of more water that causes solidification of stool.
   - Conversely, when the contents pass faster due to increased motility, **diarrhea** occurs. Secretion of water and electrolyte in large quantity can also cause diarrhea.

Transfer of electrolytes and water: Large intestine can absorb Na^+, K^+, Cl^-, glucose and certain vitamins. However, secretion of K^+ and $HCO3^-$ into the colon is more. Colon can not absorb protein, fat or Ca^{2+}. Na^+ is actively absorbed from the colon and water follows along the osmotic gradient generated by absorption of Na^+ and Cl^-.

Colonic Bacteria

Colonic bacteria resemble the intestinal flora inhabiting ileum. They produce about **8 liter of gas per day** that contributes to flatus and colonic motility. They have **trophic effects** on colonic mucosal growth. Ammonia is produced by colonic bacteria, which is detoxified in the liver. Hence, in severe liver disease, hepatic encephalopathy (suppression of brain activities) occurs.

Organisms

At birth, the colon is sterile but the colonic bacterial flora becomes established early in life. The micro-organisms habituating the colon are bacilli such as mainly **Escherchia coli and Enterobacter aerogens**. Gas gangrene bacilli may be present.

Functions of Colonic Bacteria

The physiological role of colonic bacterial flora are:

1. **Synthesis of the vitamins:** Vitamins e.g. vitamin K, number of B complex vitamins and folic acid are produced by these colonic organisms.
2. **Production of gas:** CO_2, hydrogen sulphide, hydrogen and methane which contribute to the flatus, are produced by bacterial flora (Application Box 44.1)
3. **Smell of stool:** The smell of stool is largely due to sulphides.
4. **Acidic reaction of stool:** Organic acids formed from carbohydrates by bacteria causes slightly acidic reaction of the stool (pH 5 to 7):
   a. **Production of amines:** A number of amines are formed in the colon by bacterial enzymes that decarboxylate amino acids. These amines are **histamine and tyramine** which may be harmful if produced in excess quantity. **Indole and skatole** are responsible for the odour of the faeces.
5. **Colour of stool:** Pigments biliverdin and stercobilinogen formed from the bile pigments by the intestinal bacteria are responsible for the brown colour of the stool.
6. **Decrease blood lipids:** Intestinal bacteria play some role in **cholesterol metabolism** and decrease plasma cholesterol and LDL levels.

Application Box 44.1

Excess gas production causes borborygmi: The volume of gas normally found in the human gut is approximately 200 mL, and the daily production is 500–1,500 mL. In some individuals, more gas is produced in the intestine that causes cramps, borborygmi (rumbling noise) and abdominal discomfort.

Absorption of Water

Normally, about 1.5 liters of water is ingested per day and 7 liters is added from GI secretions per day. However, only about 100 ml of water is excreted in the stool daily. Thus, **GI tract absorbs more than 99.5% of water load** presented to it per day:

1. Water is not absorbed from mouth, esophagus, and stomach.
2. As most of the nutrients are absorbed mainly in the duodenum and jejunum, the osmolality of intestinal content which is about 600 mOsm/kg H_2O, decreases to about 200 mOsm/kg H_2O in the ileum and colon.
3. Therefore, **water is absorbed mainly from terminal ileum and colon** (Fig. 44.3) by osmotic gradient as osmolality of blood is about 290 mOsm/kg H_2O.

PHYSIOLOGY OF RECTUM

Rectum stores fecal materials. Role of rectum in defecation reflex is discussed in 'Motility of Large Intestine". Though, normally absorption of water from rectum is not significant, the **absorptive capacity is more** (Clinical Box 44.1)

Clinical Box 44.1

Rectal administration of drugs: The absorptive capacity of mucosa of colon and rectum is large. Therefore, sometimes drugs are administered through rectum. Rectal administration is more preferred in children. Drugs that are administered rectally include purgatives, sedatives, anesthetics, and tranquilizers. However, care should be taken to control the volume of enema introduced into rectum in children as excess water absorption can cause water intoxication.

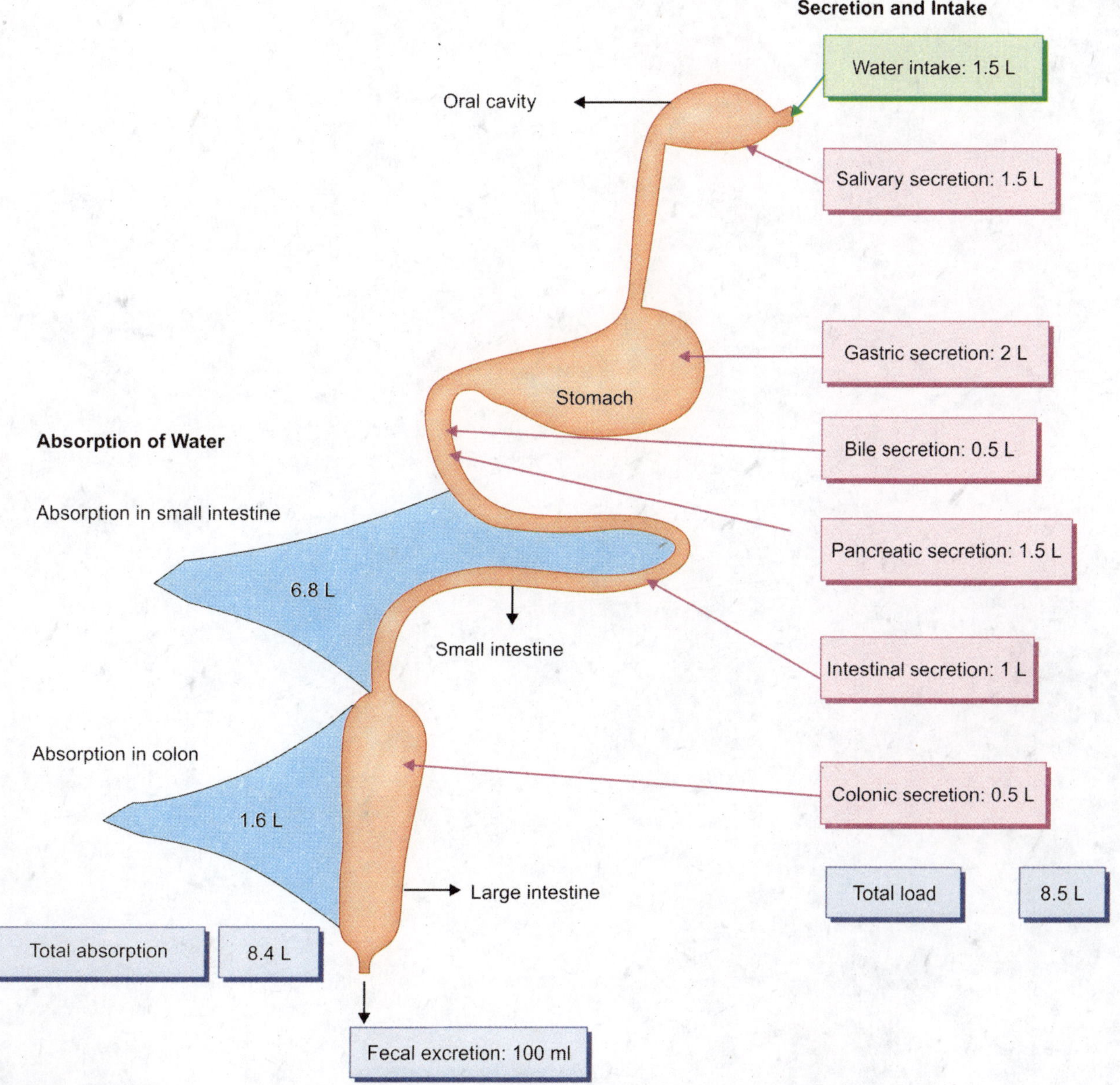

Fig. 44.3: Water absorption in small and large intestines. Note, out of 8.5 liters of load of fluid to the intestine per day, about 75% of absorption takes place in small intestine (6.8 L) and about 25% occurs in large intestine (1.6 L). Thus, total 99.5% of water presented to gut, is absorbed to blood by intestine. Thus, intestine plays an important role in water homeostasis of the body.

CHAPTER SUMMARY

Key Concepts

1. Large intestine does not produce any enzyme for digestion of nutrients. However, significant quantity of water is reabsorbed from colon.
2. Colonic bacteria are involved in gas production that facilitates the process of bowel movement by distending the bowel and also they help in synthesis of few vitamins.

Important to Know (Must Read)

1. In examinations, no **Long Question** is asked from this chapter.
2. Colonic bacterial flora, Colonic secretion, Role of colon in water and electrolyte absorption, Absorption of water by intestine, may come as **Short Questions.**
3. In **Viva**, examiner may ask… Layers of wall of large intestine, Structure of large intestinal glands, Structure of large intestinal mucosa, Mechanism and regulation of colonic secretion, Types of bacteria in bacterial flora of intestine, Functions of bacterial flora in large intestine, How is water secreted and absorbed in different parts of the colon.

CHAPTER 45

Introduction to GI Motility

Learning Objectives

On completion of study of this chapter, the student **MUST** be able to:

1. Correlate the electrophysiology of smooth muscle with GI movements.
2. Draw a labeled diagram of slow wave of GI smooth muscle.
3. List the types of GI motilities and give their functions.
4. Understand the role of VARIOUS sphincters in GI tract.
5. Appreciate the applied aspects of physiology of GI motility.

The student **MAY** also be able to:

1. Describe the electrophysiological properties of GI smooth muscle.

PHYSIOLOGY OF GI SMOOTH MUSCLES

Movements of GI tract assist in propelling foodstuffs in the forward direction, breaking down foodstuffs into smaller particles and mixing of food with GI secretions for proper digestion and absorption. This is possible due to the presence of ***smooth muscles*** in the wall of the GI tract and presence of a developed system of ***enteric motor neurons***.

1. GI smooth muscles are **unitary type** of smooth muscles.
2. The unique feature of GI smooth muscles is that they ***contract spontaneously without external neural and humoral influences***.
3. They also ***contract when stretched*** without external innervation.
4. There is no structured neuromuscular junction.
5. GI smooth muscles are long (about 500 mm) and slender (5–20 mm in width).
6. They are arranged in bundles.

Electrophysiology of GI Smooth Muscle

Types of Couplings

There are **three types** of couplings: electromechanical, pharmacomechanical, and mechanomechanical.

Electromechanical Coupling

Like skeletal muscle, smooth muscle have electromechanical coupling. That means, **depolarization of the membrane causes opening of voltage-gated Ca^{++} channels** and increases cytosolic calcium, which leads to muscle contraction.

Pharmacomechanical Coupling

In addition, smooth muscles have an additional mechanism of pharmacomechanical coupling, in which **binding of a ligand to its receptor** on the muscle membrane leads to **opening of Ca^{++} channels** and increase in cytosolic calcium without change in membrane potential.

Mechanomechanical Coupling

Stretch of smooth muscle causes muscle contraction, which is known as mechanomechanical coupling. Stretch on muscle opens **stretch-sensitive calcium channel** on the muscle cell membrane. Calcium influx causes muscle contraction.

Syncytial Tissues and Pacemaker Tissues

GI smooth muscles have numerous **gap junctions** that easily transmit electrical impulse from cell to cell. This accounts for the **syncytial nature** of smooth muscle in GI

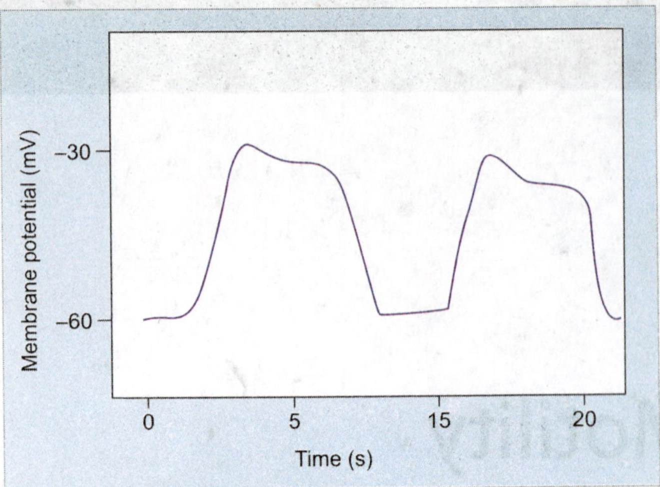

Fig. 45.1: Electrical slow waves of small intestine.

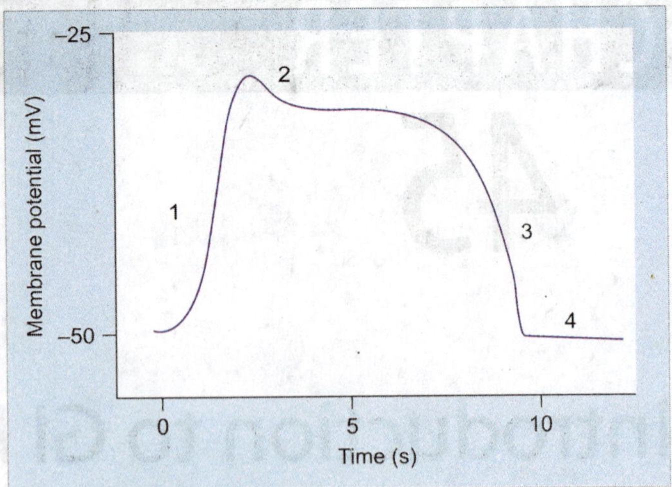

Fig. 45.2: Phases of electrical slow waves of small intestine. When action potentials are associated with slow waves, they occur on the plateau phase (phase 2).

tract. There are also **pacemaker tissues** in GI tract that generate and spread electrical impulses.

Basic Electrical Rhythm and Slow Waves

Resting membrane potential (RMP) of smooth muscle of GI tract exhibit wide range of fluctuation.

1. The electrical **slow waves** are wide spontaneous rhythmic fluctuations in the membrane potential ranging between –65 and –40 mV (Fig. 45.1).
2. The slow waves, which oscillate significantly are called **basal electrical rhythm** (BER) that occurs due to wide variation in the RMP of GI smooth muscles.
3. The BER is present in all parts of GIT **except in the esophagus.**

Slow Waves

Slow waves in many regions of GI tract represent only as BER, whereas at other places like gastric antrum and intestine, they trigger action potential.

1. Slow waves are generated by the **interstitial cells of Cajal** located between the longitudinal and circular muscle layers.
2. Interstitial cells have ***long processes that form gap junctions*** with longitudinal and circular muscle cells. This enables *easy and rapid conduction of slow waves* from the interstitial cells into the smooth muscles.
3. The slow waves spread throughout the smooth muscles of each segment of GI tract.

Phases of Slow Waves

A typical slow wave has **four phases** (Fig. 45.2).

Phase 1: This is the **rising phase *(depolarization)***, which occurs due to opening of voltage gated Ca^{++} channel.

Phase 2: This is the **plateau phase** that occurs due to balance between inward Ca^{++} current and outward K^+ current.

Phase 3: This is the **falling phase *(repolarization)*** occurring due to activation of voltage gated K^+ channel.

Phase 4: Return to membrane potential.

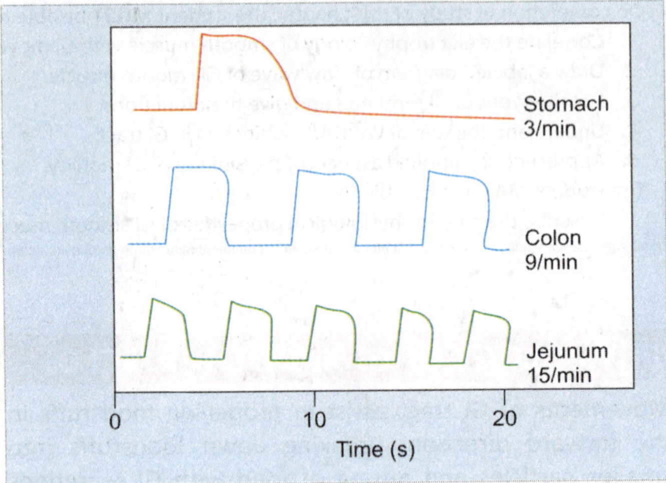

Fig. 45.3: Frequency of slow waves. Note that frequency is least in stomach (3/min) and maximum in intestine (15/min).

Frequency: The frequency of slow waves is 3/min in stomach, 6 to 10/min in colon, 15/min in jejunum and ileum, and 18/min in duodenum (Fig. 45.3).

- The amplitude and the frequency of slow waves are influenced by the activity of extrinsic and intrinsic nerves, and by hormones.
- Usually, sympathetic stimulation decreases the amplitude and parasympathetic stimulation increases the amplitude of slow waves.

Action Potentials

When the peak of a slow wave exceeds the threshold, action potential is **triggered from the peak** (Fig.45.4). These action potentials ***facilitate the force of contraction*** of smooth muscle.

1. Action potentials have longer duration (10–20 ms). Usually, they do not overshoot.
2. The **rising phase** of the action potential is caused by *influx of Ca^{++} and Na^+.*

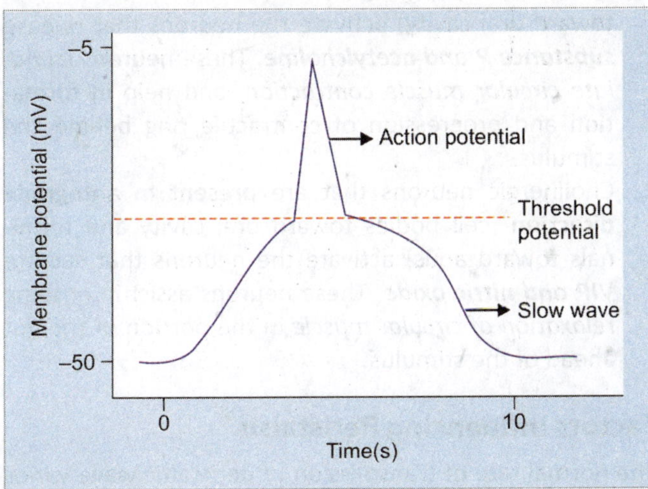

Fig. 45.4: Action potential of GI smooth muscle. Note, once the threshold is reached, action potential is generated on the peak of slow wave.

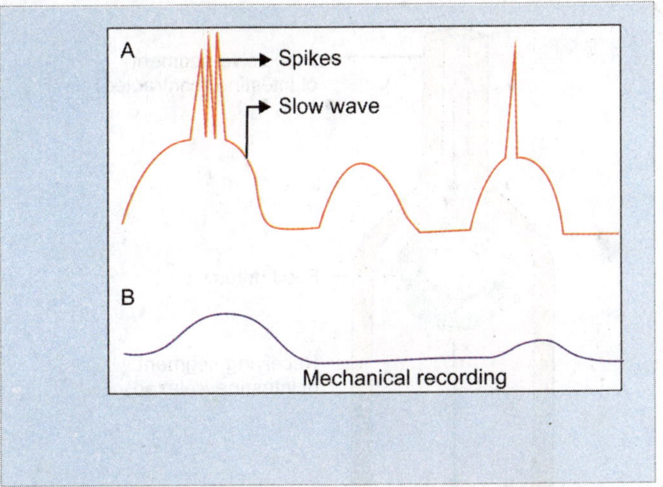

Fig. 45.5: Relationship between electrical (A) and mechanical (B) responses of GI smooth muscle. Note that with increased number of action potential on a slow wave increases the magnitude of contraction and contraction does not occur in the absence of action potential.

3. The **repolarization phase** is due to K^+ *efflux*.
4. The magnitude and frequency of action potential are enhanced by vagal stimulation and inhibited by sympathetic stimulation.

Relationship between electrical and mechanical responses: Slow waves that are not accompanied by action potentials do not elicit contraction, whereas, slow waves that are accompanied by action potentials evoke contraction. The ***greater the frequency of action potential*** (that occur at the peak of slow waves), ***the more intense is the contraction*** (Fig.45.5).

Electrical Coupling between Cells

The smooth muscle cells of the GIT are well coupled (better coordinated). Electrical charge spreads rapidly from cell to cell. However, the **electrical coupling between circular cells is better than the longitudinal cells** because the circular cells have more gap junctions.

Enteric Motor Neurons

Enteric motor neurons innervate the smooth muscles of GI tract and are the final pathway for output of information from autonomic nervous system (ANS) and enteric nervous system (ENS) to the muscle cells (Fig. 45.6).

1. They neither form regular neuromuscular junctions nor do they release neurotransmitters at their axon terminal. Rather, most of motor axons **release transmitters from varicosities** that occur all along their axon, during propagation of an action potential, and the neurotransmitter diffuses to reach the muscle or interstitial cells (refer to Fig. 36.6, Chapter 36).
2. The major **excitatory neurotransmitters** are acetylcholine and substance P, and **inhibitory neurotransmitters** are catecholamines, ATP, VIP, and NO.
3. Cell bodies of excitatory motor neurons are present in the myenteric plexus and the axons project aborally to innervate muscle fibers.

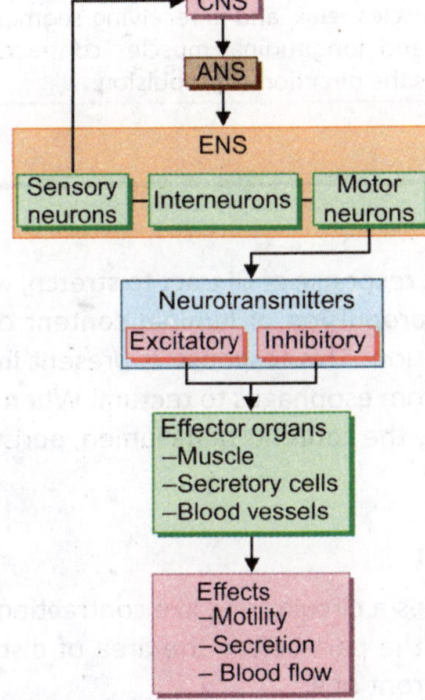

Fig. 45.6: Enteric nervous system (ENS). Note that ENS is the final common pathway for GI effector organs. (ANS: Autonomic nervous system; CNS: Central nervous system).

4. There are also **secretomotor neurons** that stimulate secretion of water, electrolytes and mucous from GI tract. The cell bodies of secretomotor neurons are present in the submucosal plexus.
5. Stimulation of secretomotor neurons release *histamine during allergic reactions* and produce **neurogenic secretory diarrhea** during stress.

BASIC PATTERNS OF GI MOTILITY

GI motility is required for **propulsion, trituration** (crushing and grinding), and **mixing** of food. Propulsion of food is achieved by **peristaltic movement**; trituration and mixing are accomplished by **retropulsive** and **segmental movements**.

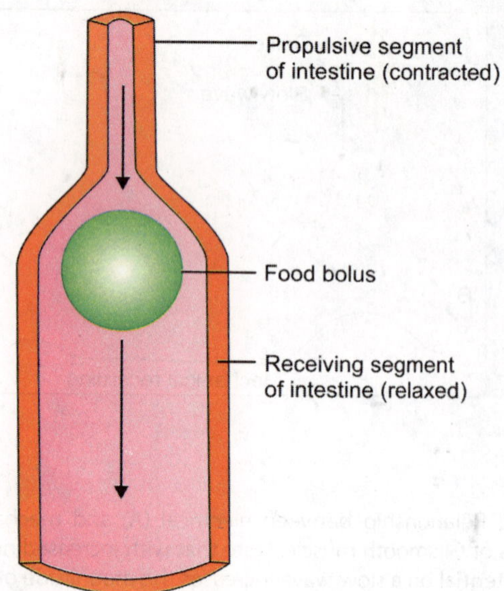

Fig. 45.7: Propulsion of food bolus in intestine by peristaltic movement. In the propulsive segment, the circular muscles contract and longitudinal muscles relax, and in receiving segment the circular muscles relax and longitudinal muscles contract. Direction of arrows indicates the direction of propulsion.

Peristalsis

Definition

This is a reflex response of GI tract to stretch, which results in organized propulsion of luminal content of the gut in forward direction. This response is present in all parts of GIT starting from esophagus to rectum. When the gut wall is stretched by the contents of its lumen, peristalsis is initiated.

Mechanism

Stretch initiates a circular ring like contraction behind the stimulus (i.e. the part before the area of distension) and relaxation in front of it.

1. The part behind the stimulus is called ***propulsive segment*** as it propels the bolus of food or chyme and the part ahead of the stimulus is called ***receiving segment*** as it receives the bolus (Fig. 45.7).
2. In the propulsive segment, the *circular muscles contract and longitudinal muscles relax*, and in receiving segment the *circular muscles relax and longitudinal muscles contract*.
3. The contraction wave then moves in forward direction, i.e. from oral to anal direction. It helps in propelling the contents aborally.

Role of Cholinergic Neurons

The local **cholinergic neurons** play an important role in the transmission of peristaltic waves.

1. Cholinergic neurons that are **present in a retrograde direction** (with cell bodies toward anus and terminals toward oral cavity) activate the neurons that release ***substance P and acetylcholine***. These neurons *stimulate circular muscle contraction*, and help in formation and progression of contractile ring behind the stimulus.
2. Cholinergic neurons that are **present in antegrade direction** (cell bodies toward oral cavity and terminals toward anus) activate the neurons that secrete ***VIP and nitric oxide***. These neurons assist in ensuing *relaxation of circular muscle* in the portion of the gut ahead of the stimulus.

Factors Influencing Peristalsis

The normal rate of transmission of peristaltic wave varies in different parts of GI tract, ranging between 2–15 cm/s. This is influenced by intrinsic and extrinsic nerve supply.

1. **Sympathetic stimulation** inhibits peristalsis and **parasympathetic stimulation** enhances it. Though the transmission of peristalsis is affected by autonomic influence, its ***genesis is independent of it***.
2. It is affected by the **hormones** secreted locally. **Serotonin**, secreted by local stretch of gut enhances peristalsis.

Migrating Motor Complex

During the interdigestive period, the electromechanical activity of GI smooth muscles is altered. A cycle of motor activity migrates from stomach to distal ileum. This is called migrating motor complex (MMC) or **long (mass) peristalsis**.

Phases

MMC has three phases:

Phase-I: The quiescent phase

Phase-II: The period of irregular electrical and mechanical activity.

Phase-III: The period of burst of electrical activities.

Usually it originates in the stomach and transmitted aborally at a rate of 5 cm/min. It occurs at an interval of 90 min, after which the cycle is repeated.

Significance

MMC occurs in the **interdigestive phase**.

1. The phase III of MMC results in long peristalsis, which starts from stomach and terminates in distal part of the ileum. Therefore, it sweeps the gastric and intestinal contents into the large intestine. Consequently, MMC is alternatively called ***sweeper of GI tract***.
2. This clears the stomach and intestine of their luminal contents, so that they are ready to receive and digest the next meal whenever ingested.
3. Characteristically, MMC immediately stops when food is ingested.

Retroperistalsis

Normally, peristalsis moves in forward direction. However, if there is an obstruction in the lumen, ***reverse peristalsis*** occurs. This is called retroperistalsis.

1. Vomiting occurs due to retroperistalsis.
2. Retroperistalsis is also initiated by emotional factors or due to stimulation of medullary vomiting centers.

Segmentation

This commonly occurs in **small intestine**.

1. It is characterized by closely spaced contraction of the circular muscle layer.
2. These contractions *divide the small intestine into many segments*. Therefore, the movement is called segmentation.
3. It is primarily meant to ***mix chyme with pancreatic and intestinal secretions*** and also bring the fresh chyme into contact with the mucosal surface.
4. Therefore, segmentation is also called **mixing movement** (for details, refer to "Intestinal Motility").

ROLE OF SPHINCTERS

Sphincters are rings of smooth muscles that remain in a state of continuous contraction. There are **anatomical and physiological sphincters**. Upper esophageal sphincter is an example of **physiological sphincter**, which prevents esophageal content to regurgitate back into oral cavity. **Anatomical sphincters** are located at gastroesophageal, gastroduodenal and ileocecal junctions, and at the opening of bile duct in the duodenum and opening of rectum into anus. Thus, sphincters:

1. Separate two specialized compartments,
2. Regulate movement of content from upper compartment to lower compartment,
3. Prevent backward movement of content from lower to upper compartment.

Usually, when wall of the gut contracts sphincters relax and when gut wall relaxes sphincters relax. Hence, sphincters regulate **coordinated propulsion of contents aborally**. They also mediate **reflex activities** like gastrocolic, gastroileal reflexes, etc.

CHAPTER SUMMARY

Key Concepts

1. Electrical slow waves that oscillate significantly in GI smooth muscles are called basal electrical rhythm (BER). BER is due to the wide variation in RMP in GI smooth muscle.
2. Number of spikes on slow waves determines the magnitude of contraction.
3. Peristalsis is the propulsive movement and segmentation is the mixing movement.

Important to Know (Must Read)

1. In examinations, no **Long Question** is asked from this chapter. However, "Describe the electrical properties of GI smooth muscles", may come as a long question.
2. Basal electrical rhythm of GI smooth muscle, Slow waves of GI smooth muscle, Enteric motor neurons, Migrating motor complex, may come as **Short Questions**.
3. In **Viva**, examiner may ask... What are the specialities of electrical activity of GI smooth muscles, What is basal electrical rhythm of GI smooth muscle, Slow waves of GI smooth muscle, Organization of enteric motor neurons, Function and mechanism of peristalsis, segmentation, retroperistalsis, and migrating motor complex.

CHAPTER 46

Chewing and Deglutition

Learning Objectives

On completion of study of this chapter, the student **MUST** be able to:

1. List the functions of mastication.
2. Understand the mechanism of deglutition.
3. Appreciate, why one should not speak while eating.

The student **MAY** also be able to:

1. Describe the mechanism of deglutition reflex.

CHEWING (MASTICATION)

Chewing or mastication is mostly a voluntary activity. The process of mastication is **initiated usually reflexly** following the arrival of food in the mouth.

Mastication has following functions:

1. Mastication ***cuts and grinds larger food particles*** into smaller particles.
2. It ***increases salivary secretion*** (Application Box 46.1).
3. It ***mixes food with saliva***.
4. It lubricates content of the oral cavity, so that swallowing becomes easier.
5. It ***breaks down starch*** and allows saliva to mix with the broken starch particles. Therefore, chewing improves the taste of starch containing foods.
6. It ***improves dental strength*** and hygiene. To keep the teeth strong and in good health, dentists always encourage chewing of food adequately before swallowing.

Chewing occurs due to forceful contraction of **four groups of muscles** of mastication.

1. **Masseter** elevates mandible and helps in clenching of teeth.
2. **Temporalis** helps in retracting mandible.
3. **Pterygoids** (external and internal) protrude mandible and depress chin. This helps in opening the mouth. Alternative contractions of right and left pterygoids help in grinding movements.
4. **Buccinator** prevents accumulation of food between cheek and mouth.

Application Box 46.1

Food should be chewed adequately before swallowing: Mastication breaks the larger food particles into smaller particles. Mastication is the major stimulus for salivary secretion. More saliva is required for a smooth swallowing. Digestion of salivary amylase takes place in the stomach. More quantity of saliva facilitates more breaking down of food particles so that the work load on stomach for grinding food becomes less, and grinding and mixing of becomes easier. This helps in easy digestion of food. Therefore, it has been said that one should chew 32 times before swallowing. As it is always not possible to chew 32 times, chewing should be done at least 10 times.

SWALLOWING (DEGLUTITION)

Swallowing or deglutition is the process by which the food material from oral cavity is transported into esophagus. Though it is initiated voluntarily, most part of it is involuntary or reflexive. Therefore, this is also called **deglutition reflex**.

1. During the reflex act of deglutition, **respiration is inhibited**, which prevents entry of food into the trachea.
2. The **receptors** for deglutition reflex are present near the opening of the pharynx.
3. The ***afferent impulses*** are transmitted to deglutition centers in medulla and pons.
4. The ***efferent impulses*** are directed to the muscles of pharynx and upper esophagus via cranial nerves.

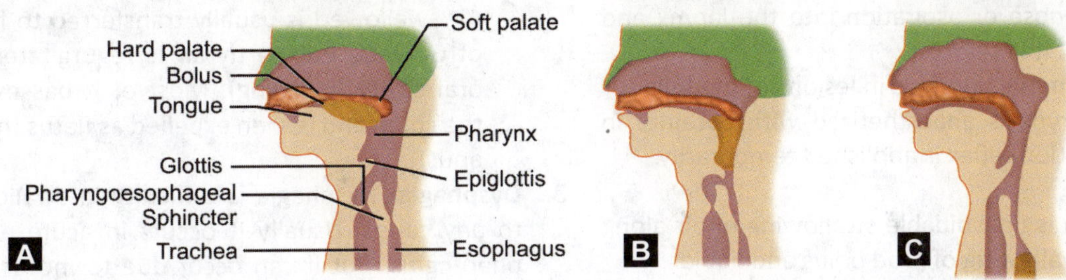

Figs. 46.1A to C: Phages of deglutition. Note the mechanism of deglutition in oral (A), pharyngeal (B), and esophageal (C) stages. In the oral phase, tongue pushes bolus of food into the back of pharynx. In the pharyngeal phase, epiglottis covers the glottis to prevent aspiration of food (prevents food to enter trachea) and soft palate is elevated to prevent food to enter nasal passage. In the esophageal phase, upper esophageal sphincter (UES) relaxes to allow food to descend into esophagus.

Stages of Deglutition

Swallowing is divided into **three stages** (phases): oral phase, pharyngeal phase, and esophageal phase. Oral phase is voluntary and pharyngeal and esophageal phases are involuntary.

Oral Phase

This is also called **buccal phase**. This is the voluntary phase of swallowing. It is initiated when the tongue separates a bolus of food from the mass of foodstuff present in the mouth. At the beginning, the tip of the tongue presses against the hard palate and then the body of tongue presses on it. This action of the tongue moves the food backward in the oral cavity. Thus, the food bolus is forced into the pharynx. Once the food touches the receptors at the pharyngeal opening, swallowing reflex is initiated.

Pharyngeal Phase

The major objective of pharyngeal phase is **to push food bolus into the esophagus** without its entry into respiratory passage.

Reflex Pathway

Receptors: Receptors are present around the pharyngeal opening.

Afferent: Impulses from pharyngeal receptors are transmitted to centers through ***trigeminal, glossopharyngeal, and vagus nerves***.

Centers: Centers for deglutition are ***nucleus tractus solitarius*** and ***nucleus ambiguous*** located in the medulla.

Efferents: Effector organs are muscles of pharynx and tongue that are innervated by ***trigeminal, glossopharyngeal, vagus and hypoglossal*** nerves.

Events

The events in pharyngeal phase occur in sequence within few milliseconds (Figs. 46.1A to C).

1. The **soft palate** is pulled in upward direction. The **palatopharyngeal folds** move in inward direction. These movements prevent entry of food into the nasopharynx. This also provides a small passage for food to enter the pharynx.
2. **Laryngeal opening is closed** by vocal cards pulled together. The larynx moves forward and upward against the epiglottis. These events **prevent entry of food into trachea** (Clinical Box 46.1).
3. The **superior constrictor muscles of pharynx** constrict, which forces food to enter deep into the pharynx and then from there into the esophagus. Simultaneously, **relaxation of upper esophageal sphincter** (UES) occurs that allows the food to easily enter the esophagus.
4. During this phase, **respiration is reflexly inhibited** due to inhibition of respiratory centers. This is called **deglutition apnea**.

Esophageal Phase

Once food enters into esophagus, which is facilitated by relaxation of UES, the peristaltic wave (**primary peristalsis**) is initiated just below the UES.

1. Reflexly, **UES contracts** that prevent regurgitation of food back into the pharynx.
2. The **peristaltic wave** travels at about 3–5 cm/s. It takes about 10 seconds for food bolus to pass through the entire esophagus.
3. If the primary peristalsis is ineffective, a second peristaltic (**secondary peristalsis**) wave is initiated to push the food bolus. Motility of esophagus is discussed in detail in next chapter "Esophageal Motility".

Clinical Box 46.1

Do not speak while eating: During, deglutition, respiration is temporarily arrested and food does not enter the respiratory passage. Laryngeal opening is closed by vocal cords pulled together. Larynx moves forward and upward against the epiglottis. Speaking or coughing during swallowing keeps the laryngeal outlet opened and therefore there is risk of food particle entering into the respiratory passage. Food or water entering into respiratory passage causes laryngeal and bronchial spasm. Sometimes it may cause sudden respiratory arrest and death. Therefore, one should eat in silence and concentrate on the universal energy that he receives through the food.

Disorders of Deglutition

1. **Decreased or Absence of deglutition reflex:** If deglutition reflex is impaired or abolished, regurgitation of

food into the nose or aspiration into the larynx and trachea occurs. It is seen in:
- IXth or Xth nerve paralysis in lesions of medulla
- When pharynx is anaesthetized with cocaine. In this deglutition reflex is abolished temporarily.

2. **Aerophagia**
   - Aerophagia is unavoidable swallowing of air along with the swallowing of food bolus and liquids.
   - It is seen in nervous individuals who have decreased tone of the upper oesophageal sphincter.
   - Air swallowed is usually transferred to lower part of GI tract, but partly air is regurgitated into the oral cavity (belching). Most of it passes down to the colon and is then expelled as flatus through the anus.
3. **Dysphagia:** Dysphagia is difficulty in swallowing due to any cause. Usually it occurs in acute and severe pharyngitis. But it can occur due to motor problems in pharynx, upper esophagus or foreign body, acute inflammation in oral cavity.

CHAPTER SUMMARY

Key Concepts

1. Though swallowing is voluntary process, most part of it is a reflex phenomenon.
2. Laryngeal opening closes during deglutition, preventing entry of food into respiratory passage. Speaking or coughing during eating allows food to enter into trachea and may cause choking in severe cases.
3. Mastication increases salivary secretion and facilitated swallowing and digestion in the stomach. Therefore, food should be chewed enough before swallowing.

Important to Know (Must Read)

1. In examinations, no **Long Question** is asked from this chapter.
2. Deglutition reflex may come as **Short Questions**.
3. In **Viva**, examiner may ask... Functions of mastication, phases of deglutition, afferent and efferent pathways and mechanism of deglutition in each phase, Problems of deglutition.

CHAPTER 47

Esophageal Motility

Learning Objectives

On completion of study of this chapter, the student **MUST** be able to:

1. Understand the functions of lower and upper esophageal sphincters.
2. Learn the mechanism of esophageal peristalsis.
3. Understand the physiological abnormalities in reflux esophagitis and achalasia cardia.

Esophagus serves as a conduit to transfer food from pharynx into the stomach. Once food enters the esophagus, reflex contraction of esophagus is initiated that transports food into the stomach.

FUNCTIONAL ANATOMY

Parts of Esophagus

Esophagus is divided into **three parts**: upper esophageal sphincter, body of esophagus and lower esophageal sphincter.

1. **In the upper part of esophagus**, the ***muscles are striated*** (like skeletal muscles) muscles, **in the lower part** the ***muscles are smooth muscles*** and **in the middle part**, there is ***mixture of smooth and skeletal muscles*** (Fig. 47.1).
2. However, all esophageal muscles are mainly **innervated by vagal fibers**. Even the striated esophageal muscles receive vagal motor fibers.

Special Features

1. Esophagus differs from other parts of GI system **for not having electrical slow waves** to trigger contraction. Therefore, **excitability of its muscle is low.**
2. Muscles in the body of the esophagus are **relaxed always**, except during deglutition.
3. All muscle fibers including striated fibers are innervated by **vagus nerve.**
4. Activation of deglutition reflex initiates **peristaltic contraction** by neural mechanism (*primary peristalsis*) or presence of food bolus locally stimulates peristalsis (*secondary peristalsis*).

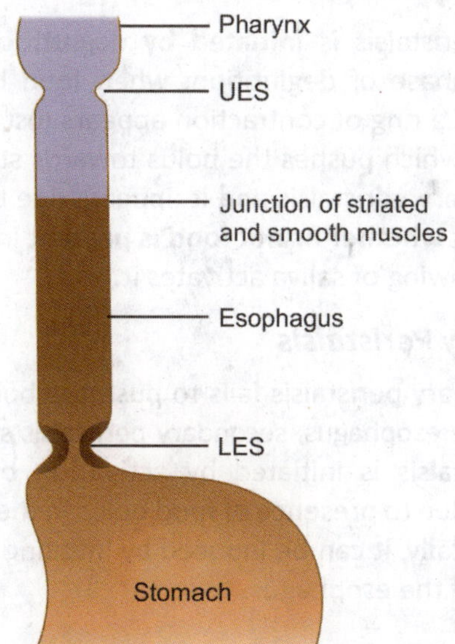

Fig. 47.1: Structure of esophagus. (UES: upper esophageal sphincter; LES: lower esophageal sphincter). Note that the muscle of upper part of the esophagus is striated and of lower part is smooth. A transitional zone of striated and smooth muscles exists between them.

Esophageal Sphincters

Upper Esophageal Sphincter

Upper esophageal sphincter is mainly a **physiological sphincter**.

1. It ***reflexly relaxes*** to allow the food from pharynx to enter the esophagus.
2. However, once food has entered the esophagus, **it constricts to prevent regurgitation of food** back into the pharynx.

Lower Esophageal Sphincter

Lower esophageal sphincter **remains tonically contracted.** It relaxes only when food from the esophagus enters the stomach. Therefore, it always prevents reflux of food back into the esophagus from the stomach.

1. The significant fraction of **basal tone of lower esophageal sphincter** is contributed by *vagal cholinergic fibers*.
2. However, vagal fibers **inhibit circular muscles of the sphincter** in response to primary peristalsis that relaxes the sphincter and allows food to enter the stomach. This inhibitory action is mediated by stimulation of other neurons through activation of cholinergic vagal neurons that ***secrete VIP and nitric oxide (NO)***.

ESOPHAGEAL PERISTALSIS

Two types of peristalsis occur in esophagus: primary and secondary.

Primary Peristalsis

Primary peristalsis is **initiated by deglutition reflex.** In the third phase of deglutition, when food bolus enters esophagus, a ring of contraction appears just cephalad to the bolus, which pushes the bolus towards stomach. This is the primary peristalsis and it appears due to the **act of swallowing whether or not food is present** in the mouth. Even swallowing of saliva activates it.

Secondary Peristalsis

When primary peristalsis fails to push the bolus from the body of the esophagus, secondary peristalsis starts. Secondary peristalsis is initiated by **activation of mechanoreceptors** due to presence of food bolus in the esophagus. Experimentally, it can be induced by inflating a balloon in the body of the esophagus.

Applied Physiology

Reflux Esophagitis and Barrett's Esophagus

Lower esophageal sphincter (LES) remains always tonically contracted except during swallowing when food in the esophagus stimulates esophageal peristalsis. The tonic contraction of LES prevents regurgitation of gastric content back into the esophagus.

1. When **LES becomes incompetent**, ***reflux of acid gastric content*** into esophagus produces esophagitis, known as ***reflux esophagitis***.
2. Popularly, it is known as **"heartburn"** as the patient describes the pain in the retrosternal area. In the long run, it can cause stricture or ulceration of esophagus.
3. It is treated by **proton pump blocker** or H_2 receptor blocker.
4. **Fundoplication** may also be tried in this condition, in which a portion of the fundus of the stomach is wrapped around the lower esophagus so that LES remains inside a narrow tunnel of the stomach.

Barrett's Esophagus

In few cases of chronic reflux esophagitis, the normal squamous epithelium of esophagus is replaced by columnar epithelium. This is called columnar metaplasia. This is a premalignant condition.

Achalasia Cardia

'Achalasia' means **failure to relax**. Normally, when food enters esophagus, esophageal peristalsis pushes food into the stomach. During this process, **LES relaxes** so that food easily passes into the stomach. However, in some individuals, ***resting tone of LES is high***. Therefore, the ***sphincter fails to relax*** completely during deglutition. This causes **inadequate emptying of esophagus** and food collects in the esophagus and the ***organ is massively dilated***. The condition is called achalasia cardia.

Causes

It occurs due to **deficiency of myenteric plexus** at LES in the esophagus. Also, the *secretion of VIP and NO*, the neurotransmitters that cause relaxation of GI muscles, *is defective* in this condition. Thus, resting tone of LES becomes high.

Diagnosis

Diagnosis is made by demonstrating **rat tail in barium meal X-ray** (body of esophagus is dilated and lower part is narrowed giving appearance of a rat) (Fig. 47.2) or by demonstrating retained food and fluid in esophagoscopy (Fig. 47.3)

Treatment

Treatment for achalasia is **mechanical pneumatic dilatation** of the sphincter.

1. In severe cases, **surgical weakening** of the sphincter by myotomy (incision of the esophageal muscle) is performed.
2. Also, **administration of drugs** that decrease tone of the sphincter has been successfully tried. For example, **injection of botulinum toxin** into LES that inhibits acetylcholine release produces relaxation of the sphincter.

Aerophagia

While eating and drinking, some volume of air is automatically swallowed. This is called aerophagia. A small volume of the swallowed air is removed by **belching** (regurgitation of air) and a volume of it enters into the intestine.

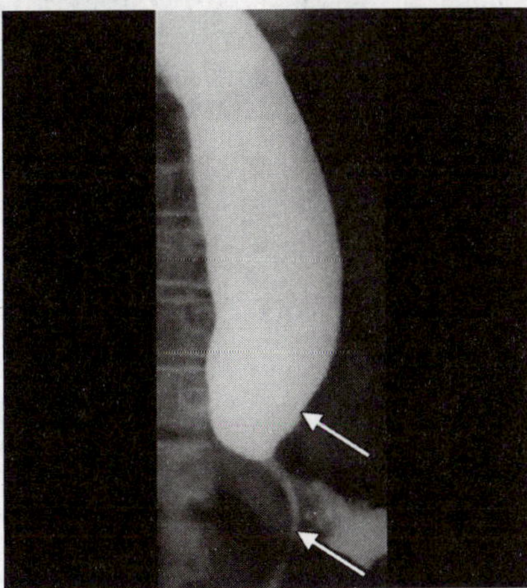

Fig. 47.2: Rat tail appearance of esophagus in barium meal X-ray. Note, the body of esophagus is dilated (upper arrow) and lower part is narrowed giving appearance of a rat tail (lower arrow).
Courtesy: Figure 45.5, Clinical Anatomy, by Neeta Kulkarni, Vol. 2, 3rd edition, 2016; Jaypee Brothers Medical Publishers (P) Ltd.

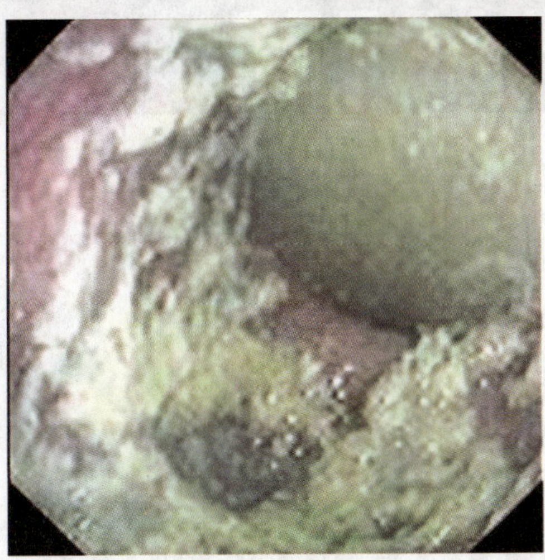

Fig. 47.3: Esophagoscopy in achalasia cardia demonstrates retained food and fluid in lower part of esophagus.
Courtesy: Figure 2.7, Gastrointestinal Surgery, by S Devaji Rao, 1st edition, 2009; Jaypee Brothers Medical Publishers (P) Ltd.

1. Intestinal and colonic bacteria add hydrogen, hydrogen sulfide, CO_2 and methane to this air that are expelled from rectum as **flatus**.
2. The daily production of gas by GI tract is about one liter.
3. The volume of gas present in GIT at any given time is about **200 mL** as a large volume of produced and swallowed air is removed regularly as flatus.
4. The smell of the flatus is mainly due to the presence of sulfides.
5. Some individuals have **more aerophagia** or more production of gas. *Disturbance in intestinal* flora also leads to more gas production. These individuals develop ***abdominal discomfort and borborygmi*** (rumbling noises in the intestine and colon).

CHAPTER SUMMARY

Key Concepts

1. Esophagus is a unique structure having both striated and smooth muscle, and both the muscle are innervated by vagus nerve.
2. Esophagus does not exhibit electrical slow waves.
3. Esophageal peristalsis is initiated by swallowing, which may be air, or saliva, and need not be food.
4. Relaxation of LES mediated by VIP and NO released from vagal neurons.

Important to Know (Must Read)

1. In examinations, no **Long Question** is asked from this chapter.
2. Esophageal peristalsis may come as **Short Questions**.
3. In **Viva**, examiner may ask...... Special features of esophageal muscles, Esophageal sphincters, Types and mechanism of esophageal peristalsis, Causes and treatment of achalasia cardia and reflux esophagitis.

CHAPTER 48

Gastric Motility

Learning Objectives

On completion of study of this chapter, the student **MUST** be able to:

1. List the gastric motilities.
2. Appreciate the electrophysiology gastric smooth muscles.
3. Name the types of gastric relaxations and give the importance.
4. Understand the mechanism and regulation of gastric emptying.
5. Correlate the electrophysiology of gastric contractions with gastric motor dysfunctions.
6. Understand the mechanism of vomiting.

The student **MAY** also be able to:

1. Describe the mechanism and regulation of gastric emptying.
2. Describe the vomiting reflex.

Functionally, stomach is divided into *two parts*: the **proximal stomach** (consisting mainly the body of the stomach), which ***acts as a reservoir***, and the **distal stomach** (consisting mainly the antrum of the stomach), which ***acts as a pump***.

1. The **proximal stomach**, for its property of ***receptive relaxation***, receives and stores food, and for its ***tonic contractions*** pushes food toward the antrum.
2. The **distal stomach** for its property of ***phasic contractions***, mixes, grinds, and breaks down food into smaller particles and regulates emptying of food into small intestine through gastroduodenal junctions.

Thus, **major objectives** of gastric motility are:

1. To allow the stomach to act as a **reservoir for storage *of large amount of food*** of a single meal.
2. To cut foodstuff into smaller particles and mix the food with gastric juice, the process in which **food is converted into chyme**.
3. To allow gastric contents to **enter the duodenum at a slow but controlled rate**, so that duodenum and jejunum being narrower tubes, handle the chyme appropriately.

Scientist contributed

William Beaumont (1785–1853) was a surgeon in the US Army who became known as the "Father of Gastric **Physiology**" following his extensive research on human digestion, gastric juice and gastric functions. He was the first scientist to systematically study the digestive processes in human beings. He was first physiologist to study gastric motility in a patient with a gastric fistula.

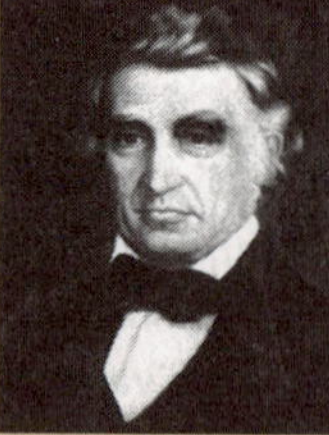

W Beaumont
(1785–1853)

Source: Mai FM. Beaumont's contribution to gastric psychophysiology: a reappraisal. Canadian Journal of Psychiatry 1988;33(7):650–3.

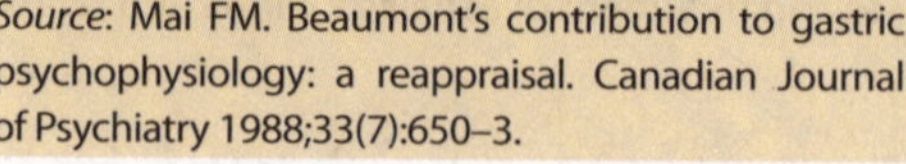

FUNCTIONAL ANATOMY

Parts of Stomach

As described above, for understanding gastric motility, stomach is divided into **two parts**: the proximal stomach and distal stomach (Fig. 48.1).

Proximal Stomach

The proximal part of stomach accommodates large volume of food (as large as 2 to 4 liters) without much increase in intragastric pressure.

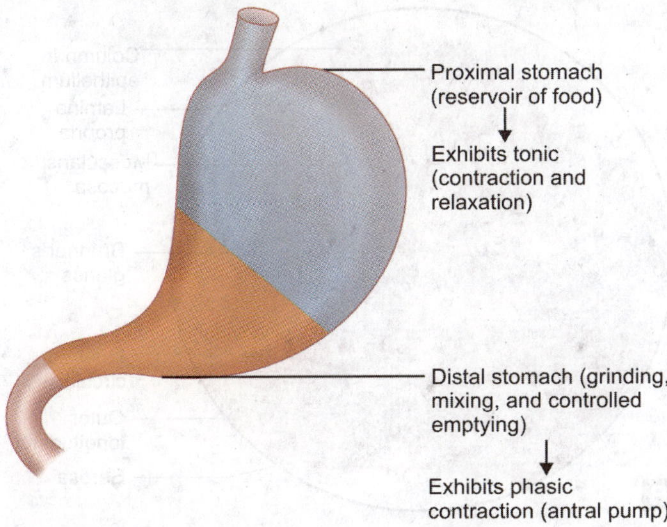

Fig. 48.1: Motor parts of stomach. The proximal stomach is formed by fundus and major portion of the body. The distal stomach is formed by antrum and lower portion of the body.

1. This becomes possible due to the phenomenon of **receptive relaxation**.
2. The contractile ability of fundus and body of stomach is normally poor. Therefore, food in fundus and body remains relatively unmixed for a longer duration.
3. Thus, the proximal stomach serves mainly as **reservoir of food**.

Distal Stomach

It consists mainly of the antrum.

1. The antrum, physiologically acts as a mechanical pump, which **propels food towards the pylorus** and helps in **grinding and mixing of food**.
2. Antral contractions break foodstuff into smaller particles and mix food thoroughly with gastric juice that help in partial digestion of food.
3. ***Pyloric sphincter remains partially closed*** and does not allow easy entry of gastric contents into the duodenum.
4. However, vigorous contractions of gastric antrum help gastric content enter the duodenum at a **slow but controlled rate**.
5. After grinding and mixing of food with gastric juice, the gastric content is now called **chyme**.

Structure of Stomach Wall

Stomach wall contains all general components of the wall of the GI tract.

1. However, the **circular muscle layer of the muscularis externa is more prominent** than the longitudinal layer.
2. In general, muscularis externa in fundus and body is thin and in antrum and pylorus is considerably thick. The **thickness of muscularis externa increases from body toward pylorus** (Figs. 48.2A and B). The highly developed muscle coat helps antrum work as **effective pump**.

Gastroduodenal Junction

The junction between the stomach and duodenum is called gastroduodenal junction. The pylorus separates antrum and duodenum. There is a sphincter in the pylorus consisting of a ring like thickening of circular muscle fibers, known as **pyloric sphincter**.

Important functions of gastroduodenal junction are:

1. To allow gastric contents to enter the duodenum at a **slow and controlled rate** (the rate at which duodenum is capable of possessing the chyme).
2. To **prevent regurgitation of duodenal contents** back into the stomach.

Gastroduodenal Mucosa

The duodenal mucosa is relatively resistant to bile acids but sensitive to gastric acid, whereas gastric mucosa is apparently resistant to gastric acid but sensitive to bile acids.

1. Therefore, in case of ***incompetent pyloric sphincter***, regurgitation of duodenal content (containing bile acids) into the stomach usually results in **gastric ulcer**.
2. On the other hand, ***rapid emptying of gastric contents*** (containing acidic chyme) into the duodenum promptly causes **duodenal ulcer**.
3. Normally, as soon as acidic chyme from stomach enters the duodenum, the acidic pH stimulates release of secretin from S cells of duodenum and upper jejunum. Secretin stimulates pancreatic secretion rich in water and bicarbonate. Therefore, immediately the **acidic chyme is neutralized** by the aqueous component of pancreatic juice. This is the physiological mechanism that prevents formation of duodenal ulcer.
4. However, when gastric emptying is faster or secretion of pancreatic juice is less, the possibility of duodenal ulcer is more. Moreover, the content in the part of the duodenum above the sphincter Oddi does not get well mixed with pancreatic secretion.

Neural Control of Pyloric Part

The pylorus is richly innervated by parasympathetic (vagal) and sympathetic fibers.

1. Normally, **sympathetic stimulation causes constriction of pyloric sphincter**.
2. However, activation of **parasympathetic fibers have both stimulating and inhibiting effects**.
3. The stimulatory effects are mediated by cholinergic vagal fibers and the inhibitory effects are mediated by the **vagal fibers** that release **VIP or nitric oxide (NO)**.
4. Constriction of pyloric sphincter also occurs in response to hormones like CCK, gastrin, GIP, and secretin. Therefore, these hormones slow gastric emptying.

Innervation of Stomach

Stomach is densely innervated by both the division of ANS and the neurons of the enteric nervous system.

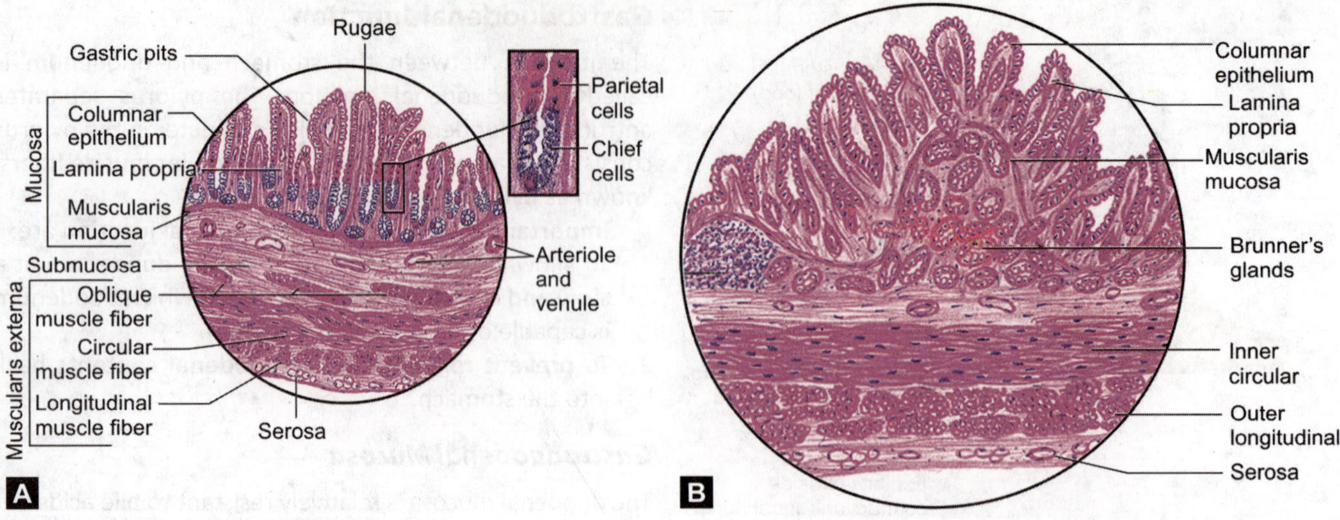

Figs. 48.2A and B: Layers of the stomach wall. (A) Fundus and body of the stomach; (B) Antrum of the stomach. Note, muscularis externa is more developed in the antrum of the stomach (B) compared to the body of the stomach (A).
Courtesy: Figures 13.17A and 13.21B. Basic Histology, by V Subhadra Devi, 1st edition, 2016; Jaypee Brothers Medical Publishers (P) Ltd.

1. **Parasympathetic innervation** (vagal fibers) stimulates whereas **sympathetic innervation** (fibers originate from celiac plexus) inhibits gastric motility and secretion.
2. Axons arising from intramural plexuses innervate smooth muscles and secretory cells.
3. **Sensory fibers** from stomach travel to CNS via vagal and sympathetic fibers. Some of the sensory fibers act as **afferent link** between the sensory receptors of the gastric mucosa and the intramural plexuses.
4. Few of these afferent fibers provide information about an **intragastric pressure, gastric distention, chemical composition and pH** of gastric content, and ***pain sensation*** originating in the stomach.
5. All these stimuli influence gastric motility.

Electrophysiology of Gastric Motility

The **peristaltic waves** in the stomach occur usually at the frequency of **gastric slow waves**. These peristaltic waves are generated by a **pacemaker zone** located in the middle of the body of the stomach. The **frequency of peristaltic wave** *is about 3 per minute* in human being and the waves are conducted from body toward pylorus.

1. The gastric slow wave has **four phases** that resemble the action potentials of cardiac muscle (Fig. 45.2; Chapter 45). However, it ***does not overshoot*** and ***last for a longer period*** (10 times that of cardiac action potential).
2. The smooth muscles of stomach contract when the depolarization of the slow wave *exceeds the threshold for contraction*.
3. **The force of contraction depends on the degree, frequency and duration of depolarization.**
4. Greater the depolarization and longer the muscle cells remain depolarized (above threshold), greater is the force of contraction.
5. **In antrum of the stomach**, action potential spikes occur in the plateau phase. The contractions that result from these action potentials are stronger than the contractions that occur in the absence of these action potentials.
6. **Acetylcholine and gastrin improve gastric contractility** *by enhancing the amplitude and duration of the plateau phase* of gastric slow waves. **Norepinephrine inhibits** by the opposite mechanism.

TYPES OF GASTRIC MOTILITY

The types of gastric movements are hunger contractions (movements of empty stomach), receptive relaxation, peristalsis, migrating motor complex and reverse peristalsis. The peristalsis of stomach results in a regulated gastric emptying.

Hunger Contractions

When, stomach is empty, motility of the stomach increases. If stomach is allowed to **remain empty for a longer duration**, contractions become **vigorous**. These contractions are called hunger contractions.

1. Usually, hunger contractions are *distressing and painful*.
2. The antral contractions are intense in such a situation and are associated with the relaxation of pyloric sphincter.

Gastric Relaxations

Receptive Relaxation

This is the relaxation of the fundus and body of the stomach **in response to chewing and swallowing of food**. Thus, stomach prepares itself to receive food (Fig. 48.3). The

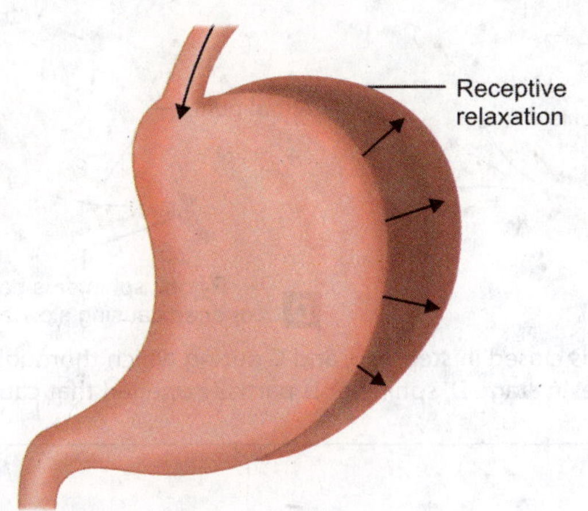

Fig. 48.3: Receptive relaxation of stomach.

relaxation continues till food continues to enter the stomach, so that a large meal is easily accommodated in it.

1. Because of receptive relaxation, the **intragastric pressure does not rise** in spite of accumulation of a large volume of food.
2. The receptive relaxation is ***mediated by vagus nerve*** (Fig. 48.4). Normally, gastric motility induced by vagal stimulation is mediated by cholinergic fibers. However, receptive relaxation mediated by vagus is due to **release of neurotransmitters like VIP and NO** (*non-cholinergic fibers*) at its nerve ending.

Adaptive and Feedback Relaxations

There are other two types of gastric relaxations: adaptive and feedback.

1. The **adaptive relaxation** is the relaxation of stomach triggered by distension of stomach. Receptive relaxation starts even before food reaches stomach whereas adaptive relaxation occurs in response to stretching of stomach wall. This is mediated by **vagovagal reflex** (Fig. 48.4) and is meant to accommodate a greater volume of food.
2. The **feedback relaxation** of stomach is a **reflexive relaxation** that occurs due to presence of food in proximal segment of small intestine. Acidic chyme and fatty acid in intestine inhibit gastric motility by both **hormonal and neural mechanisms** that cause feedback relaxation of stomach (Fig. 48.4).

Peristalsis

After about half an hour following gastric filling, gastric peristalsis starts.

1. The peristaltic movements are initiated by gastric slow waves.
2. The **pacemaker for gastric peristalsis** is located in the middle of the stomach close toward greater curvature.

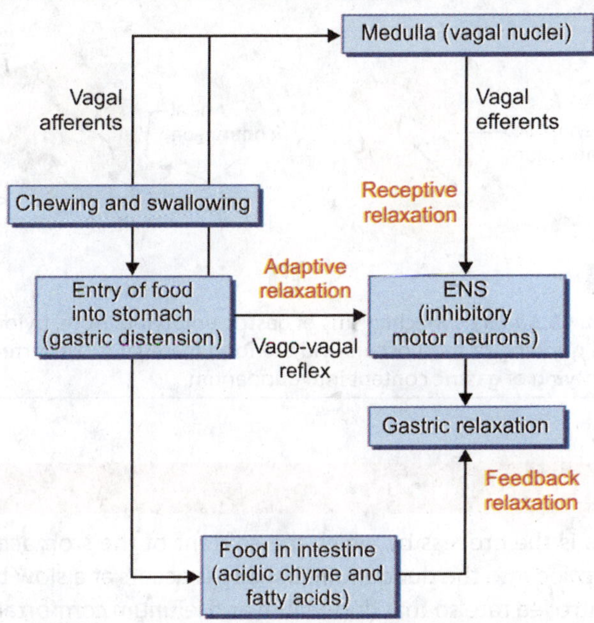

Fig. 48.4: Mechanisms of relaxations (receptive, adaptive, and feedback) of stomach. Receptive relaxation is vagally mediated and adaptive relaxation is mainly a vagovagal reflex.

3. It starts as a ring of contraction that progress slowly toward antrum.
4. It usually occurs at the rate of **3 per minute**.
5. It helps in **propelling food into the antrum and mixing of food with gastric juice**.
6. During this gastric peristalsis, pylorus usually remains closed. Therefore, food does not enter the duodenum, rather is recirculated in the stomach.

Migrating Motor Complex

During the **interdigestive phase**, antrum of the stomach remains silent for about 75–90 minutes, after which a **burst of electrical and motor activities occurs**.

1. This causes intense antral contraction with relaxation of pylorus. Therefore, the **remaining gastric content is emptied** into the duodenum.
2. The wave of contraction progresses from stomach toward terminal ileum. Thus, it helps in **cleaning the stomach and intestine** and keeps the GI tract ready for the next meal.
3. Usually, it is **repeated every 90 minutes** during interdigestive phase.

Reverse Peristalsis

Sometimes in abnormal situations, peristalsis occurs in reverse direction, which starts in the lower parts of the body and proceeds toward esophagus.

1. The **lower and upper esophageal sphincters relax** so that gastric content is **forced out** of esophagus and oral cavity.
2. This results in vomiting (described below).

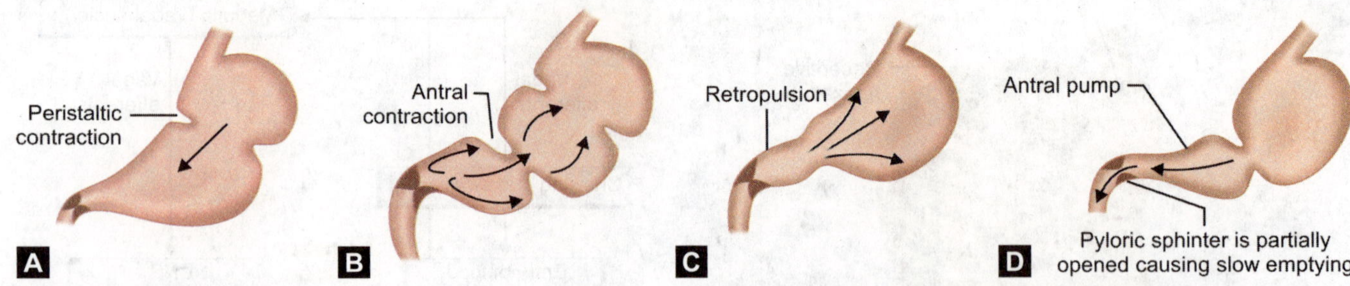

Figs. 48.5A to D: Mechanisms of gastric emptying. Note, pyloric sphincter is closed in step A, B, and C during which thorough mixing and grinding of food occurs and the food material is converted into chyme. In stage D, sphincter is partially opened that causes slow emptying of gastric content into duodenum.

GASTRIC EMPTYING

This is the process by which the content of the stomach is emptied into the duodenum. Usually, it occurs at a slow but controlled rate so that duodenum and jejunum comfortably accommodate and process the chyme at a desired rate.

Mechanism of Gastric Emptying

When food enters stomach, stomach relaxes due to receptive and adaptive relaxations. Later, after about half an hour, slowly gastric motility begins. Gastric emptying occurs by **three mechanisms**: peristaltic contraction, antral contraction, and retropulsion (Figs. 48.5A to D).

Peristaltic Contractions

The peristaltic contractions usually begin in the middle of the stomach and proceeds in a ring like fashion toward pylorus (Fig. 48.5A). These contractions **mainly push food into the antral part of the stomach.**

1. The **velocity and magnitude of contraction** *increase as the contractile waves approach pylorus*.
2. As contractions are *weak in the fundus and body of the stomach*, the proximal portion of stomach mainly serves the reservoir function. Therefore, usually proper mixing of food with gastric secretion does not occur in these parts of the stomach.
3. Major amount of **mixing takes place in the antrum**, as antrum contracts vigorously.

Antral Contractions

Antral contractions help **thorough mixing of food with the gastric juice.**

1. The forceful contraction of antrum forces gastric contents toward the pylorus. But, as the pyloric sphincter remains closed, peristaltic wave fails to push food into the duodenum, rather food **returns back into the body of the stomach** (Fig. 48.5B).
2. After few such contractions, pylorus opens partially with a narrow opening at the center.
3. Therefore, stomach *empties in small squirts with each peristaltic wave*.

Retropulsion

The terminal part of antrum exhibits rapid and forceful contractions that forces the chyme to be propelled back toward the proximal part of the antrum and body of the stomach (Fig. 48.5C). This movement is called **retropulsion.**

1. Retropulsion is very **effective in mixing and grinding** the larger food particles into smaller ones.
2. Then, pyloric sphincter partially opens and gastric pump slowly pushes food into duodenum (Fig. 48.5D).

Physiological Significance

As the muscle layers in the fundus and body are thin, contractions in these parts of the stomach are weak. Therefore, gastric content in body of stomach **settles into different layers** based on their density.

1. Fat content of the food forms an oily layer on the top of the other gastric contents. This is why **fat is emptied slower than the carbohydrate and protein** (Application Box 48.1).
2. Liquid portion of the food flow around the mass and enter the antrum, and from there into the duodenum. Therefore, **liquid is emptied faster than the solid.**

Application Box 48.1

A cup of fat is taken in cocktail party: As fat decreases gastric emptying, usually a cup of fat is ingested before drinking alcohol in cocktail party. Fat ensures slow gastric emptying and slow absorption of alcohol from intestine, and therefore the person drives his car back after the party, even after a heavy drink.

Regulation of Gastric Emptying

Gastric emptying is regulated by both **neural and hormonal mechanisms.** The upper part of the small intestine (duodenum and jejunum) contains receptors that detect change in **pH, osmotic pressure, and products of fat and protein digestion.** The chyme that enters duodenum is highly acidic and hypertonic and contains products of protein and fat digestion. All these stimuli influence gastric emptying.

1. **Acid in the duodenum:** With decrease in the pH of the duodenal content the rate of gastric emptying decreases.

- This response is mediated by both *neural and hormonal mechanisms*.
- The acidic chyme in the duodenum **releases secretin** that decreases gastric emptying by inhibiting contraction of the antrum and by stimulating the contraction of pyloric sphincter.

2. **Products of fat digestion:** Products of fat digestion like **fatty acids** and also some fat molecules in the duodenal content **inhibit gastric emptying**. This response is mediated by **CCK and GIP**.
   - CCK is secreted from duodenum and jejunum in response to fatty acids and it inhibits gastric emptying.
   - GIP, which is released in response to fatty acids also inhibits gastric emptying.
3. **Osmolality of duodenal content:** The chyme entering into duodenum has higher osmolality. There are **osmoreceptors** in the mucosa of duodenum and jejunum that detect change in osmolality of the duodenal content. **Hypertonic solutions in the duodenum** release **hormones that inhibit** the rate of gastric emptying.
4. **Products of protein digestion:** Presence of **peptides and amino acids** in the duodenum release **gastrin** from the G cells located in the duodenum.
   - Gastrin **increases antral contraction** but at the same time also causes **constriction of pyloric sphincter**. Therefore, the net effect is *decreased rate of gastric emptying*.
   - The products of protein digestion also release **CCK and GIP** from duodenum and jejunum that *inhibit gastric emptying*.
5. **Volume of the meal:** Whenever a large amount of food is taken in a meal, the time taken for gastric emptying prolongs. However, if the volume is mainly due to liquid then emptying is faster.
6. **Stretching of duodenum:** Entry of chyme into the duodenum stretches the wall of duodenum. This initiates **enterogastric reflex** that inhibits gastric emptying. Enterogastric reflex is also activated by acid in the duodenum.
7. **Neural factors**
   - **Vagal stimulation promotes** gastric emptying. Therefore, **vagotomy produces gastric stasis.** Consequently, whenever vagotomy is performed for the treatment of peptic ulcer, usually a *drainage procedure* like pyloroplasty or gastrojejunostomy is also performed to ensure proper passage of food from the stomach into the duodenum (Clinical Box 48.1).
   - **Sympathetic stimulation inhibits** gastric emptying.
8. **Hormonal factors:** Most of the hormones liberated from duodenum and jejunum like **CCK, GIP, secretin, etc., inhibit gastric emptying**.

Clinical Box 48.1

Drainage procedure is done with vagotomy: As vagotomy decreases gastric motility and produces gastric stasis, whenever vagotomy is performed as done for the treatment of peptic ulcer, usually a drainage procedure like gastrojejunostomy is also performed to ensure proper passage of food from the stomach into the duodenum.

APPLIED PHYSIOLOGY

Dysfunctions of Gastric Emptying

Delayed Gastric Emptying

1. Gastric emptying is delayed in **autonomic neuropathy** as occurs in diabetes mellitus.
2. Paralysis of propulsive movements occurs following **vagotomy**, which is called **gastroparesis**. Therefore, a drainage procedure like pyloroplasty is performed to overcome post-vagotomy gastric stasis.
3. **Hypertrophic pyloric stenosis** can cause gastric stasis.

Rapid Gastric Emptying

Normally, vagus stimulation promotes gastric emptying.

1. Therefore, states of **increased vagal activity increase emptying.**
2. Conversely, **sympathetic stimulation inhibits emptying.** Therefore, loss of appetite is a feature of acute stress, a state of sympathetic overactivity.
3. Hormones like **thyroxine** stimulate gastric emptying and intestinal motility. Hence, increased appetite and hyperdefecation are features of hyperthyroidism.
4. Increased liquid content of food increases gastric emptying.

Vomiting

Definition

Vomiting is the **expulsion of gastroduodenal content** from GIT to the external environment via mouth.

Associated Features

Vomiting is usually preceded by the feeling of **nausea, tachycardia, sweating, pallor, dizziness**, and **dilatation of pupils**. It is associated with retching that forces contents of the stomach into the esophagus.

Stimuli and Vomiting Centers

Vomiting is a reflex phenomenon, the center for which is located in the medulla (Fig. 48.6).

1. The receptors present in many parts of the body provide inputs to the **vomiting center,** in the brainstem. Vomiting center present in the reticular formation of medulla consists of various scattered group of neurons that control different aspects of vomiting.
2. **Vestibular nuclei** mediate vomiting in response to motion sickness.
3. Pharyngeal stimulation induces vomiting by activating **nucleus tractus solitarious.**
4. **Area postrema** mediate vomiting activated by drugs (opiates, chemotherapeutic agents, etc.) and hormones (as in pregnancy).
5. Vomiting activated by emotion influenced by **limbic and diencephalic** inputs.

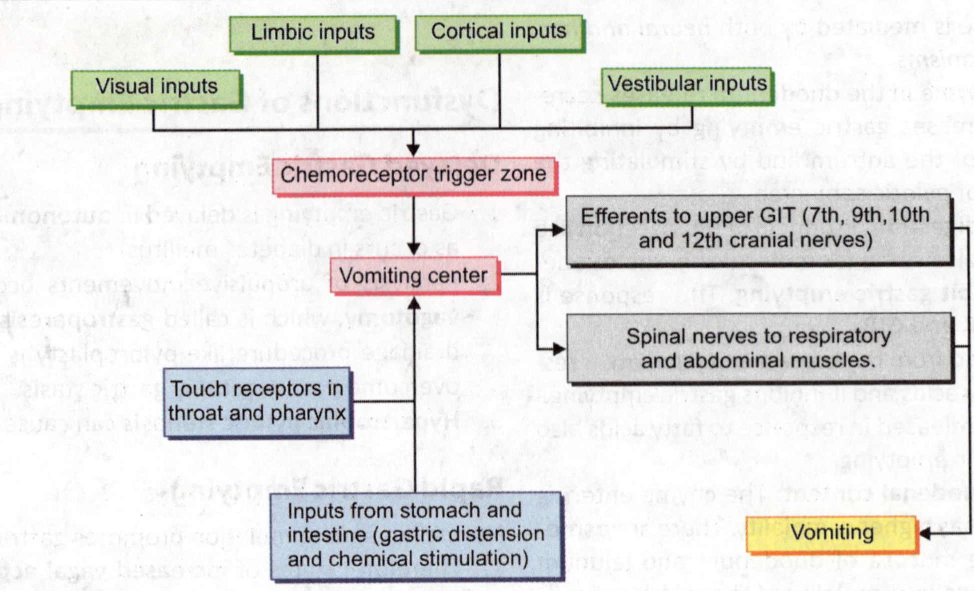

Fig. 48.6: Mechanism of vomiting reflex.

The **important stimuli** that activate these afferent fibers are:

1. Distension of stomach
2. Tickling the back of throat
3. Painful injury of the genitourinary tract
4. Conditions associated with dizziness and nausea
5. Many chemicals or drugs can elicit vomiting.

Emetics and Antiemetics

Drugs that induce vomiting are called **emetics**. The common emetics are apomorphine, ipecac, etc.

1. These chemicals stimulate the receptors that are present in the CTZ (**chemoreceptor trigger zone**), located in **area postrema**, a V-shaped band of tissue on the lateral wall of the fourth ventricle.
2. Many **antiemetics** prevent vomiting **by inhibiting CTZ**.
3. There are 5-HT$_3$ and D$_2$ receptors in area postrema. **Serotonin** stimulates vomiting through **5-HT$_3$ receptors. Ondensetron**, a 5-HT$_3$ receptor antagonist is an antiemetic.
4. **Chlorpromazine**, a D$_2$ receptor antagonist and **haloperidol** are also effective antiemetics.
5. Corticosteroids, cannabinoids, and benzodiazepines are useful antiemetics for chemotherapy-induced vomiting.

Mechanism of Vomiting

Vomiting reflex is executed in a sequence of events.

The steps of vomiting are:

1. Genesis of **reverse peristalsis** that starts from the middle of the jejunum. This sweeps the content of intestine and duodenum into the stomach.
2. **Relaxation of the pyloric sphincter** that allows the intestinal content to enter the stomach.
3. Forced inspiration occurs against the closed glottis. Lowering of the diaphragm **increases intra-abdominal pressure.**
4. This is followed by vigorous **contraction of abdominal muscles.** Thus, intra-abdominal pressure sharply increases, which **forces the gastric contents to enter the esophagus.**
5. Relaxation of the lower esophageal sphincter allows gastric content to enter the esophagus.
6. Normally, the upper esophageal sphincter remains closed and prevents regurgitation of food into the pharynx. With stronger retching and sharp rise in intra-abdominal pressure, **upper esophageal sphincter relaxes,** which allows chyme to enter the pharynx and then from there into the mouth. Entry of vomitus into the trachea is prevented by central movement of vocal cards, closure of glottis and inhibition of respiration.

Dumping Syndrome

This is a distressing syndrome consisting mainly of weakness, dizziness and sweating that develop in about **two hours after meal** in persons who have undergone gastrectomy or gastrojejunostomy (that bypasses stomach).

This occurs due to **two causes:**

1. **Hypoglycemia:** Rapid entry of food into intestine causes quick absorption of glucose from intestine and produces prompt hyperglycemia, which in turn increases **insulin secretion**. Insulin produces **hypoglycemia** that produces weakness, dizziness, and sweating.
2. **Hypovolemia:** The speedy entry of hypertonic meal from esophagus directly into intestine produces ***high osmotic load on intestine that transfers water from blood into the gut***. This produces hypovolemia, dehydration and hypotension that lead to weakness, dizziness and sweating.

CHAPTER SUMMARY

Key Concepts

1. The proximal stomach is mainly for receiving and storing food, and the distal stomach is meant for mixing and emptying food.
2. Antral contractions help in proper mixing and grinding food that finally becomes chyme.
3. LES sphincter partially opens in response to every antral pump activity so as to allow small quantity of chyme to be delivered to duodenum at a time.
4. Degree of distension and type of food mainly contribute to gastric emptying. Vagal fibers stimulate and sympathetic fibers inhibit gastric emptying.
5. Vomiting is mainly a central phenomenon initiated by stimulation of vomiting center in medulla, though local factors contribute to it.

Important to Know (Must Read)

1. In examinations, "Mechanism and factors affecting gastric emptying" may come as a **Long Question**.
2. Gastric relaxations, Reverse peristalsis of stomach, Electrophysiology of gastric smooth muscles, Gastric emptying, Vomiting, may come as **Short Questions**.
3. In **Viva**, examiner may ask... What are the parts of the stomach and what are their functions, Who is the Father of Gastric Physiology, What are the special electrophysiological properties of gastric smooth muscles, Types of gastric relaxations, What is the importance of receptive and adaptive relaxation, What is the mechanism of gastric emptying, What are the factor affecting gastric emptying, What is Retropulsion, What is the specialty of gastric peristalsis, Who is the pacemaker of gastric contractions, What is hunger contraction, What are the causes of rapid and delayed gastric emptying, Reverse peristalsis of stomach, Mechanism of vomiting, What is dumping syndrome and how is it treated.

CHAPTER

49

Small Intestinal Motility

LEARNING OBJECTIVES

On completion of study of this chapter, the student **MUST** be able to:

1. Understand the importance of intestinal movements in mixing, propelling, and absorption of food materials in GI tract.
2. Name intestinal motilities, and give their mechanisms and functions.
3. Name the intestinal reflexes and give their functions.
4. Appreciate the physiological basis of motility disorders.

The student **MAY** also be able to:

1. Describe the detailed mechanism of intestinal movements.

The main objective of the motility of the small intestine is to **thoroughly mix the chyme** with the pancreatic, bile and intestinal juices so that proper digestion and absorption of the essential nutrients can take place. Intestinal motility also **propels chyme** into the colon.

FUNCTIONAL ASPECTS

The length of small intestine is about **three-fourths of the length** of the whole of the GI tract. It measures 285 cm.

1. It takes *2–4 hours* for the chyme to traverse the small intestine.
2. Small intestine consists of duodenum, jejunum, and ileum. Duodenum is the first part of the intestine and constitutes 5% of it. Jejunum constitutes 40% and ileum constitutes more than 55% of the small intestine. However, there is no definite demarcation between jejunum and ileum.
3. The wall of small intestine have all the layers of the gut (refer to Figs. 36.3 and 36.4, Chapter 36). However, the **muscularis externa** consisting of outer longitudinal and inner circular muscles **is well developed** in small intestine (Fig. 49.1). This helps in effective intestinal motility.
4. Though the **lymphatic nodules** are less in jejunum, they are more in number in ileum, and they extend into the submucosa (Fig. 49.2).

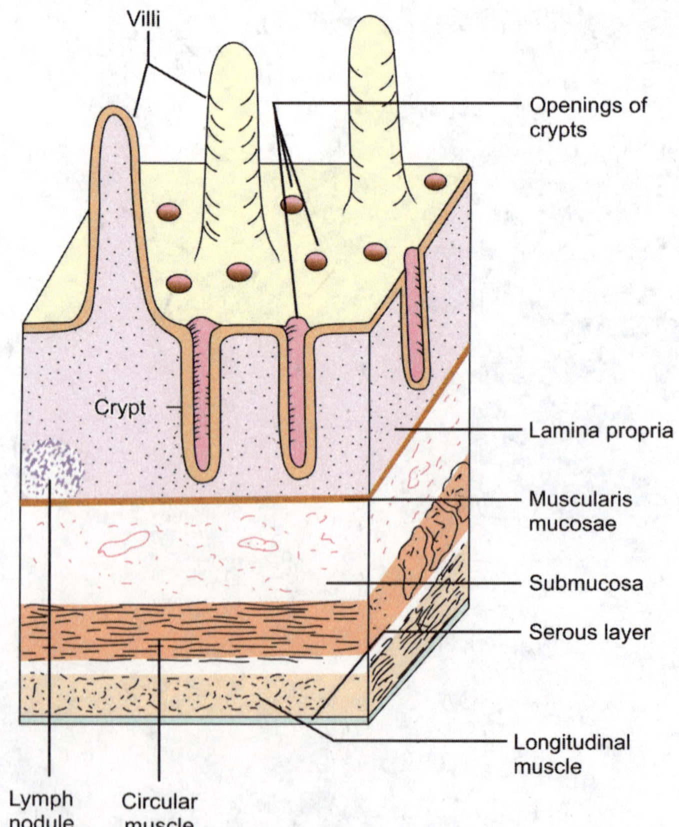

Fig. 49.1: Layers of the wall of small intestine. Note, muscle layer consisting of outer longitudinal and inner circular muscles is well developed.

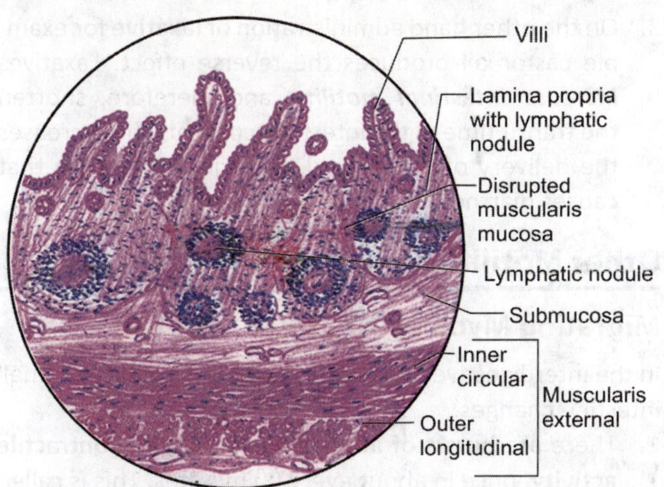

Fig. 49.2: Histology of the intestinal wall at the level of ileum. Note that the lymphatic nodules are plenty, and extend into the submucosa. The muscularis externa (outer longitudinal and inner circular muscles) is well developed.
Courtesy: Figure 13.25A, Basic Histology, by V Subhadra Devi, 1st edition, 2016; Jaypee Brothers Medical Publishers (P) Ltd.

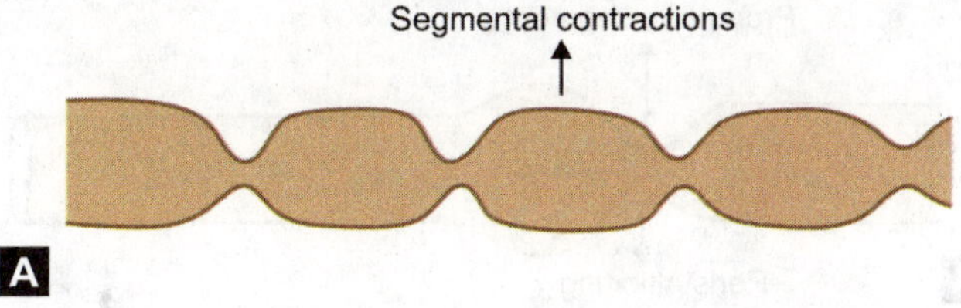

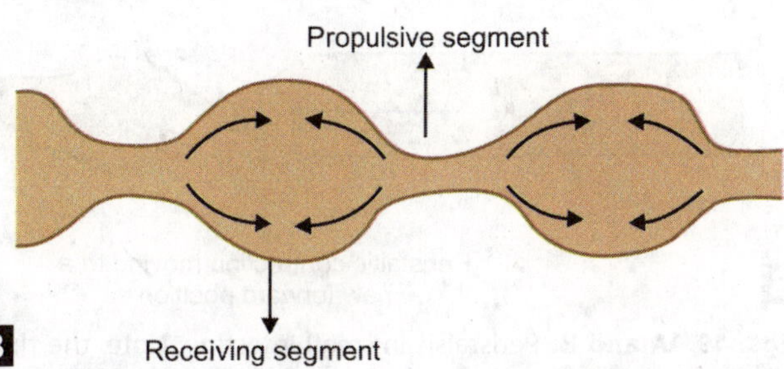

Figs. 49.3A and B: Segmentation movement of small intestine (A). Note the mechanism for mixing of food in segmental contractions (B), in a slightly enlarged view of intestine. The direction of arrows indicates the direction of movement of food particles. Note, in segmental contractions, food is grinded and thoroughly mixed between two propulsive segments.

Electrophysiology of Intestinal Smooth Muscles

The frequency of slow wave is maximum in small intestine that occurs regularly. The frequency is highest in duodenum (about 15 per minute) and decreases slowly toward ileum where it is about 8–10 per minute.

1. Slow waves are not always accompanied by bursts of action potential spikes. When slow wave is associated with spike, the contraction is stronger and in its absence (no spike), contraction is weaker or absent (refer to Fig. 45.5; Chapter 45).
2. A **characteristic feature** of slow waves of intestine is that they are *localized to a short segment of the intestine*. Therefore, contraction is also localized to the segments. This results in **segmentation type of movement** in the intestine.
3. The basic electrical rhythm is purely intrinsic.
4. The frequency of action potential spike, which determines the strength of muscle contraction, depends on **excitability of the smooth muscles**. The excitability in turn depends on autonomic innervation, activity of the enteric neurons and the circulating hormones.
5. **Parasympathetic stimulation enhances** and **sympathetic stimulation inhibits** intestinal contractility.

TYPES OF INTESTINAL MOVEMENTS

Intestinal movements carry out **three primary functions**:

1. **Mixing the chyme** with digestive secretions.
2. Bringing the chyme **in contact with the absorptive surface** of the microvilli to increase absorption.
3. **Propelling the chyme** toward colon.

These functions are achieved by various small intestinal motilities. The motilities are segmentation, peristalsis, migrating myoelectric complex, contraction of the muscularis mucosa, villus contractions, and movements due to intestinal reflexes.

Segmentation

This is the most common variety of movement of the small intestine.

1. It is characterized by **closely spaced contraction of the circular muscle layer**. These contractions divide the small intestine into many segments (Fig. 49.3A).
2. The **rate of segmental contraction is same as the frequency of slow waves**. It is about 18/min in duodenum, 15/min in jejunum, and 12/min in ileum.
3. Segmentation contractions effectively **mix chyme with pancreatic and intestinal secretions**.
4. Two nearby propulsive segments force the chyme toward each other into the receiving segment (Fig. 49.3B), which efficiently helps in mixing.
5. They also *bring the fresh chyme into the contact with the mucosal surface*.
6. Therefore, segmentation movements are also called **mixing movements**. They help in digestion and absorption of nutrients.

Peristalsis

Peristalsis is the progressive contraction of successive portions of circular smooth muscles of the small intestine.

1. The wave of contraction moves in ***orthograde direction,*** i.e. toward colon. In fact, peristaltic wave spreads in both directions. However, wave toward oral cavity (oral spread) dies out after a short distance, and wave

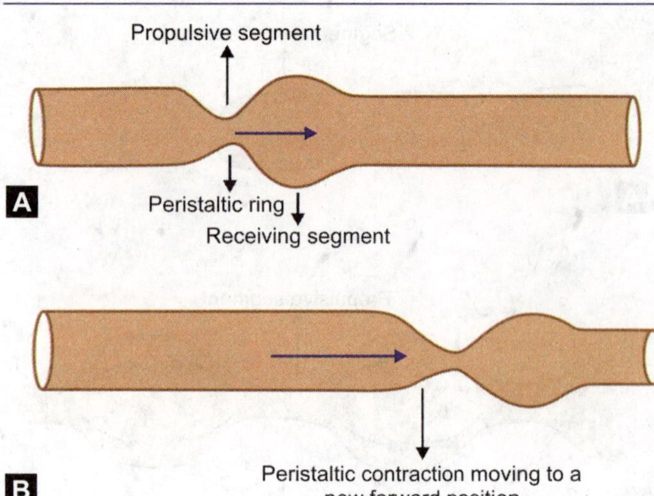

Figs. 49.4A and B: Peristalsis in small intestine. Note, the ring of peristaltic contraction moves from the initial position (A) to a new forward position (B). Thus, peristalsis moves aborally.

toward colon (**aboral spread**) continues progressively. This is called **law of the intestine**.

2. Peristaltic waves involve only a **short length of intestine**. When chyme enters the intestine, the bolus of the chyme stretches its wall. The part of the intestine behind the chyme contracts and the part of the intestine in front of the chyme relaxes and the ring of contraction proceeds in forward direction (Figs. 49.4A and B).
3. The *primary function of peristaltic movements is to propel chyme* in forward direction. Sometimes, the frequency of peristalsis increases to an extent that intestinal contents are emptied very fast (with a speed of 20 cm/s) into the colon. This is called **rush peristalsis**. This is typically seen in acute diarrhea.
4. There are also **antiperistaltic contractions** of intestine. Antiperistalsis results in vomiting.

Short Range Peristalsis

Short range peristalsis also occurs in the intestine, but less frequently.

1. Short range peristalsis along with segmentation contraction decreases the net rate of propulsion of chyme in forward direction.
2. This allows the chyme to stay more time in intestine to facilitate digestion and absorption.

Clinical Significance

1. Administration of **codeine** decreases the motility of the intestine, therefore *decreases the frequency of defecation*.
2. The decreased motility also prolongs the transit time for the intestinal contents so that more water and nutrients are reabsorbed. Therefore, this also *decreases the volume of stool*.
3. On the other hand administration of **laxative** for example castor oil produces the reverse effect. Laxatives ***increase intestinal motility***, and therefore, shorten the transit time of the intestinal content. This increases the delivery of chyme and water into the colon that causes diarrhea.

Other Motilities

Migrating Myoelectric Motor Complex

In the interdigestive phase, the pattern of motility of small intestine changes.

1. There are **bursts of intense electrical and contractile activity**, once in about every 90 minutes. This is called migrating motor complex or migrating myoelectric complex (MMC).
2. MMC **starts in the stomach** and is propagated throughout the intestine to the terminal part of the ileum. Once, a MMC reaches the distal end of the ileum, a next MMC begins in the stomach. Likewise, MMC is repeated every 75–90 minutes.
3. MMC results in **vigorous and strong propulsive contraction**; therefore, this sweeps the intestine and empties the remaining contents into the colon.
4. MMC cleans the entire lumen of the stomach and intestine, to keep the house ready for the next meal. This is why the MMC is known as **housekeeper of small intestine**.
5. MMC also ***inhibits the migration of colonic bacteria*** into the intestine.

Contraction of Muscularis Mucosa

The muscularis mucosa of small intestine contracts irregularly. These contractions alter the patterns of the mucosal folds.

1. Contractions occur at a frequency of about **3 per minute**.
2. Such contractions help in *mixing the luminal contents* and also in **bringing the fresh chyme in contact with mucosal surface.**

Villus Contraction

The villi of small intestine also contract irregularly. This is called villus contraction.

1. This is typically seen in upper part of the small intestine.
2. These contractions are especially meant for **emptying the central lacteals of the villi.**
3. They also increase intestinal lymph flow.

Intestinal Reflexes

There are two reflexes observed in the intestine: intestino-intestinal reflex and gastroileal reflex.

Intestinointestinal Reflex

When a part of the intestine is over-distended, the rest of the intestine relaxes. This is called intestinointestinal reflex. It is mediated by **local enteric neurons** and vagovagal pathways.

Gastroileal Reflex

When food enters the stomach (stretching of stomach), the **motility of the terminal part of the ileum is enhanced**. This increases entry of contents of ileum into the colon through ileocecal sphincter. This reflex is believed to be mediated **by vagus nerve**.

Law of the Intestine

When a bolus of chyme enters the intestine, the part of the intestine behind the bolus contracts and the portion of the intestine ahead of it relaxes. This helps in **propagation of ring of contraction in aboral direction**. This response is known as law of the intestine. This is meant to propel the intestinal content in the forward direction as occurs in peristalsis.

Function of the Ileocecal Sphincter

This is also known as ***ileocecal valve***. It separates terminal part of the ileum from the cecum.

1. Normally, the ileocecal sphincter is **tonically contracted**, and therefore the sphincter remains closed most of the time and prevents small intestinal emptying.
2. When a **peristaltic wave reaches the terminal part of the ileum**, the sphincter relaxes so that the ileal content enters the cecum.
3. **Distention of ileum** also causes *opening of ileocecal sphincter*. On the other hand, **distention of cecum** *causes closure of the ileocecal sphincter*.
4. Ileocecal sphincter is also controlled by *extrinsic nerve fibers*. For example relaxation of the sphincter occurs by vagal stimulation as seen in gastroileal reflex.

APPLIED PHYSIOLOGY

Adynamic Ileus

When the intestine is injured, excessively handled or mishandled, the smooth muscles of the intestine are inhibited. This decreases the intestinal motility, sometimes even resulting in paralysis of the gut. This is called adynamic ileus or **paralytic ileus**.

1. This usually occurs ***following abdominal surgery***. Following such procedures, GI tract remains paralyzed for about 6 hours to few days. Peristalsis first starts in the small intestine (6–8 hours later) followed by in the stomach (8–12 hours) and finally in the colon (2–3 days).
2. Adynamic ileus is also observed in *peritonitis*.
3. This occurs due to increased discharge of non-adrenergic fibers in the splanchnic nerves.

Intestinal Colic

Severe abdominal cramps are experienced in **localized obstruction** of small intestine.

1. The segment proximal to the obstruction dilates and gets filled with fluid and gas. This increases the pressure inside the lumen that causes compression of blood vessels in the intestinal wall. Resulting **local ischemia** of the intestinal wall produces severe cramping pain.
2. Abdominal cramps are also experienced in other diseases that result in distention of the intestine.

CHAPTER SUMMARY

Key Concepts

1. The primary function of small intestine is to adequately mix the chyme with intestinal and pancreatic juice. This is archived by Segmentation. Therefore, segmentation is called mixing movement.
2. The other important function of intestine is to push the chyme into the colon. This is achieved by peristalsis. Therefore, peristalsis is called propulsive movement.
3. The peristaltic movements move in aboral (away from oral cavity) direction. This is called the law of the gut.

Important to Know (Must Read)

1. In examinations, "Describe the mechanism and significance of intestinal motitlites" may come as a **Long Question**.
2. Segmentation, Peristalsis, MMC, Villous contraction, Intestinal reflexes, Gastroileal reflex, Law of the gut, may come as **Short Questions**.
3. In **Viva**, examiner may ask... What are the special electrophysiological properties of intestinal, Name the types of intestinal movements, What is segmentation and peristalsis and what are their functions, What is MMC, What is Villous contraction, Name the intestinal reflexes and what are their functions, What is law of the gut, What is inflammatory bowel disease.

CHAPTER 50

Motility of Large Intestine

Learning Objectives

On completion of study of this chapter, the student **MUST** be able to:

1. Understand the physiology of colonic movements, colonic reflexes, and their functions.
2. Understand the mechanism and pathway of defecation reflex.
3. Learn the physiological basis of Hirschsprung, disease, irritable bowel syndrome, diarrhea, and constipation.

The student **MAY** also be able to:

1. Describe the mechanism and significance of colonic movements.
2. Explain the physiological basis of colonic dysfunctions.

Large intestine consists of cecum, colon, rectum, and anal canal. **Colon constitutes about 90% of large intestine** and consists of **ascending, transverse, descending, and sigmoid colons**. Anatomically, cecum is considered as part of the ascending colon (refer to Fig. 44.1; Chapter 44).

1. Small intestine receives chyme of meals sequentially with no mixing of individual meals, whereas **large intestine contains mixture of chymes of many meals of one to three days.**
2. On average the total **transit time of chyme** of a meal through large intestine as recorded from passage of radiopaque markers is about **30 to 48 hours.**

The **transit time** of chyme through different parts of gut is as follows:

1. In small intestine: 4 hours
2. In ascending colon: 6 hours
3. In transverse colon: 8 hours
4. In descending and pelvic colons: 12 hours
5. From pelvic colon to rectum, the transit is very slow, which may take 2 to 3 days.

However, transit time depends on the fiber content of diet. Transit time is less in high fiber diet, sometimes may even be reduced to 6 hours through the entire gut.

MOTILITY OF COLON

The **major functions of colon** are storage of chyme that arrives from small intestine, and absorption of salt and water from the chyme. Therefore, though colon **receives about 2 liters of chyme per day** from small intestine, its **output is only about 200 mL.**

1. The **objectives** of colonic contractions are to **mix the chyme** and circulate it across the mucosal surface of the colon so that ***maximum contact occurs between the chyme and the mucosal epithelium***.
2. This, plus the slow movement of the chyme across the colon, which is about 5–10 cm/hour allows **maximum absorption of salt and water.**

Physiological Anatomy

Structure of the wall of large gut resembles the general structure of the GI tract. However, the **special features** are:

1. Longitudinal muscle layer of muscularis externa is concentrated into **three bands**, called as **tenia coli**. These bands are shorter than rest of the colon. Therefore, the wall of the colon forms **haustra** (outpouchings).
2. There are **no villi** on the mucosa. There are many goblet cells.
3. The colonic glands are small inward projections of the mucosa. They secrete mucus.
4. The **circular muscles usually do not exhibit action potentials.**
5. outer longitudinal muscle layer is specialized into tenia coli (Fig. 50.1).

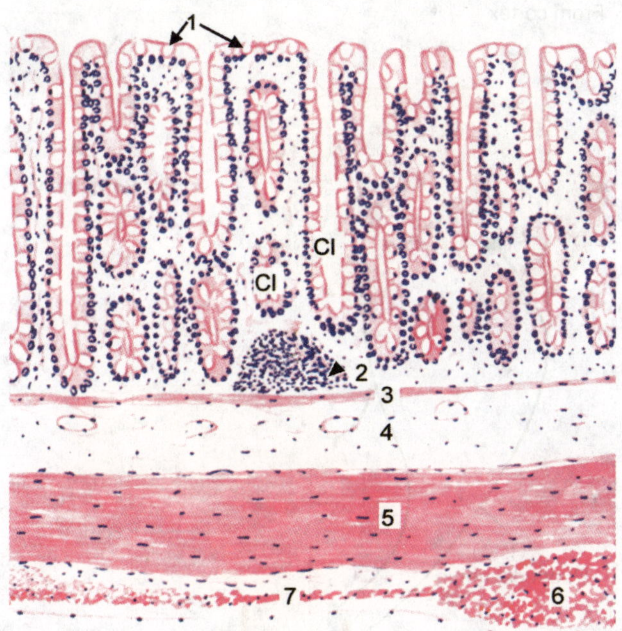

Fig. 50.1: Layers of the wall of large intestine. Note, absence of villi, many goblet cells in the mucosal epithelium, outer longitudinal muscle layer is specialized into tenia coli. 1: Columnar epithelial lining with goblet cells; 2: Lamina propria; 3: Muscularis mucosa; 4: Submucosa; 5: Muscle coat; 6: Tenia coli; 7: Longitudinal muscle laerr. (Cl: Crypts of Lieberkuhn).

Innervation of Large Intestine

1. **Parasympathetic innervation** to cecum, ascending, transverse and most part of descending colon comes via **vagus nerve**, whereas innervation to the sigmoid colon, rectum, and anal canal comes via **pelvic nerves** that arise from the sacral spinal cord.
2. **Sympathetic fibers** to large gut come via superior and inferior mesenteric plexuses, and superior and inferior hypogastric plexuses.
3. Parasympathetic stimulation increases and sympathetic stimulation decreases colonic movements.

Electrophysiology of Colonic Muscle

Colon consists of both circular and longitudinal muscle.

Circular Muscle

There are two types of pace making (rhythm generating) cells in the colon. They are made up of **interstitial cells**.

1. The one set of cells that are present near the inner border of circular muscles produce **regular slow waves of high amplitude** like that of gastric slow waves.
2. The second set of interstitial cell is present near outer border of the circular muscle that produces ***waves with low amplitude and high frequency*** oscillations called **myenteric potential oscillations** (MPO).
3. Circular muscles **do not fire action potentials**.

Longitudinal Muscle

These muscles also exhibit myenteric potential oscillations MPO. However, longitudinal muscles ***sometimes fire action potentials*** at the peak of MPO that elicit contractions of the large intestine.

Colonic Movements

Colonic movements include haustral contractions, propulsive movements, mass peristalsis, and colonic reflexes.

Haustral Contractions

These are contractions *similar to that of segmentation*. Haustra become more prominent in these contractions. Therefore, they are called haustral contractions. They help in **mixing and circulation of chyme** within the large intestine.

Propulsive Movements

These are peristaltic movements that **propel colonic contents toward the rectum.** The mechanism of colonic peristalsis is same as intestinal peristalsis.

Mass Peristalsis

Mass colonic peristalsis is a **stronger peristaltic contraction** that forcefully pushes the contents from colon into the rectum. Activation of mass peristalsis in colon finally leads to the **initiation of defecation reflex**. It also **cleans** the large intestine. It occurs **3 to 4 times a day**, and is initiated ***usually after a meal***. Mass peristalsis is not affected after colostomy (Clinical Box 50.1).

Colonic Reflexes

Colonic reflexes include colonocolonic reflex and gastrocolic reflex.

Colonocolonic Reflex

Colonocolonic reflex is the relaxation of the entire colon in response to distention of one part of the colon. This is partly mediated by sympathetic fibers.

Gastrocolic Reflex

Gastrocolic reflex is initiated when food accumulates in the stomach.

1. Distention of the stomach causes **motility of proximal and distal colon**.
2. This pushes colonic content into the rectum, which **stimulates the desire for defecation**. Therefore, usually after taking a large meal, the urge for defecation is enhanced.
3. This reflex is more developed in children.
4. Gastrocolic reflex is proposed to be **mediated by gastrin** secreted from stomach in response to gastric distension, and not by neural factors.

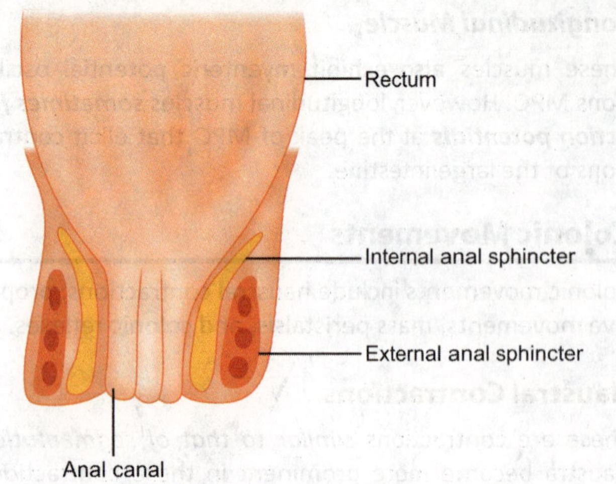

Fig. 50.2: Structure and position of external and internal anal sphincters.

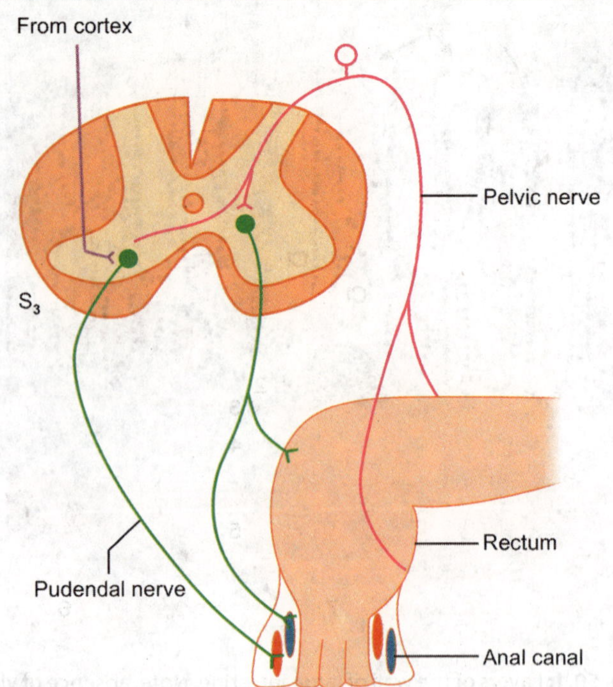

Fig. 50.3: Mechanism of defecation reflex.

Clinical Box 50.1

Colostomy: When a large part of colon is removed (*colectomy*), the terminal part of ileum or proximal part of colon is brought to the anterior abdominal wall through an opening. This is called ileostomy or colostomy. The chyme that comes out from the gut is collected in a *colostomy bag* fastened around the colostomy opening. Usually, colectomy or hemicolectomy is performed for cancer of colon. This procedure per se does not affect the health of the individual if water and electrolyte balance are maintained.

MOTILITY OF RECTUM AND ANAL CANAL

Normally, rectum remains empty. **Mass colonic peristalsis** pushes contents in the colon into the rectum.

1. Anal canal **always remains closed** by the tonic contractions of internal and external anal sphincters. The **internal anal sphincter** is made up of thickening of circular smooth muscle of the anal canal.
2. The **external anal sphincter** consists of *striated muscle* (Fig. 50.2). Thus, external sphincter is innervated by somatic motor fibers via pudendal nerves, which brings it under voluntary control.

Before initiation of the defecation reflex, colonic peristalsis pushes colonic contents into the rectum. This causes filling and distension of the rectum that initiates relaxation of internal anal sphincter and constriction of external anal sphincter.

- **With initiation of defecation reflex**, the external sphincter opens and the person defecates.
- However, the reflex relaxation of the internal sphincter in response to rectal distention is a temporary phenomenon.
- If **defecation is delayed**, the internal sphincter regains its normal tone and the ***reflex is inhibited***.

Defecation

This is a **reflex phenomenon with a voluntary control**. Thus, it has both **reflexive (automatic) and voluntary components**. The center for defecation is present in **the sacral portion of the spinal cord**, which is influenced by higher centers. The efferent pathway involves cholinergic parasympathetic fibers in the pelvic nerves.

Stimulus

Defecation reflex is initiated when **mass peristaltic movement** of the descending and sigmoid colons pushes the colonic content into the rectum (filling of the rectum).

1. As the external anal sphincter is innervated by somatic nerves, the **voluntary effort is also important** in initiating defecation.
2. However, normally defecation is inhibited by the **acute anorectal angle**, which is about 90°, and **contraction of external sphincter and puborectalis muscle.**

Pathway

1. **Receptors** for defecation reflex are stretch receptors located in the wall of rectal rectum.
2. **Afferent information** from the wall of rectum is conveyed to **sacral segment (S_3) of spinal cord** via pelvic nerve.
3. **Efferent input** from spinal cord to rectum and internal anal sphincter comes via **pelvic nerve** and to external anal sphincter via **somatic nerve** (Fig. 50.3).
4. **Higher center**, especially cortex influences spinal cord center via corticospinal pathway.
5. Relaxation of internal anal sphincter is due to inhibitory signals that originate in myenteric plexus in response to peristaltic wave approaching anus. This allows the fecal matter to press onto the anal canal.

Mechanism

The individual sits on toilet and strains. This **increases intra-abdominal pressure**, which forcefully expels the rectal contents through the anal canal. This is assisted by **relaxation of external anal sphincter**, **decreased anorectal angle** and **relaxation of puborectalis muscle**.

1. Evacuation of bladder is preceded by a **deep breathing that pushes the diaphragm downward**.
2. Contraction of respiratory muscles *increases intrathoracic and intra-abdominal pressures*.
3. Contraction of abdominal wall muscle further increases abdominal pressure.
4. When all these mechanisms elevate the intra-abdominal **pressure to about 200 cm of H_2O**, the feces is forced out through the external anal sphincter.

Applied Aspect

Defecation reflex is a **spinal reflex**. Therefore, following spinal transection, *defecation is never complete*. However, evacuation of bowel and bladder can be achieved by **activating mass reflex** in paraplegic patients.

Feces

Stool is a semisolid mass of about 200–250 mL excreted form large gut per day. It contains inorganic material, undigested fibers, bacteria, and water. Water constitutes 75% and solids 25% of the total volume. The undigested fibers include cellulose and other fibers. Bacteria and inorganic materials constitute 30% and 15% of the total solids respectively. The composition of feces is relatively not affected by diet as a large fraction of it comes from non-dietary origin. Even in fasting, a good amount of feces is passed. The **color of the stool is due to the presence of bile pigments**. The **smell of feces is due to presence of indole and skatole**, the amines that are produced by colonic bacterial flora.

Applied Physiology

Hirschsprung's Disease

Cause

This is also known as **congenital megacolon** or **aganglionosis**. In this condition, the *entire neuronal plexuses in the wall of the colon are congenitally absent*.

1. The enteric neurons are usually markedly absent in the anus and distal part of the rectum.
2. Failure of migration of neural crest from cranial to caudal region results in *absence of ganglion in both myenteric and submucosal plexuses in distal part of colon and rectum*.
3. This prevents relaxation of rectal outlet and internal anal sphincter in response to rectal filling. Thus, obstruction occurs to the outflow of feces and feces accumulate behind the obstruction.
4. Consequently, **distention of the colon** ensues.

Features

Clinically, it manifests as **abdominal distention**, anorexia and lassitude. In severe cases, symptoms appear in newborns as early as third day after birth.

Treatment

Usually, it is treated by **surgical dilation**.

Diarrhea

Diarrhea occurs in many conditions.

1. Physiologically it may be due to either **increased secretion** as occurs in cholera or **increased GI motility**.
2. In any case, acute diarrhea results in dehydration and hypovolemia.
3. **Oral rehydration therapy** is the immediate treatment to prevent volume and electrolyte loss. **Oral rehydration solution** (ORS) contains salt, electrolytes, and glucose. ORS contains both Na^+ and glucose so that Na^+ is absorbed via SGLT 1 (Na^+-glucose cotransporter). Glucose facilitates Na^+ transport.

Constipation

Constipation occurs due to many causes. However, the physiological basis is the **decreased intestinal motility** that causes stasis of chyme in the large intestine, which facilitates water absorption and dehydration of intestinal contents. The chyme hardens and feces become more solid. Usually it is treated by distending rectum by inert material.

Irritable Bowel Syndrome

This condition has been known by several synonyms such as **mucous colitis, spastic colon, irritable colon, and colonic neurosis**. In the West 20–30% of gastrointestinal disorders are constituted by IBS. In India this is very common and many cases used to be misdiagnosed as chronic amebiasis in the past.

1. IBS is a **functional disorder** of the intestine characterized by alteration of the bowel habits and abdominal pain in the absence of any detectable organic pathology.
2. There is **no morphologic, histologic, microbiologic, or biochemical abnormalities** in IBS. Changes in gut motility are observed in several studies though they poorly correlate with the symptoms.
3. In the **constipated variety** the frequency of high altitude peristaltic contraction is less whereas nonpropulsive segmentation contractions are more.
4. Moreover **food induced hypermotility** of the colon occurring normally about one hour after the meal is reduced in many patients. This may account for their **postprandial symptoms**.
5. Emotional stress is seen to aggravate the motility disorder.

Electrical Abnormalities

Normally gut has two types of myoelectrical activity, the basal electric rhythm (BER) and spike activity (SA). The BER is in the continuous wave form at the rate of 6 cycles per minute. The SA is in the form of electrical bursts superimposed on BER and this is responsible for the mechanical contraction of the gut.

1. BS patients have a slow BER at the rate of 3 cycles per minute.
2. In normal people, feeding induces SA immediately which peaks in 30 minutes and lasts for about 50 minutes. But in the IBS patients the feeding induced SA is dampened in the first 50 minutes, but it becomes stronger later on.

Clinical Features

In India the female to male ratio is 1:3, though in the West, female suffer more. The clinical spectrum is wide. The presentations include

i. Painless functional diarrhea
ii. Painless simple constipation
iii. Alternating diarrhea and constipation
iv. Bloating of abdomen
v. Pain due to spasm of colon and small intestine.

The common age group is **20–40 years.** Symptoms are vague and these include **abnormal bowel habits** ranging from constipation to diarrhea (often alternating irregularly), pallet like stools, increased gastrocolic reflex, vague abdominal pain ranging from dull ache to severe colic, flatulence relieved by belching, capricious appetite and insomnia. Around 20% of subjects complain of weight loss. All **patients are emotionally tense** and they tend to exaggerate the disability.

Inflammatory Bowel Disease (Crohn's Disease and Ulcerative Colitis)

The term "inflammatory bowel disease (IBD)" is commonly used to include 2 idiopathic bowel diseases having many similarities but the conditions usually have distinctive morphological appearances.

These 2 conditions are: Crohn's disease (regional enteritis) and ulcerative colitis.

1. **Crohn's disease or regional enteritis** is an idiopathic chronic ulcerative IBD, characterized by transmural, non-caseating granulomatous inflammation, affecting most commonly the segment of terminal ileum and/or colon, though any part of the gastrointestinal tract may be involved.
2. **Ulcerative colitis** is an idiopathic form of acute and chronic ulcero-inflammatory colitis affecting chiefly the mucosa and submucosa of the rectum and descending colon, though sometimes it may involve the entire length of the large bowel.

Both these disorders primarily affect the bowel but may have **systemic involvement** in the form of polyarthritis, uveitis, ankylosing spondylitis, **skin lesions,** and **hepatic involvement**. Both diseases can occur at any age but are more frequent in **2nd and 3rd decades** of life. **Females are affected more** than males.

CHAPTER SUMMARY

Key Concepts

1. The primary function of large intestine is to reabsorb water and electrolytes from chyme and from fecal matters. The mass peristalsis pushes feces into the rectum and initiates defecation reflex.
2. External anal sphincter is made up of striated muscle, and therefore defecation reflex can be voluntarily controlled.
3. Defecation reflex is a spinal reflex, which can be taught to spinal man to self-initiate the process.

Important to Know (Must Read)

1. In examinations, **Long Question** is not asked from this chapter.
2. Colonic movements, Mass peristalsis, Colonic reflexes, Gastrocolic reflex, Defecation reflex, may come as **Short Questions**.
3. In **Viva**, examiner may ask... What are the special electrophysiological properties of colonic muscles, Name the types of colonic movements, What is mass peristalsis & what is its significance, Name colonic reflexes, What is gastrocolic reflex & what is its significance, Details of defecation reflex, What is inflammatory bowel disease and irritable bowel syndrome, What is Hirschsprung's disease.

CHAPTER

51

Principles of Digestion and Absorption

Learning Objectives

On completion of study of this chapter, the student **MUST** be able to:

1. Understand the principle of digestion and absorption of carbohydrate, protein, fat, and other nutrients from GIT.
2. Appreciate the physiological basis of common malabsorption syndromes.
3. Learn the importance of digestion and absorption of various nutrients.

The student **MAY** also be able to:

1. Describe the mechanism of digestion and absorption of each category of nutrient.
2. Explain the physiological basis of problems in malabsorption syndrome.

PHYSIOLOGICAL ASPECTS

Digestion is the process by which foodstuff are broken down into smaller particles that can be absorbed from the GIT. **Absorption** is the process by which the products of digestion, vitamins, minerals, and water are transported from the lumen of the GI tract into the blood and the lymph draining the GI tract.

Digestion is a complex process involving breaking down of foodstuffs by many enzymes into their absorbable form. Though the major part of digestion takes place in the small intestine, digestion starts as soon as food enters the mouth. The mucosal epithelial cells of the small intestine are called enterocytes. Enterocytes have brush border, which is rich in digestive enzymes. The nutrients first pass from lumen of GI tract to the interstitial fluid and then from there into the blood or lymph.

Scientist contributed

Herman Boerhaave (1668–1738) was a Dutch botanist, physician and physiologist of European fame. He is regarded as the ***founder of clinical teaching*** and is sometimes referred to as "the father of ancient physiology", along with his pupil **Albrecht von Haller**. He is best known for demonstrating the relation of symptoms to lesions and, in addition, he was the first to isolate the chemical urea from urine. He had emphasized the **role chemical factors** in functional activity, especially in **digestive process**.

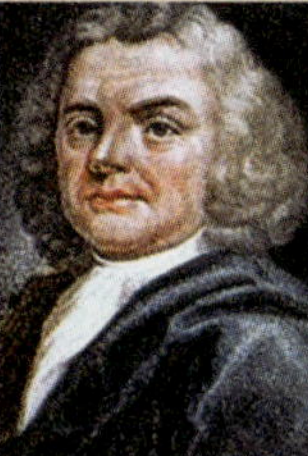

H Boerhaave
(1668–1738)

Digestion and Absorption of Carbohydrates

Digestion of Carbohydrate

The dietary carbohydrates are mainly polysaccharides, disaccharides, and monosaccharides. Starch is the polysaccharide that is usually digested in human GI tract.

1. Digestion of carbohydrate begins in the mouth by the action of **salivary amylase** which catalyses the hydrolysis of α-1, 4 linkage (but not α-1, 6 linkage) to form α-dextrins.
2. The **pancreatic amylase** also does the same function. The products of amylase digestion are maltose, maltotriose and α-dextrins.
3. The further digestion of starch is carried out by **oligosaccharidases** that are present in the ***brush border of the intestine***. These membrane enzymes are α-**dextrinase** that causes hydrolysis of α-1,6 linkage, **maltase** that causes hydrolysis of maltotriose and maltose, **lactase** that causes hydrolysis of lactose into glucose and galactose, **glucoamylase** that splits malto-oligosachharides into single glucose molecules and **sucrase** that causes hydrolysis of sucrose into fructose and glucose.
4. The end product of these membrane digestions are glucose, galactose, and fructose (monosaccharides).

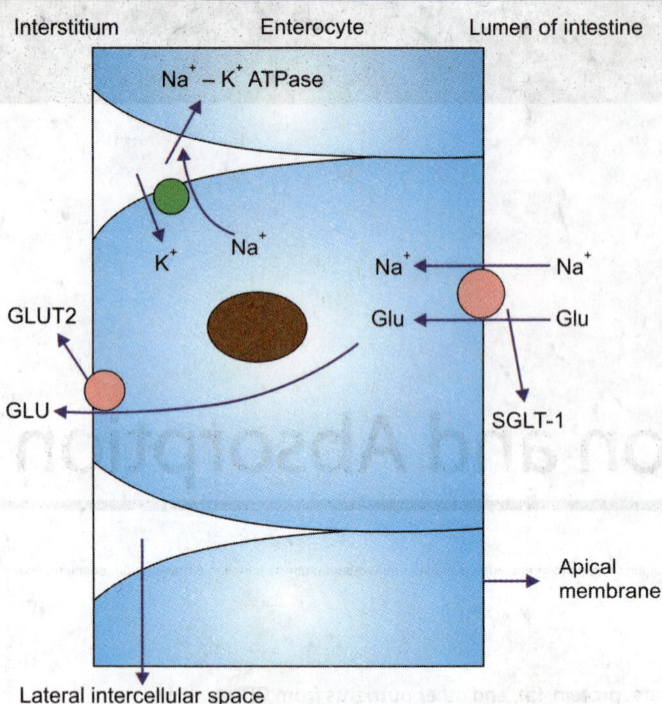

Fig. 51.1: Mechanism of glucose (GLU) absorption in intestine.

Oligosaccharidases activity is maximum in duodenum and upper jejunum and minimum toward the terminal part of ileum.

Absorption of Carbohydrates

The carbohydrate absorption is maximum in duodenum and jejunum, which progressively decreases toward the terminal part of ileum. The easily absorbable forms of carbohydrate are monosaccharides that are glucose, galactose, and fructose.

1. They are first transported from the lumen into the epithelial cells. The apical membrane of epithelial cells contains SGLT (**sodium dependent glucose transporter**).
2. The transport is greatly influenced by the concentration of Na^+ in the intestinal lumen. The higher the concentration of Na^+, the greater the degree of glucose absorption. This is because both ***glucose and Na^+ share the same transport protein***, the **SGLT**. The SGLT that transports glucose and Na^+ is SGLT 1.
3. The concentration of Na^+ is less in the enterocytes, which is **created by Na^+-K^+ pump** present on the basolateral membrane of the cells that pumps Na^+ into the lateral intercellular space from the enterocytes in exchange for K^+. Therefore, Na^+ moves into the cells along the concentration gradient (Fig. 51.1). Glucose enters along with Na^+ using the same co-transporter (SGLT 1).
4. From the cell, glucose is transported by GLUT 2 (**glucose transporter**) into the interstitium (ECF). From the ECF glucose enters the blood.
5. As the glucose transport depends on Na^+-K^+ pump present on the basolateral membrane that creates gradient for Na^+, this mechanism of glucose transport is a **secondary active transport**.
6. **Galactose uses the same carrier protein** (SGLT 1) for absorption.
7. The entry of **fructose** into the enterocytes is facilitated by GLUT 5, which is present only in the brush border of matured enterocytes.

Applied Aspects

Carbohydrate Malabsorption Syndromes

Carbohydrate malabsorption occurs due to *deficiency of oligosaccharidases*, the membrane enzymes of enterocytes.

Lactose Intolerance

This occurs due to *deficiency of lactase* in the brush border of enterocytes. Therefore, lactose is not digested and absorbed from the intestinal lumen. The lactose enters the colon where it is utilized by colonic bacteria that produce gas, and different metabolites. The metabolites increase colonic motility and diarrhea. Excess gas production results in borborygmi (gurgling sounds in the intestine) and abdominal distention.

Sucrase-Isomaltase Deficiency

Deficiency of sucrase and isomaltase in the brush border of enterocytes is an autosomal recessive disease. It is present in 10% of Eskimos (in Greenland) and few North Americans. Ingestion of fructose in this condition results in diarrhea and flatulence.

Glucose-Galactose Malabsorption Syndrome

This is a rare hereditary disorder due to *deficiency of SGLT 1* in the brush border of enterocytes. In this condition, ingestion of glucose or galactose or starch produces diarrhea and flatulence. Fructose is well tolerated.

Oral Sugar Tolerance Test

In carbohydrate malabsorption diseases oral sugar tolerance test is performed to diagnose the disease. An oral dose of sugar (in question) is given to the patient following which the concentration of the sugar in patients, blood and stool is monitored. If the patient is intolerant to the sugar, the ingestion of sugar causes diarrhea and flatulence, the concentration of sugar in stool increases, but characteristically the sugar concentration fails to increase in the blood.

Digestion and Absorption of Proteins

The quality and quantity of dietary protein depend on the socioeconomic status and food habit of the individual. Ten to thirty gram of protein is added to the intestinal content from the GI secretions and the ex-foliated intestinal cells. Normally, all ingested protein is digested and absorbed. However, excess protein intake causes excretion of protein in the stool.

Digestion of Proteins

Digestion of protein starts in the stomach.

1. **Pepsinogen secreted from chief cells** is converted to pepsin by the action of HCl. Pepsin hydrolyzes proteins into peptides and amino acids.
2. **In the duodenum and small intestine**, the proteins are digested by proteases secreted in the pancreatic secretion. The proteases are trypsin, chymotrypsin, carboxypeptidases and elastase.
3. The **enterokinase** secreted from mucosal cells of duodenum and jejunum converts trypsinogen into trypsin, which then acts as an enzyme to convert other proteases.
4. **Peptidases** are also present in the brush border of enterocytes. These enzymes hydrolyze the peptides produced by pancreatic proteases into oligopeptides and amino acids. The **brush border peptidases** are amino peptidases, and dipeptidases.
5. The **products of protein digestion** are small peptides and amino acids.

Absorption of Proteins

There are many **transport systems** (at least **seven such systems** are known) for absorption of amino acids and peptides. The five protein transport systems **require Na^+** like that of Na^+-glucose co-transporter. The other two transporters **use Cl^-** (***independent of Na^+***). Absorption of amino acid is greater in the duodenum and jejunum and slower in ileum.

Defects of Protein Digestion

Hartnup Disease

This is a hereditary disorder in which **absorption of amino acids** in the intestinal and renal epithelial cells is defective. The neutral amino acids appear in the stool and urine.

Cystinuria

This is a congenital disease in which the amino acid cystine appears in the urine. The **defect is in the protein transporter** in the mucosal cells of intestine and epithelial cells of PCT of kidney.

Prolinuria

This is a rare disorder in which proline is not reabsorbed from intestine and kidney. This causes prolinuria and hydroxyprolinuria.

Digestion and Absorption of Lipids

Digestion

Digestion of lipid starts in the mouth.

1. In oral cavity **lingual lipase** is secreted from Ebner's glands in the tongue.
2. **Gastric lipase** also helps in digestion of fat. However, deficiency of lingual and gastric lipase does not result in malabsorption of fat as pancreatic lipase is actually important for lipid digestion.
3. Principal fat digestion starts in the duodenum by the **pancreatic lipase**, which hydrolyses 1 and 3 bonds of triglycerides that results in formation of free fatty acid and 2-monoglycerides (2-monoglycerols). Pancreatic lipase acts on lipids that **have been emulsified** (emulsification by bile acids).
4. Fat digestion is facilitated by *pancreatic co-lipase*.
5. There is another lipase secreted from pancreas called as **bile salt activated lipase**, which also assists in lipid digestion.
6. The dietary cholesterol is hydrolyzed by **cholesteryl ester hydrolase**.

Absorption

Lipids are absorbed by passive diffusion and carrier mediated transport. As soon as lipids enter the cell they are esterified, therefore a gradient is maintained for their entry into the cell.

1. For their absorption, fats are **emulsified in the intestine** by detergent action of bile salts, lecithin, and monoglycerides. With the help of bile salt, lipids form micelles.
2. **Micelles** are cylindrical aggregates of lipids like fatty acids, monoglycerides, and cholesterol with their hydrophobic ends at the center.
3. Micelle solubilizes the lipids and provides a medium for their transport to the intestinal epithelial cells. Thus, micelles help in transport of lipids to the enterocytes, where they disintegrate into the individual lipids and passively diffuse into the cells.

Short chain fatty acids are produced in the colon by the colonic bacteria and absorbed there. About 60% of short chain fatty acid is acetate, 25% propionate, and 15% butyrate. Short chain fatty acids are absorbed in exchange for H^+, therefore help in acid base balance. They also promote the absorption of Na^+.

Cholesterol is easily absorbed from the intestine in the presence of bile, fatty acid and pancreatic juice. The absorbed cholesterol is incorporated into the chylomicrons that enter circulation via lymphatics.

The **vitamins A, D, E, and K** are fat soluble vitamins. Their absorption is facilitated by presence of bile acids and products of lipid digestion in the intestine. Therefore, in the absence of bile acids or malabsorption of fat, deficiency of these vitamins occurs.

Disorders of Fat Digestion

Steatorrhea

This is a condition in which there is passage of **fatty, bulky, and clay colored stool**.

1. This occurs due to **deficiency of exocrine pancreas.** *Pancreatic lipase deficiency* results in impairment of fat digestion.
2. This is also sometimes seen in patients with **excess secretion of gastric acid** in which decreased duodenal pH ***inhibits pancreatic lipase***. Acid also **precipitates bile salt.**
3. Another cause of steatorrhea is **impaired reabsorption of bile salts in the distal ileum.**
4. Steatorrhea can also occur due to **intestinal diseases.**

Tropical Sprue

In this condition, the **enterocytes are distorted** and the **density of microvilli is decreased**. This causes lipid malabsorption probably due to decreased surface area for absorption of lipids.

Absorption of Water and Electrolytes

Absorption of Water

Normally, about 1–2 liters of water is ingested per day and 7 liters is added from GI secretions. However, only about 100 mL of water is excreted in the stool. Thus, GI tract absorbs more than 99.5% of water load presented to it per day.

1. Water is not absorbed from mouth, esophagus, and stomach.
2. Due to hyperosmolality of duodenal contents, **water is secreted from blood into duodenum.** As most of the nutrients are absorbed mainly in the duodenum and jejunum, the **osmolality of intestinal content** which is about 600 mosm/kg H_2O, decreases to about 200 mosm/kg H_2O in the ileum and colon.
3. Water is absorbed from intestinal lumen into blood as osmolality of blood is about 290 mosm/kg H_2O. Thus, **water is mainly absorbed in the small intestine and colon.**
4. The absorption of water depends on the absorption of electrolytes, especially that of Na^+ and Cl^-.
5. In the colon, part of water absorption occurs against an osmotic pressure gradient, the mechanism is known as ***standing gradient osmosis***.

Absorption of Sodium

Sodium is absorbed along the entire length of the intestine. Sodium absorption is mainly a **secondary active transport** in which, Na^+–K^+ ATPase on the basolateral surface pumps sodium out of the enterocytes, which creates low concentration of sodium in the cell. Therefore, **sodium enters the enterocytes by facilitated diffusion** and via SGLT.

Physiological Importance

The sodium and glucose reabsorption are facilitatory to each other. This physiological process is utilized in **oral rehydration therapy** (ORT). ORT is commonly prescribed for condition of acute dehydration. ORT includes solution containing sugar (glucose), salt (sodium chloride), and lime juice (Application Box 51.1).

Application Box 51.1

Sodium and glucose facilitate absorption of each other in ORT: The glucose in ORT helps in absorption of sodium and sodium helps in the absorption of glucose. Thus, glucose and sodium content in ORT facilitate each others absorption in the intestine.

Absorption of Other Nutrients

Absorption of Potassium

The average intake of K^+ per day is 4 g. K^+ is absorbed mainly passively in the intestine (jejunum and ileum).

1. In small intestine, as water is reabsorbed, the concentration of K^+ increases in the lumen. This causes **diffusion of potassium** across the concentration gradient.
2. The mechanism for **active transport of K^+ is absent in the intestine.**
3. In the **large intestine**, potassium is both secreted and reabsorbed. Hypokalemia produces cardiac abnormalities (Clinical Box 51.1)

Clinical Box 51.1

Prolonged diarrhea can cause cardiac arrhythmias: As the K^+ absorption is dependent on water absorption, significant K^+ loss occurs in diarrhea. Therefore, prolonged diarrhea, especially in infants and children makes them susceptible to hypokalemia (low plasma K^+), which may be life threatening. Hypokalemia can cause cardiac complications such as arrhythmias, and muscular dysfunctions.

Absorption of Cl^- and HCO_3^-

HCO_3^- is secreted mainly in pancreatic juice into duodenum. Cl^- is secreted in gastric, pancreatic and intestinal juices.

1. Cl^- and HCO_3^- are **reabsorbed mainly in the jejunum.**
2. In ileum, HCO_3^- is secreted and Cl^- is absorbed.
3. In colon, Cl^- absorption occurs through special Cl^- channels in the enterocytes.

Physiological Significance

1. In acute diarrhea like **cholera** (secretory diarrhea), Cl^-, Na^+ and water are secreted into the lumen. The cholera toxin produced by *Vibrio cholerae* activates adenylate cyclase, therefore increases cAMP concentration in the mucosal cells. The cAMP in turn activates Cl^- channels and Cl^- is actively secreted into the lumen. This facilitates the secretion of Na^+ and water resulting in profuse watery diarrhea (Clinical Box 51.2).
2. In cystic fibrosis, an autosomal disorder, the defective gene for Cl^- channel causes reduction in these channels in the mucosal cells of intestinal epithelium. Therefore, such patients suffer from less severe secretory diarrheas as compared to normal individual.

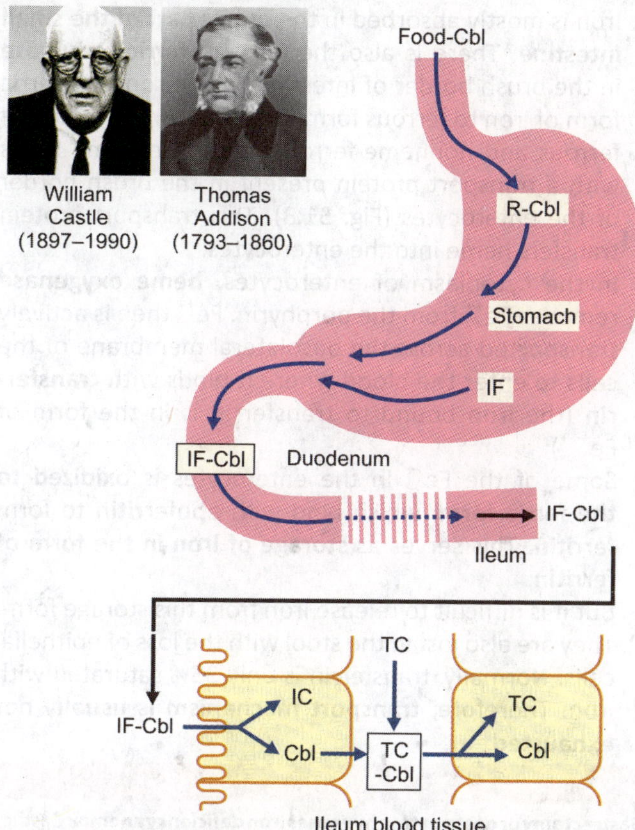

Fig. 51.2: Absorption and storage of vitamin B_{12}. (R: Cobalophilin; Cbl: Cobalamin; IF: Intrinsic factor; TC: Transcobalamin).
Courtesy: Figure 38.8, Textbook of Biochemistry, by DM Vasudevan, 7th Edition; 2013; Jaypee Brothers Medical Publishers (P) Ltd.

Clinical Box 51.2

Cholera is a secretory diarrhea: The cholera toxin activates adenylate cyclase, and increases cAMP concentration. The cAMP activates Cl^- channels and Cl^- is actively secreted. This facilitates the secretion of Na^+ and water into lumen resulting in profuse watery diarrhea.

Absorption of Vitamins

Absorption of Water Soluble Vitamins

Water soluble vitamins are absorbed mostly by simple diffusion though there are specific transport mechanisms available for them, especially for absorption of B_{12}.

Absorption of Vitamin B_{12}

Vitamin B_{12} present in food is mostly bound to proteins.

1. In the stomach, low pH and pepsin release vitamin B_{12} from the protein. The free B_{12} then binds with **R protein (Cobalophilin** secreted in the saliva), which is a glycoprotein, forming **R-B_{12} complex** (Fig. 51.2).
2. However, vitamin B_{12} also **binds with intrinsic factor** (IF) in the stomach, though it has less affinity for IF than the R proteins.
3. **In the intestine,** pancreatic proteases degrade the R-B_{12} complex and decrease the affinity of vitamin B_{12} for R proteins. This facilitates the binding of vitamin B_{12} with IF, forming **B_{12}-IF complex.**
4. B_{12}-IF complex resists degradation by pancreatic proteases. Therefore, **in pancreatic deficiency,** vitamin B_{12} absorption is impaired as degradation of R protein is not adequate.
5. Binding of IF with B_{12}, brings structural change in IF resulting in formation of **dimers**.
6. Each dimer of IF binds two vitamin B_{12} molecules. There are **specific receptors** on the brush border of the epithelial cells of terminal ileum for IF-B_{12} complex that do ***not recognize free vitamin B_{12} or IF alone.***
7. The binding of IF-B_{12} complex to the receptor is facilitated by **cubilin**, a high affinity apolipoprotein component of receptor. Then the complex is absorbed by **endocytosis.**
8. The transport of vitamin B_{12} from the epithelial cells into the blood is a remarkably slow process. Therefore, vitamin B_{12} concentration in plasma **rises after 6–8 hours after a meal.**
9. Vitamin B_{12} then dissociates from IF and enters the mitochondria of epithelial cells where it binds with transcobalamin II (TC II) forming **TC II-B_{12} complex.** This complex is rapidly cleared from portal blood by the liver by receptor mediated endocytosis.

Absorption of vitamin B_{12} is very less (2%) in the absence of IF. However, the IF-independent absorption of B_{12} is faster and there is no saturation in this absorption process (Clinical Box 51.3).

Clinical Box 51.3

IF-independent absorption of B_{12}: IF-independent absorption of B_{12} is faster. Therefore, for treatment of **pernicious anemia** (megaloblastic anemia due to IF deficiency), a high dose of orally administered vitamin B_{12} (1 mg/day) can be given in addition to IV/IM B_{12} therapy.

Clinical Significance

Deficiency of IF causes impaired absorption of vitamin B_{12} from distal ileum. As vitamin B_{12} is essential for maturation of red cells, IF deficiency results in **pernicious anemia**, a type of **megaloblastic anemia.**

There are three types of pernicious anemia.

1. **Autoimmune pernicious anemia:** This is caused by autoimmune atrophy of gastric mucosa that decreases secretion of IF from parietal cells. In most patients, antibodies against parietal cells are detected in the serum.
2. **Congenital IF deficiency pernicious anemia:** In this condition, IF secretion is deficient inspite of normal secretion of HCl from parietal cells.
3. **Congenital vitamin B_{12} deficiency pernicious anemia:** This is due to congenital problem in malabsorption of vitamin B_{12}, in which gastric function and IF secretions are normal. The disease occurs due to deficiency of ileal receptors that recognize IF-B_{12} complex.

Absorption of Fat Soluble Vitamins

The fat soluble vitamins are A, D, E, and K. Most of these vitamins are absorbed in the upper small intestine. Absorption of these vitamins requires intactness of the mechanisms for absorption of fat, which depends on

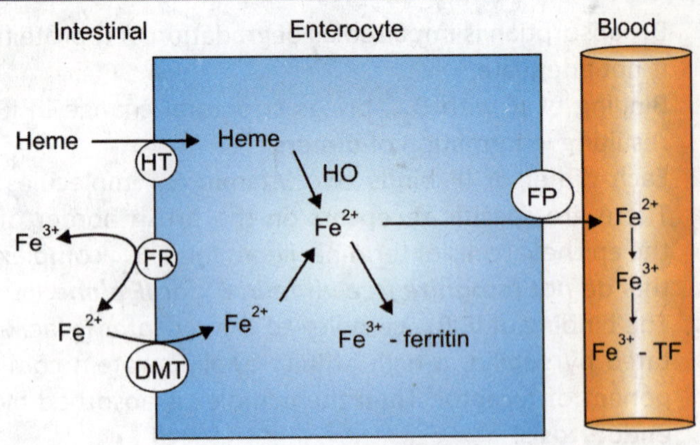

Fig. 51.3: Mechanism of iron reabsorption in intestine. (HT: Heme transporter; FR: Ferric reductase; DMT: Membrane iron transporter; HO: Heme oxygenase; FP: Ferroprotein transporter; TF: Transferrin).

normal pancreatic secretion and bile secretions. Therefore, deficiency of A, D, E, and K are seen in pancreatic deficiency or biliary obstruction that prevents flow of bile into the intestine.

Absorption of Minerals

Absorption of Calcium

About 50% of dietary calcium is absorbed. Absorption occurs primarily in the upper segments of small intestine.

1. The absorption is mostly by an **active transport**, which is **facilitated by 1,25-dihydroxycholecalciferol** that increases expression of calcium binding protein in the mucosal cells.
2. Decreased serum calcium concentration increases 1,25-dihydroxycholecalciferol and increased serum calcium decreases it. This **feedback mechanism** controls calcium absorption according to the need of the body.
3. Calcium absorption is inhibited by phosphates and oxalates, as they form insoluble salts with calcium in the intestine.

Absorption of Iron

The normal plasma level of iron is 130 μg/100 mL in males and 110 μg/100 ml in females. Normally, absorption of iron ranges from 3–6% of the iron ingested.

1. Iron is absorbed in the **ferrous (Fe^{++}) form**.
2. The iron ingested in the diet is present in the ferric (Fe^{+++}) form. In the stomach, ferric form is converted to ferrous form by the **action of hydrochloric acid**. Gastric secretion dissolves the iron and allows it to form soluble complexes with ascorbic acid, which facilitates iron absorption. Therefore, iron deficiency anemia occurs in chronic gastric disease (Clinical Box. 51.4).
3. Iron is mostly absorbed in the **upper part of the small intestine**. There is also the enzyme **ferric reductase** in the brush border of intestine, which converts ferric form of iron to ferrous form. Iron is absorbed in heme-ferrous and nonheme-ferrous form. The heme binds with a transport protein present in the brush border of the enterocytes (Fig. 51.3). This transport protein transfers heme into the enterocytes.
4. In the cytoplasm of enterocytes, **heme oxygenase** removes Fe^{++} from the porphyrin. Fe^{++} then is actively transported across the basolateral membrane of the cells to enter the blood where it binds with **transferrin** (the iron bound to transferrin is in the form of Fe^{+++}).
5. Some of the Fe^{++} in the enterocytes is **oxidized to the ferric form**, which bind with **apoferritin** to form **ferritin**. This serves as **storage of iron in the form of ferritin**.
6. But it is difficult to release iron from this storage form. They are also lost in the stool with the loss of epithelial cells. Normally, transferrin is only 35% saturated with iron. Therefore, **transport mechanism is usually not exhausted**.

Clinical Box 51.4

Gastrectomy or gastric atrophy causes iron deficiency anemia: Gastric secretion dissolves the iron and allows it to form soluble complexes with ascorbic acid, which facilitates iron absorption. Therefore, though iron is not actually absorbed in the stomach, *gastrectomy or gastric atrophy causes iron deficiency anemia.*

Hemosiderosis and Hemochromatosis

Absorption of iron increases when body iron store is less or when there is increased demand for iron like increased erythropoiesis. In conditions of ***iron overload***, more ferritin is formed in the enterocytes, which is then excreted in the stool.

1. Ferritin is the principal storage form of iron in the tissue. In the tissue, ferritin molecules aggregate in the lysosomal membranes, which is called *hemosiderin*. Hemosiderin accumulates in the tissue when iron overload is prolonged. The condition is called **hemosiderosis**.
2. Deposition of large of hemosiderin in the tissue causes damage to the tissue. This condition is called **hemochromatosis**, which is characterized by skin pigmentation, diabetes (due to damage to the pancreatic tissue; bronze diabetes), cirrhosis of liver, and gonadal atrophy (testicular atrophy in males).

Iron present in the body is mainly in the form of hemoglobin (70% of the total iron). About 23% is present in the ferritin (in the store form) and only 3% is present in the form of myoglobin.

CHAPTER SUMMARY

Key Concepts

1. The major part of absorption of nutrients takes place in the small intestine. Therefore, chronic intestinal disease or intestinal resection leads to malabsorption syndrome.
2. Though the mechanisms are specific for specific nutrient, few of them facilitate each other.

Important to Know (Must Read)

1. In examinations, "Describe the mechanism of digestion and absorption of carbohydrate, fat and proteins from intestine" may come as a **Long Question**.
2. Mechanism of digestion and absorption of carbohydrate, Mechanism of digestion and absorption of fat, Mechanism of digestion and absorption of proteins, Mechanism of absorption of water, Mechanism of absorption of sodium, Mechanism of absorption of chloride and bicarbonate, Mechanism of absorption of Vit.B_{12}, Mechanism of absorption of iron may come as **Short Questions**.
3. In **Viva**, examiner may ask… mechanism of digestion and absorption of each nutrient and clinical conditions that occur due to their deficiencies.
4. Usually questions are asked about malabsorption syndrome, in oral.

SECTION–6

Endocrine Physiology

52. Introduction to Endocrinology
53. Mechanisms of Hormone Action
54. Hypothalamus and Hypothalamo-pituitary Axis
55. Pituitary Gland: The Anterior Pituitary
56. Posterior Pituitary
57. Thyroid Gland
58. Adrenal Gland: The Adrenal Medulla
59. Adrenal Cortex
60. Endocrine Pancreas
61. Calcium and Phosphate Metabolism and Physiology of Bone
62. Parathyroid Gland, Calcitonin and Vitamin D
63. Pineal Gland
64. Local Hormones

"But when the hour of the Divine draws near
The Mighty mother shall take birth in Time
And God be born into the human clay
In forms made ready by your human lives.
Then shall the Truth supreme be given to men."

Sri Aurobindo (in 'SAVITRI')

CHAPTER 52

Introduction to Endocrinology

Learning Objectives

On completion of study of this chapter, the student **MUST** be able to:

1. Appreciate the importance of learning endocrine physiology in understanding medicine.
2. Classify hormones and give examples.
3. Understand the principles of hormone synthesis.
4. Understand regulation of hormone secretion, especially the feedback mechanisms.
5. Learn the physiological importance of binding of hormones to plasma proteins.
6. Know different mechanisms of hormone signaling and intercellular communications, and give examples for each.

The student **MAY** also be able to:

1. Describe the principle of synthesis, secretion and metabolism of hormones.
2. Understand how are the hormones are degraded in the body.
3. Briefly describe the procedure of estimation of hormones.

Endocrine physiology is the branch of physiology that deals with the study of processes involved in regulation and integration of cells and organ systems by specialized chemical substances called hormones. The word '**hormone**' is derived from *"hormaein"* a Greek word, which means 'to excite':

1. **Hormone** is defined as *specialized organic molecules that are synthesized by endocrine glands or tissues in response to specific stimuli and exert their precise effects on particular target cells*.
2. An endocrine gland is a **ductless gland** that pours its secretion directly into general circulation. Hormones circulate in blood to reach the target tissues on which they act.

Scientist contributed

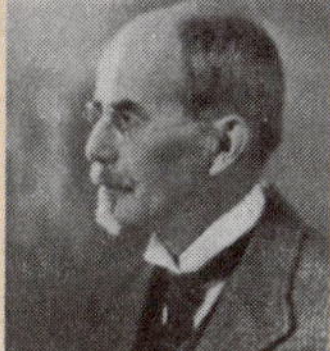
JJ Abel
(1857–1938)

John Jacob Abel (1857–1938) was pioneered in the study of endocrine secretions. He received his PhD in physiology from Johns Hopkins University and studied in Germany under Carl Ludwig. His works on the blood pressure-raising constituent of the adrenal medulla led to the identification and synthesis of **catecholamines**, and further to the development of many derivatives of catecholamines. Similarly, his studies on the **anterior pituitary** gland resulted in the isolation of its ***oxytocic, pressor and diuretic principles***. He also pioneered with crystalline **insulin**. With Leonard G Rowntree, he introduced kidney and liver function tests.

3. Target cells are conferred with **receptors that are specific in their affinity** for hormones. Actions of hormones on the target tissues are diverse in nature. Broadly, **functions of hormone** include:

1. Change in cell function
2. Control of growth and development
3. Alteration in body mass and its composition
4. Reproductive functions
5. Digestion, utilization and storage of nutrients
6. Regulation of volume and composition of fluid compartments
7. Behavioral changes
8. Control of senescence.

Hormones to accomplish their functions, **bind to receptors** on the target tissues. **Activation of these receptors** leads to alteration in multiple intracellular mechanisms and signaling pathways that change cell functions.

ENDOCRINE GLANDS

Types

Endocrine structures can broadly be divided into major endocrine glands (Fig. 52.1) and other endocrine organs:

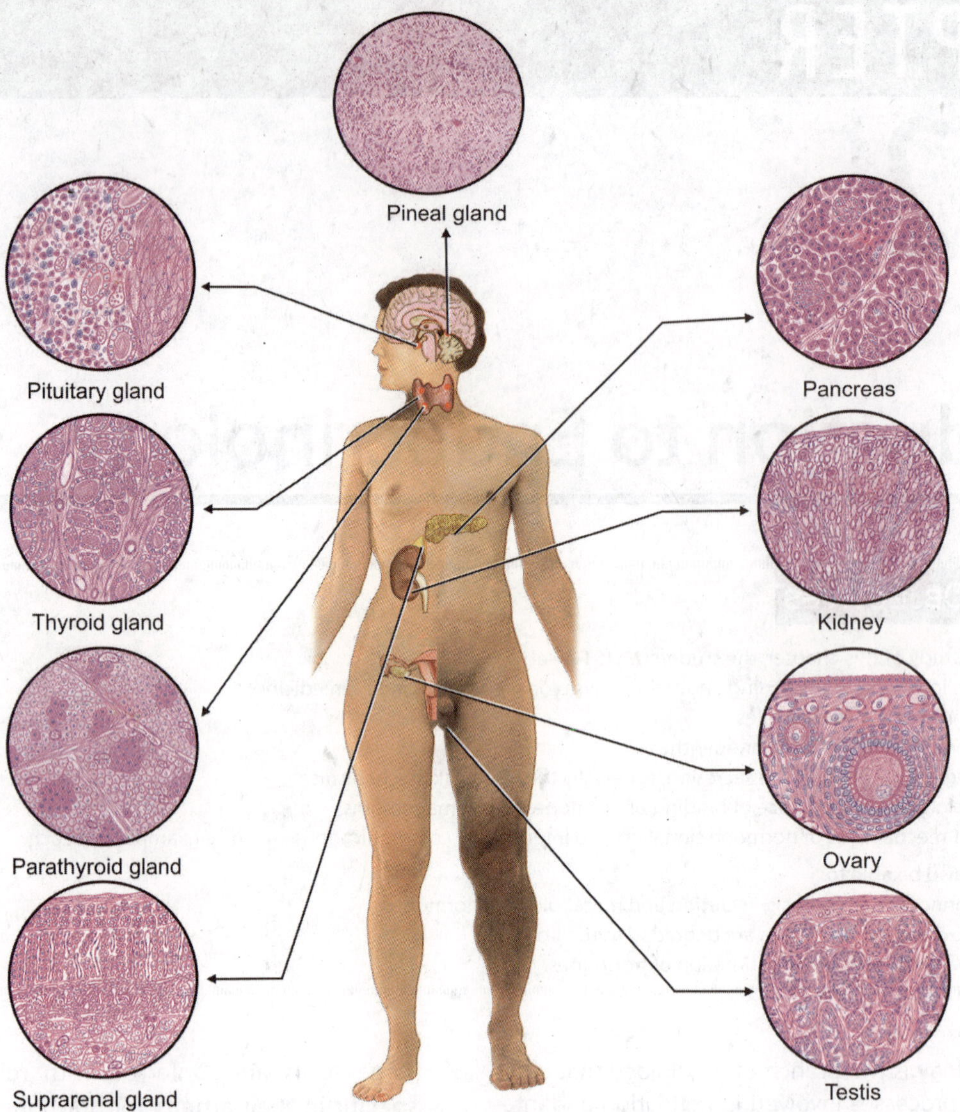

Fig. 52.1: Major endocrine glands in the body.
Courtesy: Figure 18.1, Basic Histology, by V Subhadra Devi, 1st edition, 2016; Jaypee Brothers Medical Publishers (P) Ltd.

A. **Major endocrine glands**
   1. Hypothalamus
   2. Pituitary (anterior and posterior pituitaries)
   3. Thyroid
   4. Adrenals (adrenal cortex and medulla)
   5. Parathyroid
   6. Endocrine pancreas
   7. Gonads (testis and ovary)
   8. Pineal gland.

B. **Other endocrine organs**
   1. Thymus (secretes thymosin, especially in childhood)
   2. Kidney (secretes erythropoietin, renin, etc.)
   3. Heart (secretes ANP)
   4. Lungs (secrete prostaglandins and activate angiotensin)
   5. GI tract (secretes many GI hormones)
   6. Placenta (secretes many hormones during pregnancy).

Analogy with Nervous and Immune Systems

The endocrine system is closely associated with the nervous and immunes systems of the body and also resembles them in many aspects.

Similarity with Nervous System

Endocrine system like that of nervous system is a major system of communication. In its various physiological aspects, it is analogous to the nervous system:

1. Nervous system requires signaling by a stimulus that evokes a response and a feedback mechanism that controls the response. Similarly, endocrine system needs signaling for hormone secretion and feedback mechanisms for regulation of secretion. The control mechanisms that regulate hormone secretion operate mainly on **feedback principle**.
2. Moreover, neurons secrete chemicals at their axon terminals, **the neurotransmitters**, which are basically

hormones in their chemical structure. In fact, many hormones act locally as neurotransmitters in the nervous system.

Thus, nervous and endocrine systems integrate with each other to bring about desirable effects in response to changes in external or internal environment. Even some of the hormones are called neurohormones.

Similarity with Immune System

The immuno-competent cells (immunocytes or immune cells) secrete many chemicals that are grouped as 'cytokines':

1. Cytokines resemble hormones in structure and functions. Like hormones, cytokines act on specific receptors on the target tissues to achieve desirable changes.
2. In fact, many hormones are synthesized and secreted by immune cells, though they act locally.
3. Also, cytokines modulate functions of endocrine glands and hormones modulate functions of immunocytes.

Types of Hormones

Hormones are broadly classified into **three types**: peptides, amino acids and steroids.

Proteins or Peptides

Peptide hormones include a large group of hormones secreted from a variety of endocrine tissues. These hormones are made up of peptide chains:

1. Depending on the number of amino acids in the chain, they may be **oligopeptides** (less than 10 amino acids) like oxytocin and ADH, and **polypeptides** (10 or more amino acids) like insulin and growth hormone.
2. They originate from a common ancestral gene during evolution.
3. Based on their structure and functions, they are grouped into a **number of families** like insulin, glycoprotein, growth hormone and secretin families (Table 52.1).

Amino Acids

These hormones are amines. Many of them are derived from a **common amino acid**, for example dopamine, epinephrine, norepinephrine and thyroxine are derived from tyrosine. They are usually hydrophilic.

Steroids

Steroid hormones are **synthesized from cholesterol**, and are lipid soluble and hydrophobic:

1. This group includes hormones of **adrenal cortex and many gonadal hormones**.
2. The biological activities of this group are determined by **modification of their side chains, hydroxylation and ring aromatization** at various sites.

Table 52.1: Classification of hormones.

A. Peptide Hormones

1. Insulin family
   - Insulin
   - Insulin like growth factors
   - Relaxin
2. Glycoproteins
   - LH
   - FSH
   - TSH
   - hCG
3. Growth hormone family
   - GH
   - Prolactin
   - Human placental lactogen
4. Secretin family
   - Secretin
   - Glucagon
   - VIP
   - GIP
5. Others
   - ANP
   - Calcitonin
   - CCK
   - ADH
   - Inhibin
   - Somatostatin
   - ACTH
   - Parathormone

B. Amino Acid Derivative

1. Amines
   - Epinephrine
   - Norepinephrine
   - Dopamine
   - Serotonin
2. Iodinated amino acid
   - Thyroxine (T_4)
   - Triiodothyronine (T_3)

C. Steroid Hormones

- Glucocorticoids
- Mineralocorticoids
- Estrogen
- Progesterone
- Testosterone
- 1,25-dihydroxycholecalciferol

GENERAL PHYSIOLOGY OF HORMONES

Principles of Synthesis and Secretion

Peptide Hormone Synthesis

In general, protein hormones are synthesized in the **rough endoplasmic reticulum** of endocrine cells:

1. They are first synthesized as a signal peptide called **preprohormone**, which is then cleaved to form **prohormone**.

Flowchart 52.1: General outline of peptide hormone synthesis.

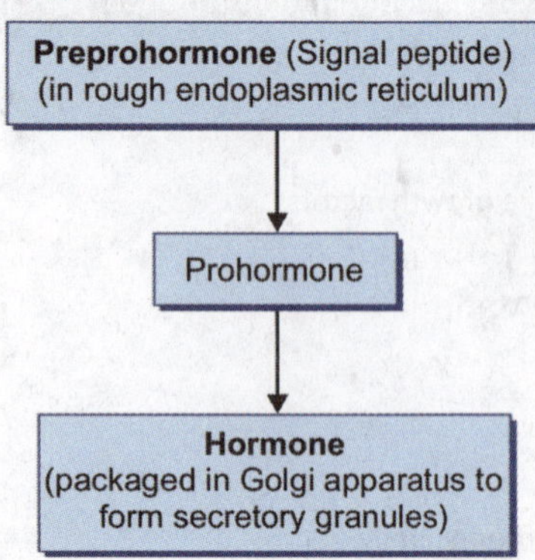

2. Prohormone is then transported into the Golgi apparatus, where it is converted into **hormone**. Hormone is packaged in the secretory granules for storage (Flowchart 52.1).
3. The hormone is secreted from **stored granules** on appropriate stimulation. Granules are released by ***calcium-mediated exocytosis***.
4. Hormones are also secreted from **neoplastic tissues** (Application Box 52.1).

Application Box 52.1

Ectopic Hormone Secretion: Sometimes in pathological conditions, nonendocrine tissues secrete hormones. For example, **neoplastic tissues of lungs** like small cell pulmonary carcinoma produce several hormones. The condition is called **paraneoplastic syndrome**. The hormones usually secreted in such syndromes are ACTH, ADH and parathormone, resulting in Cushing syndrome, water retention and hypercalcemia respectively. Hormones are also secreted from **gastrointestinal tumors** and the condition is called **carcinoid syndrome**. Carcinoid tumors are also associated with melanoma, lymphoma and neural tumors.

Pathways of Synthesis

Peptide Hormone Synthesis

Synthesis and secretion of peptide hormones occur in **two pathways**: the regulated and constitutive pathways.

Regulated Pathway

In regulated pathway, external stimuli trigger release of hormone which is already synthesized and **stored in secretory granules**, and also promote synthesis of some additional hormones. For example, GnRH from hypothalamus stimulates release of gonadotropins and additional synthesis of gonadotropins from anterior pituitary.

Constitutive Pathway

In constitutive pathway, secretion of hormones occurs more directly from endoplasmic reticulum or vesicles formed from the Golgi apparatus, in which additional hormones are formed simultaneously.

Thus, **regulated pathway is capable of secretion of large amount of hormones**, whereas ***constitutive pathway promotes secretory reserve***. In any case, stimuli that trigger secretion also increase synthesis of hormones.

Amine Hormone Synthesis

All amine hormones except serotonin are synthesized from the amino acid tyrosine that requires a series of enzymatic reactions. Serotonin is synthesized from 5-HT. Catecholamines are **stored in granules** and secreted by calcium mediated exocytosis of granules in which they are stored.

Steroid Hormone Synthesis

Steroid hormones are synthesized from cholesterol. Many enzymatic reactions are involved in the process of steroid hormone synthesis:

1. These hormones are **not stored in the cell as granules.**
2. They are usually present in the cytosol **bound to proteins.**
3. On stimulation, the hormones become free form intracellular proteins and are transported outside the cell usually by diffusion.

Regulation of Hormone Secretion

Normally, concentration of a hormone in circulation is maintained within a narrow range. Increase or decrease in hormone concentration for a longer period results in major dysfunctions. Alteration in hormone concentration is mainly checked by regulation of hormone secretion. Hormone secretion is principally controlled by **four mechanisms**:

1. Feedback control,
2. Neural control,
3. Rhythmic or chronotropic control, and
4. Humoral control.

Of these control processes, feedback control is the most common and developed mechanism for regulation of hormone secretion. However, many factors arriving from variety of stimuli play simultaneously to achieve an integrated response of hormone secretion. This is called **multiplicity of regulation of hormone secretion.**

Feedback Control

When the change in concentration of a hormone in plasma alters its rate of secretion, the mechanism is called feedback control. There are **two feedback mechanisms**: The positive and the negative feedbacks.

Negative Feedback

When increased concentration of a hormone and its metabolites provide feedback inhibitory signal to the gland that secretes the hormone, the mechanism is called negative feedback mechanism. This is the **common mechanism of hormone homeostasis.** Depending on the circuit or the pathway involved in the feedback control, the mechanism may be simple feedback or complex feedback.

Simple Feedback Control

This is the **first order of feedback control** in which the hormone secreted from a gland controls its secretion through

Flowchart 52.2: Simple feedback system in the regulation of hormone secretion. Endocrine gland senses biological activity of the hormone and accordingly modulates its secretion.

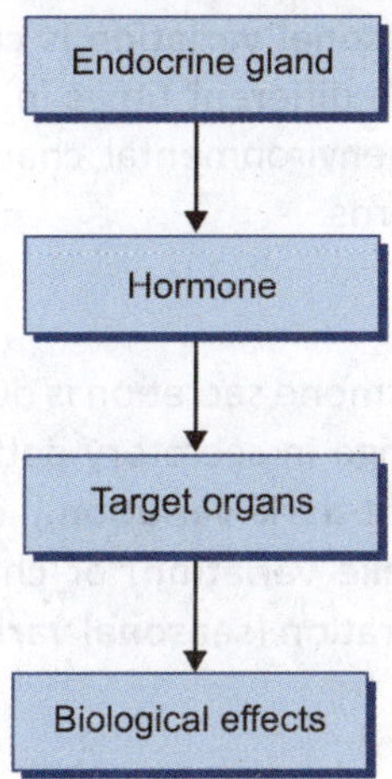

the physiological effects. The endocrine cells that secrete the hormone also **sense the biological activity** produced by the hormone:

1. When the biological effects are more, the hormone secretion decreases appropriately to maintain normal function of the hormone (Flowchart 52.2). For example, β cells of pancreas secrete insulin that acts on liver and skeletal muscles to regulate blood glucose concentration. β cells in turn sense the alteration in plasma glucose and accordingly adjust their insulin secretion to maintain the plasma glucose concentration within normal range.

Complex or Hierarchical Feedback Control

When the feedback regulation involves **second or third order feedback loop** or both, the control mechanism is called complex or hierarchical control. This multiorder or complex control system is the usual mechanism for regulation of many hormone secretions:

1. In this system, the hormone secreted by **first (upper) order gland** stimulates secretion of **second (middle) order gland**.
2. Secretion (usually, trophic hormones) of middle order gland stimulates secretion of **final (lower) order gland** or *target gland*.
3. Secretion of target gland (**target gland hormone**) inhibits the secretion of first order or middle order glands (Flowchart 52.3).
4. Also, secretion of middle order gland (**trophic hormone**) inhibits secretion of first order gland.
5. This system operates mainly for control of **hypothalamo-pituitary-target endocrine gland axis.**
6. As this is an integrated system of control of endocrine functions, disorder at any level of hierarchy influences the function of other levels.

The major hormone axes regulated by **hierarchial system of feedback control** are:

Flowchart 52.3: Hierarchical or complex feedback system in the regulation of endocrine functions. This system operates mainly for control of hypothalamo-pituitary-target endocrine gland axis.

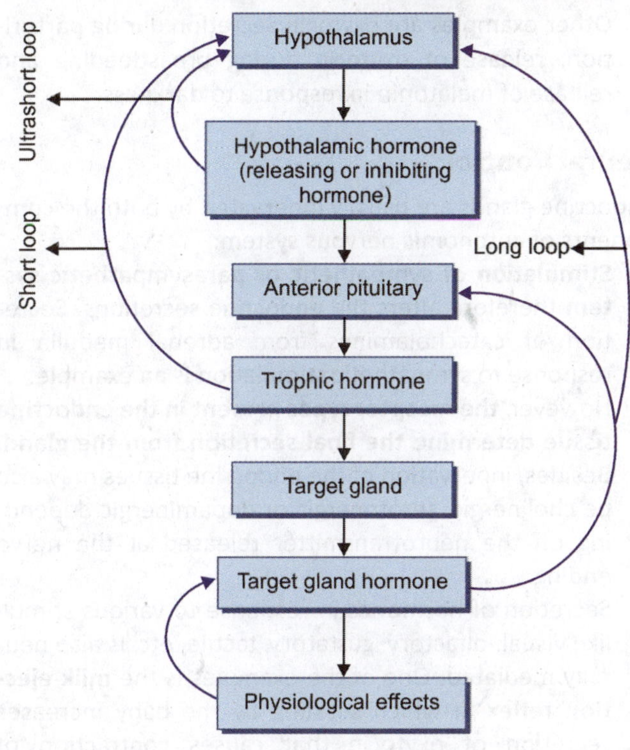

- Hypothalamo-pituitary-thyroid axis
- Hypothalamo-pituitary-adrenal axis
- Hypothalamo-pituitary-gonadal axis.

For example, in hypothalamo-pituitary-adrenal axis, excess cortisol in plasma inhibits secretion of adrenal cortex by decreasing ACTH secretion from anterior pituitary or by inhibiting hypothalamic release of CRH.

Loops of Negative Feedback Control

Depending on the distance from which the hormone of the target gland inhibits the upper order glands, the inhibition is classified into **long loop, short loop and ultrashort loop**. For example, in the same hypothalamo-pituitary adrenal axis, cortisol inhibiting CRH release is the **long loop** of negative feedback, ACTH inhibiting CRH release is the **short loop** of negative feedback and CRH inhibiting its own release is the **ultrashort loop** of negative feedback (Flowchart 52.3).

Positive Feedback

This is a less common mechanism of regulation of hormone secretion. In this control system, increase in hormone concentration in plasma stimulates further secretion of that hormone so that the hormone concentration **increases steadily to reach a peak plasma level**:

1. The best example of positive feedback regulation is the **LH surge** that occurs just before ovulation. Normally, estrogen inhibits LH secretion; however, just before ovulation, increased estrogen concentration

in plasma provides a positive feedback for LH release from anterior pituitary that results in LH surge (for details, refer 'Menstrual Cycle').

2. Other examples are oxytocin secretion during parturition, release of oxytocin during breastfeeding and release of melatonin in response to darkness.

Neural Control

Endocrine glands are usually innervated by both the components of autonomic nervous system:

1. **Stimulation of sympathetic or parasympathetic system** therefore alters the endocrine secretions. Secretion of catecholamines from adrenal medulla in response to sympathetic stimulation is an example.
2. However, **the receptor types present in the endocrine tissue determine the final secretion from the gland.** Besides, innervation of the endocrine tissues may also be cholinergic, serotonergic or dopaminergic depending on the neurotransmitter released at the nerve ending.
3. Secretion of hormones in response to various stimuli like visual, olfactory, gustatory, tactile, etc. is also neurally mediated. One of the examples is the **milk ejection reflex** in which suckling by the baby increases secretion of oxytocin that causes contraction of myoepithelial cells of the mammary gland.

Rhythmic or Chronotropic Control

Chronotropic control of hormone secretion is the regulatory mechanism operated by **various rhythms of biologic phenomena** that either cycle at regular intervals like **circadian rhythm, sleep-wake cycle, seasonal rhythm and menstrual cycle**, or appear at **different phases of development** like hormonal changes occurring in pre-pubertal children.

Influenced by chronotropic control mechanism, hormones are secreted in a definable and rhythmic pattern, which may be:

1. episodic or **pulsatile** lasting for few minutes to hours
2. **diurnal** lasting for several hours in a light-dark cycle
3. **periodical** lasting for many days
4. **developmental** occurring at different phases of development
5. **seasonal,** in different seasons.

Examples of chronotropic control:

1. **Example of episodic (pulsatile) hormone secretion** is the secretion of GnRH. Normally, GnRH is secreted in episodic bursts that cause circhoral peaks of LH secretion (for details, refer, "Female Reproduction").
2. **Example of diurnal hormone secretion** is the change in ACTH or cortisol at different times of day and night. Another example of day-night variation is melatonin secretion.
3. **Example of periodical secretion** is alteration in sex hormones or gonadotropins in different phases of menstrual cycle.
4. Alteration in secretion of gonadal hormones at puberty in both boys and girls is the **example of developmental hormonal secretion.**
5. **Example of seasonal variation** is change in hormone concentration in different times in a year that mostly occurs due to environmental changes. This is more prominent in birds.

Mechanisms

The variation in hormone secretion is due to many mechanisms such as change in secretory pattern influenced by photic stimuli (**light-dark variation**), change influenced by sleep (**sleep-wake variation**) or change subjected to environmental alteration (**seasonal variation**).

Humoral Control

Humoral control is the control by hormones and chemicals.

Hormonal Control

Many hormones influence secretion of other hormones. Examples are glucagon stimulating insulin secretion, angiotensin stimulating aldosterone secretion, somatostatin inhibiting growth hormone secretion and so on.

Chemical Control

Secretion of hormone is influenced by various chemical stimuli such as concentration of blood gasses, acids, ions and osmolality. Examples are hypokalemia inhibiting insulin secretion, hyperkalemia or hyponatremia stimulating aldosterone secretion, etc.

Hormone Signaling

The chemical signaling of hormone occurs through **three pathways**: endocrine, paracrine, and autocrine.

Endocrine Signaling

Hormone secreted from the endocrine gland reaches distant target tissues via bloodstream. Most of the hormones signal target tissues located far away from the gland via this route. Thus, cells of hormone secreting tissue communicate with cells of other tissues of the body via endocrine signaling. Hence, this type of intercellular communication is called **endocrine communication.**

Paracrine Signaling

Hormone secreted from endocrine tissue diffuses into extracellular space and **signals the neighboring tissue.** This is called paracrine signaling. For example, **somatostatin secreted from D cells** of pancreatic islets influences the secretion of insulin and glucagon from same islet cells (Flowchart 52.4).

Flowchart 52.4: Paracrine and autocrine mechanism of hormone signaling.

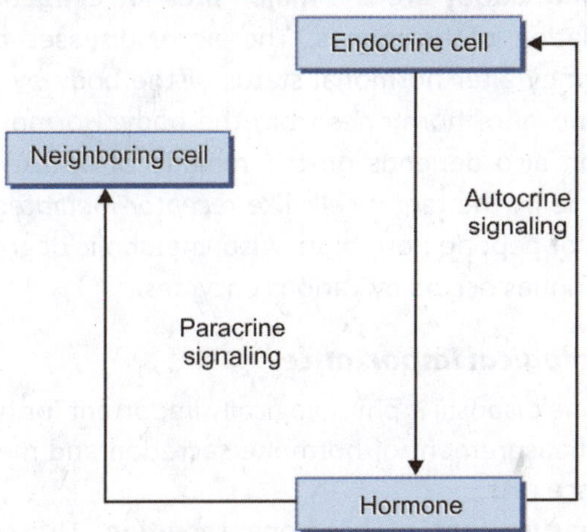

Autocrine Signaling

Hormone secreted from an endocrine cell binds with the **receptor located in the same cell** that secretes the hormone. Thus, hormone modifies the function of its parent cell. The example of autocrine **signaling is the platelet activating factor** secreted from platelet, which activates the platelet.

Intercellular Communications

Cells communicate with each other by **five major mechanisms**: direct, neural, endocrine, paracrine and neurocrine (Table 52.2). Autocrine and juxtacrine communications are strictly not part of the intercellular communications, as in these two systems cells influence their own activities or the other cells in the vicinity:

1. **Direct communication** occurs between cells via gap junction (electrical synapses). Example is rapid transmission of impulse between cardiac myocytes via gap junctions.
2. **Neural communication** is the major mechanism of intercellular communication. Examples are neurons communicating through synapses.
3. **Endocrine, paracrine and autocrine communications** are described above in 'Hormone signaling'.
4. **Juxtacrine communication** is the communication through cell adhesion to growth factors expressed on cell surface. For example, many cells having receptors for ***transforming growth factor*** α (TGFα) interact with each other by attaching themselves to the transforming growth factor α (TGFα) present on their cell surface.
5. **Neurocrine communication** is via secretion of chemicals at nerve ending. For example, ***cholinergic vagal fibers*** to oxyntic cells in stomach influence parietal cell function by releasing **acetylcholine** at their terminals, and ***non-cholinergic vagal fibers*** to G cells in the antrum of stomach influence G cell function by releasing gastrin releasing peptide (**GRP**) at their terminals.

Table 52.2: Intercellular communications.

Types	Mechanism
Direct communication	Via gap junctions between cells
Neural communication	Via synapses (synaptic transmission)
Endocrine communication	Via circulating hormones
Paracrine communication	Via locally released hormones from neighboring endocrine cells
Autocrine communication	Hormone secreted from the same cell
Juxtacrine communication	Through growth factors expressed on the cell surface
Neurocrine communication	Through chemicals released at nerve terminal

Transport of Hormones

By definition, hormones are secretions of ductless glands, transported via blood stream to reach their target tissues. After entering the blood they **either remain in free form or bind with a specific carrier protein**. Usually, *amine and protein hormones remain in unbound* (circulate in free) form, and *thyroxine and steroid hormones* (and vitamin D) *circulate in the bound form*.

Transport of Amine and Peptide Hormones

Amino acid-derived and peptide hormones **readily dissolve in the plasma** and do not require special mechanism for their transport.

Transport of Steroid Hormones

Thyroxine, steroid hormones and vitamin D are **relatively insoluble in plasma** and circulate in the **bound form**. In blood, more than 90% of thyroid and steroid hormones are bound to plasma proteins. The transport proteins are specific for hormones (Table 52.3). However, few nonspecific proteins are also involved in the process of hormone transport.

Importance of Hormone Binding

Binding of hormone with carrier proteins influences important biological properties of hormones, especially, hormone action, metabolism, storage and removal:

1. **Hormone action:** The intensity of the hormone action depends on the extent to which hormone is bound to the proteins. Usually, hormones that bind to transport proteins remain 1 to 10% only in the free form, which is called as the **biologically active hormone**. Thus, about 90% of these hormones, i.e. the hormone in bound form constitutes the **inactive pool of hormone**. Any condition that decreases hormone binding by decreasing the concentration of proteins available for binding or by any other mechanism, increases the hormone

Table: 52.3: Transport proteins for hormones.
A. Specific proteins
1. Thyroxine binding globulin (TBG) – Transports T3 and T4
2. Corticosteroid binding globulin (CBG) – Transports cortisol and aldosterone
3. Sex-hormone binding globulin (SHBG) – Transports testosterone and estrogen
B. Nonspecific proteins
1. Serum albumin – Transports many steroid and thyroid hormones
2. Prealbumin – Transports thyroxine

activity as plasma level of free hormone rises; and conversely, condition that increases binding decreases hormone activity.

2. **Hormone reservoir:** Transport proteins also provide reservoir of hormones that is essential for **buffering rapid change in hormone concentration** in plasma.
3. **Hormone metabolism and clearance:** Binding with carrier protein influences metabolism and removal of hormone from circulation. This **determines the half-life of the hormone.** For example, the plasma half-life of thyroxine is 6 days as it is 99.9% protein bound, whereas half life of aldosterone is 25 minutes as only 15% of it is bound to protein.
4. **Diagnostic importance:** Form diagnostic view-point, it is important to know the both free and bound form of the hormone. Assay of total hormone concentration may sometimes be misleading as total concentration may be normal in the presence of actual hormonal deficiency or excess. For example, binding proteins may be increased in various conditions such as pregnancy, drug therapy, etc. that decrease the free form, and therefore lead to functional hormone deficiency though the total concentration of hormone remains normal. Therefore, free concentration of hormone (**free hormone index**), or the **ratio of free form to bound form** of hormone reflects the actual physiological state of hormone. Hence, often, in the diagnosis of hormonal disorder, measurement of free hormone index is preferred to total hormone estimation to evaluate the degree of dysfunction.

Hormone Alteration, Degradation, and Disposal

Alteration of Hormone

Some of the hormones are transformed in the peripheral blood, which is **required for their full biological activity**. Examples are the conversion of T_4 to T_3 and testosterone to dihydrotestosterone.

Degradation and Disposal of Hormone

Liver and kidney are the major sites for extraction and degradation of hormones. Therefore, diseases of liver and kidney alter hormonal status of the body by impairing removal of hormones from the body. Hormone degradation also depends on the rapidity of uptake of the hormone by the target cells like *receptor-mediated endocytosis* of peptide hormones. Also, metabolic degradation of hormones occurs by various enzymes.

Physiological Importance

Hormone disposal is physiologically important for two reasons: measurement of hormone secretion and metabolic clearance rate.

1. **Measurement of hormone secretion:** Urine is the major route of excretion for many hormones, and few hormones are excreted in bile. Therefore, for many hormones, measurement of hormone metabolites in urine is a better indicator of the rate of production of hormones. For example, *urinary excretion of metanephrine or VMA is an index of catecholamine secretion*, which provides a simple and noninvasive test for assessment of adrenomedullary function.
2. **Estimation of metabolic clearance rate (MCR):** Sometimes estimation of rate of metabolism is clinically useful for assessing hormone dysfunction. The rate at which the hormone is removed from the body is one of the indices of MCR. MCR is the hormone removed per unit time divided by the plasma concentration of the hormone.

$$\text{MCR} = \frac{\text{Hormone removed per unit time (mg/min)}}{\text{Plasma conc. of hormone (mg/mL)}}$$

MCR is reported as ml of plasma per min. Half-life of hormone and MCR are inversely related. Thus, *shorter the half life, greater is the MCR.*

Estimation of Hormone Concentration

Measurement of concentration of hormone in biological fluids is often performed for confirmation of clinical diagnosis. Hormone estimation can be done by bioassay, radioimmunoassay (RIA) and enzyme-linked immunosorbent assay (ELISA).

Bioassay

Bioassay is the assay of hormone's ability to produce a characteristic biological response:

1. In this method, hormone is estimated in terms of **units**, which is defined as an amount sufficient to produce a response of specified magnitude under standard conditions.
2. Bioassay was the earlier method of assessment of hormone concentrations.

3. After the discovery of RIA and ELISA, bioassay is rarely used at present for the purpose.
4. Also, the method is slow and often expensive.

Radioimmunoassay (RIA)

RIA is usually used for estimation of hormones, proteins, drugs and vitamins in body fluids like plasma, urine and CSF. RIA is a type of **competitive binding assays**. It is based on the theory of competitive binding. In RIA, **two components** are used: a ***specific antibody*** (Ab) that is produced against the hormone to be assayed, and a ***radioactively labeled hormone*** (H^r):

1. When the hormone to be measured is a peptide, the molecule is commonly labeled with a radioactive iodine atom (^{125}I or ^{131}I) that can be easily attached to the tyrosine residue of peptide chain, and if the hormone is a steroid (that lack tyrosine residue), labeling is done by radioactive carbon (^{14}C) or hydrogen (^3H).
2. The **principle of RIA** is that the labeled and unlabeled hormones compete for a limited number of antibody binding sites. The quantity of each hormone bound to antibody is the ratio of that present in solution. The hormone and the radioactive hormone bind to antibody, and the amount of radioactivity present as Ab-H^r is determined.
3. The response produced by the standards is used to generate a standard curve and the response produced by the unknown samples is then compared to the standard curve to determine the amount of hormone present in the unknowns.
4. The **major drawback** of the RIA is that it measures immunoreactivity, not the biological activity of the hormone.
5. Therefore, recently RIA is modified to **radioreceptor assay** (RRA), in which specific receptors of hormone instead of antibodies are used as hormone-binding reagent. In RRA, as the receptor binding (the hormone that binds to its own receptors) is assessed, it measures ***biologically active hormone***.

Enzyme-linked Immunosorbent Assay (ELISA)

This is an enzyme-based colorimetric or fluorometric assay of hormones that does not produce radioactive wastes. Therefore, the **environmental hazard is reduced**. Moreover, as it is a solid-phase assay, it is automated to a large extent.

Hormone Actions

Most of the hormones have several effects on target tissues that are called as **pleiotropic effects of hormones**. For example, acting on liver, cortisol not only decreases glucose uptake, but also influences glycogenolysis, glycogenesis, neoglucogenesis, lipolysis, protein synthesis, etc. Similarly, many hormones have **multiple actions** on several other tissues simultaneously. For example, the same cortisol apart from acting on liver, also acts on other tissues like skeletal muscle, intestine, heart, brain, bones, blood cells etc for various other functions:

1. As hormones act on different body systems for different actions, some of the actions are complementary and some are antagonistic.
2. However, both complementary and antagonistic actions of hormones are meant for integration of body functions in normal conditions as well as in different other situations.

Complementary Actions

When actions of different hormones ***facilitate a function of the body in a particular situation***, it is called complementary actions of hormone. Complementary actions may be for a **short-term regulation** or for a **long-term modification**:

1. The example for **short-term complimentary action** is the acute physical exercise, during which secretion of epinephrine, cortisol and glucagon contributes to defend plasma glucose concentration. Deficiency of one or more hormones in such a condition results in severe hypoglycemia.
2. The example of **long-term complementary actions** is the regulation of growth by growth hormone, thyroxine, insulin like growth factors and sex steroids.

Antagonistic Actions

When the action of a hormone on a target organ **is opposed by another hormone**, the process is called antagonistic action. The example is the effect of insulin and glucagon on liver to regulate plasma glucose concentration. Insulin lowers plasma glucose by inhibiting hepatic glycogenolysis and gluconeogenesis, whereas glucagon increases blood glucose by stimulating glycogenolysis and gluconeogenesis. Thus, glucose homeostasis depends on the balance of actions of insulin and glucagon and other hyperglycemic hormones. Therefore, antagonistic actions of hormones, is an important regulatory process of the nature to fine-tune the physiological activities of the body.

CHAPTER SUMMARY

Key Concepts

1. Regulation of hormone secretion occurs mainly by feedback control mechanism, in which negative feedback system is the usual process.
2. Hormone concentration in the blood depends mainly on the free hormone available (the quantity of the hormone not bound to binding proteins).

3. Also, the concentration remains elevated when the degradation of the hormone is less, in addition to increased production.
4. Paracrine signaling is for controlling of neighboring cells, and endocrine signaling is for control of all the cells including the distant cells.

Important to Know (Must Read)

1. In examinations, 'Mechanism of regulation of hormone secretion' may come as a **Long Question**.
2. Classification of hormones, Pathways of hormone synthesis, Types of feedback control of hormone secretion, Negative feedback mechanism of hormone control, Hormone signaling mechanisms, Intercellular communications, Types of hormone actions, are usual **Short Questions** in exams.
3. In **Viva**, examiner may ask... Define hormone, Classify hormones and give example of each category, Name the endocrine glands, How is endocrine system analogous with nervous and immune system, What is the basic principle of hormone synthesis, What are the pathways of hormone synthesis, What is the meaning of ectopic hormone secretion, In what conditions ectopic hormone secretion occurs, What is paraneoplastic syndrome, What is the meaning and role of a feedback system, What are types of feedback control of hormone secretion, and give example for each, What is negative and positive feedback mechanism of hormone control, give examples, What are the hierarchial systems of negative feedback process, What are the hormone signaling mechanisms and give example for each, What are the intercellular communications and give example for each type of communication, How are the hormones transported, What are importance of hormone binding, What are the processes of hormone degradation, How are hormones estimated, What are types of hormone actions.

CHAPTER 53

Mechanisms of Hormone Action

Learning Objectives

On completion of study of this chapter, the student **MUST** be able to:

1. Understand the concept of receptor up-regulation and down-regulation.
2. Appreciate the role of G proteins in hormone action.
3. List the second messengers produced by first messengers (hormones).
4. List the important hormones that act through different second messengers.
5. Describe the mechanism of hormone action via adenylyl cyclase-cyclic AMP system, membrane phospholipid-phospholipase system, cyclic-GMP system and transcription of mRNA system.

The student **MAY** also be able to:

1. Explain the role of G proteins in health and disease.
2. Describe the effects of various second messengers on cells and tissues.

RECEPTORS

Hormones to exert their effects on tissues bind with the **specific receptors** located in the target cell. The receptor may be present on the **surface of the cell**, in the **cytoplasm** or **nucleus of the cell**.

1. The binding of hormone with the receptor that forms **hormone-receptor complex** (HR complex), activates a series of **signal generating mechanisms** via a cascade of enzymatic reactions in the target cell.
2. The generated signal molecules increase in number in each step leading to manifold increase in final effect of the hormone on the cell. This is called **signal amplification.**
3. Normally, concentration of hormones in the body fluid is exceedingly low, which is usually in the range of 10^{-9} to 10^{-12} mol/L. In-spite of their very low concentration, hormones effectively alter cell functions through the process of signal amplification.
4. The ***peptide hormones*** *bind to the cell surface receptors* and activate a series of intracellular signal transduction systems.
5. **Amine hormones** also act via surface receptors.
6. *Steroid and thyroid hormones bind to the intracellular receptors* that regulate gene transcription.

Scientist contributed

The **Nobel Prize in Physiology or Medicine 1971** was awarded to American physiologist and endocrinologist, **Earl W Sutherland, Jr** *"for his discoveries concerning the mechanisms of the action of hormones"*. He worked extensively on the physiology of **cyclic AMP.**

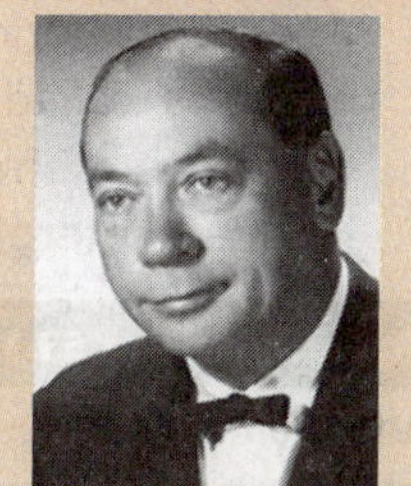

Earl W Sutherland, Jr
(Born 1915)

Receptor Functions

The receptors located on the membrane are usually **large glycoproteins** with molecular weight of 50,000–200,000 dalton. They usually span the membrane seven times. Following binding of hormone with the receptor, **HR complex** is formed, which is **internalized by endocytosis.** Inside the cell, **HR complex is degraded by lysosomal enzymes.**

1. Usually, the receptor molecule is **recycled back to the cell membrane.** However, degradation of the receptor within the cell is not uncommon.
2. Mutation of receptors produces receptor diseases (Application Box 53.1).

Quantity and Sensitivity of Receptor

The receptor quantity and sensitivity are usually regulated by the ***concentration of the hormone*** that acts specifically on that set of receptors. Accordingly, there is **up-regulation, down-regulation, and desensitization** of receptors.

Up-regulation

When, concentration of a **hormone decreases in plasma for a longer period**, the *number of receptors* for that hormone usually increases in the target tissue. Also, *sensitivity of receptor* to the hormone increases. This is called up-regulation.

1. The exact mechanism by which deficiency of hormone results in increased recruitment of its own receptors is not clearly understood.
2. Up-regulation of receptors forms the **physiological basis of denervation hypersensitivity**.

Down-regulation

When, a **hormone is present in excess** in blood for a longer period, the *number of receptors for that hormone in the target tissue decreases*. This is called down-regulation.

Desensitization

When cells are ***chronically exposed to the excess concentration*** of a hormone, they become **less responsive on subsequent exposures**. The process is called desensitization. In this process, the sensitivity of receptors for the hormone decreases.

1. Chronic exposure to one hormone can also cause desensitization of receptors ***to other hormones***.
2. If, desensitization occurs for the same hormone, the effect is called **homologous desensitization**, and if desensitization occurs for other hormones, the effect is called **heterologous desensitization**.

Application Box 53.1

Mutation of receptors: Receptor diseases are produced by mutation of receptors. Examples are Hirschsprung disease due to mutation of endothelin B receptors, familial hypothyroidism due to mutation of TSH receptors, color blindness due to mutation of receptors for cone opsins, X-liked nephrogenic diabetes insipidus due to mutation of V_2 vasopressin receptors and so on.

G PROTEINS

Peptide hormones with the exception of IGF I and IGF II usually circulate freely as they do not have binding proteins for them in plasma. They bind with surface receptors on the target cells. Receptors are **coupled with G proteins** in the cell membrane.

1. G proteins belong to **several families** of intrinsic membrane proteins that link receptors to the nearby effector molecules in the membrane. Also, there are **different subunits of each family** of G proteins. In fact, specific subunit of G protein of a family relay specific signal from the receptors to the effectors that are usually specific ion channels or enzymes.
2. The effector molecules in turn generate second messengers that produce changes in cell functions when hormone binds with the receptors. Thus, **G proteins convert the signal into biological activities.**
3. These membrane proteins are called G proteins **as they are attached to GDP**. When the signal binds with the G protein, G protein **exchanges GDP for GTP**.
4. The **GTP-protein complex** influences subsequent signal transductions that results in **generation of many intracellular signals**, which mediate physiological effects of the hormone (Flowchart 53.1).
5. G protein has the **inherent GTPase activity**, which *converts GTP to GDP*. Therefore, once the hormone action is over, resting state of the G protein is restored.

Flowchart 53.1: Function of G protein.

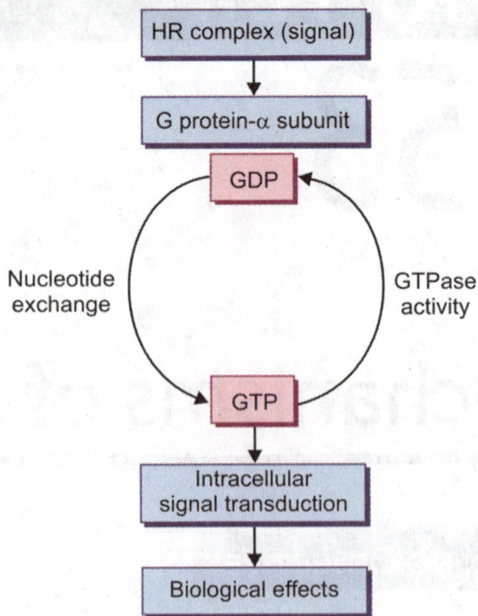

Scientists contributed

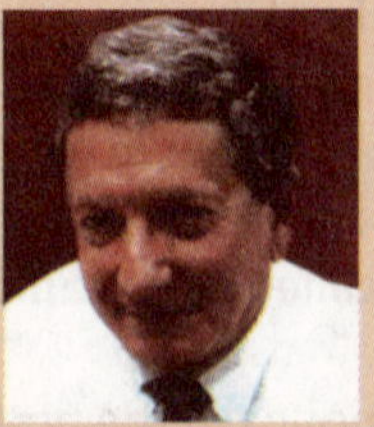

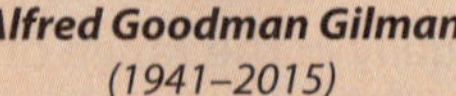

Alfred Goodman Gilman
(1941–2015)

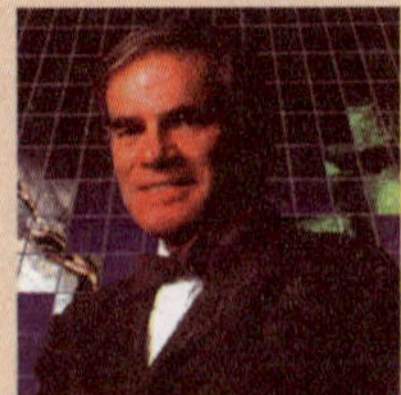

Martin Rodbell
(1925–1998)

Alfred Goodman Gilman (1941–2015) was an American pharmacologist and biochemist. He and Martin Rodbell shared the **1994 Nobel Prize in Physiology or Medicine** "for their **discovery of G-proteins** and the role of these proteins in signal transduction in cells". **Martin Rodbell** (1925–1998) an American biochemist and molecular endocrinologist discovered that ATP could reverse the binding action of glucagon to the cell receptor. He then noted that traces of GTP (guanosine triphosphate) could reverse the binding process almost one thousand times faster than ATP. This GTP, he found, stimulated the activity in the guanine nucleotide protein (later called the G protein), which, in turn, produced profound metabolic effects in the cell.

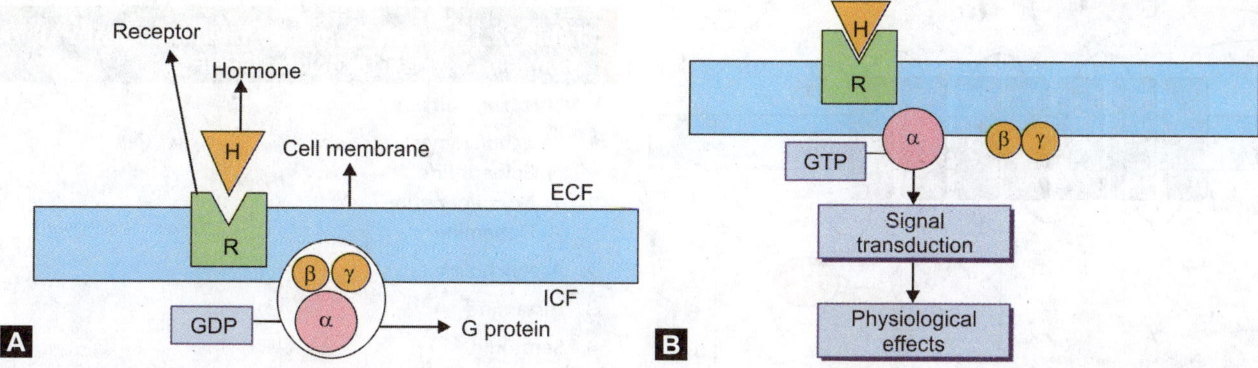

Figs. 53.1A and B: Mechanism of action of hormone through G proteins. (A) Note that G protein has three subunits (α, β, and γ) and GDP is normally attached to the α subunit of G protein, which is a larger subunit; (B) When HR complex is formed (following binding of hormone with receptor), GTP replaces GDP and α subunit is separated from β–γ subunits that remain attached to each other. This separation leads to generation of intracellular signals that in turn mediate hormone action.

Types of G Proteins

Broadly, G proteins are classified into two categories based on their molecular size: **small G proteins and large G proteins.**

Small G Proteins

There are **six different subfamilies** of small G proteins. The major categories among them are **Rab, Rac, and Ras families**. A number of small G proteins contain lipid modifications that help them to adhere to membranes, whereas other small G proteins diffuse throughout the cytosol.

GAPs and GEFs

The GTPase activating proteins (GAPs) inactivate small G proteins by facilitating the hydrolysis of GTP to GDP in the central binding site. Guanine exchange factors (GEFs) activate small G proteins by facilitating exchange of GDP for GTP in the active site.

Functions of Small G Proteins

The small G proteins **regulate many cellular activities**.

The **Rab family** regulates rate of vesicle movement between cell organelles and the cell membrane.

The **Rho/Rac family** mediates interaction between cytoskeleton and the cell membrane.

The **Ras family** controls growth by regulating transmission of signals from the cell membrane to the nucleus.

Large G Proteins

These are the membrane proteins coupled to the receptors. Presently, **five families** of large G proteins have been discovered: G_s, G_i, G_t, G_q, and G_{13}. In addition, there are **three genes** for G proteins: 20α, 6β, and 12γ genes. Therefore, a **large number of subunits** of G protein families are produced. Usually, G proteins are trimeric proteins consisting of three subunits. Therefore, they are called **heterotrimeric G proteins**. The subunits are called α, β, and γ subunits. Normally, α *subunit* is bound to GDP.

Mechanism of Action

When HR complex binds to the **G protein couple receptors** (GPCR), GDP is exchanged for GTP and α subunit is separated from β *and* γ *subunits* of the G protein. This separation of α subunits from β-γ subunits bring about physiological activities (Figs. 53.1A and B). The β and γ subunits do not separate from each other. The α **subunit has the intrinsic GTPase activity** that converts GTP to GDP. This results in reassociation of α subunit with the β and γ subunits of the G proteins. The GTPase activity of α subunit can be facilitated by **regulators of G protein signaling (RGS).**

The α subunit of three types of G proteins (G_s, G_i, and G_q) are physiologically most important. They are **α_s, α_i, and α_q subunits**. Their activation produces following effects:

1. **Activation of α_s subunit** activates the membrane enzyme adenylyl cyclase that promotes cAMP formation.
2. **Activation of α_i subunit** inhibits the membrane enzyme adenylyl cyclase that decreases cAMP formation.
3. **Activation of α_q subunit** activates membrane bound phospholipases like phospholipase C.

G Protein Coupled Receptors

G protein coupled receptors **(GPCR)** are membrane proteins that span the membrane seven times (Fig. 53.2). Hence, they are called **serpentine receptors (seven-helix receptors)**. A large number of GPCR have been cloned recently. They have many diverse functions.

1. When a ligand binds with GPCR, conformational change occurs in GPCR that activates the large G protein attached to the cytoplasmic surface of the cell membrane.
2. Activation of a single GPCR can lead to activation of multiple large G proteins that transduces and amplifies the action of first messenger.

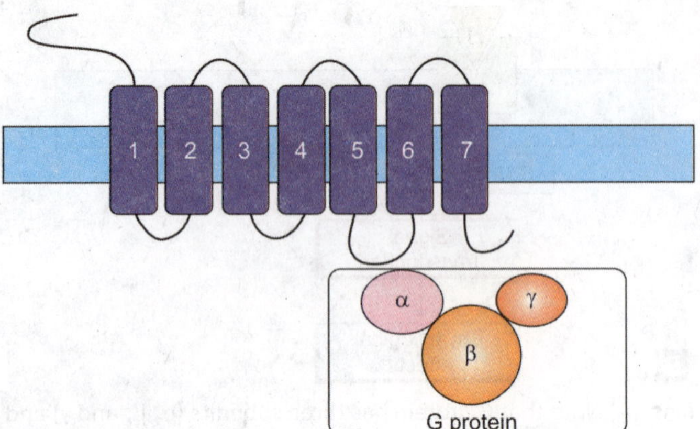

Fig. 53.2: Structure of G-protein coupled receptor (GPCR).

Scientists contributed

Robert Joseph Lefkowitz *(Born 1943)*

Brian Kobilka *(Born 1955)*

Robert Joseph Lefkowitz (1943) is an American physician (cardiologist). He was awarded the **2012 Nobel Prize for Chemistry** with American Physiologist **Brian Kobilka.** Lefkowitz studies receptor biology and signal transduction and is most well known for his detailed characterizations of the sequence, structure and function of the β-adrenergic and related receptors and for the discovery and characterization of the two families of proteins which regulate them, the **G protein-coupled receptor** (GPCR) **kinases and β-arrestins**.

3. The GPCR bound to a ligand can be inactivated by phosphorylation of cytoplasmic side of the receptor to limit the process of cellular signaling.

There are many ligands (hormones/chemicals) for receptors coupled to G proteins (Table 53.1).

G Protein Diseases

Mutation of G protein resulting in diseases is not uncommon. G protein responses may be increased or decreased by mutations.

Dysfunction due to Increased G Protein Responses

An example of increased G protein activity is **somatotroph tumor** causing **acromegaly**, in which mutation of $G\alpha_s$ **decreases its intrinsic GTPase activity**, therefore G protein activity is prolonged and **more cAMP is produced**. This leads to hyperplasia of somatotrophs of anterior pituitary producing acromegaly in about 40% of patients.

Another example is **McCune-Albright syndrome**, in which mutation of $G\alpha_s$ increases G protein activity producing *areas of skin with hyperpigmentation and the state of hypercortisolism*.

Table 53.1: Ligands (hormones/chemicals) that act through G proteins coupled receptors (GPCRs).

A. Neurotransmitters
1. Catecholamines – Epinephrine – Norepinephrine – Dopamine
2. Acetylcholine
3. Histamine
4. Serotonin
5. Adenosine
6. Opioids
B. Other peptides
1. Angiotensin II
2. ADH, Oxytocin
3. GRP, VIP, PTH, TRH
C. Glycoprotein hormones
1. TSH, FSH, LH
2. hCG
D. Arachidonic acid derivative
– Thromboxane A2
E. Tachykinins
1. Neuropeptide K
2. Neurokinin A
3. Substance P
F. Other ligands
1. Endothelins
2. PAF
3. Testants, Odorants

Dysfunction due to Decreased G Protein Responses

An example of decreased G protein responses is **type 1 pseudohypoparathyroidism**, in which **mutation of $G\alpha_s$** leads to failure of G protein to respond to parathyroid hormone. This results in features of hypoparathyroidism without actual decrease in parathyroid hormone.

SECOND MESSENGERS (Signal Transduction Pathways)

Hormones are considered as **first messengers** that bind with the receptors. The hormone (or the ligand) binding with receptors forms the complex called **hormone-receptor (HR) complex**. Formation of HR complex is the first step in the hormone action that eventually leads to formation of second messengers.

In general, the processes of second messenger formation are broadly categorized into **4 types** (Table 53.2):

1. Activation of ion channels
2. Activation of G proteins

Table 53.2: Broad mechanisms of ligands bringing about change in cell functions.
A. Opening or closure of ion channels
1. Ach on nicotinic receptors
2. NE on K^+ channel in heart
B. Via adenylate cyclase (cAMP formation)
1. NE via β_1 receptor (↑ cAMP)
2. NE via α_2 receptor (↓ cAMP)
C. Activation of phospholipase C (DAG, IP_3 formation)
1. Angiotensin II
2. NE via α_1 receptor
3. ADH via V_1 receptor
D. Via cyclic GMP
– ANP, NO
E. Via tyrosine kinase activity
– Insulin, PDGF, M-CSF, EGF
F. Via serine or threonine kinase
– Inhibin, Activin, TGF-β
G. Via nuclear receptors (m-RNA transcription)
– Steroid hormones
– Thyroid hormones

3. Activation of intracellular or membrane enzymes
4. Activation of transcription process.

Role of phosphorylation: Phosphorylation is an important ***post-translational event*** in the cell signaling pathway. Phosphorylation in the cell is controlled by ***two group of proteins*** namely kinases and phosphatases.

1. **Kinases** catalyze the phosphorylation of tyrosine or threonine residues in proteins and **phosphatases** remove phosphates from proteins.
2. More than 300 protein kinases have been described (Table 53.3).
3. The process of phosphorylation-dephosphorylation of cellular proteins is important in control of some ligand signaling pathway, which is referred to as **phosphate timer**.

Second Messengers

The intracellular signal molecules that are formed by a series of enzymatic reactions subsequent to the formation of HR complex are designated as **second messengers**.

1. Second messengers are formed depending on the hormone signaling of the effector cells.
2. The signal transduction pathways are activated depending on G protein activation of membrane enzymes (Table 53.4).
3. **The major second messengers are:** cyclic AMP, diacylglycerol (DAG), inositol triphosphate (IP_3), cyclic GMP, phosphoproteins, transcripted new mRNAs, and intracellular calcium.

Table 53.3: Important protein kinases in the cell.
A. Kinases that phosphorylate serine or threonine residues or both
1. Calmodulin-dependent kinases – Myosin-light cahin kinase – Phosphorylase kinase – Ca^{++}-calmodulin kinase I, II and III
2. Calcium-phospholipid dependent kinases – Protein kinase C
3. Cyclic nucleotide dependent kinase – Protein kinase A (cAMP dependent) – cGMP dependent kinase
B. Kinases that phosphorylate tyrosine residues
– Insulin receptor
– EGF receptor
– PDGF receptor
– M-CSF receptor

Second messengers are formed by activation of **four main transduction systems**:

1. Adenylyl cyclase–cyclic AMP system
2. Membrane phospholipase–phospholipid system
3. Guanylyl cyclase–cyclic GMP system
4. Transcription of mRNAs.

Cyclase–Cyclic AMP System

Cyclic adenosine monophosphate (cAMP) is an important **second messenger for many peptide and amine hormones.** It also causes *lymphocyte activation and mast cell degranulation*. Formation of cAMP and alteration in cell functions by it involve a series of events following interaction of hormone with receptor on the cell membrane (Fig. 53.3).

Steps of Signal Transduction

The steps of signal transduction are as follows:

1. The hormone binds with the receptor present on the cell membrane and forms hormone-receptor complex (**HR complex formation**).
2. HR complex is formed that results in **activation of G proteins** (either α_s or α_i).
3. The membrane enzyme **adenylyl cyclase is activated** (*if α_s is stimulated*).

   Adenylyl cyclase is a membrane protein that spans the membrane 12 times. When the binding of hormone to receptor stimulates the stimulatory G protein (α_s subunit), adenylyl cyclase is activated. If the hormone binding with receptor stimulates the inhibitory G protein the (α_i subunit), adenylyl cyclase is inhibited. (Accordingly, in the next step, cAMP formation is either increased or decreased in the cell).
4. Adenylyl cyclase catalyzes the **conversion of ATP to cyclic AMP**.

Table 53.4: Signal transduction pathways for hormones.

Hormones	Membrane or G proteins	Enzyme activated in the process	Second messenger
PTH, NE (β receptor)	$G\alpha_s$	Adenylyl cyclase (AC)	cAMP
A II, NE (α_2 receptor)	$G\alpha_i$	Inhibition of AC	Decreased cAMP
A II, NE (α_1 receptor), ADH (V_1 receptor), TRH	$G\alpha_q$	Phospholipase C	IP_3, DAG
ANP, EDRF	......	Guanylyl cyclase	cGMP
Insulin, IGF I and II PDGF, EGF, M-CSF	......	Tyrosine kinase (TK)	Phosphoproteins
GH, Erythropoietin	......	JAK/STAT family of TK	Phosphoproteins
TGF, MAPKs	......	Serine or threonine kinase	Phosphoproteins
T3, T4, steroid hormones	......	Transcription process	mRNAs
NE (on K^+ channels)	Membrane ion channels		K^+ (influx or efflux)
Ach (nicotinic receptor)	Ligand gated Ca^{++} channels		Intracellular Ca^{++}

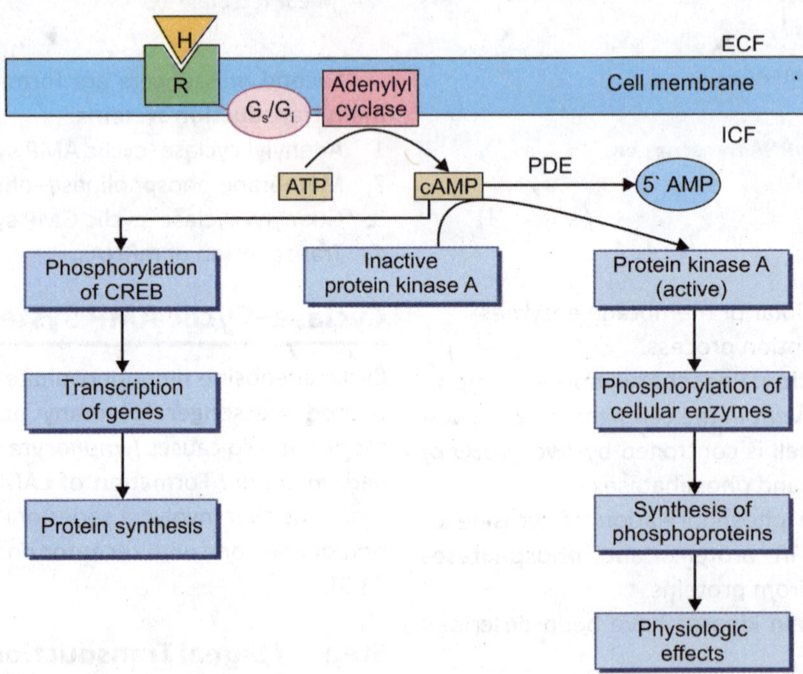

Fig. 53.3: Mechanism of hormone action through adenylyl cyclase-cyclic AMP system. (H: Hormone; R: Receptor; Gs/Gi: Stimulatory G protein or inhibitory G protein; PDE: Phosphodiesterase; CREB: cAMP-responsive element-binding protein).

5. The cAMP **activates protein kinase A** (PKA).
   Protein kinase A (PKA) has two catalytic and two regulatory subunits. cAMP separates catalytic from regulatory subunits. This separation of subunits leads to activation of PKA.
6. Free catalytic subunits **phosphorylate the serine and threonine residues** on many cellular enzymes and other proteins. This process of phosphorylation of intracellular proteins results in **formation of various phosphoproteins.**
7. New phosphoproteins **induce cell functions** (mediate the physiological effects of hormone).

The PKA also migrates to the nucleus where it **phosphorylates CREB** (cAMP-responsive element-binding protein). CREB binds to DNA and influences **transcription of a number of genes**. Thus, cAMP also *alters genetic functions of the cell*.

Termination of cAMP Actions

Actions of cAMP in the cell are terminated in two ways.

1. cAMP is **degraded to 5'–AMP** in the cell by the cytoplasmic enzyme *phosphodiesterase* (PDE).
2. Serine or threonine specific phosphatases **dephosphorylate the proteins** already phosphorylated by PKA.

Clinical Importance

Not only, many hormones act through cAMP (Table 53.5), but also, toxins released by various pathogens produce toxic features by altering cAMP concentration in the cell. **Cholera and pertussis toxins** are examples of stimulation and inhibition of cAMP respectively.

Stimulation of cAMP

In cholera, the highly infective acute diarrheal disease caused by Vibrio cholerae, the **cholera toxin** (especially, subunit A_1 of the toxin) irreversibly transfers ADP-ribose from NAD to its specific target protein, the GTP-binding regulatory component of adenylate cyclase in intestinal epithelial cells. The ADP-ribosylated G protein **up-regulates activity of adenylate cyclase.** Therefore, cAMP production is increased. In intestinal epithelial cells, cAMP **decreases Na^+ absorption and increases Cl^- secretion**. Increased NaCl content in the intestinal lumen osmotically retains water and produces **isotonic fluid diarrhea**. Tea and coffee stimulate cyclic AMP formation (Application Box 53.2).

Table 53.5: Important hormones that act by altering cAMP concentration in the cell.

A. Hormones that act by increasing cAMP formation
1. GHRH
2. CRH
3. GnRH
4. FSH
5. LH
6. Norepinephrine via β_1 receptor
7. ADH via V_2 receptor
B. Hormones that act by inhibiting cAMP formation
1. Norepinephrine via α_2 receptor
2. Somatostatin

Inhibition of cAMP

In pertussis (whooping cough), an acute respiratory tract infection caused by *Bordetella pertussis*, a variety of toxins are produced by the pathogen. A component of pertussis toxin decreases adenylyl cyclase activity **by activating inhibitory G protein.** This impairs the host's defense ability.

Application Box 53.2

Tea and coffee is good for heart: Normally, PDE degrades cAMP in the cells. Therefore, the agents that inhibit the action of PDE like caffeine and theophylline increase the concentration of intracellular cAMP. These chemicals increase myocardial contractility by increasing intracellular cAMP. Caffeine and theophylline are active principles in coffee and tea. Hence, moderate intake of tea and coffee is good for heart, and tea is considered better than coffee in this regard.

Membrane Phospholipid-Phospholipase System (via IP_3 and DAG)

This is an important system for transduction of hormone signals into physiological activities. In this system, binding of hormone with the receptor initiates the following cascade of reactions (Fig. 53.4).

1. Hormone binding with receptor results in **HR complex formation.**
2. HR complex **activates $G\alpha_q$**.
3. Activated $G\alpha_q$ **activates the membrane enzyme phospholipase C.**

   Phospholipase C (PLC) is attached to protein $G\alpha_q$ and is located on the inner surface of the membrane. There are eight isoforms of PLC. Usually, **PLC β_1 and β_2 isoforms** are activated by $G\alpha_q$. They catalyze the cleavage of membrane phosphatidylinositols, the phospholipids present in the inner lamella of cell membrane.

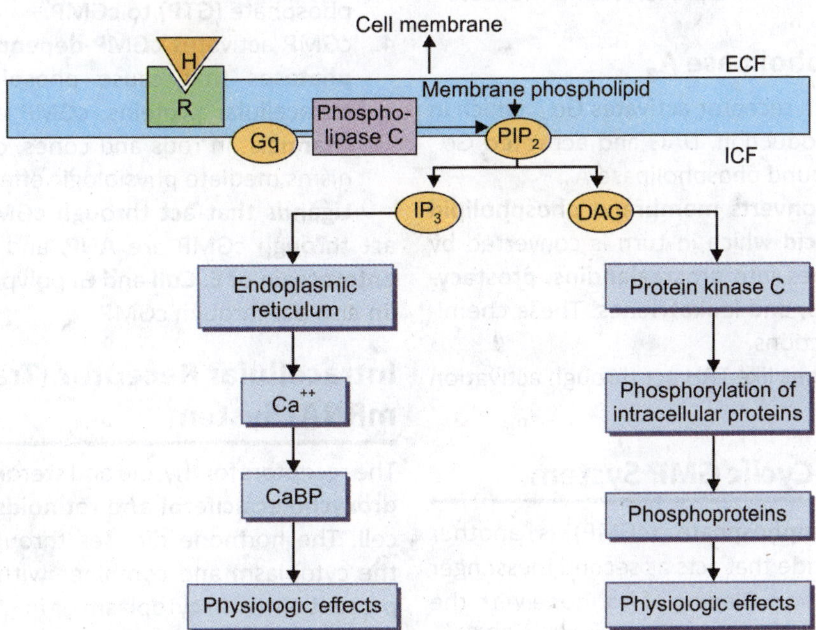

Fig. 53.4: Mechanism of hormone action through membrane phospholipid-phospholipase system. (H: Hormone; R: Receptor; Gq: Gαq protein; PIP_2: Phosphatidyl inositol biphosphate; IP_3: Inositol triphosphate; DAG: Diacylglycerol; CaBP: Calcium binding proteins).

4. PLC β_1 or β_2 causes hydrolysis of phosphatidylinositols 4-5,bisphosphate (PIP_2) that **generates two important signal molecules: *inositol 1,4,5-triphosphate (IP_3) and diacylglycerol (DAG).***
   – IP_3 releases calcium from endoplasmic reticulum.
   – DAG stimulates intracellular (submembrane) enzyme protein kinase C.
5. The **increased protein kinase C activity** activates many intracellular enzymes that bring about change in cell functions. Thus, two subsystems are formed in this pathway: the IP_3 subsystem and the DAG subsystem.

In IP_3 Subsystem:

5a. IP_3 binds with its receptors located on cytosolic surface of endoplasmic reticulum (ER). This binding facilitates **release of Ca^{++} from ER**, which causes cytosolic Ca^{++} to increase several-fold.

6a. Increased intracellular Ca^{++} facilitates **binding of Ca^{++} with calcium-binding proteins** (CaBP) like calmodulin, and also activates CaBP. Ca^{++}-calmodulin dependent protein kinases are also activated in this process.

7a. CaBP alters cell functions.

In DAG Subsystem:

5b. DAG **stimulates the enzyme protein kinase C** (PKC).

6b. PKC causes **phosphorylation of a variety of intracellular proteins** leading to formation of phosphoproteins.

7b. Phosphoproteins alter cell functions.

Examples of hormones that **act via IP_3 and DAG** are: norepinephrine acting via α_1 receptors, ADH acting via V_1 receptors, angiotensin II, TRH, etc.

When the hormone action is over, **IP_3 is metabolized** by dephosphorylation process to inositol, and **DAG is converted** first to phosphatidic acid and then to cytosine diphosphate (CDP). CDP combines with inositol to form **phosphatidylinositol** to be reused in future for hormone action.

Activation of Phospholipase A_2

Binding of hormone with receptor activates $G\alpha_q$, which in turn stimulates DAG production. DAG and activated $G\alpha_q$ stimulate membrane bound phospholipase A_2.

1. Phospholipase A_2 **converts membrane phospholipid into acrachidonic acid** which in turn is converted by a number of enzymes into **prostaglandins, prostacyclins, thromboxanes, and leukotrienes**. These chemicals change cell functions.
2. Few peptide hormones like TRH act through activation of phospholipase A_2.

Guanylyl Cyclase-Cyclic GMP System

Cyclic guanosine monophosphate (cGMP) is another important cyclic nucleotide that acts as second messenger for peptide hormone action. Binding of hormone with the receptor initiates following cascade of events (Fig. 53.5):

1. The hormone binds with the receptor on the surface of the cell.

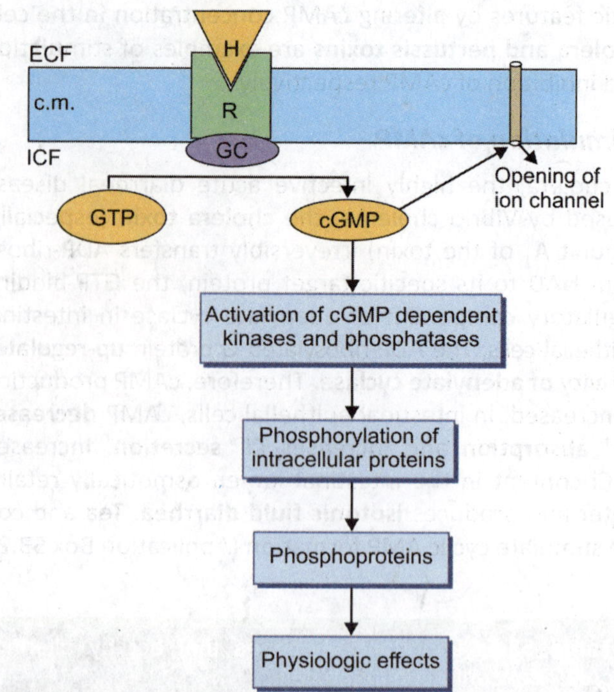

Fig. 53.5: Mechanism of hormone action through GC-cGMP system. (H: Hormone; R: Receptor; GC: Guanylyl cyclase; c.m.: Cell membrane).

2. The HR complex **activates guanylyl cyclase** in the membrane.
   Guanylyl cyclase is the sub-membrane enzyme that forms part of the receptor. In fact, it is the **cytoplasmic domain of the receptor**. Therefore, binding of hormone with receptor automatically activates this enzyme. There are various isoforms of the guanylyl cyclase.
3. Guanylyl cyclase converts cytoplasmic guanosine triphosphate **(GTP) to cGMP**.
4. cGMP activates **cGMP-dependent kinases and phosphatases** that cause phosphorylation of different intracellular proteins. cGMP also **directly opens ion channels.** In rods and cones, cGMP operated mechanisms mediate physiologic effects.
   Ligands that act through cGMP: The hormones that act through cGMP are **ANP,** and **nitric oxide** (NO). The **enterotoxin of E. Coli** and GI polypeptide hormone **guanylin** also act through cGMP.

Intracellular Receptor (Transcription of mRNA) System

The receptors for thyroid and **steroid hormones, 1,25-dihydroxycholecalciferol and retinoids** are located inside the cell. The hormone diffuses through cell membrane into the cytoplasm and combines with the receptor, which is present either in cytoplasm or in nucleus. The receptor for glucocorticoid is present in cytoplasm, whereas the receptor for thyroxine and other steroid hormones are located in nucleus.

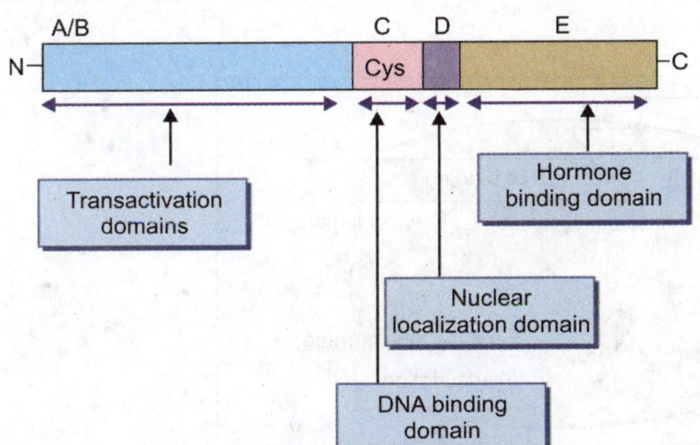

Fig. 53.6: Structure of steroid receptor. C and N at both end of the receptor depict carboxy terminal and amino terminal, respectively.

Receptors

The receptors for steroid hormones are **monomeric phosphoproteins**. They have amazing resemblance with the receptors for 1,25-dihydroxycholecalciferol, thyroid hormones, and retinoic acids. Receptors for all these diverse hormones are considered to be part of a single gene superfamily.

1. They have five domains (A to E), and the **homology is mainly seen for the C domain**, especially C1 subdomain (Fig. 53.6). The estrogen receptor has an extra domain called F domain. The *C1 sub-domain of the receptor is responsible for binding to DNA*.
2. The receptors dimerize when they bind with DNA, which is essential for gene transcription.
3. The receptors have an amino terminal and a carboxy terminal.
4. The **hormone binding domain** is present close to the carboxy terminal.
5. A cysteine-rich **DNA binding domain** is located close to the hormone-binding domain.
6. When hormone binds with receptor, C1 DNA binding domain binds with DNA through two zinc fingers.

Steps of Signal Transduction

Binding of hormone with the receptor triggers following series of events:

1. The binding of hormone with the receptor causes **conformational change** in the receptor protein. The DNA binding domain of the receptor is exposed.
2. The hormone and active-receptor complex then moves to the DNA and **binds with the enhancer elements** (also called hormone response elements or steroid response elements; SRE) in the DNA.
   Normally, steroid receptors are bound to **heat shock protein** (HSP) that covers the DNA binding domain (Fig. 53.7). When hormone binds with receptors, the conformational change in receptor releases the heat shock protein from it, which exposes the DNA binding domain. Heat shock proteins are intracellular proteins and they are so named as their concentration increases on exposure of cells to heat and stress. Therefore, they are also called **stress proteins**. They protect cells from various stresses.
3. The binding of active HR complex to DNA facilitates transcription of mRNAs.
4. The mRNAs are then translated in the ribosomes to form new proteins.
5. Formation of new proteins in the cell alters cell function.

Other Mechanisms of Signal Generation

Tyrosine Kinase Activation

Some peptide hormones do not require G protein for inducing the signal transduction system. The hormone binds with the receptor, which has **intrinsic tyrosine kinase activity**. The receptor has three domains: extracellular, membrane and intracellular domains. The extracellular domain possesses the binding site for hormone and the intracellular domain possesses tyrosine kinase activity.

The **steps of signal induction** are as follows:

1. The binding of hormone with the receptor causes **conformational change in the receptor** that exposes the intracellular sites of the receptor for autophosphorylation (Fig. 53.8).
2. The kinase **autophosphorylates** tyrosine residue within the receptor and tyrosine residues on intracellular protein substrates.
3. The phosphorylation of tyrosine residue initiates cascade of phosphorylation reactions that **phosphorylates various enzymes** like serine and threonine kinases, and phosphatases. Phosphorylated enzymes change cellular activities.

The hormones that act through tyrosine kinase are insulin, IGF I, IGF II, other growth factors like PDGF, and EGF, and M-CSF.

JAK-STAT Pathway

The other method of tyrosine kinase activation is that the hormone binding causes conformational change in the intracytoplasmic tip of the receptor that exposes the sites to which cytoplasmic tyrosine kinase binds.

1. The activation of tyrosine kinase such as Jannus tyrosine kinase (**JAK**) phosphorylates signal transducers and activator of transcription proteins (**STAT proteins**).
2. Activation of **JAK-STAT pathway** further activates intracellular enzymes that change cell function. Example of the hormone acting through JAK-STAT pathway is the growth hormone (for details of mechanism, refer "Growth Hormone").

Calcium–Calmodulin System

This is the system of transduction of the hormone signal in which binding of hormone to a receptor on the cell

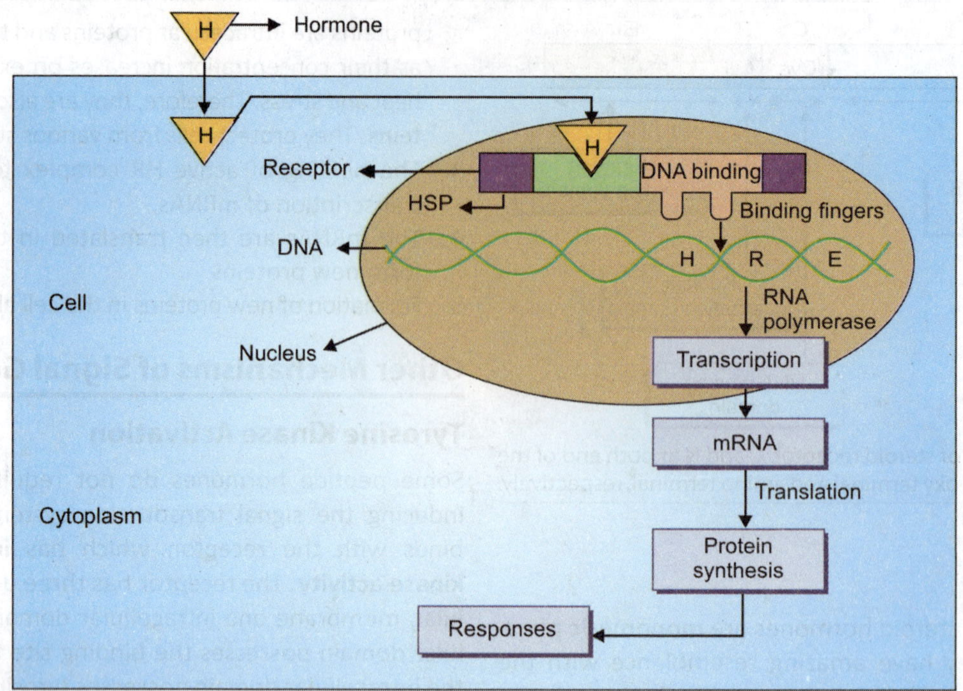

Fig. 53.7: Mechanism of hormone action through intracellular receptor system. The receptor is present either in the cytoplasm or in the nucleus. Note, binding of hormone with receptor exposes DNA binding-domain of the receptor, which interacts with hormone response element (HRE) on DNA.

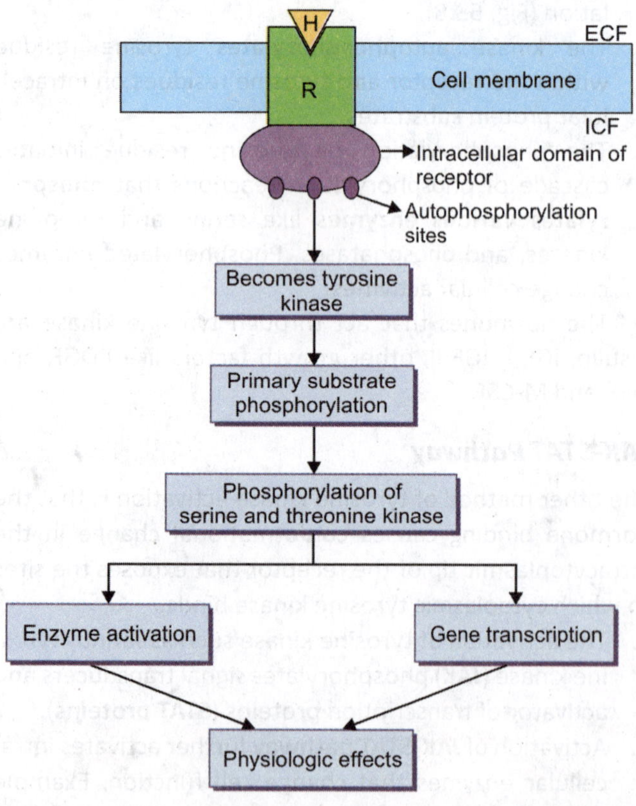

Fig. 53.8: Mechanism of hormone action through tyrosine kinase system. (H: Hormone; R: Receptor).

membrane stimulates G protein to activate a specific membrane channel (for example, **ligand-gated calcium channel**) through which ***calcium from the ECF enters into the cell***. Increased intracellular calcium changes cell function by various mechanisms.

1. Thus, in this system, **calcium is the second messenger** for hormone action.
2. Calcium is also **mobilized from the intracellular storage sites** like mitochondria and endoplasmic reticulum (Fig. 53.9).
3. In many tissues, the secretion of calcium from the intracellular storage sites triggers opening of calcium channels in the cell membrane. This is called **store-operated calcium influx**. This further increases the calcium concentration in the cell and ***replaces calcium in endoplasmic reticulum and mitochondria***. Store-operated calcium influx is mediated through IP_3.
4. Calcium then binds with many intracellular **calcium binding proteins**. One of the important calcium binding proteins is the **calmodulin**.

Calmodulin-dependent Kinases

Calmodulin is a polypeptide containing 148 amino acids and has four calcium binding domains. When calcium binds with calmodulin, it activates different calmodulin-dependent kinases. There are various **calmodulin-dependent kinases** in the cell. The important kinases are:

1. **Myosin light change kinase** that causes phosphorylation of myosin.
2. **Phosphorylase kinase** that causes phosphorylation of many intracellular proteins.
3. Other important kinases are **calcium-calmodulin kinase I, II, and III.** Kinases I and II are concerned with synaptic function and kinase III is involved in protein synthesis.

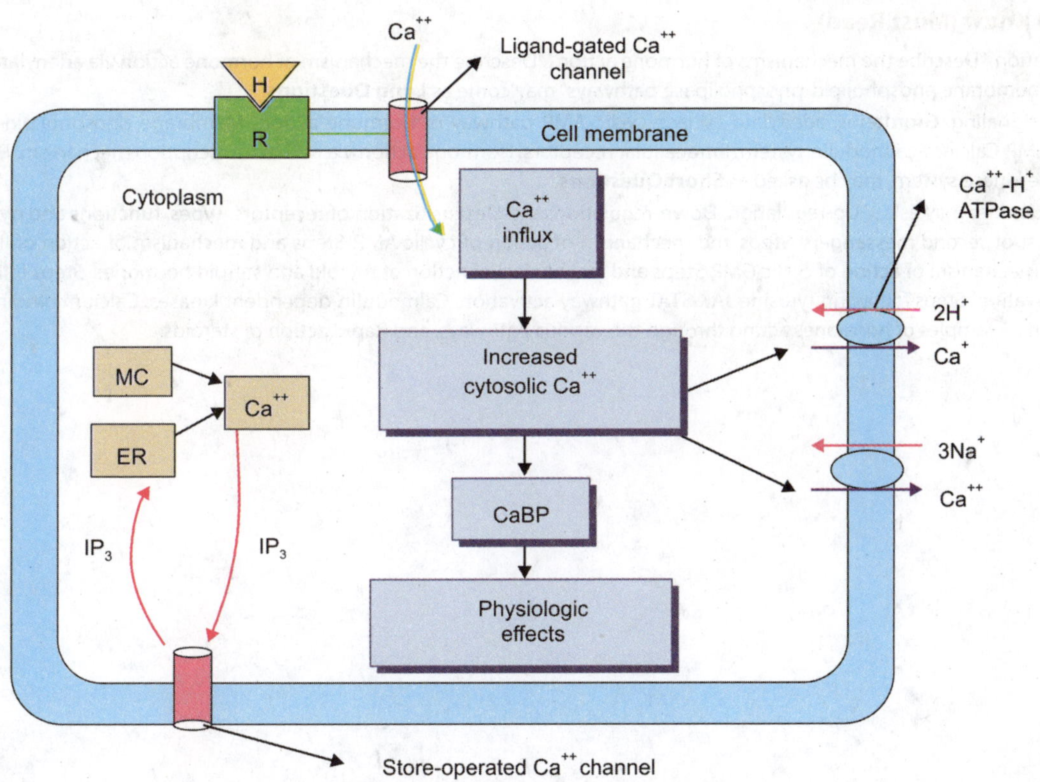

Fig. 53.9: Mechanism of hormone action through calcium-calmodulin system. (H: Hormone; R: Receptor; MC: Mitochondria; ER: Endoplasmic reticulum; IP_3; Inositol triphosphate; CaBP: Calcium binding proteins).

Likewise, there are many kinases that are involved in various cell functions.

Calcium Binding Proteins

The calcium binding proteins in the cells are **calmodulin, troponin, and calbindin.**

1. The troponin is the calcium binding protein present in the skeletal muscle involved in muscle contraction.
2. **Calcineurin**, a calmodulin-activated protein, is a phosphatase, which inactivates calcium channels through dephosphorylation. Calcineurin also participates in immunity by activating T cell.

Rapid Actions of Steroids

Usually steroids act through the intracellular receptor that causes translation and transcription of mRNA to form new proteins. As transcription of mRNA is a time-consuming process, actions (**genomic actions**) of steroids are normally delayed. However, some actions of steroid hormones manifest more rapidly than the transcription process. These are categorized as **nongenomic actions** of steroids.

1. **For nongenomic actions**, the hormone binds with the surface receptors that either changes membrane permeability to ***calcium or other ions***, or stimulates **formation of second messengers** like cAMP in the cell. An example of nongenomic action is the **rapid neuronal changes induced by steroid.**
2. Thus, steroids also act through **intracellular second messengers** that are activated by other hormones.
3. This forms the physiological basis of interaction of steroid hormones with other hormones. For example, ***estrogen and dopamine*** interact at the second messenger level for nongenomic actions of estrogen.

CHAPTER SUMMARY

Key Concepts

1. Protein and amino acid hormones act by altering intracellular levels of cAMP, cGMP, IP_3, DAG, and Ca^{++}. Few hormones act directly by altering ion channels in the membrane and many through the G proteins.
2. Steroid hormones and thyroid hormones act by altering cellular transcription and translation mechanisms.
3. Few hormones like insulin do not require G proteins. Binding with the receptor, activate the intrinsic tyrosine kinase activity of the receptor that triggers the induction of intracellular signaling pathway.
4. Up-regulation and down-regulation of receptors occurs with sustained decrease or increase in the level of hormone in the blood.

Important to Know (Must Read)

1. In examination, "Describe the mechanisms of hormone action", "Describe the mechanism of hormone action via adenylate cyclase-cyclic AMP and membrane phospholipid-phospholipase pathways" may come as **Long Questions**.
2. Hormone signaling, G proteins, adenylate cyclase-cyclic AMP pathway of hormone action, Membrane phospholipid-phospholipase system, cGMP, Calcium-calmodulin system, Intracellular receptors, Hormone action via mRNA transcription mechanism, Hormone action via tyrosine kinase system, may be asked as **Short Questions**.
3. In **Viva**, examiner may ask... Up-regulation, Down-regulation, and Desensitization of receptors, Types, functions and dysfunctions of G proteins, list of second messengers, Steps and mechanism of action of cyclic AMP, Steps and mechanism of action of IP_3-DAG system, Steps and mechanism of action of cyclic GMP, Steps and mechanism of action of thyroid and steroid hormones, Steps following tyrosine kinase activation, Steps following tyrosine JAK-STAT pathway activation, Calmodulin-dependent kinases, Calcium binding proteins and their actions, Examples of hormones acting through the various pathways, and Rapid action of steroids.

CHAPTER 54

Hypothalamus and Hypothalamo-pituitary Axis

Learning Objectives

On completion of study of this chapter, the student **MUST** be able to:

1. Appreciate the importance of hypothalamus as an endocrine organ.
2. List the hormones secreted from hypothalamus and mention their functions.
3. Understand the functional organization of hypothalamo-pituitary axis (HPA).
4. Brief the role of HPA in the regulation of pituitary functions.

The student **MAY** also be able to:

1. Describe the functions of hypothalamic hormones.
2. Explain the function of HPA in the control of pituitary function.

HYPOTHALAMUS

Hypothalamus plays a vital role in the regulation of visceral functions. For its central location in the brain, hypothalamus is closely connected with the limbic system, autonomic nervous system and pituitary gland. Therefore, hypothalamus is the main neural structure for the integration of visceral homeostatic mechanisms. Through the regulation of pituitary secretions, hypothalamus plays a master role in the control of many endocrine functions of the body. As the hormones secreted from hypothalamus (especially to posterior pituitary) are synthesized in hypothalamic neurons, they are called as **neurohormones**.

Scientists contributed

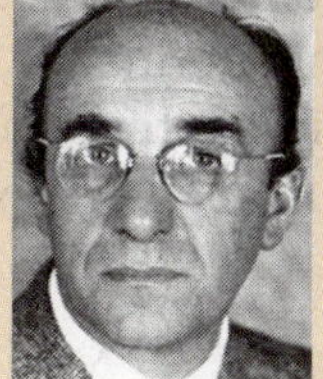

RC Louis Guillemin
(Born, 1924)

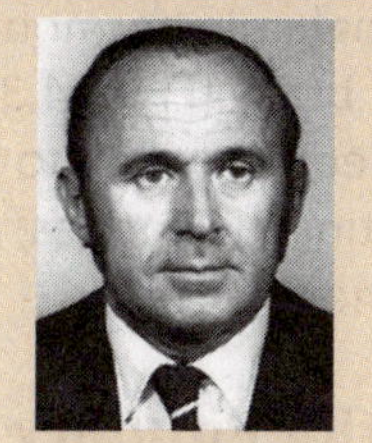

Andrew V Schally
(Born, 1926)

Roger Charles Louis Guillemin received the National Medal of Science in 1976, and the **Nobel prize in Physiology and Medicine for the year 1977** for his work on **neurohormones** (peptide hormones produced in the brain), sharing the prize with **Andrew V Schally**. Guillemin and Schally discovered the structures of TRH and GnRH in separate laboratories.

Hypothalamus as an Endocrine Gland

The hypothalamus plays an important role in the regulation of endocrine functions. It controls all the secretions from pituitary gland.

1. Through its connection with anterior pituitary gland, it controls:
   - thyroid functions (**hypothalamo-pituitary-thyroid axis**),
   - adrenocortical secretions (**hypothalamo-pituitary-adrenocortical-axis**), and
   - gonadal functions (**hypothalamo-pituitary-gonadal axis**).
2. Via its influence on sympathetic output, hypothalamus controls secretions of adrenal medulla (**hypothalamo-sympatho-adrenal-axis**).
3. It directly controls the secretions from posterior pituitary.

Thus, hypothalamus regulates functions of major endocrine glands. Therefore, hypothalamus is apparently designated as the ***"master of endocrine orchestra"***.

Integration with Neural Structures

Anatomically and physiologically, hypothalamus is situated at the center of the brain, below the corpus callosum and thalamus (Fig. 54.1). Therefore, hypothalamus collects and integrates information from various parts of

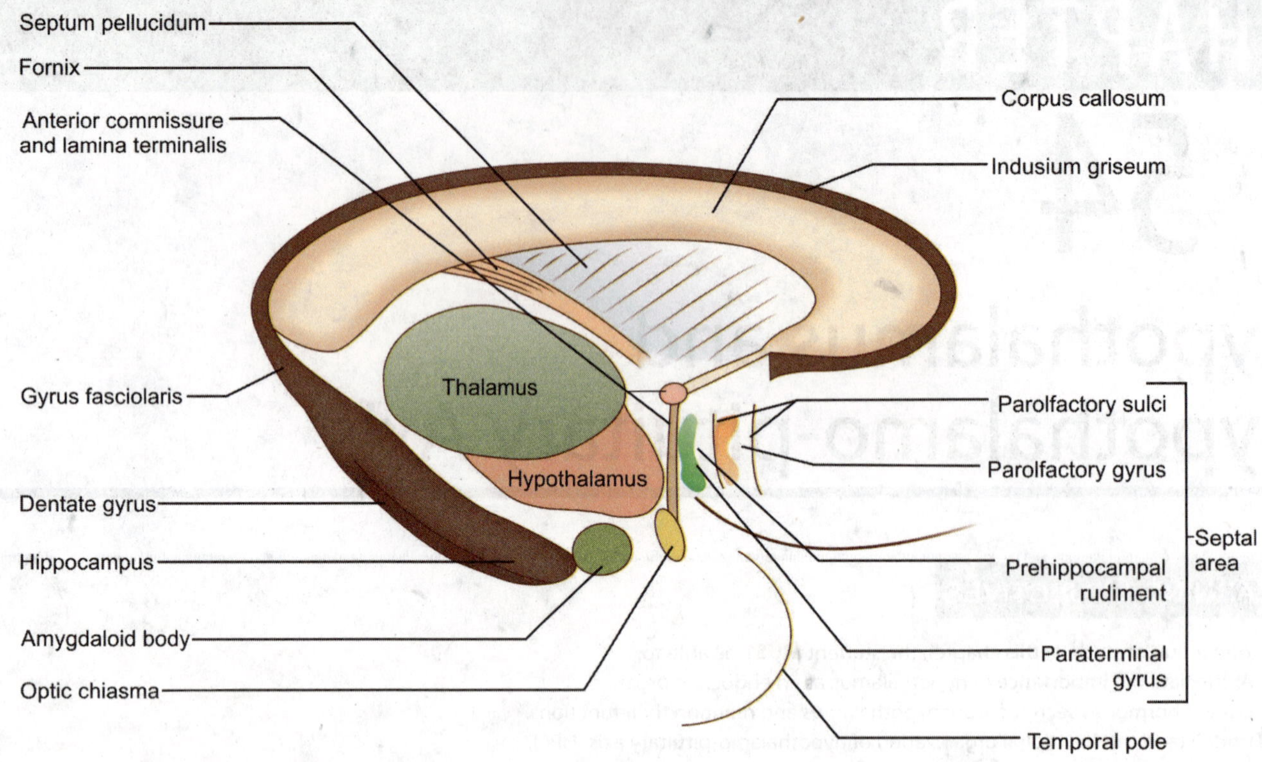

Fig. 54.1: Location of hypothalamus in the brain.

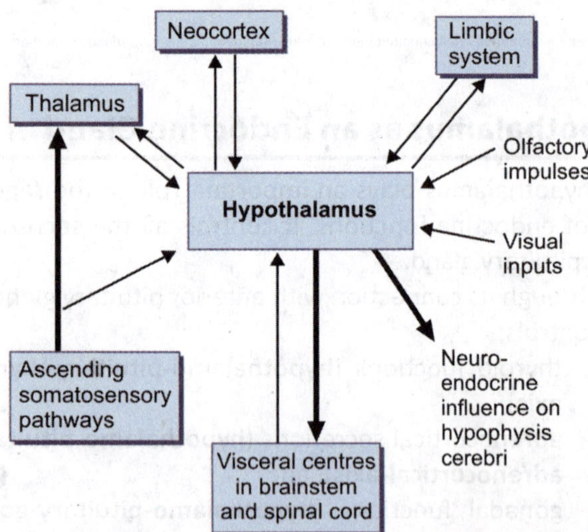

Fig. 54.2: Connection of hypothalamus with other brain centers. Note, after receiving inputs from all these structures hypothalamus funnels these inputs to brainstem and pituitary for regulation of visceral functions.

the brain and funnels them through the pituitary gland for modification of endocrine functions. Thus, hypothalamus is the primary link between nervous and endocrine systems. It receives afferent signals from:

1. Reticular activating system
2. Thalamus
3. Neocortex
4. Eyes
5. Limbic system, especially from amygdala, septum, olfactory bulb, and hippocampus (Fig. 54.2).

These neural inputs convey the information regarding alertness, application of nociceptive stimuli, sleep-wakefulness, changes in environment, emotion, visual, olfactory and gustatory sensations and so on. After gathering these information, hypothalamus appropriately alters body functions partly through its influences on endocrine secretions and partly through its control on major neural outputs from brain like projections from brainstem cardio-respiratory centers, and autonomic and limbic outputs (Flowchart 54.1).

Hypothalamus, via its endocrine influences also controls thirst, appetite, energy store, body fat composition, immunity, behavior and visceral functions. Thus, hypothalamus through its extensive neuroendocrine connections, controls major body functions. Hence, diseases affecting hypothalamic nuclei result in many pathological syndromes.

Hypothalamic Hormones

Hypothalamic hormones are secreted from various nuclei of the brain (Fig. 54.3). Hypothalamic hormones can be classified broadly into **three categories**: anterior pituitary regulating hormones, posterior pituitary hormones and other hormones.

Anterior Pituitary Regulating Hormones

Hypothalamic hormones that regulate anterior pituitary secretions are known as releasing or release inhibiting hormones as they stimulate or inhibit the release of various hormones from this part of the pituitary. The hormones are: Thyrotropin releasing hormone, gonadotropin releasing hormone, corticotropin releasing hormone, growth hormone releasing and inhibiting hormones, and prolactin

Flowchart 54.1: Hypothalamic integration of neural and endocrine functions.

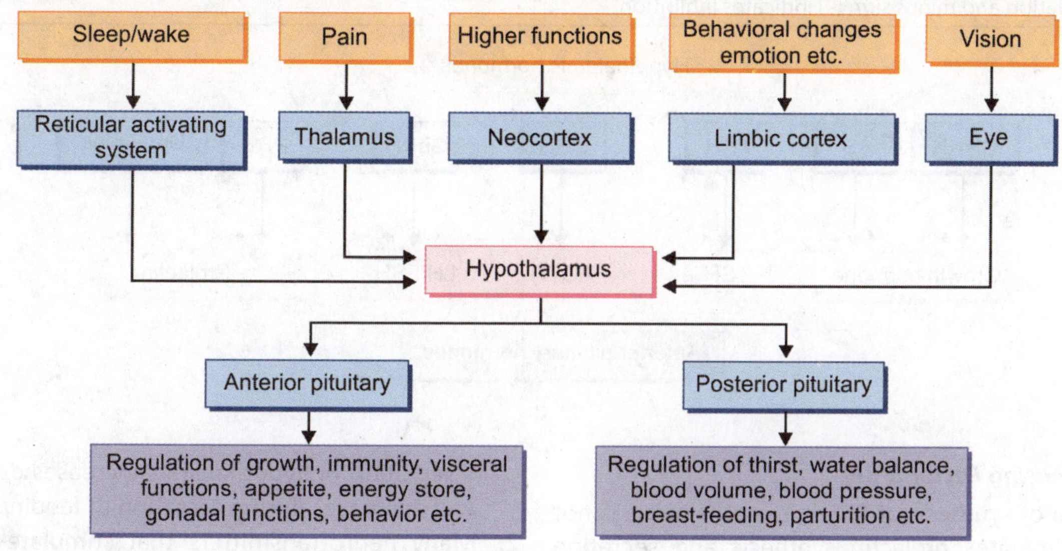

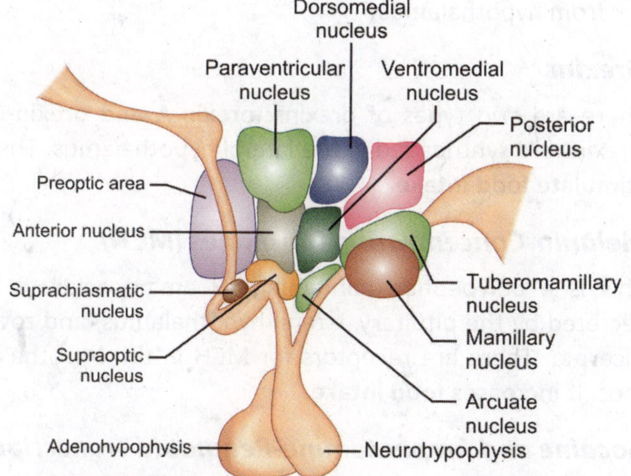

Fig. 54.3: Hypothalamic nuclei.
Courtesy: Figure 84.4, Clinical Anatomy, Vol. 2, 3rd edition, by Neeta Kulkarni, 2016; Jaypee Brothers Medical Publishers (P) Ltd.

releasing and inhibiting hormones (Flowchart 54.2). These are peptide hormones that act on target cells mostly through cyclic AMP and IP3 or DAG as second messengers. They regulate secretions from anterior pituitary.

A. Releasing Hormones

Thyrotropin Releasing Hormone (TRH)

TRH is an oligopeptide containing 3 amino acids.

Source: TRH is secreted from **paraventricular nucleus of hypothalamus.**

Functions:

1. TRH stimulates secretion of thyroid stimulating hormone (TSH) or thyrotropin from thyrotrophs of anterior pituitary.
2. It stimulates expression of genes for α and β subunits of TSH in thyrotrophs.
3. It also promotes secretion of prolactin and growth hormone (GH).

Gonadotropin Releasing Hormone (GnRH)

GnRH is a peptide containing 10 amino acids.

Source: GnRH is secreted from the **arcuate nucleus of hypothalamus.**

Functions:

1. GnRH stimulates secretion of luteinizing hormone (LH); therefore, GnRH is known as luteinizing hormone releasing hormone (LHRH). It also stimulates secretion of follicular stimulating hormone (FSH). Together, it is known as gonadotropins releasing hormone as it stimulates secretion of both LH and FSH.
2. GnRH also stimulates secretion of GH.

Corticotropin Releasing Hormone (CRH)

CRH is a polypeptide having 41 amino acids.

Source: CRH is secreted from **paraventricular nucleus of hypothalamus.**

Functions:

1. CRH stimulates the secretion of adrenocorticotropic hormone (ACTH) or corticotropin from corticotrophs of anterior pituitary.
2. It also stimulates the expression of proopiomelanocortin (POMC) gene in corticotrophs.
3. CRH promotes secretion of β- and γ-lipotropin and β-endorphins.

Growth Hormone Releasing Hormone (GHRH)

GHRH appears in two forms in humans, one containing 40 and other 44 amino acids.

Source: GHRH is secreted from the **arcuate nucleus of hypothalamus.**

Functions:

1. GHRH stimulates secretion of growth hormone from somatotrophs of anterior pituitary.
2. It also stimulates the expression of GH gene in corticotrophs.

Flowchart 54.2: Hypothalamic control of anterior pituitary secretions. PRF: prolactin releasing factor; SS: somatostatin. Plus sign (+) indicates stimulation and minus sign (–) indicates inhibition.

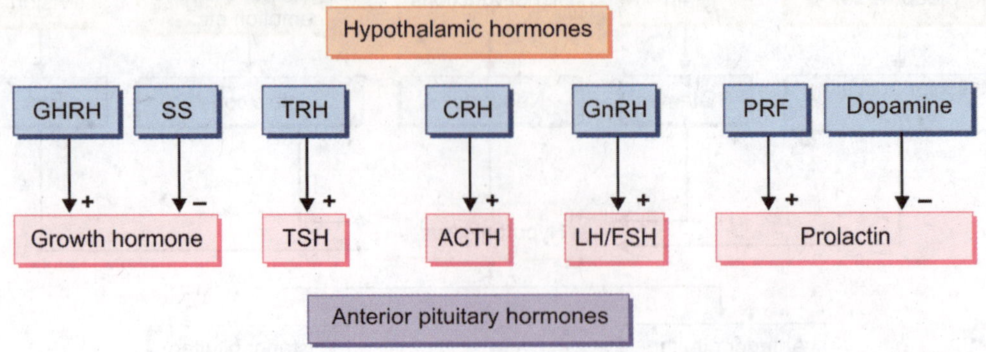

Prolactin Releasing Factor (PRF)

The exact site of synthesis of PRF in hypothalamus is not known. It stimulates prolactin synthesis and secretion from lactotrophs of anterior pituitary.

B. Release Inhibiting Hormones

Growth Hormone Inhibiting Hormone (Somatostatin)

Somatostatin is a peptide having 14 amino acids. It is secreted from **anterior periventricular nucleus** of hypothalamus. It inhibits secretion of growth hormone, prolactin and TSH.

Prolactin Inhibiting Hormone (PIH)

PIH is the **dopamine**, which is secreted from **arcuate nucleus of hypothalamus**. It inhibits secretion of prolactin, TSH, and growth hormone from anterior pituitary.

Posterior Pituitary Hormones

ADH and oxytocin secreted from posterior pituitary are actually not formed in this gland. They are synthesized in supraoptic and paraventricular nuclei of hypothalamus and stored in posterior pituitary (for details, see below and refer the chapter on "posterior pituitary").

Other Hypothalamic Hormones

Other hormones of hypothalamus are **neuropeptide Y, orexins, MCH, ghrelin, MSH and CART**. They are mainly involved in the control of ingestive behaviors and regulation of body weight and composition. Ghrelin is secreted mainly from GI tract, and less from hypothalamus.

Neuropeptide Y

This polypeptide hormone containing 36 amino acids is secreted from hypothalamus. The cell bodies of neurons that synthesize neuropeptide Y are present in the **arcuate nucleus,** and the axons ***project to the paraventricular nucleus***.

1. It is the principal neurohormone that **stimulates food intake**. It has also been observed that neuropeptide Y secretion in hypothalamus increases during feeding and decreases during cessation of feeding (satiety).
2. Many neurotransmitters that stimulate food intake increase neuropeptide Y release and neurochemicals that inhibit feeding decrease neuropeptide Y release from hypothalamus.

Orexins

There are two types of orexins: **orexin-A and orexin-B**. Orexins are synthesized in the lateral hypothalamus. They **stimulate food intake.**

Melanin-Concentrating Hormones (MCH)

This is a polypeptide containing 19 amino acids. It is secreted by the pituitary, lateral hypothalamus, and zona incerpta. There are receptors for MCH in the hypothalamus. It **increases food intake.**

Cocaine and Amphetamine-Regulated Transcript

The hypothalamic hormone CART (cocaine and amphetamine-regulated transcript) **inhibits food intake.**

Applied Physiology

Endocrine hypothalamic dysfunctions lead to abnormalities of hypothalamo-endocrine axes described above. This results in irregularities in anterior and pituitary secretions and many target organ dysfunctions. These are called **hypothalamic syndromes** (for details, refer the Chapter "Hypothalamic Functions" in Neurophysiology).

HYPOTHALAMO-PITUITARY AXIS

The hypothalamus is closely linked with pituitary gland both anatomically and functionally. The connection between hypothalamus and pituitary is called hypothalamo-pituitary axis. Hypothalamus is connected separately and differently with anterior and posterior pituitaries. The connection with anterior pituitary is by means of blood vessels (**portal-hypophyseal vessels**) and with posterior pituitary is through the neurons (**hypothalamo-hypophyseal tract**).

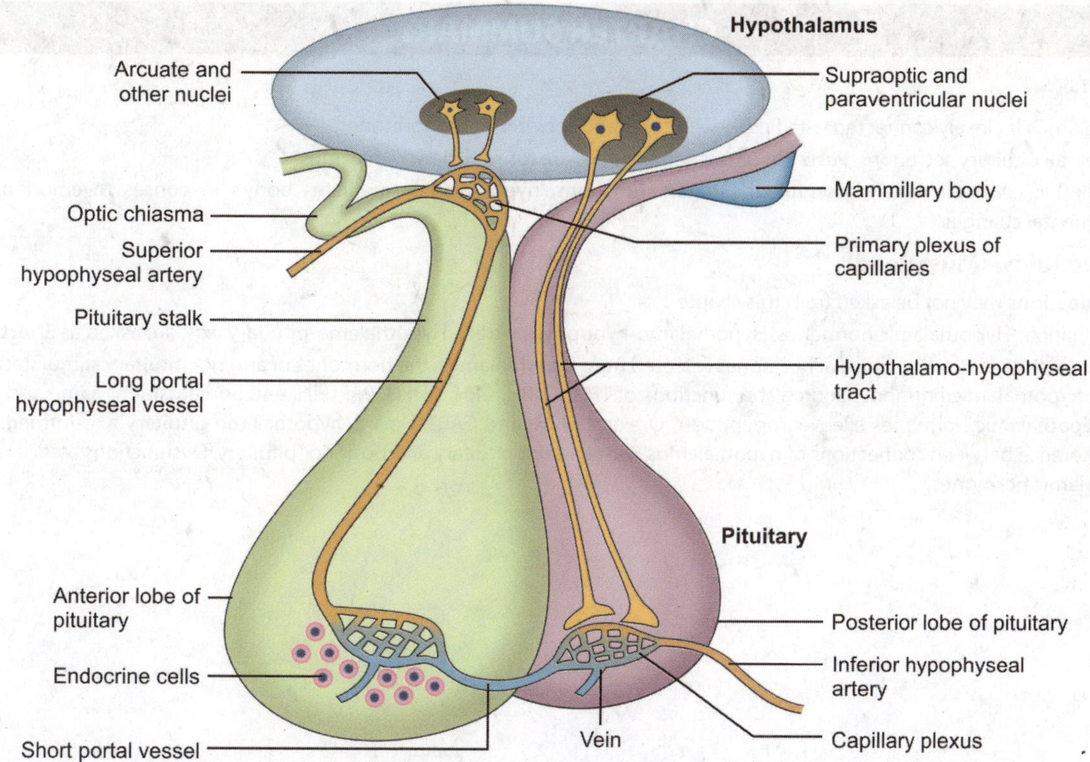

Fig. 54.4: Hypothalamo-pituitary axis. Note, hypothalamus is connected to anterior pituitary via blood vessels (long hypophyseal portal vessel) and to posterior pituitary via neurons (hypothalamo-hypophyseal tract).

Portal Hypophyseal Vessels

The connection between the anterior pituitary and hypothalamus is vascular. Anterior pituitary develops from the **Rathke's pouch**, an evagination from the roof of the pharynx. The portal hypophyseal vessels directly connect between hypothalamus and anterior pituitary.

1. The blood vessels **arise from capillaries** on the ventral surface of hypothalamus (***primary capillary plexus***) that derive blood from **superior hypophyseal artery** (Fig. 54.4).
2. The capillaries drain into the sinusoidal **portal hypophyseal vessels**. These ***long portal hypophyseal vessels*** carry blood down the pituitary stalk to the anterior lobe of the pituitary where they *end in another set of capillaries*. Thus, the system of blood vessels begins with capillaries and ends with capillaries without passing through the heart. Therefore, they are examples of **true portal system of blood vessels** (a portal vessel starts and ends with capillaries without traversing through the heart).
3. The releasing hormones secreted from hypothalamus reach anterior pituitary via hypophyseal portal circulation. Therefore, these hormones are also called **hypophysiotropic hormones.**
4. Hypophysiotropic hormones are synthesized in small hypothalamic neurons (**parvocellular neurons**), the axon terminals of which contact the capillary network in the median eminence and infundibulum in hypothalamus that give rise to long portal vessels in the pituitary stalk.
5. Thus, hypophysiotropic hormones are transported to anterior pituitary via hypophyseal portal blood.
6. **Short portal hypophyseal vessels** communicate the capillaries of anterior pituitary with capillaries of posterior pituitary, which derives blood from **inferior hypophyseal artery**.

Hypothalamo-hypophyseal Tract

The connection between hypothalamus and posterior pituitary is neural. Posterior pituitary develops as an evagination of the floor of the third ventricle. It is formed by the terminals of the nerves, the cell bodies of which are present in the **supraoptic and paraventricular nuclei of hypothalamus**.

1. The cell bodies of these neurons are larger than the cell bodies of other hypothalamic neurons. Therefore, they are called **magnocellular neurons**.
2. The axons arise from these cell bodies and descend down to terminate on the capillary bed in the posterior pituitary. They form the **hypothalamo-hypophyseal tract** (Fig. 54.4).
3. Because of its neural origin and connections, posterior pituitary is known as **neurohypophysis**.
4. Most of the fibers **originating from supraoptic nucleus** *terminate in the posterior pituitary* whereas some of the fibers **originating from the paraventricular nucleus** in addition to their termination on posterior pituitary *also terminate in the median eminence*.

CHAPTER SUMMARY

Key Concepts

1. Hypothalamus is closely connected with limbic structures and secretes neurohormones.
2. It controls all pituitary secretions. Posterior pituitary hormones are formed in hypothalamus.
3. For its limbic connections, and control of pituitary functions, hypothalamus mediates body's responses to emotion, stress and environmental changes.

Important to Know (Must Read)

1. **Long Questions** may not be asked from this chapter.
2. In examination, 'Hypothalamic hormones, Hypothalamo-hypophyseal tract, Hypothalamo-pituitary axis', are asked as **Short Questions**.
3. In **Viva**, examiner may ask… name of hormones secreted from hypothalamus, the hormones of anterior pituitary stimulated or inhibited by each hypothalamic hormone, Source and functions of TRH, GnRH, CRH, GHRH, PRF, PIH, and Somatostatin, name and functions of other hypothalamic hormones like Neuropeptide Y, Orexins, MCH, and CART, How is hypothalamo-pituitary axis formed, What is the main difference between connections of hypothalamus with anterior pituitary and posterior pituitary. Dysfunctions associated with each hypothalamic hormones.

CHAPTER

55

Pituitary Gland: The Anterior Pituitary

Learning Objectives

On completion of study of this chapter, the student **MUST** be able to:

1. Appreciate the importance of anterior pituitary as an important endocrine gland and its role in regulation of body functions.
2. List the hormones secreted from anterior and name the cells that produce them.
3. Describe the regulation, mechanism of action, functions and dysfunctions of growth hormone (GH).
4. Understand the role of GH in regulation of growth and development.
5. Mention the functions and dysfunctions of other anterior pituitary hormones.

The student **MAY** also be able to:

1. Describe the regulation of GH secretion.
2. Explain the mechanism of action of GH.
3. Describe the details of the functions and diseases of GH.

PITUITARY GLAND

The pituitary gland or **hypophysis** controls many aspects of human physiology starting from the birth (delivery of the fetus) and feeding of the baby to the growth and development of the individual to adulthood and reproduce. It controls various aspects of metabolism. It contributes to regulation of blood volume and pressure and body's reaction to stress. Therefore, dysfunctions of pituitary gland result in various clinicopathological disorders.

Scientist contributed

Bernardo Alberto Houssay (1887–1971) was an Argentine physiologist who, in 1947, received one-half of **Nobel Prize for Physiology or Medicine** for his discovery of the role played by anterior pituitary in regulating the amount of blood sugar (glucose) in animals. He shared the prize with *Carl Ferdinand Cori* and *Gerty Cori*, who won for their discoveries of catalytic conversion of glycogen in carbohydrate metabolism. The animals used for pituitary related experiments are called as '**Houssay animals**'.

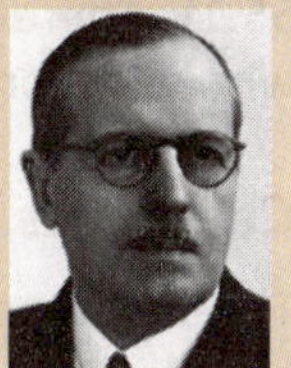

BA Houssay
(1887–1971)

Functional Anatomy

Pituitary gland is situated at the base of the brain in **sella turcica**, a small cavity on sphenoid bone. It consists of **two lobes**: ***anterior and posterior lobes*** (Fig. 55.1). Though,

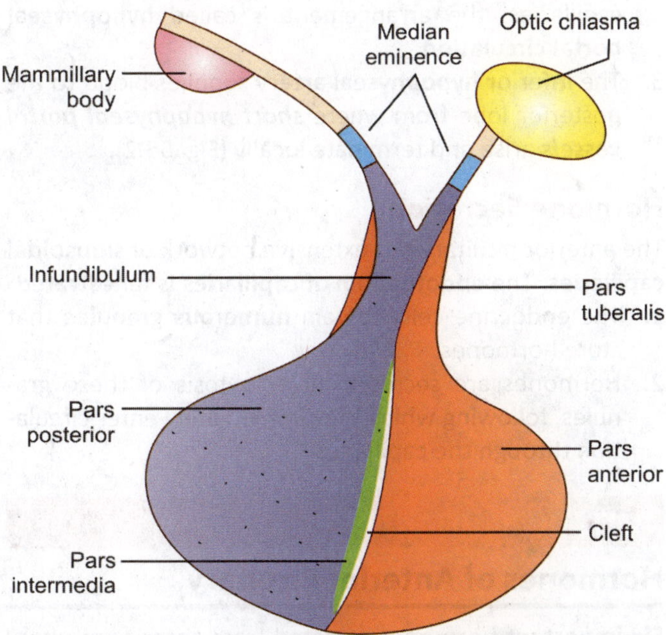

Fig. 55.1: The pituitary gland. Note that intermediate lobe (pars intermedia) is rudimentary. The posterior pituitary (pars posterior) is connected to hypothalamus through infundibulum, and anterior pituitary (pars anterior) is connected to hypothalamus through pars tuberalis.

intermediate lobe of pituitary is present in many species, in human beings, it is rudimentary. Anterior and posterior lobes of pituitary are two separate and distinct glands.

1. The anterior pituitary is rich in various ***endocrine cells***. Hence, anterior pituitary is called **adenohypophysis**.
2. The posterior pituitary contains ***neurons that secrete hormones***. Hence, posterior pituitary is called **neurohypophysis**.

Development

Embryologically, anterior and posterior pituitaries develop from different sources:

1. Anterior pituitary develops as an **evagination from Rathke's pouch** and neurohypophysis develops as part of developing hypothalamus that later merges with Rathke's pouch.
2. Later, endocrine tissue of **anterior lobe becomes purely glandular** (adenohypophysis) and **posterior lobe becomes neuroendocrine** (neurohypophysis).

Blood Supply

Blood supply to pituitary is achieved by means of **superior and inferior hypophyseal arteries**:

1. The **superior hypophyseal artery** terminates in rich capillary network in the median eminence, from where *long hypophyseal portal vessel* arises and descends down the pituitary stalk to end in capillaries in the anterior lobe.
2. As the major hypophyseal vessels start and end with capillaries, the arrangement is called **hypophyseal portal circulation**.
3. The **inferior hypophyseal artery** supplies blood to the posterior lobe from where ***short hypophyseal portal vessels*** arise and terminate locally (Fig. 55.2).

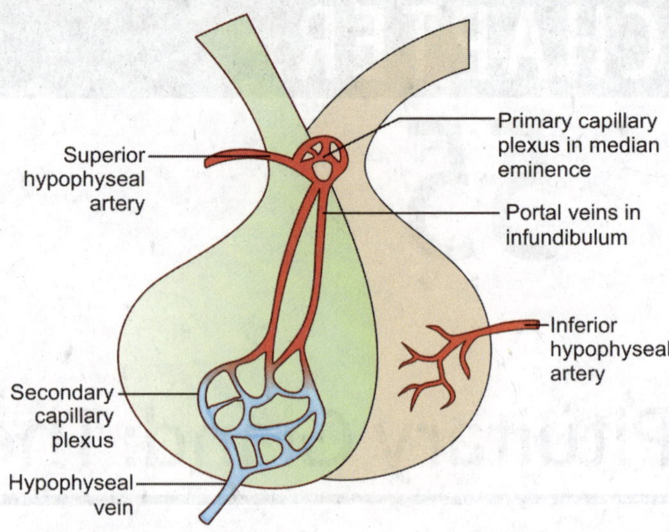

Fig. 55.2: Special arrangement of blood supply of pituitary gland. Note the portal circulation of anterior pituitary and short portal vessels originating from inferior hypophyseal artery for posterior pituitary.

Hormone Secretion

The anterior pituitary has extensive network of **sinusoidal capillaries.** The **endothelium of capillaries is fenestrated**:

1. The endocrine cells contain **numerous granules** that store hormones.
2. Hormones are secreted by exocytosis of these granules, following which they immediately enter circulation through the capillaries.

ANTERIOR PITUITARY

Hormones of Anterior Pituitary

Six important hormones secreted from anterior pituitary are:

1. Growth hormone (GH) or somatotropin
2. Thyroid-stimulating hormone (TSH) or thyrotropin
3. Adrenocorticotropic hormone (ACTH) or corticotropin
4. Follicle-stimulating hormone (FSH) or gonadotropin
5. Luteinizing hormone (LH) or gonadotropin
6. Prolactin

Other hormones are: β-lipotropin (β-LPH), α-melanocyte-stimulating hormone (α-MSH) and interleukins.

Structure

Anterior pituitary hormones are **polypeptides**. LH, FSH, and TSH are glycoproteins containing two subunits: **the α and β subunits**, similar to that of hCG secreted from placenta. The α subunit of these hormones have similar amino acid pattern. Therefore, the β **subunit confers specificity** to the hormones.

Control of Secretion and Major Effects

Secretion of anterior pituitary is controlled **by hypothalamic hormones** (Fig. 55.3). Anterior pituitary hormones in turn control secretion of major endocrine glands of the body except pancreas. They also control growth and development and all aspects of metabolism (Flowchart 55.1). Therefore, diseases of anterior pituitary manifest with widespread and extensive abnormalities.

Cell Types of Anterior Pituitary

The cell types of anterior pituitary are divided into two broad categories: **chromophobes and chromophils.**

Chromophil Cells

The chromophil cells are subdivided into **acidophils** (α cells) **and basophils** (β cells):

1. The *acidophils* are the cells that stain with acidic dyes, and *basophils* are the cells that stain with basic dyes (Fig. 55.4).
2. There are **five types of chromophil cells** (Table 55.1):

- **somatotrophs** that secrete growth hormone,
- **lactotrophs** (or mammotrophs) that secrete prolactin,
- **corticotrophs** that secrete ACTH and β–lipotropin,
- **thyrotrophs** that secrete TSH, and,
- **gonadotrophs** that secrete LH and FSH.

Chromophobe Cells

The chromophobic cells are usually less active and therefore, have few secretory granules.

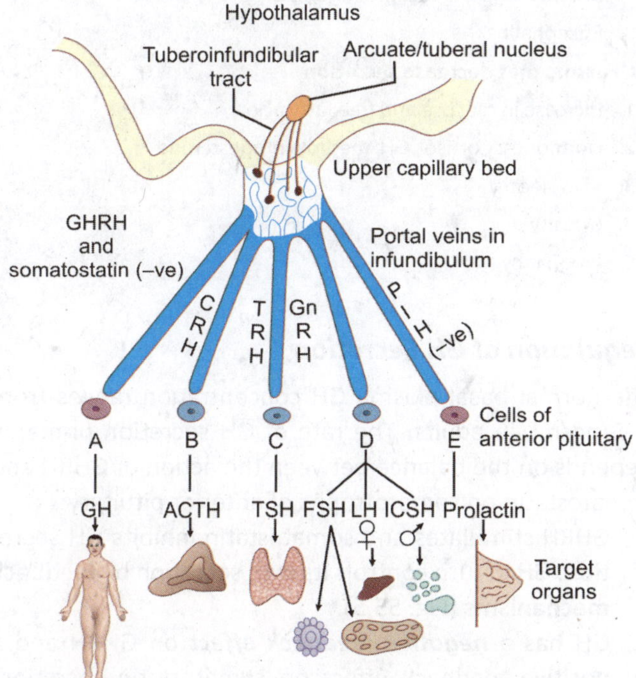

Fig. 55.3: Schematic diagram representing control of pituitary hormones by hypothalamic hormones and major effects of pituitary hormones.
Courtesy: Figure 80.13, Clinical Anatomy, by Neeta Kulkarni, Vol. 2, 3rd edition, 2016; Jaypee Brothers Medical Publishers (P) Ltd.

Folliculostellate Cells

Recently, **folliculostellate cells** have been identified in the anterior pituitary that secrete cytokines, especially IL-6.

GROWTH HORMONE

Growth hormone (GH) is secreted from **somatotrophs** that constitute about 50% of the total endocrine cells of the anterior pituitary. As GH promotes postnatal somatic growth, it is also known as **somatotropin**. It does not stimulate fetal growth. It maintains normal lean body and bone mass in adults. It has many metabolic effects.

Structure

Human GH is a polypeptide containing 191 amino acids. It has structural resemblance with human prolactin and placental lactogen.

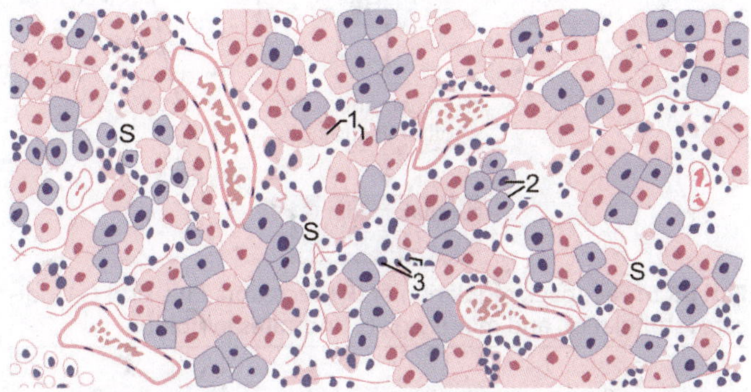

Fig. 55.4: Histology of anterior pituitary gland showing, [1: Acidophil cells (light pink cytoplasm and pink nucleus); 2: Basophil cells (light violet cytoplasm and violet nucleus); 3: Chromophobe cells (small cells in between acidophils and basophils)].

Flowchart 55.1: Hypothalamic-pituitary-target organ axis. Plus sign (+) indicates stimulation and minus sign (–) indicates inhibition.

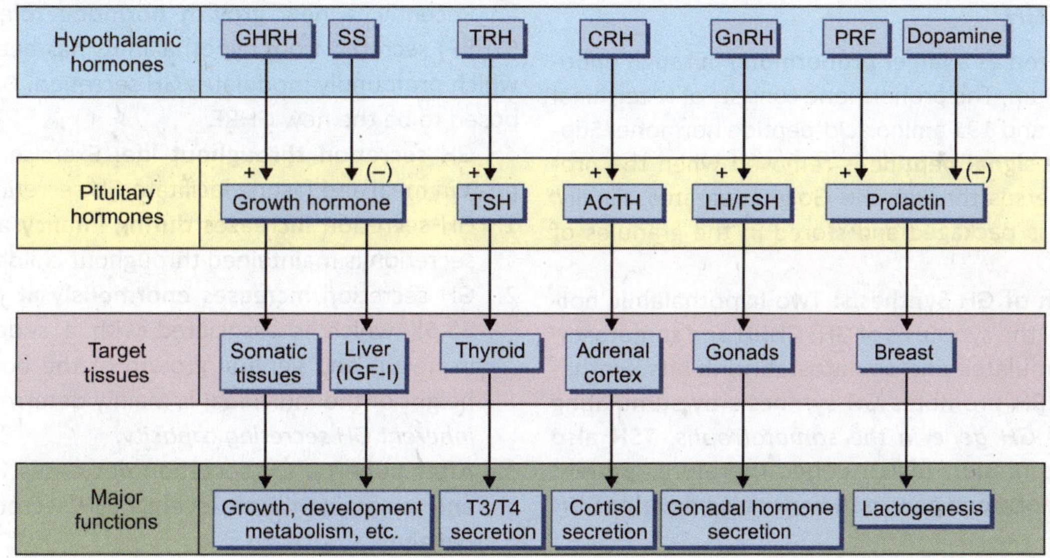

Table 55.1: Hormone-secreting cells of the human anterior pituitary gland.

Cell type	% of total cells	Staining property	Hormone secreted
Somatotrophs	40–50	Acidophilic	Growth hormone
Lactotrophs	10–25	Acidophilic	Prolactin
Corticotrophs	10–20	Basophilic	ACTH
Thyrotrophs	3–5	Basophilic	TSH
Gonadotrophs	10–15	Basophilic	LH and FSH

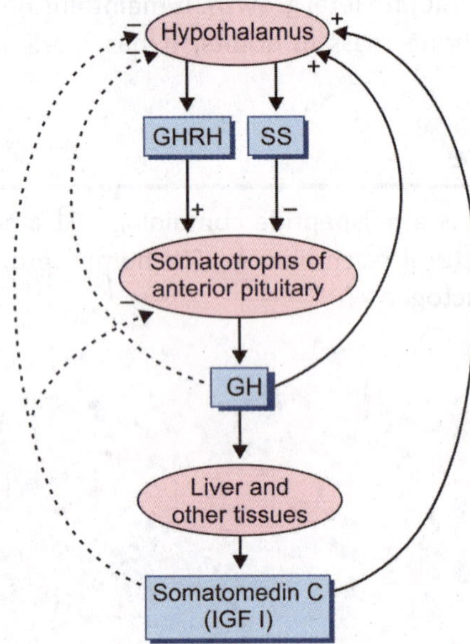

Fig. 55.5: Feedback regulation of GH secretion. Plus sign (+) indicates stimulation and minus sign (–) indicates inhibition.

Table 55.2: Factors affecting GH secretion.

A. Factors that increase secretion
1. Hypoglycemia, as occurs in exercise and fasting
2. Hyperaminoacidemia, as occurs after a high protein meal.
3. Hormones: Estrogens, androgens, acetylcholine, serotonin and glucagon
4. Stress like fever, surgery, etc., or any psychological trauma
5. Puberty
6. Stage IV sleep
7. Drugs: L-dopa, α-receptor agonists, apomorphine
8. Enkephalins
B. Factors that decrease secretion
1. Increase in glucose and free fatty acid
2. Hormones: Cortisol, GH, medroxyprogesterone
3. REM sleep
4. Obesity
5. Pregnancy

Types, Secretion and Metabolism of GH

There are **two forms** of GH: **22 K GH** (molecular weight of 22000) that constitutes 90%, **20 K GH** (molecular weight of 20000) that constitutes 10% of the total circulating GH.

Synthesis of GH

GH is synthesized as a **larger prohormone** in rough endoplasmic reticulum. The prohormone consists of N-terminal signal peptide and 191 amino acid-peptide hormone. Subsequently, the **signal peptide** is removed when the prohormone traverses through the Golgi apparatus. Finally, the hormone is packaged and stored in the granules of somatotrophs.

Regulation of GH Synthesis: Two hypothalamic hormones control the synthesis of GH: GHRH and somatostatin. GHRH stimulates and somatostatin inhibits synthesis of GH. GHRH promotes GH synthesis by stimulating expression of *GH gene in the somatotrophs*. **TSH also stimulates** expression of GH gene. Therefore, **patient with thyroid hormone gene deficiency also develops GH deficiency**.

Regulation of GH Secretion

The normal basal plasma GH concentration ranges from 0–5 ng/mL in adults. The rate of GH secretion primarily depends on the balance between the action of GHRH and somatostatin on somatotrophs of anterior pituitary:

1. GHRH stimulates and somatostatin inhibits GH secretion. GH in turn controls its own secretion by **feedback mechanisms** (Fig. 55.5).
2. GH has a ***negative feedback effect*** on GHRH and a positive feedback effect on somatostatin secretion. GH stimulates production of **insulin like growth factor I** (IGF-1) or **somatomedin C**, which in turn has a negative feedback effect on GH secretion.
3. **IGF I** has effects both at pituitary and hypothalamus levels. Various factors regulate GH secretion (Table 55.2) by influencing secretion of GHRH, somatostatin and IGF I.

Recently, a new **growth hormone releasing factor** (GHRF) secreted from hypothalamus has been identified, which profoundly modulates GH secretion. **Ghrelin** is proposed to be the new GHRF.

GH secretion throughout life: Exercise, stress, high protein meal and fasting facilitate GH secretion:

1. GH secretion **increases during infancy** and then the secretion is maintained throughout childhood.
2. GH secretion **increases enormously at puberty** (Fig. 55.6), which is associated with a sudden increase in height and general growth of the body. The final height of the individual is mainly determined by their *inherent GH secreting capacity*.
3. **After puberty,** GH secretion decreases to adult level and maintains till senescence. GH secretion is less in old age.

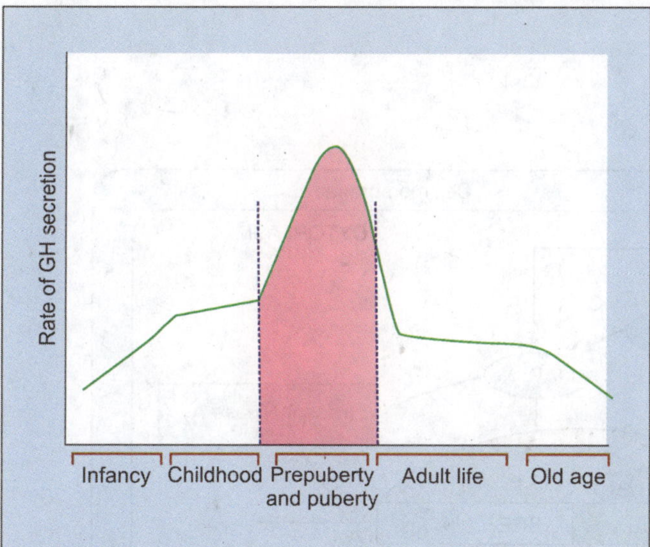

Fig. 55.6: Rate of GH secretion throughout life. Note that secretion is maximum during pubertal life.

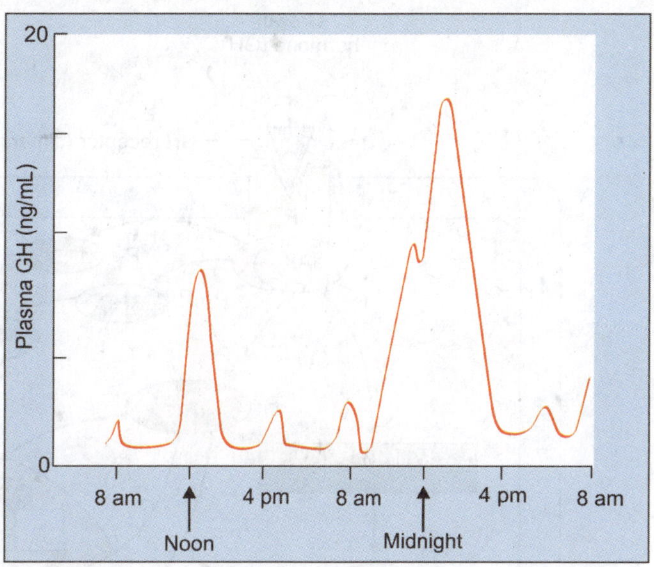

Fig. 55.7: 24-hour fluctuations in plasma GH level. Note, about two-thirds of secretion occurs in the midnight.

GH secretion in sleep: It is not clearly known why GH secretion occurs in episodes or bursts throughout the day when growth occurs slowly over months and years. The pulsatile secretion becomes more prominent in the midnight, especially within first few hours of deep sleep (Fig. 55.7). Approximately, 70% of total 24 hours GH secretion occurs during slow wave sleep (stages 3 and 4) (Application Box 55.1).

Application Box 55.1

Adequate sleep promotes growth: In a normal sleep, maximum time is spent in slow wave sleep. As GH secretion is maximum in slow wave sleep, individuals who sleep adequate usually remain healthy and those who sleep less do not gain weight. Especially, children (this is the growing phase of life) are advised to sleep more to attain normal growth. Those who have sleeplessness, they do not gain weight.

Metabolism

GH binds with a **plasma protein**, which is a **fragment** of the extracellular domain of GH receptor. The concentration of this plasma protein **(GH receptor fragment)** is therefore ***an index of the number of GH receptors in the tissue***:

1. About 50% of the GH is bound to this protein that provides a reservoir of GH in the plasma.
2. GH is metabolized rapidly by the liver.
3. The half life of GH is about 6–20 minutes.
4. Normally, in adult, less than **3 ng/mL** of GH is present in the plasma in basal conditions.
5. Though, only a small quantity of GH is excreted unaltered in urine, **daily urinary output of GH reflects its 24 hours profile.**

Mechanisms of Action

Growth hormone binds with the receptor called **growth hormone receptor,** which is a membrane polypeptide containing 620 amino acids. This receptor neither resemble any of the G protein-linked receptor, nor is it similar to receptors with intrinsic tyrosine kinase activity. Rather, it is a **tyrosine kinase associated receptor** that belongs to the member of ***cytokine receptor superfamily***:

1. It has **three domains**: a large extracellular domain, a transmembrane domain, and a large cytoplasmic domain.
2. GH receptor has **two subunits** and there is binding site on each subunit.
3. When GH binds to one receptor subunit, the binding site on other subunit is attracted and subunits come close to each other. This produces a **homodimer of GH receptor**.
4. This **dimerization is an essential component of receptor activation** as it initiates the activation of a number of enzyme cascades including JAK-STAT pathway of hormone action (Fig. 55.8).
5. The hormone binding with receptor activates following ***four signaling pathways***:
   a. **JAK-STAT pathway: JAK-2** is the member of the family of cytoplasmic tyrosine kinases, known as Jannus kinase. It is associated with but not an integral part of GH receptor. **STAT** is the signal transducers and activators of transcription, which belongs to a family of inactive cytoplasmic transcription factor:
      - Binding of GH with GH receptor activates cytoplasmic domain of it, which induces JAK kinase.
      - STAT on **phosphorylation by JAK kinases** migrate to the nucleus.
      - This results in **induction of various genes** that mediate hormone action.
      - Prolactin and other growth factors also act through the JAK-STAT pathway.
   b. **SHC-Grb pathway:** JAK 2 phosphorylates intracellular protein SHC which in turn activates Grb2 proteins. **Grb2 proteins** stimulate MAP kinase that induces various gene transcriptions.

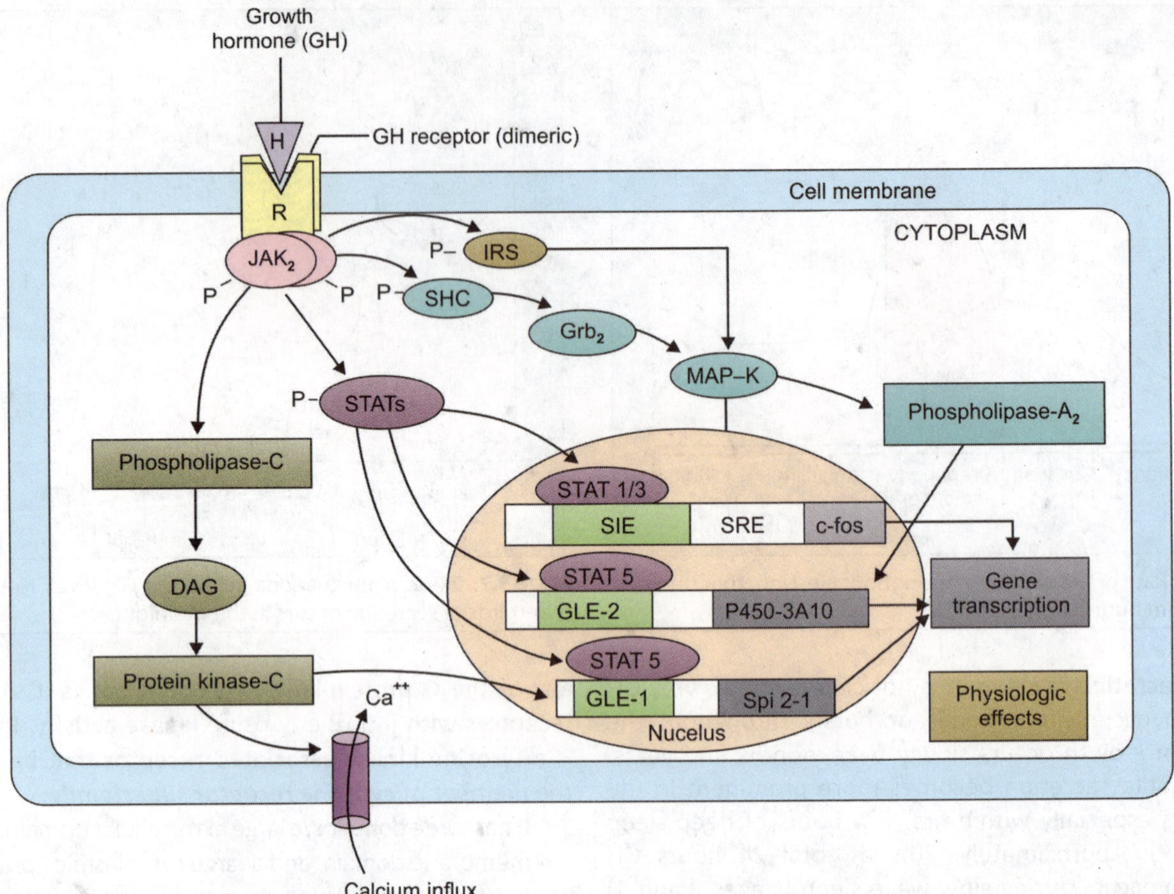

Fig. 55.8: Mechanism of action of GH. Binding of GH with its receptor causes dimerization of the receptor. Dimerization activates JAK 2 (intracellular portion of the receptor), which in turn activates gene transcription via various pathways. (JAK: Jannus kinase; STATs: Signal transducer and activator of transcription factors; IRS: Insulin receptor substrate; SIE: Sis-induced element; SRE: Serum response element; GLE: Interferon-activated response element; SHC and Grb2: Intracellular proteins; MAP-K: Mitosis activated protein kinase; DAG: Diacylglycerol).

c. **TK-IRS pathway:** Activation of JAK-tyrosine kinase causes **phosphorylation of IRS** (insulin receptor substrate) which in turn induces various intracellular enzymes.

d. **Phospholipase-C pathway:** HR complex also stimulates membrane enzyme **phospholipase C**, which results in production of DAG. **DAG initiates calcium influx** into the cell and probably, also initiates gene transcription.

Physiological Actions of GH

Growth hormone is an anabolic hormone with profound **short-term metabolic effects** and **long-term growth promoting effects**:

1. **Acute metabolic effects** of GH like lipolysis in adipose tissue, decreased glucose uptake by muscle and stimulation of gluconeogenesis by hepatocytes are due to its **direct actions** on target tissues.
2. Whereas, many **long-term effects** of GH are mediated by **somatomedins** (IGF-1 and IGF-2) produced by it. Growth promoting effects are also part of the direct effects of GH (Flowchart 55.2).

Direct Actions of GH

Effects on Growth

The most striking and specific effect of GH is the **stimulation of linear growth**, which occurs due to its action **on the epiphyseal cartilage of long bones**. GH stimulates *all aspects of metabolism of chondrocytes* (the cartilage forming cells). The major actions of GH on chondrocytes include:

1. Incorporation of **proline into collagen** and its conversion into **hydroxyproline** (Application Box 55.2).
2. Incorporation of sulfate into the proteoglycan chondroitin. The hydroxyproline and chondroitin together form the extracellular matrix of cartilage. Thus, GH **promotes cartilage matrix formation**.
3. Increased amino acid uptake and **protein synthesis**, and increased RNA and DNA synthesis in chondrocytes.
4. Increase in **size and number of chondrocytes**.
5. GH also acts directly on progenitor or stem cells such as **prechondrocytes** in growth plates of bone. It facilitates the **differentiation of prechondrocytes to chondrocytes**.

All these actions result in **growth of epiphyseal cartilage** that increases the length of the bone and consequently promotes linear growth of the body. Thus, GH increases the height of the individual before closure of epiphysis.

Flowchart 55.2: Direct and indirect (mediated through IGF-I) actions of GH.

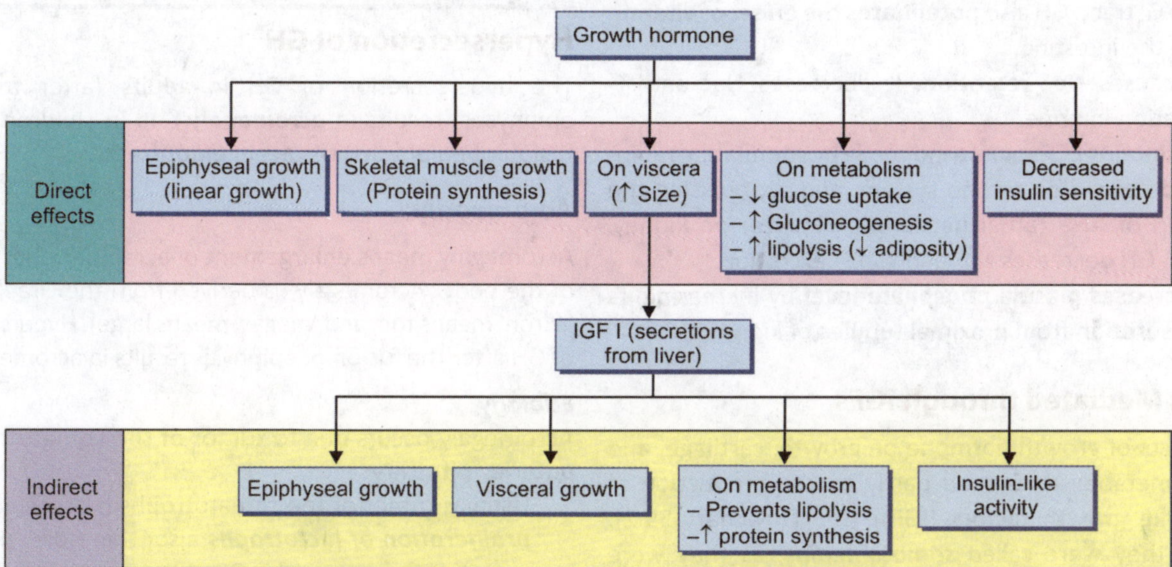

Application Box 55.2

Hydroxyprolinuria reflects GH activity: Increased secretion of GH manifests as hydroxyprolinuria (excretion of hydroxyproline in the urine). Hydroxyproline is derived from collagen. As GH increases the soluble collagen synthesis, hydroxyproline is formed and excreted. Thus, hydroxyprolinuria is an index of GH activity. However, hydroxyprolinuria is also associated with diseases that cause collagen destruction.

Other growth promoting effects of GH include:

1. **On bone:** GH stimulates the activity of bone modeling units. It increases activity of both osteoclasts and osteoblasts. However, **osteoblastic activity predominates**, and therefore bone formation becomes more. The total bone mass and mineral content of bone increase.
2. **On skeletal muscle:** GH increases the growth of skeletal muscle by increasing protein synthesis and causing hypertrophy of skeletal muscle cell. It also *promotes activity of satellite cells* of skeletal muscle. **Satellite cells** are progenitor cells in skeletal muscles.
3. **On visceral organs:** GH also **stimulates growth of many visceral organs** like liver, kidney, heart, pancreas, intestine, etc., many endocrine organs, skin, and connective tissue. All these organs **increase in size and function** due to *hypertrophy and hyperplasia* in response to GH. Organs grow in size due to:
   - increased protein synthesis,
   - increased RNA and DNA synthesis and
   - increase in cell size and number.

   The general visceral functions like digestion and specific visceral functions like cardiac output and GFR improve.
4. **Pubertal and gonadal growth:** GH increases height during puberty. It also sensitizes gonads to the actions of LH and FSH. Thus, GH promotes *prepubertal sexual maturation*.

Effects on Protein Metabolism

The effects of GH on general somatic growth are primarily due to the **protein anabolic effects**. These include:

1. Positive nitrogen and phosphorus balance.
2. **Increased amino acid entry** into the cells in many tissues.
3. Increased **RNA and DNA synthesis** in the cell.
4. Increased **protein synthesis.**
5. Decreased plasma level of amino acid and urea that occur secondary to amino acid entry into the cells and increased protein synthesis.

Effects on Carbohydrate Metabolism

Growth hormone is a **prodiabetogenic hormone** as it causes hyperglycemia by following actions:

1. It increases release of glucose from liver by **facilitating hepatic neoglucogenesis.**
2. It **decreases glucose uptake** by skeletal muscle.
3. Decreases insulin sensitivity.

However, GH **stimulates insulin secretion** indirectly by increasing the ability of pancreas to various insulinogenic stimuli. IGF-I, secreted mainly from liver under the influence of GH has insulin like activity. Thus, indirectly GH also promotes growth, as insulin is a growth stimulating hormone.

Effects on Fat Metabolism

Growth hormone causes **lipolysis and increases plasma level of FFA**. By increasing FFA, it **promotes ketogenesis.** As it increases FFA and ketoacids in plasma, GH provides energy in various conditions of hypoglycemia and stress.

Effects on Electrolyte and Water Metabolism

Growth hormone influences concentration of various electrolytes by following mechanisms:

1. GH **increases plasma Ca^{++}** by increasing its absorption from GI tract. GH also **potentiates the effect of vitamin D** on the intestine.
2. GH causes **Na^+ retention.** It decreases Na^+ and K^+ excretion in urine.
3. It **maintains ECF volume** indirectly by stimulating renin-angiotensin-aldosterone system, and suppressing the action of ANP (atrial natriuretic peptide) on kidney. Thus, GH decreases Na^+ and water excretion.
4. It **increases plasma phosphate level** by increasing its reabsorption from proximal tubules of kidney.

Effects Mediated through IGFs

The effects of growth hormone on growth, cartilage, and protein metabolism depend partly on the production of **insulin-like growth factors** (IGFs) (*see* Flowchart 55.2). Initially, they were called ***somatomedins***, as they were found to mediate the somatic effects of GH:

1. The principal circulating somatomedins are **insulin-like growth factors-I** (IGF-I, which is also called as ***somatomedin C***) and **insulin like growth factors-II** (IGF-II).
2. IGF-1 and II have similar actions as insulin and therefore, are called insulin like growth factors.
3. IGFs are **polypeptide** growth factors synthesized mainly in the liver.
4. They are also formed in cartilages and other tissues.

IGF-I

IGF-I is more potent in mediating the effects of GH than IGF-II. It is a **polypeptide** containing 70 amino acids:

1. **IGF-I receptor** is very similar to insulin receptor.
2. IGF-I is secreted independent of GH before birth. However, after birth, IGF-I secretion and actions are dependent on GH. Its **plasma concentration is 10–700 ng/mL**, which peaks at puberty. The concentration of IGF-I rises in childhood, attains peak at puberty and declines in old age.
3. It binds with plasma protein called **insulin-growth factor binding proteins** (IGFBP). There are **six IGFBPs.** ***IGFBP-3 is the most prevalent*** IGFBP, which serves as reservoir for IGFs in plasma.
4. IGF-I mainly causes **skeletal and cartilage growth.**

IGF-II

IGF-II is independent of GH action and plays an **important role in the fetal growth**. It is a polypeptide containing **67 amino acids**:

1. IGF-II receptor is a mannose-6-phosphate receptor.
2. In adults, IGF-II genes are expressed only in the choroid plexus and meninges.
3. The plasma concentration of IGF II is 300–800 ng/mL.

Applied Physiology

Hypersecretion of GH

The hypersecretion of GH in adults (after fusion of epiphyses) results in ***acromegaly*** and in children (before fusion of epiphyses) results in ***gigantism***.

Acromegaly

Acromegaly means enlargement of acral (peripheral) parts of the body. 'Acromegaly' is derived from the Greek words, 'akron' means top, and 'megas' means large). Hypersecretion of GH **after the fusion of epiphysis** results in acromegaly.

Etiology

Acromegaly occurs due to **tumor of the somatotrophs of anterior pituitary**:

1. Usually, tumor of the somatotrophs is associated with ***proliferation of lactotrophs*** also; therefore, **prolactin secretion is increased** in 20–40% of patients.
2. Acromegaly can also occur due to **extra-pituitary causes** like increased hypothalamic secretion of GRH (in *hypothalamic tumors*).

Features

Enlargement of acral parts of the body, especially of hands and feet, **prognathism** (protrusion of lower jaw), **acromegalic facies** (overgrowth of malar, frontal and facial bones), increased amount body hair, **osteoarthritis** (due to skeletal changes), glucose intolerance, hirsutism, gynecomastia and lactation, increased heel pad thickness, and **visual field changes** (bitemporal hemianopia) are common features (Fig. 55.9).

1. **Visceromegaly** increases the size and function of the viscera. Macroglossia may be seen.
2. Enlargement of acral parts and skeletal deformities occur as ***bones enlarge in width***. Bones cannot grow in length as epiphyses are already closed.
3. The **visual defects** are due to the effect of the pituitary tumor that enlarges the sella turcica and *compresses on optic chiasma*. This also causes **headache.**

Management

Disease is diagnosed by typical clinical presentation, demonstration of pituitary tumor by CT scan or MRI and demonstration of high GH level in plasma by estimation of the hormone. **Surgical removal** of tumor is the best option to cure the disease.

Gigantism

Hypersecretion of GH **before fusion of epiphysis** results in gigantism.

Causes

Pituitary tumor (of somatotroph) during childhood resulting in increased GH secretion causes gigantism. ***Hypothalamic tumor*** causing excess GHRH secretion can also produce the disease.

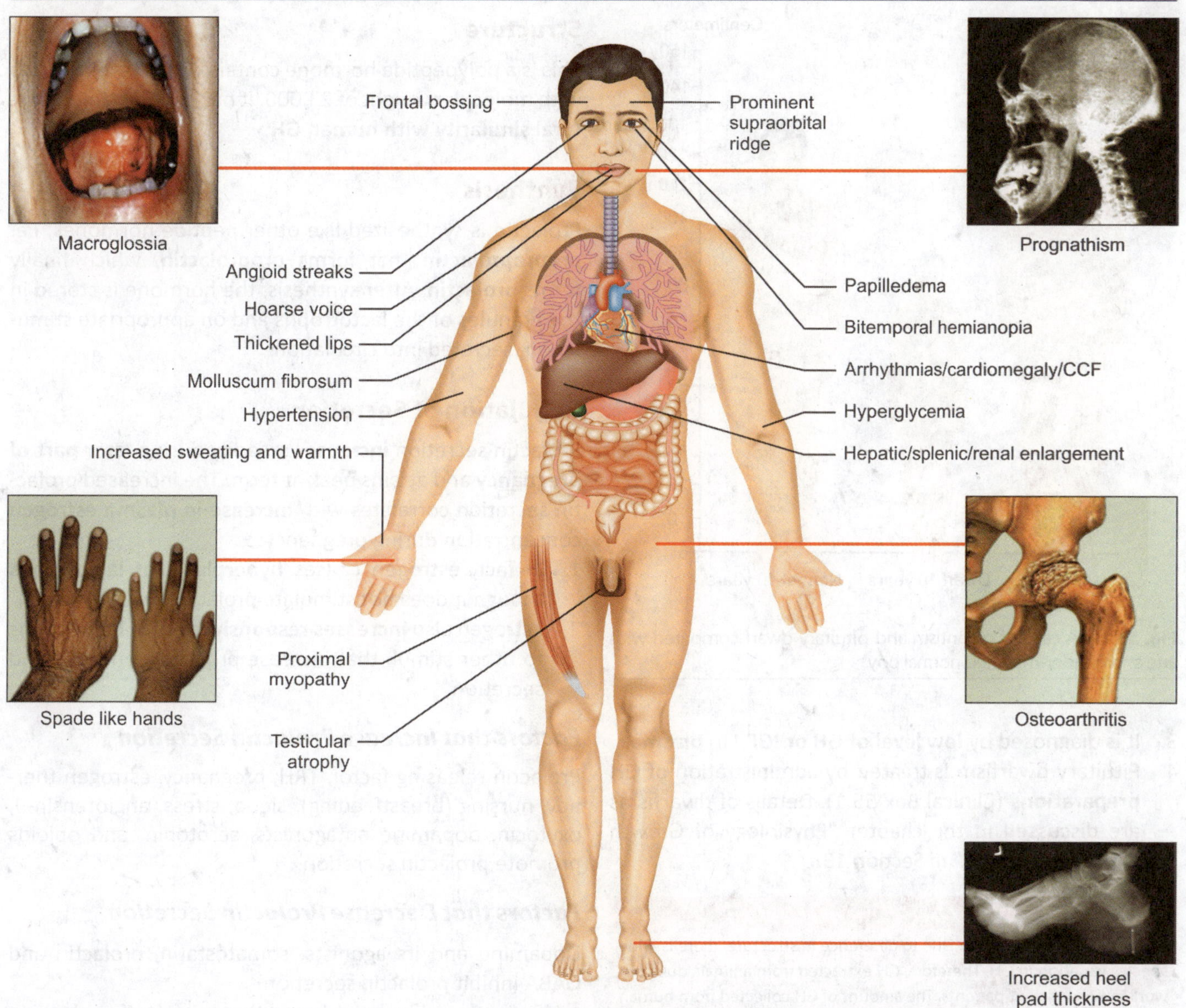

Fig. 55.9: Features of Acromegaly. Note the presence of acromegalic facies (malar and frontal prominence) and prognathism (enlarged and protruded mandible as shown in skull X-ray), enlarged acral parts of the body (increased hand and finger size as compared with a normal hand), osteoarthritis, macroglossia, increased heel pad thickness and increased size of visceral organs (visceromegaly).
Courtesy: Figure 10.1, page 757, Manual of Practical Medicine, by R Alagappan, 5th edition, 2014; Jaypee Brothers Medical Publishers (P) Ltd.

Features

Increased GH secretion before closure of epiphysis **increases the epiphyseal growth of long bones**. Therefore, the patient becomes **abnormally tall**, with giant stature (Fig. 55.10). Other features are same as acromegaly except the acromegalic facies.

Management

Disease is diagnosed by typical clinical presentation, demonstration of pituitary tumor by CT scan or MRI and demonstration of high GH level in plasma by estimation of the hormone. Surgical removal of tumor at the earliest cures the disease.

Hyposecretion of GH

Deficiency of GH results in **dwarfism**.

This may occur due to four causes:

1. Decreased GRH deficiency (hypothalamic failure)
2. Decreased GH secretion (pituitary failure)
3. Decreased IGF synthesis by the liver (as seen in African pygmies)
4. Decreased or unresponsive GH receptors (**Laron dwarfism**).

Pituitary Dwarfism

A pituitary dwarf (dwarfism due to **GH deficiency**) is characterized by **short stature** and correspondingly delayed bone and sexual maturation (Fig. 55.10):

1. **Decreased muscle and total body mass**, decreased cardiac function and decreased bone density are common.
2. **Mental power relatively remains normal** in a pituitary dwarf, which helps in differentiating from a **thyroid dwarf** in whom mental retardation is an outstanding feature.

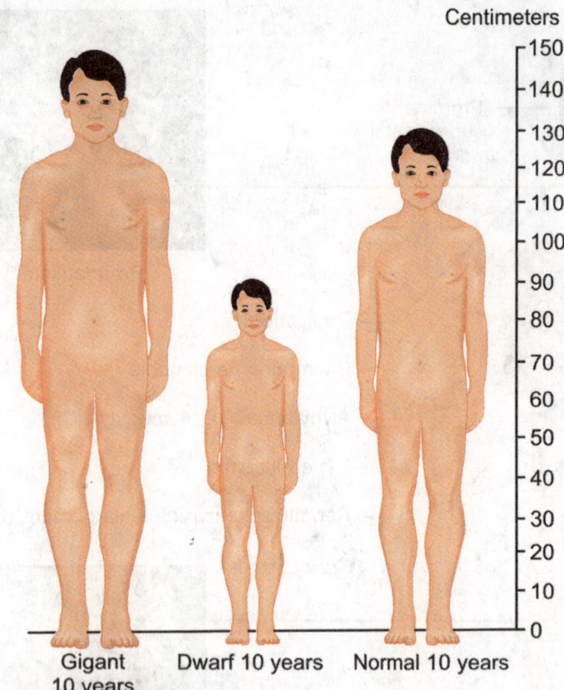

Fig. 55.10: A case of gigantism and pituitary dwarf compared with age and gender-matched normal boy.

3. It is diagnosed by **low level of GH or IGF-I in plasma.**
4. Pituitary dwarfism is treated by administration of **GH preparations** (Clinical Box 55.1). Details of dwarfisms are discussed in the chapter "Physiology of Growth and Development" in Section 13.

Clinical Box 55.1

Recombinant human GH: Due to difference in structure, there is wide species variation in GH. Therefore, GH extracted from animals does not work in GH deficient patients. The amount of GH collected from human pituitaries at the time of autopsy is not adequate for treatment of GH deficient dwarfs. Presently, large quantity of human GH is produced by recombinant DNA technology that meets the need of the GH deficient children.

OTHER HORMONES

Prolactin

Prolactin is the hormone for milk synthesis. The term 'prolactin' refers to a hormone that favors lactogenesis ('pro' favoring, and 'lactin' lactogenesis). It also influences development of the mammary gland, reproductive functions and immune responses.

Source

Prolactin is secreted from the **lactotrophs of anterior pituitary,** which constitutes 10–25% of the total secreting cells of the gland. However, lactotroph population **increases during pregnancy, lactation, and estrogen therapy.**

Structure

This is a polypeptide hormone containing **198 amino acids** with molecular weight of 23,000. It has considerable structural **similarity with human GH**.

Synthesis

Prolactin is synthesized like other peptide hormones, i.e. **preproprolactin** that forms **proprolactin**, which finally forms **prolactin**. After synthesis, the hormone is stored in the granules of the lactotrophs and on appropriate stimulation, secreted into circulation.

Regulation of Secretion

Prolactin secretion **increases steadily during later part of pregnancy** and attains peak at term. The increased prolactin secretion correlates with **increase in plasma estrogen** concentration during pregnancy:

1. In fact, **estrogen causes hyperplasia of lactotrophs** though it does not stimulate prolactin synthesis.
2. Estrogen also **increases responsiveness of lactotrophs** to other stimuli that increase prolactin synthesis and secretion.

Factors that Increase Prolactin Secretion

Prolactin releasing factor, TRH, pregnancy, estrogen therapy, nursing (breastfeeding), sleep, stress, angiotensin-II, oxytocin, dopamine antagonists, serotonin, and opioids promote prolactin secretion.

Factors that Decrease Prolactin Secretion

Dopamine and its agonists, somatostatin, prolactin and GABA inhibit prolactin secretion.

Recently, it has been found that a **prolactin releasing factor** is secreted from hypothalamus. However, the exact nature of the chemical is not yet known. **TRH stimulates prolactin secretion**. Dopamine has been identified as **the prolactin inhibiting factor** (PIF) secreted from hypothalamus (Clinical Box 55.2). Somatostatin also inhibits prolactin secretion. Prolactin stimulates secretion of dopamine and somatostatin, those in turn inhibit prolactin secretion. Thus, prolactin **controls its own secretion** by this feedback mechanism (Fig. 55.11).

Clinical Box 55.2

Dopamine is used in hyperprolactinemia: Dopamine is a potent inhibitor of prolactin secretion. Therefore dopamine is used in the treatment for conditions of hyperprolactinemia and dopamine antagonists are used in conditions of hypoprolactinemia.

Mechanism of Action

Prolactin binds with the prolactin receptors that are homologous with GH receptors in their extracellular domain. Binding of hormone with the receptor activates the cytoplasmic domain of the receptor, which in turn

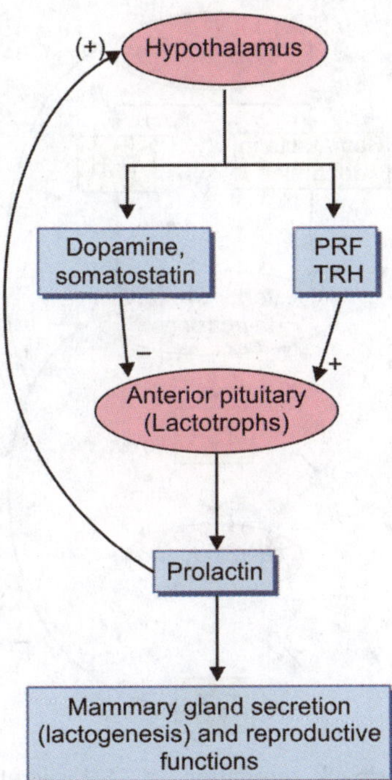

Fig. 55.11: Feedback regulation of prolactin secretion. Plus (+) indicates stimulation and minus (–) indicates inhibition. Note, prolactin stimulates secretion of dopamine and somatostatin from hypothalamus that are known to inhibit prolactin secretion. Thus, prolactin inhibits its own secretion by negative feedback mechanism.

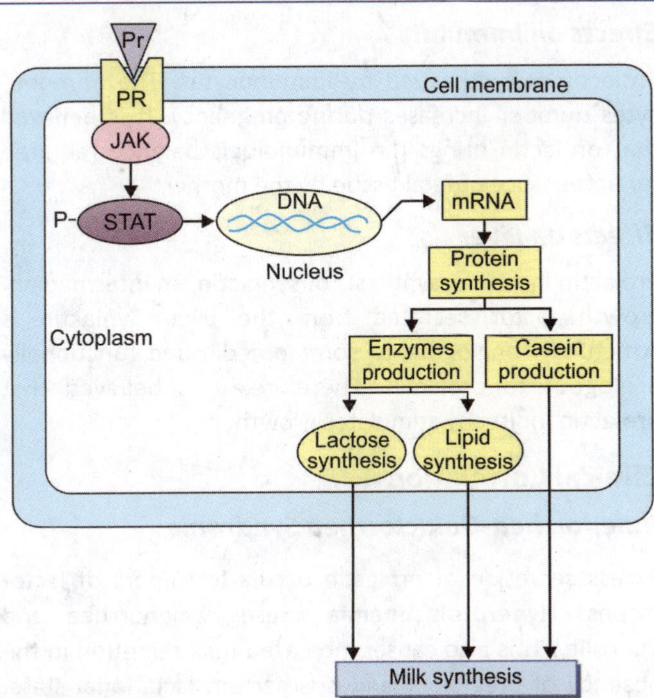

Fig. 55.12: Mechanism of prolactin action. Prolactin (Pr) binds with prolactin receptor (PR) on cell membrane of lobular cells (in which lactogenesis takes place) of alveoli of mammary gland that activates intracellular JAK-STAT pathway for gene transcription. (JAK: Jannus kinase; STATs: Signal transducer and activator of transcription factors).

activates cytoplasmic tyrosine kinases (Fig. 55.12). Activation of **JAK-STAT signal induction pathway** stimulates formation of transcription factors that induces DNA and mRNA synthesis. Increased formation of mRNA promotes **specific protein synthesis** in the ribosomes, which in turn causes formation of casein, lipid and lactose, the ingredient of milk. Thus, milk production is stimulated.

Physiological Effects

Effects on Milk Synthesis and Secretion

The primary function of prolactin is to **stimulate milk synthesis and secretion** (therefore, the name pro-lactin). Therefore, prolactin secretion increases during lactation.

Effects on Breast Development

Prolactin causes **hyperplasia of breast tissue** before and after puberty. It also causes hyperplasia of breast tissue **during pregnancy and lactation**:

1. Together with estrogen, progesterone, cortisol and GH, it stimulates development (**branching and proliferation of ducts**) of the female mammary gland.
2. Along with estrogen and progesterone, especially during pregnancy, it **increases the lobules of alveoli** of the mammary gland in which milk is produced.
3. During lactation, together with insulin and cortisol, it **increases milk synthesis and secretion** in the mammary gland.

Effects on Reproduction

In Females

Increased prolactin concentration in plasma ***inhibits hypothalamic GnRH secretion***. Therefore, the concentration of LH and FSH decreases during lactation:

1. This ***prevents ovulation*** and causes **amenorrhea in lactating mothers** (Clinical Box 55.3). This is called **lactational amenorrhea.**
2. Prolactin also controls some reproductive behaviors such as **inhibition of libido** in human beings and stimulation of **maternal behavior** (love, affection and protective behavior of the mother for the newborns).

In Males

In males, prolactin **decreases spermatogenesis.**

Clinical Box 55.3

Lactation prevents pregnancy: After delivery, pregnancy does not occur till active breast feeding continues. Lactation prevents pregnancy by maintaining high prolactin concentration that in turn inhibits GnRH secretion. Decreased GnRH **inhibits ovulation**. Therefore, conception does not occur till breastfeeding continues **(physiological contraception during lactation)**. Breastfeeding has **two important objectives**: First, to provide best food for the baby, and second, to prevent pregnancy, so that automatically adequate spacing occurs between two children. The first one is important for the educated mothers as now-a-days breastfeeding is practiced less amongst them, the second one is essential for uneducated mothers.

Effects on Immunity

Prolactin is synthesized by immunocytes. The immunocytes number increases during pregnancy. It is believed that prolactin brings the immunologic balance required for acceptance of fetal tissue by the mother.

Effects on Liver

Prolactin increases synthesis of **synlactin**, an intermediary growth factor secreted from the liver. Synlactin is structurally analogous to somatomedin and functionally analogous to prolactin. Therefore, it is believed that prolactin indirectly stimulates growth.

Clinical Correlation

Amenorrhea-Galactorrhea Syndrome

Excess secretion of prolactin occurs in tumors of lactotrophs. **Hyperprolactinemia** causes amenorrhea and infertility. This also causes increased milk secretion in the absence of pregnancy and postpartum lactational state. Therefore, the condition is called **amenorrhea-galactorrhea syndrome**:

1. This is seen in **hypothalamic or pituitary tumors** that increase prolactin secretion.
2. The **diagnosis is established by detecting high plasma prolactin level** or by demonstrating tumor of lactotroph by CT scan or MRI.
3. The disease is treated by **dopaminergic drugs** that inhibit the secretion of prolactin. This restores fertility and libido.

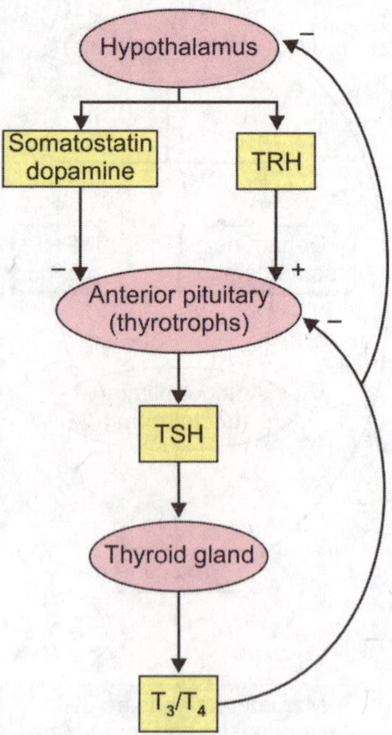

Fig. 55.13: Feedback regulation of TSH secretion. Note, TSH stimulates thyroid gland to secrete T_3 and T_4 that in turn provide negative feedback to anterior pituitary and hypothalamus to inhibit TSH and TRH secretion respectively. Plus (+) indicates stimulation and minus (–) indicates inhibition.

Thyroid Stimulating Hormone

Structure

Thyroid stimulating hormone (TSH) is a **glycoprotein hormone** that controls the growth and function of thyroid gland. It mainly controls the secretion of thyroid hormones especially T_4 and T_3. It has two subunits: α and β. **The α subunit** is nonspecific as it is similar in structure with that of the LH and FSH because it is derived from the same gene for these hormones. It contains 96 amino acids. **The β subunit** contains 110 amino acids and **provides specificity to TSH**. The molecular weight of TSH is 28,000.

Source

Thyroid stimulating hormone is secreted from the **thyrotrophs of anterior pituitary** that account for 3–5% of the cell population of the gland. These cells develop at about **13 weeks of gestation**. Fetal thyroid gland starts secreting hormones in response to TSH almost during the same time in pregnancy.

Synthesis

Like other peptide hormones, TSH is synthesized as **preprohormone**, which is converted to **prohormone**. The α and β subunits are synthesized separately from separate mRNA molecule:

1. **Separate genes** on different chromosomes code for synthesis of α and β subunits.
2. The peptide chains of α and β subunits **undergo glycosylation** in rough endoplasmic reticulum. The carbohydrate moiety, which is **rich in mannose**, is added to the prohormone molecule.
3. During packaging in the Golgi apparatus the carbohydrate unit undergoes modification by **addition of sialic acid and sulphate** to it, which allows two subunits to combine to form TSH molecule.
4. The TSH molecule is stored in the secretory granules of thyrotrophs.

Thyrotrophs normally **synthesize more α subunits than β subunits**. Therefore, secretory granules of thyrotrophs contain **extra α subunits** along with TSH, which is released into circulation along with the hormone at the time of secretion.

Regulation of Secretion

The normal plasma concentration of TSH is 0.3 to 5 μU/mL. The secretion of TSH is mainly controlled by two factors:

1. TRH, secreted from hypothalamus is the major stimulant for TSH secretion.
2. Somatostatin, released from hypothalamus inhibits TSH secretion.

The secretion of TRH is **inhibited by T_3 and T_4** secreted from thyroid gland, by **negative feedback mechanism** (Fig. 55.13). **Dopamine**, another hypothalamic hormone also inhibits TSH secretion. TSH secretion exhibits some diurnal variation with maximum secretion occurring in the night, which may be influenced by **cortisol** that inhibits both TRH and TSH secretion. **Growth hormone** also inhibits TSH secretion.

Mechanism of Action

TSH exerts its effects on thyroid cells by increasing concentration of intracellular cyclic AMP.

Functions

Thyroid stimulating hormone **promotes growth of the thyroid gland** and **stimulates thyroid hormone synthesis and secretion**. TSH acts almost in all the steps of thyroid hormone synthesis:

1. It **facilitates iodide uptake** and its organification in the thyroid gland. **Iodide trapping** is increased in few hours of TSH injections.
2. It **enhances intermolecular coupling** (coupling reaction), and thyroglobulin synthesis and secretion into the colloid.
3. It stimulates **release of thyroid hormones** and iodotyrosines from the gland.
4. It **promotes endocytosis** of colloid.
5. It increases blood flow to the thyroid gland.
6. It causes growth and hypertrophy of the thyroid gland.

Applied Physiology

Decreased secretion of TSH due to pituitary diseases results in thyroid atrophy and decreased secretion of thyroid hormones (***secondary hypothyroidism** or **hypopituitary hypothyroidism***). Chronic increase in TSH secretion results in hypertrophy of thyroid gland, called goiter.

Adrenocorticotropic Hormone

Adrenocorticotropic hormone (ACTH) is an important hormone that controls growth and secretion of adrenal cortex. It mainly influences the secretion of cortisol. ACTH plays vital role in physiology of **stress** and pathophysiology of stress disorders.

Source and Structure

Adrenocorticotropic hormone is secreted from **corticotrophs of anterior pituitary** that constitute 10–20% of its total cell population. ACTH is the smallest peptide hormone of anterior pituitary containing **39 amino acids**. It has molecular weight of 4500.

Synthesis

Like other peptide hormones ACTH is synthesized as a preprohormone. It is synthesized in the corticotrophs as part of a larger molecule called **pro-opiomelanocortin** (POMC), which cleaves to form **β-lipotropin**, and **ACTH** in human beings (Fig. 55.14). In other species, POMC also forms **β-endorphins**. In the intermediate lobe of pituitary, POMC forms **α-MSH** (melanocyte stimulating hormone), especially in lower vertebrates. Intermediate lobe is rudimentary in humans. However, in humans, ACTH contains α-MSH sequence at its N-terminal, and therefore, it possesses **intrinsic α-MSH activity**.

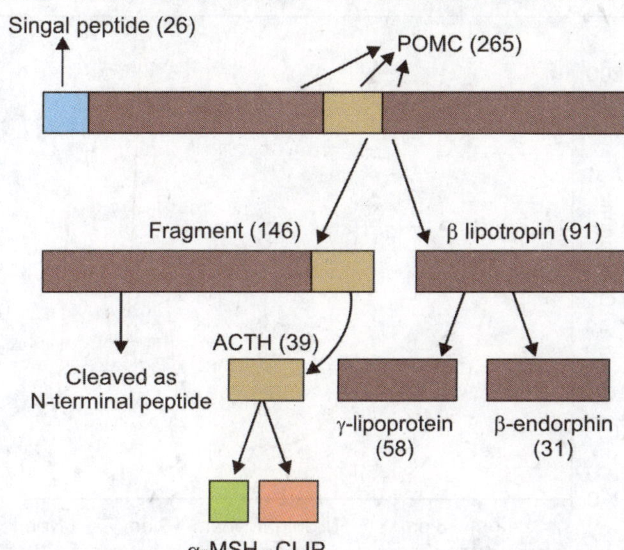

Fig. 55.14: Synthesis of ACTH from proopiomelanocortin (POMC). (CLIP: Corticotropin-like intermediate peptide; MSH: Melanocyte stimulating hormone).

Circadian Rhythm of ACTH Secretion

Normally, ACTH secretion occurs in irregular bursts. The pulsatile secretion of ACTH is due to several bursts of CRH (corticotropin releasing hormone) secretion in 24 hours. However, there is a prominent diurnal rhythm for ACTH secretion, in which **secretion is more in the early morning**, which constitutes about **75% of the total 24 hours secretion**:

1. The secretion begins to rise at about 4 am and reaches a **peak between 7 and 10 am** and then falls slowly to basal level by noon (Fig. 55.15). Another **small peak** occurs in the evening between 4 and 6 pm.
2. The secretion is **minimal when the person sleeps**, especially in the midnight when the individual is in deep sleep. Again, ACTH secretion starts increasing at about 2 hours before awakening.
3. This diurnal variation in ACTH secretion is due to the natural sleep-wake cycle, controlled by inherent **biological rhythm of suprachiasmatic nucleus of hypothalamus**.
4. The pattern of secretion is reversed in individuals who sleep in the day and remain awake during night. The pattern of glucocorticoid secretion closely follows the ACTH secretion (for details, refer the chapter "Adrenal Cortex").

Regulation of ACTH Secretion

Adrenocorticotropic hormone secretion from anterior pituitary is controlled by various factors. However, **the**

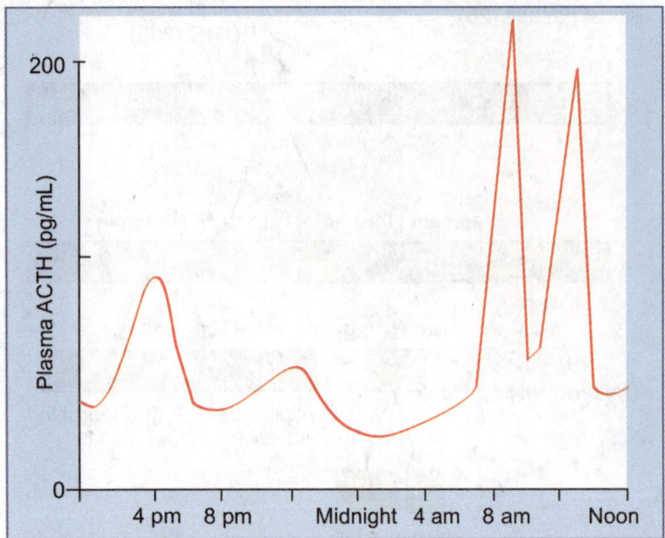

Fig. 55.15: Diurnal variation in secretion of ACTH. Note, maximum secretion occurs in the early morning between 4 am and 10 am. ACTH secretion is minimum in the midnight when person sleeps.

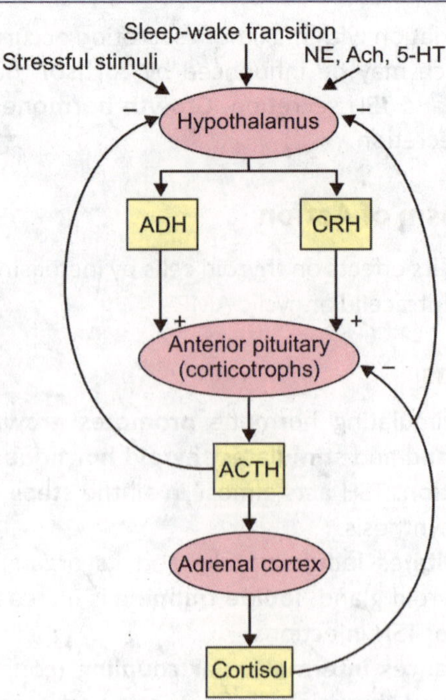

Fig. 55.16: Feedback regulation of ACTH secretion. Note, ACTH stimulates adrenal cortex to secrete cortisol that in turn provides negative feedback to anterior pituitary and hypothalamus to inhibit ACTH and CRH secretion respectively. ACTH also inhibits hypothalamic secretion of corticotropin releasing hormone (CRH). (NE: Norepinephrine; 5-HT: 5-hydroxytryptamine (serotonin). Plus (+) indicates stimulation and minus (–) indicates inhibition).

primary factor controlling the ACTH secretion is CRH secreted from hypothalamus. Many factors influence ACTH secretion by regulating CRH secretion from hypothalamus (Fig. 55.16). CRH in addition to its stimulation of ACTH secretion, also stimulates sympathetic activity, increases blood pressure and activates brainstem reticular activating system (causes arousal). Also, **ADH is an important regulator of ACTH secretion.**

Factors that Increase ACTH Secretion

Corticotropin releasing hormone, ADH, sleep-wake transition, stress (hypoglycemia, surgery, anesthesia, injury, infection, fever, etc.), anxiety, depression, α receptor agonist, β receptor antagonist, serotonin, acetylcholine, interleukins, and GI hormones.

Factors that Inhibit ACTH Secretion

Cortisol, ACTH, somatostatin, GABA, brain natriuretic peptide and opioids.

ACTH and Stress

Stress and hypothalamo-pituitary-adrenocortical axis are closely associated. Stress profoundly influences this neuroendocrine axis. Increased ACTH secretion is an immediate response of the body to any form of stress. Therefore, stress is defined as a condition that results in **increased ACTH level in plasma.**

1. Due to increased ACTH secretion, **glucocorticoid secretion increases** rapidly. Inspite of increased cortisol secretion, ACTH secretion continues to remain high due to ***direct stimulation of hypothalamo-pituitary-adrenocortical axis*** by neurally mediated stimulation of hypothalamic paraventricular nucleus that secretes CRH.
2. In stress, higher brain centers stimulate hypothalamic nucleus to secrete CRH at a higher rate. Thus, **stress induced CRH release overrides the negative feedback control of ACTH secretion.**
3. If stress continues, glucocorticoid concentration remains high and mechanism of negative feedback control operates at a higher set point.

Mechanism of Action

ACTH acts primarily by increasing cAMP in the target cells.

Functions

1. ACTH **stimulates synthesis and secretion of cortisol and other steroid hormones** from adrenal cortex by stimulating growth of specific zone of the adrenal cortex. ACTH increases adrenocortical secretion by producing hypertrophy rather than hyperplasia of adrenal cells. The impact of ACTH is more on glucocorticoid secretion than on other steroids.
2. ACTH has **intrinsic MSH activity**; therefore, it stimulates growth and activity of melanocytes. This results in **hyperpigmentation of the skin** due to increased synthesis of melanin (Clinical Box 55.4).
3. The receptors for ACTH are also present in the GI tract and brain, where it acts as a **local neurotransmitter**.
4. ACTH influences immunity by controlling **secretion of cytokines from lymphocytes**. Cytokines also stimulate ACTH secretion.

Clinical Box 55.4

High ACTH level causes Hyperpigmentation: Patients with high ACTH level, which may be due to either Addison's disease or ACTH secreting tumor of anterior pituitary, are hyperpigmented (appear black). In Addison's disease, hyposecretion of cortisol increases ACTH production by negative feedback mechanism. ACTH promotes melanocyte activity as it has inherent MSH actions, and therefore causes skin hyperpigmentation.

LH and FSH

Luteinizing hormone (LH) and follicle-stimulating hormone (FSH) are called **gonadotropins** as they regulate growth and development of gonads, pubertal maturation and secretion of sex steroids.

Source and Structure

Gonadotropic hormones are secreted from **gonadotrophs of anterior pituitary** that constitute 10–15% of cell population of the gland. LH and FSH are **glycoproteins**. Both of them have α **and** β **subunits**.

1. The α **subunit is nonspecific** as it is similar to the α subunit of TSH and hCG.
2. The β **subunit confers specificity** to LH and FSH. The peptide chain of β subunit of FSH contains 111 amino acids and of LH contains 121 amino acids.
3. The carbohydrate moiety constitutes 15–25% of the hormones.
4. The molecular weight of LH is 28,000 and of FSH is 38,000.

Synthesis

Both LH and FSH are produced by the same gonadotrophs. There are separate genes that code the synthesis of α and β subunits of gonadotropins. The addition of **carbohydrate moiety to the molecules allows variation in biological activity** of LH and FSH in different conditions.

Regulation of Secretion

The regulation of LH and FSH is a complex phenomenon. The secretion of gonadotropins is **pulsatile, periodic, diurnal, cyclic, and seasonal**. However, secretion of both the hormones is mainly controlled by gonadotropin releasing hormone (GnRH) secreted from hypothalamus. GnRH secretion is influenced by various psychological, emotional and chemical factors. Among chemicals, important are norepinephrine that stimulates, and dopamine and endorphins that inhibit GnRH secretion.

LH and FSH secretion is regulated by **feedback inhibition through gonadal hormones** such as estrogen, testosterone, activin, inhibin, and follistatin (Clinical Box 55.5):

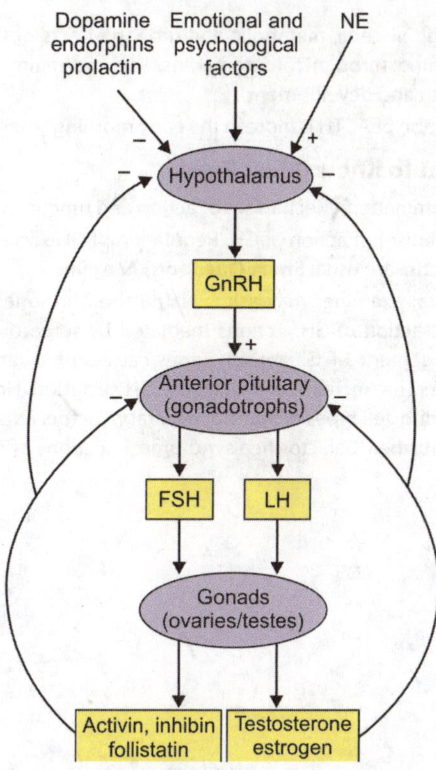

Fig. 55.17: Feedback regulation of LH and FSH secretion. Note, LH and FSH stimulate gonads to secrete various gonadal hormones that in turn provide negative feedback to hypothalamus and anterior pituitary to inhibit GnRH and LH/FSH secretions respectively. [NE: Norepinephrine; Plus (+) indicates stimulation and minus (–) indicates inhibition].

1. Testosterone in males and estrogen in females provide negative feedback signal to inhibit gonadotropin secretion from anterior pituitary (Fig. 55.17).
2. **Inhibin,** a hormone secreted by gonads inhibits GnRH and gonadotropin secretion.
3. **Activin** which is structurally similar to inhibin stimulates FSH synthesis and secretion.
4. **Follistatin** inhibits FSH secretion.
5. **Prolactin** inhibits LH and FSH secretion by inhibiting GnRH secretion from hypothalamus.

Clinical Box 55.5

Oral contraceptives: Oral contraceptives (estrogen and progesterone preparations) use negative feedback influence of gonadal hormones to interfere with LH and FSH secretion in both timing and concentrations. This prevents ovulation by interfering in balanced action of LH and FSH on ovary.

Functions

Luteinizing hormone and FSH exert their effects by increasing cyclic AMP concentration in the target cells.

CHAPTER SUMMARY

Key Concepts

1. Secretion of interior pituitary hormones is controlled primarily by hypothalamic hormones. Therefore, disorders of anterior pituitary hormones can occur in hypothalamic diseases.

2. Though visceral, metabolic and growth effects of GH are due to direct action of GH on target tissues, many of these effects are also mediated through somatomedins, that are mainly produces in liver. Therefore, liver diseases in childhood may considerably affect growth and development.
3. Secretion of ACTH is more in the early morning. Therefore, getting up early in the morning and do activities, help in keeping good health.

Important to Know (Must Read)

1. In examination, 'Mechanism of action and functions growth hormone (GH)' comes as a **Long Question**.
2. Mechanism of action of GH, Regulation of GH secretion, Insulin-like growth factors, Somatomedins, Acromegaly, Gigantism, Dwarfism, Prolactin, are usual **Short Questions** in exam.
3. In **Viva**, examiner may ask... Name the hormones secreted anterior pituitary, What is hypothalamopituitary axis, functions of GH, Direct action of GH, Actions mediated by somatomedins, Etiology, features and management of Acromegaly, Etiology, features and management of Gigantism, Types/causes of dwarfism and its treatment, Differences between pituitary dwarf and thyroid dwarf, Factors that increase and decrease GH secretion, Hormones of anterior pituitary and their target gland and major functions, Hormone secreting cell types of anterior pituitary, Factors affecting prolactin secretion, Functions of prolactin, How lactation prevents pregnancy, Amenorrhea-Galactorrhea syndrome, Functions of TSH and Functions of ACTH.

CHAPTER 56

Posterior Pituitary

Learning Objectives

On completion of study of this chapter, the student **MUST** be able to:

1. Name the hormones secreted from posterior pituitary.
2. Describe the mechanism of action, physiological effects and dysfunctions of ADH and oxytocin.
3. Understand the meaning and importance of a neurohumoral reflex.
4. Understand the pathophysiological basis of diabetes insipidus.

The student **MAY** also be able to:

1. Describe the synthesis, metabolism and regulation of posterior pituitary hormones.
2. Explain the detailed mechanisms of milk ejection reflex, parturition reflex and SIADH.

Posterior pituitary secretes two important hormones: **ADH and oxytocin**. These hormones are formed in **supraoptic and paraventricular nuclei of hypothalamus** and released into posterior pituitary. They are called **neurohormones** as they are synthesized and secreted by neurons into the circulation.

ANTIDIURETIC HORMONE

Antidiuretic hormone (ADH) plays an important role in regulation of blood volume and pressure.

Structure, Synthesis and Secretion

Structure and Source

ADH, also known as arginine-vasopressin (AVP) or **vasopressin**, is an oligopeptide containing **nine amino acids**. It is synthesized in the **magnocellular cells of supraoptic and paraventricular nuclei of hypothalamus**. The synthesis of ADH largely occurs in the supraoptic nucleus.

Important Note

Roger CL Guillemin received **Nobel Prize in Physiology and Medicine for the year 1977** for his discovery of and extensive work on **neurohormones** (For details, refer to Chapter 54).

Synthesis of ADH

The hormone is synthesized in the cell bodies of the **supraoptic and paraventricular nuclei of hypothalamus** (Fig. 56.1). It is synthesized as preprohormone which becomes prohormone and then forms the hormone. The genes that cause ADH synthesis are located on **chromosome 20**. They code for synthesis of a larger molecule that includes a distinct larger protein called as **neurophysin**:

1. There are two neurophysins: **neurophysin I**, meant for oxytocin, and **neurophysin II**, meant for ADH. The neurophysins are almost identical.
2. The precursor molecule for ADH is **prepropressophysin** having 19 amino acids that contains ADH, neurophysin II and a glycoprotein (Fig. 56.2).

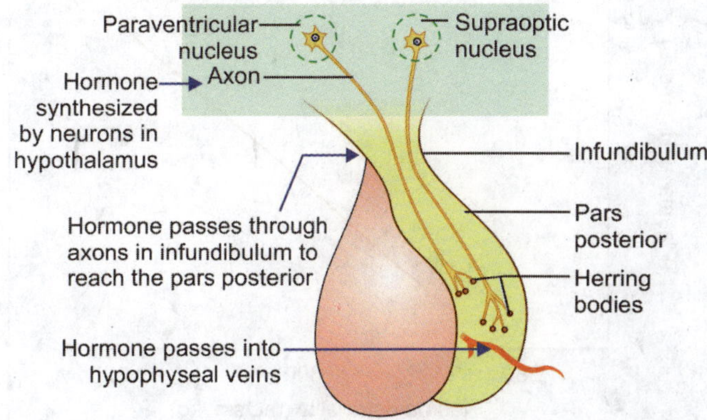

Fig. 56.1: Hypothalamic nuclei (supraoptic and paraventricular) synthesize and secrete posterior pituitary hormones (ADH and oxytocin). Note the Herring bodies at the end of these neurons in posterior pituitary.

3. Prepropressophysin is cleaved enzymatically to release ADH, neurophysin II and glycoprotein molecules.
4. The glycoprotein and ADH are packaged in the Golgi apparatus as secretory granules along with the neurophysin II.
5. **Neurophysin serves as carrier protein** to transport the hormone from the cell body to the axon terminals. The secretory granules are called as **Herring bodies** that are transported to axon terminal by slow axoplasmic flow. The axon terminals of the neurons are located in the posterior pituitary.

Regulation of Secretion

ADH secretion is primarily controlled by **two important stimuli**: plasma osmolality and ECF volume.

Plasma Osmolality

Increased plasma osmolality above 285 mOsm/kg increases ADH secretion proportionate to the osmolality rise (Fig. 56.3):

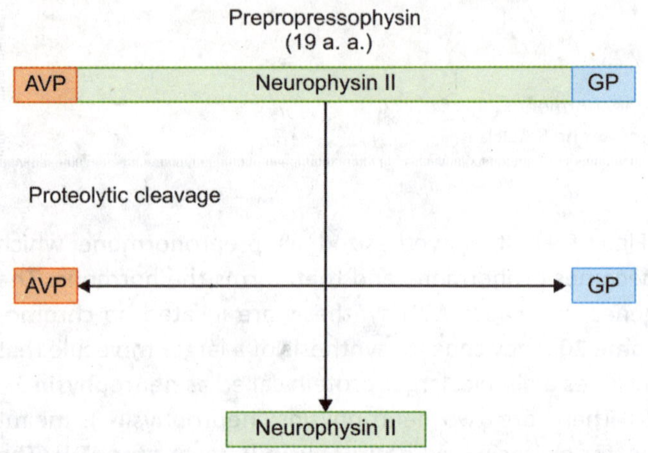

Fig. 56.2: Synthesis of ADH. The other name of ADH is AVP (arginine vasopressin). (GP: Glycopeptide).

1. The increased osmolality is sensed by **hypothalamic osmoreceptors** that increases the synthesis of ADH in supraoptic and paraventricular nuclei and increase ADH release from posterior pituitary. ADH causes water retention and brings osmolality back to normal.
2. Osmolality of plasma is a very **sensitive regulator** of ADH secretion. Even, **change in 1% osmolality** leads to appreciable increase in plasma ADH level.
3. The hypothalamic osmoreceptors are located in the anterior hypothalamus.

Blood Volume and Pressure

Decrease in blood pressure and blood volume stimulates ADH secretion:

1. Percentage **fall in mean arterial pressure** (MAP) causes linear increase in ADH release (Fig. 56.4).
2. **Decreased ECF volume** also stimulates ADH secretion. However, change in osmolality is a stronger stimulus than the change in volume of plasma. Hypovolemia sensitizes ADH response to hyperosmolality (Fig. 56.5).
3. Effect of hypovolemia on blood volume and blood pressure is partly mediated by activation of *renin-angiotensin system* (RAS).
4. Angiotensin II (AII) formed by stimulation of RAS acts on **subfornical organ** (SFO) and **organum vasculosum of lamina terminalis** (OVLT) that are part of thirst center to stimulate thirst and water intake. SFO, OVLT, area postrema and posterior pituitary are **circum ventricular organs** that are located outside blood-brain barrier.

Factors Affecting ADH Secretion

Factors that Increase ADH Secretion

Increased plasma osmolality, decreased ECF volume, decreased blood pressure, angiotensin II, pain, nausea and vomiting, emotion, hypoglycemia, standing, increased temperature and stress increase ADH secretion.

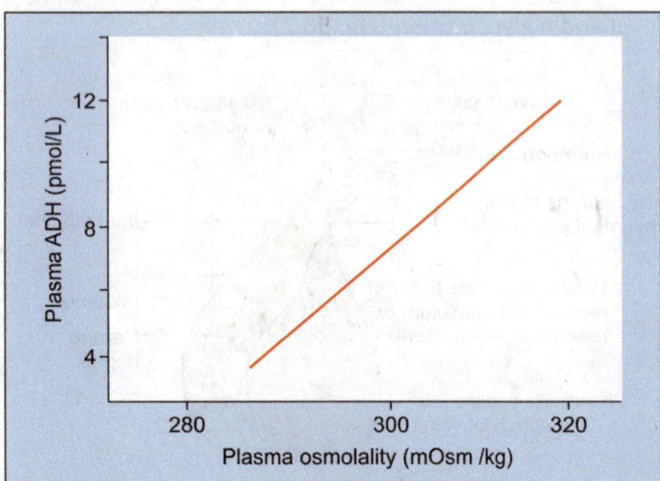

Fig. 56.3: Effect of plasma osmolality on ADH secretion. Note, increase in plasma osmolality above 285 mOsm/kg results in linear increase in plasma ADH concentration.

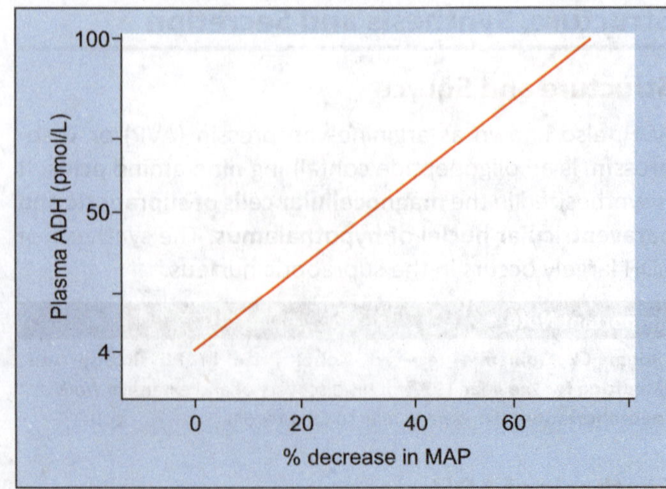

Fig. 56.4: Effect of fall in blood pressure on ADH secretion. Note, % decrease in mean arterial pressure (MAP) results in linear increase in plasma ADH concentration.

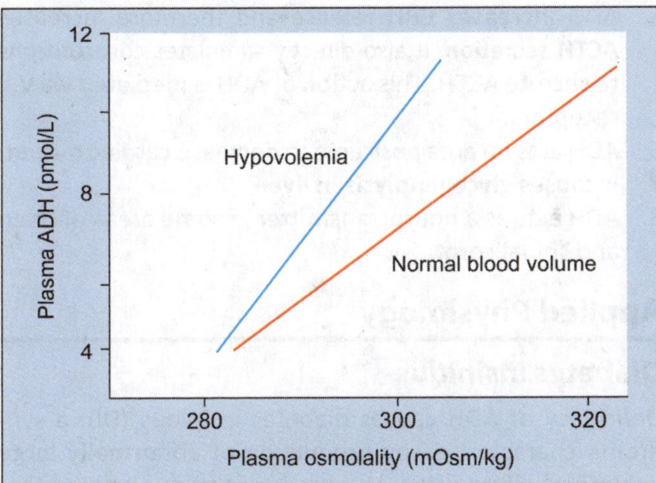

Fig. 56.5: Effect of hypovolemia on osmotically-induced change in ADH secretion. Note, hypovolemia potentiates the osmotic effect on plasma ADH level. In hypovolemia, the effect is shifted to left (compared with normal) indicating early and more ADH secretion at the osmolality of plasma.

Stimuli that Inhibit ADH Secretion

Decreased plasma osmolality, increased ECF volume, decreased temperature, ethanol, cortisol, ANP, thyroxine and α-adrenergic agonist decrease ADH secretion.

Metabolism

ADH is rapidly inactivated in kidneys and liver. In humans, the **biologic half-life** of ADH is about 18 min

Mechanism of Action

ADH acts on kidney to conserve water and on blood vessel to regulate blood pressure. There are receptors for ADH on these organs:

ADH Receptors

There are **two types of ADH receptors**: V_1 and V_2.

V_2 Receptors

V_2 receptors are located on the kidney tubules. ADH increases permeability of the tubular cells by acting on the V_2 receptors.

1. It acts by **increasing the cyclic AMP concentration** on the target cells. Cyclic AMP **activates protein kinase**, which causes **phosphorylation** of different membrane and cellular proteins.
2. This leads to **transport of vesicles or endosomes** by the microfilaments and microtubules from the cytosol to the luminal membrane of the epithelial cells of the tubule.
3. The **endosomes contain water channels** (aquaporins). Thus, *water channels are incorporated into the cell membrane* of epithelial cells on the luminal side of the tubules. This increases the **permeability** of the collecting duct (CD) and distal convoluted tubule (DCT) to water (Flowchart 56.1). The water channels are called **aquaporins**.
4. **Aquaporin 2** is responsible for water reabsorption from DCT by ADH.

Flowchart 56.1: Steps of ADH action on kidney tubular cells.

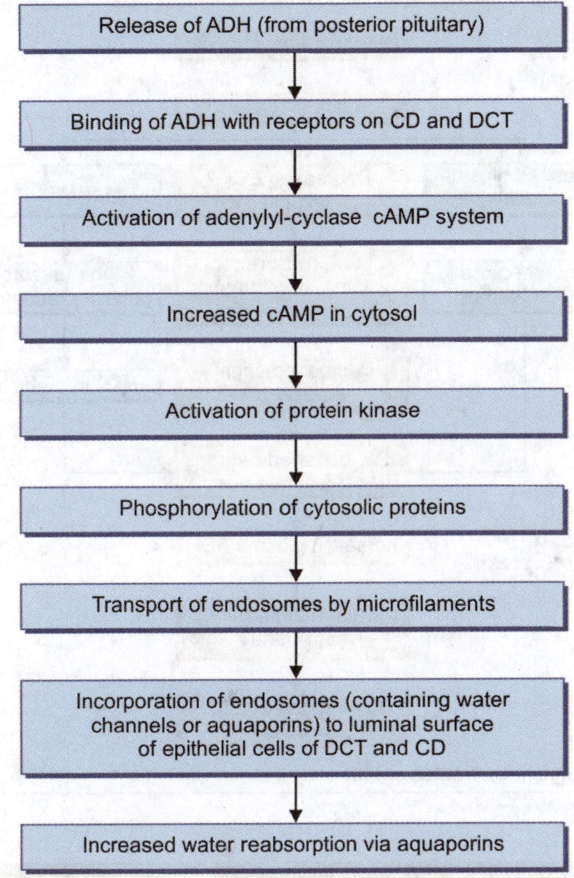

Aquaporins

13 types of aquaporins have been identified till date: AQP0 to AQP12. Aquaporins 1, 2 and 3 are found in kidney, aquaporin 4 is found in brain and aquaporin 5 is present in salivary and lacrimal glands and in respiratory tract. Aquaporin 9 has been described in human leucocytes. According to recent observations, aquaporins are distributed in all tissues of the body.

V_1 Receptors

For its vasoconstriction effect, ADH acts on **V_1 receptors** present in the smooth muscles of blood vessels. There are **two types of V_1 receptors**: V_{1A} and V_{1B}. The **V_{1A} receptors** cause constriction of smooth muscles of blood vessels. ADH increases calcium concentration in the smooth muscles by activating the membrane enzyme phospholipase C that causes hydrolysis of phosphatidylinositol (increases intracellular Ca^{++} concentration). Via its action through **V_{1B} receptors** (that are also called **V_3 receptors**), ADH increases CRH and ACTH secretions.

Flowchart 56.2: Restoration of fluid volume of the body by ADH in volume depletion state.

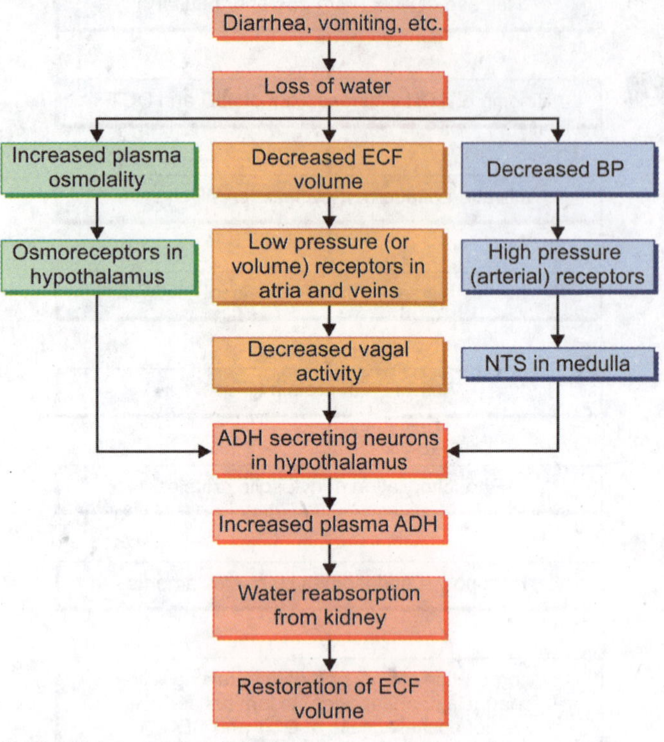

(NTS: Nucleus tractus solitarious).

Scientist contributed

The **Nobel Prize in Chemistry 2003** was awarded to **Peter Agre** *"for the discovery of water channels"* called **aquaporins** that revolutionized the mechanism of water absorption by many cells, tissues and organs in the body, including the process in the renal tubules.

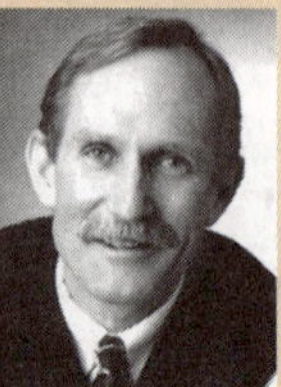

Peter Agre
(Born, 1949)

Functions of ADH

1. ADH acts mainly on DCT and collecting duct of renal tubule to **increase water reabsorption**. It is secreted in conditions of hypovolemia, hypotension and hyperosmolality. It is an important hormone for **restoration of ECF volume** in conditions of depletion like acute diarrhea, vomiting, etc. (Flowchart 56.2).
2. Acting on blood vessels, ADH causes **vasoconstriction**. Thus, in higher concentration it increases blood pressure. However, water conservation occurs at physiological concentration whereas vasoconstriction occurs at supraphysiological concentration of ADH.
3. ADH **facilitates memory** by acting as a neurotransmitter in memory areas of the brain.
4. It causes **contraction of smooth muscles of spermatic cord**. Therefore, it facilitates ejaculation of sperm. This action is mediated via V_1 receptors.
5. ADH **increases CRH release** and therefore increases **ACTH secretion**. It also directly stimulates corticotrophs to secrete ACTH. This action of ADH is mediated via V_{1B} receptors.
6. ADH acts on area postrema to **decrease cardiac output**.
7. It causes **glycogenolysis in liver**.
8. ADH acts as a **neurotransmitter** in some areas of brain and spinal cord.

Applied Physiology

Diabetes Insipidus

Deficiency of ADH causes diabetes insipidus (DI), a syndrome characterized by production of **abnormally large volume of dilute urine**. Usually, it occurs due to hypothalamic or posterior pituitary dysfunctions:

1. The main clinical features are **polyuria and polydipsia**. **Polyuria** occurs due to ADH deficiency that promotes water diuresis. **Polydipsia** occurs secondary to dehydration caused by polyuria.
2. Polyuria and polydipsia *are also features of diabetes mellitus*. However, the main distinguishing characteristic is the difference in osmolality of the urine; in diabetes insipidus urine is dilute (**pure water loss**) and urine osmolality is <300 mOsm/L, whereas in diabetes mellitus the urine is hyperosmolal due to loss of glucose in urine (>1200 mOsm/L). In diabetes insipidus, the urine is tasteless (*insipidus*, means tasteless), whereas in diabetes mellitus urine is tasty due to presence of more glucose in it (*mellitus*, means sweet taste).

There are **two types** of DI: **nephrogenic** (kidneys fail to respond to ADH) and **neurogenic** (deficiency of ADH secretion). Neurogenic DI is also called **central DI**.

Nephrogenic DI

Etiology and Types

In nephrogenic DI, ADH secretion is normal, but **kidney is unresponsive to it** due to receptor deficiency or abnormality. It may be acquired or genetic:

1. **Acquired causes** are **usually due to drugs** such as demeclocycline, rifampicin, aminoglycoside, lithium, cisplantin and amphotericin B. Other acquired causes are ischemia resulting in acute tubular necrosis, metabolic disorders such as hypercalcemia and hypokalemia, and infiltrative diseases like neurosarcoidosis and amyloidosis.
2. **Genetic disorders** are X-linked recessive defect in which V_2 receptor gene is deficient and autosomal defect in which aquaporin gene is deficient.

Treatment

Chlorpropamide is used for treatment of the disease as it increases the renal response to ADH.

Neurogenic DI

Etiology and Types

This occurs in **diseases of CNS** in which hypothalamus, hypothalamo-hypophyseal tract or posterior pituitary are affected. Accordingly, the disease is referred to as, **central, neurohypophyseal or pituitary DI**. It occurs in head injury, tumors such as craniopharyngeoma and suprasellar pituitary tumors, infections such as meningitis and encephalitis, vascular lesions such as Sheehan's syndrome and aneurysm of internal carotid artery, and congenital or genetic defects. ADH secretion is deficient in these conditions.

Treatment

Uncomplicated pituitary DI is cured completely by **treatment with DDAVP**, a synthetic analogue of AVP that acts selectively on V_2 receptors to increase water reabsorption from tubular fluid. Injection of vasopressin is useful. **Clofibrate therapy** also improves the condition.

Syndrome of Inappropriate ADH Secretion

Excessive secretion of ADH occurs in a clinical syndrome called as SIADH (syndrome of inappropriate ADH secretion). The term SIADH is used as ADH secretion is inappropriately high relative to serum osmolality.

SIADH is seen in:

1. Head injury
2. **Ectopic production of ADH** by some malignant tumors such as carcinoma of lungs, pancreas, ovary and bladder.
3. **Neurologic diseases** like multiple sclerosis, Guillain-Barré syndrome, brain abscess, meningitis, encephalitis, etc.
4. **Drugs** such as desmopressin, chlorpropamide, high dose of oxytocin, vincrisitine, phenothiazine, carbamazepine, etc.

In SIADH, not only there is **dilutional hyponatremia** due to increased absorption of large quantity of water from kidney, but also there is **natriuresis** (loss of sodium in urine) secondary to decreased aldosterone secretion activated by expansion of ECF (Application Box 56.1). If SIADH is due to brain diseases, the condition is called **cerebral salt wasting**, and if due to lung diseases the condition is called **pulmonary salt wasting**.

Application Box 56.1

Vasopressin escape: In lung cancers and other malignant tumors, ADH secretion is very high. In such conditions, the water retaining action of ADH is counteracted by a process called vasopressin escape that limits the degree of hyponatremia. This escape phenomenon occurs due to **down regulation of aquaporins production** in collecting duct. Thus, urine output increases despite high ADH levels in plasma, which indicates that the kidney has escaped from the effects of vasopressin (hence, the term 'vasopressin escape').

OXYTOCIN

Structure, Synthesis and Secretion

Source and Synthesis

Oxytocin is an oligopeptide containing nine amino acids. The hormone is synthesized in magnocellular neurons of hypothalamus. Oxytocin is mainly synthesized in the **paraventricular cells of hypothalamus** though synthesis also occurs in supraoptic nucleus (*see* Fig. 56.1):

1. After synthesis, oxytocin is **secreted into the posterior pituitary** where it is stored.
2. The precursor molecule is **prepro-oxyphysin** that contains oxytocin, neurophysin I and a glycoprotein. Otherwise, the steps of synthesis and secretion of oxytocin are similar to that of ADH, as described above.

Regulation of Secretion

Oxytocin secretion occurs in response to **two important physiological stimuli**:

1. **Suckling** at the time of breastfeeding, and
2. **Cervical dilatation** at the time of parturition.

Genital stimulation in females during coitus increases oxytocin release. **Stressful stimuli** facilitate oxytocin release. Oxytocin secretion is inhibited by alcohol.

Functions

Oxytocin mediates two physiological reflexes: 1. milk ejection reflex and 2. parturition reflex.

Milk Ejection Reflex

Discharge or expulsion of milk from the breast of the mother into mouth of the baby when baby suckles during breastfeeding, is called milk ejection reflex.

Receptors

Tactile receptors in and around the nipple.

Reflex Arc

Nipple is stimulated by suckling of the baby:

1. The afferent neural impulses are transmitted from the nipple to the spinal cord and from there via **spinothalamic tract to the brainstem** (Fig. 56.6).
2. In the midbrain, the information reaches paraventricular nucleus of hypothalamus via collaterals arising from the ascending sensory pathway. The neurons terminating on hypothalamus **are cholinergic**.
3. These fibers stimulate oxytocin secreting magnocellular neurons of hypothalamus.
4. Via hypothalamopituitary axis, oxytocin is released from posterior pituitary and enters circulation.
5. Oxytocin causes **contraction of myoepithelial cells** of the milk-laden alveoli of the mammary gland. Therefore, milk is forced from the alveoli into the ducts and from there to the mouth of the infant.

Effects

Due to initiation of this reflex, milk from the mother's breast ***is forcefully discharged*** into the mouth of the baby. Therefore, the reflex is called milk ejection reflex.

Physiological Significance

This is an example of **neurohumoral reflex** (Application Box 56.2). Ovulation that occurs during mating in some animals like rabbit is also an example of neurohumoral reflex.

Application Box 56.2

A neurohumoral reflex: Normally, a reflex is purely a neural phenomenon, the reflex arc having neurons in both afferent and efferent limbs. When, a hormone forms part of the efferent limb, the reflex becomes a neurohumoral reflex. Thus, the neurohumoral reflex involves both neurons and hormones in the reflex pathway. Therefore, milk ejection by oxytocin is a neurohumoral reflex.

Parturition Reflex

Oxytocin causes contraction of uterine muscle:

1. Toward term, oxytocin secretion gradually increases and reaches its peak just before parturition. Also, **number of oxytocin receptor** increases in the uterine muscle.
2. Due to increased plasma level of oxytocin and **increased sensitivity of uterus to oxytocin**, uterus contracts vigorously leading to expulsion of the fetus.
3. Thus, oxytocin initiates and completes parturition. Parturition reflex is also a **neurohumoral reflex**.

Other functions of oxytocin are as follows:

1. Oxytocin receptors are also present in the ovary. It is believed that oxytocin facilitates **degeneration of corpus luteum** at the end of the menstrual cycle.
2. Oxytocin **secretion increases in males during orgasm**, though the exact physiological significance of it is not known. At the time of ejaculation in male, possibly oxytocin causes contraction of smooth muscles of vas deferens that helps in propelling sperms toward the urethra.
3. In females, following ejaculation of sperms into female genital tract, oxytocin **causes contraction of nonpregnant uterus to facilitate sperm transport** into fallopian tubes. Though sperm transport to the fallopian tube for fertilization depends on motility of sperm, uterine contraction facilitates the process.

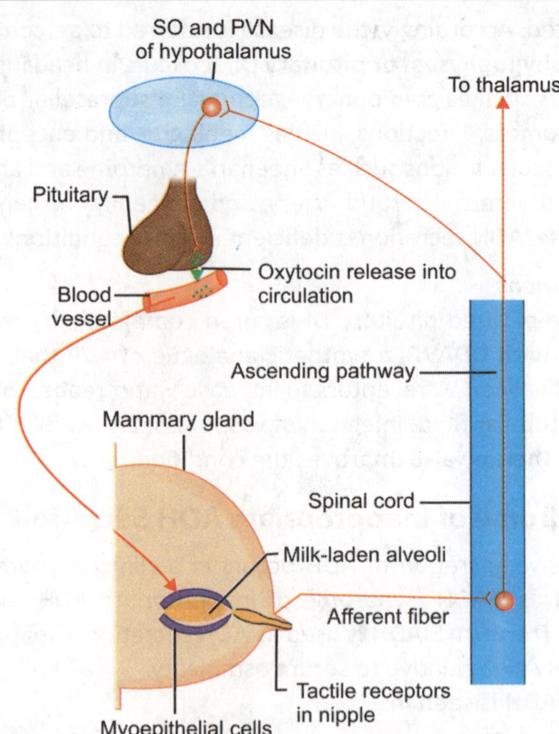

Fig. 56.6: Milk-ejection reflex. Note, afferent limb is the ascending spinothalamic tract that gives collateral to supraoptic and paraventricular nuclei (SO and PVN) of hypothalamus. The efferent limb is mainly humoral, in which oxytocin from posterior pituitary released into circulation causes contraction of myoepithelial cells of alveoli to eject milk into the milk duct.

Applied Physiology

Oxytocics (preparations of oxytocin) are used routinely for:

1. **Induction of labor**, if labor pain does not start effectively at term.
2. Oxytocic infusion is given to **facilitate the progress of labor**.
3. It is routinely injected immediately following delivery of placenta, to **prevent excessive postpartum hemorrhage**, in which uterus contracts severely in response to oxytocic and bleeding vessels are compressed in the contracted uterus that prevents bleeding.

CHAPTER SUMMARY

Key Concepts

1. Hormones of posterior pituitary are synthesized in hypothalamic neurons. Therefore, they are called neurohormones. Therefore, the reflexes caused by ADH and oxytocin are called neurohumoral reflex.
2. Osmolality is a better stimulus than hypotension and hypovolemia for secretion of ADH.
3. SIADH occurs in paraneoplastic syndrome.

Important to Know (Must Read)

1. In examination, 'Mechanism of action, and function of hormones of posterior pituitary/ may come as a **Long Question**.
2. In examination, ADH, Oxytocin, Diabetes insipidus, Neurohumoral reflex, may be asked as **Short Questions**.
3. In **Viva**, examiner may ask... Hormones secreted from posterior pituitary, Source, structure and synthesis of ADH, Functions of ADH, Mechanism of action of ADH, Regulation of secretion of ADH, Types, features and management of Diabetes insipidus, Syndrome of Inappropriate ADH secretion, Sources of ADH and Oxytocin, Functions of Oxytocin, regulation of secretion of Oxytocin, Milk ejection reflex, Parturition reflex, Neurohumoral reflex, Vasopressin escape, and Uses of oxytocics.

CHAPTER 57

Thyroid Gland

Learning Objectives

On completion of study of this chapter, the student **MUST** be able to:

1. Appreciate the role of thyroid hormones in the integration of various body functions.
2. Name the hormones secreted from thyroid gland.
3. Briefly describe the steps of thyroid hormone synthesis.
4. Comprehend the role of TSH in regulation of thyroid hormone secretion.
5. Know the important aspects of thyroid hormone metabolism.
6. Describe the mechanism of action and physiological effects of thyroid hormones.
7. Understand physiological basis of dysfunctions in hyperthyroidism and hypothyroidism.
8. Learn the physiological basis of thyroid function tests.

The student **MAY** also be able to:

1. Describe the synthesis of thyroid hormones.
2. Explain the mechanisms of action of thyroid hormones
3. Describe the regulation of thyroid hormone secretion.
4. Describe the thyroid function tests.

Thyroid is an important endocrine gland that primarily governs the rate at which metabolism occurs in the individual cells. Thyroid hormones profoundly influence normal growth and development of the individual. They are essential for mental and psychological development in infancy and early childhood. Though, thyroid hormones are not very essential for immediate maintenance of vital functions of life, their deficiency causes severe deficit in mental and physical growth, and extreme decrease in body metabolism. Thyroid gland also influences calcium metabolism by secreting calcitonin from its parafollicular cells.

Scientist contributed

Emil Theodor Kocher (1841–1917) was a Swiss surgeon, medical researcher and physiologist who, in 1909, received **Nobel Prize in Physiology and Medicine** for his outstanding contribution in ***physiology, pathology and surgery of the thyroid gland***. His studies on goiter began the systematic work on the functions of thyroid. Among his many accomplishments are the introduction and promotion of aseptic surgery and scientific methods in surgery, specifically ***reducing the mortality of thyroidectomies below 1% in his operations***. He was the first Swiss citizen and the first surgeon to ever receive a Nobel Prize.

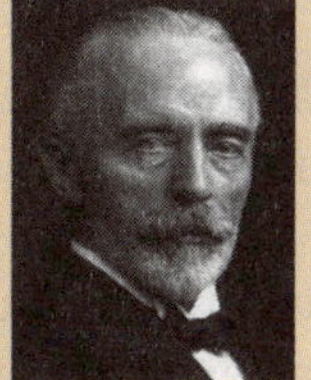

ET Kocher
(1841–1917)

FUNCTIONAL ANATOMY

General Aspects

Development

Thyroid gland develops from the **floor of primitive pharynx** during ***third week*** of gestation. Along with thyroglossal duct, it migrates ***from floor of the tongue*** to the neck. Therefore, **ectopic thyroid** gland may be located at the base of the tongue, which is called as **lingual thyroid**. Normally, thyroid hormone synthesis **begins at about 11th week of gestation.**

Location

Thyroid gland is present on the anterior aspect of the neck. It is located **anterior to trachea**, between the cricoid cartilage and the suparasternal notch. It consists of **two lobes** that are connected by a band of thyroid tissue called **isthmus**. Sometimes an extra thyroidal tissue arises from the isthmus, which is known as ***pyramidal lobe***. The weight of thyroid gland in a healthy adult is between **15 and 20 g**. Four tiny **parathyroid glands** are located posteriorly at each pole of thyroid gland (Clinical Box 57.1).

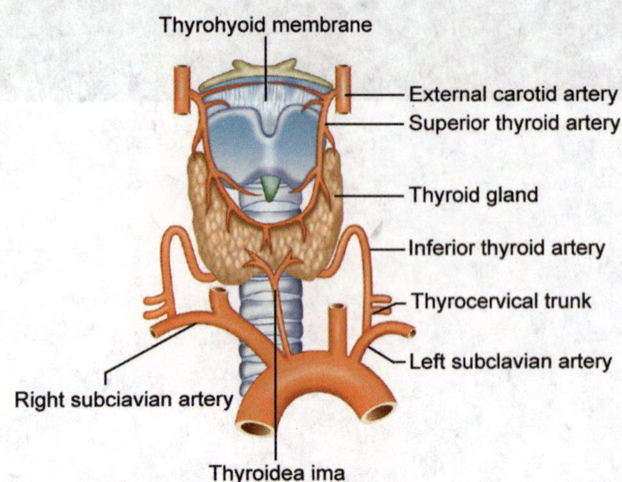

Fig. 57.1: Location and blood supply of thyroid gland. Note, blood supply to thyroid gland is derived from superior and inferior thyroid arteries that originate from external carotid and subclavian arteries respectively.

Courtesy: Figure 63.1, Clinical Anatomy, by Neeta Kulkarni, Vol. 2, 3rd edition, 2016; Jaypee Brothers Medical Publishers (P) Ltd.

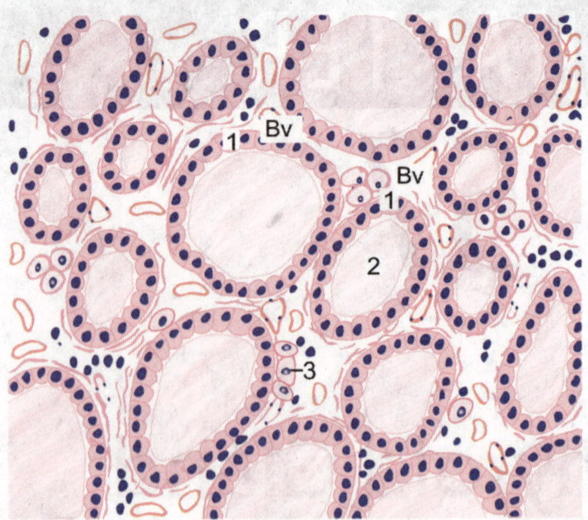

Fig. 57.2: Histology of thyroid gland. Note the follicles lined by cuboidal epithelium (1), colloid in the follicle (2), and parafollicular cells between the follicles (3).

Clinical Box 57.1

Surgical precautions: During thyroid surgeries, utmost care is taken not to remove parathyroid glands that are embedded in thyroid tissue; otherwise that leads to acute hypoparathyroidism (**hypocalcemic tetany**) following thyroidectomy. Also, **recurrent laryngeal nerves** traverse beneath the lateral borders of the thyroid gland on both sides. Therefore, care is also taken to prevent damage to this nerve **to avoid vocal cord paralysis** during thyroid surgery.

Blood Supply

Thyroid gland has rich blood supply, which is maximal among all endocrine organs. Blood flow per gram is even more than that of kidneys. The blood supply to thyroid gland is derived from superior and inferior thyroid arteries that originate from external carotid and subclavian arteries respectively (Fig. 57.1). Thyroid veins drain into external jugular and innominate veins.

Innervation

Thyroid gland is innervated by autonomic nerves. The fibers for **sympathetic innervation** originate from cervical ganglia and fibers for **parasympathetic innervation** travel in vagus nerve. Autonomic innervation ***regulates delivery of TSH and iodide*** to the gland by controlling vasomotor tone. Sympathetic innervation plays important role as it has direct influence on functions of thyroid cells.

Histology

Thyroid gland is formed by aggregates of acini or **follicles** (Fig. 57.2). The **thyroid follicles** are spherical in shape and are formed by a single layer of epithelial cells that surround a central thick solution called **colloid**, which is a viscous-gel like substance containing thyroglobulin in it.

1. The apical membrane of the follicular cells that face the colloid is covered with microvilli. The cells contain numerous granular endoplasmic reticulum, lysosome, Golgi complex (Fig. 57.3).
2. The basal membrane of the follicular cells is in close contact with the **numerous capillaries** present in the interfollicular space.
3. **Parafollicular cells** or C cells that secrete calcitonin are present close to follicles.
4. Size of the follicle and the quantity of colloid varies with the **state of activity of the gland**. The follicles are large in size containing more colloid when the **gland is inactive**. In the **active gland**, follicles are small, cells are cuboidal, and colloid is present in small quantity (Fig. 57.4).

SYNTHESIS, SECRETION AND METABOLISM OF THYROID HORMONES

The principal hormones synthesized and secreted by thyroid gland are:

1. T_4 (thyroxine)
2. T_3 (triiodothyronine).
3. RT_3 (reverse-triiodothyronine), secreted in small quantity.
4. Calcitonin

T_4, T_3, and RT_3 are secreted from thyroid follicles and calcitonin is secreted from the parafollicular cells (C cells) of thyroid gland.

Normally, T_3 is more active than T_4, though T_4 is secreted in more quantity from thyroid gland. T_4 is converted to T_3 in the peripheral blood and tissues. Therefore, T_4 is **mainly a prohormone**. RT_3 is physiologically inactive.

The raw materials required for thyroid hormone synthesis are the iodine and tyrosine. Therefore, iodine

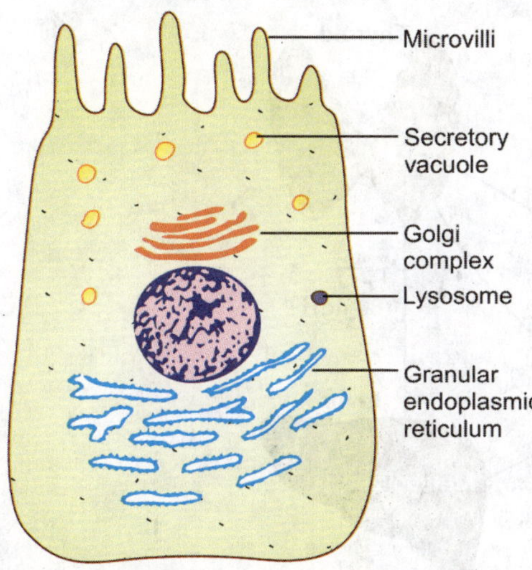

Fig. 57.3: Structure of thyroid follicular cells. Note the presence of microvilli toward apical surface. The cells contain numerous granular endoplasmic reticulum, lysosome, and golgi complex.

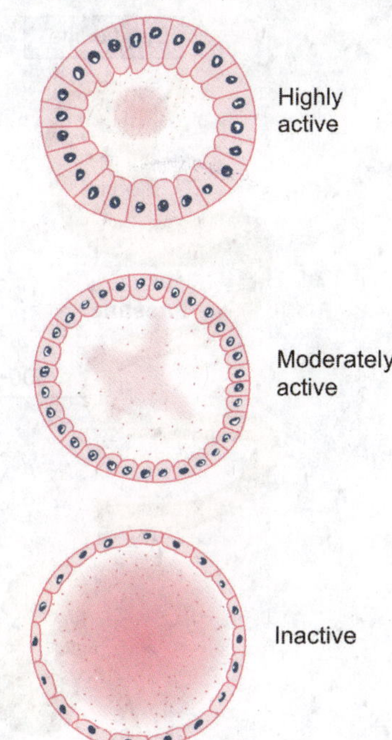

Fig. 57.4: Appearance of thyroid follicles in different levels of activity.

deficiency or excess produces thyroid dysfunction. Before discussing thyroid hormone synthesis, it is desirable to know the basics of iodine metabolism.

Iodine Metabolism

Iodide uptake is the first and crucial step in the thyroid hormone synthesis.

1. About **500 µg of iodine is ingested daily** in the food, which is converted to iodide and absorbed from GI tract.
2. Ingested iodine binds with albumin and unbound iodine is mainly excreted in urine.
3. However, **daily ingestion of 150 µg of iodine** in an adult maintains normal thyroid function. The normal plasma concentration of iodide is **0.3 µg/dL.** Thyroid gland is the principal organ that takes up iodine to form thyroid hormone.
4. Normally, about 120 µg of iodide is taken up by the thyroid gland per day for thyroid hormone synthesis.
5. Kidney is the principal organ that excretes iodide in the urine.
6. The thyroid gland secretes **80 µg of iodine in the form of T_3 and T_4**, and 40 µg of iodine directly into ECF per day (Fig. 57.5).
7. T_3 and T_4 are primarily metabolized in liver. Daily, liver releases about 60 µg of iodine into the ECF and 20 µg of iodine into bile, which is excreted in stool.
8. On average, 480 µg of iodine is excreted in the urine and 20 µg is excreted in the stool.

Iodine deficiency is prevalent in developing countries and ***in mountainous regions*** all over the world. When iodine intake is less than 50 µg per day, thyroid hormone synthesis decreases. The consequent increase in TSH results in goiter, hypothyroidism and cretinism.

Thyroid Hormone Synthesis

Steps of Thyroid Hormone Synthesis

The thyroid hormone synthesis involves following steps:

1. Iodide trapping
2. Conversion of iodide into iodine
3. Thyroglobulin synthesis
4. The coupling reaction
5. Proteolysis of thyroglobulin
6. Secretion of thyroid hormones

Iodide Trapping

Thyroid gland takes up iodide by **active mechanisms.** The active transport of iodide from circulation into the colloid of the thyroid follicles is known as iodide trapping or **iodide pump.**

1. The transport process is a secondary active transport. Na^+ and I^- are co-transported into the thyroid cell by means of **Na^+-I^- symporter (NIS) or cotransporter** (Clinical Box 57.2). NIS can cause 20 to 40 times intracellular iodine accumulation, compared to the concentration of iodine in plasma.
2. **TSH induces expression and retention of NIS** in the basolateral membrane of thyrocytes where it facilitates sustained iodine uptake.
3. The **Na^+ is pumped back** into the interstitium by Na^+-K^+ pump (Fig. 57.6).
4. The RMP of thyroid cell is –50 mV and iodide is negatively charged. Therefore, iodide is pumped into the cells **against the electrical gradient.**

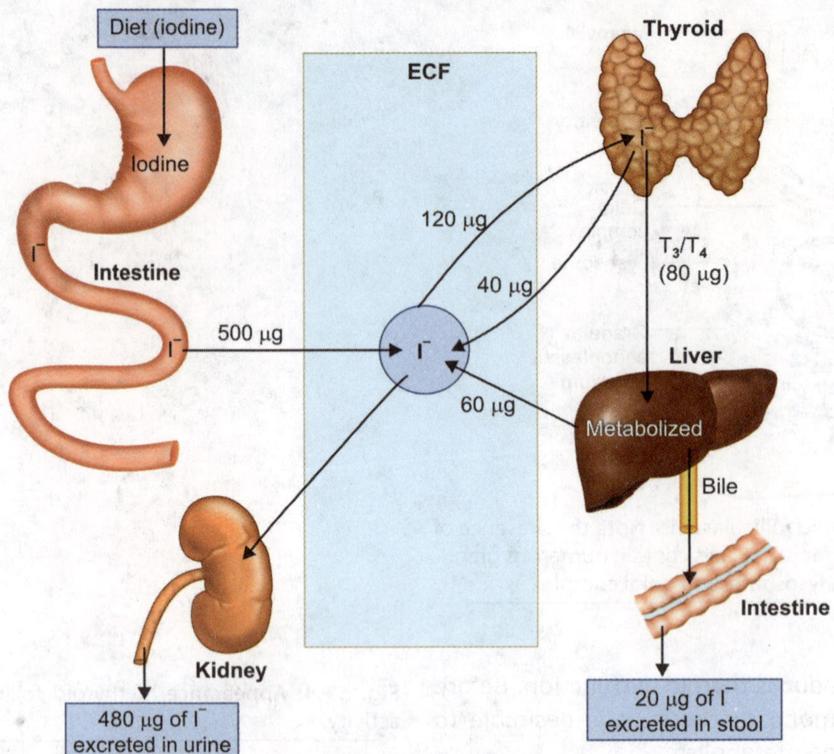

Fig. 57.5: Metabolism of iodine. Note, normally a balance is maintained between the amount of iodide presented to extracellular fluid from intestine and the amount excreted from the body (in urine and stool).

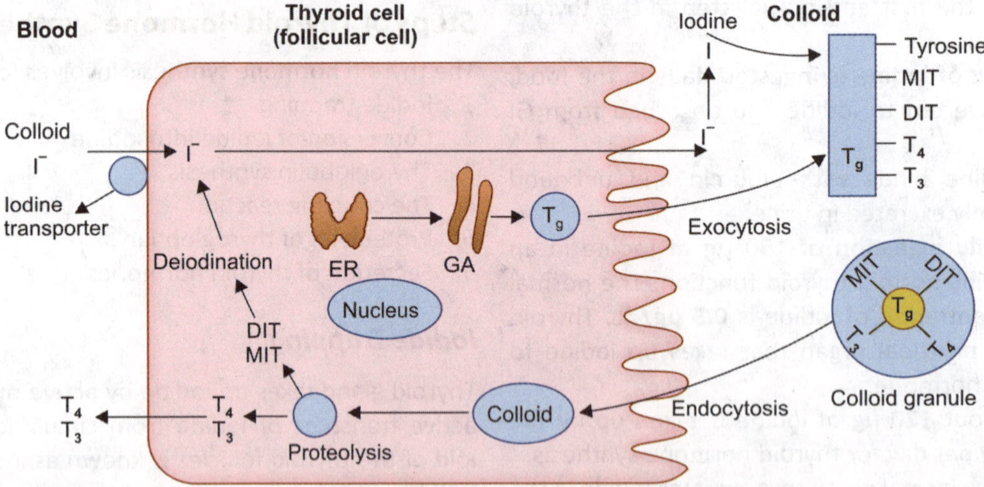

Fig. 57.6: Steps of synthesis of thyroid hormones. (Tg: Thyroglobulin; ER: Endoplasmic reticulum; GA: Golgi apparatus; MIT: Monoiodotyrosine; DIT: Di-iodotyrosine).

5. The iodide concentration inside the colloid is usually very high. Therefore, iodide is also pumped **against its own chemical gradient**.
6. ATP is used in iodide uptake by thyroid cells. This enables the follicular cells to accumulate more iodide than its concentration in blood.
7. The **other tissues that accumulate iodide** are salivary gland, placenta, choroid plexus, mammary gland, gastric mucosa, and ciliary body; however, *they do not form thyroid hormones*. Iodide trapping is **stimulated by TSH**.

Clinical Box 57.2

NIS deficiency: Mutation of NIS (Na$^+$-iodide symporter) gene, an autosomal recessive condition results in decreased thyroid uptake and causes congenital hypothyroidism.

Conversion of Iodide into Iodine

Iodide that is actively transported into the colloids of thyroid follicles is **immediately converted to iodine** by means of oxidation. This oxidation of I$^-$ to I, also known as **organification** (Clinical Box 57.3) is facilitated by the enzyme **thyroid peroxidase**.

Clinical Box 57.3

Pendred syndrome: An iodine transporter called **pendrin** is located on the apical surface of the thyroid cells that transports iodine actively from thyroid cells into the colloid. Pendrin is an **anion exchanger** (Cl^--I^- exchanger). Mutation of pendrin gene leads to **Pendred syndrome,** which is characterized by ***defective organification of iodine, goiter and sensorineural deafness.***

Thyroglobulin Synthesis

Thyroglobulin is the glycoprotein with two subunits and the molecular weight of 660,000. It contains 123 tyrosine residues. It is synthesized in the endoplasmic reticulum of thyroid cells, packaged in Golgi apparatus and then, **secreted into the colloid by exocytosis.** This secretion is **facilitated by thyroid peroxidase.** The thyroid hormones are synthesized in the thyroglobulin molecule and remain bound with the thyroglobulin till they are secreted.

Binding of Iodine to Thyroglobulin

Once reactive iodine is formed (by **oxidation of iodide to iodine**), it binds immediately with the tyrosine molecule, which is attached to thyroglobulin molecule at 3 position. This binding of iodine to thyroglobulin is **facilitated by thyroid peroxidase.**

Coupling Reaction

Binding of iodine with tyrosine at 3 positions forms **monoiodotyrosine** (MIT), which is again iodinated in the 5 position to form **diiodotyrosine** (DIT). Two DIT molecules undergo oxidative condensation to form **thyroxine** (T_4). This is called coupling reaction. There are **two theories of coupling reaction**: intramolecular coupling and intermolecular coupling.

Intramolecular Coupling

In this process, coupling occurs with both DIT molecules attached to thyroglobulin.

Intermolecular Coupling

In this process, DIT that forms the outer ring is detached from the thyroglobulin.

The coupling reaction is also **facilitated by thyroid peroxidase.** The condensation of MIT with DIT forms **triiodothyronine** (T_3). When condensation of DIT occurs with MIT, **reverse-T_3** (RT_3) is formed. Normally, distribution of MIT, DIT, T_4, and T_3 in the thyroid cell is 23%, 33%, 35%, and 7% respectively. RT_3 is present in very minor quantity.

Secretion of Thyroid Hormones

The thyroid cells **ingest colloid by endocytosis.**

1. The **lysosomal enzymes** digest the peptide bonds between iodinated residues and thyroglobulin. This is called **proteolysis of thyroglobulin molecule.**
2. This results in formation of free T_4, T_3, DIT, and MIT in the cytoplasm. The iodinated tyrosines are deiodinated by the microsomal enzyme **iodotyrosine deiodinase.**

Fig. 57.7: Structure of T_3 and T_4. Note, thyroxine contains four iodine atoms, at 3, 5, 3′ and 5′ positions, and triiodothyronine contains three iodine atoms at 3, 5 and 3′ positions of the thyronine ring structures.

3. The T_3 and T_4 are then released from thyroid cells into the general circulation.
4. The iodine released by deiodination of MIT and DIT is usually **reutilized by the gland** for further synthesis of thyroid hormone.
5. This *provides more supply of iodine* for thyroid hormone synthesis in comparison to the iodine available by iodide pump.
6. MIT and DIT are not secreted by the thyroid gland.

Thus, thyroid cells serve **three important functions**:

1. They **actively accumulate iodide** from blood for synthesis of thyroid hormones.
2. They **synthesize thyroglobulin molecules** and secrete them into the colloid.
3. They **digest the colloid** and **free thyroid hormones** from thyroglobulin molecules to secrete them into the circulation.

Structure of T_3 and T_4

Thyroxine contains four iodine atoms, each one at 3, 5, 3′ and 5′ positions, whereas triiodothyronine contains three iodine atoms, each one at 3, 5 and 3′ positions of the thyronine ring structures (Fig. 57.7). For the positions of iodine atoms in thyroid hormones, thyroxine and triiodothyronine are abbreviated as T_3 and T_4 respectively.

Metabolism of Thyroid Hormones

Normal Concentration

In a normal individual, total plasma T_4 concentration is about 8 μg/dL, and plasma T_3 is about 0.15 μg/dL. In circulation, most of the thyroid hormones bind with the plasma proteins. About 99.9% of T_4 and 99.8% of T_3 are bound to plasma proteins. Therefore, the **free T4 level in plasma is about 2 ng/dL**, and **free T3 is about 0.3 ng/dL** (Application Box 57.1).

Application Box 57.1

Measurements of free and bound forms: Concentration of thyroid hormone is measured by RIA. As physiological effects of thyroid hormones **depend on their free-form level in plasma**, and the free hormone component influences feedback control of hypothalamo-pituitary-thyroid axis, in thyroid dysfunctions, mainly the free hormone concentrations are measured. However, it is ideal to measure both total and free level of hormones in blood for diagnosing thyroid dysfunctions.

Protein Binding

Thyroid hormones bind with three types of plasma proteins:

1. Thyroxine binding globulin (TBG)
2. Thyroxine binding prealbumin (TBPA), also called transthyretin.
3. Albumin.

Normally, T_4 binds mainly with TBG and TBPA, and T_3 binds with albumin and TBG.

TBG

TBG is a glycoprotein synthesized by liver. Its molecular weight is 54000. Each TBG molecule has a single binding site on it for a molecule of thyroid hormone.

1. About **70% of T_4 and 45% of T_3 are bound to TBG**.
2. TBG level in plasma **increases in pregnancy** and in patients receiving **estrogen, major tranquilizers, clofibrate,** etc.
3. Plasma **TBG level decreases** in patients receiving glucocorticoids, androgens, danazol and L-asparaginase (cancer chemotherapeutic drug). Salicylates, phenytoin (anticonvulsant), mitotane (cancer chemotherapeutic drug) and 5-fluorouracil inhibit binding of T_3 and T_4 to TBG.

TBPA

TBPA, though named as prealbumin is not an albumin, rather a globulin. Recently, TBPA has been designated as **transthyretin**. The binding of T_3 with TBPA is very less (less than 1%), whereas about 20% of T_4 binds to it.

Albumin

T_3 mainly binds with albumin. About 55% of T_3 and 10% of T_4 bind with albumin.

The concentration of free T_3 and T_4 depends on the concentration of plasma proteins that bind these hormones.

1. When, *concentration of thyroid binding proteins increases in plasma*, the ***free level of thyroid hormones decreases***. However, the decreased hormone level provides **feedback signals** to secrete more TSH, which in turn **increases secretion of thyroid hormones**.

Flowchart 57.1: Daily secretion and fate of thyroxine.

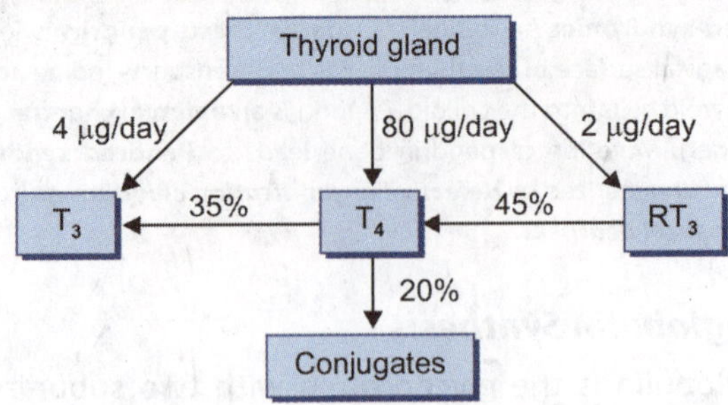

2. The opposite phenomenon occurs when level of plasma binding protein decreases in plasma.
3. Thus, initial change observed in thyroid hormones due to change in plasma proteins is a **temporary effect**. Therefore, thyroid activity remains normal (*euthyroid state*) in patients with altered binding proteins.

Importance of protein binding:

1. Protein-bound forms of T_3 and T_4 **serve as reservoir** of these hormones. This can replenish the circulating hormone, when due to some reasons or the other, the secretion is decreased or metabolism is increased suddenly and temporarily.
2. Protein binding **protects the hormone against metabolic degradation**. Therefore, the half-lives of circulating T_3 and T_4 are more (1 day for T_3 and 7 days for T_4).
3. Circulating free form concentration provides **feedback effect on regulation** of hormone secretion.

Peripheral Conversion

The major product of thyroid gland secretion is T_4.

1. Normally, about 35% of secreted T_4 is converted to T_3 in the circulation by the enzyme **5′-deiodinase** (Flowchart 57.1) present in liver and kidney, and this accounts for about 85% of circulating T_3.
2. T_3 mainly acts on the target cells. Therefore, physiologically T_3 is considered as the most **active hormone**.
3. About 45% of T_4 is also converted to RT_3 by the enzyme **5-deiodinase**, which accounts for 95% of circulating RT_3. However, **RT_3 is physiologically inert**.
4. As 5′-deiodinase is present in high concentration in pituitary and cerebral cortex, the ratio of T_3/T_4 is very high in these structures. Remaining about 20% is conjugated with sulphates and glucuronides.

Effect of Diet

Fasting decreases conversion of T_4 to T_3. Therefore, T_3 concentration in plasma decreases in fasted individuals. However, conversion of T_4 to RT_3 is facilitated. Therefore, RT_3 is increased and T_4 remains normal in fasting. **In starvation** (chronic and severe fasting), RT_3 returns to normal, but T_3 continues to remain low. **In overfeeding,** opposite happens; T_3 is increased and RT_3 is decreased.

Flowchart 57.2: Metabolism of thyroxine.

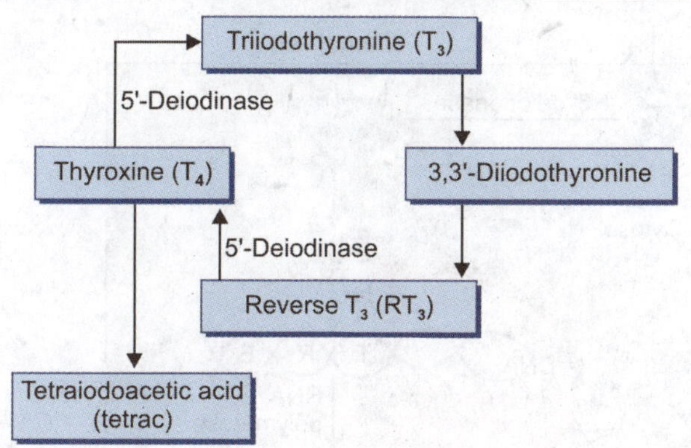

Effect of Drugs

Various drugs inhibit deiodinase, and therefore, they decrease T_3 and increase RT_3 level in plasma.

Effects of Diseases

In many **nonthyroidal conditions** such as chronic febrile illness, trauma, burns, liver and kidney failure, myocardial infarction, selenium deficiency, advanced stage of cancers and other cachectic states, activity of deiodinases is suppressed. Therefore, **level of T_3 decreases** in these conditions. However, *T_3 becomes normal when patient recovers*.

Peripheral Degradation

Thyroid hormones are metabolized mainly by enzymes **deiodinases** (Flowchart 57.2).

1. There are **three types of deiodinases**: Type 1 (D_1), type 2 (D_2) and type 3 (D_3).
2. All the deiodinases contain a special amino acid **selenocysteine**. This rare amino acid makes the enzyme potent **to catalyze oxidoreductive reactions**. In fact, the *selenium in the amino acid* is essential for their enzyme activity.
3. **D_1** is present in liver, kidney, thyroid and pituitary. **D_2** is present in skeletal muscle, brain, pituitary gland, placenta and brown fat. **D_3** is present in brain and reproductive tissues.
4. **D_1 and D_2 are 5′-deiodinase** that convert T_4 to T_3 and *maintain the intracellular T_3* in their target tissues.
5. **D_3 promotes conversion of T_4 to RT_3**.
6. Especially in brain, D_2 maintains the supply of T_3 to the neurons. T_3 is degraded to diiodothyronines by deiodinases that are present in the liver and kidney.
7. In liver, T_4 and T_3 are metabolized by **conjugation with sulphates and glucuronic acid**. The conjugated forms are **secreted in the bile into the intestine** to reenter the *enterohepatic circulation*. Thus, iodine is lost minimally, about 4% in stool.
8. In many tissues, T_4 is also metabolized to **tetraiodoacetic acid (tetrac)**.

Regulation of Secretion

Secretion of thyroid hormones is regulated by a **feedback control mechanism**. Hypothalamus secretes **thyrotropin releasing hormone** (TRH), which stimulates thyrotrophs of anterior pituitary to secrete thyroid stimulating hormones (TSH). TSH stimulates thyroid gland to secrete T_3 and T_4.

1. The plasma concentration of **free T_3 and T_4 provides feedback signal** for regulated release of TRH and TSH (refer to, Fig. 55.17; Chapter 55).
2. When **thyroid hormones decrease** in plasma, TSH secretion increases, and conversely, when **thyroid hormones increase**, TSH secretion decreases.
3. This counter regulation of TSH by thyroid hormones is partly attributed to their *inhibitory effect on thyrotrophs* to directly inhibit TSH secretion and partly to their *effects on hypothalamus* to inhibit the secretion of TRH.
4. Thus, **concentration of TSH is a better index of thyroid activity**. Dopamine, somatostatin and glucocorticoid also inhibit TSH secretion from the anterior pituitary.

TSH

Structure and Secretion

TSH is a glycoprotein containing **211 amino acids**. It has two subunits: α **and** β.

1. **The α-subunit** of TSH is structurally similar to the α-subunits of LH, FSH, and hCG (Application Box 57.2).
2. Therefore, the **specificity of TSH is conferred by its β-subunit**.
3. Normally, TSH is secreted at the rate of 110 µg/day and its plasma concentration is about 2 µU/mL.
4. Secretion of TSH is usually **pulsatile**. The mean secretion starts increasing at about 9 PM, reaches its peak at midnight and then decreases slowly. The secretion is ***less during the day***.

Functions of TSH

TSH stimulates thyroid hormone synthesis and secretion by **influencing almost all the steps involved in it**.

1. This includes iodide trapping, iodide binding, synthesis of T_3 and T_4 (coupling reaction), secretion of thyroglobulin into the colloid and endocytosis of colloid.
2. TSH also **increases blood supply** to the thyroid gland.
3. TSH **increases the size and number of follicles**. Therefore, chronic rise in TSH causes **thyroid hypertrophy** or **goiter** (for details of TSH, refer Chapter "Anterior Pituitary").

TSH Receptor and Other Receptors

The receptor for TSH on thyroid cells is a **glycoprotein receptor** with an extended *glycosylated extracellular domain*. It is a **G protein-coupled receptor** having typical seven transmembrane segments.

1. It activates adenylyl cyclase via Gs protein.
2. It also acts via phospholipase-C pathway.

Apart from having TSH receptors, thyrocytes also have **receptors for IGF-1, EGF, TNF-α and γ-interferon** and other growth factors.

1. IGF-1 and EGF promote growth and TNF-α and γ-interferon inhibit growth of thyroid tissue.
2. Cachexia in chronic inflammation could be due to decreased thyroid activity mediated by action of inflammatory cytokines (TNF-α and γ-interferon) on thyrocytes.

Application Box 57.2

Placental tumors can cause hyperthyroidism: As α-subunit of hCG is identical to the α-subunit of TSH, the hypersecretion of hCG stimulates thyroid activity. Major source of hCG is placenta. Therefore, mild to moderate hyperthyroidism is observed in tumors of placental origin like choriocarcinoma.

PHYSIOLOGICAL EFFECTS OF THYROID HORMONES

Mechanism of Action

The mechanism of action of thyroid hormones is **similar to that of steroid hormones**. They act by binding with the intracellular receptors. With few exceptions like adult brain and gonads, receptors for thyroid hormones are present in all tissues and organs. Though the developing neurons in infants and children are highly sensitive to thyroid hormones, it is not clear why the adult neurons are not so sensitive.

The **steps of mechanism** of action are as follows:

1. T_3 and T_4 enter the cells of the target organs by **carrier mediated** (energy dependant) transport.
2. Inside the cell, most of the **T_4 is converted to T_3**, which then binds with the thyroid-hormone receptors (TR) present on nucleus. The thyroid receptor protein binds to thyroid-hormone response elements (TRE) in the DNA via zinc fingers.
3. Binding of T_3 with thyroid hormone receptor-TRE elements cause **translation of DNA** that in turn increases the **transcription of mRNA** (Fig. 57.8).
4. Increased mRNA causes increased **intracellular protein synthesis** that stimulates cellular growth and maturation, increases intracellular enzyme synthesis, increases mitochondria formation and respiratory enzyme synthesis, and increases Na^+-K^+ ATPase activity.
5. The increased Na^+-K^+ ATPase activity increases cellular oxygen consumption and increased mitochondrial activity increases general metabolism of the cell.

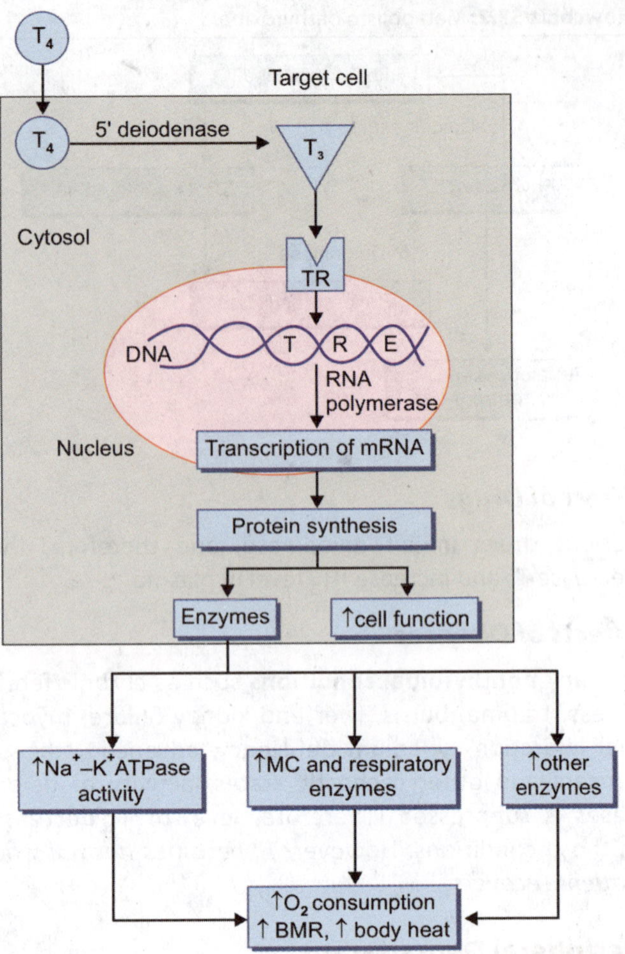

Fig. 57.8: Mechanism of action of thyroxine. Note, the mechanism of thyroxine action is similar to steroid hormones. (TR: Thyroid-hormone receptor; TRE: Thyroid-hormone response element; MC: Mitochondria).

Thyroid-Hormone Receptors (TR)

There are two human TR genes: α and β. The α **receptor gene** is located on chromosome 17 and β **receptor gene** is located on chromosome 3.

1. Each of them synthesizes two different mRNAs. Therefore, two different receptor proteins are formed: **TRα1, TRα2, TRβ1 and TRβ2**. TRα1, TRβ1 and TRβ2 bind with T_3.
2. TRα1 and TRβ1 are widely distributed in tissues.
3. TRα2 does not bind with T_3, though widely distributed and its function is not clearly known. TRβ2 is found only in the brain.
4. There are many activators and repressors of TR, which makes thyroid hormones, exert their diverse effects in various tissues. ***T_3 binds more rapidly and avidly*** to TR. Therefore, **T_3 is more potent than T_4**.
5. In myocytes, especially in heart T_3 is not formed from T_4. However, T_3 directly enters myocyte to combine with nuclear receptors and promotes expression or inhibition of genes.

Physiological Actions

In general, thyroid hormones control basal energy metabolism, and development of CNS and normal body growth in childhood.

General Effects on Basal Metabolism

The metabolism of a cell depends on the rate of its oxygen consumption. Oxygen is essential for oxidative phosphorylation of ADP to ATP that takes place in mitochondria.

1. Thyroid hormones **increase the basal rate of oxygen consumption** and therefore, the basal metabolism of the tissues. This **increased metabolism increases the rate of heat production**. This is called **calorigenic** or **thermogenic actions** of thyroid hormones.
2. The cellular metabolism is also activated by **increased Na^+-K^+ ATPase activity**. Increased oxygen consumption by the cells ***parallels their increase in Na^+-K^+ ATPase activity*** and in some of the tissues, inhibition of Na^+-K^+ pump decreases oxygen consumption.
3. T_3 also stimulates the **transcription of genes** for both α and b subunits of Na^+-K^+ pump. Therefore, it is strongly perceived that increased oxygen consumption stimulated by thyroid hormones is mediated by Na^+-K^+ ATPase activity, at least partly.

Target tissues: The increased consumption of oxygen by thyroid hormone is observed in **all tissues of the body**, which is prominent especially **in skeletal muscle, liver, heart, kidney and connective tissues**. However, **exceptions are** anterior pituitary, adult brain, gonads (testis and ovary), uterus, lymph nodes, and spleen that show little thermogenic response. Receptors for thyroid hormones are *almost absent in adult brain*.

Basal metabolic rate: In the resting stage, oxygen consumption in human is about 250 mL/min. In hyperthyroid state, it increases to about 400 mL/min. Therefore, the **basal metabolic rate** (BMR) **increases to about +80%** in hyperthyroidism. Conversely, in hypothyroidism BMR decreases to **as low as –40%.** Increased BMR increases body temperature.

Mitochondrial mechanism: Metabolism is increased by thyroid hormones not only by increased oxygen consumption and Na^+-K^+ ATPase activity, but also by increase in **synthesis of mitochondrial cytochromes** and promote **cytochrome oxidase activity**.

1. Thus, thyroid hormones regulate the number of respiratory unit in each cell and their capacity to carry out **oxidative phosphorylation**.
2. Thyroid hormones also stimulate **synthesis of uncoupling protein 1** (UCP-1) that contributes significantly to oxidation of nutrients and heat production.
3. The tissue expression of UCP-2, and UCP-3 are also increased by thyroid hormones.

Effects Secondary to Metabolic or Thermogenic Actions

Increased body metabolism **increases nitrogen excretion**. Therefore, increased food intake should be associated with hypermetabolic states to prevent catabolism of endogenous protein and fat. Thus, **significant weight loss** occurs promptly in increased thyroid activity, without adequate nutrient supplementation.

1. Increased metabolism **increases body temperature**.
2. This causes vasodilation that **decreases peripheral resistance** and consequent changes occur in hemodynamics.
3. Increased metabolism also **increases the requirement for vitamins**. Therefore, **vitamin deficiency** is common in increased thyroid activity.

Effects on Nervous System

Thyroid hormones are essential for **development of the central nervous system**, especially **during infancy and early childhood**. Development of brain occurs maximally in last six months of fetal life and first six months of postnatal life. During this period, thyroid hormones initiate and facilitate the process of **differentiation and maturation of brain cells**.

Thyroid hormones are required for following neural functions:

1. Growth of cerebral and cerebellar cortices, and basal ganglia.
2. Proliferation of axons and branching of dendrites.
3. Development of **synaptic connections**.
4. Development of neurotransmitter systems in CNS. Thyroid hormones induce formation of enzymes essential for **neurotransmitter synthesis.**
5. Increase in number of receptors on different brain tissues for various neurotransmitters in the brain.
6. **Myelination of neurons**. Thyroid hormones stimulate galactosyl sialyl transferase activity, which is essential for myelin formation.
7. Synthesis of proteins and various enzymes like succinic dehydrogenase that are required for energy generation in neurons.
8. Cell migration during brain development.
9. General alertness and responsiveness to various stimuli.
10. Speed and amplitude of stretch reflexes.
11. Memory, learning and intellectual capacities.

Deficiency of thyroid hormones during infancy results in irreversible retardation in CNS development (Clinical Box 57.4). This is why thyroid deficiency in newborn should be detected early and treated promptly.

Cerebral blood flow, glucose and oxygen utilization by brain remains normal in adult hypothyroidism and hyperthyroidism. Thyroid hormones enter the brain in adults and found in gray matter of various parts of the brain. Also, T_4 is converted to T_3 by astrocytes in brain. After thyroidectomy, D_2 type 2 deiodinase activity in brain increases enormously, which is reversed in 3 to 4 hours following injection of T_3.

Flowchart 57.3: Mechanisms of increased cardiac output by thyroid hormones.

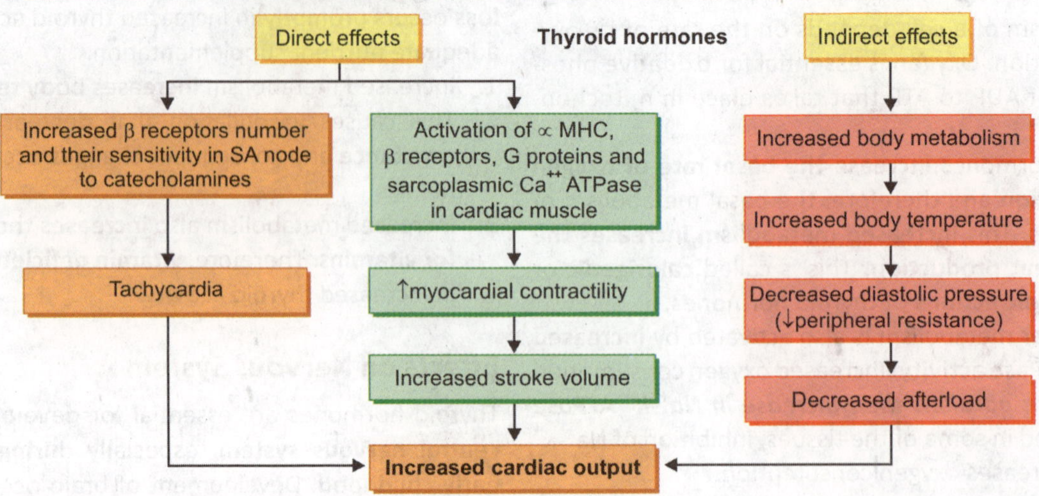

Clinical Box 57.4

Mental retardation in hypothyroid children: Thyroid hormones are essential for normal mentation. Therefore, mental retardation is an important feature of a thyroid deficiency in infancy and early childhood (thyroid dwarf). This differentiates it from a pituitary dwarf in whom mental activities are apparently normal. Decreased stretch reflex activities, especially decreased reaction time of **Achilles tendon reflex** (ankle jerk) is diagnostic in hypothyroidism.

Effects on Growth and Development

Thyroid hormones are essential for **normal growth and musculoskeletal maturation**.

1. Thyroid hormones promote **expression of gene for growth hormone** (GH) in somatotrophs of anterior pituitary.
2. They facilitate the effect of GH on tissues.
3. They stimulate linear growth of bones, and **endochondral ossification and maturation** of epiphyseal bone centers.
4. They enhance the **activity of chondrocytes** in cartilage.
5. They increase **osteoid activity** and bone remodeling.
6. They cause eruption and development of teeth.
7. They promote epidermal growth, and growth of nails and hairs.
8. They stimulate synthesis of structural and enzymatic proteins

In hypothyroid children, bone growth is slowed and epiphyseal closure is delayed.

On tissues: Thyroxine causes alteration in the characteristics of mucopolysaccharides in the subcutaneous tissue. It decreases synthesis and promotes degradation of glycosaminoglycans (mucopolysaccharides).

Cardiovascular Effects

Thyroid hormones increase heart rate and myocardial contractility. Therefore, they increase the cardiac output.

1. **Heart rate:** Thyroid hormones **increase the number of β receptors** on the nodal tissues (SA and AV nodes) of the heart and also increase the **sensitivity of β receptors to catecholamines**. Thus, thyroid hormones **increase the heart rate**. Tachycardia is a common feature of hyperthyroidism (Clinical Box 57.5).
2. **Myocardial contractility:** Myocardial contractility increases by following mechanisms:
   i. Thyroid hormones induce **myosin heavy chain** (MHC) expression in the cardiac muscle. Especially, the α-MHC activity is increased, which has more actin and calcium-activated ATPase activity.
   ii. Thyroid hormones increase the **expression of β receptors, G proteins and Na^+-K^+ ATPase** in myocardial cells.
   iii. They also increase the **calcium-ATPase activity** of the sarcoplasmic reticulum in cardiac muscle, which facilitates sequestration of calcium.

   All these factors increase the force of contraction that in turn **increase stroke volume.**

   MHCs in heart muscle: Normally, heart muscle contains two MHCs: α and β MHCs. The α MHC has high myosin ATPase activity, and β MHC has low myosin ATPase activity. Thyroid hormones **stimulate α MHC and inhibit β MHC activities.** In hyperthyroidism, expression of α MHC gene is enhanced and of β MHC gene is suppressed. However, in myocytes, thyroid hormones inhibit phospholamban, adenylyl cyclase, T_3 nuclear receptor and Na^+-Ca^+ exchanger, in addition to its inhibition of β MHC.
3. **Systolic pressure:** Increased heart rate and stroke volume result in increase in cardiac output (Flowchart 57.3). Thus, **systolic blood pressure increases** significantly.
4. **Diastolic pressure:** Via its calorigenic action, thyroid hormones increase body temperature that causes **thermogenic cutaneous vasodilation** and decreases peripheral resistance. Thus, **diastolic pressure decreases**.

5. **Pulse pressure and circulation time:** The net effect on blood pressure is **increased pulse pressure**. Wide pulse pressure is a prominent feature of hyperthyroidism. Increased cardiac output and vasodilation makes the circulation hyperdynamic. Therefore, **circulation time is shortened**.

Clinical Box 57.5

Tachycardia in sleep: Tachycardia is an important feature of hyperthyroidism. Tachycardia due to other causes (anxiety, tension, etc.) usually disappears during sleep or heart rate falls significantly. In thyroid excess, tachycardia persists even during sleep. **Sleeping tachycardia is an important diagnostic feature of thyrotoxicosis.** Sometimes atrial arrhythmias such as flutter or fibrillation are also seen in hyperthyroidism, especially in elderly people.

Effects on Intermediary Metabolism

Thyroid hormones by increasing oxygen consumption of tissues **increase oxidation of substrates** in general. They also **increase the supply of substrates** for metabolism by increasing their absorption from GI tract. By activating genes encoding enzymes of various metabolic pathways, thyroid hormones amplify all intermediary metabolisms.

On Carbohydrate Metabolism

Thyroid hormones **increase absorption of glucose** from intestine.

1. They **increase hepatic glucose output** by inducing **gluconeogenesis**. They also stimulate **hepatic glycogenolysis**. Therefore, plasma glucose level increases.
2. However, thyroid hormones **increase the turnover of glucose** by increasing its uptake and oxidation. Therefore, the net effect is **no substantial change** in plasma glucose concentration.
3. In hyperthyroidism, though plasma glucose level rises fast after a carbohydrate meal, it **decreases rapidly**.
4. Thus, sustained hyperglycemia or *glucose intolerance is not a usual feature* of hyperthyroidism. However, some patients develop **glucose intolerance or even diabetes** in the long run.

On Fat Metabolism

Thyroid hormones **stimulate lipolysis**.

1. Thus, thyroxine increases **release of free fatty acids and glycerol** from adipose tissues. Glycerol is utilized for gluconeogenesis.
2. Thyroid hormones also **increase turnover of lipids,** by facilitating their oxidation.
3. They **stimulate synthesis of cholesterol** and simultaneously promote its oxidation and biliary excretion.
4. Hepatic uptake of cholesterol is increased by increased expression of LDL receptors in liver.
5. Therefore, the net effect is **significant decrease in plasma cholesterol** and total lipid.

On Protein Metabolism

Thyroid hormones **promote proteolysis** in skeletal muscle, increasing the release of amino acid. They ***increase protein turnover*** by promoting protein degradation.

On Metabolic Actions of Other Hormones

Thyroid hormones **potentiate the metabolic actions of catecholamines, glucagons, cortisol and growth hormone**, especially their **gluconeogenic and lipolytic** effects.

Effects on Sympathetic Nervous Systems

Thyroid hormones increase the rate of metabolism, heat production, heart rate and neuromuscular functions; the features that are **similar to the effects of sympathetic stimulation** (Clinical Box 57.6).

1. They also synergize the metabolic effects of catecholamines like lipolysis, glycogenolysis, and gluconeogenesis.
2. In fact, they do not increase the release of catecholamines; rather **increase the expression and sensitivity** of β receptors in various tissues like heart, skeletal muscle and adipose tissues to catecholamines.
3. Recently, it has been observed that T_3 **stimulates the production of thermogenin**, a protein in the brown adipose tissue that partly mediates the thermogenic action of catecholamines.

Clinical Box 57.6

Hypersympathetic state: The features of hyperthyroidism mimic the features of sympathetic stimulation like increased metabolism, increased body temperature, nervousness, increased motor activity, and excessive sweating. Use of sympathetic blockers such as **propranolol** that blocks β receptors alleviates many features of hyperthyroidism. β blockers have some degree of inhibitory effects on conversion of T_4 to T_3; and therefore, mildly decrease plasma T_3 level.

Effects on Respiratory System

Thyroid hormones **increase oxygen utilization** of tissues. Therefore, the demand for oxygen also increases.

1. Thyroxine meets this demand by **stimulating the rate of respiration, minute ventilation, and ventilatory responses** to hypercapnia and hypoxia.
2. Thus, **arterial PO_2 increases** that increase the ***supply of oxygen to tissues***.
3. Thyroid hormones **stimulate erythropoiesis** by increasing the synthesis of erythropoietin. Thus, the supply of oxygen to the tissues is also increased.

Effects on GI Tract

Thyroid hormones **enhance the motility** GI tract. Therefore, ***hyperdefecation*** is a feature of hyperthyroidism and constipation is a feature of hypothyroidism. Thyroid hormones also **increase appetite and food intake, and reabsorption of glucose** from GI tract.

Effects on Skeletal Muscle

Thyroid hormones increase the **expression of MHC genes** in the skeletal muscle. Therefore, hypothyroidism is associated with **muscle cramp and weakness**. However, muscle weakness also occurs in hyperthyroidism, which may partly be due to increased protein catabolism in the muscle. **Myopathy** occurs in chronic hyperthyroidism (**thyrotoxic myopathy**).

Effects on Reproductive System

In both males and females, thyroid hormones play an important role in the regulation of reproductive functions.

1. **In women**, they cause **follicular maturation and ovulation.** Thyroid abnormalities in woman result in irregularities in menstrual cycle, such as menorrhagia (increased menstrual loss) in hypothyroidism and oligomenorrhea (decreased menstrual loss) in hyperthyroidism.
2. **In males**, they **promote spermatogenesis.** T_3 promotes differentiation of prepubertal testicular Sertoli cells.

Effects on Kidney

Thyroid hormones increase kidney size and promote growth of renal tubular epithelial cells. They **increase renal blood flow and GFR**. Tubular **reabsorption of electrolytes, glucose and water** is also increased by thyroid hormones. Increased water reabsorption increases blood volume.

In summary, thyroid hormones have widespread effects on metabolism, growth and development and control of many systemic functions (Table 57.1)

Table 57.1: Summary of physiologic effects of thyroid hormones.

Target system	Functions
Metabolism	Increase in BMR (↑ O_2 consumption in all tissues except testes, uterus, lymph node, spleen and anterior pituitary)
CVS	1. Tachycardia (increased no. and sensitivity of β receptors) 2. Increased myocardial contractility (increased MHC and myosin ATPase) 3. Increased SBP (↑ cardiac output) 4. Decreased DBP (↓ peripheral resistance)
CNS	Brain development
Bone	Skeletal development and ↑ growth
Muscle	↑ expression of MHC gene, Protein catabolism
Adipose tissue	↑ Lipolysis
GIT	Stimulates GI motility, ↑ appetite, ↑ Carbohydrate absorption
Reproduction	Follicular maturation and ovulation

APPLIED PHYSIOLOGY

Hyperthyroidism

Hyperthyroidism occurs due to hypersecretion of thyroid hormones from thyroid gland or from extrathyroidal tissues, which may be broadly divided into primary and secondary varieties.

Primary Hyperthyroidism

When hyperthyroidism occurs due to pathology of the thyroid gland, the condition is called primary hyperthyroidism. The common causes are:

1. Adenoma of thyroid
2. Multinodular goiter
3. Metastatic carcinoma of functioning thyroid gland
4. Graves' disease
5. Activating mutation of TSH receptors
6. Iodine excess (**Jod-Basedow phenomenon**)

Secondary Hyperthyroidism

When hyperthyroidism occurs due to the pathology outside thyroid gland, the condition is called secondary hyperthyroidism, which may be due to a **tumor of the pituitary gland or of extrathyroidal tissue.**

Pituitary Causes

Tumor of thyrotrophs of anterior pituitary (secretes excess of TSH).

Extrathyroidal Causes

Chronic excess administration of thyroid hormones (iatrogenic), tumor of ectopic thyroid tissue (lingual thyroid), hCG secreting tumors such as choriocarcinoma.

Features of Hyperthyroidism

Features of hyperthyroidism in descending order of frequency are:

Symptoms

Hyperactivity and irritability, heat intolerance, fatigue, tremor, sweating, palpitation, nervousness, hyperphagia (due to increased appetite), weight loss in spite of hyperphagia, hyperdefecation (due to increased GI motility), loss of libido, and oligomenorrhea (in females).

Signs

Sinus tachycardia, atrial fibrillation, systolic hypertension and increased pulse pressure, fine tremor, thyroid swelling (goiter), increased body temperature (warm and moist skin), muscle weakness (proximal myopathy), protrusion of eyeball with retracted lid (exophthalmos) (Fig. 57.9), periorbital edema, and gynecomastia (in males).

Increased BMR to as high as +100 is an important and diagnostic laboratory finding of hyperthyroidism.

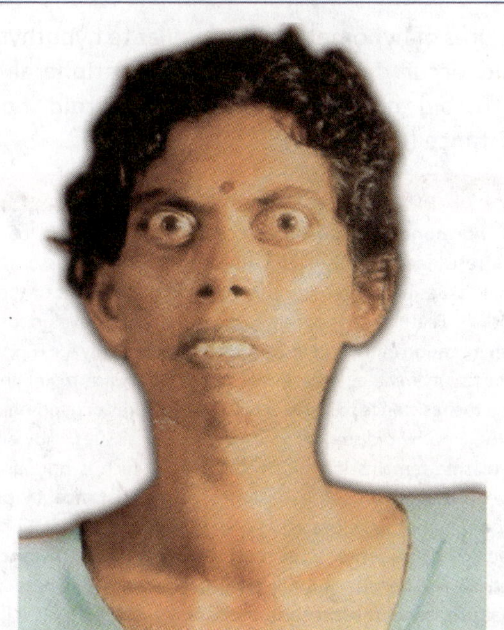

Fig. 57.9: A hyperthyroid patient. Note the presence of exophthalmos.
Courtesy: Dr. Abdoul Hamide, Professor of Medicine, Endocrinology Clinic, JIPMER, Puducherry.

Diagnosis of Hyperthyroidism

Diagnosis is made by estimation of T_3, T_4, and TSH in plasma.

1. Typically, in **primary hyperthyroidism,** ***T_3 and T_4 are*** *high* and ***TSH is low***.
2. **In secondary hyperthyroidism** due to pituitary cause, **TSH is high** along with high T_3 and T_4.

Physiological Basis of Treatment

Administration of **antithyroid drugs** is the mainstay of treatment of hyperthyroidism. They usually inhibit iodide trapping mechanism or binding of iodide with the tyrosine molecule.

Antithyroid drugs are thionamides, anions, high dose of iodides, nonspecific beta-blockers and radioiodines.

Thionamides

These are thioureylenes, a group of **compound related to thiourea**. The commonly used thionamides are propylthiouracil, carbimazole and methimazole (active metabolite of carbimazole). The mechanisms of action of thionamides are:

1. They inhibit the function of thyroid peroxidase.
2. They inhibit oxidation and organification of iodide. Thus, they inhibit iodination of monoiodotyrosine and coupling reaction.
3. They reduce the level of thyroid stimulating antibodies.
4. Propylthiouracil reduce the rate of conversion of T_4 to T_3 by inhibiting D_2–deiodinase activity.

Anions

These are chlorate, perchlorate, pertechnetate, periodate, biiodate, etc. They are monovalent anions that compete with iodide for transport into the thyroid via NIS (Na^+-I symporter). Thus, **they prevent iodide trapping**. Thiocyanate is also an anion that **inhibits iodide transport**, but is less potent.

High Dose of Iodide

Iodide is essential for thyroid hormone synthesis. However, in very high dose it **prevents organic binding** by itself, and therefore, prevents thyroid hormone synthesis. This inhibition is called **Wolff-Chaikoff effect**. High dose of iodide also inhibits the effect of TSH on the gland by decreasing cAMP production in the cell, and by inhibiting proteolysis of thyroglobulin.

Propranolol

It is a nonspecific β-blocker. By preventing the action of catecholamines on β receptors, propranolol ameliorates many of the hyperthyroid features. It decreases heart rate, cardiac output, nervousness etc. and is very helpful in the early stages of the disease.

Radioiodine

It causes progressive destruction of thyroid cells and achieves euthyroid state. The dose should be appropriately adjusted to prevent development of hypothyroidism.

However, from the above-listed drugs, most commonly used drugs are propylthiouracil, methimazole and perchlorate.

Special States of Hyperthyroidism

Thyrotoxicosis

Thyrotoxicosis is not synonymous with hyperthyroidism. It is a state of thyroid hormone excess that occurs due to severe hyperthyroidism as seen in **Graves' disease**, toxic **multinodular goiter** and **toxic adenoma**. This can also occur without hyperthyroidism as seen in **thyroiditis** or due to excess administration of thyroid hormones (***thyrotoxicosis factitia***).

Graves' Disease

Graves' disease is a condition in which there is diffuse enlargement of thyroid gland, which is usually associated with exophthalmos.

1. This is an **autoimmune disease** that occurs due to development of **autoantibodies against TSH receptors**. The antibodies formed against the TSH receptors activate the receptors. Therefore, thyroid gland **becomes hypertrophied and hyperactive.**
2. There is marked stimulation of secretion of thyroid hormones. Therefore, plasma level of **T_3 and T_4 is very high.**

3. **TSH concentration is less** as excess thyroid hormones inhibit TSH secretion.
4. **Exophthalmos** occurs due to swelling of extraocular muscles and proliferation of connecting tissue within the bony walls of the orbit that pushes the eyeball forward.
5. **The disease is treated by** using antithyroid drugs, by decreasing thyroid hormone synthesis, or by reducing the amount of thyroid tissue (with treatment of radioactive iodine like ^{131}I or by subtotal thyroidectomy).

Thyroid Storm

A patient suffering from hyperthyroidism becomes **suddenly extremely ill** with features like high fever, profound tachycardia, restlessness, and sometimes circulatory collapse. This is called thyroid storm. It usually develops when a hyperthyroid patient **undergoes major surgery, or experiences a major trauma or illness**. This is a medical emergency that requires immediate fluid replacement and steroid therapy with antithyroid drugs.

Hypothyroidism

Hypothyroidism in Adult

Hypothyroidism in adult is usually known as **myxedema**.

Etiology

Hypothyroidism, according to the cause may be classified into two categories: Primary and secondary.

Primary Hypothyroidism

When hypothyroidism develops due to the diseases or causes that primarily affect thyroid gland, is classified under primary hypothyroidism. The common causes are:

1. Autoimmune hypothyroidism: for example, Hashimoto's thyroiditis.
2. Iatrogenic: Excess use of radioiodine (^{131}I), thyroidectomy, etc.
3. Iodine deficiency
4. Drugs: Excess of iodine, excess use of antithyroid drugs, lithium, etc.
5. Congenital hypothyroidism

Secondary Hypothyroidism

When hypothyroidism develops primarily due to a defect outside the thyroid gland, the condition is called secondary hypothyroidism. Usually, it occurs due to a defect either in the pituitary or in the hypothalamus.

1. **Pituitary hypothyroidism:** Pituitary resection, pituitary tumors affecting thyrotrophs, and Sheehan's syndrome (**postpartum necrosis of pituitary**). Hypothyroidism *occurs due to decreased TSH secretion.*
2. **Hypothalamic hypothyroidism:** Brain injury involving hypothalamus, tumors of hypothalamus, etc. in which *secretion of TRH is less.*
3. Features of hypometabolism similar to hypothyroidism could occur due to resistance of peripheral tissues to thyroid hormones, called as **thyroid hormone resistance** (Clinical Box 57.7).

Clinical Box 57.7

Thyroid hormone resistance: Recently, the condition of thyroid hormone resistance has been described, in which the tissues (usually peripheral tissues and anterior pituitary) become resistant to the effects of T_3 and T_4. Features of hypothyroidism may not develop, as in this condition mutation of thyroid receptor gene occurs only for TRβ, whereas TRα remains unaffected. Also, levels of T_3 and T_4 are maintained that overcome the resistance to some extent. But, features of hypometabolism similar to hypothyroidism occur in peripheral tissues. However, TSH level of plasma remains inappropriately high, which is not suppressed by exogenous thyroxine. The **patients with resistance in pituitary** have hypermetabolism, elevated T_3 and T_4 and normal nonsuppressible TSH level. The **patients with peripheral tissue resistance** have hypometabolism despite normal levels of T_3 and T_4. These patients require large doses of thyroid hormone to maintain their BMR. It has been observed that the **attention deficit hyperactive disorder** in children is more associated with thyroid hormone resistance.

Features of Hypothyroidism

Following are the features in descending order of frequency:

Symptoms

Cold intolerance, weakness and easy-tiredness, dry-thick skin, loss of hair, poor memory and inability to concentrate, constipation (due to decreased GI motility), weight gain in spite of poor appetite, thick and husky voice (typical hoarse voice that helps physician to **diagnose the disease over phone**), yellow skin (occurs due to carotenemia, as thyroxine causes conversion of carotene to vitamin A; therefore deficiency of it causes deposition of carotene), alopecia, psychosis (myxedema madness) menorrhagia (in females), galactorrhea and infertility (Fig. 57.10).

Signs

Cool extremities with dry coarse skin, dry hair, bradycardia, puffy face, with edematous hands and feet (**myxedema**), diffuse alopecia, goiter, bradycardia, hypertension (diastolic), anemia, decreased reaction time of tendon reflexes (especially, delayed Achilles tendon reflex relaxation), carpal tunnel syndrome and periorbital edema.

BMR decreases to about –40, and plasma cholesterol is usually elevated.

Diagnosis of Hypothyroidism

In primary hypothyroidism, **T_3 and T_4 levels are decreased,** but **TSH is increased** by feedback mechanism. In hypopituitary or hypothalamic hypothyroidism, the TSH concentration is less, in addition to decreased T_3 and T_4. The TSH response to TRH is usually normal in hypothalamic hypothyroidism, whereas it is increased in hypothyroidism caused by thyroid disease.

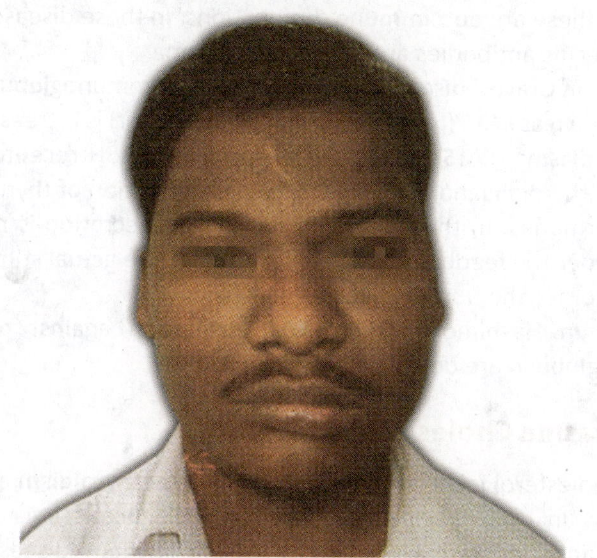

Fig. 57.10: A hypothyroid patient. Note pronounced myxedema in face (puffy face) with coarse hair on head.
Courtesy: Dr. T. Kadhiravan, Associate Professor of Medicine, JIPMER, Puducherry.

Treatment of Hypothyroidism

Thyroid hormone replacement is the mainstay of treatment. T_4 is instituted at a dose (usually 10 to 15 µg/kg/day) to maintain its normal level in plasma.

Hashimoto's Thyroiditis

It is a chronic form of **autoimmune thyroiditis** in which antibodies are formed against the thyroglobulin and thyroid peroxidase. Therefore, thyroid cells are damaged and hypothyroidism develops. Fine needle aspiration cytology (FNAC) demonstrates sheet of Hürthle cells with lymphoid infiltrate.

Hypothyroidism in Children (Cretinism)

Cretinism is the hypothyroidism in children. When hypothyroidism develops from or before birth, the patients are called **cretins.**

Causes

Maternal iodine deficiency during pregnancy, maldevelopment of thyroid gland during fetal life, inborn errors of thyroid hormone synthesis, antithyroid antibodies in mother that crosses placenta and enters fetal circulation, and hypopituitarism in fetal life are usual causes of cretinism.

Features

Patients are **dwarf** and **mentally retarded**. Typically, they have potbelly and protrusion of tongue (Fig. 57.11). Other features of hypothyroidism are also present.

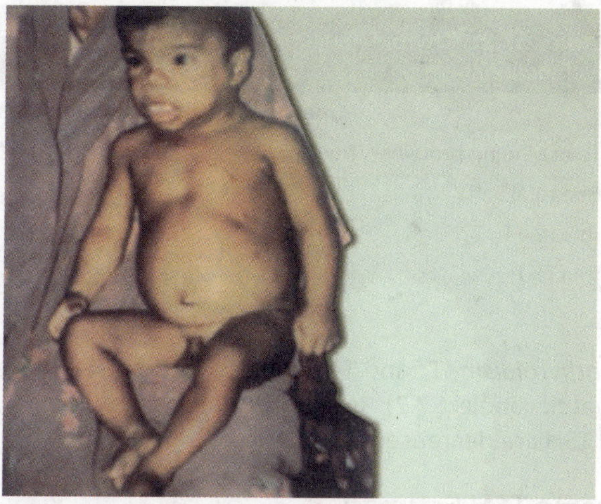

Fig. 57.11: A child with cretinism. Note the potbelly and protrusion of tongue of the child.
Courtesy: Figure 10.14, Page 771, Manual of Practical Medicine by R Alagappan's, 5th edition, 2014; Jaypee Brothers Medical Publishers (P) Ltd.

Treatment

Hypothyroidism is an important cause of mental retardation, which can be prevented if the disease is diagnosed and treated immediately after birth. **Thyroid hormone replacement early in infancy** can totally cure the disease. The usual treatment is the *prompt replacement of thyroxine* as soon as the diagnosis is made.

THYROID FUNCTION TESTS

Thyroid function tests include measurement of hormones in plasma, estimation of plasma TSH, measurement of binding proteins, TRH response test, radioactive iodine uptake, thyroid scanning, detection of thyroid antibodies, and determination of cholesterol level in blood.

Classification

A. Isotopic tests:

a. Estimation of T_3 and T_4
b. Estimation of free T_3 and free T_4
c. TRH stimulation test
d. Thyroid scan
e. ^{125}I uptake studies, TSH stimulation and T_3 suppression tests. These are seldom done at present.

B. Non-isotopic tests:

a. Demonstration of thyroid autoantibodies
b. Imaging procedures of the neck. USS, CT and MRI
c. Biopsy of thyroid: fine needle aspiration cytology (FNAC) or open biopsy.

Measurement of Thyroid Hormones

T_3 and T_4 concentration in plasma are usually measured by RIA or sometimes by ELISA test. In *primary hyperthyroidism*, the thyroid hormone levels are increased, but typically the TSH is reduced due to feedback inhibition. In *primary*

Table 57.2: Thyroid function tests in primary thyroid dysfunctions.

	Hyperthyroidism	Hypothyroidism
Conc. of binding proteins	Normal	Normal
Plasma total T_3, T_4	High	Low
Plasma free T_3, T_4	High	Low
Plasma TSH	Low	High

hypothyroidism, T_3 and T_4 are decreased but TSH level is elevated (Table 57.2). In *pituitary hypothyroidism* T_3, T_4 and TSH are decreased.

Plasma TSH Estimation

Measurement of plasma TSH is an important diagnostic tool for the detection of thyroid abnormalities. In *primary hypothyroidism* TSH label is high but, in secondary hypothyroidism TSH as well as T_3 and T_4 are low. In *primary hyperthyroidism*, TSH is low. But, in hyperthyroidism due to pituitary causes, TSH, T_4 and T_3 are high.

Measurement of Binding Proteins

Usually, T_3 uptake by the resin is measured. The **T_3 resin uptake** indicates the free binding sites on the TBG.

1. In this test, radioactive iodine labeled-T_3 is added to the patient's serum. The labeled-T_3 occupies the free binding sites on TBG.
2. Then, a resin is added to the tube, which absorb the excess of labeled-T_3. The amount of labeled-T_3 absorbed by the resin (T_3 resin uptake) is directly proportional to the amount of thyroid hormones present in the serum and is inversely proportional to the free binding sites on the TBG.
3. When the hormone level is high as *in hyperthyroidism, the free binding site on TBG is less.*
4. Therefore, more T_3 is taken up by the resin. *In hypothyroidism*, due to more of free binding sites on the TBG, *T_3 resin uptake is low.*

TRH Response Test

This is a useful test for diagnosing both hypo- and hyperthyroidism. Normally, administration of TRH increases TSH production and therefore, the secretion of T_3 and T_4. An **abnormal response** is seen in hyperthyroidism because the negative feedback effect of high T_4 overrides the stimulant effect of TRH. In hypopituitarism in which pituitary cannot respond to TRH, the TRH response test is also abnormal. An *exaggerated response* is observed in primary hypothyroidism because the negative feedback effect of T_4 is reduced.

Detection of Thyroid Antibodies

Detection of antibodies against thyroid glands is essential for diagnosing Graves' disease and Hashimoto's thyroiditis, as these are autoimmune dysfunctions. In these diseases, specific antibodies are detected in plasma.

In Graves' disease thyroid stimulating immunoglobulin known as **LATS** (long acting thyroid stimulator) is increased in plasma. **LATS mimic TSH** by binding to TSH receptors on thyroid gland and stimulates more secretion of thyroid hormones. In this condition, the thyroid secretion is not under the feedback control as TSH is not the actual stimulator for the hormone secretion.

In Hashimoto's thyroiditis, antibodies against thyroglobulin are detected in circulation.

Plasma Cholesterol Estimation

Cholesterol level in plasma is **high in hypothyroidism** and low in hyperthyroidism. This is not diagnostic because change in plasma cholesterol occurs in many diseases. However, plasma cholesterol level is a useful index for monitoring the effectiveness of therapy in thyroid diseases, especially in hypothyroidism. Moreover, hyperlipidemic complications such as coronary artery disease are common in hypothyroidism.

Estimation of BMR

BMR is invariably **high in hyperthyroidism** and **low in hypothyroidism**. Though BMR determination is not performed now-a-days, and it is also not diagnostic, its alteration is highly suggestive of thyroid dysfunctions.

Thyroid Scintiscanning

Scintiscanning offers a **visual display** of the size and shape of the thyroid gland. It is employed in following situations.

1. It provides an objective assessment of the morphology of the gland.
2. It locates ectopic foci of the thyroid tissue.
3. The functional activity of the thyroid nodules (hot or cold nodules) (hot or cold nodules) can be evaluated.
4. In the investigation of masses in the neck or mediastinum, scintiscanning is useful to detect their nature (e.g: retrosternal thyroid).
5. Metastasis from thyroid carcinoma can be visualized.

Originally ^{131}I was used for visualizing the thyroid, the scan being done after 24 hours of administration. At present **technetium pertechnetate,** which has a half life of 6 hours is used for this purpose. With technetium scanning it can be done soon after the injection of the radioisotope.

Additional laboratory investigations include hematological tests and estimation of the levels of serum calcium, sodium, CPK and proteins.

Fine-Needle Aspiration Cytology

This biopsy of FNAC is a very **valuable preoperative procedure** done routinely. A correct diagnosis can be obtained in over 80% of cases. False negative results occur more frequently than false positive ones. The diagnosis accuracy of FNAC is about 95%, specificity 92% and sensitivity is around 83%.

Ultrasound/CT/MRI

Ultrasound scanning provides an accurate indication of the size and is useful for ***differentiating cystic from solid lesions***. **CT and MRI** are useful in the evaluation of retrosternal and retrotracheal extension of the gland, compression of trachea, extent of intrathoracic extensions of thyroid malignancy and infiltration to adjacent structures. **MRI** gives better delineation of soft tissue involvement like infiltration of nerves.

Achilles Tendon Reflex

Decreased relaxation time of Achilles tendon reflex is an important clinical assessment to suspect hypothyroidism.

CHAPTER SUMMARY

Key Concepts

1. Thyroid hormone is the key hormone for body metabolism. In hyperthyroidism there is substantial increase in BMR. Most of the features of hyperthyroidism are due to increased BMR and secondary to increased BMR. Opposite phenomena happens in hypothyroidism.
2. Thyroxine is highly essential for brain development in first year of life. Hypothyroidism in early infancy leads to severe mental retardation. Therefore, thyroxine deficiency if present in newborn, should be detected and treated immediately after birth.
3. Thyroxine profoundly increases body metabolism and HR. Therefore, heat intolerance and tachycardia even during sleep (sleeping tachycardia) are highly indicative of hyperthyroidism.

Important to Know (Must Read)

1. In examination, Steps of thyroid hormone synthesis, mechanism of action and physiological actions of thyroid hormone, is usually asked as a **Long Question**.
2. Mechanism of action of thyroxine, Synthesis and regulation of secretion of thyroxine, Actions of thyroxine on the cardiovascular system, nervous system and general effects on basal metabolism, Hyperthyroidism, Graves' disease (Features and Physiological basis of treatment) Hypothyroidism (Etiology, features, diagnosis and treatment), Cretinism (Causes, features and treatment), and Thyroid function tests, can come as **Short Questions** in exam.
3. In **Viva**, examiner may ask... Name of hormones secreted from thyroid gland, Actions of Thyroxine, specially on the cardiovascular system, nervous system and general effects on basal metabolism, Steps of thyroid hormone synthesis, specially mechanism of Iodide trapping, role of Na^+-I^- cotransporter, Pendred syndrome, Synthesis and secretion of thyroglobulin, Intramolecular and Intermolecular coupling, Proteins binding to T_4 and importance of protein binding, Factors affecting peripheral conversion of T_4, Regulation of thyroxine secretion, Mechanism of action of thyroid hormone, Functional anatomy of thyroid gland especially blood supply and histology of thyroid follicles, Surgical precautions during thyroid surgery, Functions of TSH, Features of Hyperthyroidism, Diagnosis of hyperthyroidism, Graves' disease, Thyrotoxicosis, Hashimoto's thyroiditis, Mechanism of action/ Physiological basis of different antithyroid drugs like Thionamides group (Propylthiouracil, Carbimazole, Methimazole), Anions, Iodide in high dose, Radioiodine, Propranolol etc., Etiology, features, diagnosis and management of Hypothyroidism, Etiology, features and management of cretinism, and Classify thyroid function tests and explain few important tests.

CHAPTER

58

Adrenal Gland: The Adrenal Medulla

LEARNING OBJECTIVES

On completion of study of this chapter, the student **MUST** be able to:

1. Give the structural organization of adrenal glands.
2. Name the hormones secreted from adrenal glands.
3. List the hormones secreted from adrenal medulla.
4. Give the steps of synthesis of catecholamines.
5. Apply the knowledge of understanding metabolism of catecholamines in diagnosing the excess or deficiency of catecholamines.
6. Describe the functions of catecholamines.
7. Give the differences between the functions of epinephrine and norepinephrine, especially their cardiovascular effects.
8. Learn the physiological basis of features, diagnosis, and treatment of pheochromocytoma.

The student **MAY** also be able to:

1. Describe the synthesis, secretion, and regulation of secretion of adrenomedullary hormones.
2. Explain the differences between the functions of epinephrine and norepinephrine.
3. Explain the role of catecholamines in acute and chronic stress.

ADRENAL GLAND

General Features

There are two adrenal glands, each one located at the upper pole of each kidney (Fig. 58.1). The adrenals consist of **two distinct endocrine glands**, one surrounding the other: the inner **adrenal medulla**, surrounded by the outer **adrenal cortex** that consists of three layers (Fig. 58.2).

1. The outer zone of adrenal gland, i.e. the **adrenal cortex forms about 80–90%** of the total gland, the inner zone, i.e. the **adrenal medulla consists of 10–20%** of the gland.
2. Developmentally and functionally, these glands are **two separate endocrine organs**. Adrenal cortex develops from the mesodermal tissue and secretes steroid hormones.
3. Adrenal medulla develops from **neuroectodermal tissue related to sympathetic ganglia**, and therefore secretes catecholamines.

Blood Supply

Weight of each adrenal gland is about 5–10 g. The gland is **highly vascular** and receives blood from **three sources**: branches of aorta, renal arteries, and phrenic arteries. The arterial blood enters the sinusoidal capillaries in the cortex and then drains into the medullary venules. This arrangement exposes the medulla to the high concentration of corticosteroids secreted from the cortex.

General Importance

The adrenal glands are essential for survival. In general, they play important role in following physiological processes of the body:

1. Homeostasis of energy stores
2. Control of fluid volume and extracellular environment of cells
3. Supply of substrates for generation of ATP in the cells
4. Regulation of intermediary metabolisms
5. Control of immunological mechanisms
6. Regulation of functions of various organ systems.

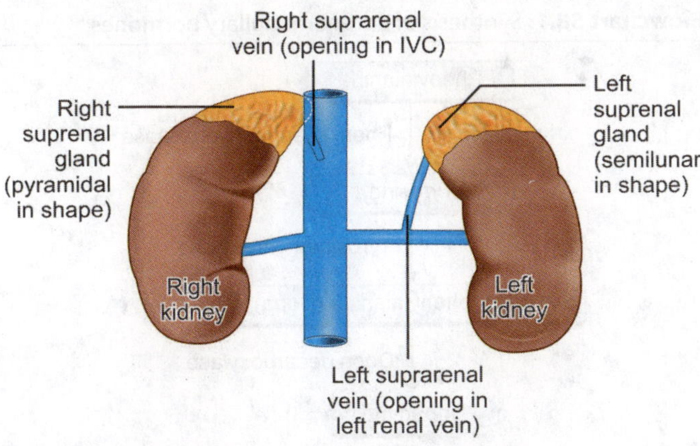

Fig. 58.1: Location of adrenal (suprarenal) gland.

Therefore, an adrenalectomized animal unlike its normal counterpart, **cannot survive prolonged fasting and stress**, and dies due to hypoglycemia, inadequate ATP generation in the cells and inefficiency to maintain fluid volume and composition (circulatory collapse). However, the adrenocortical hormones are essential for survival of the being. Though, adrenomedullary hormones are not essential for immediate survival, they help **prepare the individual to deal with emergencies**.

ADRENAL MEDULLA

Unlike hormones of adrenal cortex, adrenomedullary hormones are not very essential for survival. However, they help the individual to cope with emergencies. Adrenal medulla, by secreting catecholamines assist the individual to prepare for Fight or flight responses and also assist in meeting the metabolic requirements of the body in hypoglycemic emergencies in addition to their effects on other systemic functions.

Scientist contributed

John Jacob Abel (1857–1938), a German scientist, who later worked in USA, was pioneer in the study of endocrine secretions, especially on adrenal medulla. His outstanding works on the blood pressure-raising constituents of the adrenal medulla led to the identification and synthesis of catecholamines, and further to the development of many derivatives of catecholamines. Similarly, his studies on pituitary gland resulted in the isolation of its oxytocic, pressor and diuretic principles. He also pioneered with crystalline insulin. With *Leonard G. Rowntree* he introduced kidney and liver function tests.

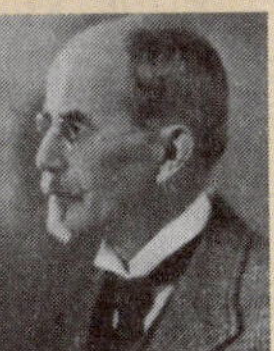

JJ Abel
(1857–1938)

Cell Types

Adrenal medulla is the **inner zone of the adrenal gland**, which constitutes about 20–30% of its mass. Essentially, adrenal medulla represents an enlarged and specialized **sympathetic ganglion** in which the postganglionic fibers are embedded and modified to become the endocrine cells. The tissue of adrenal medulla weighs about 1 g in adults.

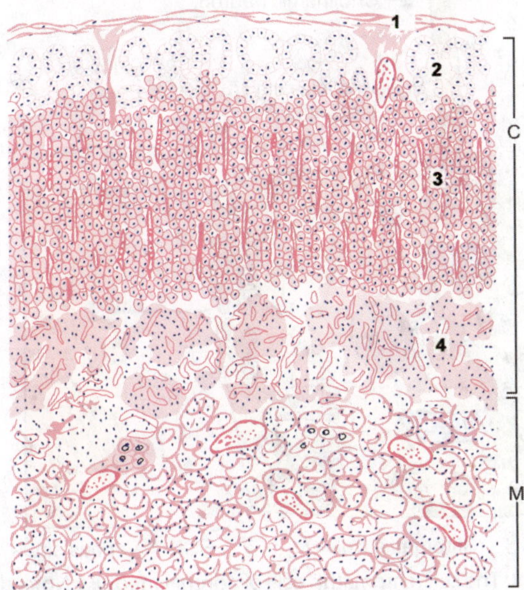

Fig. 58.2: Structure of different layers of adrenal gland: (C: Cortex; M: Medulla; 1: Capsule; 2: Zona glomerulosa; 3: Zona fasciculata; 4: Zona reticularis).

The gland consists of clumps and strands of **chromaffin cells**, interspersed with venous sinuses. The cells are called chromaffin cells as they have greater affinity for chromium stains. They contain numerous granules that are present in the vesicles that store catecholamines (Fig. 58.3).

There are **two types of endocrine cells** in the adrenal medulla: epinephrine-secreting and norepinephrine-secreting,

1. **Epinephrine-secreting type:** In humans, **90% of cell types** in adrenal medulla are epinephrine-secreting type. The granules in these cells are **lager and less dense**. Granules completely fill the vesicles.
2. **Norepinephrine-secreting type:** They constitute **10% of the cell mass** of adrenal medulla. The granules in these cells are **small and very dense**. The granules do not fill the vesicles in which they are present.

The types of **cells that secrete dopamine** are not known, but are believed to be very less in number. Chromaffin cells receive **sympathetic preganglionic cholinergic innervation** and on stimulation discharge their content into venous sinuses. Small group of chromaffin cells are present near abdominal sympathetic ganglia. These are called **paraganglia**. They also secrete catecholamines.

ADRENOMEDULLARY HORMONES

The major hormones secreted from adrenal medulla are catecholamines:

1. Epinephrine
2. Norepinephrine
3. Dopamine.

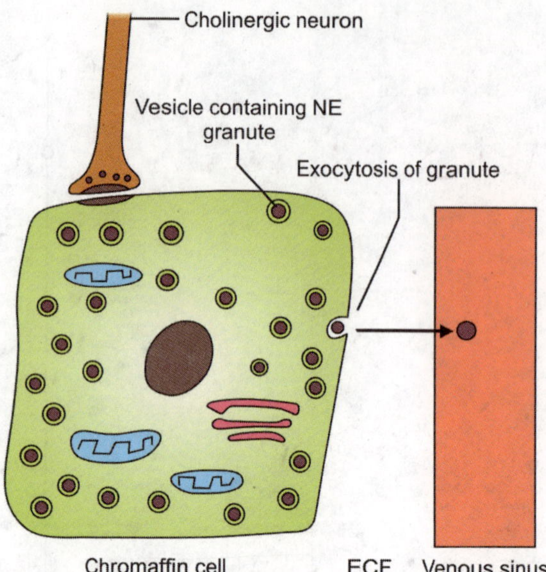

Fig. 58.3: The cell (chromaffin cell) of adrenal medulla. Note, the cell is innervated by sympathetic preganglionic cholinergic neuron. The granules containing hormone is discharged into extracellular space by exocytosis and from there the hormone enters sinusoidal vein.

In addition to secretion of catecholamines, the gland also secretes following peptides:

1. Adrenomedullin
2. Enkephalins
3. β-endorphin
4. Neuropeptide-Y
5. Chromogranin

Epinephrine secreting cells secrete **opioid peptide**. Most of the circulating **metenkephalins** are secreted from adrenal medulla.

The major secretion from adrenal medulla in human is epinephrine. About 85% of adrenomedullary secretion is epinephrine, 10–12% is norepinephrine and 1–3% dopamine, whereas secretion from sympathetic noradrenergic nerve ending is almost entirely norepinephrine.

Effect of Sympathetic Stimulation

Adrenal medulla is stimulated with the activation of sympathetic system. Therefore, sympathetic stimulation not only ***increases norepinephrine secretion from its nerve endings*** that slowly enters circulation, but also directly increases ***epinephrine secretion from adrenal medulla*** that rapidly enters circulation. Thus, sympathetic activation increases the level of **both epinephrine and norepinephrine** in blood.

Synthesis, Secretion, and Metabolism of Catecholamines

Synthesis and Secretion

Catecholamines are synthesized from the amino acid **phenylalanine and tyrosine** (Flowchart 58.1).

Flowchart 58.1: Synthesis of adrenomedullary hormones.

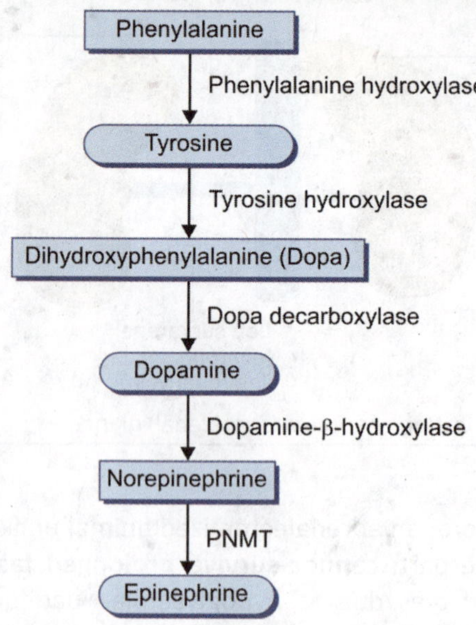

1. Conversion of tyrosine to Dopa is catalyzed by *tyrosine hydroxylase* and dopa to dopamine by *dopa decarboxylase*.
2. Norepinephrine is formed by hydroxylation and decarboxylation of tyrosine and epinephrine is formed by methylation of norepinephrine by *phenylethanolamine-N-methyltransferase* (PNMT).
3. After synthesis, the hormones are **stored in the granules** of chromaffin cells before they are secreted into venous blood.

Effects of Glucocorticoid

The enzyme **PNMT is induced by glucocorticoid** at higher concentration. It may be noted that, the concentration of **glucocorticoids is normally high in blood bathing adrenal medulla** as blood from cortex drains into medulla before entering general circulation. Therefore, **in adrenocortical deficiency, epinephrine synthesis is also reduced**. Also, glucocorticoid promotes normal growth of adrenal medulla.

Effects of 21β-hydroxylase

During fetal life, the adrenocortical enzyme, **21β-hydroxylase** stimulates development of adrenal medulla. Therefore, **fetal deficiency of 21β-hydroxylase** results in dysplasia of adrenal medulla, and if enzyme deficiency is not corrected promptly after birth, circulating catecholamines remain permanently low.

Regulation of Secretion

Catecholamine secretion from adrenal medulla increases in following conditions.

1. Exercise
2. Hypoglycemia
3. Trauma (Physical injury)

Flowcharts 58.2A and B: Metabolic degradation of epinephrine (A) and norepinephrine (B).

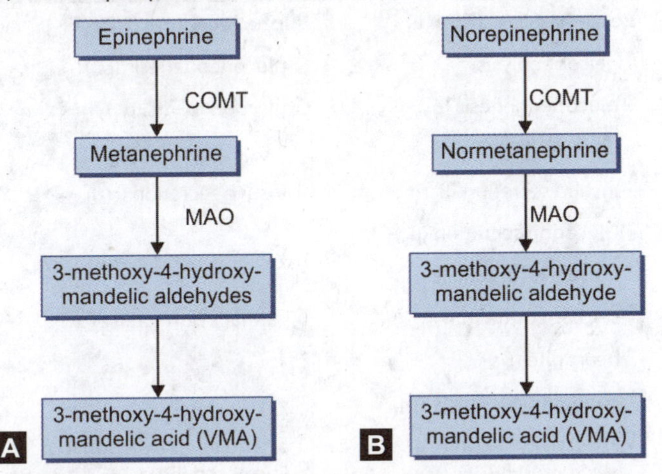

(COMT: Catecholamine-O-methyltransferase; MAO: monoamine oxidase).

4. Anger and anxiety
5. Pain
6. Cold

The main mechanism of secretion in these conditions is **sympathetic stimulation**. **Hypoglycemia** is a strong stimulus for catecholamine release. When **blood glucose is less than 60 mg%**, CNS receptors monitoring plasma glucose are activated. They stimulate the neural pathways that activate sympathetic fibers to release norepinephrine and adrenal medulla to release mainly epinephrine. These catecholamines in turn increase plasma glucose level.

Metabolism

The normal **plasma concentration of free hormone** in recumbent posture is as follows:

Norepinephrine : 300 pg/mL
Epinephrine : 30 pg/mL
Dopamine : 35 pg/mL

On standing, the hormone level increases by 50–100%. The circulating epinephrine is mainly derived from adrenal medulla and norepinephrine from the sympathetic nerve endings, whereas dopamine is derived equally from adrenal medulla and autonomic nerve endings.

1. About 70% norepinephrine and epinephrine, and 90% of dopamine are conjugated to sulfate. They have very short life span. Half-life is about 1–3 minutes.
2. They are metabolized primarily in the liver and kidney. The key enzymes of metabolism are catecholamine-O-methyltransferase (**COMT**), and monoamine oxidase (**MAO**).
3. Metabolism of epinephrine forms **metanephrine** and norepinephrine forms **normetanephrine**.
4. Epinephrine and norepinephrine are also commonly degraded to form dihydroxymandelic acid which is further metabolized to form **vanillylmandelic acid (VMA)** and **methoxyhydroxy-phenylglycol (MOPG)**.

Flowchart 58.3: Steps of metabolic degradation of dopamine.

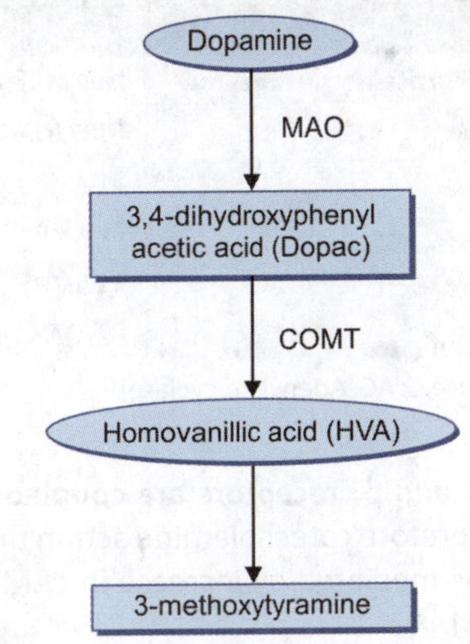

Degradation

The **steps of degradation** of epinephrine and norepinephrine are summarized in Flowcharts 58.2A and B respectively. Only 2–3% of catecholamines are excreted unchanged in urine. About 50% of secreted catecholamines appear in urine as metanephrine and normetanephrine, and 35% as 3-methoxy-4-hydroxy-mandelic acid, also called as VMA (Application Box 58.1).

The steps of degradation of dopamine are listed in Flowchart 58.3.

24 h urinary excretion: The normal daily urinary excretion of catecholamines and their metabolites are as follows:

Metanephrine plus normetanephrine : 300 µg
VMA : 400–600 µg
MOPG : 200 µg
Norepinephrine : 30 µg
Epinephrine : 6 µg

Application Box 58.1

VMA is the index of sympathetic activity: Urinary excretion of VMA and MOPG reflect activity of sympathetic nervous system as they are mainly derived from norepinephrine. Epinephrine contributes relatively less to the production of VMA and MOPG. Therefore, the activity of adrenal medulla is assessed primarily by measurement of plasma epinephrine or free urinary epinephrine.

Mechanism of Action

Catecholamines act on α **and** β **receptors.** There are **three types of** β **receptors**: β_1, β_2, and β_3, and **two types of** α **receptors**: α_1 and α_2.

1. The α_1 and α_2 **receptors** have *three subtypes each*. Epinephrine and norepinephrine act on both α and β receptors.
2. However, in general, epinephrine acts more on β receptors and norepinephrine on α receptors. β_1, β_2, and α_2 are structurally similar.

Table 58.1: Mechanism of action at various catecholaminergic receptors.

Receptors	G proteins	Enzyme	2nd Messengers
α_1	$G\alpha_q$	PLC	↑ IP3, DAG, Ca^{++}
α_2	$G\alpha_i$	AC	↓ cAMP
β_1	$G\alpha_s$	AC	↑ cAMP
β_2	$G\alpha_s$	AC	↑ cAMP
β_3	$G\alpha_s$	AC	↑ cAMP

(PLC: Phospholipase C; AC: Adenylate cyclase).

3. The β_1, β_2, and β_3 **receptors are coupled to adenylyl cyclase**; therefore catecholamine action through these receptors is mediated by increase in cAMP in the cell (Table 58.1).
4. The α_2 **receptor is coupled to inhibitory G protein**; therefore, binding of catecholamines with this receptor decreases cAMP in the cells.
5. The α_1 **receptor is coupled to phosphatidylinositol** in the membrane. Therefore, hormones acting on this receptor exert their action through DAG and IP_3 as second messengers.

Physiological Actions of Catecholamines

Catecholamines have profound effects on carbohydrate and fat metabolisms. They supply energy at the time of emergency and prepare the individual for either Fight or flight responses. They also control many autonomic and visceral functions.

Effects on Intermediary Metabolism

On Carbohydrate Metabolism

Catecholamines act on liver to increase glucose production by following mechanisms:

1. Catecholamines **stimulate hepatic glycogenolysis** by activating the key enzyme **glycogen phosphorylase**, which causes hydrolysis of stored glycogen. They, also activate glycogenolysis in the skeletal muscle.
2. They **stimulate gluconeogenesis** from lactate and amino acids in the liver.
3. They also **inhibit glycogen synthesis** by inhibiting glycogen synthase enzyme complex.
4. Epinephrine **inhibits insulin mediated glucose uptake** by the skeletal muscle and adipose tissue.
5. Catecholamines also **stimulate glucagon and inhibit insulin** secretion from pancreas.

All these effects are primarily aimed to increase plasma glucose concentration.

On Fat Metabolism

Catecholamines promote lipolysis.

1. Epinephrine **activates hormone sensitive lipase** in the adipose tissue that causes hydrolysis of triglycerides and **increases plasma FFA**. FFA provides an alternative substrate for energy metabolism.
2. Catecholamines also *promote β oxidation of FFA* in muscle and liver to **form ketone bodies.**
3. Catecholamines are therefore ***prodiabetogenic and proketogenic*** hormones.

Table 58.2: Various major actions of catecholamines.

Beta receptors (E > NE)	Alpha receptors (NE > E)
↑ glycogenolysis	↑ gluconeogenesis (α_1)
↑ gluconeogenesis (β_2)	↑ glycogenolysis (α_1)
↑ lipolysis (β_3,β_2)	
↑ insulin secretion (β_2)	↓ insulin secretion (α_2)
↑ Glucagon secretion (β_2)	
↑ muscle K^+ uptake (β_2)	
↑ cardiac contractility (β_1)	↑ cardiac contractility (α_1)
↑ heart rate (β_1)	
↑ conduction velocity (β_1)	
↑ arteriolar dilation (β_2) (decreased BP)	↑ arteriolar constriction (α_1) (increased BP)
↑ muscle relaxation (β_2) (GI, urinary and bronchial)	↑ sphincter contraction (α_1) Pupillary dilation (α_1)

On Thermogenesis

Epinephrine is more potent than norepinephrine in most of the metabolic effects. Epinephrine **increases BMR** by 10–15%. It increases **nonshivering thermogenesis** and **diet-induced thermogenesis**. Therefore, epinephrine plays an important role in body adjustment mechanisms in response to cold.

During Hypoglycemia

Secretion of catecholamines increases in profound hypoglycemia, as occurs during strenuous exercise or fasting.

1. Catecholamines induce **glycogenolysis and gluconeogenesis** to combat hypoglycemia.
2. **Lipolysis-induced release of FFA** is used as alternative fuel.
3. In such situation, catecholamines also stimulate secretion of glucagon and inhibit insulin release.

Various metabolic effects of catecholamines mediated though different receptors are summarized in Table 58.2.

Fight or Flight Response

Norepinephrine and epinephrine have widespread effects on cardiovascular, respiratory and gastrointestinal systems, and intermediary metabolisms to prepare the individual to Fight or flight at the time of emergency.

1. They increase cardiac output, promote blood flow to organs, increase ventilation, stimulate energy supply, relax the smooth muscle of GI tract and urinary

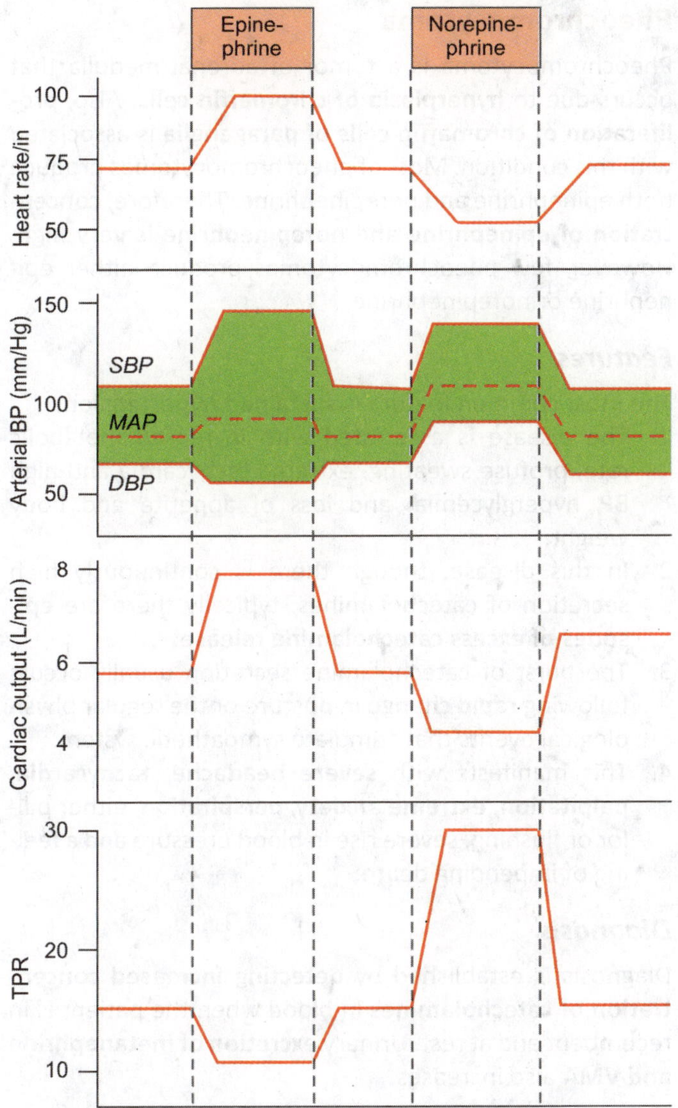

Fig. 58.4: Cardiovascular changes following i.v. administration of epinephrine and norepinephrine. (SBP: Systolic pressure; MAP: Mean arterial pressure; DBP: Diastolic pressure; TPR: Total peripheral resistance).

system, and cause piloerection; all these effects are intended to either Fight with the enemy to finish or escape fast from the enemy to protect.

2. This is called Fight or flight response, which is exclusively mediated by **sympathetic stimulation and catecholamines released** from adrenal medulla (for details, refer Chapter "Sympathetic System").

Effects on Cardiovascular System

Both epinephrine and norepinephrine increase force and rate of contraction of the heart that are mediated by β_1 receptors. Catecholamines also increase cardiac excitability and conductivity.

Effects of Epinephrine

1. Epinephrine **increases heart rate and force of myocardial contraction**, and therefore, causes adequate **increase in cardiac output**. Due to increased cardiac output **systolic pressure increases.**
2. It causes ***selective arteriolar constriction*** in renal, splanchnic and cutaneous vascular bed. However, epinephrine **produces vasodilation** in the skeletal and hepatic circulation via β_2 receptors. The ***vasodilation effect of epinephrine overrides the vasoconstriction effect*** and therefore, **total peripheral resistance falls.** Consequently, the **diastolic pressure decreases mildly**.
3. Thus, **pulse pressure widens**. This occurs especially during sympathetic stimulation that takes place during exercise.
4. The primary aim of all these changes is to divert blood from splanchnic and cutaneous circulation to the exercising (active) muscles, while maintaining the cerebral and coronary blood flow.
5. This also occurs during stress. These changes ensure delivery of substrate for energy production to the vital organs during Fight or flight situations (Application Box 58.2).

Effects of Norepinephrine

1. Norepinephrine produces **vasoconstriction** in most of the organs via α_1 receptors that **increases peripheral resistance** and therefore, **diastolic blood pressure rises.**
2. Norepinephrine also produces some degree of tachycardia and increases myocardial contractility; therefore, **systolic blood pressure also increases.**
3. However, hypertension produced by norepinephrine stimulates baroreceptors in the carotid sinus and aortic arch (activates baroreceptor reflex) that causes **reflex bradycardia,** and **overrides cardioacceleratory effects.**
4. Therefore, the net effect is **decrease in heart rate and cardiac output** inspite of increased peripheral resistance (Fig.58.4).

Application Box 58.2

Chronic catecholamine secretion is not good: In shock or circulatory failure, sympathetic stimulation that causes catecholamines secretion benefits the individual. However, if secretion of catecholamine is prolonged, then the effect on the body is deleterious, because renal vasoconstriction decreases kidney blood flow and compromises kidney function. Also, decreased splanchnic circulation impairs visceral functions. Chronic sympathetic stimulation may even result in intestinal paresis or hepatic failure.

Effects on Other Systems

GI System

Catecholamines **inhibit gastric secretion** and motility.

Respiratory System

Catecholamines cause **bronchial dilation** (prevent expiratory airway obstruction) so that gas exchange improves. They also stimulate respiration.

On Eye

They cause **pupillary dilation**; therefore vision for distant objects improves. This helps to see the surroundings clearly that helps the endangered individual.

On Endocrine Glands

Catecholamines **stimulate ADH release** through β receptors. They also increase renin secretion from the JG apparatus of kidney. Catecholamines **increase thyroid hormone** secretion and promote peripheral **conversion of T_4 to T_3** which is mediated by β_2 receptors.

On Kidney

Catecholamines **increases Na^+ reabsorption** from kidney. Catecholamines also redistribute renal blood flow. They **increase renin formation** that causes angiotensin and aldosterone synthesis and secretion, which in turn increases Na^+ and water retention.

On Electrolyte Balance

Catecholamines **stimulate the entry of K^+ into the muscle cell**. Therefore, they decrease plasma K^+ (prevent hyperkalemia). Catecholamines also increase plasma Na^+ concentration.

Effects of Dopamine

1. It produces **renal and mesenteric vasodilation.**
2. It causes vasoconstriction in other parts of the body.
3. It has **positive inotropic effects (via β_1 receptors),** increases cardiac output.
4. It increases systolic pressure, whereas diastolic pressure does not change significantly.
5. It causes **natriuresis,** by inhibiting Na^+-K^+ ATPase in proximal tubule.

As dopamine increases systolic pressure and at the same time maintains kidney functions, it is very useful for the treatment of **traumatic and cardiogenic shocks.**

Applied Physiology

Clinical Uses of Catecholamines

Agonists and antagonists of catecholamines are widely used in clinical practice.

1. The agonists are used as nasal decongestant, appetite inhibitor, and for stimulation of general body functions.
2. The antagonists (both α and β receptor antagonists) are also used for the treatment of hypertension.
3. The antagonists (β receptor blockers) are also used for the treatment hyperthyroidism, especially to prepare the patient before thyroid surgery to decrease the heart rate.
4. Catecholamines are used for the treatment of shock.
5. Dopamine is used for treatment of traumatic and cardiogenic shock.

Pheochromocytoma

Pheochromocytoma is a tumor of adrenal medulla that occurs due to **hyperplasia of chromaffin cells**. Also, **proliferation of chromaffin cells of paraganglia** is associated with this condition. Most of pheochromocytomas produce both epinephrine and norepinephrine. Therefore, **concentration of epinephrine and norepinephrine is very high**. However, few pheochromocytomas produce either epinephrine or norepinephrine.

Features

The most common feature is **sustained hypertension**.

1. The disease is associated with increased metabolic rate, profuse sweating, extreme tachycardia and high BP, hyperglycemia, and loss of appetite and body weight.
2. In this disease, though there is continuously high secretion of catecholamines, typically there are **episodes of excess catecholamine release.**
3. The burst of catecholamine secretion usually occurs following **rapid change in posture** or the regular physiological events that stimulate sympathetic system.
4. This manifests with **severe headache, tachycardia, palpitation, extreme anxiety, perspiration**, either pallor or flushing, severe rise in blood pressure and a feeling of impending death.

Diagnosis

Diagnosis is established by **detecting increased concentration of catecholamines** in blood when the patient is in recumbent and at rest. Urinary **excretion of metanephrine and VMA** also increases.

Treatment

Treatment is by surgical removal of the tumor. The systematic improvement occurs with administration of α blockers.

Role of Catecholamines in Stress

Stress activates **CRH and ADH secreting neurons** of hypothalamus.

1. CRH in turn increases adrenergic discharge. Adrenergic stimulation **increases plasma catecholamine** concentration.
2. All these hormones together **increase glucose concentration** in plasma. **Catecholamines increase glycogenolysis** and **cortisol promotes gluconeogenesis.**
3. They also shift glucose utilization from peripheral tissues to the neural tissue.
4. Epinephrine **increases supply of FFA** to the heart.
5. Catecholamines increase cardiac output and blood pressure and promote supply of substrate to the tissue.

During acute stress, a **general state of arousal and vigilance** is maintained by catecholamines. **In chronic stress,** reproductive functions, sexual activity, and feeding are suppressed that are also mediated by catecholamines. A variety of **cytokines** are secreted during stress. The **hypothalamic-pituitary-adrenal axis** works in adaptation to stress. They generally activate the lifesaving mechanisms.

OTHER ADRENOMEDULLARY PEPTIDES

Adrenomedullin

Adrenomedullin is a polypeptide hormone. It is synthesized from *proadrenomedullin*. It is also formed in other tissues like brain and kidney.

Functions

1. Adrenomedullin decreases blood pressure by causing vasodilation, which is due to the increased production of EDRF by it.
2. It inhibits aldosterone secretion, and therefore, decreases ECF volume.
3. It, along with proadrenomedullin decreases peripheral sympathetic activity.

Chromogranin

This is a granular protein present in the secretory granules of chromaffin cells. The protein makes the dense core vesicles denser. The dominant chromogranin in human is **chromogranin B**.

1. Chromogranins are secreted along with catecholamines from the granules.
2. Therefore, measurement of their concentration in plasma **indicates the secretory activity of chromaffin cells** and indirectly the rate of catecholamine secretions.

Other Hormones

Enkephalins, endorphins, and neuropeptide Y are discussed elsewhere in the book.

CHAPTER SUMMARY

Key Concepts

1. Adrenal medulla is a neuroendocrine gland, a modified sympathetic postganglionic tissue. Therefore, sympathetic stimulation results in instantaneous increase in catecholamines level in plasma.
2. Though, epinephrine and norepinephrine act on both α and β receptors, in general, epinephrine acts more on β receptors and norepinephrine on α receptors.
3. Increased level of urinary VMA is an index of increased sympathetic activity.
4. Though sympathetic activation is essential in stressful situations to maintain energy metabolism and cardiovascular parameters, chronic stress (sustained sympathetic stimulation) is not good for body as it leads to depletion and degeneration.

Important to Know (Must Read)

1. In examination, "Describe the synthesis, metabolism and physiological effects of adrenaline and noradrenaline" may come as a **Long Question**.
2. In examination, Fight or flight response, Pheochromocytoma, Difference in the effects of adrenaline and noradrenaline on cardiovascular system, Effects of catecholamines on intermediary metabolism can be asked as **Short Questions**.
3. In **Viva**, examiner may ask… List the hormones secreted from adrenal medulla, Why VMA is an index of sympathetic activity, What is Fight or flight response, Cause, features, diagnosis, and treatment of Pheochromocytoma, Why chronic catecholamine secretion is not good, Types of catecholaminergic receptors, Which catecholamine act more on which receptor, Mechanism of action of catecholamine on different receptors, Effects of catecholamines on cardiovascular system, Effects of catecholamines on intermediary metabolism, Effects of catecholamines on other systems, Effects of Dopamine, Clinical uses of catecholamines, Mechanism of action of catecholamines, Steps of synthesis of adrenomedullary hormones, Factors regulating secretion of catecholamines, Names of other adrenomedullary hormones, Functions of adrenomedullin, and Functions of chromogranin.

CHAPTER 59

Adrenal Cortex

LEARNING OBJECTIVES

On completion of study of this chapter, the student **MUST** be able to:

1. Correlate the histological specialization of different layers of adrenal cortex and medulla for secretion of specific hormones.
2. List the hormones secreted from different layers of adrenal cortex.
3. Give the steps of synthesis of different adrenocortical hormones.
4. Understand the deficiency of adrenocortical enzymes causing a specific dysfunction or syndrome.
5. Describe the regulation of secretion, mechanism of action and functions of glucocorticoids.
6. Describe the regulation of secretion, mechanism of action and functions of mineralocorticoids.
7. Appreciate the physiological importance of cortisol, and indications & contraindication of cortisol use in clinical medicine.
8. Understand the physiological basis of dysfunctions caused by excess or deficiency of glucocorticoids and mineralocorticoids.
9. Outline the functions and dysfunctions of adrenal sex steroids.

The student **MAY** also be able to:

1. Describe the steps of synthesis and regulation of secretion of adrenocortical hormones.
2. Explain the mechanism of action of glucocorticoids and mineralocorticoids.
3. Describe the role of cortisol in stress.
4. Describe the functions and dysfunctions of adrenal sex steroids.

The adrenals consist of **two distinct endocrine glands**, one inside the other. The inner **adrenal medulla** is surrounded by the outer **adrenal cortex** that consists of three layers (Figs. 59.1A to C). The outer zone of adrenal gland, i.e. the adrenal cortex forms about 80–90% of the total gland, the inner zone, i.e. the adrenal medulla consists of 10–20% of the gland. Developmentally and functionally, these glands are **two separate endocrine organs**. Adrenal cortex develops from the mesodermal tissue and secretes steroid hormones. Adrenal medulla develops from neuroectodermal tissue related to sympathetic ganglia, and, therefore, secretes catecholamines.

Scientists contributed

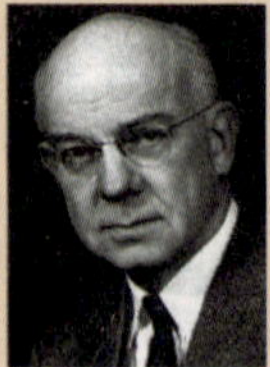

EC Kendall
(1886–1972)

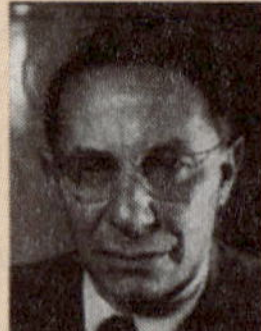

T Reichstein
(1897–1996)

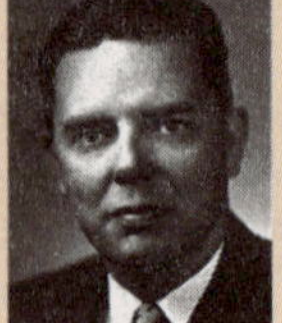

PS Hench
(1896–1965)

The **Nobel Prize in Physiology or Medicine 1950** was awarded jointly to American biochemist and endocrinologist **Edward Calvin Kendall**, Swiss biochemist and endocrinologist **Tadeus Reichstein**, and Jamaican biochemist and endocrinologist **Philip Showalter Hench** *"for their discoveries relating to the **hormones of the adrenal cortex**, their structure and biological effects"*.

FUNCTIONAL ANATOMY

Adrenal cortex, the outer zone of the adrenal gland constitutes 80–90% of the gland. **In fetus,** adrenal cortex is larger in size in which **fetal adrenal cortex constitute 80%** of the gland and the future permanent adrenal cortex makes only 20% of the gland.

1. At term, the fetal adrenal cortex *undergoes rapid degeneration* and almost disappears in early infancy.
2. The remaining permanent cortex remains and constitutes **postnatal adrenal cortex.**
3. During fetal life, the **fetal adrenal cortex synthesizes and secretes sulfate conjugates of androgens** that

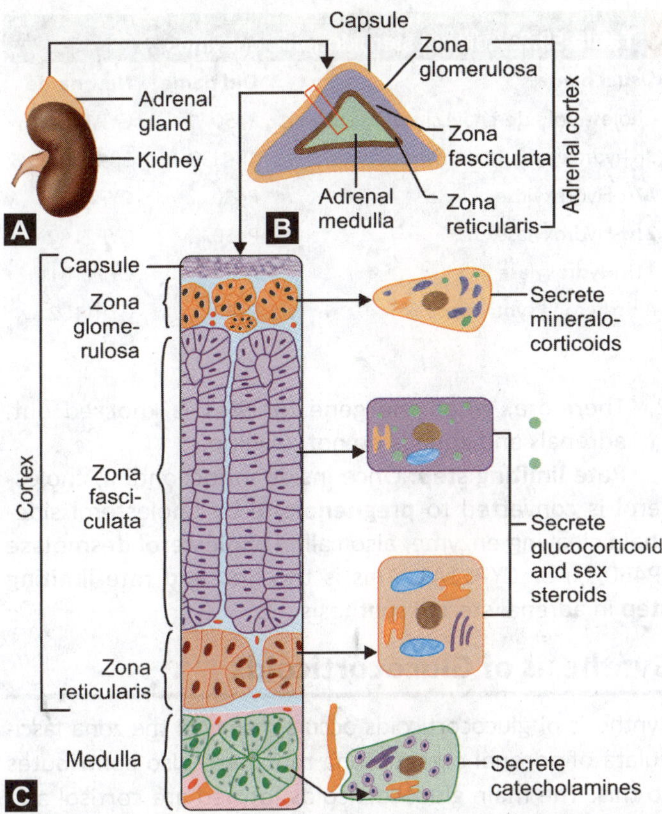

Figs. 59.1A to C: (A) Location of adrenal gland; (B) Parts of adrenal gland as seen in cross-section of the gland; (C) Histology of adrenal gland. Note, zona fasciculata constitutes more than 80% of adrenal cortex.

are **converted to estrogens and progesterone** in the placenta, which is ***essential for maintenance of pregnancy*** (*see* below).

Hormones and their major functions: Adrenal cortex secretes **three categories of hormones**: glucocorticoids, mineralocorticoids and sex hormones (Table 59.1).

1. The **glucocorticoids** are important for their metabolic, permissive, anti-inflammatory and immunosuppressive effects.
2. **Mineralocorticoids** are important for their role in extracellular fluid volume and electrolyte balance.
3. The **sex steroids** contribute to establish and maintain secondary sexual characteristics.

Of adrenocortical hormones, glucocorticoids and mineralocorticoids are the indispensable hormones.

Histology

Adrenal cortex consists of **three layers:** the outer zona glomerulosa that secretes mineralocorticoids, the middle zona fasciulata that secretes glucocorticoids and sex steroids, and the inner zona reticularis that secretes sex steroids and glucocorticoids (Figs. 59.1A to C).

Zona glomerulosa: This is the outermost and thinnest layer of the gland. It constitutes 20% of the adrenal cortex and consists of ***small clumps of cells*** that contain numerous mitochondria. It ***secretes mineralocorticoids***, mainly aldosterone.

Table 59.1: Hormones secreted from adrenal cortex.

1. Mineralocorticoids a. Aldosterone b. Deoxycorticosterone
2. Glucocorticoids a. Cortisol b. Corticosterone
3. Sex steroids a. Dehydroepiandrosterone b. Androstenedione

Zona fasciculata: This is the middle and **widest layer** of the adrenal cortex. It constitutes 80% of the adrenocortical mass. It consists of ***columnar cells that form long cords***. The cytoplasm is loaded with vacuoles and lipid droplets. The mitochondria are large and contain numerous vesicular cristae. Cells of this layer ***secrete glucocorticoids*** (mainly cortisol and corticosterone) and sex steroids.

Zona reticularis: This is the innermost layer of the adrenal cortex and constitutes about 10% of its mass. It contains ***network of intercalated cells***. The mitochondria are large and have vesicular cristae. There are no vacuoles and fat droplets. Cells of this layer ***secrete sex steroids*** like androgens and estrogens, and to some extent also glucocorticoids.

SYNTHESIS OF ADRENOCORTICAL HORMONES

Adrenocortical steroid hormones are synthesized from **cholesterol**. Cholesterol used for synthesis of steroid hormones in the adrenal cortical cells, are made available from **two sources**:

1. From blood, and,
2. Synthesized de novo.

From blood: Most of the cholesterol used for biosynthesis of steroid hormones are derived from cholesterol esters attached to the LDL (*LDL-cholesterol*) in circulating blood. Cells of adrenal cortex **actively take up cholesterol** from plasma by **endocytosis of LDL molecules.**

1. There are abundant LDL receptors on adrenocortical cells. In the cytoplasm, the cholesterol is esterified immediately and then stored as cholesterol esters in the lipid droplets (Fig. 59.2).
2. Whenever required for synthesis of hormones, cholesterol ester is converted to free cholesterol by the action of the cytosolic enzyme **cholesterol ester hydrolase**.
3. Cholesterol is then transported to mitochondria by a carrier protein, called **sterol carrier protein 2.** Sterol carrier protein 2 facilitates entry of cholesterol into mitochondria for hormone synthesis.

From the cell itself (de novo synthesis): Cholesterol is synthesized de novo in the cytosol of adrenocortical cells from acetate by the action of the enzyme **HMG CoA reductase**.

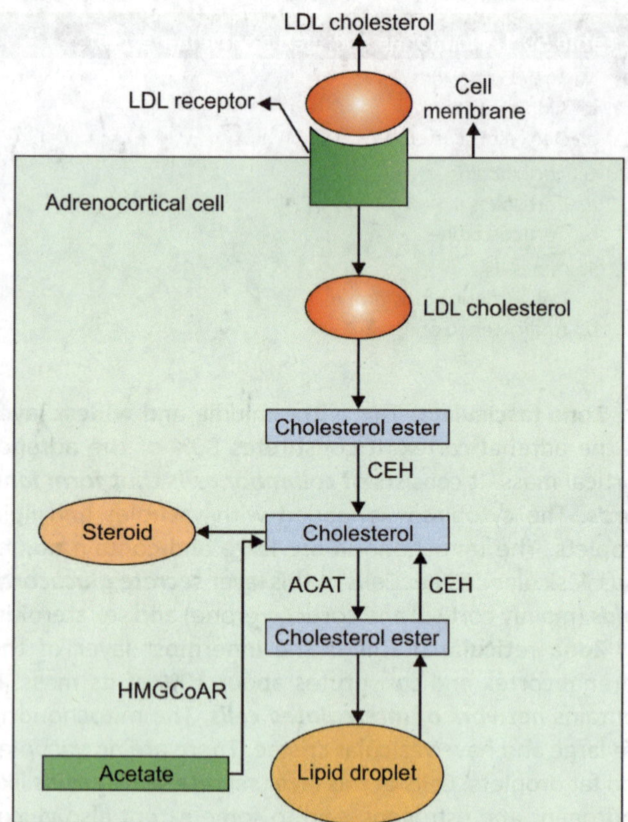

Fig. 59.2: Synthesis of steroid hormone in adrenocortical cells from cholesterol. (CEH: Cholesterol ester hydrolase; ACAT: Acyl-CoA-cholesterol acyltransferase). Note, excess cholesterol in the cell forms cholesterol ester, which is deposited as lipid droplet. De novo synthesis of cholesterol in the cells occurs from acetate by the action of HMGCoA reductase (HMGCoAR).

1. Formed cholesterol is then converted to **cholesterol ester** by the action of ***acyl-CoA-cholesterol acyltransferase*** (ACAT).
2. **Cholesterol ester** is then stored in the lipid droplet, to be used later for hormone synthesis.

Though, cells of the adrenal cortex can synthesize cholesterol *de novo*, under basal conditions **plasma cholesterol is the major source** for adrenocortical hormone synthesis. However, **when hormone synthesis is stimulated by ACTH**, the stored cholesterol in the cytosol of adrenocortical cells and newly formed cholesterol in the cytosol become the important source for hormone synthesis. In such conditions, plasma cholesterol without undergoing esterification directly enters mitochondria for biosynthesis of hormones.

Cytochrome P-450 enzymes: The synthesis of hormones from cholesterol involves ***cytochrome P-450 enzymes***, also known as CYPs (Table 59.2). These are the enzymes that ***catalyze hydroxylation of steroids***. They are located in the membranes of endoplasmic reticulum and mitochondrial cristae.

1. Cytochrome P-450 enzymes for their steroid synthetic actions depend on an extra nuclear receptor, called **steroid factor 1** (SF 1).

Table 59.2: Adrenal steroidogenic enzymes.

Usual name	Old name	New name
Cholesterol side-chain cleaving enzyme	$P450_{SCC}$	CYP11A1
3β hydroxysteroid dehydrogenase	3β-HSD	3β-HSD11
17α-Hydroxylase	$P450_{C17}$	CYP17
21α-Hydroxylase	$P450_{C21}$	CYP21A2
11β-Hydroxylase	$P450_{C11}$	CYP11B1
Aldosterone synthase	$P450_{C11AS}$	CYP11B2

2. Therefore, when the gene for SF-1 is knocked out, adrenals and gonads do not develop.

Rate limiting step: Once inside mitochondria, cholesterol is converted to **pregnenolone** by Cholesterol side-chain cleaving enzyme, also called **cholesterol desmolase** ($P450_{SCC}$) or CYP11A1. This is the **first and rate limiting step** in adrenal steroid synthesis.

Synthesis of Glucocorticoids

Synthesis of glucocorticoids occurs mainly in the zona fasciculata of adrenal cortex. Zona reticularis also contributes to this. The main glucocorticoids formed are cortisol and corticosterone (Application Box 59.1).

Application Box 59.1

Glucocorticoid secretion varies in different species: The **ratio of cortisol to corticosterone** varies from species to species. In rats, mice and birds, corticosterone is the major glucocorticoid. In humans, monkeys and cats, the major glucocorticoid is cortisol. In dogs, cortisol and corticosterone are secreted in equal proportions.

Steps of Cortisol Synthesis

Steps of **cortisol synthesis** are depicted in Flowchart 59.1.

In the mitochondria, pregnenolone forms 17-hydroxypregnenolone by the enzyme 17α-hydroxylase. 17-hydroxypregnenolone then moves into endoplasmic reticulum, where it is converted to 17-hydroxyprogesterone by 3β-hydroxysteroid dehydrogenase, which in turn hydroxylated to 11-deoxycortisol by 21β-hydroxylase. 11-deoxycortisol then moves back to mitochondria to be hydroxylated to form cortisol by mitochondrial enzyme 11β-hydroxylase (Fig. 59.3). ACTH facilitates cortisol synthesis by increasing the supply of cholesterol and by converting the cholesterol to pregnenolone.

Steps of **corticosterone synthesis** are depicted in Flowchart 59.2.

The cholesterol is converted to pregnenolone by the mitochondrial enzyme cholesterol desmolase. Pregnenolone then moves to endoplasmic reticulum where it is dehydrogenated to form progesterone by the enzyme 3β hydroxysteroid dehydrogenase. Progesterone is hydroxylated by the 21β-hydroxylase to form 11-deoxycorticosterone, which then moves back to mitochondria to form corticosterone by the enzyme 11β-hydroxylase.

Flowchart 59.1: Steps of cortisol synthesis.

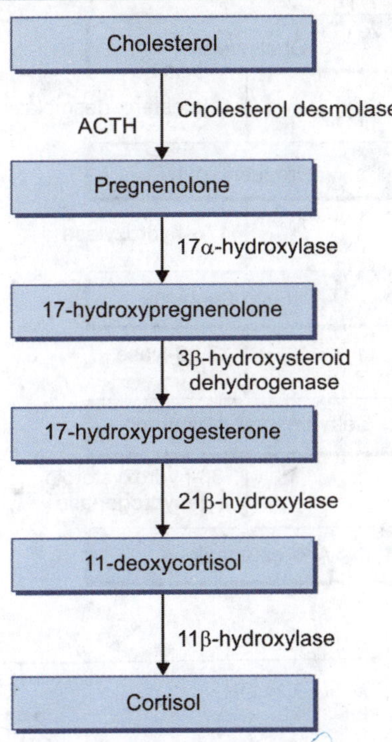

Flowchart 59.2: Steps of corticosterone synthesis.

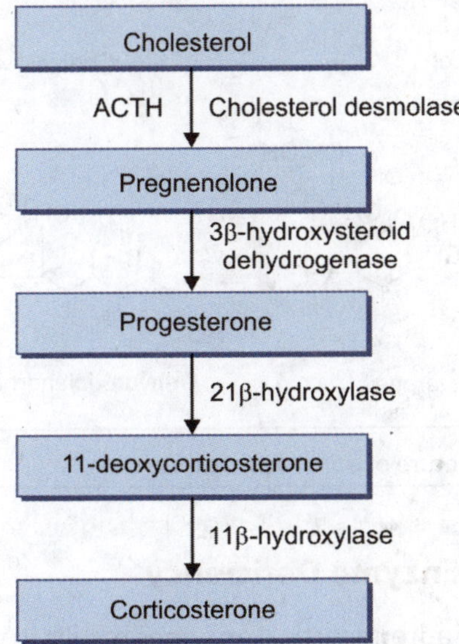

Synthesis of Mineralocorticoids

Mineralocorticoids are formed in the zona glomerulosa of adrenal cortex. Aldosterone is the major mineralocorticoid synthesized in humans.

The steps of **aldosterone synthesis** are depicted in Flowchart 59.3.

The conversion of cholesterol to pregnenolone is **stimulated by ACTH and A II.** The steps till the formation of 11-deoxycorticosterone is same as described above in glucocorticoid synthesis. The rest of the steps of aldosterone synthesis are catalyzed by the enzyme **aldosterone synthase.**

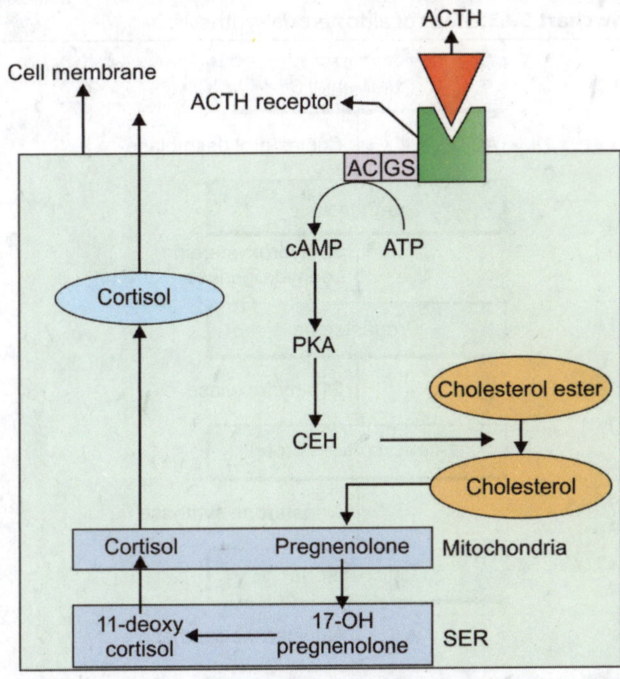

Fig. 59.3: Mechanism of cortisol synthesis. Note, ACTH facilitates cortisol synthesis by activating the enzyme cholesterol ester hydrolase (CEH) that converts cholesterol ester in the cell into cholesterol that enters mitochondria for cortisol synthesis. (GS: Stimulatory G protein; AC: Adenylyl cyclase; PKA: Protein kinase A; SER: Smooth endoplasmic reticulum).

1. *Aldosterone synthase is found only in the cells of zona glomerulosa* of adrenal cortex.
2. Therefore, aldosterone synthesis is limited to the zona glomerulosa. Zona glomerulosa lacks the enzyme 17α-hydroxylase. Hence, synthesis of glucocorticoid and sex steroid does not occur in this layer of adrenal cortex.

Synthesis of Sex Steroids

In adrenal cortex, sex steroids are formed mainly in the zona reticularis. However, zona glomerulosa also contributes to it. The major sex steroids formed are dehydroepiandrosterone and androstenedione. The steps of **androstenedione synthesis** are depicted in Flowchart 59.4.

1. Dehydroepiandrosterone is converted to dehydroepiandrosterone sulfate by the enzyme sulfokinase. Though, androstenedione is synthesized from dehydroepiandrosterone, it can also be formed from 17-OH-progesterone.
2. Androstenedione is then converted to testosterone, which later forms estradiol.

The steps of **estradiol synthesis** are depicted in Flowchart 59.5.

In woman, adrenal gland supplies about 50–60% of the androgenic hormones. The **adrenal androgen is not important in males** because the testes produce testosterone. Similarly, the conversion of androgen to estrogen in the adrenal cortex in females is not important because ovaries secrete estrogen. However, **after menopause** secretion

Flowchart 59.3: Steps of aldosterone synthesis.

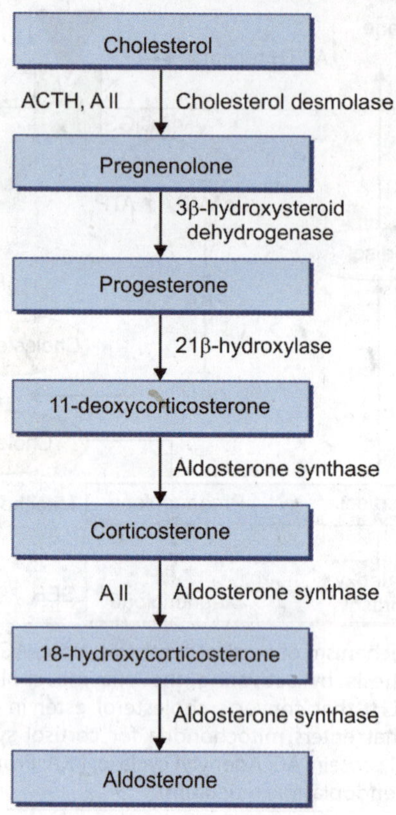

Flowchart 59.5: Steps of estradiol synthesis.

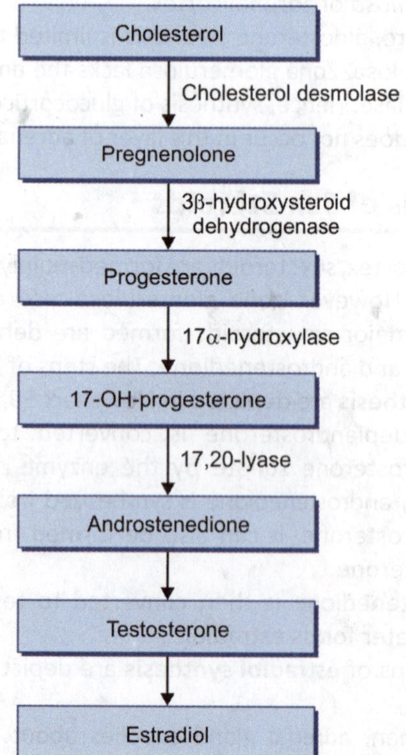

of *estrogen from adrenal gland in females* becomes the important ***source of estrogenic activity***.

Structure of adrenocortical steroids is given in Figure 59.4.

Flowchart 59.4: Steps of androstenedione synthesis.

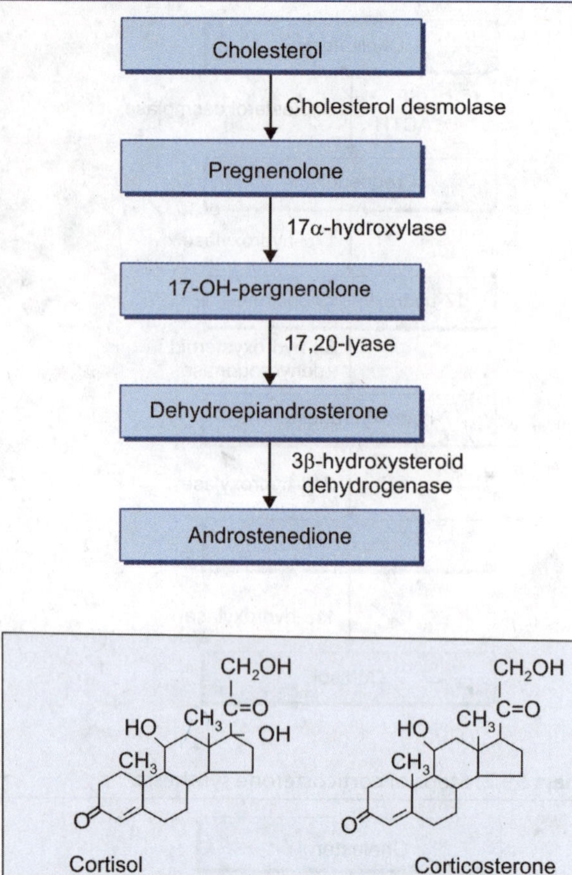

Fig. 59.4: Structure of adrenocortical steroids.

Effects of Enzyme Deficiency

Deficiency of adrenocortical enzymes results in various syndromes. The congenital deficiency of the adrenal enzymes results in decreased cortisol secretion. Decreased level of cortisol in plasma stimulates ACTH secretion. As the ACTH has growth promoting (trophic) effects on cells of adrenal cortex, the gland size increases. Therefore, the conditions are called **congenital adrenal hyperplasia**. Deficiency of 21β-hydroxylase and 11β-hydroxylase are common.

Deficiency of 21β-Hydroxylase

Deficiency of 21β-hydroxylase accounts for **90% of the cases of congenital adrenal hyperplasia**. Deficiency of 21β-hydroxylase decreases the production of glucocorticoids and mineralocorticoids. Decreased cortisol level in plasma increases the production of ACTH, which **facilitates the production of pregnenolone** from cholesterol. Surplus pregnenolone is diverted for the excess production of androgens. Therefore, the condition is mainly characterized by **virilization**.

1. This leads to characteristic **adrenogenital syndrome in females.** The **features of this syndrome are** hirsutism, small breasts, male escutcheon, heavy arms and legs, enlarged clitoris (Clitromegaly), and receding hairline.
2. In severe cases, genitalia of genetic females are masculinized (**female pseudohermaphroditism**).
3. Many of them develop hyponatremia (**salt losing form of congenital virilizing adrenal hyperplasia**). Hyponatremia occurs due to urinary loss of Na^+, which occurs due to lack of mineralocorticoid activity.
4. Hyponatremia causes hypovolemia and hypotension.

Deficiency of 11β-hydroxylase

In 11β-hydroxylase deficiency, **increased production of androgen** is associated with increased secretion of 11-deoxycortisol and 11-deoxycorticosterone. The 11-deoxycorticosterone is a mineralocorticoid. Thus, excess mineralocorticoid activity increases **retention of Na^+ and water**. Therefore, patient develops **hypertension** in addition to virilization (**hypertensive form of congenital virilizing adrenal hyperplasia**).

In all virilizing forms of adrenal hyperplasia, **glucocorticoid therapy** is preferred. Exogenously administered glucocorticoid fills the endogenous cortisol deficit, and also suppresses the production of ACTH. Thus, ACTH induced excess production of sex steroid is decreased.

Deficiency of 17α-hydroxylase

This is a rare condition. It results in **decreased production of sex steroids**. Therefore, **female external genitalia** are present. However, as the production of aldosterone and corticosterone is normal, elevated level of mineralocorticoids result in **hypertension and hyperkalemia**.

3β-hydroxysteroid Dehydrogenase

This is also a rare condition, in which **production of dehydroepiandrosterone is increased**. There is some degree of masculinization in females. But, as dehydroepiandrosterone is a weak androgen, it does not cause full masculinization of the genitalia in genetic males. Therefore, **hypospadias** (urethral opening on the undersurface of the penis) develops.

Cholesterol Desmolase Deficiency

Deficiency of the cholesterol side-chain cleaving enzyme **decreases production of all adrenocortical hormones** as it converts cholesterol to pregnenolone, the first step in steroidogenesis. The condition is **fatal during fetal life**. The production of placental progesterone depends on fetal adrenocortical production of androgen. Progesterone is essential for pregnancy to continue. Thus, deficiency of this enzyme results in **termination of pregnancy**. However, this condition is very rare.

Table 59.3: Daily secretion and plasma concentration of adrenocortical steroids.

Hormone	Daily secretion (mg/24 h)	Average plasma conc. (μg/dL)
Cortisol	10–15	14
Corticosterone	2–4	0.5
Aldosterone	0.1–0.2	0.0006
Deoxycorticosterone	0.2–0.25	0.0006
Dehydroepiandrosterone	20–25	175

Metabolism of Adrenocortical Hormones

Normal Secretion

The daily secretion and plasma concentration of adrenocortical hormones are listed in Table 59.3.

Plasma Protein Binding

Adrenocortical steroids usually bind with proteins, such as transcortin and albumin.

Transcortin Binding

About 80% of adrenal steroids, especially cortisol and corticosterone bind with a plasma protein called **transcortin**, or **corticosteroid binding globulin** (CBG). The transcortin is a glycoprotein produced by liver. The normal plasma concentration of transcortin is **3 mg/dL.**

1. The concentration **increases in pregnancy and estrogen therapy**. When transcortin level increases, the quantity of hormone binding to it increases that in turn **decreases free cortisol level.**
2. The decreased free hormone increases ACTH secretion, which consequently increases cortisol secretion. However, a new state is reached at which the bound form is increased, but the free form remains normal.
3. Thus, the *total hormone concentration increases without changing the concentration of the free form*. Therefore, **in pregnancy features of cortisol excess do not appear** inspite of increased total cortisol level.

Albumin Binding

About 10–15% of cortisol is bound to albumin. Thus, only 5–10% of cortisol is free in the plasma.

Because of its protein binding, the **half life of cortisol is more** (60–90 mins), its concentration as free hormone in plasma is less and its excretion in urine is less. As binding of aldosterone to protein is less, the **half life of aldosterone is less** (about 20 minutes).

Metabolic Degradation

Cortisol is **metabolized in liver**, where it is reduced to **dihydrocortisol and tetrahydrocortisol glucuronides**. The

Flowchart 59.6: Steps of metabolic degradation of cortisol.

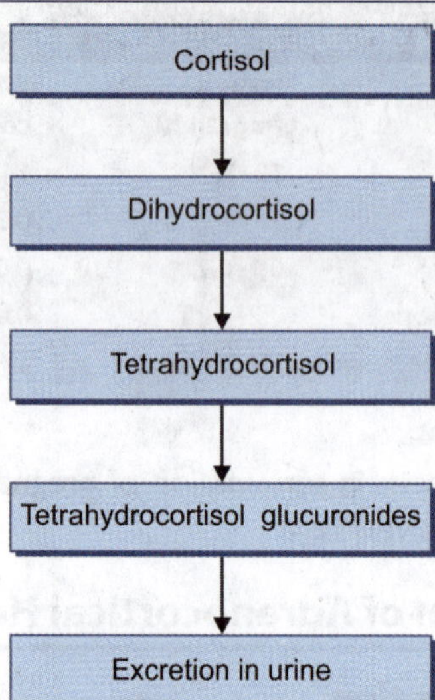

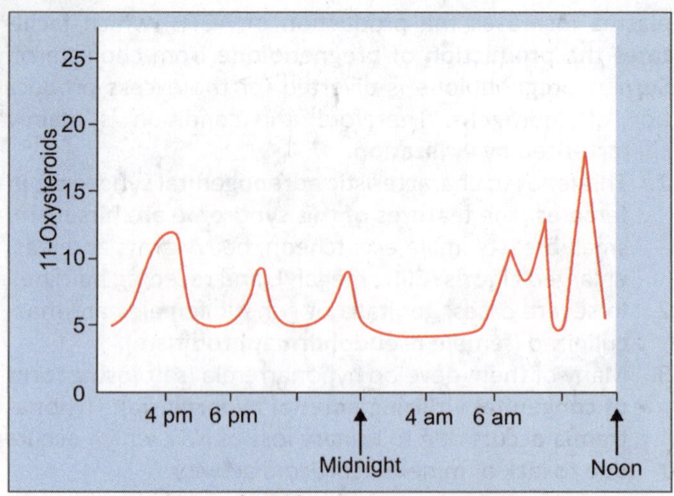

Fig. 59.5: Circadian variation in cortisol secretion. Note, it closely follows the pattern of ACTH secretion as depicted in Figure 55.19 (in Chapter 55). 11-Oxysteroid is the plasma cortisol estimated (Duration of the night is truncated in the time scale).

tetrahydroglucuronide derivative cortisol and corticosterone are **water soluble**, and therefore is rapidly excreted in urine (Flowchart 59.6).

1. The free cortisol circulating in the plasma is filtered by kidney and about 50 μg is excreted in the urine. The measurement of **urinary metabolite of cortisol provides a reliable index of cortisol secretion**.
2. The excretion of **17-hydroxycorticoids** represents about 50% of the total daily cortisol secretion. Normally 2–12 mg of 17-hydroxycorticoids is excreted per day.
3. The precursors of cortisol (progesterone and 17-OH-progesterone) are metabolized to *pregnanediol and pregnanetriol*.
4. **In adult females,** urinary excretion of these metabolites reflects the *activities of ovarian-adrenal axis*. However, their increased urinary concentration **in prepubertal girls** indicates specific *congenital defect in cortisol secretion* (due to disease of the adrenal cortex, not the ovary).

17-Ketosteroids

17-Ketosteroid derivative is formed in the liver from cortisol. However, corticosterone does not form 17-ketosteroid. Dehydroepiandrosterone, the major adrenal androgen is a 17-ketosteroid. Testosterone is converted to 17-ketosteroid.

1. **Etiocholanolone,** a metabolite of adrenal androgens and testosterone, forms 17-ketosteroid.
2. 17-ketosteroid is **excreted in the urine**. Normally, 5–10 mg of 17-ketosteroids in women, and 8–20 mg of 17-ketosteroids in men is excreted in urine per day.
3. About 70% of this amount excreted is normally derived from adrenal cortex and 30% from the gonadal androgens.
4. When they accumulate in blood, they cause episodic fever known as **etiocholanolone fever**.

Regulation of secretion, mechanism of action, functions and dysfunctions of each category of adrenocortical hormones are discussed separately in the following sections:

GLUCOCORTICOIDS

Regulation of Secretion

Glucocorticoid secretion is controlled mainly by **feedback mechanisms of ACTH secretion**. Angiotensin II and other hormones also contribute.

Role of ACTH

ACTH is the polypeptide hormone containing 39 amino acids secreted from anterior pituitary. This is the major stimulator of glucocorticoid secretion. ACTH is secreted in **irregular burst**s throughout the day. Accordingly, the concentration of cortisol alters in the plasma.

1. The bursts are more frequent and prominent in the early morning (4–10 AM), which accounts for about 75% of the total ACTH secreted in a day (for details, refer chapter "Anterior Pituitary").
2. This **circadian rhythm** (the diurnal variation) of ACTH secretion is an important regulator of cortisol secretion. Therefore, **cortisol secretion also has a definite pattern** that follows the pattern of ACTH secretion (Fig. 59.5).

Feedback Control

Glucocorticoid secretion is controlled by feedback release of **ACTH** from the anterior pituitary.

1. ACTH secretion is stimulated by **CRH** (corticotropin releasing hormone) secreted from the hypothalamus CRH secretion is influenced by various stimuli originating

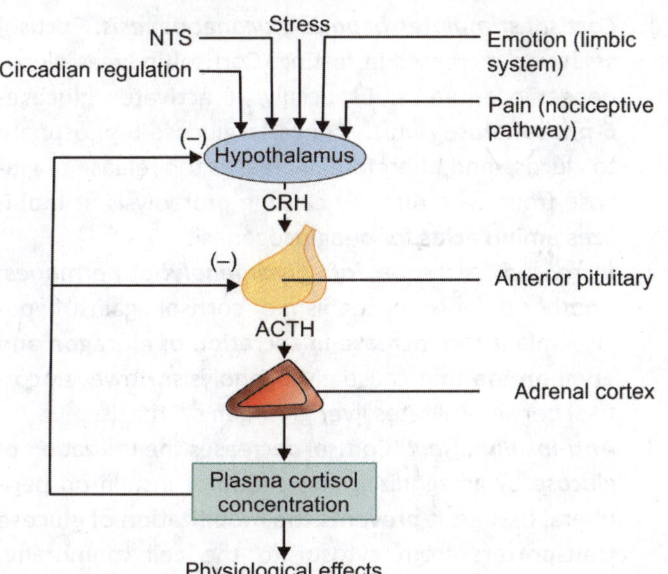

Fig. 59.6: Regulation of cortisol secretion. (NTS: Nucleus tractus solitarius. Minus sign indicates inhibition).

from the limbic system, pain pathways, NTS, reticular formation and suprachiasmatic nucleus (Fig. 59.6).

2. CRH increases ACTH secretion, which in turn increases glucocorticoid secretion from the adrenal cortex.
3. Increased glucocorticoid level in plasma provides **negative feedback signal to the hypothalamus and anterior pituitary** to inhibit the secretion of CRH and ACTH respectively.
4. Thus, cortisol secretion returns to normal.
5. Conversely, decreased glucocorticoid secretion increases CRH and ACTH release by feedback mechanisms that tend to increase the secretion of cortisol (Clinical Box 59.1).

Clinical Box 59.1

Steroid therapy should not be stopped abruptly: A patient receiving steroid for a long time should not stop the medicine abruptly. This is because, after a prolonged treatment with steroid, the adrenal cortex atrophies and becomes unresponsive to the ACTH for about six months. Also, pituitary secretes less ACTH initially, due to its diminished synthesis. However, pituitary recovers and secretes more ACTH thereafter. Increased level of ACTH slowly stimulates adrenal cortex to secrete glucocorticoids and it takes about 8 to 10 months for cortisol level to return to normal plasma level (Fig. 59.7). ACTH, from its level also returns to normal in about 10 months. Thus, **pituitary-adrenocortical axis takes about 10 months** to recover from the suppressive effect of prolonged steroid therapy. During this period, an individual fails to cope with stress and **may succumb to stressful situations**. To prevent such a dangerous complication, steroids should not be stopped abruptly after a prolonged therapy; rather the dose should be decreased gradually over weeks before finally stopping the treatment.

In Stress

In stress, increased cortisol secretion occurs mainly due to **increased hypothalamic release of CRH**. Fibers projecting from limbic system, especially from amygdala to

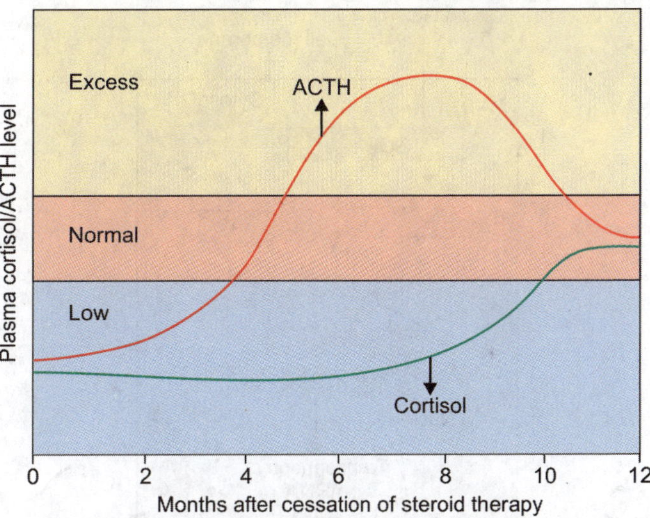

Fig. 59.7: Pattern of plasma level of cortisol and ACTH following cessation of high dose steroid therapy given for a longer duration. Note, cortisol takes about 8 to 10 months to return to normal, though ACTH secretion recovers early. This is the period during which the subject is vulnerable to collapse on exposure to stress; therefore, steroid therapy is advised to be withdrawn slowly over a period of months instead of stopping abruptly.

hypothalamus (amygdalohypothalamic pathway) mediate the responses to **emotional stress**, fear, and anxiety. Ascending nociceptive fibers give collaterals to hypothalamus and they mediate the **stress response to painful stimuli** or injury.

Angiotensin II

Normally, angiotensin II is an important stimulator for aldosterone secretion. However, it also induces glucocorticoid secretion.

Other Hormones

ADH, serotonin, and VIP also stimulate glucocorticoid secretion. But their role in the physiologic regulation of glucocorticoid secretion is not clearly known.

Mechanism of Action

Cortisol takes few hours to days to exert its effect.

1. It diffuses into the cell and binds with the **glucocorticoid receptors (GR) present in the cytoplasm.**
2. Binding of cortisol with the receptor displaces the inhibitory heat shock protein complex from the receptor.
3. This results in alteration in the receptor configuration and causes **hyperphosphorylation** of the receptor.
4. Then, the hormone-receptor complex enters the nucleus, where it binds with the specific **glucocorticoid regulatory elements** (GRE) on the target DNA molecule (Fig. 59.8).
5. This leads to **transcription of mRNAs** that regulate expression of various genes.

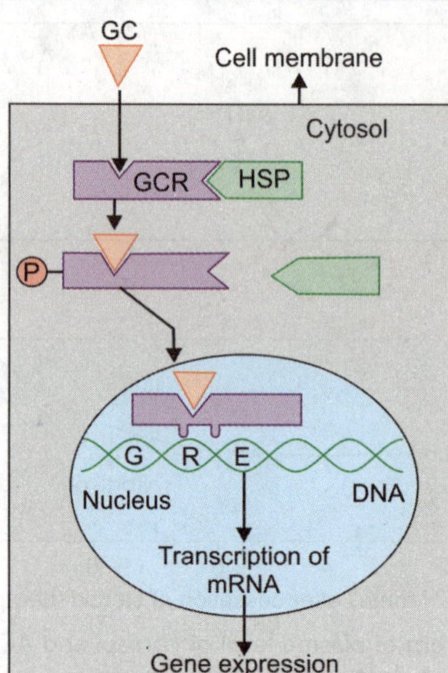

Fig. 59.8: Mechanism of cortisol action. (GC: Glucocorticoid; GCR: Glucocorticoid receptor; HSP: Heat shock protein; P: Phosphorylation of hormone-receptor complex; GRE: Glucocorticoid response element).

Functions of Glucocorticoids

There are receptors for glucocorticoids in almost all tissues of the body and glucocorticoids influence many physiological processes of the body. Cortisol influences metabolisms profoundly, facilitates action of other hormones (permissive actions), influences functions of important organ systems, controls inflammation and immunity, and mediates responses of the body to stress. For its all-around physiological and pharmacological effects, cortisol is used widely in clinical practice.

Effects on Intermediary Metabolisms

On Carbohydrate Metabolism

Glucocorticoid is **essential for survival during fasting**. In prolonged fasting, the liver glycogen store is depleted and unless there is gluconeogenesis, death occurs due to hypoglycemia. **Cortisol increases blood glucose** by various mechanisms and, thus, plays an **important defensive role in fasting** (Clinical Box 59.2), and also against *hypoglycemia induced by insulin*.

Clinical Box 59.2

Adrenal-deficient patients should not fast: Cortisol increases blood glucose, and therefore is an important defense against hypoglycemia in fasting. In adrenal insufficiency, blood glucose remains normal so long as the food intake is normal. However, fasting induced hypoglycemia becomes fatal in such patients, as cortisol defense of hypoglycemia is lacking. Therefore, patients suffering from adrenocortical insufficiency are advised not to fast.

Cortisol **increases plasma glucose** by following mechanisms:

1. ***Cortisol stimulates hepatic gluconeogenesis***: Cortisol secretion increases in fasting. Cortisol induces gluconeogenic enzymes. Especially, it **activates glucose-6-phosphatase**, which converts glucose-6-phosphate to glucose and, therefore, increases the release of glucose from liver. Also, by causing proteolysis, it **mobilizes amino acids** for neoglucogenesis.
2. ***Increased secretion of glycogenolytic hormones***: Another defense mechanism of cortisol against hypoglycemia is the **increase in secretion of glucagon and epinephrine** that cause glycogenolysis. However, cortisol per se facilitates liver glycogen synthesis.
3. ***Anti-insulin effect***: Cortisol **decreases the utilization of glucose** by antagonizing the action of insulin on peripheral tissues. It **prevents the mobilization of glucose transporters** from cytosol to the cell membrane. Especially, it *inhibits the insulin stimulated glucose uptake* in skeletal muscle and adipose tissue. This adds to the hyperglycemic effects of cortisol and makes diabetes worse (Clinical Box 59.3). It also reverses insulin suppression of hepatic glucose production.

Clinical Box 59.3

Cortisol complicates diabetes: In normal individuals, rise in blood glucose by cortisol increases insulin secretion, which counteracts ketone bodies and lipids raised by the cortisol. In diabetes, cortisol effects on ketone body and lipid remain unaffected as insulin is lacking. Thus, excess cortisol makes the diabetes worse by promoting ketoacidosis.

On Protein Metabolism

Cortisol **facilitates proteolysis**, especially in skeletal muscle, and *inhibits protein synthesis*. It mobilizes muscle protein for gluconeogenesis. The overall action is to **facilitate the conversion of protein to glycogen**. The chronic administration of cortisol or excess secretion of glucocorticoid causes **depletion of protein storage** in the body, especially in the muscle, bone, skin, and connective tissue.

On Fat Metabolism

Cortisol causes lipolysis. In fact, the lipolytic effect of epinephrine and growth hormone requires cortisol. During fasting, by **promoting lipolysis**, cortisol causes rapid release of free fatty acid and glycerol from adipose tissues, which are utilized for gluconeogenesis. Increased free fatty acid formation **promotes ketogenesis**, especially in diabetes.

On Food Intake and Fat Distribution

Cortisol **increases appetite** and food intake by *stimulating neuropeptide Y secretion* from the hypothalamus.

1. It stimulates differentiation of pre-adipocytes to adipocytes in the adipose tissue.
2. It also **stimulates lipogenesis** by activating lipoprotein lipase and glucose-6-phosphate dehydrogenase activity of the adipocytes in some other parts of the body.

Flowchart 59.7: Summary of metabolic actions of cortisol

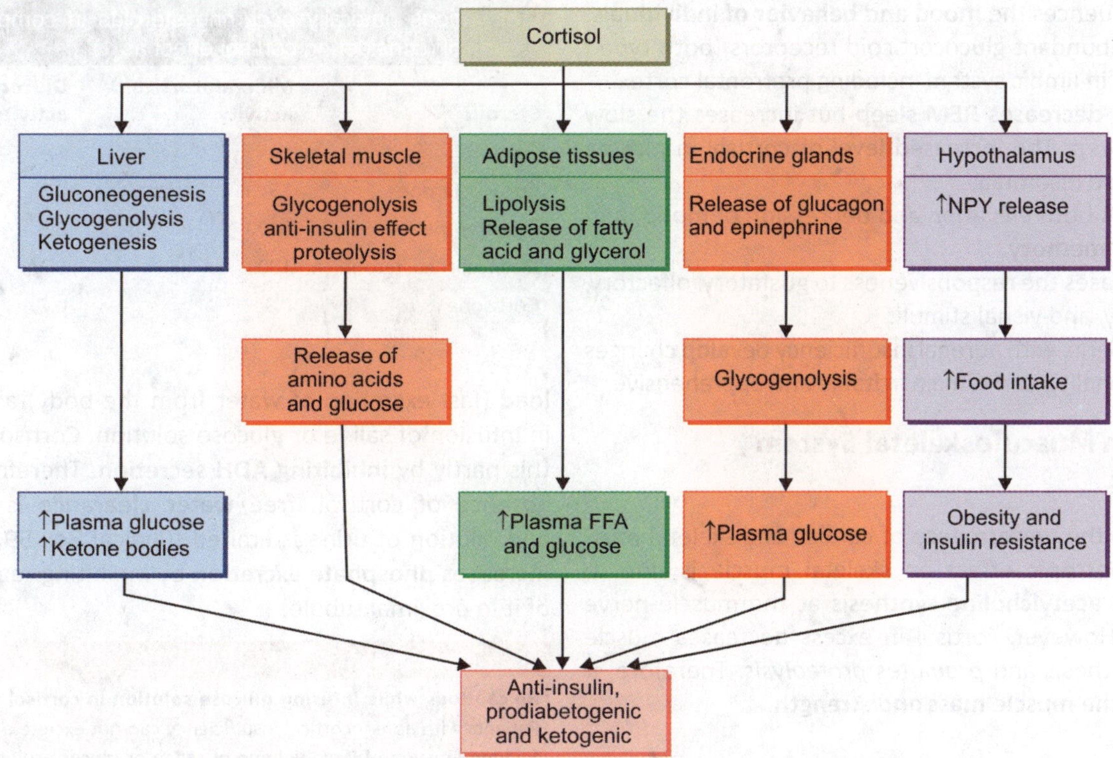

3. Therefore, the action of cortisol varies from tissues to tissues. Thus, cortisol excess causes **maldistribution of fat** in the body that result in **truncal obesity, moon face and buffalo hump** with thinning of extremities. The exact cause of peculiar distribution of fat is not known, but it is ***associated with insulin resistance*** and/or increase in insulin level.
4. Cortisol also **increases leptin synthesis** in adipose tissue. Therefore, obesity is restricted by the ***negative feedback actions of leptin*** (leptin inhibits feeding).

To summarize the effect of cortisol on metabolisms, it is an important diabetogenic, ketogenic, and anti-insulin hormone (Flowchart 59.7).

Permissive Actions of Cortisol

Glucocorticoid is essential (even in small quantity) for some **physiological actions of other hormones to take place.** This is called permissive action of cortisol (as cortisol allows the specific actions of these hormones to occur, though it does not produce these effects by itself).

Permissive actions of cortisol include the following:

1. **Vasopressor and bronchodilator effects** of catecholamines.
2. **Calorigenic effects** of glucagon and catecholamines.
3. **Lipolytic effects** of catecholamines.
4. Development of ***mammary gland*** during puberty in females.
5. Development of **hepatic enzyme systems** during fetal life.
6. **Surfactant synthesis** in the fetal lung and maturation of lungs during intrauterine life.
7. Development of **bacterial flora and enzyme** systems in the intestine.

Effects on Cardiovascular System

On Heart

Cortisol **increases myocardial performance** by increasing Na^+–K^+ ATPase activity and also by increasing expression of β-adrenergic receptors in the heart.

On Blood Vessels

Cortisol maintains **vascular reactivity**. This is an important action of cortisol. It increases the **responsiveness of arterioles to catecholamines and angiotensin II**.

1. Probably, this action is mediated by *inhibition of* Na^+-Ca^{++} *exchanger* in the cell membrane so that the Ca^{++} concentration is maintained in the blood vessel smooth muscle cells. Cortisol also **decreases the release of vasodilators** like prostaglandins.
2. In adrenal insufficiency, blood vessels become unresponsive to catecholamines (Clinical Box 59.4). This ***promotes vascular collapse***, as already hypovolemia exists in such patients.

Clinical Box 59.4

Injection of cortisol is a must in shock: Injection of catecholamines in hypovolemic shock is required to restore blood pressure, as they cause vasoconstriction and increase cardiac output. However, it is desirable to inject cortisol along with catecholamines as it maintains vascular reactivity. Also, cortisol mediates responsiveness of catecholamines to vasoconstrictors by its permissive action. Catecholamine injection without administration of cortisol in shock does not ensure adequate vasoconstriction and blood pressure continues to remain low.

Effects on Central Nervous System

Cortisol influences the **mood and behavior of individuals**. There are abundant glucocorticoid receptors (both type I and type II) in limbic system including prefrontal cortex.

1. Cortisol **decreases REM sleep** but increases the slow wave sleep. The increased level of cortisol in plasma can cause insomnia.
2. It causes both elevation and depression of mood, and **impairs memory**.
3. It decreases the responsiveness to gustatory, olfactory, auditory, and visual stimuli.
4. The patients with adrenal insufficiency develop changes in personality, and remain irritable and apprehensive.

Effects on Musculoskeletal System

On Muscle

It increases the performance of cardiac and skeletal muscle. The **inotropic effect** on skeletal muscle is due to **increase in acetylcholine synthesis** at the muscle-nerve terminals. However, cortisol in excess decreases muscle protein synthesis and *promotes proteolysis*. Therefore, it **decreases the muscle mass and strength**.

On Bone

Cortisol **inhibits bone formation** by various mechanisms:

1. It **decreases the synthesis of type-I collagen**, which is a fundamental component of bone matrix.
2. It **inhibits the conversion** of *osteoprogenitor cells to the osteoblasts*.
3. It **decreases absorption of** Ca^{++} from GI tract (by inhibiting the effect of vitamin D on GIT). It also ***decreases the synthesis of active vitamin D***. Thus, it decreases supply of Ca^{++} to the bones, which is essential for bone mineralization.
4. Cortisol also **facilitates bone resorption**.

The overall effects are **decreased bone mass and mineralization**. Therefore, prolonged administration of cortisol may cause **osteoporosis** (Clinical Box 59.5).

Clinical Box 59.5

Bone X-ray should be done to check complications: Cortisol decreases bone mass and promotes osteoporosis. Even, vertebral collapse may occur. Therefore, patients receiving steroid for a longer period should be checked for osteoporotic changes by taking bone X-rays or MRI, especially in elderly patients.

Effects on Connective Tissue

Cortisol **inhibits collagen synthesis**. Therefore, it decreases skin thickness and causes thinning of capillary walls. The **capillaries become fragile** (susceptible to rupture). Thus, intracutaneous hemorrhage occurs in cortisol excess.

Effects on Kidney and Water Metabolism

Cortisol **increases GFR** by increasing glomerular blood flow. It is essential for the **rapid clearance of a water load** (fast excretion of water from the body) as happens in infusion of saline or glucose solution. Cortisol achieves this partly by **inhibiting ADH secretion**. Therefore, in the absence of cortisol, **free water clearance is impaired** and dilution of urine is limited (Clinical Box 59.6). It also **increases phosphate excretion** by inhibiting reabsorption of it in proximal tubule.

Table 59.4: Mineralocorticoid and glucocorticoid activities of various naturally occurring steroids in comparison to cortisol (considering cortisol effect as 1).

Steroid	Mineralocorticoid activity	Glucocorticoid activity
Cortisol	1	1
Corticosterone	15	0.3
Aldosterone	3000	0.3
Deoxycorticosterone	100	0.2
Cortisone	0.8	0.7

Clinical Box 59.6

Be cautious while infusing glucose solution in cortisol deficiency: Patients with adrenocortical insufficiency can not excrete a water load. Sudden infusion of large volume of saline or glucose solution in such patient may result in **water intoxication**. Following infusion of glucose saline, the glucose is metabolized, but the body can not remove water as cortisol is lacking. Therefore, plasma becomes hypoosmolar due to hemodilution. The cells in the brain swell, that impairs the hypothalamic thermoregulatory centers. Patient develops high fever and collapses. Therefore, such patients **should receive cortisol while receiving a water load.**

Apparent Mineralocorticoid Excess

In the absence or deficiency of 11β-OH-steroid dehydrogenase type-2 (that converts cortisol into cortisone), **cortisol has marked mineralocorticoid activity** (Table 59.4), which causes hyperaldosteronism like situation due to action of cortisol on mineralocorticoid receptors.

1. The patient develops clinical features of hyperaldosteronism, though the plasma aldosterone and plasma renin activity remains low. Hence, the condition is called **apparent mineralocorticoid excess.**
2. It may occur due to congenital deficiency of the hormone or ingestion of licorice.
3. Licorice contains glycyrrhetinic acid that inhibits 11β-OH-steroid dehydrogenase type-2. Persons consuming large quantity of licorice may also develop hypertension as sodium absorption through ENaC (epithelial sodium channel) in kidney is high.

Effects on Fetus

Cortisol imparts profound influence on fetal maturation.

1. Cortisol causes **maturation of CNS** during intrauterine life.
2. It causes growth of retina, GI tract, lungs, and skin of the fetus.

3. The intestinal enzyme system of fetal pattern to the postnatal or adult pattern is altered by cortisol, which is essential for disaccharides to be digested by the infants.
4. Cortisol causes **lung development**. It promotes growth of alveoli and causes flattening of alveolar epithelial cells. Cortisol also facilitates pulmonary surfactant synthesis. All these actions allow the fetal lung to satisfactorily expand at the first breath.

Effects on Blood Cells

Though, cortisol influences all the three formed elements of blood, the impact is more on leucocytes.

On Leucocytes

Cortisol causes leucocytosis. Though it causes mild neutrophilia and monocytosis, it causes profound **lymphocytopenia, eosinopenia and basopenia**.

Causes of Lymphocytopenia

1. Cortisol decreases circulating lymphocyte count by **decreasing mitotic activity of lymphocyte precursors.**
2. It decreases the size of lymph nodes and thymus.
3. It decreases the ability of lymphocytes and monocytes to secrete cytokines that are essential for proliferation of lymphocytes.

Causes of Eosinopenia

1. Cortisol causes eosinopenia by **stimulating apoptosis** (programmed cell death) of eosinophil.
2. By inhibiting the release of cytokines, it prevents eosinophil growth.
3. It facilitates sequestration of eosinophil in spleen and lungs (thus, decreases the peripheral eosinophil count).

On RBC

It causes **mild erythrocytosis** by stimulating erythropoietin production.

On Platelets

It produces **mild thrombocytosis**.

Effects on Inflammation

Cortisol has profound **anti-inflammatory and anti-allergic actions**. Inflammation is the response of tissue to injury. The inflammatory responses include: dilation of capillaries, increased capillary permeability, migration of granulocytes to the site of injury and killing of the organisms or the insulting agents by the granulocytes, mainly neutrophils (for details, refer Chapter 19). These responses are mediated by various chemicals like prostaglandins, thromboxanes, leukotrienes, kinins, histamine, serotonin, lymphokines, EDRF and PAF (platelet activating factor) (refer to Tables 19.2 and 19.5, Chapte 19). Cortisol interferes in most of the mechanisms of inflammation.

1. Cortisol **inhibits synthesis of chemical mediators** of inflammation. It stimulates synthesis of **lipocortins** (a family of phosphoproteins) in the target cells. Lipocortin **inhibits the activity of phospholipase A_2**; therefore, **decreases the release of arachidonic acid**, which is the precursor for many mediators of inflammation like prostaglandins, thromboxanes, leukotrienes, etc. Thus, cortisol prevents the formation of these mediators of inflammation.
2. Cortisol **stabilizes the lysosomal membrane**. Therefore, it ***decreases release of proteolytic enzymes*** *and hyaluronidase* from lysosomes that are required for inflammatory reactions to occur.
3. Cortisol **inhibits mast cells**. It prevents differentiation and proliferation of mast cells. Consequently, it ***decreases the release of histamine***, an important mediator of inflammation (histamine causes vasodilation and increases capillary permeability).
4. Cortisol **inhibits leucocyte functions**. It prevents migration of leucocytes to the site of inflammation or infection. It **prevents the margination of leucocytes and adherence of leucocytes** to the capillary endothelial wall. Cortisol ***inhibits the expression of receptors*** in the endothelial cells that normally causes chemotactic peptides to interact with leucocytes to stick to the vessel endothelium.
5. Cortisol **inhibits phagocytic and bactericidal activity of neutrophils**. Though cortisol causes mild neutrophillia, it actually decreases the activity of leucocytes.
6. Cortisol **inhibits proliferation of fibroblasts**. Thus, it ***decreases the synthesis and deposition of fibrils*** at the site of inflammation. This forms the basis of chronic anti-inflammatory action of cortisol to injury. Cortisol **prevents walling off of a chronic infection**.
7. Recent evidences suggest that a transcription factor, called **nuclear factor-$_k$B** (NF$_k$B), plays an important role in inflammation. Normally, NF-$_k$B is bound to another cytoplasmic protein called I_kB_α, and this binding keeps NF-$_k$B in an inactive state. Viruses and cytokines that induce inflammation separate NF-$_k$B from I_kB_α by activating I_kB kinase. NF-$_k$B then migrates to nucleus and attaches with the DNA. This induces the transcription of genes for formation of various chemicals that participate in inflammation. Thus, NF-$_k$B stimulates synthesis and secretion of mediators of inflammation. Glucocorticoids increase the production of I_kB_α in the cell, and, therefore, **prevent the activation of NF-$_k$B**. This is suggested to be the *primary mechanism of anti-inflammatory actions* of cortisol (Flowchart 59.8).

Nevertheless, the physician has to be cautious for use of cortisol to prevent inflammation (Clinical Box 59.7)

Flowchart 59.8: Mechanism of anti-inflammatory actions of cortisol.

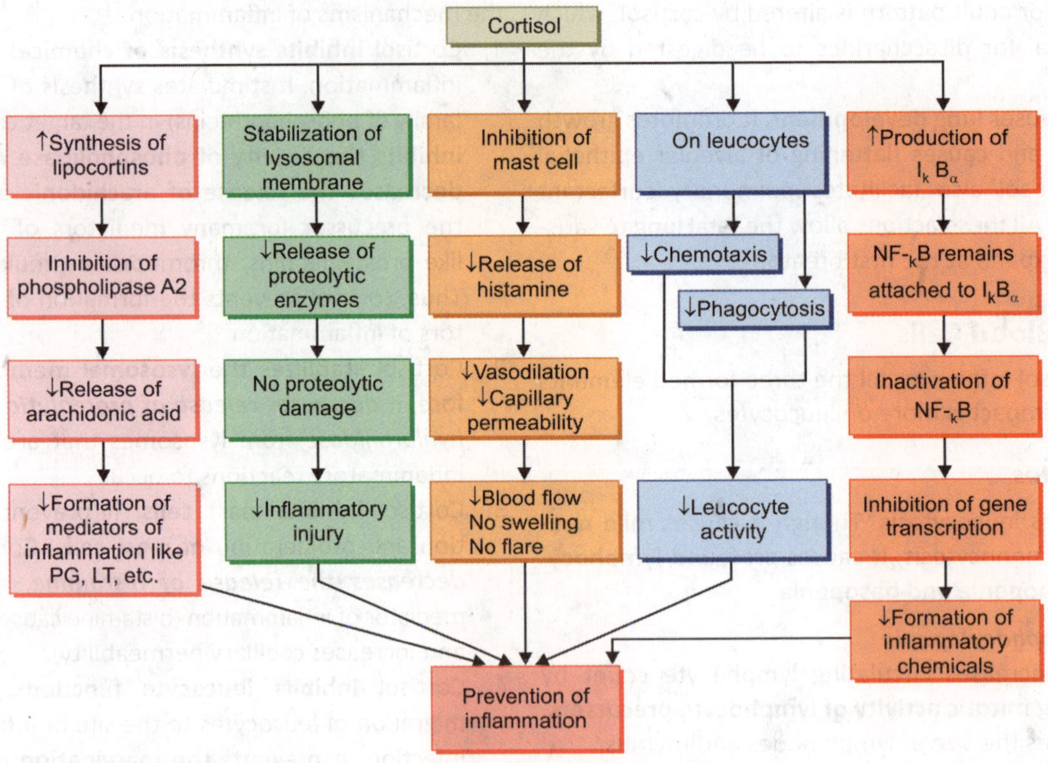

(PG: Prostaglandins, LT: Leukotrienes; I_kB_α: A cytoplasmic protein; NF_kB: Nuclear factor-$_kB$).

Clinical Box 59.7

Cortisol should be given with antibiotics: For its strong anti-inflammatory properties, cortisol is very often prescribed for the treatment of inflammatory diseases. However, it should not be prescribed for treating acute inflammations due to infections. If cortisol is given in infections, the toxic features of infection dramatically disappear due to its anti-inflammatory actions. This may give the wrong impression that the infection has subsided. But, actually infection spreads as cortisol suppresses immunity (discussed below). Thus, cortisol in such conditions masks the actual disease and delays the diagnosis. Moreover, it also aggravates the disease, which may become fatal. Therefore, cortisol should not be prescribed in acute infections like pneumonia, cholecystitis, pancreatitis, active tuberculosis etc. If situation warrants cortisol treatment in such conditions, it should always be prescribed with appropriate and adequate antibiotics.

Effects on Allergy

Cortisol has intense **anti-allergic effects**. Allergy occurs due to antigen-antibody reaction that stimulates the release of histamine from mast cells. There are two types of allergies: local and systemic.

1. **In local allergy,** release of histamine locally causes redness, itching and swelling.
2. **In systemic allergy** (anaphylaxis), histamine released into circulation inhibits heart that decreases cardiac output, and causes vasodilation that decreases blood pressure. Most of the effects of allergy are mediated through histamine.

   The **antiallergy effects** of cortisol include the following:

1. Cortisol inhibits degranulation of mast cells and, therefore, **prevents release of histamine.**
2. It also **prevents the growth of mast cells.**

   Thus, cortisol strongly prevents allergic reactions. Therefore, cortisol is used frequently for the treatment of allergy both locally and systemically (Clinical Box 59.8).

Effects on the Immune System

Cortisol has **profound immunosuppressive effects**. The influence is **more on cellular immunity**. When an antigen enters the body, antigen presenting cells (APCs) take it up and present to the T cells. This causes proliferation and activation of T cells. The activated T cells kill organisms, secrete interleukins and activate type 1 helper-T cells that mediate immunological responses. Cortisol suppresses immunity by following mechanisms.

1. Cortisol **decreases circulating lymphocytes** by inhibiting lymphocyte mitotic activity. It mainly decreases T cell population, especially ***type-I helper T cells by stimulating their apoptosis.***
2. Immature T cells in thymus and immature B and T cells in lymph nodes are destroyed by high level of plasma cortisol, which in turn decreases the size of thymus and lymph nodes.
3. Cortisol **inhibits the cytotoxic effects of T cells** by ***inhibiting the transport of lymphocytes*** to the site of antigenic stimulation and by ***decreasing the production of cytokines*** from them. Cortisol inhibits cytokine secretion by **inhibiting the NF-$_k$B activity** of the cells.

Flowchart 59.9: Immunosuppressive mechanisms of cortisol.

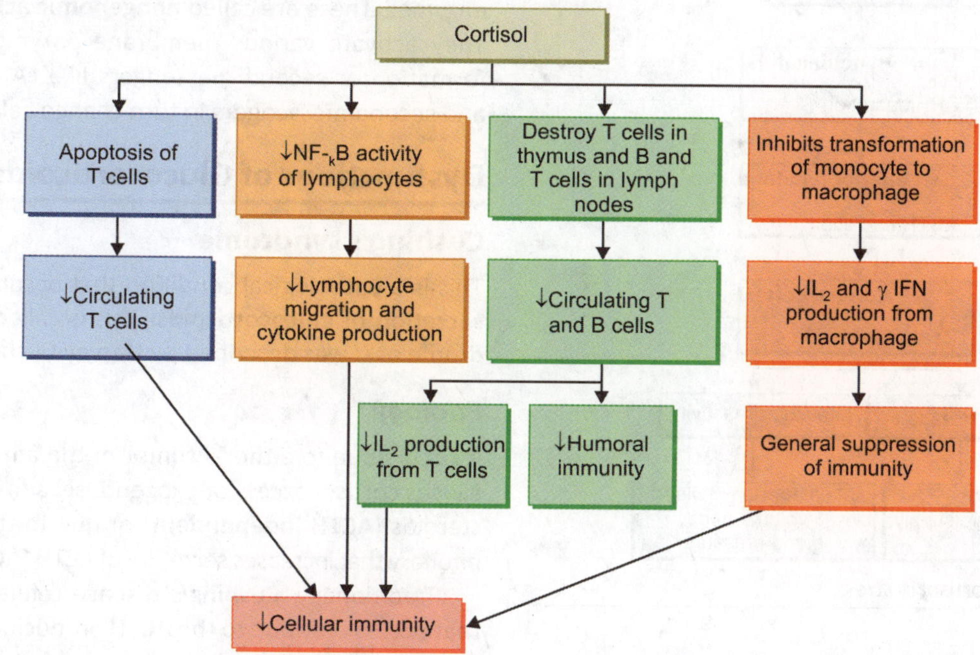

4. Cortisol **inhibits production of interleukins** (IL-1, IL-2, and IL-6) from the helper T cells, and inhibits synthesis of γ interferon from macrophage and lymphocytes. IL-2 and γ interferon are essential for cellular immunity.
5. Cortisol inhibits both resting as well as activated lymphocytes. It **inhibits lymphocyte proliferation**. It also inhibits differentiation of monocytes to macrophages (Flowchart 59.9).

Important Note

Indications and contraindications of cortisol use: Cortisol is used in the treatment of many diseases and also contraindicated for other diseases.

1. Cortisol is used for the treatment of **inflammatory diseases** like rheumatoid arthritis, etc. When an inflammatory process is life-threatening, administration of cortisol provides immediate relief.
2. Cortisol is frequently used for **prevention of transplant rejection** as it inhibits cellular immunity. However, cortisol given for a long time decreases body immunity and, therefore, increases the susceptibility to various bacterial fungal and viral infections. Therefore, cortisol treatment is supplemented with antibiotics.
3. Cortisol is used in the **treatment of both local and systemic allergy**. For example, in the management of bronchial asthma, to ensure effective bronchodilation, inhalation of both cortisol and salbutamol is advised. In acute exacerbation of asthma, systemic steroid is very helpful.
4. Cortisol prevents fibroblastic growth. Therefore, it is used in the treatment of **keloid** (the tumor of scar tissue) by local injections.
5. A person suffering from acute infection **should not be treated with steroids without antibiotics**, though it suppresses inflammation and dramatically improves the condition. This is because cortisol suppresses immunity and spreads infection (person may die due to severe infection).

Thus, cortisol has **profound inhibitory effects on cellular immunity**, for which it is frequently **used for prevention of transplant rejection**. However, in large doses, it also suppresses production of antibodies and, therefore, inhibits humoral immunity. Cortisol does not facilitate degradation of antibodies nor does it interfere in the interaction of antigen and antibodies. The decreased production of interleukin-1 by cortisol suppresses the febrile responses to inflammation.

Clinical Box 59.8

Use and misuse of steroids: Steroids are used in the treatment of various diseases for their anti-inflammatory, immunosuppressive, metabolic and permissive actions. However, they are **also misused** by some sportspersons and others. The usual **synthetic steroids in use** are:

1. **Prednisolone:** It has predominantly glucocorticoid activity and less mineralocorticoid activity. Its glucocorticoid activity is about **four times that of cortisol**.
2. **Dexamethasone:** It has only glucocorticoid activity. Its glucocorticoid activity is about **six times that of prednisolone**.
3. **9α-Flurocortisol:** It has predominantly mineralocorticoid activity and less glucocorticoid activity. Its glucocorticoid activity is about **two-and-half times that of prednisolone**.

Effects on GI tract

1. It **stimulates HCl secretion** from parietal cells of the stomach. Thus, it causes **hyperacidity and gastritis**. Given for a long period, it produces gastric ulceration. Therefore, cortisol is prescribed cautiously in patients already having history of peptic ulcer.
2. Cortisol **decreases Ca^{++} absorption** from GI tract.

Effects on Endocrine Function

1. Cortisol inhibits growth hormone secretion. Therefore, it **inhibits growth**.
2. Cortisol inhibits TSH secretion. Therefore, it **inhibits thyroid functions**.

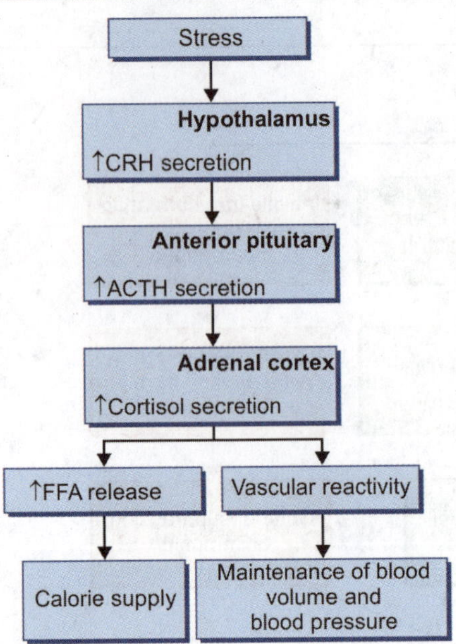

Fig. 59.9: Role of cortisol in stress.

3. Glucocorticoids **inhibit ACTH secretion**. In cortisol excess ACTH secretion is less and in cortisol deficiency ACTH secretion is more. This helps in the diagnosis of adrenocortical dysfunction by estimating plasma ACTH concentration.
4. Cortisol **induces expression of PNMT** (phenylethanolamine-N-methytransferase), the enzyme that catalyzes the formation of epinephrine from norepinephrine.

Role in Stress

The most important function of cortisol is to protect the body against stress. In absence of glucocorticoids, body can not cope with stress even in mild intensity.

1. The glucocorticoid secretion increases due to **increased ACTH secretion**, which exclusively occurs due to increased **release of CRH from hypothalamus**.
2. In fact, stress is defined as the condition in which plasma ACTH secretion is high. The stimuli that increase ACTH secretion are called **stressors**.
3. In stress, glucocorticoid is essential for catecholamines to exert their FFA mobilizing action (FFA is an important source of energy supply in emergency situations) and for maintenance of vascular reactivity to catecholamines (Fig. 59.9).
4. Therefore, in absence of cortisol, the individual succumbs to stress.

Rapid Actions of Steroid

As steroids act though transcription of genes in the cells, it takes hours to days for their full actions to manifest. These are called **genomic actions**. However, recently, it has been observed that some of the steroid actions occur within few minutes. These rapid actions of steroid are due to their direct action on the membrane channels or enzymes. These are called **nongenomic action** of steroids. They activate various membrane enzymes that lead to formation of second messengers like cAMP in the cells, and second messengers in turn change cell functions.

Dysfunctions of Glucocorticoids

Cushing's syndrome

This is a pathological condition that occurs due to **hypersecretion of glucocorticoids**. This is called Cushing's syndrome as it was described by Harvey Cushing.

Etiology

It occurs due to either a tumor of the adrenal cortex that causes cortisol excess or exogenously administered excess steroids (**ACTH independent**) or due to the tumor of the pituitary that increases secretion of ACTH (**ACTH dependent**).

Traditionally, **Cushing's disease** refers to the disease that occurs only due to the ACTH producing tumor of pituitary, whereas **Cushing's syndrome** refers to all the causes of cortisol excess.

Scientist contributed

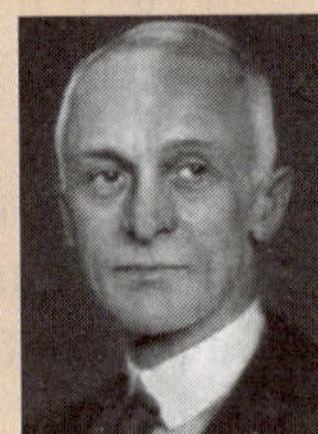

HW Cushing (1869–1939)

Harvey William Cushing (1869-1939) was an American Neurosurgeon, developed neurosurgery as a branch of medicine, and he is often called as the *'Father of modern neurosurgery'*. He had pioneered in the study of functions hypothalamus, pituitary and the hypothalamo-pituitary-adrenocortical axis. During his experiments with Kocher, he first encountered the **Cushing reflex** which describes the relationship between blood pressure and intracranial pressure. He described the cortisol excess is due to increased pituitary activity, which was later named after him as **Cushing's disease** and the cortisol excess is due to adrenocortical tumor as **Cushing's syndrome**.

Source: Papers relating to pituitary body, hypothalamus and parasympathetic nervous system. Springfield Publ. Thomas: 1932.

The **common causes** of Cushing's syndrome are:

1. Adrenal hyperplasia secondary to pituitary ACTH producing tumors, hypothalamo-pituitary dysfunctions, and ectopic ACTH or CRH producing tumors, such as bronchogenic carcinoma.
2. Adrenal tumors (adenoma or carcinoma)
3. Adrenal macronodular hyperplasia
4. Familial adrenal dysplasia (**Carney syndrome**)
5. Prolonged and excess use of ACTH or cortisol (iatrogenic)

Features

The features of Cushing's syndrome according to their frequency of occurrences are:

1. **Centripetal obesity and overweight:** This is due to peculiar distribution of body fat in which fat is deposited more in the abdomen and upper back. Fat pad in lower neck and interscapular region gives the typical appearance of **buffalo hump** (Fig. 59.10).

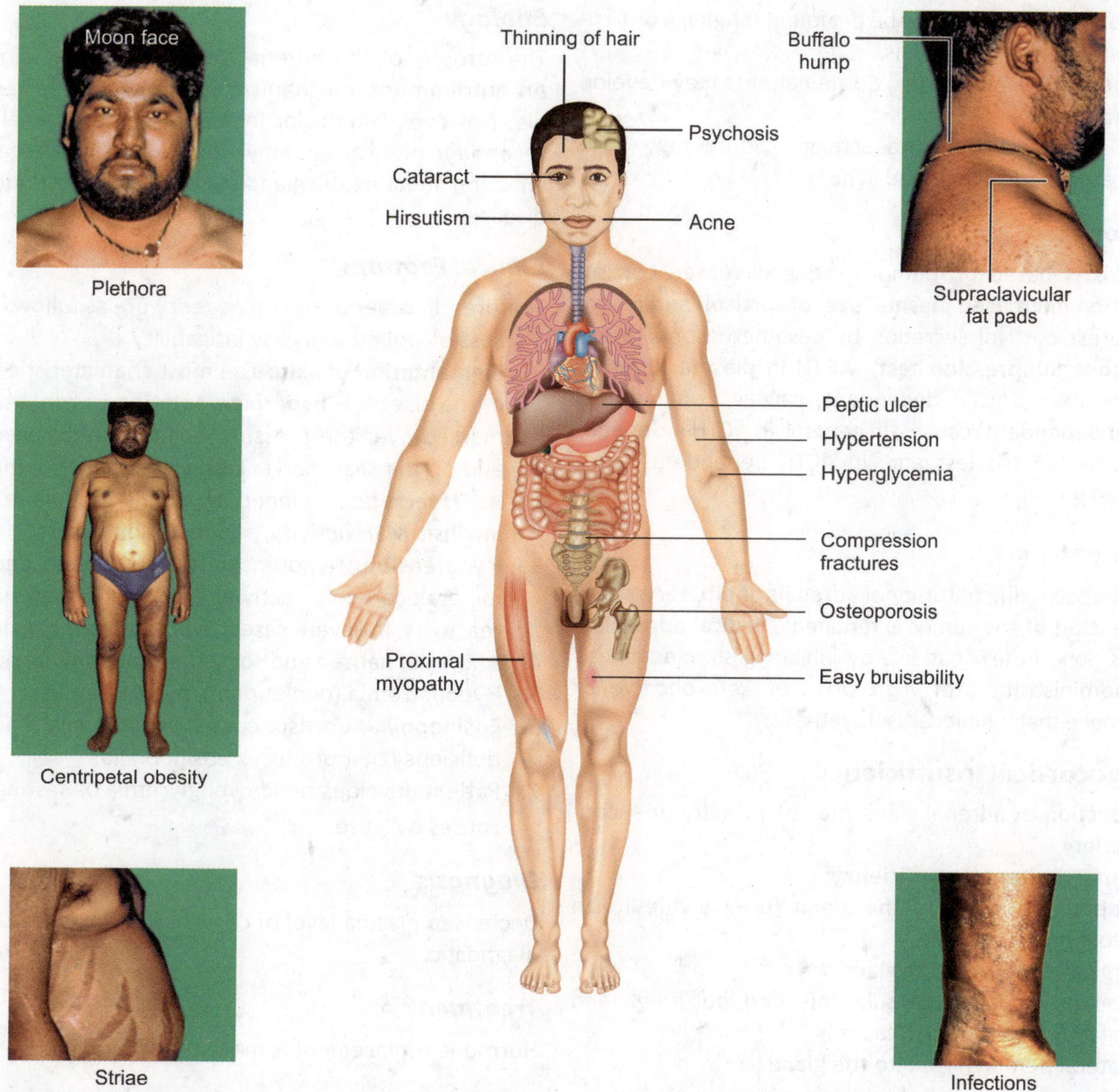

Fig. 59.10: Features of Cushing syndrome. Note the presence of centripetal obesity, moon face, buffalo hump, pendulous abdomen with stria over it, poor muscle development and thin limbs, easy bruisability, poor wound healing (infections).
Courtesy: Figure 10.26, page 786, Manual of Practical Medicine, by R Alagappan, 5th edition, 2014; Jaypee Brothers Medical Publishers (P) Ltd.

2. **Moon face:** The face becomes round with red cheeks due to fat deposition. Salt and water retention contribute to it.
3. Fatigability and weakness. Thin limbs.
4. **Hypertension:** Patient develops hypertension due to water accumulation as glucocorticoid in excess has significant mineralocorticoid activity. Increased angiotensinogen secretion by cortisol and direct action of cortisol on blood vessel contribute to it.
5. **Hirsutism and amenorrhea:** Occurs due to associated increased adrenal androgens.
6. **Reddish purple striae:** Striae develop on the abdomen. Excess fat deposition in abdomen causes rapid stretching of the skin that results in formation of striae.
7. **Ecchymoses:** The skin and subcutaneous tissue are thin as a result of protein catabolism. Capillaries of the skin become thin and fragile. Therefore, minor injury causes ecchymoses and bruises (subcutaneous and intracutaneous hemorrhages).
8. **Proximal myopathy:** The ***legs become thin*** due to proteolysis in the skeletal muscle and reduced bone mass. The muscle development is poor.
9. **Poor wound healing:** Hyperglycemia promotes growth of the organism at the wound site. Also, decreased immunity favors growth of the organism. Cortisol prevents walling off of a chronic infection.
10. Many patients develop **hyperglycemia** and glucose intolerance, and about 20% of patients develop insulin resistant ***diabetes mellitus***.
11. **Osteoporosis** develops due to decreased bone mineralization and decreased bone mass. This may cause collapse of vertebral bodies and pathologic fractures of bones.

12. **Emotional changes** may be profound ranging from irritability to frank **psychosis**.
13. **Hyperacidity** is common. Some patients may develop **peptic ulcer**.
14. The hairs are thin and scraggly. Some may have increase in facial hair and acne.

Diagnosis

Diagnosis is based on demonstrating increased cortisol production (**increased plasma level of cortisol**) and failure to suppress cortisol secretion by dexamethasone (**dexamethasone suppression test**). ACTH in plasma differentiates pituitary (ACTH dependent) causes from adrenal (ACTH independent) causes. In general, in ACTH independent cases, ACTH is less and, in ACTH dependent cases, ACTH is high.

Treatment

If the disease is due to tumor of adrenals or pituitary, **surgical resection** of the tumor is required. **Medical adrenalectomy** is done in few patients by inhibiting steroidogenesis with administration of *high dose of ketokonazole or metyrapone* that inhibit cortisol synthesis.

Adrenocortical Insufficiency

Hypofunction of adrenal gland may be primary or secondary variety.

Primary adrenal insufficiency:

1. Idiopathic atrophy of the gland (usually due to an autoimmune process).
2. Surgical removal of the gland
3. Infection (usually tubercular infection, but fungal and viral infection may also cause)
4. Bilateral hemorrhage into the gland
5. Metastatic invasion of the gland
6. Drugs: ketokonazole, metyrapone, mitotane, etc.

Primary adrenocortical insufficiency is called **Addison's disease.**

Secondary adrenal insufficiency:

1. Pituitary disease that decreases ACTH secretion
2. Hypothalamic disease that decreases CRH secretion

Addison's Disease

This is the condition of **hyposecretion of glucocorticoid** that results from progressive destruction of the adrenals.

Scientist contributed

Thomas Addison (1793–1860) was an English Physician and Scientist. Addison first gave a clue to the significance of the adrenal glands by giving the details of their deficiencies. He was first to study the details of adrenocortical deficiency. Adrenocortical deficiency is named after him as **Addison's disease**. He had also pioneered in the study of blood disorders.

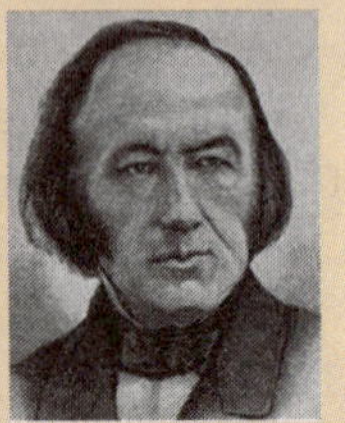

Thomas Addison
(1793–1860)

Source: On the constitutional and local effects of disease of suprarenal capsules. S. Highley Publ. London: 1855.

Etiology

The atrophy of the adrenal cortex is usually idiopathic. An **autoimmune mechanism** is thought to be responsible. However, tubercular infection of the adrenal gland, secondary metastasis, amyloidosis and cytomegalovirus infection affecting the gland may destroy and produce the disease.

Clinical Features

Features, in order of their frequency are as follows:

1. Loss of weight and easy fatigability
2. **Pigmentation of skin:** The most characteristic feature of the disease is **hyperpigmentation** of skin, especially marked over the pressure points, sun-exposed areas and on the scar marks. Less plasma cortisol ***increases ACTH secretion*** by feedback mechanism. As ***ACTH has intrinsic MSH activity***, pigmentation occurs.
3. **Hypotension:** Hypotension occurs due to decreased mineralocorticoid activity and decreased vascular reactivity. In severe cases, *hypotensive shock* occurs.
4. Anorexia, nausea and sometimes abdominal pain.
5. Hyponatremia (depletional), hyperkalemia.
6. **Eosinophilia:** Cortisol causes eosinopenia. Therefore, deficiency of it produces eosinophilia.
7. Patient develops rapid hypoglycemia on fasting; stress causes collapse.

Diagnosis

Decreased plasma level of cortisol with increased ACTH is diagnostic.

Treatment

Hormone replacement is mainstay of therapy.

Adrenogenital Syndrome

Etiology

This occurs due to **21β-hydroxylase deficiency**, which decreases the synthesis of glucocorticoids and mineralocorticoids. Decreased plasma level of cortisol increases secretion of ACTH by feedback mechanism that increases the production of pregnenolone. Excess pregnenolone is diverted for the production of androgen. Thus, steroids in this syndrome are converted to excess of androgen that produces **virilization.**

Features

Excess androgen secretion in females causes **masculinization** and **precocious pseudopuberty** or **female pseudohermaphroditism**. The usual features are:

1. Hirsutism
2. Small breast
3. Receding hairline
4. Heavy arms and legs
5. Enlarged clitoris (clitoromegaly)

Table 59.5: Conditions that alter aldosterone secretion.

A. Conditions that increase secretion
1. Hemorrhage
2. Hypovolemia
3. Hyperkalemia
4. Hyponatremia
5. Standing
6. Anxiety
7. Physical trauma and surgery
8. Secondary hyperaldosteronism: Aldosterone secretion may increase in congestive heart failure, cirrhosis of liver, and nephritic syndrome.
B. Conditions that decrease secretion
1. Expansion of ECF volume
2. Hypernatremia
3. Hypokalemia

6. Male escutcheon (male distribution of suprapubic hair)
7. Androgenic flush.

MINERALOCORTICOIDS

Aldosterone is the major mineralocorticoid in humans.

Regulation of Aldosterone Secretion

Aldosterone secretion is regulated mainly by ***three important stimuli:* angiotensin-II, ACTH, and plasma K$^+$** concentration. Many conditions alter aldosterone secretion (Table 59.5) by influencing these stimuli.

Angiotensin II

Angiotensin II is an important stimulator of aldosterone synthesis and secretion. It is formed from angiotensinogen, an α_2-globulin secreted from liver.

1. Renin, a circulating protease enzyme secreted from JG cells of kidney catalyzes the conversion of angiotensinogen to angiotensin I (A I).
2. A I is converted to angiotensin II (A II) by the action of angiotensin converting enzyme (ACE), present in the endothelial cell of blood vessels, especially in the pulmonary vasculature.
3. A II is further degraded to angiotensin III (A III). A II and A III stimulate the formation of aldosterone (Flowchart 59.10).

Thus, this system of aldosterone formation is called **renin-angiotensin-aldosterone system** (Details of RAS is described in first chapter of Renal System). A III is as potent as stimulator of aldosterone synthesis and secretion as A II. A I has no such activity. A II also stimulates ***synthesis of aldosterone***. A II causes vasoconstriction and has many other functions (for details, refer to Chapter 75).

Flowchart 59.10: Renin-angiotensin system controlling aldosterone secretion.

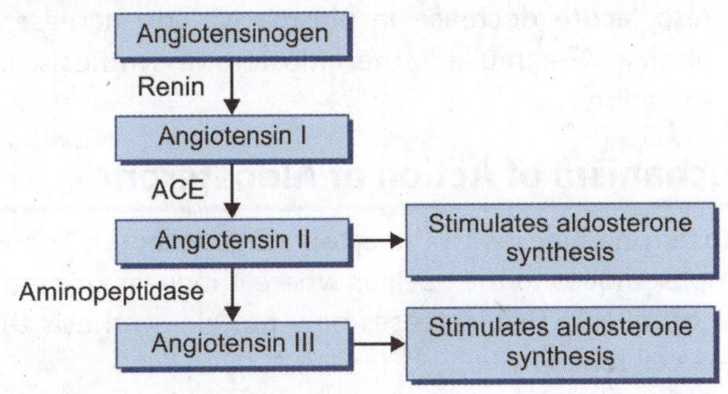

Angiotensin Receptors

There are two types of angiotensin receptors: AT_1 and AT_2. **AT_1 receptors** are present on the zona glomerulosa cells of adrenal cortex. A II binds with AT_1 receptors and increases intracellular **IP_3 and DAG** production that in turn increase intracellular calcium. **Rise in calcium facilitates aldosterone secretion.**

ACTH

Cells of zona glomerulosa of adrenal cortex have ACTH receptors.

1. ACTH stimulates aldosterone synthesis and secretion, mediated by cyclic AMP and protein kinase.
2. However, the quantity of ACTH required to stimulate aldosterone secretion is more than the concentration required to stimulate cortisol secretion.
3. Moreover, the effect of ACTH on aldosterone secretion is **temporary** (Application Box 59.2). **Aldosterone secretion declines**, even if ACTH secretion is elevated, which is partly due to ***decreased renin secretion*** secondary to hypervolemia. Interestingly, deoxycorticosterone (another mineralocorticoid) secretion remains high.

Application Box 59.2

ACTH stimulated aldosterone secretion is not transient in GRA: Though ACTH-mediated aldosterone secretion is a temporary phenomenon; it is persistent in **glucocorticoid-remediable aldosteronism** (GRA). This is an autosomal dominant disorder, in which ACTH causes persistent hypersecretion of aldosterone that leads to hypertension. GRA occurs due to fusion of genes coding for 11β-hydroxylase and aldosterone synthase (as they are 95% identical and remain close together on chromosome 8) forming a hybrid gene called **ACTH-sensitive aldosterone synthase**. Therefore, ACTH effect on aldosterone secretion becomes a prolonged phenomenon. Hypertension in GRA is treated by glucocorticoid, as this decreases the production of ACTH, which in turn decreases the synthesis of aldosterone. Hence, this syndrome is called **glucocorticoid-remediable** aldosteronism.

Hyperkalemia

Aldosterone secretion is stimulated by increase in K$^+$ in ECF.

1. Rise in ECF K$^+$ ***activates voltage gated calcium channels*** that increases intracellular calcium.
2. **Increased cytosolic calcium** increases aldosterone synthesis and secretion.

3. Aldosterone, in turn promotes excretion of K^+. Thus, **aldosterone is a natural regulator of K^+ level in ECF**. Also, **acute decrease in plasma Na^+** or increase in plasma K^+ stimulates the aldosterone synthesis and secretion.

Mechanism of Action of Aldosterone

Aldosterone binds with the cytoplasmic receptor. The HR complex moves to the nucleus where it induces transcription of mRNA. This increases new protein synthesis that alters cell function.

Aldosterone has both genomic and nongenomic actions:

Genomic Action

The gene activated by aldosterone is **sgk gene** (serum and glucocorticoid regulated kinase gene).

1. This is an early response gene that increases **ENaC** (Epithelial Na^+ Channels) activity.
2. Aldosterone also increases mRNA for synthesis of proteins that form subunits of ENaC.
3. Aldosterone increases **insertion of these channels** on cell membrane and also **increases their activity**.

Nongenomic Action

Nongenomic action occurs rapidly. This is due to stimulation of the **activity of Na^+-K^+ exchanger**, which increases intracellular accumulation of Na^+. The second messenger that mediates this action is IP_3.

Physiological Actions of Aldosterone

Electrolyte and Water Balance

The main function of aldosterone is to **increase Na^+ and water reabsorption** and to **promote K^+ and H^+ excretion** from the kidney. Na^+ reabsorption is the primary function, and other effects are mostly secondary to Na^+ reabsorption. For Na^+ reabsorption, aldosterone acts primarily on **P cells** (principal cells) of **collecting duct and distal tubule** of kidney. In fact, aldosterone controls only 3% of total Na^+ reabsorption from the kidney. However, aldosterone deficiency results in significant hyponatremia.

Aldosterone increases Na^+ and water reabsorption by following mechanisms:

1. It increases the **number of Na^+ channels** in the epithelial cells of the kidney tubule.
2. It **stimulates Na^+-K^+ ATPase activity**, therefore, Na^+ is reabsorbed and K^+ is excreted.
3. It **stimulates enzymes of Krebs cycle** that facilitate ATP generation and provide energy for removal of Na^+ from the interstitial fluid into the capillary.

Thus, aldosterone increases plasma Na^+ concentration and decreases K^+ concentration. Therefore, in aldosterone deficiency, hyponatremia is associated with hyperkalemia.

As Na^+ is reabsorbed, **Cl^- is transported** in the same direction to maintain electroneutrality. The reabsorption of NaCl causes **osmotic reabsorption of water**. Thus, reabsorption of salt and water leads to **ECF expansion**.

Aldosterone Escape Phenomenon

Increased reabsorption of salt and water by aldosterone causes ECF expansion.

1. Increased ECF volume **increases venous return** to the heart that causes further **distention of atria** during their filling.
2. Atrial stretching **increases synthesis and secretion of ANP** from atrial myocytes.
3. ANP causes profound **natriuresis and diuresis**.
4. Therefore, ECF volume returns back to normal. This is called aldosterone escape phenomenon as kidney escapes from the effect of aldosterone.

Dysfunctions of Aldosterone

Hypersecretion of Aldosterone

Hyperaldosteronism can be divided broadly into **two categories**: primary and secondary.

Primary Hyperaldosteronism

The cause of excess aldosterone secretion is due to adrenal disease. The usual causes are aldosterone-producing adrenal adenoma (*Conn's syndrome*), adrenal hyperplasia and adrenal carcinoma. **Renin secretion is decreased** in primary hyperaldosteronism (Fig. 59.11A).

Conn's Syndrome

This is the major cause of primary hyperaldosteronism. It occurs due to the **tumor (adenoma) of zona glomerulosa of adrenal cortex**.

1. The disease manifests with **hypertension** (due to sodium retention and ECF expansion), **muscle weakness** and fatigue (due to potassium depletion), and **polyuria** (due to impairment of urinary concentrating ability).
2. Edema is usually not a feature of primary hyperaldosteronism.
3. **Hypokalemia**, hypernatremia and low renin in plasma, and **metabolic alkalosis** are usual laboratory findings.

Secondary Hyperaldosteronism

Increased aldosterone secretion due to **activation of renin-angiotensin system** is called secondary hyperaldosteronism.

1. It is associated with **increased renin in plasma** (Fig. 59.11B), as decreased volume is the initiating stimulus for renin secretion. This is a *major differentiating feature* from primary hyperaldosteronism, in which renin secretion is less.
2. It occurs in congestive heart failure, cirrhosis of liver and nephritic syndrome. Renin secreting tumor (primary reninism) can also cause it.

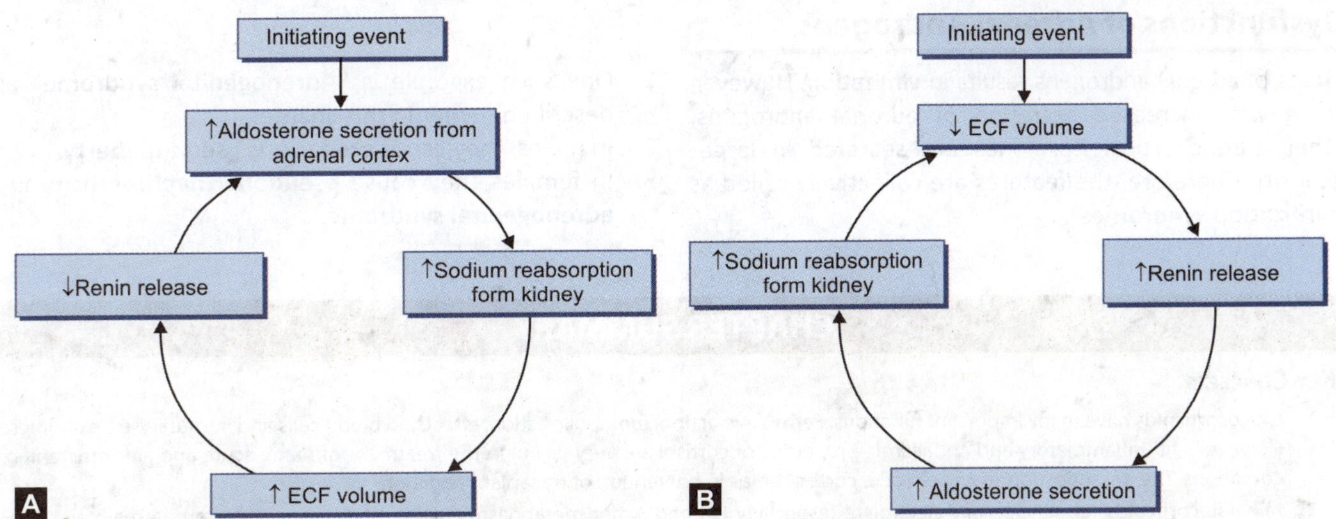

Figs. 59.11A and B: Renin secretion in primary (A) and secondary hyperaldosteronism (B). Note, decreased renin secretion occurs (hence, no activation of renin-angiotensin-aldosterone axis) in primary aldosteronism; therefore, edema is not a feature. In secondary aldosteronism, renin secretion is more (activation of renin-angiotensin-aldosterone axis) hence, edema is usually a feature.

3. **Edema is a usual feature** in secondary hyperaldosteronism. However, secondary hyperaldosteronism in *Bartter syndrome* and *Gitelman syndrome* occurs without edema.

Bartter Syndrome

It is a condition of hyperplasia of JG cells (**juxtaglomerular hyperplasia**).

1. The disease occurs due to **mutation in the Na^+-K^+-$2Cl^-$ cotransporter gene**, which results in ***high renin activity*** and increased aldosterone synthesis.
2. Hyperaldosteronism produces **K^+ depletion.**
3. Major features are **hypokalemic alkalosis and hypercalciuria.**
4. However, **blood pressure remains normal and there is no edema.**

Hyposecretion of Aldosterone

Hyposecretion of mineralocorticoid is usually associated with **adrenal insufficiency**. However, **isolated hypoaldosteronism** with normal cortisol production occurs in following conditions:

1. Inherited defect of biosynthesis of aldosterone.
2. Decreased renin production (**hyporeninemic hypoaldosteronism**).
3. Surgical removal of aldosterone secreting adenoma causing more resection of normal adrenocortical tissue.
4. During protracted heparin administration.
5. Selective unresponsiveness of Zona glomerulosa to angiotensin II (**hyperreninemic hypoaldosteronism**).
6. Pretectal disease of nervous system.
7. Severe postural hypotension.

SEX STEROIDS

Sex steroids secreted from adrenal gland are called **adrenal androgens**. The major adrenal androgens are **dehydroepiandrosterone and androstenedione.**

1. Androstenedione is **converted to estrogen** in the peripheral blood and tissues.
2. The secretion of adrenal androgen increases at puberty, reaches peak at about 20 years of age and then declines slowly to reach a low level in old age. These changes correlate with the change in 17 α-hydroxylase activity.
3. The secretion of adrenal androgen is **controlled by ACTH**, not by gonadotropins.

Functions of Adrenal Androgens

Adrenal androgens have less than 20% of activity of testicular androgen.

1. **Adrenarche:** At the onset of puberty in both boys and girls, in the **stage 1** (before the physical development of puberty), *secretion of adrenal androgen becomes high* before the gonadal secretions are significantly elevated. This is called **adrenarche**. It is proposed that adrenarche *initiates the process of puberty* in which **adrenal androgen sensitizes the gonads** to secrete more sex hormones and **sensitizes the sex organs** to the effects of sex hormones.
2. They exert **masculinizing effect:** However, the masculinizing effect is less in normal concentration of adrenal androgens. These effects are prominent only when the hormones are secreted in excess amount.
3. **Promote protein synthesis:** They are protein anabolic, **increase protein synthesis**.
4. **Facilitate growth:** They **facilitate growth**. In adult males, they accentuate the already developed sex characteristics. However, in prepubertal boys, in excess, they develop secondary sex characteristics precociously. This is called **precocious pseudopuberty**.
5. **Source of estrogen:** Adrenal androgens are converted to estrogen in the peripheral tissue and serve as the **major source of estrogen in males and postmenopausal females.**

Dysfunctions of Adrenal Androgens

Excess of adrenal androgens results in **virilization**. However, along with increased secretion of adrenal androgens, other adrenocortical hormones are secreted in larger quantity. Therefore, the features are collectively called as "**virilization syndromes**".

1. One such example is "**Adrenogenital syndrome**" as described earlier in this chapter.
2. In males, they cause **precocious pseudopuberty.**
3. In females they cause **pseudohermaphroditism** and **adrenogenital syndrome**.

CHAPTER SUMMARY

Key Concepts

1. Glucocorticoids have many important functions. Permissive action, metabolic action, effects on blood cells and immunity are examples. However, anti-inflammatory and antiallergic properties of cortisol are very useful in the treatment of many acute and life-threatening conditions. The immunosuppressive effect of cortisol helps in prevention of transplant rejection.
2. Mineralocorticoids regulate serum electrolyte (especially K^+) and water metabolisms of the body. Thus, aldosterone maintains ECF volume and blood volume. Cortisol maintains vascular reactivity to assist in control of blood volume and pressure.
3. Sex hormones, especially adrenal androgens (mainly DHEA) sensitize gonads for secretion of sex hormones at the time of puberty. Therefore, adrenocortical deficiency leads to delayed puberty or dysfunctions of puberty.

Important to Know (Must Read)

1. In examination, Describe the functions of glucocorticoids (or cortisol) usually comes as a **Long Question.** Regulation of secretion, mechanism of action, physiological actions and dysfunctions of aldosterone may come as a **Long Question**.
2. Regulation of cortisol synthesis and secretion, Mechanism of action of cortisol, Effects of cortisol on inflammation, Effects of cortisol on allergy, Effects of cortisol on immunity, Effects of cortisol on blood cells, Permissive actions of cortisol, Cushing's syndrome (etiology, features diagnosis and treatment), Addison's disease (etiology, features diagnosis and treatment), Conn's syndrome, Adrenogenital (Virilization) syndrome, Aldosterone (physiological actions, regulation of secretion, mechanism of action), Mechanism of action of glucocorticoids, Aldosterone escape phenomenon, are usual **Short Questions** in exam.
3. In **Viva**, examiner may ask… List the hormones of adrenal cortex and the layer from where they are secreted, Specific enzymes involved in synthesis of adrenocortical steroids and the diseases produced by their deficiencies, Functions of cortisol especially permissive actions of cortisol, effects of cortisol on inflammation, allergy, immunity and blood cells, Why steroid therapy should not be stopped abruptly? Why adrenal deficient patients should not fast? How cortisol excess complicates diabetes mellitus? Why injection of cortisol is a must during treatment of shock? Why bone X-ray should be checked in patients receiving steroid therapy for a prolonged period? Why one should be cautious while infusing glucose solution in cortisol deficiency? What are the indications and contraindications for cortisol use? Name some important synthetic steroids and their glucocorticoid activity, What is rapid action of steroids? What is the role of cortisol in stress? Effects of cortisol on intermediary metabolism (carbohydrate, protein and fat), Effects of cortisol on cardiovascular system and central nervous system, Effects of cortisol on bone, connective tissue and musculoskeletal system, Effects of cortisol on fetus, Effects of cortisol on gastrointestinal tract and endocrine system, What is Cushing's syndrome and what are its features? Also, how these features develop? What is Addison's disease and what are its features? Physiological actions of aldosterone, What are the conditions that increase or decrease aldosterone secretion? What is aldosterone escape phenomenon? What is Conn's syndrome and what are its features? Functions of adrenal androgens, What is adrenogenital (Virilization) syndrome and what are its features? Regulation of glucocorticoids secretion, Mechanism of action of glucocorticoids, Regulation of aldosterone secretion, Mechanism of action of aldosterone, What is apparent mineralocorticoid excess? Cause and features of hyposecretion of aldosterone, Why ACTH stimulated aldosterone secretion is not transient in GRA (Glucocorticoid-remediable aldosteronism), Steps of synthesis of Cortisol, Steps of synthesis of Corticosterone, Steps of synthesis of Aldosterone, Steps of synthesis of Androstenedione, Steps of synthesis of Estradiol, and effect of deficiency of key enzymes like 21 β-hydroxylase, 11 β-hydroxylase, 17 α-hydroxylase and 3 β-hydroxysteroid dehydrogenase and cholesterol desmolase.

CHAPTER 60

Endocrine Pancreas

Learning Objectives

On completion of study of this chapter, the student **MUST** be able to:

1. List the hormones secreted form endocrine pancreas, and name the cells secreting them.
2. Understand the synthesis, regulation of secretion and metabolism of insulin.
3. Describe the mechanism of secretion of insulin.
4. Classify GLUTs and give their functions.
5. Describe the functions of insulin.
6. Give the etiological classification of diabetes, understand the important differences between type I and type II diabetes.
7. Explain the physiological basis of features and treatment of diabetes.
8. Give the important functions of glucagon, somatostatin and pancreatic polypeptide.
9. Understand the importance of insulin-glucagon ratio.

The student **MAY** also be able to:

1. Describe the synthesis and regulation of insulin secretion.
2. Describe the functions of glucagon, somatostatin and pancreatic polypeptide.
3. Describe the physiological basis of metabolic abnormalities in diabetes.

The digestion, storage and utilization of nutrients are processes that require higher degree of regulation. Pancreas plays a crucial role in controlling these processes. Pancreas has two parts: **the exocrine pancreas,** which constitutes about 80% of the pancreatic tissue that controls digestion, and **the endocrine pancreas**, which constitutes 1–2% of the pancreatic tissue that controls storage and utilization of nutrients. Endocrine pancreas is an important endocrine organ as it secretes insulin, the **only antidiabetogenic and antiketogenic hormone** in the body.

Importance of insulin-glucagon ratio: Pancreas secretes another **three hormones**: glucagon, somatostatin and pancreatic polypeptide. Glucagon has metabolic actions that are opposite to that of insulin:

1. **Insulin is anabolic and promotes storage of nutrients** (glucose, fatty acids and amino acids), whereas **glucagon is catabolic and promotes mobilization of nutrients** from their storage depots into the blood stream.
2. Insulin and glucagon, by their opposing effects, control metabolism of carbohydrate, fat and protein to ensure energy supply during basal and active states. As insulin and glucagon have reciprocal physiological actions, the **ratio of insulin to glucagon** is more important than their individual concentrations in the regulation of intermediary metabolisms.

Scientists contributed

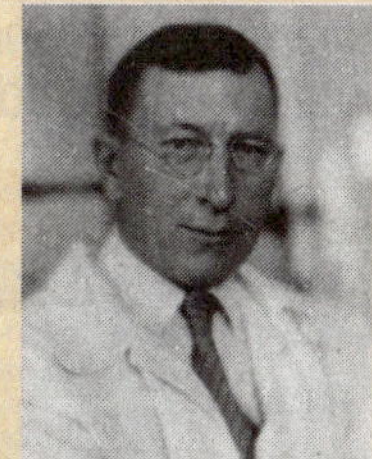

FG Banting
(1891–1941)

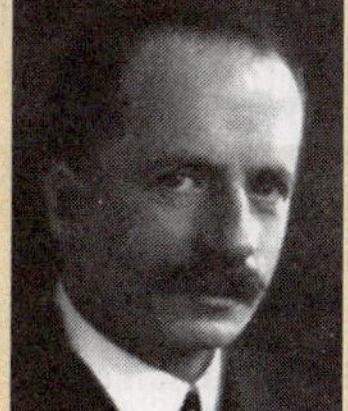

JJ Rickard Macleod
(1876–1936)

The **Nobel Prize in Physiology or Medicine 1923** was awarded jointly to American endocrinologist and physiologist **Frederick Grant Banting** and Canadian endocrinologist and physiologist **John James Rickard Macleod** *"for the discovery of insulin".* They studied the role of insulin for the control of carbohydrate metabolism. They acknowledged and shared the prize with ***Charles H Best*** and ***James Bertram Collip***, who had also worked with them.

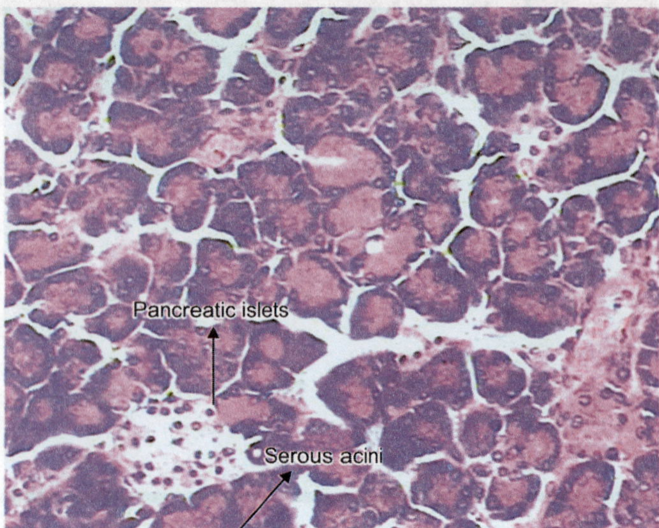

Fig. 60.1: Histology of pancreas showing islets of Lnagerhans. *Courtesy*: Figure 13.50B, Basic Histology, by V Subhadra Devi, 1st Edition, 2016; Jaypee Brothers Medical Publishers (P) Ltd.

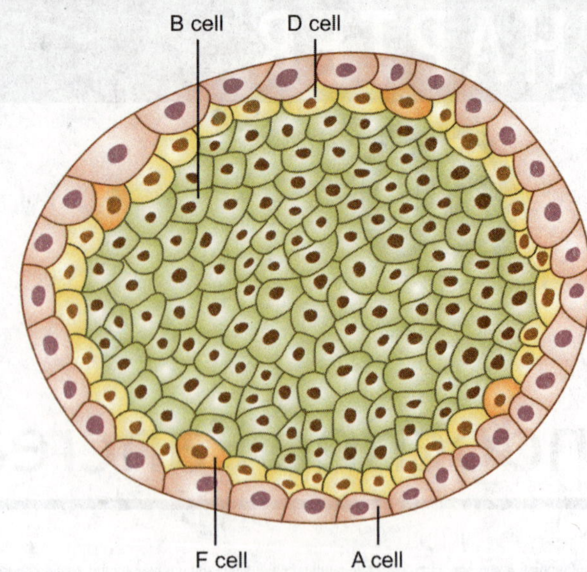

Fig. 60.2: Structure of islet of Langerhans. Note, beta cells constitute majority of cell mass of the islet.

3. Usually, the conditions that stimulate secretion of one inhibit the secretion of other, because when one is essential for the body the other is usually not.
4. **Deficiency of insulin produces diabetes mellitus** and its excess results in hypoglycemia. On the contrary, **deficiency of glucagon produces hypoglycemia** and its excess worsens diabetes mellitus.
5. Usually, insulin deficiency is associated with glucagon excess.

PHYSIOLOGICAL ANATOMY

Islets of Langerhans

The endocrine pancreas, which constitutes less than 2% of the total pancreatic tissue, is formed by **islets of Langerhans** (named after the German medical student, Paul Langerhans who first described it in a dog pancreas in 1869). Islets are more abundant in the tail than the head and body of the pancreas. There are about **1 million islets** in the human pancreas. Islets are oval in shape with diameter ranging from 50 to 300 µm (Fig. 60.1). Each islet contains about **2,500 cells.**

Scientist contributed

Paul Langerhans Jr (1847–1888), a German pathologist and physiologist was born into a family of physicians and scientists, known for two medical eponyms. He made his first major contribution before he finished his medical school, with the discovery of epidermal nonpigmentary dendritic cells that are derived from the bone marrow and play a role in cell-mediated immunity. These cells are known as **Langerhans cells**. Second, Langerhans made the first detailed description of the pancreas during his studies for his doctorate degree at the Berlin Pathological Institute in 1869. He described different types of cells in the pancreatic islets, that later became known as the **islets of Langerhans**.

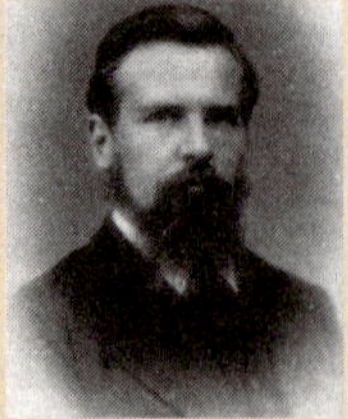

Paul Langerhans *(1847–1888)*

Four type of cells present in the islets:

1. β **cells** (B cells): Secrete **insulin.**
2. α **cells** (A cells): Secrete **glucagon.**
3. δ **cells** (D cells): Secrete **somatostatin.**
4. **F cells** (PP cells): Secrete **pancreatic polypeptide**.

β Cells

They constitute 70–80% of islet cells that **secrete insulin**. The cells are placed centrally in the islet (Fig. 60.2):

1. The diameter of each cell is 10–20 µm.
2. Packets of insulin are present in the form of **secretory granules** in the cell cytoplasm that measure about 0.25 µm.
3. Each packet of insulin is present in a vesicle and a clear space or halo exists between the wall of the vesicle and the packet.
4. A developed system of microtubules and microfilaments are present in the cytoplasm that facilitates the exocytosis of vesicles.

α Cells

They constitute 15–20% of islet cells that **secrete glucagon**. They are present in the periphery of the islet.

δ Cells

They constitute about 10% of the islet cells that **secrete somatostatin**. The cells are typically located toward the periphery between the β and α cells.

F Cells

They constitute 1–2% of islet cells that **secrete pancreatic polypeptide**. The cells are distributed randomly among the D cells.

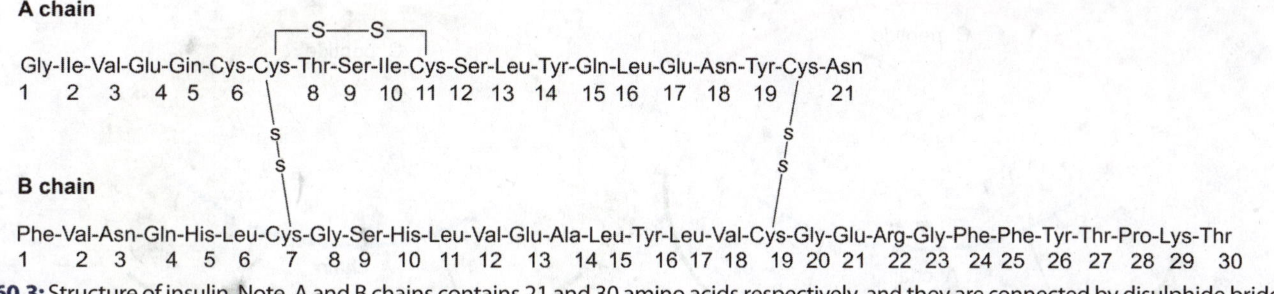

Fig. 60.3: Structure of insulin. Note, A and B chains contains 21 and 30 amino acids respectively, and they are connected by disulphide bridges.

Fate of islet hormones: The hormones secreted from islets are released into the *pancreatic vein* from where they are transported into the *portal vein* and from there they enter general circulation:

1. This special arrangement provides **liver the first and maximum access** to the proper concentrations of islet hormones as they are secreted, and then to other tissues in the body.
2. Thus, liver being the primary site of substrate metabolism avails maximum advantage of actions of islet hormones, especially of insulin and glucagon.

Islet blood supply: Islets are **highly vascular**:

1. They receive about 10% of the total pancreatic blood supply though they constitute only about 1% of the pancreatic tissue.
2. There is a ***portal arrangement*** of the blood vessels of pancreas, which allows hormones secreted from a cell group to reach the other islet cells.
3. This arrangement is essential for paracrine regulation of hormone secretion from the islet cells.

Innervation: Islet cells are **neuroectodermal in development**:

1. They receive both parasympathetic and sympathetic innervations.
2. Usually, stimulation of β **adrenergic receptor increases** insulin secretion and α **adrenergic receptor decreases** it.
3. Increased **vagal (cholinergic) activity increases insulin secretion.**

INSULIN

Structure of Insulin

Insulin is **a peptide hormone** consisting of two chains, A and B, which are connected by disulfide bridges. The molecular weight of insulin is 6,000:

1. The **A chain** contains 21 amino acids and **B chain** 30 amino acids (Fig. 60.3).
2. The final structure of insulin is determined by the N-terminal and C-terminal amino acids of A chain, and the hydrophobic character of the amino acids at the C-terminal of B chain.
3. However, the hydrophobic character of the amino acids at the C-terminal of B chain is important for biological activity of insulin.
4. Insulin is synthesized as monomers that immediately form the crystalline hexamer unit within two zinc atoms (Application Box 60.1).

Application Box 60.1

Synthetic insulin: Insulin is synthesized in pharmaceuticals usually as crystalline zinc insulin. This preparation is the fast acting insulin. Usually, insulin is injected subcutaneously as it is absorbed slowly to provide a slow rise in insulin concentration that resembles basal insulin secretion from pancreas.

Scientist contributed

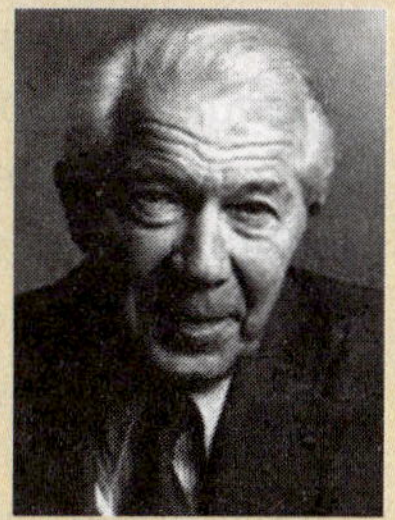
Christian de Duve
(Born, 1917)

Christian de Duve (born, 1917) a Belgian cytologist and biochemist, was awarded the **Nobel Prize for Physiology or Medicine in 1974**, for his research work on **lysosomes** (the cell's digestive system) and **peroxisomes** (cell metabolic system), and shared his Nobel honors with Albert Claude and George E. Palade. He won Nobel Prize for his research in the field of **diabetes mellitus** and how his revelations led to the **discovery of lysosomes.** de Duve demonstrated that hepatectomized dogs needed considerably less glucose to be kept normoglycemic after injection of a supramaximal dose of insulin than did an intact animal. He proved that the **liver is the major site of insulin action.**

Synthesis, Secretion and Metabolism

Synthesis of Insulin

Like other peptide hormones, insulin is synthesized as **preproinsulin**, containing 110 amino acids. The insulin gene belongs to the superfamily of genes that encode synthesis of a variety of insulin like growth factors. The **insulin gene** is located on the **short arm of the chromosome 11**. Insulin is first formed as **preproinsulin** in the ribosome of rough endoplasmic reticulum. The preproinsulin contains four sequential peptides:

1. An N-terminal signal peptides
2. The B chain of insulin
3. A connecting peptide (C peptide), and
4. The A chain of insulin.

The N-terminal signal peptide is immediately cleaved from the preproinsulin molecule to form the **proinsulin**, a 86 amino acid peptide, which then enters the Golgi apparatus.

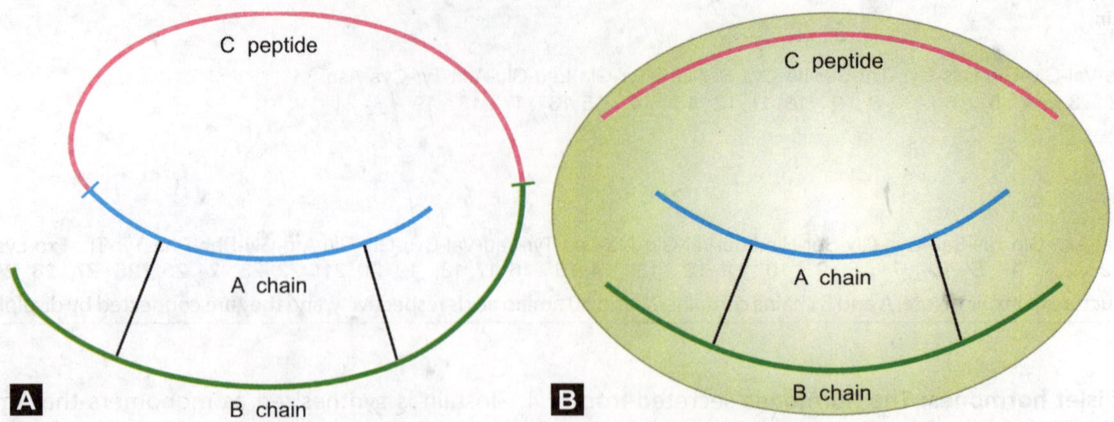

Figs. 60.4A and B: (A) Structure of proinsulin as formed in endoplasmic reticulum (ER). Note, the molecule containing A and B chains and connecting peptide (C peptide) is folded. The A and B chains are connected by C peptide. (B) Insulin molecule in packaged in the granule in Golgi apparatus (GA), after its synthesis. The granules contain insulin and C peptide.

1. In the Golgi apparatus, the disulfide bridges are established that allows the proinsulin molecule to be folded (Figs. 60.4A and B). The A and B chains of insulin are linked by the *connecting peptide* (**C peptide**). The C peptide **not only connects, but also facilitates folding of A and B chains.**
2. During packaging in the Golgi apparatus into the granules, the proinsulin is cleaved to form insulin molecules, and C peptides are retained in the granules.
3. When insulin is secreted, the C peptide is also released in *equimolar concentration with insulin*.
4. Insulin is associated with zinc as molecule matures. The zinc insulin crystals form the **dense central core** of the granule with a ***clear space around***.
5. The C peptide is present in the clear space between the membrane of the granule and the central dense core.
6. Also, during insulin secretion, some amount of proinsulin is secreted from the granules.

Thus, **β-cell granules secrete** the following substances:

1. **Insulin:** Insulin constitutes about 95% of secretion from β-cell.
2. **Proinsulin:** Proinsulin is a 86 amino acid peptide. It has about 10% of biological activity of insulin. It is secreted as only about 3% of the amount of secreted insulin. However, as plasma clearance is slower (half life 15-30 min) than insulin, the plasma concentration in fasting state is about 10-15% of insulin concentration.
3. **C peptide:** It is a 31 amino acid peptide. The amount of C-peptide secreted is about 7% of the insulin secreted from the gland:
   - It has **no biological activity of insulin**. Its importance lies in the fact that it is **secreted in equimolar ratio with insulin.**
   - Measurement of C-peptide has advantages over measurement of insulin. Hepatic metabolism of C-peptide is negligible; therefore its **concentration in plasma directly reflects the β-cell activity**.
   - Moreover, C-peptide assay does not measure exogenous insulin and do not cross-react with insulin antibodies, whereas insulin measurements have these fallacies.
   - Therefore, C-peptide assay is the **better index of β-cell activity** (Application Box 60.2).

Substances Having Insulin Like Activity

There are few substances present in human plasma having insulin like activity. However, their insulin activity is very poor. Therefore, insulin deficiency or insulin resistance leads to diabetes. Important among them are **nonsuppressible insulin like activities** (NSILAs) that are mainly **somatomedins** (IGF I and II). NSILAs are not suppressed by anti-insulin antibodies. Following are the insulin like activities in human plasma:

1. Insulin
2. Proinsulin
3. NSILA (IGF I, IGF II and IGF bound proteins).

> **Application Box 60.2**
>
> **C peptide measurement:** As C peptide is secreted in equimolar concentration with insulin, and is least degraded in liver, its concentration in plasma provides a good index of beta cell secretory capacity. It is measured by RIA.

The major regulator of insulin synthesis is the plasma glucose concentration. Glucose stimulates insulin secretion. Therefore, feeding (hyperglycemia) increases and fasting (hypoglycemia) decreases insulin synthesis and secretion. Glucose increases insulin synthesis by increasing translation of insulin mRNA and transcription of insulin gene.

Secretion of Insulin

Insulin secretion is greatly influenced by plasma glucose concentration. Elevation of glucose level in plasma is an important stimulator of insulin secretion. Factors that control insulin secretion are listed in Table 60.1.

Table 60.1: Important factors that regulate insulin secretion.

A. Factors that increase insulin secretion
1. Carbohydrates: Glucose, galactose, mannose, and glyceraldehydes (Hyperglycemia is the important stimulator).
2. Amino acids: Arginine, lysine, leucine, alanine.
3. Ketoacids
4. Free fatty acids, especially long chain FFA
5. Hormones: GIP, gastrin, secretin, glucagon, GLP1, cholecystokinin.
6. Increased vagal activity, acetylcholine
7. β adrenergic receptor agonists
8. K^+, Ca^{++}
9. Theophylline
B. Factors that decrease insulin secretion
1. Hypoglycemia as occurs in fasting, exercise
2. Somatostatin
3. Leptin
4. Interleukin I
5. α adrenergic agonists, and β blockers
6. Hypokalemia
7. β cell poisons: Streptozotocin, alloxan
8. Inhibitors of microtubules like colchicine

Regulation of Insulin Secretion

Insulin secretion is mainly regulated by the feedback control signal provided by nutrients level in plasma. When the nutrients are more, insulin secretion increases to facilitate their metabolism and use, and when nutrients are less, insulin secretion is less.

Plasma Glucose

Glucose is the **most important stimulator** of insulin secretion. With the rise in plasma glucose level, there is almost a linear rise in plasma insulin concentration in the range of 50–300 mg% of plasma glucose (Fig. 60.5). Insulin secretion is almost nil below 50 mg% and no extra secretion above 300 mg% of plasma glucose. The secretion of insulin in response to rise in plasma glucose concentration occurs in **two phases.**

First Phase Response

Immediately following the rise in plasma glucose (in response to i.v. glucose infusion), insulin secretion increases rapidly to reach a **peak within 1–2 minutes** and then **decreases to basal level in another 2 to 3 minutes** (Fig. 60.6).

1. This is the ***first and rapid phase*** of insulin secretion in response to sudden increase plasma glucose concentration.
2. The first phase response is due to **release of already synthesized and stored insulin** from granules of β cells.

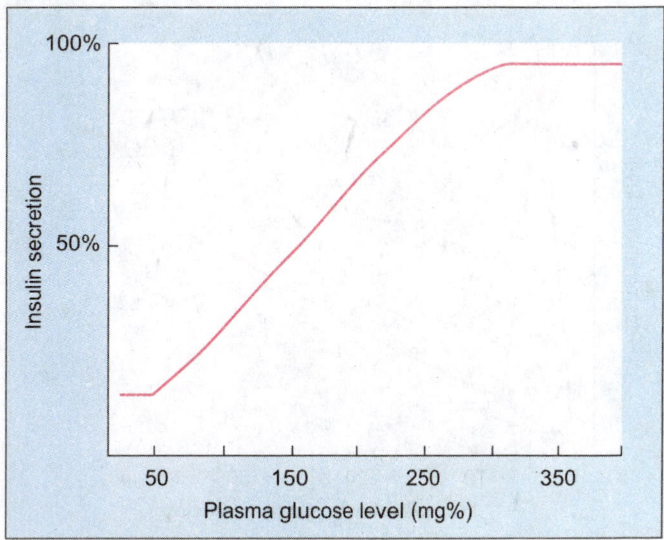

Fig. 60.5: Relationship between plasma glucose and the rate of insulin secretion. Note, a linear relation exists between 50 and 300 mg% of plasma glucose concentration.

Second Phase Response

In the next phase, the rise in plasma insulin concentration **occurs slowly** that reaches a **peak in about 60 minutes** and then **remains elevated for 3–5 hours**. The second and slow phase insulin response is due to **stimulation of insulin synthesis and secretion.**

Mechanism of Glucose-induced Insulin Secretion

Glucose enters β-cells of pancreas via GLUT 2:

1. In the β-cells, glucose is utilized by glycolytic enzymes (*see* below) to pyruvate that enters TCA cycle to **produce ATP**.
2. Increased intracellular ATP **inhibits ATP-sensitive K^+ channels**, which ***increases cytosolic K^+*** by decreasing K^+ efflux (Fig. 60.7).
3. This depolarizes the β cells, which in turn **opens the Ca^{++} channels.** ***Ca^{++} influx*** increases cytoplasmic Ca^{++} that facilitates **Ca^{++}-mediated exocytosis** of insulin granules.
4. Plasma K^+ is a natural regulator of insulin secretion. **Hypokalemia decreases insulin secretion** (Application Box 60.3).

Response depends on route of administration: The insulin response to plasma glucose depends on the **route of glucose administration:**

1. The response of insulin secretion **to orally administered glucose is more** than the glucose administered intravenously.
2. When given orally, glucose stimulates secretion of hormones from gastrointestinal tracts. Many **GI hormones** such as gastrin, secretin, enteroglucagon, GLP1, and GIP are insulinogenic.
3. They stimulate insulin secretion in addition to its secretion that occurs due to rise in plasma glucose.

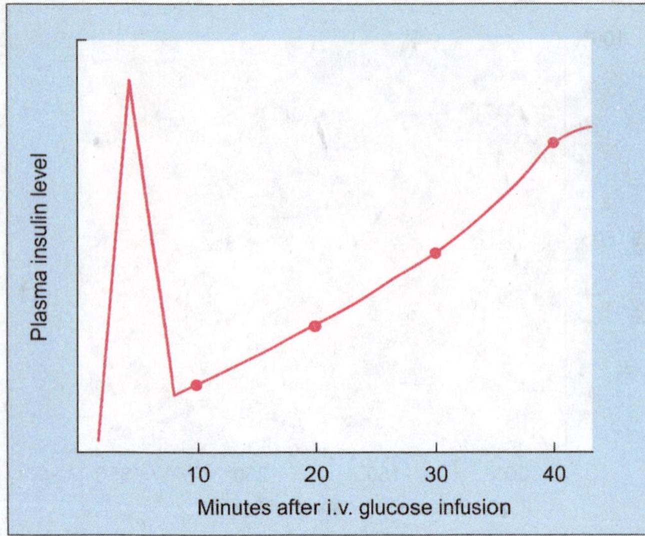

Fig. 60.6: Level of plasma insulin following i.v. infusion of plasma glucose. Note, a biphasic response is observed in which, there is a sharp increase in plasma glucose within five minutes of infusion, which falls immediately, and then a slow rise occurs in the plasma glucose.

Therefore, **insulin response is higher when glucose is given orally than intravenously**.

Application Box 60.3

Effects of hypokalemia: Hypokalemia decreases insulin secretion. Therefore, patients with hypokalemia as seen in primary hyperaldosteronism develop impaired glucose tolerance. Similarly, patients receiving thiazide diuretics develop glucose intolerance as thiazide causes hypokalemia and may also produce damage to pancreatic islets.

Other Stimuli

Insulin secretion is also stimulated by **products of protein digestion**. Arginine, leucine, lysine and alanine are potent stimulator of insulin release:

1. **Glucose and amino acids** facilitate the insulinogenic action of each other.
2. **Triglycerides and fatty acids** also stimulate insulin secretion.
3. **Ketoacids** are also insulinogenic.
4. **Cholinergic vagal stimulation** strongly increases insulin secretion, which provides the basis of secretion in the cephalic phase of digestion.
5. Catecholamines via β **receptors stimulate** and via α **receptors inhibit** insulin secretion.
6. **During exercise**, sympathetic stimulation causes α-adrenergic inhibition of insulin secretion that tries to prevent hypoglycemia during exercise.

Obesity significantly increases insulin secretion and activity of insulin receptors. However, down-regulation of receptor causes insulin resistance (*see* below). Therefore, obesity contributes to development of type II diabetes mellitus (NIDDM), which can be prevented by regular physical exercises and maintaining normal weight.

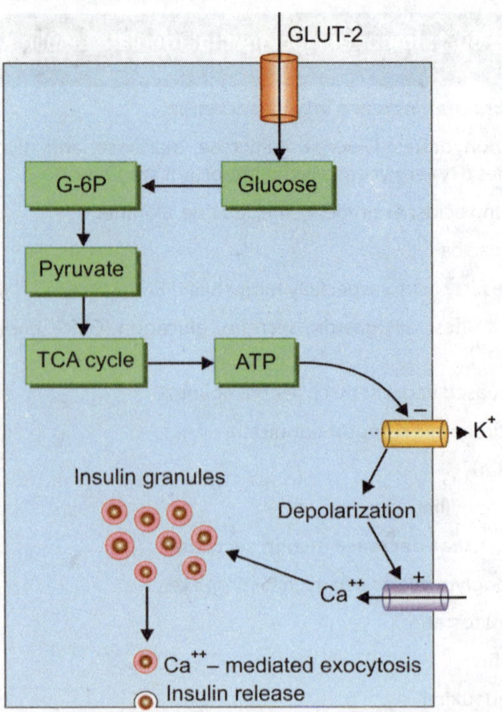

Fig. 60.7: A: Mechanism of insulin secretion from beta cells in response to glucose. Note, glucose enters the cell through GLUT 2 and is immediately converted to glucose-6-phosphate (G-6P) by glucokinase (GK), which undergo metabolism to generate ATP. ATP inhibits K^+ efflux (depicted by minus sign) that causes depolarization of the cell. Voltage gated Ca^{++} channels open (depicted by + sign) and calcium influx increases intracellular Ca^{++} concentration. Ca^{++}-mediated exocytosis of insulin granules leads to secretion of insulin.

Metabolism of Insulin

Insulin circulates freely (unbound to carriers) in the plasma, therefore, its **half-life is 5–8 minutes**. The metabolic clearance rate of insulin is about 800 mL/min.

1. The basal insulin release to the circulation is about 0.5 – 1 unit/h (20–40 µg/h).
2. Following food intake, release of insulin increases to about 10 times.
3. The total release of insulin into peripheral circulation in a day is about 30 units.
4. Insulin is **metabolized mainly in the liver and kidney**.

C peptide Activity

C peptide is secreted in equimolar concentration to that of insulin. However, the basal plasma concentration of C peptide is 5 times more than insulin (1 ng/mL). This is because the **metabolic clearance of C peptide is slower** than insulin. Therefore, the concentration of **C peptide in plasma is a better index of β cell activity than the insulin (Clinical Box 60.1).**

Clinical Box 60.1

C Peptide is a better marker β **of cell activity:** C peptide is secreted in equimolar concentration with insulin. But, as the metabolic clearance of C peptide is slower than insulin, its concentration in plasma provides better knowledge **of** β **cell activity than the insulin.** Therefore, **C peptide assessment** is done in good laboratories to assess β cell functional status.

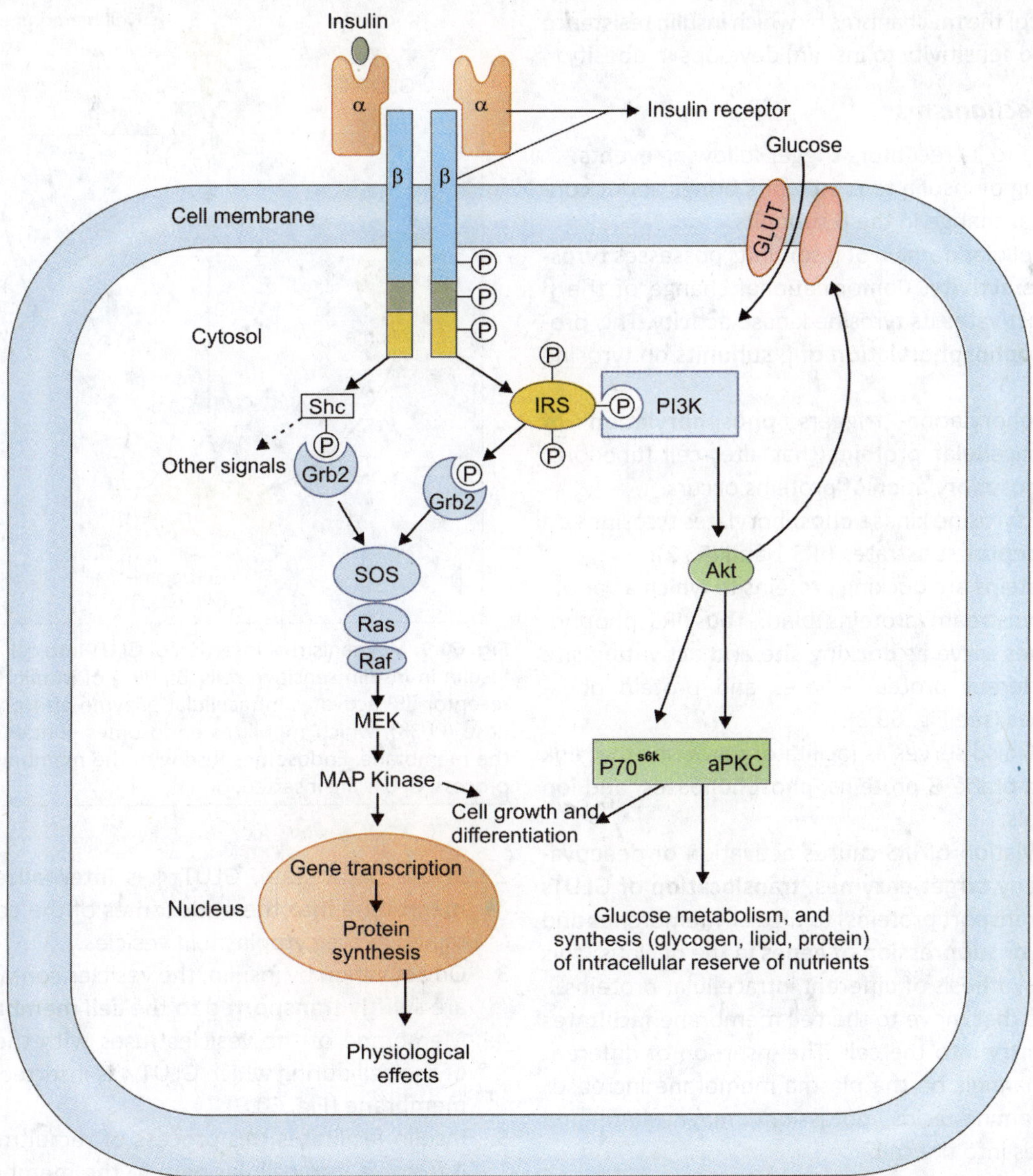

Fig. 60.8: A: Mechanism of action of insulin. Binding of insulin with α-subunit causes autophosphorylation of intracellular part of β-subunit of the insulin receptor. This causes phosphorylation of intracellular proteins like IRS and Shc that in turn activate phosphorylation cascades and generate other signals. Phosphorylation of Grb 2 proteins activates a series of signals that finally activate mitogen activated protein (MAP) kinase, which induces gene transcription. Phosphorylation of IRS activates intracellular enzymes that alter cell metabolisms, and transfers GLUT from cell to the cell surface. Increased GLUT on cell surface increases glucose uptake of the cell.

Mechanism of Action

Insulin acts on insulin receptors present on various cells. The major target tissues of insulin are liver, skeletal muscle and adipose tissues.

Insulin Receptor

Insulin receptor (IR) is a **glycoprotein tetramer** consisting of **two α and two β subunits**. The α subunits are present on the membrane extracellularly, whereas the β subunits traverse the membrane. Thus, β subunits have extracellular domain, membrane domain, and intracellular domain (Fig. 60.8). The α and β subunits are glycosylated. They are bound to each other by disulfide bridges. The insulin **receptor gene is located on the chromosome 19**, which belongs to the superfamily of genes that code for other growth factors also.

Down regulation of IR: Insulin binds with α subunits of the insulin receptor, which results in conformational change of the receptor. The **HR complex is then internalized** by endocytosis:

1. The hormone is degraded in the cytoplasm, whereas the ***receptor is either degraded, or stored or recycled back*** to the membrane.
2. Therefore, excess insulin activity **down-regulates the insulin receptors**.

3. This is one of the mechanisms by which **insulin resistance** (decreased sensitivity to insulin) develops in obesity.

Hormone Mechanisms

Insulin binding to its receptors trigger following events:

1. The binding of insulin to α subunits brings about conformational change in the β subunits.
2. The intracellular domain of β subunits possesses **tyrosine kinase activity**. Conformational change of the β subunits activates its tyrosine kinase activity. This produces **autophosphorylation of β subunits** on tyrosine residues.
3. Autophosphorylation triggers **phosphorylation of many intracellular proteins** that alter cell functions. Also, dephosphorylation of proteins occurs.
4. The active tyrosine kinase phosphorylates tyrosines on **insulin receptor substrates** (IRS 1 and IRS 2):
   - IRS proteins are docking proteins to which a variety of downstream proteins bind. Thus IRS phophotyrosines serve as **docking site and activating site** for different protein kinases and protein phosphatases (*see* Fig. 60.8).
   - The IRS also serves as facilitatory proteins that link to membrane G proteins, phospholipases, and ion channels.
5. Phosphorylation of IRS causes activation or deactivation of many **target enzymes**, **translocation of GLUTs** (glucose transport proteins) to the cell membranes and **induction or suppression of genes** in the nucleus. This results in synthesis of different intracellular proteins.
6. The GLUTs that move to the cell membrane **facilitates glucose entry** into the cell. The insertion of different protein channels on the plasma membrane increases entry of amino acids, potassium, magnesium, and phosphates into the cell.
7. Activation of mitogenic proteins **increases transcription of various factors** that are essential for stimulation of gene expression, especially concerned with cell growth.
8. IRS also activates **growth receptor binding protein-2** (GRB 2), which stimulates binding of GTP to **ras oncogene** (a proto-oncogene present in plasma membrane). This activates the enzyme glycogen synthase, a key enzyme that modulate the metabolic effects of insulin.

Action through GLUT 4

Binding of insulin with receptors rapidly mobilizes glucose transport into the muscle and adipose tissue cells. This process of glucose entry in to the cell is **increased by about 20 times** by the activation of a glucose carrier system in the plasma membrane:

1. Insulin **rapidly recruits the glucose transporter 4** (GLUT-4), which is specifically meant for insulin-stimulated glucose uptake in skeletal and cardiac muscle, adipose tissue and other tissues.

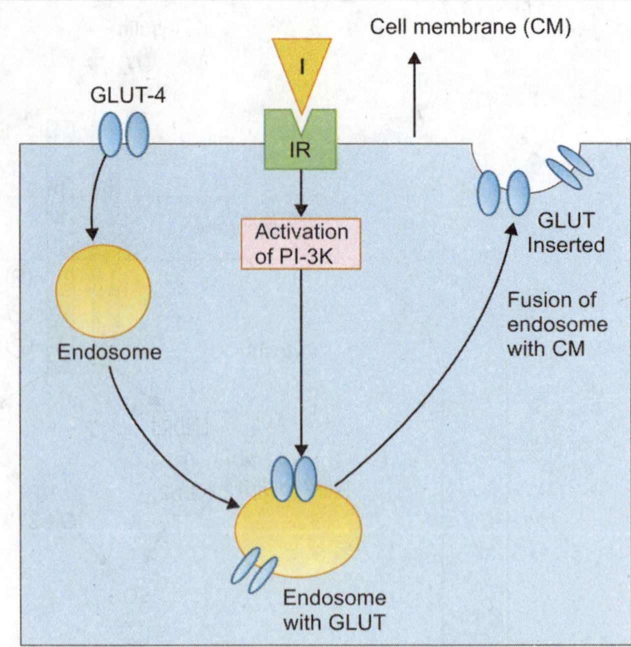

Fig. 60.9: Mechanism of insertion of GLUT into cell membrane by insulin in insulin sensitive cells. Binding of insulin (I) with insulin receptor (IR) activates intracellular enzyme phosphoinositol-3-kinase (PI-3K), which mobilizes endosomes containing GLUT-4 to the membrane. Endosomes fuse with the membrane, and in the process, GLUTs are inserted.

2. In the basal state, GLUT 4 is **internalized from cell membrane into the endosomes** of the cell and maintained in the cytoplasm in vesicles.
3. On activation by insulin, the vesicles containing GLUT 4 are **swiftly transported to the cell membrane**.
4. Membrane of the vesicles fuses with the membrane of the cell during which GLUT 4 is inserted into the cell membrane (Fig. 60.9).
5. Insulin facilitates this process of recruitment of GLUT 4 from its intracellular pool to the membrane pool by activating the enzyme **phosphoinositol-3-kinase**, and perhaps this is the **most important function of insulin** (Application Box 60.4).

Application Box 60.4

Regular exercise prevents diabetes: Exercise facilitates the recruitment of GLUT 4 from its cytoplasmic pool into the cell membrane in all tissues of the body, especially in the skeletal muscle and adipose tissues. Thus, exercise promotes glucose uptake by the cells and decreases blood glucose level. The increased glucose entry into the cell persists for many hours after exercise. Moreover, exercise-induced glucose entry **does not depend on insulin**. It is likely that **5´-AMP-activated kinase** facilitates GLUT 4 insertion from endosomes into membrane in exercise. Thus, to check the rise in plasma glucose, one should perform regular exercise. Also, regular exercise can cause prolonged increase in insulin sensitivity. However, **diabetic patients should be careful during exercise**. As acute exercise significantly decreases blood glucose level by facilitating glucose uptake by skeletal muscles, and during exercise absorption of injected insulin is more rapid, **hypoglycemia may be precipitated** in diabetic patients during exercise. Therefore, diabetic patients should decrease their insulin dose when they exercise or they should take extra calorie just prior to exercise.

Table 60.2: Types of glucose transporters and their functions.

Types of GLUT	Functions
A. Secondary active transport (Na^+–Glucose cotransport)	
SGLT 1	Increases absorption of glucose in the intestine and kidney tubules
SGLT 2	Increases reabsorption of glucose in the kidney tubules
B. Facilitated diffusion via GLUTs (Na^+ independent)	
GLUT 1	Basal glucose uptake in the placenta, brain, RBC, colon, kidney and other organs
GLUT 2	Acts as a glucose sensor in the β cells of pancreas
GLUT 3	Same as GLUT 1, i.e., basal glucose uptake in the placenta, brain, kidney and in other tissues
GLUT 4	Causes ***insulin stimulated glucose uptake*** in the skeletal and cardiac muscle, adipose tissue, and other tissues
GLUT 5	Facilitates transport of fructose in the jejunum and into the sperm
GLUT 6	Acts as a pseudogene
GLUT 7	Increases transport of glucose 6-phosphate into the endoplasmic reticulum in hepatic and other tissues

6. Once insulin action is over, again they are internalized into the vesicles. In liver, insulin facilitates glucose uptake by activating the enzyme glukokinase not by GLUT 4.

Glucose Transporters

Glucose enters the cell by means of facilitated diffusion or by secondary active transport with sodium in intestine and kidney. In skeletal and cardiac muscle, adipose tissue and other tissues, entry of glucose into the cell is facilitated by insulin by **increasing the number of glucose transporters** (GLUTs) in the cell membrane. GLUTs **promote the facilitated diffusion of glucose** into the cell:

1. Glucose transporters are different from sodium dependent glucose transporters (SGLT 1 and SGLT 2) that mediate secondary active transport of glucose in the kidney and GIT.
2. GLUTs are expressed in different tissues. GLUTs are membrane proteins that **span membrane 12 times**.
3. About **14 different types** of glucose transporters have been described (GLUT 1 – GLUT 14). However, the first 7 types have been extensively studied.
4. **GLUT 1 and GLUT 3** are meant for ***basal glucose uptake*** by the cells.
5. **GLUT 4** is primarily meant for ***insulin stimulated glucose uptake*** especially in the skeletal and cardiac muscle and adipose tissues (Table 60.2).
6. **GLUT 2** acts as the **β cell glucose sensor**.
7. **GLUT 5** facilitates ***fructose transport*** in jejunum and sperm.
8. **GLUT 7** acts as ***glucose-6-phosphate transporter*** in the endoplasmic reticulum of liver and other tissues.
9. GLUT 6 is a pseudogene.

Physiological Actions of Insulin

Insulin is secreted in fed state, i.e. at the time of nutrient abundance. Therefore, insulin is known as the **hormone of abundance**. Insulin **facilitates storage of nutrients** when nutrients are present in excess of the energy need. It also ***suppresses mobilization of endogenous substrates***. The stored nutrients are made available at the time of need like exercise, fasting, etc. Insulin produces its target effects by acting mainly on the **liver, adipose tissue, and skeletal muscle**.

On Carbohydrate Metabolism

Insulin increases glucose entry into the cell, stimulates its oxidation and promotes also its storage. At the same time insulin inhibits glucose production. Therefore, the primary function of insulin is to **lower the plasma glucose concentration**. It is the ***only hormone that decreases plasma glucose level*** (decreases basal glucose level and also prevents rise in plasma glucose following feeding). Insulin is the **only effective anti-diabetogenic hormone**. The antidiabetogenic functions of insulin are mediated by its action on liver, adipose tissue and muscle.

In general, insulin **increases glucose entry** into cells of almost all tissues of the body except brain (excluding ventromedial hypothalamus), RBCs, epithelium of GI tract, and renal tubules.

In Liver

In liver, insulin promotes glucose storage and prevents its production by following mechanisms (Flowchart 60.1):

1. Insulin **facilitates glucose entry** into the hepatic cell by inducing the action of the enzyme ***glucokinase***. Glucokinase catalyzes phosphorylation of glucose to glucose-6-phosphate. Thus, by facilitating glucose entry into the cells and also simultaneously **converting glucose into glucose-6 phosphates**, insulin keeps cytoplasmic glucose concentration at lower level. Therefore, facilitated diffusion of glucose into the cell continues.
2. It **stimulates glycolysis** by activating the enzymes ***phosphofructokinase*** and ***pyruvate kinase***. These actions convert glucose into pyruvic and lactic acids. **Pyruvate and lactate are also oxidized** by insulin as it stimulates *pyruvate dehydrogenase* activity. Thus, insulin decreases the cellular concentration of glucose and consequently helps in its facilitated diffusion into the cell.
3. It **promotes glycogen synthesis** in liver. In the liver cells, it ***activates the enzyme glycogen synthase complex*** that promotes formation of glycogen. Thus, it promotes storage of glucose in the form of hepatic glycogen.
4. It **inhibits hepatic glycogenolysis**, and therefore it decreases hepatic glucose output. Insulin achieves it by inhibiting the activity of the enzymes *glycogen phosphorylase* and *glucose-6-phosphatase*.

Flowchart 60.1: Summary of insulin actions on carbohydrate metabolism.

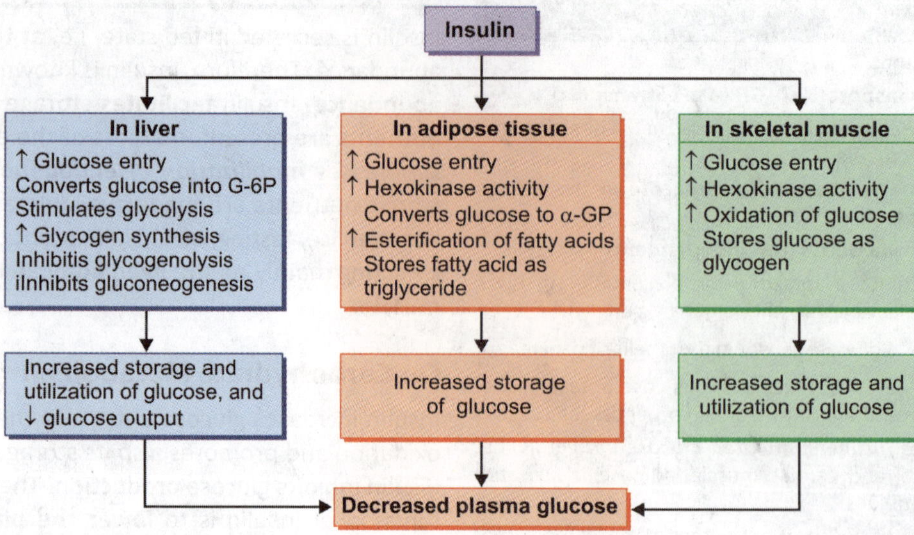

(G-6P: Glucose-6-phosphate; α-GP: α-glycerophosphate).

5. It also **inhibits gluconeogenesis**. This is achieved by two mechanisms: (i) insulin inhibits gluconeogenic enzymes (*pyruvate carboxylase, phosphoenolpyruvate carboxykinase, and fructose-1, 6-diphosphatase*), and (ii) insulin decreases hepatic uptake of gluconeogenic amino acids.

In Adipose Tissue

Insulin **stimulates entry of glucose** into the adipose tissue cells by ***activating GLUT 4 and hexokinase activity***:

1. In fat cells, glucose is then **converted into α-glycerophosphate** (α-GP). The α-GP is used for the **esterification of fatty acids**.
2. It also promotes storage of fatty acids as triglycerides.

In Skeletal Muscle

Insulin **facilitates transport of glucose** into the muscle cells by ***activating GLUT 4 and hexokinase activity***:

1. In muscle cell, **glucose is oxidized** by activation of the enzyme ***pyruvate dehydrogenase***.
2. Glucose is also **stored as muscle glycogen**, which is stimulated by insulin.

On Fat Metabolism

Actions of insulin on fat metabolism are as profound as its influences on carbohydrate metabolism. Insulin **increases storage of fat** and inhibits mobilization and oxidation of fatty acids from fat depots. It decreases the level of free fatty acids and ketoacids in the plasma. Insulin is the **only anti-ketogenic hormone** in the body. The functions of insulin on fat metabolism are achieved by its actions on adipose tissue and liver.

In Adipose Tissue

Insulin **promotes storage of fat** in the adipose tissues in various ways:

1. **By inhibiting lipolysis:** It **inhibits the activity of hormone sensitive lipase** (HSL) in adipose tissues:
   - HSL causes breakdown of triglycerides into free-fatty acids (FFA) and glycerol. Thus, insulin inhibits lipolysis and **decreases release of stored FFA.**
   - Decreased plasma FFA decreases the formation of ketoacids. Insulin also facilitates the use of ketoacids by peripheral tissues. Thus, insulin **profoundly decreases ketoacid level** in the plasma (*see* below).
2. **By promoting lipogenesis:** Lipids absorbed from intestine circulate in plasma in the form of triglycerides. Triglycerides cannot enter adipose tissue as such. They must be split by lipoprotein lipase, which is present in the vascular endothelium to FFA and glycerol. Then, FFA can enter adipose tissue and form TG there:
   - Insulin **promotes the enzyme lipoprotein lipase**, therefore makes FFA available from blood stream for formation of triglyceride in the adipose tissue cell (Fig. 60.10).
   - FFA is immediately **esterified to α-glycerophosphate** in adipose tissue, which is also induced by insulin.

In Liver

Insulin is **anti-ketogenic and lipogenic** in liver:

1. The anti-ketogenic function of insulin is achieved by *its* **stimulation of malonyl-CoA formation.** Normally, acetyl-CoA is converted to malonyl-CoA by the enzyme *acetyl-CoA carboxylase*. Insulin stimulates the activity of acetyl-CoA carboxylase and thus increases malonyl-CoA formation. Malonyl-CoA inhibits the enzyme *carnitine-acyl transferase* (CAT). CAT transfers FFA from cytoplasm into mitochondria for oxidation and then conversion into ketoacids. Thus, insulin by inhibiting CAT through malonyl-CoA prevents ketoacid formation (Fig. 60.11).

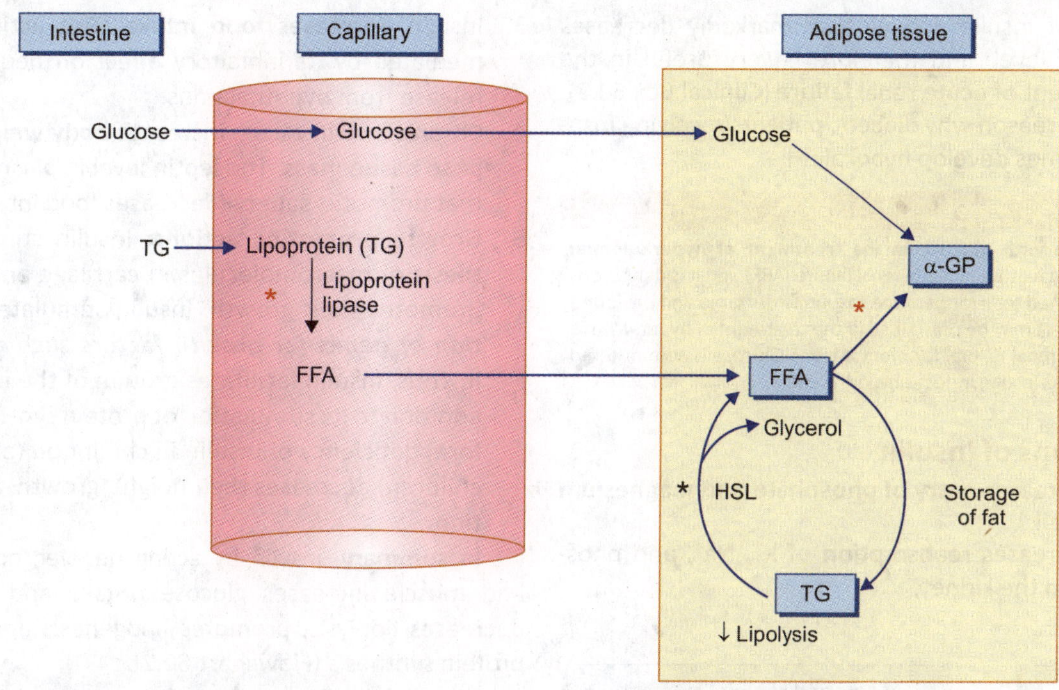

Fig. 60.10: Actions of insulin on adipose tissue. Note, insulin activates lipoprotein lipase in capillary and therefore, splits triglyceride into free fatty acid (FFA) and glycerol. FFA enters adipose tissue and form TG there. In adipose tissue, insulin inhibits hormone-sensitive lipase (HSL) and therefore, prevents breakdown of TG into FFA and glycerol. Thus, insulin prevents lipolysis and promote storage of fat. Insulin also promotes formation of α-glycerophosphate (-GP). (Red star: Stimulation by insulin; Black star: Inhibition by insulin).

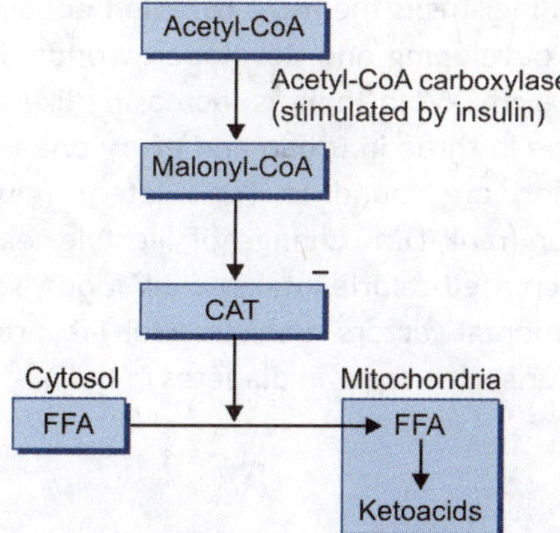

Fig. 60.11: Inhibition of ketoacid formation by insulin. Normally, carnitine acyl transferase (CAT) transfers FFA from cytoplasm to mitochondria, where FFA is converted to ketoacids. Insulin inhibits CAT (as depicted by minus sign) by promoting formation of malonyl CoA. Thus, insulin inhibits ketogenesis.

2. Fatty acid is also synthesized from glucose by insulin. Insulin achieves this by **three mechanisms**:
   i. The rate-limiting step in fatty acids synthesis is the *conversion of acetyl-CoA to malonyl-CoA* by the action of *acetyl-CoA carboxylase,* which is activated by insulin. ***Malonyl-CoA is used as substrate for FFA synthesis***.
   ii. Insulin also induces *fatty acids synthase*, the final step in fatty acid synthesis.
   iii. Insulin **activates the HMP shunt** by activating the enzyme *glucose-6-phosphate dehydrogenase*. HMP shunt increases the supply of reduced triphosphopyridine nucleotide, which is required for fatty acid synthesis. Thus, from circulation, FFA is shunted away from oxidation and ketogenesis to be stored in the liver.
3. Insulin facilitates **synthesis of cholesterol** in the liver from acetyl-CoA by activating the enzyme *HMG-CoA reductase*, the rate-limiting step in the process.

On Protein Metabolism

Insulin is an **anabolic hormone**. It **facilitates protein synthesis** in the muscles and liver by following mechanisms:

1. It **facilitates amino acid entry** into the muscle cells. Therefore, it decreases plasma amino acid concentration. Thus, supply of amino acids for gluconeogenesis is also decreased.
2. It promotes **protein synthesis** in ribosomes. This is achieved by *induction of gene transcription* for various proteins by insulin (Fig. 60.12).
3. Insulin also *decreases degradation of RNA*.
4. Insulin **inhibits proteolysis** by decreasing lysosomal activity. Thus, it decreases release of amino acid from muscle and inhibits their oxidation.

On Plasma K^+ Concentration

Insulin facilitates the **rapid entry of K^+ into the cell** by stimulating Na^+–K^+ ATPase activity in the membrane. Thus, it **decreases plasma K^+ level**:

1. Insulin is considered as a **physiological regulator of plasma K^+ concentration**.

2. Infusion of insulin and glucose markedly decreases plasma K^+ level; and therefore is very useful in the management of **acute renal failure** (Clinical Box 60.2).
3. This is the reason why diabetic patients receiving insulin sometimes develop hypokalemia.

Clinical Box 60.2

Insulin is given with glucose in the treatment of hyperkalemia: Hyperkalemia is a feature of acute renal failure (ARF) and it is dangerous if remains untreated for a longer time. Insulin for its rapid and profound hypokalemic effect may be prescribed in the treatment of hyperkalemia as seen in acute renal failure, for prompt relief. Glucose is administered simultaneously, as insulin induces hypoglycemia.

Other Actions of Insulin

1. Insulin increases **entry of phosphate and magnesium into the cell**.
2. It also **increases reabsorption of K^+, Na^+,** and phosphate from the kidney.

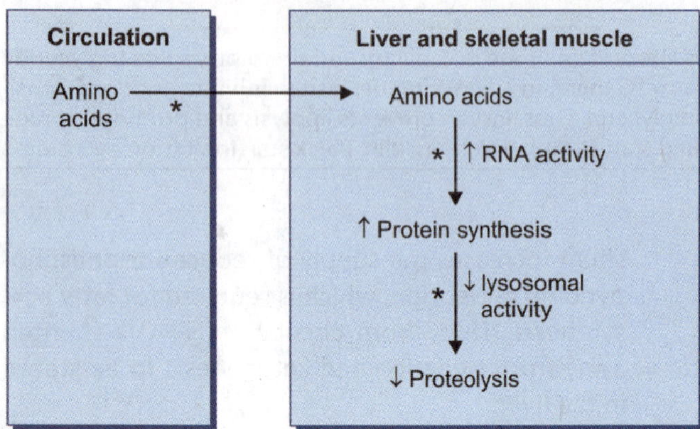

Fig. 60.12: Effects of insulin on protein metabolism. Note, insulin promotes transfer of amino acids into the cells and increases protein synthesis. Insulin also inhibits proteolysis. Star indicates site of action of insulin.

3. Insulin **decreases food intake**. This action is partly mediated by its inhibitory effect on neuropeptide Y release from hypothalamus.
4. Chronic insulin excess **increases body weight and adipose tissue mass**. The leptin level in plasma increases that promotes satiety (decreases food intake).
5. **Growth promoting actions:** Insulin stimulates synthesis of macromolecules in cartilage and bone that promotes their growth. Insulin stimulates ***transcription of genes for growth factors*** such as IGF-I and II. Thus, insulin facilitates growth of the individual, in addition to its stimulation of protein synthesis. Therefore, deficiency of insulin in childhood (as in diabetic children) decreases their height, growth, and maturation.

In summary, insulin by acting on liver, adipose tissue and muscle increases glucose uptake and its storage, decreases lipolysis, promotes lipogenesis and stimulates protein synthesis (Flowchart 60.2).

Applied Physiology

Insulin Deficiency (Diabetes Mellitus)

Deficiency of insulin results in diabetes mellitus (DM). Diabetes mellitus is the **most common endocrine disorder** in both developing and developed worlds. Recently, the incidence of DM in India is increasing like an epidemic. Every one in three in urban and every one in five in rural population are found to have latent (glucose intolerance) or frank DM. Change of lifestyle, easy access to food (increased calorie intake), junk foods, sedentary life, environmental factors and stressful life are among the causes for such a spurt in diabetes in India.

Flowchart 60.2: Summary of insulin actions.

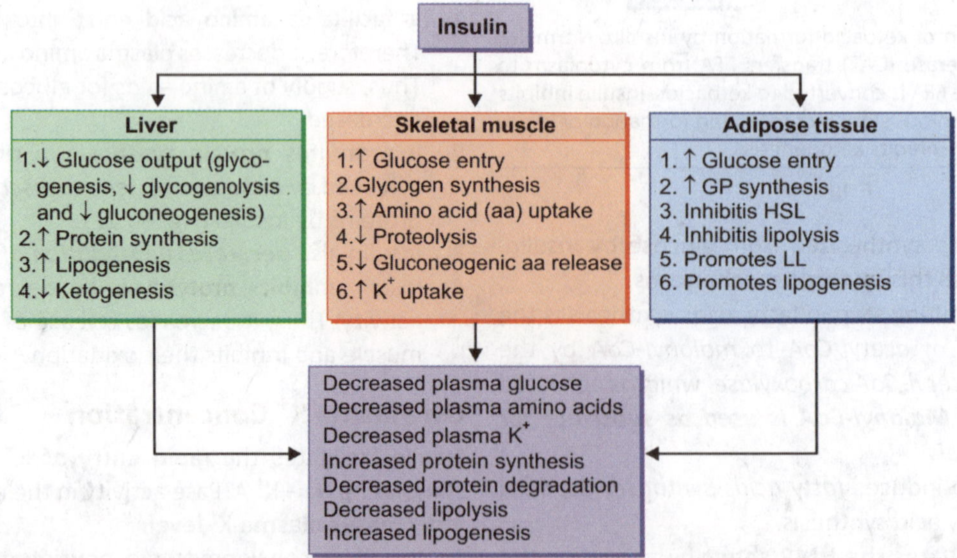

(GP: Glycerophosphate; HSL: Hormone sensitive lipase; LL: Lipoprotein lipase).

Table 60.3: Etiological classification of diabetes.

I. Type 1 diabetes
- Immune mediated
- Idiopathic

II. Type 2 diabetes
- Insulin resistance
- Pancreatic β cell failure

III. Other specific types of diabetes
1. Genetics defects of β cell function (MODY)
2. Genetics defects of insulin action
3. Pancreatic diseases (pancreatits, panceatectomy cystic fibrosis, hemochromatosis, neoplasia)
4. Excess endogenous production insulin antagonists, for example GH (acromegaly), cortisol (Cushing syndrome), NE (pheochromocytoma), thyroxine (thyrotoxicosis), glucagon (glucagonoma), etc
5. Drug-induced (corticosteroids, thiazide diuretics phenytoin)
6. Viral infections (congenital rubella, mumps, etc.)
7. Genetic syndromes (Turner, Klinefelter, Down, etc.)

IV. Gestational diabetes

Scientist contributed

Oscar Minkowski (1858–1931) was the first to demonstrate the pituitary enlargement in acromegaly. Along with Joseph von Mering, he demonstrated the role of pancreas in sugar metabolism and diabetes. The experiment famously showed ***pancreatic diabetes following pancreatectomy*** in dogs. For his exceptional contribution to diabetes research, The European Association for the Study of Diabetes has, since 1966, in his name is awarding outstanding contributions to the advancement of knowledge in the field of diabetes mellitus.

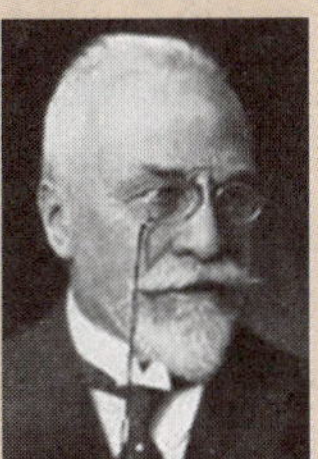

Oscar Minkowski (1858–1931)

Causes of DM

In humans, diabetes occurs usually due to **destruction of β cells of pancreas** or due to **decreased sensitivity of insulin receptors** to insulin. In animal models, diabetes is produced experimentally by administration of alloxan or streptozotocin (**experimental diabetes**).

A state of starvation in the midst of plenty: In untreated diabetes, plasma glucose concentration is always high. In spite of hyperglycemia, the ***tissue cannot utilize glucose*** either due to insulin deficiency or due to insulin resistance. In this condition, cells cannot utilize glucose though they are surrounded by a high concentration of glucose. Therefore, diabetes is called a disease of "**starvation in the midst of plenty**".

Insulin only matters: Though there are few more chemicals (**insulin like substances**) in the body having insulin activity, they are *not adequate to fulfill metabolic actions of insulin* in states of insulin deficiency. These substances are ***proinsulin and somatomedins*** (IGF I and IGF II). These chemicals have only about 10% of insulin activity. Therefore, insulin deficiency leads to DM.

Type of DM: Etiologically diabetes has been traditionally classified into two:

1. **Type I DM** or insulin-dependent DM (IDDM) as it is associated with profound insulin deficiency and requires insulin replacement therapy.
2. **Type II DM** or non-insulin-dependent DM (NIDDM) as it is associated with normal insulin level in plasma and patient is usually treated without insulin replacement therapy.

However, recently it has been observed that more than 25% of type 2 DM **ultimately develop insulin deficiency** requiring insulin replacement therapy. Therefore, the classification of IDDM and NIDDM has become obsolete. Etiological classification of diabetes is depicted in Table 60.3.

Major Types of DM

Diabetes is primarily classified into two types: type-1 and type-2.

Type-1 Diabetes Mellitus

Type 1 DM is characterized by insulin deficiency, which is usually caused by selective **autoimmune destruction of β-cells** of pancreas. Therefore, the disease has traditionally been called ***insulin dependant diabetes mellitus*** (IDDM):

1. The disease starts with insulitis. Many patients demonstrate **antibodies against β-cell surface antigens**.
2. If one of the twins develops the disease the other twin has more chance of developing the disease than people in the general population (the concordance rate is < 50%).
3. The disease usually **starts early in childhood**, and **ketoacidosis is common** (Table 60.4).
4. The disease is treated by insulin replacement.
5. Sometimes it occurs due to **mutation of proinsulin gene** that decreases insulin synthesis.

Type-2 Diabetes Mellitus

Type 2 DM is characterized by impaired ability of the target cells to respond to insulin. This is usually caused by **insulin receptor resistance**. The insulin secretion may be normal or even more. Therefore, the disease has traditionally been called ***non-insulin dependant diabetes mellitus*** (NIDDM):

1. The chance of identical twin developing the disease (concordance rate) is 100%.
2. The disease **usually starts late**, in third or fourth decade of life.
3. The patients are **usually overweight** and sedentary in their habit.
4. Feeding habit and environment also contribute.
5. **Chronic stress** is usually associated with it.
6. Usual complication is hyperosmolal coma.
7. Oral antidiabetic drugs are usually preferred for treatment. However, insulin may also be prescribed.

Table: 60.4: Major differences between Type 1 and Type 2 diabetes mellitus.

	Type I	Type II
1. Age of onset	Before the age of 40 (Juvenile onset diabetes)	After the age of 40 (Maturity onset diabetes)
2. Body fat mass	Not obese	Obese
3. Incidence	10% of the total diabetes	90% of the total diabetes
4. Genetic susceptibility	Concordance rate is < 50%	Concordance rate is > 50%
5. Incidence of ketoacidosis	High	Low
6. B cell mass of pancreas	B cells destroyed	B cells morphology is normal
7. Nature of onset	Rapid	Gradual
8. Usual complication	Ketoacidotic coma	Hyperosmolal coma

Mechanism of insulin resistance: The exact mechanism of insulin resistance in type II DM is not known. However, insulin resistance has been highly correlated with body weight gain and few other factors. The ***following factors contribute to insulin resistance***:

1. **Obesity:** In obesity, insulin fails to transport glucose into the tissues. Obesity eventually leads to hyperinsulinemia, hyperlipidemia and accelerated atherosclerosis that are part of metabolic syndrome (Clinical Box 60.3). These are combinely called as **metabolic syndrome** of obesity. With reduction in body weight, insulin resistance and dyslipidemia decrease.
2. **Adipokines:** The chemical signals originating from adipose tissue are recently proposed to be contributing factors for insulin resistance. Fat cells secrete a group of hormones called ***adipokines*** that influence insulin resistance. The known adipokines are:
   - Leptin
   - Adiponectin
   - Resistin
   - Tumor necrosis factor (TNF α) Usually, leptin and adiponectin decrease, and resistin and TNF α increase insulin resistance. ***Resistin and TNF α are increased significantly*** in NIDDM.
3. **Decreased second messengers:** Knockout of intracellular second messengers that are usually formed following autophosphorylation of tyrosine kinase has been recently reported to be the major factor in insulin resistance.

Clinical Box 60.3

Metabolic syndrome: A number of metabolic abnormalities are common in type 2 DM, especially dyslipidemia and hypertension. The constellation of abnormalities classified as metabolic syndrome include: hyperinsulinemia/insulin resistance, type II DM or impaired glucose tolerance, low HDL cholesterol and elevated triglyceride, central obesity and hypertension. These patients invariably have microalbuminuria, increased fibrinogen, increased plasminogen activator inhibitor 1, elevated plasma uric acid and increased sympathetic activity. Metabolic syndrome is also called **Raven syndrome**, and **Syndrome X**, and is strongly associated with macrovascular disease such as coronary artery and cerebral artery disease. The mortality rate is high in metabolic syndrome.

4. **Decreased GLUT:** Knock out of glucose transporters in skeletal muscles and adipose tissue has been suggested as a contributing factors.
5. **Free fatty acids:** Increased FFA contributes to insulin resistance.

Secondary Diabetes Mellitus

Diabetes also occurs due to the **diseases of pancreas** like pancreatitis, or following pancreatectomy. Diabetes can also occur in **Cushing's syndrome** (cortisol increases plasma glucose) and **acromegaly** (growth hormone increases plasma glucose). These forms of diabetes are included under the category of *secondary diabetes mellitus*. This category constitutes about 5% of the total diabetes.

Maturity Onset Diabetes of the Young (MODY)

MODY constitutes about 5% of all cases of diabetes. This is a **form of Type II** (maturity-onset) DM in younger individuals:

1. Six types of MODY have recently been described, **MODY 1 to MODY 6.** Commonest among them is **MODY 3** that accounts for 20–75% of all MODYs.
2. It occurs due to **mutation of HNF1-α gene** (gene for hepatic nuclear factor 1 alpha).
3. Patients with MODY 3 are mostly in their adolescence, diabetic complications are frequent, but they have a greater hypoglycemic response to sulphonylureas than the patients with type II DM.
4. MODY 2 is the next common (10–65%) group that occurs due to mutation of glukokinase gene. They present with mild hyperglycemia from birth, but they are stable and managed by diet alone. Other forms of MODYs are rare.

Gestational DM

This refers to the **hyperglycemia occurring for the first time during pregnancy**. 80% of women with gestational diabetes develop diabetes permanently.

Features of DM

Diabetes mellitus is characterized by **polyphagia, polyuria, polydipsia, weight loss in spite of increased food intake,**

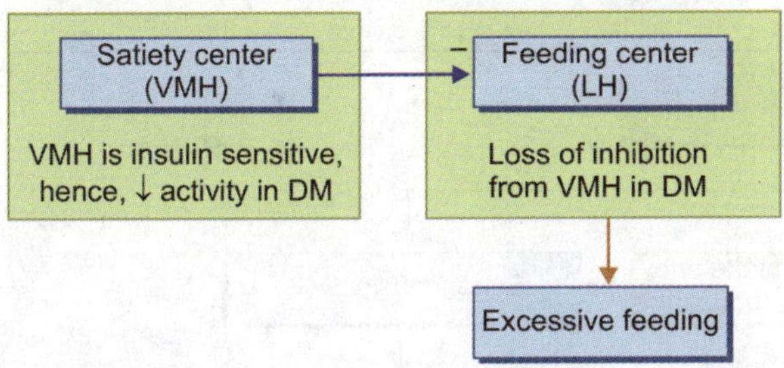

Fig. 60.13: Mechanism of polyphagia in diabetes. Normally, VMH inhibits LH (depicted by minus sign). In diabetes, loss of inhibitory control of VMH on LH leads to excessive feeding. (VMH: Ventromedial hypothalamus; LH: Lateral hypothalamus; DM: Diabetes mellitus).

hyperglycemia, and glycosuria. If not treated, the disease leads to ketosis, acidosis, and coma. In chronic cases, there may be diabetic retinopathy, neuropathy and nephropathy.

Polyphagia

Glucose entry into cells of brain except in ventromedial hypothalamus (VMH) is independent of insulin. Thus, VMH depends on insulin for its glucose uptake:

1. VMH is the *satiety center* that normally inhibits the lateral hypothalamus (LH), the *feeding center*.
2. As VMH depends on insulin for glucose uptake and utilization, **insulin deficiency in diabetes decreases the activity of VMH**.
3. Decreased VMH activity **removes its inhibitory effect on LH** (Fig. 60.13).
4. Therefore, LH activity increases due to **disinhibition** (abolition of inhibition from VMH).
5. **Facilitation of feeding center** (increased LH activity) increases feeding (polyphagia).

Polyuria

In diabetes, when plasma glucose concentration increases **above renal threshold** (above 180 mg%), glucose appears in urine. Filtration of more glucose increases its tubular load. Increased concentration of glucose in the tubular fluid causes **osmotic diuresis** that result in polyuria.

Polydipsia

In diabetes, because of polyuria water is lost in excess from the body. This decreases plasma and ECF volumes. **Dehydration stimulates thirst center** that causes polydipsia.

Weight Loss

In diabetes, food intake is more due to stimulation of feeding center. However, in spite of more food intake, **glucose is not utilized by the cells** due to deficiency of insulin. Insulin is essential for entry and utilization of glucose in the tissue. Insulin also facilitates growth. Therefore, insulin deficiency causes weight loss and growth retardation.

Hyperglycemia and Glycosuria

Insulin is the only hormone that decreases plasma glucose concentration. Therefore, deficiency of insulin results in hyperglycemia. When plasma glucose concentration exceeds renal threshold (180 mg%) glucose appears in urine (glycosuria).

Ketosis

Insulin **prevents lipolysis**, and therefore, decreases release of free fatty acids into the circulation. Insulin also facilitates **utilization of ketone bodies** (acetoacetate, acetone, and β-hydroxybutyrate) by the tissue. Therefore, ketosis occurs in insulin deficiency diabetes (IDDM). Presence of **excess acetyl-CoA** also facilitates conversion of acetoacetyl-CoA to acetoacetate in the liver.

Acidosis

The **hydrogen ions liberated from ketone bodies** (acetoacetate and β-hydroxybutyrate) are usually buffered:

1. When ketosis becomes severe, the **buffering capacity decreases**. This causes plasma acidic.
2. Decreased pH of plasma stimulates respiration (**Kussmaul breathing**).
3. Urine also becomes highly acidic.
4. Normally, insulin increases Na^+, K^+ and phosphate reabsorption from kidney. Therefore, in diabetes, there is **loss of electrolyte and water**.
5. This causes **dehydration, hypovolemia, and hypotension**.
6. Diabetic acidosis is a **medical emergency** that requires immediate and appropriate replacement of electrolyte and fluid.

Coma

Coma in diabetes is of two types: **Acidotic coma** (due to acidosis) and **hyperosmolar coma** (due to hyperosmolality of plasma):

1. **In acidosis**, loss of water and electrolyte ***causes dehydration*** that results in coma (Flowchart 60.3). Accumulation of lactate (lactic acidosis) also causes coma.
2. **Increased glucose concentration** in plasma to a very high level increases its osmolality to the extent that it causes ***dehydration of brain cells*** that results in coma without affecting pH.

Diagnosis

Diagnosis of diabetes is done by **demonstrating persistent hyperglycemia** and glycosuria. Estimation of fasting and post-prandial blood glucose is performed to demonstrate hyperglycemia, and estimation of glucose in urine is carried out to demonstrate glycosuria. This is done by GTT, estimation of fasting blood glucose (FBG), and estimation of glycated hemoglobin (HbA1c).

GTT: In the past, **glucose tolerance test** was usually performed for the diagnosis of diabetes:

1. The **oral GTT** was preferred to intravenous GTT. The ***GTT curve in diabetes*** typically exhibits persistent rise in blood glucose above the normal value (Fig. 60.14).
2. Abnormal GTT also occurs in few other conditions like renal disease, intestinal problems, etc.

FBG: Recently, **estimation of fasting blood glucose** (FBG) has been recommended to be the main criterion to diagnose DM. FBS more than 126 mg% in more than

Flowchart 60.3: Mechanism of development of coma in diabetes mellitus.

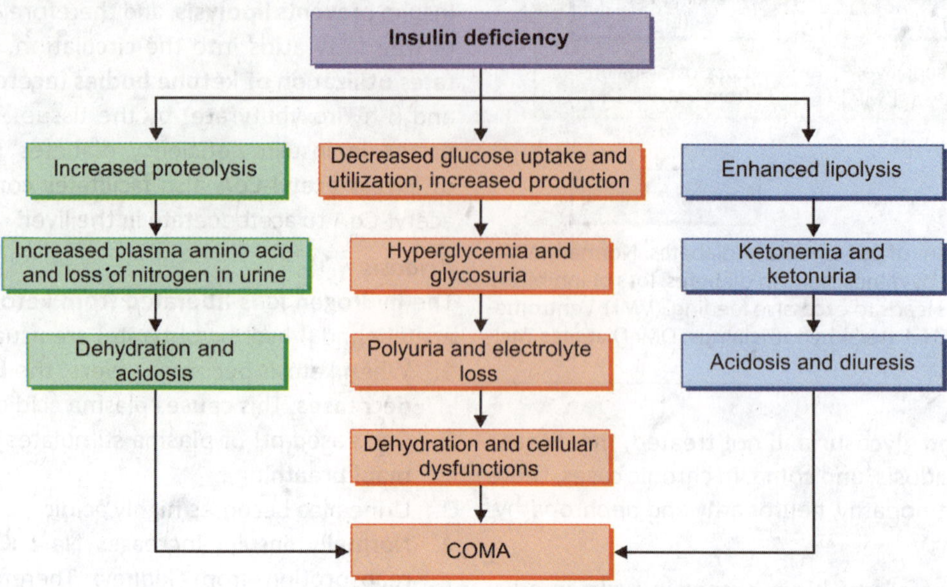

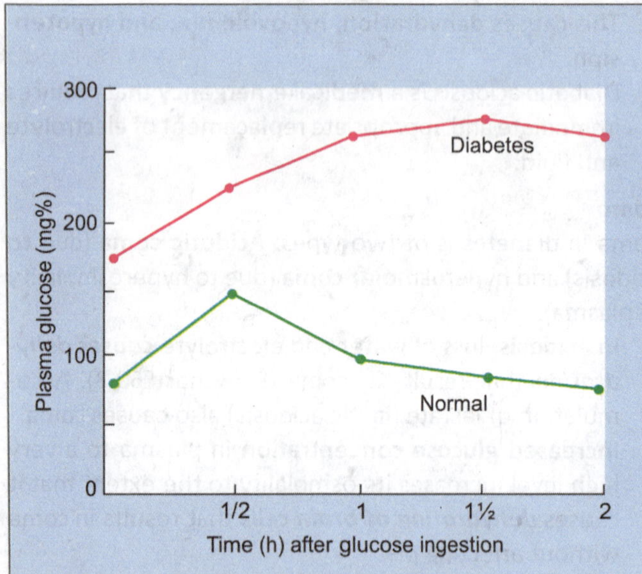

Fig. 60.14: Plasma glucose response to oral glucose tolerance test (GTT). Note, plasma glucose level remains always above the normal GTT value in diabetic patients and does not come into the normal range of plasma glucose (60 to 90 mg%).

two occasions confirms DM. The blood glucose levels are classified into 3 types (Table 60.5).

HbA1c: This is the **glycated hemoglobin**. HbA1c indicates the state of ***persistent hyperglycemia*** at least more than three months. The normal range is 4 to 5.6%. The values between 5.7 and 6.4% indicate prediabetes, and 6.5% or above indicates diabetes.

Treatment

Diabetes is usually treated by insulin and oral hypoglycemic agents. However, change in life style improves the condition to a greater extent as recently diabetes has been found to be closely associated with chronic stress.

Table 60.5: Categories of glucose tolerance based on the levels of fasting and post-prandial blood glucose (mg%), and HbA1c.

	Fasting blood glucose	Post-prandial blood glucose	HbA1c
Normal blood glucose	60–99	< 140	4 to 5.6%
Impaired fasting glucose or Impaired glucose tolerance (Prediabetes)	100–125	140 – 199	5.7 to 6.4%
Diabetes	126 or more	200 or more	6.5% or high

Insulin Therapy

Insulin replacement is the cornerstone of **treatment of type 1 DM**. The maximum decline in plasma glucose occurs following 30 minutes after IV injection of crystalline insulin. Insulin is also injected subcutaneously, but decrease in plasma glucose concentration occurs in 2–3 hours.

Different types of insulin preparations are commercially available. Generally, **insulin preparations** are divided into three categories depending on their duration of action:

1. Rapid acting insulin,
2. Intermediate acting insulin, and
3. Long acting insulin.

Pork insulin differs from human insulin only by one amino acid and therefore, has low antigenicity. Therefore, pork insulin is preferred to beef and other insulins. However, **human insulin** is produced nowadays from bacteria by recombinant DNA technology.

Oral Hypoglycemic Agents

These are usually used for the treatment of type II diabetes mellitus. The usually administered drugs are:

1. **Sulphonylurea derivatives,** like tolazamide, glipizide, glyburide, etc. These drugs are usually prescribed for

the ***treatment of type-2 (NIDDM) diabetes***. They act by **binding to the ATP-inhibited K^+ channels** in the membrane of B cells of pancreas. This **increases Ca^{++} influx and increases insulin secretion**.

2. Other oral hypoglycemic agents are **biguanides** (phenformin and metformin). **Metformin** acts mainly by decreasing gluconeogenesis; therefore, it decreases hepatic glucose output.
3. Other group of drugs like **thiazolidine-diones** (troglitazone is an example of this group) are also used. They increase insulin mediated peripheral glucose disposal. Hence, they decrease insulin resistance (used in NIDDM). Troglitazone also binds with peroxisomes proliferator-activated receptor γ (PPAR γ) in the nucleus of the cell. It **activates PPAR** γ, which induces nuclear transcription that in turn regulate metabolic functions of the cell.

Change in Lifestyle

In addition to drugs, it is important to assure lifestyle modification and proper calorie intake in the long-term management of DM:

1. **Calorie intake:** Food intake should be adjusted to ensure appropriate nutritional requirements. Excess intake should be avoided. Diet should have less carbohydrate and fat, more fibers and adequate proteins and vitamins.
2. **Regular exercise:** Morning walk and freehand exercises improve insulin release and decreases insulin resistance.
3. **Relaxation of body and mind:** Healthy body and mind without stress will not only cure diabetes, but also prevent other diseases.
4. **Practice of yoga:** Yoga is very helpful in reducing the intensity of diabetes, and reducing the complications.

Complications

Improperly treated or untreated chronic diabetes results in various complications. The disease affects small and larger vessels:

1. The **microangiopathy** causes retinal edema and scarring, which is often associated with hard exudates in retina, the condition known as **diabetic retinopathy,** which also occurs due to neovascularization of retina, especially in the advanced stages (Fig. 60.15).
2. The microangiopathy in kidney is known as **diabetic nephropathy**.
3. The macrovascular complications are primarily due to increased atherosclerosis. **Atherosclerosis** is accelerated due to increased plasma LDL. This increases the incidence of **heart attack** (myocardial infarction) and **stroke**.
4. Autonomic nervous system and peripheral nerves are also involved in the disease process. This results in **autonomic neuropathy** (diabetic neuropathy).
5. Hyperglycemia and neuropathy decrease the resistance to infection. This results in **chronic ulcer and gangrene** formation especially in the foot, called as diabetic foot.

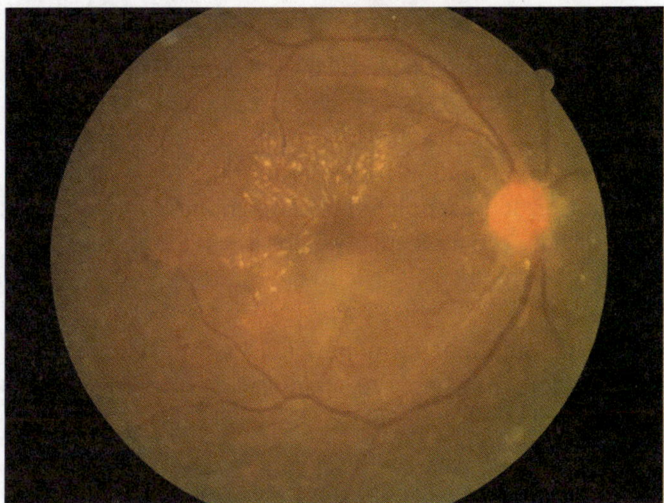

Fig. 60.15: Funduscopic view of proliferative diabetic retinopathy in chronic diabetes. Note the prominent neovascularization of retina, dot-blot hemorrhages and hard exudates in macula.
Courtesy: Dr. Subashini Kaliaperumal, Associate Professor of Ophthalmology, JIPMER, Puducherry.

Scientist contributed

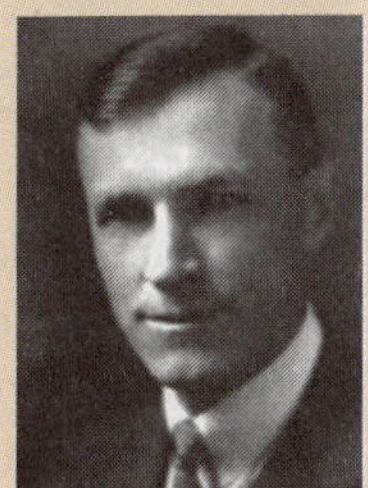

WP Murphy
(1892–1987)

William P Murphy (1892–1987) was an American physician who shared the **Nobel Prize in Physiology or Medicine** in 1934 with George Richards Minot and George Hoyt Whipple for their combined work in devising and treating macrocytic anemia (specifically, pernicious anemia). From 1923 onwards, Murphy practiced clinical medicine and engaged in **research on diabetes mellitus** and diseases of the blood. Though he got Nobel prize for his work on anemia, his contribution to diabetic research and practice is monumental.

Insulin Excess

Insulin excess occurs in insulin secreting tumor of pancreas (insulinoma). This causes hypoglycemia:

1. **Chronic hypoglycemia** causes incoordination of movement and slurring of speech. This is usually ***misdiagnosed as drunkenness***. It is typically most common in the morning, as toward the early morning blood glucose concentration decreases and hepatic glycogen store is depleted.
2. Hypoglycemia also occurs in **excess administration of insulin** in the treatment of diabetes. But in this condition hypoglycemia is acute and manifest in the form of sweating, palpitation, anxiety, and other autonomic functions.

OTHER PANCREATIC HORMONES

Glucagon

Glucagon has opposite metabolic action to that of insulin. It is a prodiabetogenic and ketogenic hormone.

Source and Structure

Glucagon is secreted from α-**cells of pancreas** which constitutes about 20–25% of the islet cell mass. Glucagon is also secreted in the intestine (enteroglucagon) as local hormone and found in some parts of the brain as neurotransmitter. It is a **polypeptide hormone** containing 29 amino acids. The molecular weight is 3,485.

Synthesis

Like other peptide hormones, it is synthesized as preproglucagon that has 179 amino acids. Preproglucagon is found in α-cells of pancreas, L cells in terminal part of intestine and in the brain. **Preproglucagon** molecule in α-cells contains glucagon, **major proglucagon fragment** (MPGF) and glicentin related polypeptide (GRPP), whereas preproglucagon molecule in L-cells of intestine contains glicentin, glucagon like polypeptides (GLP 1 and 2), oxyntomodulin and MPGF. Accordingly, preproglucagon molecule forms different hormones in α-cells and L cells. In α-cells, it forms **proglucagon** that finally forms **glucagon.**

Both glucose and insulin inhibit glucagon synthesis by suppressing transcription of preproglucagon gene.

Functions of products of preproglucagon molecule are as follows:

1. Glicentin has some glucagon activity.
2. GLP-1 and GLP-2 are found in the brain and intestine. GLP1 stimulates insulin secretion and facilitates glucose utilization. GLP 1 is a neurotransmitter in nerve terminals projecting from NTS in the medulla to the dorsomedial hypothalamus.
3. GLP 2 inhibits food intake.
4. Oxyntomodulin inhibits HCl secretion from stomach.
5. Function of GRPP is not clearly known.

Secretion

Glucagon secretion is regulated by following factors:

Factors that increase secretion: Amino acids (especially gluconeogenic amino acids), cortisol, CCK, gastrin, stress, exercise, infection, β receptor agonist and theophylline.

Factors that decrease secretion: Glucose, somatostatin, insulin, secretin, ketone bodies, FFA and α receptor agonist.

Metabolism and Mechanism of Action

It is mainly degraded in the liver. It circulates freely in blood. Its half-life in circulation is about 5–10 minutes. Glucagon acts by **increasing cyclic AMP** in the cell. It also **increases IP_3** in the cell.

Physiological Actions

Physiological actions of glucagon are almost opposite to that of insulin. It facilitates mobilization of nutrients by decreasing their storage. It especially facilitates hepatic glucose output and ketogenesis.

On Carbohydrate Metabolism

Glucagon increases blood glucose by following mechanisms:

1. **Stimulates glycogenolysis:** It causes immediate and profound **glycogenolysis in the liver** by *activating glycogen phosphorylase*. This causes release of **glucose 6-phosphate**:
   - Glucagon increases cAMP in the cell. cAMP stimulates protein kinase A that in turn activates phosphorylase and other enzymes.
   - Activated protein kinase A also inhibits conversion of fructose-6-phosphate to fructose 1,6-biphosphate, which helps in increasing glucose 6-phosphate in the cell.
   - Accumulated glucose 6-phophate is converted to glucose.
   - Thus, more glucose is released from liver. It does not cause glycogenolysis in muscle.
2. **Gluconeogenesis:** It also ***stimulates gluconeogenesis*** by activating gluconeogenic enzymes, especially *phosphoenolpyruvate carboxykinase*. It also promotes hepatic proteolysis and supplies more amino acids for gluconeogenesis.
3. **Inhibition of glycogenesis:** Glucagon ***inhibits glycogen synthase***. Therefore, conversion of glucose to glycogen is inhibited.

All these actions result in increased output of glucose from the liver. Normally, the metabolic actions of glucagon on muscle and adipose tissue are not significant.

On Fat Metabolism

Glucagon promotes lipolysis and ketogenesis in liver:

1. **Lipolysis:** In hepatic cells, glucagon facilitates lipolysis. Thus, it increases release of FFA from liver. However, the fat store of liver is not more unlike in adipose tissue. Therefore, the degree of lipolysis is moderate.
2. **Ketogenesis:** Glucagon increases ketone body formation in liver cells by decreasing the level of malonyl-CoA. Increased FFA also promotes ketogenesis. Glucagon facilitates entry of FFA into mitochondria for their β-oxidation and production of ketone bodies.

On Calorigenesis

Glucagon increases calorigenesis. Calorigenic action of glucagon is not due to increased blood glucose, rather to the hepatic deamination of amino acids.

On Heart

Glucagon in supraphysiological concentration **increases myocardial contractility** by increasing cyclic AMP level in myocardial cells. Therefore, glucagon is advocated *for the treatment of heart disease*.

On Other Hormones

Glucagon stimulates secretion of growth hormone, insulin, and pancreatic polypeptide.

Insulin-Glucagon Ratio

Insulin is glucopenic, glycogenic, anti-gluconeogenic, anti-lipolytic, and anti-ketotic (anti-diabetogenic and anti-ketogenic). Therefore, insulin is the hormone of energy storage. Glucagon is prodiabetogenic and proketogenic. Therefore, glucagon is the hormone of energy release. Because of their opposing effects, a balance should be maintained between the secretion of insulin and glucagons for maintaining normal metabolic functions. Therefore, **insulin-glucagon molar ratio** (I/G ratio) in plasma is more important than their individual concentration. Normally, the **I/G ratio following a balance diet is approximately 3**. Following overnight fasting, it decreases to 1, and after prolonged fasting the ratio may be as low as 0.4. Following glucose infusion, the ratio may rise up to 30.

Physiological Significance:

1. **During starvation**, the low I/G ratio favors glycogen break down and gluconeogenesis that increases nutrient supply. Conversely, during high-fed state, the ratio is high favoring deposition of nutrients in the form glycogen, protein and fat.
2. **During neonatal period** (immediately after birth), a low I/G ratio is critical for the survival of the neonate. In first few hours to days, the abrupt cessation of maternal fuel supply during which neonate does not receive required amount of fuel from its own GI tract, a low I/G ration maintains internal supply of nutrients.
3. **In diabetes,** inappropriate I/G ratio influences metabolic status. Secretion of glucagon is inappropriately elevated in insulin deficiency. The metabolic derangements are affected by this abnormal ratio.

Applied Physiology

Glucagon excess is produced by tumor of α-cells of pancreas. This is called **glucagonoma**. It causes hyperglycemia, ketosis and other metabolic derangements that mimic diabetes mellitus. In fact, insulin deficiency in diabetes is associated with glucagons excess. Glucagon deficiency occurs rarely.

Somatostatin

Source and Structure

Somatostatin is secreted from **D cells of pancreas**. It is also secreted in **hypothalamus and gastrointestinal tract**. Somatostatin is a **peptide hormone**. It has two forms. One contains 14 amino acids and the other 28 amino acids. The 14 amino acid somatostatin is mostly synthesized in pancreas and 28 amino acid peptide in GI tract.

Synthesis and Secretion

Like other pancreatic hormones it is synthesized as preprosomatostatin, which becomes prosomatostatin. Prosomatostatin is converted to somatostatin. Somatostatin secretion is stimulated by glucose, amino acids, free fatty acids, GI hormones, glucagon, vagal stimulation and sympathetic stimulation via β receptors.

Functions

1. Somatostatin **profoundly inhibits the secretion of insulin and glucagon** from pancreas, by neurocrine and paracrine fashions.
2. It decreases the rate of assimilation of all nutrients from GI tract.
3. It inhibits gastric, duodenal and gallbladder motility.
4. It inhibits HCl and pepsin secretions from stomach, and intestinal secretions.
5. It inhibits secretion of secretin and gastrin.
6. It inhibits pancreatic exocrine secretion.
7. It inhibits absorption of glucose, and triglycerides from the mucosal epithelial cells of intestine.
8. It regulates feedback control of gastric emptying (entry of food from stomach into the intestine). When food enters intestine, somatostatin inhibits gastric emptying. Therefore, it prevents rapid overload of intestine by gastric content.

Clinical Significance

Treatment of Diarrhea: Somatostatin preparations are used in medical practice for the **treatment of diarrhea** as somatostatin inhibits GI motility.

Somatostatinoma: In tumor of D cells of pancreas (somatostatinoma), excess somatostatin secretion decreases nutrient absorption from GI tract. Therefore, excess of **undigested food appear in the stool**. This causes weight loss. Moderate hyperglycemia is observed due to low insulin level in the plasma. These patients also develop **dyspepsia** due to decreased gastric emptying and decreased gastric secretion. They also develop **gallstone,** which is precipitated by decreased gallbladder contraction as somatostatin inhibits CCK secretion.

Pancreatic Polypeptide

Source and Structure

Pancreatic polypeptide is secreted from **F cells of pancreas**. It is a polypeptide containing 36 amino acids. It has a characteristic C terminal tyrosine-amide residue. Structurally, it is similar to the **neuropeptide Y** (NPY) secreted from hypothalamus and polypeptide YY, a GI hormone. However, in functions, it is not very similar to them.

Synthesis and Secretion

It is synthesized like other peptide hormones. It is secreted **primarily in response to food intake**. When food is ingested and food passes through the GI tract, the GI hormones and vagal stimulation stimulate the secretion of pancreatic polypeptide. It is also **stimulated by hypoglycemia and inhi-**

polypeptide. It is also **stimulated by hypoglycemia and inhibited by hyperglycemia**. Its secretion is also **inhibited by somatostatin**. As pancreatic polypeptide secretion is under the influence of cholinergic control, its secretion decreases after atropine administration. Its secretion is stimulated by protein rich food, fasting and exercise.

Functions

1. It **inhibits exocrine pancreatic secretion**. This is partly due to its inhibition of uptake of precursor amino acids by the acinar cells.
2. It slows the absorption of food from the GI tract. Recent research works suggest that it inhibits food intake.

Clinical Significance

1. Increased secretion of pancreatic polypeptide is invariably **associated with islet cell tumors**. Therefore, its increased level in plasma serves a **tumor marker** for the tumors of endocrine pancreas.
2. Failure of pancreatic polypeptide concentration in plasma to rise in response to hypoglycemia suggests loss of cholinergic innervation of pancreatic islets.

CHAPTER SUMMARY

Key Concepts

1. Insulin has prominent effects on fat metabolism, as it has effects on carbohydrate metabolism. Therefore, in diabetes, in addition to hyperglycemia, there are hyperlipidemia and ketonemia. Diabetic complications are considerably linked to hyperlipidemia.
2. HbA1c reflects the chronicity of hyperglycemia. Therefore, HbA1c should be assessed in all diabetic patients to assess their level of hyperglycemia for last few months, rather than to check FBG or PPBG, which indicates the current blood glucose level.
3. For assessing insulin sensitivity, C peptide estimation should be done, which is a more reliable marker of β cell activity.

Important to Know (Must Read)

1. In examination, 'Describe the functions of insulin' usually comes as a **Long Question.**
2. Mechanism of insulin secretion in response to plasma glucose, Mechanism of action of Insulin, Physiological actions of Insulin on fat metabolism, Physiological actions of Insulin on carbohydrate metabolism, Glucose transporters (GLUT), Explain the physiological basis of features of DM, Differences between type I and type II DM, Glucagon, Effect of life style changes including exercise on DM, Insulin-glucagon ratio (I/G ratio), Somatostatin, Pancreatic polypeptide are usual **Short Questions** in exam.
3. In **Viva**, examiner may ask… List the hormones secreted from pancreas and the cell type from which they are secreted, Physiological actions of Insulin especially on carbohydrate, fat and protein metabolism, List the factors that increase or decrease insulin secretion, What are the types of GLUTs and what are their functions, What is the mechanism of insertion of GLUT into cell membrane by insulin in insulin- sensitive cells, How is insulin secreted from beta cells in response to glucose, What is the relationship between increase in plasma glucose and rate of insulin secretion, What is first phase response and what is second phase response, Why the secretion of insulin is greater in response to orally administered glucose compared to intravenously administered glucose, Why is insulin given with glucose in the treatment of hyperkalemia, What is the effect of insulin on growth, Classify diabetes mellitus based on etiology, What are IDDM and NIDDM? List the differences between type I and type II DM, What is metabolic syndrome and what are its components, What is secondary DM, What is gestational DM, What is Maturity onset Diabetes of the Young (MODY), Explain the physiological basis of polyphagia in DM, Explain the physiological basis of polydipsia in DM, Explain the physiological basis of polyuria in DM, Explain the physiological basis of hyperglycemia and glycosuria in DM, Explain the physiological basis of weight loss in DM, Explain the physiological basis of ketosis, acidosis and coma in DM, What is the normal blood glucose level, in fasting and post prandial, What do you mean by impaired fasting glucose or impaired glucose tolerance, What is the fasting and post prandial blood glues level in DM, List some oral hypoglycemic agents and give their mechanism of action, What are the types of insulin preparation used in the treatment of DM, What is the plasma glucose response to oral glucose tolerance test (OGTT), Explain how does regular exercise prevent diabetes, What is the effect of healthy life style on DM, What are the complications of DM, What are the physiological actions of glucagon, What is insulin-glucagon ratio, What are the physiological significances of /G ratio, What are the functions of somatostatin, What are the functions of pancreatic polypeptide, What is the structure of insulin, How insulin is synthesized, What is C-peptide, What is the importance/ functions of C-peptide, List the substances having insulin like activity, What is the structure of insulin receptor, What is the physiological and clinical significance of Somatostatin, What is the physiological and clinical significance of pancreatic polypeptide.

CHAPTER

61

Calcium and Phosphate Metabolism and Physiology of Bone

Learning Objectives

On completion of study of this chapter, the student **MUST** be able to:

1. Learn the basics of calcium and phosphate metabolism.
2. Understand the importance of learning calcium and phosphate metabolism to learn bone physiology.
3. List the functions of calcium and phosphate.
4. Appreciate various aspects of bone physiology.
5. Understand the mechanism of bone formation and bone resorption.
6. Describe the hormonal regulation of calcium metabolism.
7. Learn the physiological basis of osteoporosis and osteomalacia.

The student **MAY** also be able to:

1. Describe the role of calcium and phosphate in pone physiology.
2. Describe the mechanism and regulation of bone formation and resorption.

The major hormones involved in the regulation of plasma calcium and phosphorous metabolisms are **parathormone** (PTH) secreted from parathyroid gland, **calcitonin** secreted from parafollicular cells of thyroid gland, and **vitamin D**. Other hormones like glucocorticoids, growth factors, insulin, etc. also influence calcium metabolism. These hormones control calcium metabolism by primarily acting on three structures: GI tract, kidney, and bones. While regulating calcium concentration, many of these factors also influence phosphate level in the plasma. A balance between calcium and phosphate is always maintained in our body and abnormalities in this balance result in severe dysfunctions. To understand the regulation of plasma calcium, it is important to understand the basics of calcium and phosphate metabolisms and also the physiology of bone dynamics.

CALCIUM AND PHOSPHATE METABOLISM

Calcium Metabolism

The normal **plasma calcium concentration is 9–11 mg%** (average 10 mg%). This is among the most tightly regulated physiological parameters of the body. The regulation of plasma calcium concentration within a narrow range of 1–2% indicates the importance of this ion in controlling critical body functions.

Functions of Calcium

Calcium ions are involved in many key physiological processes of the body. These are:

1. Genesis and **maintenance of action potentials**, especially in cardiac and smooth muscles.
2. Genesis of **pacemaker potential** in various pacemaking tissues.
3. **Excitation-contraction coupling** during muscle contractions.
4. **Excitability of nerve and muscle:** Calcium influences sodium permeability; therefore, influences the ease with which action potentials are triggered. Especially in nerves, low calcium can cause generation of spontaneous action potentials. This causes the characteristic muscle spasm in hypocalcemic tetany.
5. Cell division.
6. Bone formation (**mineralization of bone**).
7. Secretion of endocrine and exocrine glands (**calcium-mediated exocytosis** causes release of hormones and enzymes from the gland cells).

8. **Neurotransmitter release** from nerve terminals.
9. **Blood coagulation:** Calcium is coagulation factor IV and is highly essential for clotting of blood. Many anticoagulants chelate calcium to prevent clotting.
10. Modulation of various enzyme activities (enzymes use calcium as cofactor).
11. Calcium acts as a **second or third messenger** in various intracellular signaling pathways for hormone actions.
12. GI motility and motility of many other structures.

Therefore, it is essential to maintain calcium concentration within its normal range. A minor deviation in calcium level results in alteration in many physiological functions of the body.

Distribution of Calcium in the Body

In the cell, calcium is **stored in mitochondria and endoplasmic reticulum.** A transient alteration in plasma calcium is balanced by entry or extrusion of calcium from the intracellular or extracellular reservoirs. The total **intracellular free calcium is about 0.2 mg**, whereas about 9 g is present in the bound form or in the storage sites such as in mitochondria and endoplasmic reticulum. This intracellular calcium provides an immediate source of calcium for cell functions.

Table 61.1: Distribution of calcium in the body.

Total body content	: 1200 g (average)
In bones and teeth	: 99% of total
In intracellular fluid	: 0.9% (11 g approx.)
In extracellular fluid	: 0.1% (1 g approx.)

1. Normally, a healthy adult contains 1 to 1.5 kg of calcium in his body.
2. About 99% of the total calcium is present in **bones and teeth** (Table 61.1).
3. The total extracellular pool of calcium is about 1 to 1.5 g and intracellular pool is about 10 – 15 g.
4. The half of total plasma calcium (about **50%) is ionized** and present in the ***biologically active form***.
5. About 10% of the plasma calcium is in the non-ionized form like calcium bicarbonate, and about 40% is bound to albumin.
6. The **pH of blood affects ionization of calcium.** ***In alkalosis***, ionized calcium concentration decreases, and ***in acidosis***, it increases.

Metabolism

Daily dietary intake of calcium ranges from 200 mg to 2 g. In an adult, the ***recommended daily intake*** is about 800 mg.

1. Calcium absorption from the intestine is **inversely proportional to its intake.** This *prevents calcium overload when intake is high* or maintains calcium concentration even with low intake.
2. With a daily intake of 1 g of calcium, generally 30% (300 mg) of it is absorbed in the intestine and about **70% (700 mg) is excreted in the stool.**
3. About 150 mg of calcium is secreted into the intestine, which makes a total of about **850 mg excreted daily in the stool.**
4. About 150 mg is excreted in the urine.
5. Thus, about 1 g of calcium is excreted daily from the body to maintain the balance between input and output (Fig. 61.1).

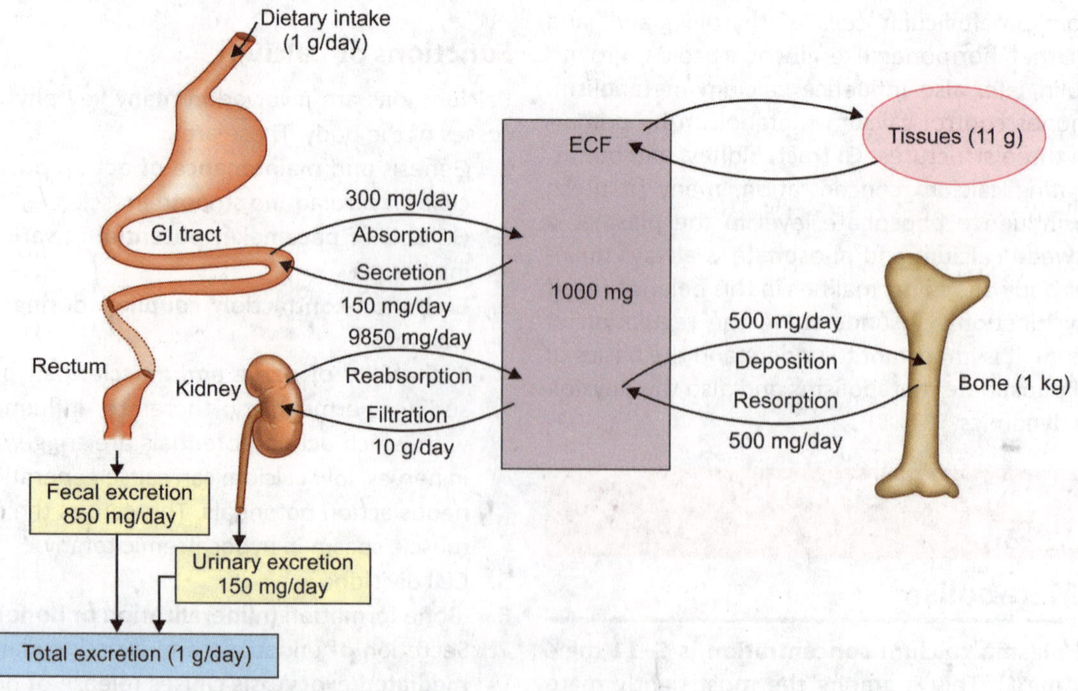

Fig. 61.1: Summary of calcium metabolism.

6. Calcium absorption from the intestine is *diminished with advancement of age, which* **contributes to the development of osteoporosis.**

Calcium absorbed from intestine enters the ECF pool of calcium which is about 1000 mg. This is in equilibrium with the rapidly exchangeable pool (4000 mg) of the body. From the rapidly exchangeable pool of plasma, 500 mg of calcium enters bones for normal bone remodeling and from bone about 500 mg of calcium extrudes back into the plasma.

Phosphate Metabolism

The normal **plasma phosphate concentration** ***is 2.5 to 4.5 mg%***.

Functions of Phosphorus

Phosphorus (usually as phosphate) is important as calcium for biological activities.

1. Phosphate is present in the ATP, creatine phosphate, various co-factors like NAD, NADP, and thiamine pyrophosphate.
2. It is an **integral part of second messengers** in the cells like cyclic AMP and inositol triphosphate.
3. It is also found in DNA and RNA.
4. It is required for **phosphorylation of many intracellular proteins**, for formation of phosphoproteins. Phosphoproteins mediate many intracellular metabolic activities.
5. Phosphate acts as covalent modifier of many enzymes.
6. It is a **major constituent of the bone and teeth** like that of calcium.
7. It serves as an important component of **intracellular pH buffering system.**

Like calcium metabolism, phosphate metabolism is also closely regulated in the body.

Distribution of Phosphate in the Body

Total body phosphate content is roughly half of the calcium content. Out of 600 g of total phosphate in the body, about 86% is present in the bones, 14% in intracellular fluid and 0.08% in extracellular fluid (Table 61.2). About 6% is present in the muscle and 8% in other cells.

Table 61.2: Distribution of phosphate in the body.

Total body content	: 600 g (average)
In bones and teeth	: 86% of total
In intracellular fluid	: 14% (about 84 g)
In extracellular fluid	: 0.08% (1.2 g)

Metabolism

The daily phosphate intake is about 1400 mg, of which **75% is absorbed from the intestine** and 25% is excreted in the stool.

1. The phosphate pool in the ECF is about 700 mg, from where about 200 mg is exchanged with the bones for bone remodeling.
2. Normally, about 1000 mg is excreted in urine.
3. Regulation of renal excretion of phosphate mainly controls the concentration of plasma phosphate.
4. Renal (1 g) and fecal (0.4 g) excretion balances the daily intake with daily output of phosphate (Fig. 61.2).
5. **Phosphate deficiency** results in muscle weakness, cardiac and respiratory dysfunction, abnormal bone formation, and loss of red cell membrane integrity.

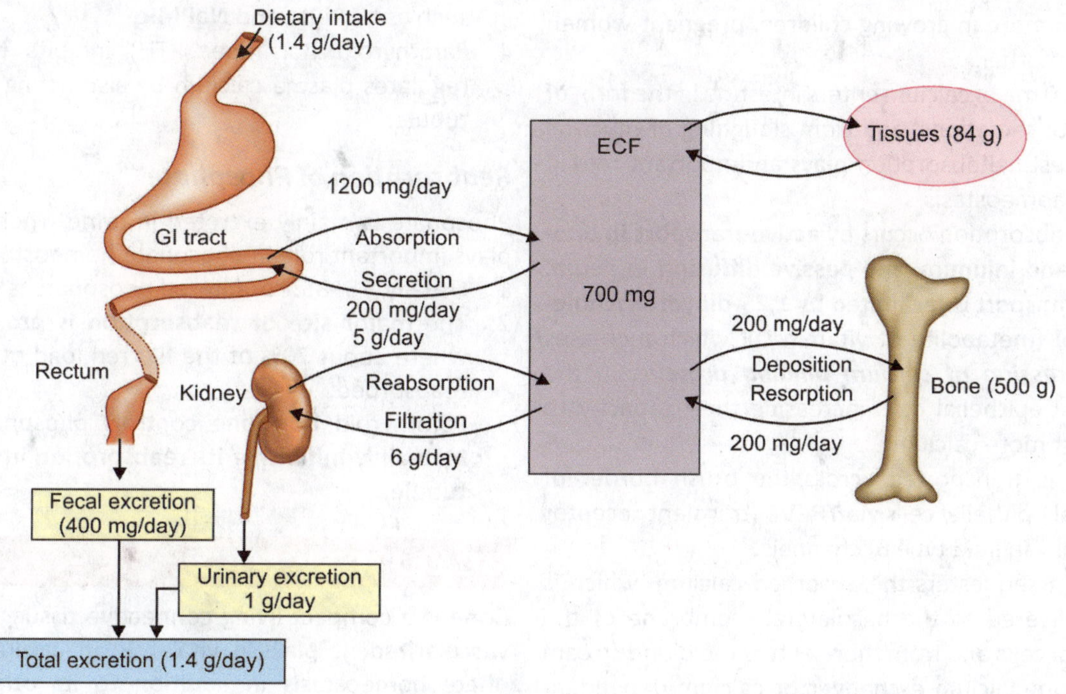

Fig. 61.2: Summary of phosphorus metabolism.

Magnesium: Magnesium is closely related with the calcium and phosphate metabolisms.

1. It is essential for **neuromuscular transmission** and it serves as **cofactor for many enzymatic activities**.
2. The normal *plasma concentration of magnesium is 1.5–2.5 mg%.*
3. About 35% of it is bound to protein.
4. There is about 25 g of magnesium in our body of which about 50% is present in the bones and rest 50% in the intracellular fluid.
5. The magnesium depletion causes neuromuscular dysfunction and ventricular arrhythmias.

Regulation of Calcium and Phosphate Homeostasis

Homeostasis of calcium and phosphate is influenced mainly by exchange of these ions between plasma and bone. Also, absorption of calcium and phosphate from intestine and kidney that determines their fecal and urinary excretion respectively greatly contributes to their homeostasis. In general, **calcium is excreted more in the stool (850 mg/day) and less in urine (150 mg/day),** whereas ***phosphate is excreted more in urine (1000 mg/day) and less in stool (400 mg/day)***.

Intestinal Control of Calcium and Phosphate

Absorption of calcium and phosphate from intestine significantly contributes to their plasma concentration.

Absorption of Calcium

About one third of ingested calcium is absorbed from GI tract and remaining two-third is excreted. The percentage absorption is more in growing children, pregnant women and nursing mother.

1. About 150 mg of calcium enters intestine in the form of various GI secretions, and from sloughing of mucosal cells. Intestinal absorption plays an important role in calcium homeostasis.
2. Calcium absorption occurs by **active transport in duodenum and jejunum**, and **passive diffusion in ileum.** Active transport is **facilitated by 1,25-dihydroxycholecalciferol** (metabolite of vitamin D), which increases the ***expression of calcium binding proteins*** in the intestinal epithelial cells increasing their capacity to transport more calcium.
3. Calcium is transported across the brush border of intestinal epithelial cells via **TRPV6** (transient receptor potential vanilloid type 6) channels.
4. **Calbindin** sequesters the absorbed calcium, which is then delivered to the basolateral membrane of the epithelial cells and from there enters the blood stream via sodium-calcium exchanger or calcium-dependent ATPase.
5. However, some degree of intestinal calcium uptake persists in the absence of TRPV6 and calbindin. **Cholecalciferol and calcitonin** influence calcium absorption either directly or indirectly through vitamin D.

Absorption of Phosphate

In contrast to calcium, most of the ingested phosphorous (about 75–85%) is absorbed from intestine as inorganic phosphate (Pi).

1. Pi absorption occurs by a transporter called **NaPi-IIb**, which is related to the transporter in kidney.
2. Though absorption occurs by both active and passive processes, **active transport is the primary mechanism** of absorption.
3. However, the regulatory mechanism for phosphate absorption is not well developed. To some extent, it is **coupled to calcium absorption**.

Renal Control of Calcium and Phosphate

Reabsorption of calcium and phosphate from kidney contributes significantly to their plasma concentration.

Reabsorption of Calcium

About 60% of plasma calcium is filtered in the glomeruli and 40% is bound to plasma proteins.

1. Of the filtered calcium, 1–5% is excreted in urine and about **95% is reabsorbed back into the plasma**. Therefore, the total urinary excretion is less.
2. Of the filtered load of calcium, about 65% is reabsorbed in proximal tubule, 25% in loop of Henle and 8% in distal tubule.
3. In proximal tubule, the transport process is active that involves two **sodium-dependent Pi co-transporters** such as **NaPi-IIa and NaPi-IIc.**
4. Parathyroid hormone (PTH) inhibits NaPi-IIa. PTH regulates plasma calcium by also acting on the distal tubule.

Reabsorption of Phosphate

Phosphate is mainly excreted in urine. Therefore, kidney plays important role in phosphate homeostasis.

1. Usually, 75–85% of filtered phosphate is reabsorbed.
2. The **major site of reabsorption is proximal tubule,** where about 70% of the filtered load of phosphate is reabsorbed.
3. Parathyroid hormone controls phosphate excretion by mainly **inhibiting its reabsorption in the proximal tubule**.

BONE PHYSIOLOGY

Bone is a compact living connective tissue, which is well vascularized. It plays a vital role in calcium and phosphate homeostasis in addition to its other important functions.

Table 61.3: Constituent of bone.

A. Inorganic components	
Calcium	: 99% of total body content
Phosphate	: 86% of total body content
Carbonate	: 80% of total body content
Magnesium	: 50% of total body content
Sodium	: 35% of total body content
Water	: 8% of total body content
B. Organic components	
Type I collagen (95% of the bone matrix)	
Ground substance (5% of the bone matrix)	
– Proteoglycans	
– High molecular weight substance	

The major functions of bones are as follows:

1. They form the **skeletal framework of the body**, which is crucial for changing and maintaining various body postures.
2. By providing stable postural background, bones allow movements to occur.
3. They play important role in metabolism of various minerals, especially, contribute to **calcium, phosphate and magnesium homeostasis.**
4. Bones **protect important structures** and viscera in the thoracic and pelvic cavities and in the skull.
5. Bone (bone marrow) is the primary **site of hemopoiesis.** They produce and supply formed elements of blood.

Composition of Bone

Bone is simply a collagen framework in which inorganic minerals are deposited on an organic matrix.

Inorganic Components

Inorganic component consists of various minerals such as calcium, phosphate, carbonate, magnesium and sodium. Minerals constitute about 25% of the bone volume, but they comprise half the bone weight because of their high density.

1. Bone is the major reservoir of these minerals in the body.
2. About **99% of calcium, 86% of phosphate, 80% of carbonate and 50% of magnesium** of their total body content are present in bones (Table 61.3).

Organic Matrix

Organic matrix of the bone is called **osteoid.**

1. It is formed mainly by the **Type I Collagen,** which forms 95% of the matrix.
2. The remaining 5% noncollagen part is called the **ground substance,** which is a mixture of various proteoglycans and high molecular weight compounds, consisting mainly of polysaccharides.

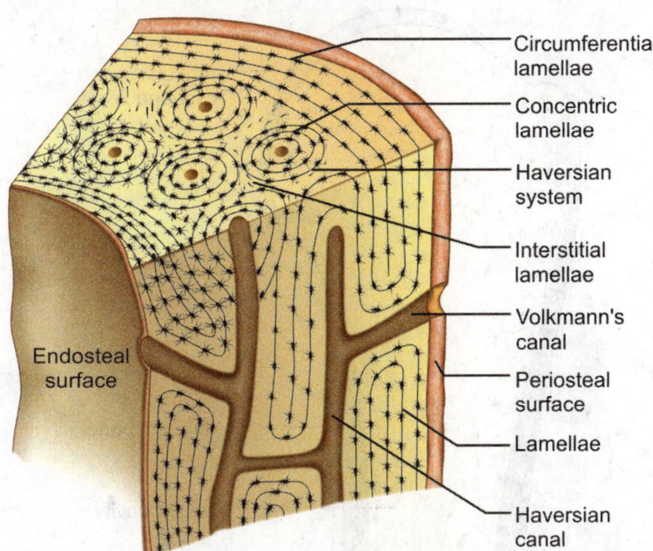

Fig. 61.3: Transverse section and longitudinal section through a compact bone. Note the arrangement of concentric lamellae and Haversian system.

3. **In compact bone** (see below), the collagen is arranged in concentric layers around **haversian canals** forming cylinder like structures called **osteons** or **haversian systems** (Fig. 61.3).

The mineral component of calcium and phosphate in the bone forms **hydroxyapatite crystals.** The hydroxyapatite crystals are microscopic needle like structures that lie in parallel alongside the collagen fibers and this arrangement provides strength and hardness to the bone. **Demineralization of bone** causes loss of hydroxyapatite crystals and makes the organic matrix (collagen framework) weak, and loss of organic matrix makes the bone brittle.

Structure of Bone

Bone consists of **two parts**: the outer cortex and the inner trabeculae.

1. **The cortical bone**, also called ***compact bone*** constitutes 80% of the total bone mass of the body. It consists of **dense concentric outer layers of the long bones** and a ***thinner outer layer of the flat bones*** (Fig. 61.4).
2. The **trabecular bone**, also called ***spongy bone*** constitutes 20% of the bone mass. It consists of **bone spicules** that make up the inner part of the axial skeletons and the smaller interior of the long bones.

Parts of Bone

Long bones consist of **epiphysis,** the both ends, and **diaphysis**, the shaft which is separated from epiphyses by **epiphyseal plates** (Fig. 61.5).

1. The linear growth of the bones occurs at the end of long bones by **replacement of cartilage at the epiphyseal plates.**

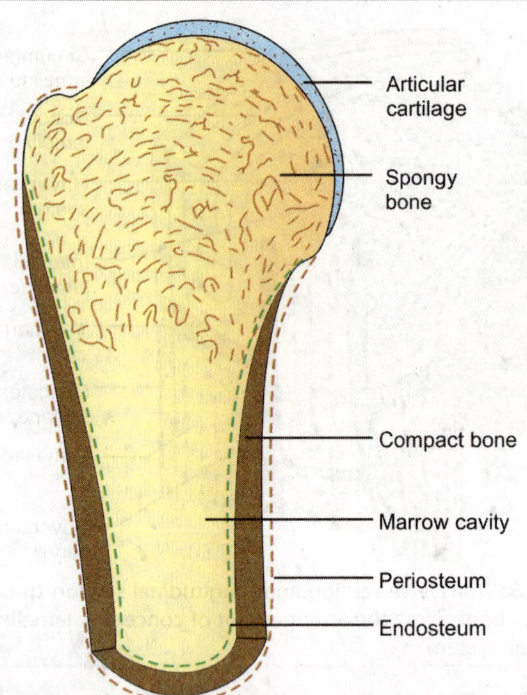

Fig. 61.4: Features of a bone. The compact bone is the cortical bone and spongy bone is the trabecular bone.

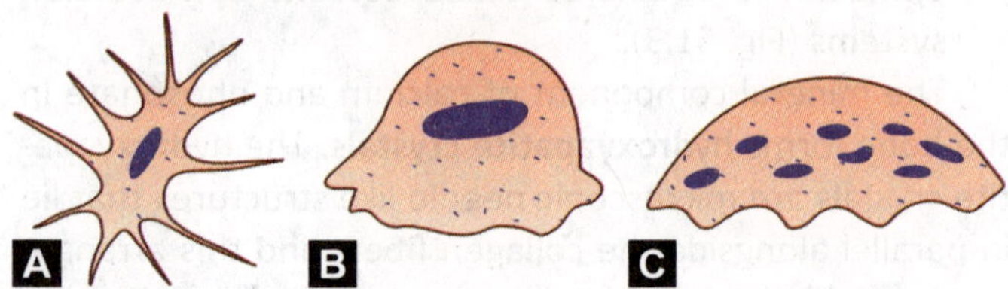

Figs. 61.6A to C: Bone cells. (A) Osteocytes; (B) Osteoblast; (C) Osteoclast.

2. Closure of epiphyseal plates occurs towards the end of puberty. This causes cessation of further increase in height of the individual.
3. However, width of the bone continues to increase due to addition of cells to the **periosteum**, the outer surface of the bone.

   The nutrients from ECF diffuse into the trabecular bone via **canaliculi** (see below). In compact bone, nutrients are supplied by Haversian canal that contains blood vessels.

Remodeling of Bone

Bone is continuously remodeled throughout the life, which is synchronized by bone formation and resorption (bone destruction).

1. **During the growth period**, bone formation exceeds bone resorption so that the bone mass increases.
2. **During the adulthood**, rate of formation and resorption is almost balanced so that the bone mass remains unchanged.
3. **After the age of 40 to 50**, bone resorption exceeds formation so that bone mass slowly decreases.

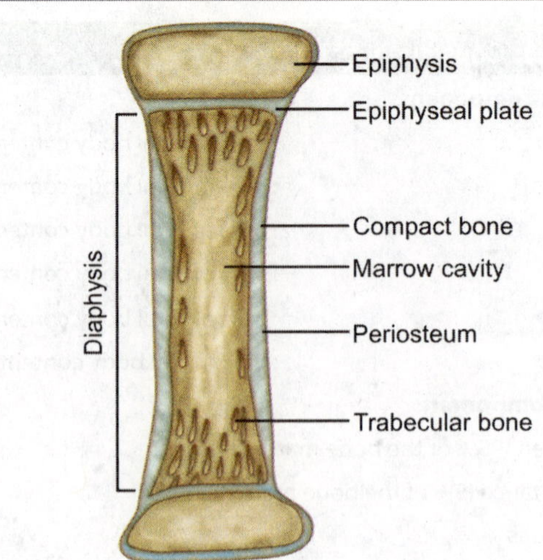

Fig. 61.5: Structure of a bone.

4. The process of bone turn over is known as **remodeling** and this is a *major mechanism of maintaining calcium homeostasis* in the body.
5. Normally, turnover of about 10% of the total bone mass occurs in a year in adults.

Cell Types in Bone

There are **three types of cells** in the bone: these are **osteoblasts, osteoclasts,** and **osteocytes** (Figs. 61.6A to C). Osteoblasts and osteocytes are called **osteoprogenitor cells** as they develop from primitive cells. Osteoclasts develop from the precursors such as monocytes and tissue macrophages.

Osteoblasts and Osteocytes

Osteoblasts are bone forming cells. They are modified fibroblasts.

1. **Osteoblasts** synthesize **osteoid**, the organic matrix of the bone. They have numerous endoplasmic reticulum and Golgi apparatus. They are present towards the periphery of the bone and their cytoplasmic processes connect osteocytes that are present deeper in the bone.
2. Osteoid produced by osteoblasts is secreted towards the interior of the bone. Slowly the osteoblasts are surrounded by osteoid and osteoid is mineralized.
3. Osteoblasts surrounded by mineralized osteoid gradually lose their ability to form bones and they become **osteocytes**.
4. The cytoplasmic connection between osteoblasts and osteocytes become **canaliculi** (Fig. 61.7).
5. The canaliculi are the anatomical link for transfer of nutrients, chemicals and waste products between the surface and interior of the bone.

Osteoclasts

Osteoclasts are **cells of mononuclear phagocyte system** in the bone. Therefore, they are large, multinucleated cells located towards the periphery of the bone.

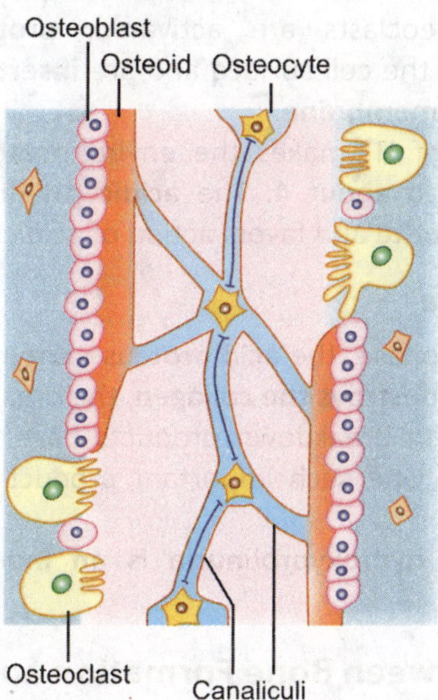

Fig. 61.7: Arrangement of cells in the bone. Note, canaliculi connect between osteocytes and osteocytes with osteoblast.

1. They **cause bone resorption** by secreting proteolytic enzymes into the surroundings.
2. The chemicals secreted by osteoclasts make the environment acidic that enhances the solubility of bone minerals and the enzymes secreted cause *degradation of the organic matrix.*

Mechanism of Bone Formation

Formation of bone is the **function of osteoblasts** (Figs. 61.8A to E).

1. Osteoblasts synthesize **collagen** and extrude it into the adjacent extracellular space (Fig. 61.8A). The *collagen fibrils* form the organic matrix of the bone, which is called as **osteoid** (Fig. 61.8B).
2. In the osteoid, calcium-phosphate is deposited which is called as **mineralization** of bone. Thereafter, to the organic matrix, hydroxides and bicarbonates are added to form the **hydroxyapatite crystals** (the *complete mineralization*). Osteoid converted into lamella of the bone (Fig. 61.8C).
3. The mineralized matrix **slowly accumulates and surrounds the osteoblasts**. As this process of mineralization of matrix continues, the osteoblasts decrease their synthetic activity and become **osteocytes** (Fig. 61.8D).
4. Osteoblastic activity is seen along the surface of the bones. Lamellae of the bones are formed with osteocytes remaining inside the lamellae (Fig. 61.8E).
5. **Vitamin D** is essential for bone mineralization. It profoundly influences the availability of calcium and phosphate to the bone matrix.
6. The canaliculi that connect osteocytes from bone interior to the surface ***transfer calcium from the interior to the exterior bone units*** and then from there to the ECF.

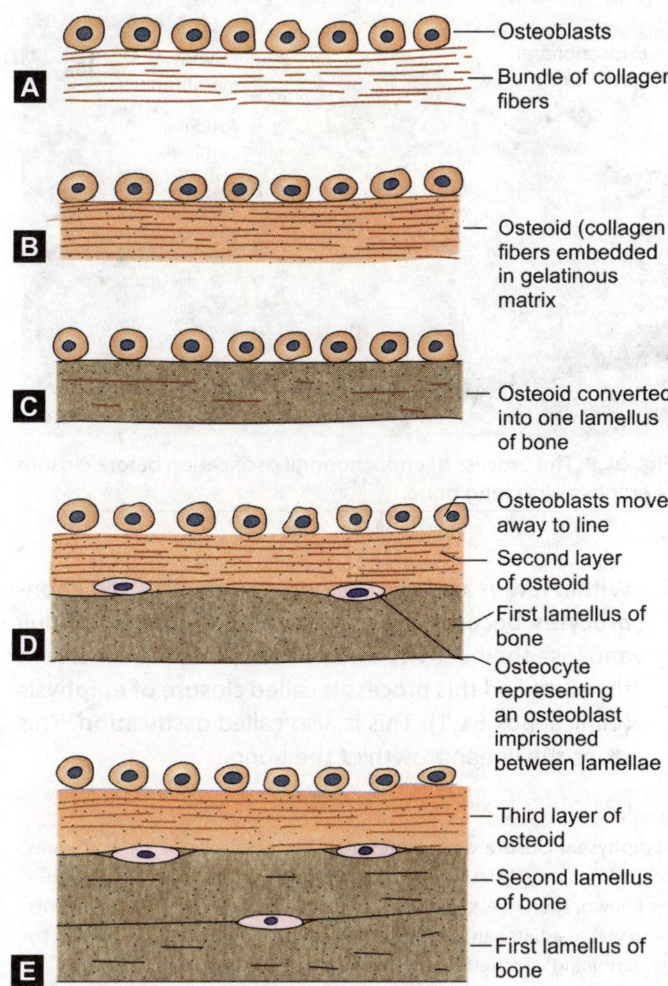

Figs. 61.8A to E: Stages of bone formation.

7. This process of transfer of calcium carried out by osteocytes is known as **osteocytic osteolysis.**
8. Normally, this process does not decrease the bone mass rather removes calcium from the recently formed bone crystals.

Role of Chondrocytes and Endochondral Ossification

Before epiphyseal closure, the leading edge of the epiphyseal plate contains **chondrocytes.**

1. The active chondrocytes synthesize cartilage that gradually embeds the chondrocytes.
2. The embedded chondrocytes die and are replaced by new chondrocytes and the formation of cartilage continues.
3. The cartilage is slowly calcified and osteoblasts migrate into it.
4. Osteoblasts secrete osteoid that ultimately mineralize and the new bone is formed.
5. Thus, the bone increases in length as the **epiphyseal plate lays down new bone** on the end of the shaft. This is called **endochondral ossification** (Fig. 61.9).
6. IGF I, insulin and thyroid hormones stimulate chondrocyte activity.

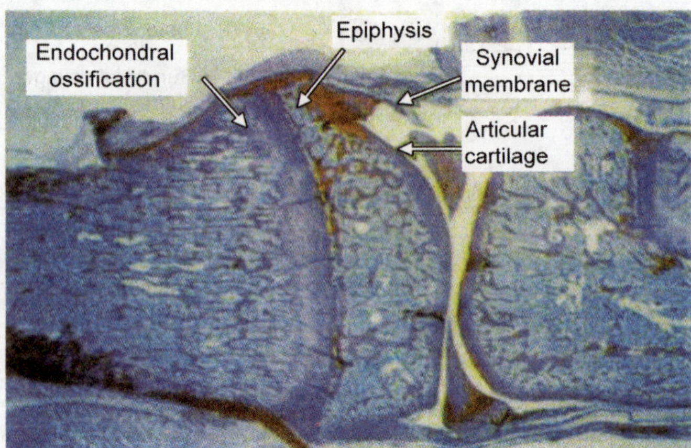

Fig. 61.9: The process of endochondral ossification before closure of epiphysis in a long bone.

7. Within few years from the onset of puberty, the **chondrocytes become unresponsive** to hormonal stimuli and lose their activity. Finally the epiphyses unite with the shaft and this process is called **closure of epiphysis** (Clinical Box 61.1). This is also called **ossification**. This stops the linear growth of the bone.

Clinical Box 61.1

Epiphyseal closure determines age: The epiphyses of various bones close in an orderly fashion in sequence and the age at which they close is known. Therefore, the age of an individual especially in adolescents and young adults can be determined easily by taking x-rays of bones by determining whether the epiphysis is closed or still open.

Bone Resorption

This is process of **destruction of the bone matrix**. Therefore, resorption of bone decreases bone mass. It also removes calcium from the bone. But, it *differs from osteocytic osteolysis* in which the calcium is removed without bone destruction. Bone resorption is carried out by ***osteoclasts***.

1. Osteoclasts contain many mitochondria and lysosomes.
2. The **phosphatases, type 4-collagenase and lysosomal enzymes** cause dissolution of bone matrix.
3. During the process of resorption, the calcium, phosphate, hydroxyproline, and hydroxylysine are released into ECF.
4. Therefore, the rate of excretion of these organic compounds, especially **hydroxyproline indicates the rate of bone resorption.**

Phases of Bone Resorption

Bone resorption occurs **in two phases.**

First Phase

In the first phase, H^+ is secreted by osteoclasts. There are proton pumps (**H^+—dependent ATPases**) in the endosomes present in the cytosol of the osteoclasts.

1. When osteoclasts are activated, **proton pumps migrate** to the cell surface and are **inserted into the osteoclast membrane**.
2. Secretion of H^+ makes the environment acidic; pH decreases to about 4. The **acidic pH dissolves the hydroxyapatite** and favors action of acidic enzymes.

Second Phase

In the second phase, the **acid protease enzyme** secreted by osteoclasts **destroys the collagen**, the organic matrix.

1. The collagen breakdown products have pyridinoline structures. One such important product is **hydroxyproline**.
2. Therefore, **hydroxyprolinuria is an index of bone resorption**.

Balance Between Bone Formation and Resorption

Normally, balance is maintained between the bone resorption and formation within its bone modeling units so that bone mass is maintained within the normal range.

1. Possibly, the balance is due to release of chemicals (some **paracrine signals**) from the osteoblasts or osteoclasts. For example, when osteoclasts cause destruction of bone matrix, the chemicals released from the osteoclasts attract osteoblasts to the site.
2. Osteoblasts then form bone matrix and fill the resorption cavity.
3. The flux of calcium into and out of bone reflects the remodeling, i.e. the **turnover and formation of bone tissue**.

Factors that Control Bone Formation and Resorption

Factors that stimulate bone formation: Growth hormone, growth factors, insulin, estrogen, testosterone, vitamin D, PDGF, transforming growth factors (TGF-β) and calcitonin.

Factors that inhibit bone formation: Cortisol.

Factors that stimulate bone resorption: Parathormone, cortisol, thyroxine, prostaglandins, interleukin 1 and 6, and TNF.

Factors that inhibit resorption: Estrogen, androgen, calcitonin, γ interferon, and TGF-β.

APPLIED PHYSIOLOGY

Osteoporosis

Osteoporosis is **decrease in bone mass and density**. All human beings gain bone early in life. The peak of total bone mass is attained between 25–35 years of age.

1. Usually, after the age of 40, bone mass gradually decreases. This is called **involutional osteoporosis**.
2. In females, the process of bone resorption is facilitated at the time of menopause due to cessation of estrogen secretion (**postmenopausal osteoporosis**).

3. In fact, the rate of bone remodeling increases with age. However, **with increased osteoclastic activity**, bone matrix is lost and ***more cavities are formed***, which is not refilled by the osteoblastic activity. Also, the mineralization decreases. This causes **reduction in bone density and bone mass**. The process is known as *osteoporosis*.

Causes

Osteoporosis is commonly seen in **following conditions**:
1. Hyperparathyroidism,
2. Hyperthyroidism,
3. Cushing's syndrome
4. Ovarian diseases reducing estrogen secretion,
5. Cigarette smoking
6. Alcoholism reducing calcium absorption
7. Deficiency of vitamin C (vitamin C causes collagen synthesis)
8. Inadequate dietary calcium.

Features

Osteoporosis increases the **susceptibility of bones to fractures**, especially in elderly. Osteoporosis is more common in **vertebra, hip bones and in distal forearms**, because these bones have **more trabecular component**. As trabecular bones are metabolically more active, they are lost rapidly.

Treatment

The **treatment is by administration of calcium** or vitamin D tablets, or in worst case estrogen therapy.

Osteopetrosis

Defective increase in bone formation is called osteopetrosis.
1. The bone resorption is defective due to **decreased osteoclastic activity**. Therefore, **osteoblastic activity is unopposed**. This results in unusual increase in bone formation.
2. **Bone density is increased** and bones are deformed.
3. Neurologic deficits occur due to bones compressing on nerves and hematologic abnormalities occur due to decreased marrow cavity.

CHAPTER SUMMARY

Key Concepts

1. Calcium, phosphate and magnesium are essential for bone formation and mineralization.
2. Calcium absorption from the intestine is inversely proportional to its intake, which prevents calcium overload when intake is high or maintains calcium concentration in low calcium intake.
3. Osteoblasts are meant for bone formation ad osteoclasts are for bone resorption. A balance between the two cells is essential for maintenance of bone mass.

Important to Know (Must Read)

1. In examination, **Long Questions** may not be asked from this chapter.
2. Osteoporosis, Functions of calcium and calcium metabolism, Mechanism of bone formation and bone resorption, Regulation of calcium and phosphate homeostasis, & Osteoblasts and osteoclasts, may be asked as **Short Questions** in exam.
3. In **Viva**, examiner may ask... List the functions of calcium, List the functions of phosphorous, How calcium and phosphorous are distributed in the body, How ECF calcium pool is exchanged with GIT, bone, kidneys and tissues, How ECF calcium pool is exchanged with GIT, bone, kidneys and tissues, How ECF phosphorous pool is exchanged with GIT, bone, kidneys and tissues, What are the types of bones, What is the composition of bone, What is the structure of bone, Functions of osteoblasts and osteocytes, Mechanism of bone formation, Mechanism of bone resorption, What are the factors that control bone formation and bone resorption, What are the cells in the bone, What are the functions of osteoblasts and osteoclasts, What are the stages of bone formation, Name the hormones that influence bone functions, Cause, features and treatment of osteoporosis, What is osteopetrosis and what are its symptoms, How epiphyseal closure determines age.

CHAPTER

62

Parathyroid Gland, Calcitonin and Vitamin D

LEARNING OBJECTIVES

On completion of study of this chapter, the student **MUST** be able to:

1. Name the cell types in parathyroid gland and give their functions.
2. Describe the mechanism of action and functions of parathyroid hormone.
3. Describe the mechanism of action and functions of calcitonin.
4. Describe functions of vitamin D.
5. Understand the physiological basis of dysfunctions of PTH.

The student **MAY** also be able to:

1. Explain the role of calcitonin and vitamin D in calcium metabolism.
2. Describe the hormonal regulation of calcium metabolism.

Parathormone (PTH) secreted from parathyroid gland, **calcitonin** secreted from parafollicular cells of thyroid gland, and **cholecalciferol** (vitamin D_3)are the major hormones involved in the regulation of plasma calcium and phosphorous metabolisms and bone physiology. Therefore, usually functions of these three hormones are discussed together.

PARATHYROID GLAND

Parathyroid gland secretes hormone called **parathyroid hormone** or **parathormone** (PTH). PTH is the major regulator of calcium and phosphate metabolism. PTH **increases plasma calcium and decreases plasma phosphate** level.

Scientist contributed

Marcel Eugène Émile Gley (1857–1930) was a French physiologist and endocrinologist. Gley was the first to show the importance of the **parathyroid glands** for the maintenance of life in mammals. He had demonstrated tetany in animal models after removal of parathyroids. Because of his discovery, parathyroid glands have sometimes been referred to as **'Gley's glands'**.

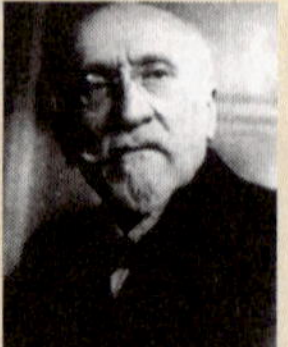

ME Émile Gley
(1857–1930)

Fig. 62.1: Location parathyroid glands. Note that these are 4 small glands (2 superior parathyroids and 2 inferior parathyroids) located behind the thyroid gland. They receive blood supply from thyroid arteries.
Courtesy: Figure 67.11, Clinical Anatomy, Vol. 2, 3rd edition, by Neeta Kulkarni, 2016; Jaypee Brothers Medical Publishers (P) Ltd.

Physiological Anatomy

In human beings, there are four parathyroid glands present in the anterior aspect of the neck embedded posteriorly at four poles in the thyroid tissue (Fig. 62.1). The glands develop at about 10th week of pregnancy from the 3rd and 4th branchial pouches. The total weight of the four glands is about 200 mg, each gland weighing approximately 50 mg. Parathyroid glands derive blood supply from the thyroid arteries.

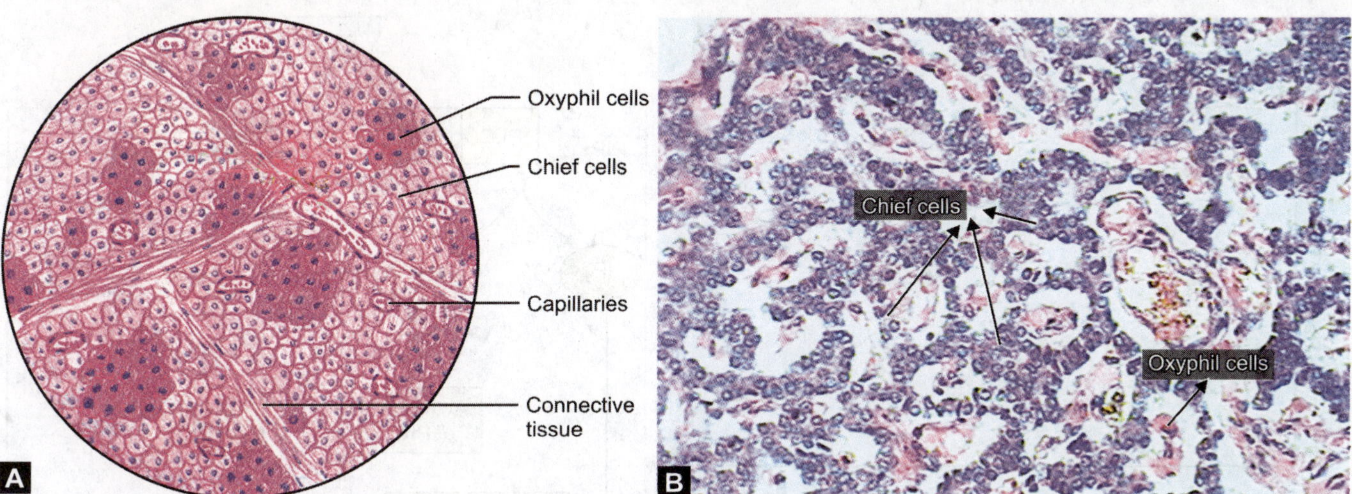

Figs. 62.2A and B: Histology picture and photomicrograph of parathyroid gland. Note the presence of chief cells and oxyphil cells.
Courtesy: Figure 18.6 A & B, Basic Histology, by V Subhadra Devi, 1st edition, 2016; Jaypee Brothers Medical Publishers (P) Ltd.

Cell Types

Parathyroid glands contain **two types of cells**: chief cells and oxyphil cells (Figs. 62.2A and B).

Chief Cells

The chief cells are the **predominant cells** in the parathyroid gland that are present throughout life.

1. They have **bigger Golgi apparatus** in their cytoplasm.
2. They also contain **numerous vesicles and endoplasmic reticulum**.
3. Chief cells **secrete PTH.**

Oxyphil Cells

Oxyphil cells are less plentiful in parathyroid gland. They **appear in the glands during puberty** and then the number increases with the advancement of age.

1. They contain numerous **oxyphil granules**.
2. Normally, they do not secrete PTH. However, **sometimes they secrete PTH** and contribute to parathormone excess.

Parathyroid Hormone (PTH)

Structure

PTH is a single chain polypeptide containing **84 amino acids**. The molecular weight is 9,500. The biological activity, especially the calcium regulating ability of PTH **resides in the N-terminal portion** of the molecule (within amino acids 1–27). The C-terminal portion is not related to its action on calcium metabolism.

Synthesis, Secretion and Metabolism

Like other peptide hormones, PTH is synthesized from the larger precursor molecule called **prepro-PTH** that contains 115 amino acids. The leader sequence containing 25 amino acids is removed from amino terminal in endoplasmic reticulum to form **pro-PTH**, which contains 90 amino acids. In the Golgi apparatus, another six amino acids are removed from the amino terminal to from **PTH** containing 86 amino acids. PTH is then packaged and stored in the granules of chief cells.

Regulation of Secretion

PTH secretion is regulated mainly by **plasma calcium and vitamin D. Other factors** also influence PTH secretion.

Plasma Calcium Level

The major regulator of PTH secretion is the plasma calcium level and they have **inverse relationship.**

1. With increased plasma concentration of ionized calcium, PTH secretion decreases. The relationship is **linear** between 3–6 mg% of the ionized plasma calcium (Fig. 62.3). It may be remembered that about 50% of the total plasma calcium is present in the ionized form. Conversely, with decreased plasma calcium, PTH secretion increases.
2. Recently, the receptors for sensing plasma calcium, the **calcium sensing receptors (CaSR)** have been identified on the membrane of chief cells. The CaSR is a **G-protein coupled receptor** attached to **phospholipase C** and on binding with calcium generates **IP_3 and DAG**.
3. IP_3 and DAG **release calcium** from cytosolic stores and activate protein kinase C that *inhibits PTH secretion*.
4. Another example of increase in calcium inhibiting hormone secretion is **decreased renin release** from JG cells of kidney.

Vitamin D

Vitamin D **inhibits PTH secretion** by decreasing the formation of preproPTH mRNA.

Other Factors

1. **Plasma phosphate:** Usually phosphate does not affect parathormone secretion. However, a rise in plasma

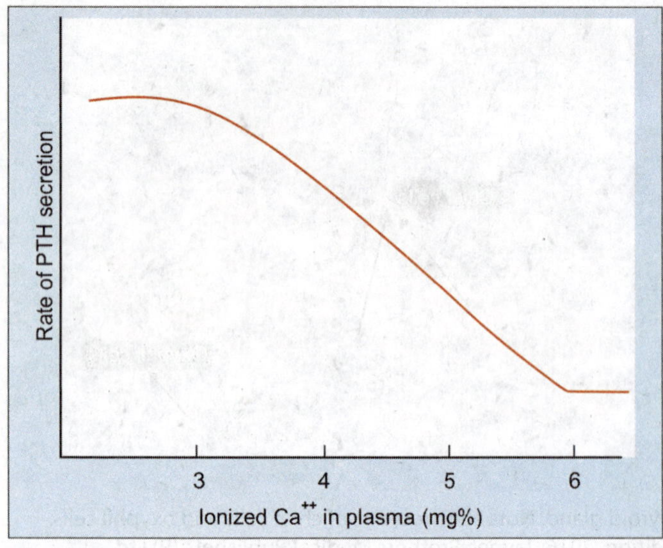

Fig. 62.3: Relation of plasma-ionized calcium with the rate of PTH secretion. Note, from 3 and 6 mg%, the relationship is linear.

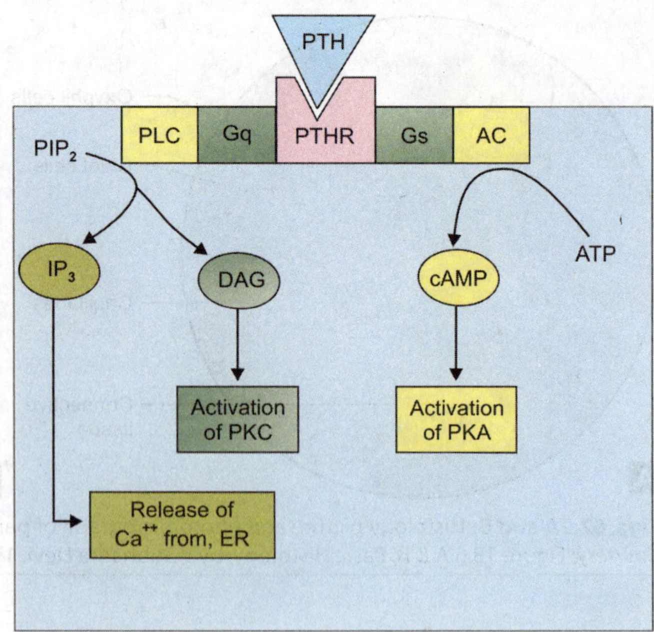

Fig. 62.4: Mechanism of action of PTH. Note, binding of PTH with its receptor (PTHR) activates two signaling pathways (cAMP and IP3-DAG) in the cell. (PK: Protein kinase; PLC: Phospholipase C; AC: Adenylyl cyclase).

phosphate stimulates PTH secretion by lowering plasma calcium and inhibiting formation of 1,25-dihydroxycholecalciferol.

2. **Cyclic AMP, β receptor agonists, dopamine, magnesium and histamine** (H_2 receptor) *stimulate* PTH secretion. **Prostaglandins and α receptor agonists** *inhibit* PTH secretion by decreasing cyclic AMP.

Metabolism of PTH

The normal plasma PTH level is **10–60 pg/mL.**

1. As PTH is **rapidly degraded by Kupffer cells** in liver to carboxy terminal and mid-region fragments, the **half life of PTH is about 10 minutes.**
2. The fragments are cleared by kidneys.
3. However, the **synthetic PTH** which has only 34 amino acid sequence of amino terminal of the natural PTH, possesses all the biological effects of the hormone.

Mechanism of Action

PTH Receptors

There are **three types of PTH receptors.**

Type 1 Receptor (PTH 1R)

It binds to PTH and **PTH related proteins** (PTHrP). The action of PTH to regulate plasma calcium is **mediated via PTH 1R.**

Type 2 Receptors (PTH 2R)

It **binds to PTH**, but not to PTHrP. It is found in brain, pancreas and placenta.

Type 3 Receptor (CPTH)

It reacts only with carboxy terminal of PTH (therefore called **CPTH**) and not with the amino terminal of the hormone.

G Proteins for PTH

PTH 1R and 2R are coupled to two types of G proteins **G_s and G_q**. Therefore, the binding of PTH with the receptors activates both adenylate cyclase and phospholipase C in the membrane. This results in activation of two signaling systems (Fig. 62.4):

1. Activation of **adenylate cyclase-cyclic AMP system** that increases cAMP. cAMP activates protein kinase A that causes phosphorylation of intracellular proteins. Formation of phosphoproteins increases transport of calcium and other ions.
2. Activation of phospholipase C that **increases IP_3 and DAG** in the cell. IP_3 causes intracellular calcium mobilization and DAG causes activation of protein kinase C.

Physiological Actions

The primary action of PTH is to **increase the level of calcium** and **decrease the level of phosphate** in the plasma. This is achieved by the action of PTH on three major target organs: **kidney, bone, and GIT** (Flowchart 62.1). PTH increases the influx of calcium into the plasma. By acting on bone and intestine, it increases phosphate influx but this is counter balanced by its action on kidney where it increases phosphate efflux. Therefore, finally plasma phosphate concentration decreases.

Actions on Kidney

PTH receptors are present on basolateral membrane of the **epithelial cells of proximal and distal tubules.** PTH has **three major effects** on kidney:

1. Increased reabsorption of calcium
2. Decreased reabsorption of phosphate
3. Stimulation of 1, 25-dihydroxycholecalciferol formation.

Increased reabsorption of calcium

Normally, 65% of filtered calcium is reabsorbed in proximal tubule, 25% in thick ascending limb of loop of Henle and 5–10% in distal tubule. About 1–2% of filtered load is excreted in urine.

1. PTH increases calcium reabsorption from kidney by **mainly acting on distal tubule and thick ascending limb of loop of Henle**. Thus, PTH action on kidney *decreases the calcium excretion to a very minimal quantity*.
2. PTH action on kidney is relatively rapid that plasma calcium increases within minutes following its injections.
3. PTH also increases the formation of **1,25-dihydroxycholecalciferol,** which in turn increases calcium absorption from distal tubule of kidney.

Decreased reabsorption of phosphate

PTH decreases reabsorption of phosphate by **mainly acting on proximal tubule**.

1. This causes **phosphaturia.**
2. By decreasing plasma phosphate concentration, PTH prevents calcium-phosphate salts to precipitate.

Stimulation of 1, 25-dihydroxycholecalciferol formation

In kidney, in the mitochondria of proximal tubule, PTH **facilitates the hydroxylation** of 25-hydroxycholecalciferol to **1,25-dihydroxycholecalciferol**, the active form of vitamin D. 1,25-dihydroxycholecalciferol increases calcium reabsorption from kidney, calcium absorption from intestine and calcium mobilization from bone.

Actions on Bone

PTH acts on the **receptors present in osteoblasts and osteoclasts.** Thus, it activates both bone synthesis and resorption. However, the net effect is increased bone resorption and excess mobilization of calcium and phosphates from bones into plasma.

1. **Stimulation of osteoclastic activity:** This is a slower effect of PTH in which **it stimulates osteoclasts** to resorp mineralized bones. In this process both calcium and phosphate are transferred into the ECF. The bone matrix is hydrolyzed by the collagenase and lysosomal enzymes.
   - PTH increases the number and size of osteoclasts and also the synthesis of RNA in the osteoclast.
   - PTH also stimulates the **differentiation of precursor cells** (monocytes, macrophages, etc.) into the osteoclasts. Under the influence of PTH **giant osteoclasts** (osteoclasts of bigger size) are formed that cause resorption of the larger areas of bone (creates large resorption cavity).
   - The **products of bone resorption** are released into the plasma. These include ***calcium, phosphate, hydroxyproline and hydroxylysine***.
   - Excretion of these substances in the urine especially that of **hydroxyproline is an index of osteoclastic activity**.
2. **Stimulation of osteolysis:** PTH activates the process of **osteocytic osteolysis**.
   - In this process, calcium is transferred from the bone fluid into the osteocyte and then from osteocytes into osteoblasts.
   - Osteoblasts then pump calcium into the extracellular matrix.
   - Calcium is also pumped into the ECF.
3. **PTH also acts on osteoblasts:** PTH **inhibits the synthesis of collagen** by osteoblasts at higher concentration.
   - However, **at lower doses**, *PTH increases osteoblastic activity* and increases collagen synthesis. Especially, **trabecular bone mass is increased.**
   - This anabolic effect is mediated by increased secretion of insulin like growth factors and transforming growth factors.
   - Therefore, the **net effect** of PTH on bone is ***increase in the bone mass in lower concentration*** and ***decrease in bone mass in higher concentration.***

In primary hyperparathyroidism (due to parathyroid adenoma), hypercalcemia, hypophosphatemia, hypercalciuria (due to increased filtered load of calcium), and renal calculi are usually seen. Areas of ***osteoclastic hyperactivity*** and ***bone resorption*** are present along with excessive and ***disorganized trabecular bone formation***. In hypoparathyroidism, generally bone mass is increased.

Actions on GI tract

Acting on intestine, PTH **increases absorption of calcium**. However, this effect is **mostly indirect**, mediated through *1,25-dihydroxycholecalciferol*, which is formed in kidney by PTH.

Thus, the overall effects of PTH are to increase plasma level of calcium and decrease plasma level of phosphate (Flowchart 62.1).

Applied Physiology

Hyperparathyroidism

Hyperparathyroidism or PTH excess is divided into **two main categories:**

1. Primary hyperparathyroidism
2. Secondary hyperparathyroidism.

Primary Hyperparathyroidism

Primary hyperparathyroidism occurs due to the tumor of parathyroid gland such as parathyroid adenoma that secretes excess PTH. It may be part of multiple endocrine neoplasia (MEN) syndrome. It is common in MEN type 1.

1. The disease is characterized by hypercalcemia, hypophosphatemia, demineralization of bone, hypercalciuria, and renal stone formation.
2. The chronic effect of parathyroid excess results in the bone disease called osteitis fibrosa. There will be features of osteopenia and fracture.

Flowchart 62.1: Summary of effects of PTH.

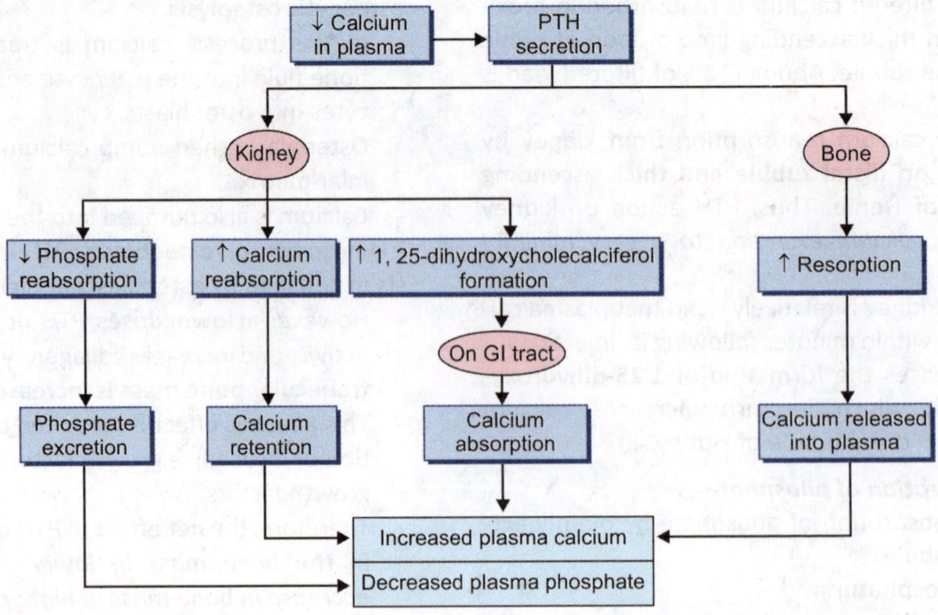

3. In this disease, the bone marrow is fibrosed and bone resorption exceeds the bone formation.

Secondary Hyperparathyroidism

Secondary hyperparathyroidism occurs in chronic renal disease and rickets.

1. In these diseases, the chronic hypocalcemia causes increased secretion of PTH.
2. This results in secondary hypertrophy of parathyroid glands.
3. Neonatal primary hyperparathyroidism has also been described that occurs due to a genetic defect.

In malignancy: *Hypercalcemia* occurs in malignancies.

- This is mainly due to the **bone metastases** by the cancer cells that cause **local osteolysis** which results in hypercalcemia.
- Hypercalcemia also occurs in malignancy due to **ectopic secretion of PTH** or PTH related proteins (PTH rP).
- Usually, it is seen in the **cancers of breast, kidney, lungs, ovary, and skin.**

Hypoparathyroidism

Hypoparathyroidism is rarely seen as a disease of parathyroid gland. Rather, the common entity is **pseudohypoparathyroidism** in which symptoms of PTH deficiency are observed in the presence of normal PTH level in plasma.

There are **two types** of pseudohypoparathyroidism:

1. A **congenital variety**, in which the PTH does not increase the cyclic AMP and IP_3 formation in the target cells due to a receptor defect.
2. Another variety in which cyclic AMP synthesis by PTH remains normal but PTH **fails to produce phosphaturic effect.**

In hypoparathyroidism, hypocalcemia and increased bone density are main feature.

Hypocalcemic Tetany

Hyposecretion of parathyroid is rather common **following thyroid surgery** in which parathyroid glands are usually removed by mistake along with thyroid tissue. This causes severe hypoparathyroidism that leads to acute hypocalcemic tetany.

Effects of Parathyroidectomy

PTH is essential for maintenance of plasma calcium concentration. Acute deficiency of PTH results in neuromuscular defects that endanger life. Therefore, PTH is essential for survival. The symptoms of tetany following thyroid surgery develop in 24 to 48 hours postoperatively.

The features of tetany are:

1. **Chvostek's sign:** This is the quick contraction of facial muscles of the same side by tapping over the facial nerve at the angle of jaw.
2. **Trousseau's sign:** The spasm of the muscles of the upper extremity that causes flexion of the wrist and thumb (i.e. flexion at metacarpophalangeal joints) with extension of fingers (i.e. extension of interphalangeal joints).
3. **Carpopedal spasm:** There is also spasm of muscles at the wrist joints (carpal spasm) (Fig. 62.5). The changes at wrist and ankle joints together called as carpopedal spasm.
4. **Laryngospasm:** In hypocalcemic tetany, usually patients die due to hypoxia that occurs due to laryngospasm. The muscles of larynx contract and occlude the laryngeal passage.
5. **Hypocalcemia:** Significant hypocalcemia occurs.
6. Hyperphosphatemia.

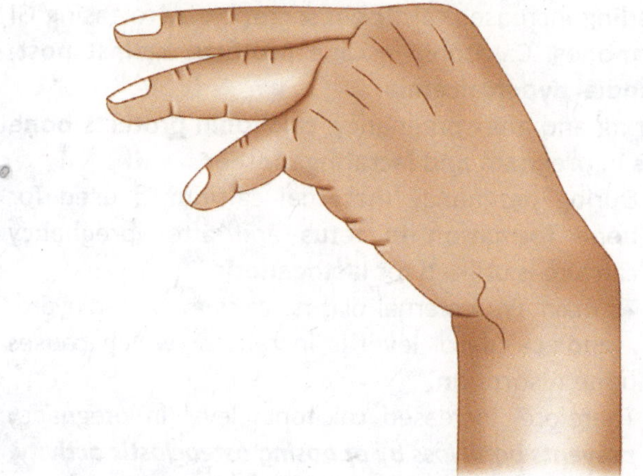

Fig. 62.5: Carpal component of carpopedal spasm.
Courtesy: Figure 8.16, Physiology Preparatory Manual for Undergraduates, by Sanoop KS et al, Jaypee Brothers Medical Publishers (P) Ltd.

The **treatment** of hypocalcemic tetany includes immediate administration of ionized calcium and parathormone.

Parathyroid Hormone-related Protein

The protein with PTH activity has been described recently. This is called parathyroid hormone related protein (**PTHrP**). This is produced by many tissues in the body. It is a **polypeptide containing 140 amino acids**. The gene that encodes the formation of PTHrP is present on the human **chromosome 12** (it should be noted that the gene for PTH is present on chromosome 11). PTHrP has marked homology with the PTH.

Functions of PTHrP

1. PTHrP stimulates **proliferation of chondrocytes** in developing cartilage and inhibits their mineralization.
2. It also **acts as a growth factor** for the development of skin, hair follicle, and breast.
3. PTHrP is produced in large quantities in the lactating breast tissue and secreted in the milk. However, the plasma concentration of PTHrP does not increase during lactation.
4. PTHrP has also been described in kidney (renal glomeruli) and in the brain (cortex, hippocampus and cerebellum). But, functions of PTHrP in these organs are not clearly known.
5. It also causes calcium transport in placenta.
6. PTHrP is elevated in hypercalcemia of malignancy (Clinical Box 62.1)

Clinical Box 62.1

Hypercalcemia of Malignancy: Hypercalcemia is common in malignancy. In 80% cases, it is due to elevated PTHrP. This is known as **humoral hypercalcemia of malignancy**. That commonly occurs in malignancy of ovary, breast, kidney and skin. In rest 20% cases, hypercalcemia is due to secondary metastasis of bones that erodes the bone and release calcium. This is called **local osteolytic hypercalcemia**.

Calcitonin

Source and Structure

Calcitonin is secreted from **parafollicular cells (C cells)** of the thyroid gland. The parafollicular cells develop from ultimobranchial bodies, a pair of glands that develop from 5th branchial pouch.

1. Calcitonin is a polypeptide hormone containing **32 amino acids**. The molecular weight is 3,500.
2. The **calcitonin gene** that transcribes mRNA to form calcitonin is processed to form a different mRNA in the nervous system where it forms **calcitonin gene-related peptides** (CGRP).
3. CGRP is a potent vasodilator.

Synthesis, Secretion and Metabolism

Synthesis and Secretion

The **major stimulus** for calcitonin secretion is the **rise in plasma calcium level**. Above the concentration of 9 mg% of plasma calcium, the secretion of calcium becomes directly proportional to the calcium concentration.

Other stimuli: The β receptor agonists, dopamine, GI hormones (CCK, glucagons, gastrin, secretin), and estrogen stimulate calcitonin secretion. ***Gastrin*** is a strong stimulus for calcitonin release (Clinical Box 62.2).

Clinical Box 62.2

Calcitonin is more in Zollinger-Ellison syndrome and in pernicious anemia: Gastrin stimulates calcitonin secretion. Therefore, plasma calcitonin concentration is raised in Zollinger-Ellison syndrome and in pernicious anemia as gastrin concentration increases in these diseases.

Metabolism

The concentration of calcitonin in plasma is 10–20 pg/mL. The concentration increases to almost 10 fold in hypercalcemia. The hormone is degraded in the liver. The half life of calcitonin is 5–10 minutes.

Mechanism of Action

Calcitonin acts on calcitonin receptors present on the target cells. The receptors are coupled to G_s proteins and therefore, stimulate the **adenylate cyclase–cyclic AMP system**.

Physiological Actions

Calcitonin decreases the plasma calcium level by acting mainly on bones and kidney (Flowchart 62.2).

Effects on Bone

Calcitonin mainly acts on the osteoclasts.

1. It **decreases osteoclastic activity**. Thus, it **inhibits the bone resorption**. The number and size of osteoclasts decrease.
2. The action of calcitonin on bone is just opposite to that of PTH with respect to the calcium turnover in the bone.

Flowchart 62.2: Summary of effects of calcitonin.

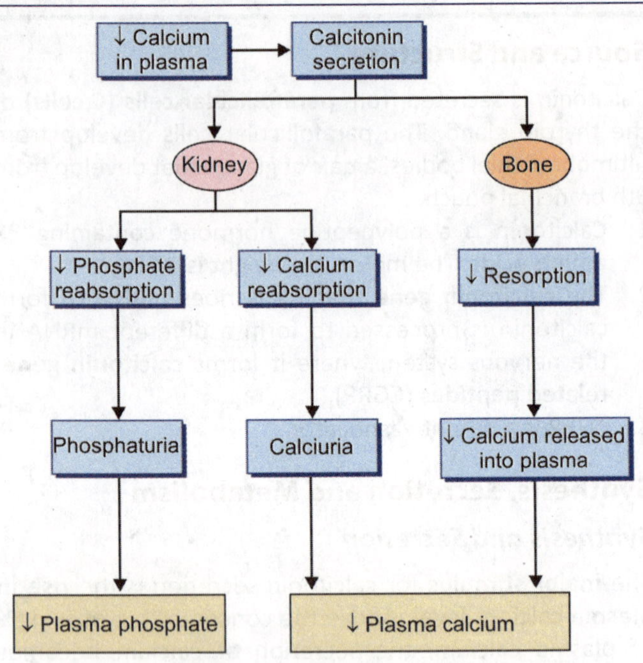

3. However, the effect on phosphate turnover is same as that of PTH. It **decreases plasma phosphate level**. This is due to inhibition of bone resorption, facilitation of phosphate entry into the bone, and also mild increase in urinary phosphate excretion.
4. Thus, the hypophosphatemic effect of calcitonin is independent of hypocalcemic effect.

Effects on Kidney

It **decreases calcium reabsorption** from kidney. Therefore, it produces calciuria. It also causes mild phosphaturia by acting on proximal tubule.

Calcitonin Escape

Injection of calcitonin produces hypocalcemia mainly **by antiosteoclastic activity**. However, this antiresorptive action of calcitonin begins to **wane within hours**.

1. The body escapes from hypocalcemic effects of calcitonin. This is called **calcitonin escape**, the exact mechanism of which is not known.
2. It is probably due to **rapid down regulation of calcium receptors**. Therefore, calcitonin is effective in decreasing plasma calcium only for a short duration.
3. This **limits the use of calcitonin** in long-term management of hypercalcemia.

Physiological Significance

1. Due to calcitonin escape phenomenon, the **bones remain essentially normal** in conditions of hypersecretion of calcitonin like medullary carcinoma of thyroid.
2. Calcitonin is **secreted more in young individuals**, which is believed to play some role in skeletal development.
3. **Feeding** increases calcitonin secretion by releasing GI hormones. Calcitonin escape **protects against post-prandial hypercalcemia**.
4. During and after pregnancy, **calcitonin protects bone loss in pregnant and lactating mother**.
   - During pregnancy maternal calcium is used for bone **formation in fetus** and after pregnancy calcium is utilized for **lactogenesis.**
   - To maintain maternal plasma calcium, 1,25-dihydroxycholecalciferol level is increased, which causes bone resorption.
   - Therefore, increased calcitonin level in pregnancy ***prevents bone loss by opposing osteoclastic activity***.
5. Calcitonin and CGRP are found together in some brain regions like pituitary, hypothalamus, limbic system etc, where they **act as co-transmitters**. They inhibit transmission of pain impulses in CNS independent of opioid system.

Applied Aspects

Clinical Use of Calcitonin

Calcitonin is used in the treatment of hypercalcemia, and in the diseases in which osteoclastic activity needs to be reduced, for example in **Paget's disease.** Calcitonin is sometimes used as a *central analgesic* as it blocks the transmission of pain impulses in CNS.

Paget's Disease

In this disease, increased osteoclastic activity of unknown etiology results in **localized regions of bone resorption** followed by a compensatory osteoblastic activity causing **patchy new bone formations**.

1. Thus, pagetic bones are structurally **disorganized and susceptible to deformities.**
2. **X-ray** pictures show areas of increased density and resorptive cavities.
3. Though most of the patients are initially asymptomatic, bone deformities resulting in compressive neuropathy and subsequent neuromuscular dysfunctions are not uncommon.
4. The disease is **treated by daily injections of calcitonin.**
5. **Bisphosphonates** like ***etidronate and pamidronate*** are more useful in preventing bone resorption.

Vitamin D

Vitamin D increases plasma calcium level by increasing calcium absorption from GI tract, calcium reabsorption from kidney and mobilization of calcium from bone. It has similar effects on phosphate.

Synthesis of Vitamin D

Vitamin D is acquired from **two sources** in human being. 1. Skin (ultraviolet irradiation of skin produces vitamin D), and 2. Diet.

From Skin

Vitamin D_3 is **synthesized in keratinocytes** present in the epidermis.

1. When the skin is exposed to sunlight (**ultraviolet radiation at 290–315 nm**), 7-dehydrocholesterol in the skin is converted to previtamin-D_3. For this conversion to occur, **minimum 20 mJ radiation energy** per sq-cm of skin is required.
2. Previtamin-D_3 is then ***automatically converted to vitamin D_3*** in another 3 days.
3. However, **continuous exposure** to sun light ***prevents*** this conversion.
4. Thus, mild to **moderate exposure to sunlight induces**, whereas ***excessive exposure prevents*** vitamin D synthesis.

From Diet

In food, minimum of 2.5 µg vitamin D should be ingested daily (**daily dietary recommendation** is 10 µg or 400 units). The **important sources** of vitamin D are liver, fish, cod liver oil and milk. Vitamin D ingested in the diet has very little biological activity.

1. It undergoes activation in the body to be converted into the active vitamin D. This requires successive **hydroxylations** in the liver and kidney.
2. In the liver, it is hydroxylated at position 25 by microsomal and mitochondrial enzyme, to form **25-hydroxycholecalciferol** which undergoes further hydroxylation in the kidney at 1 position to form **1, 25-dihydroxycholecalciferol** (Flowchart 62.3).
3. This occurs mainly in the mitochondria in epithelial cells of **proximal and straight tubules**.
4. The 1, 25-dihydroxycholecalciferol is the active metabolite of vitamin D.

Flowchart 62.3: Steps of synthesis of active Vitamin D_3.

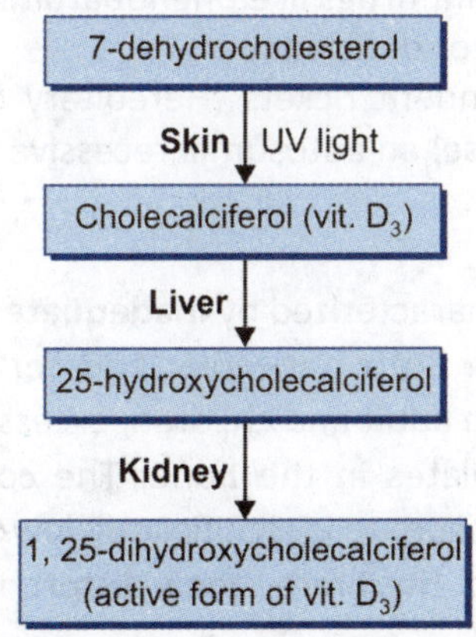

Mechanism of Action

There are vitamin D receptors in the GIT, bone, and kidney. Mechanism of Vitamin D action is **like that of steroid hormones**.

1. It binds with the **nuclear receptors** and induces receptor phosphorylation, which targets DNA molecules.
2. The major product of vitamin D action is the increase in intracellular calcium binding protein called **calbindin**.

Physiological Actions

Vitamin D increases plasma calcium level by acting on intestine, kidney and bone (Flowchart 62.4).

On small intestine: Vitamin D mainly acts on the intestine to **facilitate calcium absorption** against the concentration gradient.

1. It combines with the receptors on the brush border of the intestinal epithelial cells and **increases number of calcium pumps** (Ca^{++}-H^+ ATPase molecules) and **calcium channels** in the basolateral membrane and

Flowchart 62.4: Summary of physiological effects of vitamin D.

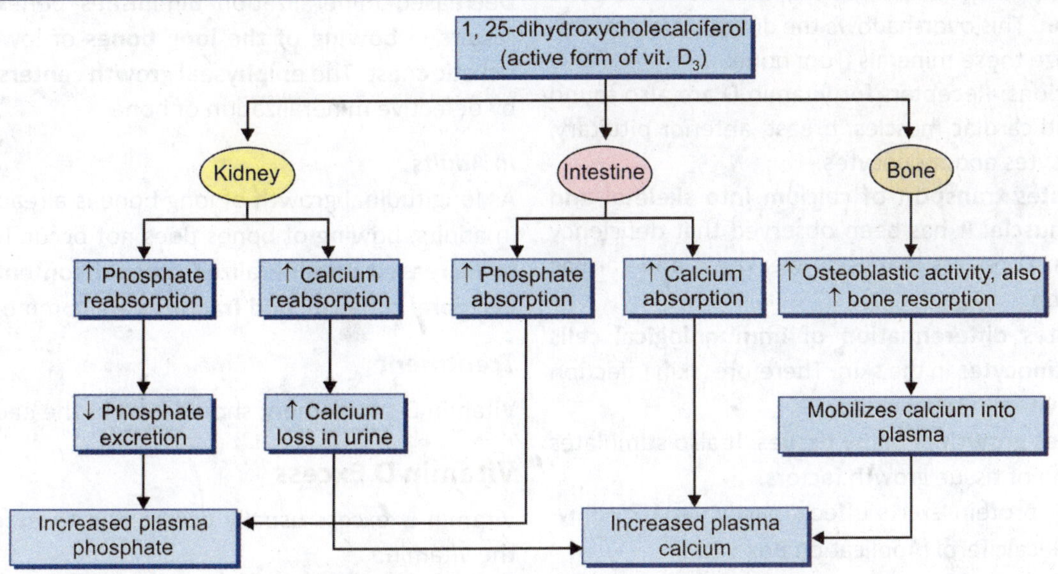

calbindin in the cytosol of the epithelial cells of the intestine.

2. Thus, **calcium is actively pumped** from the cell into the ECF.
3. It also facilitates the **absorption of phosphate and magnesium** across the intestinal epithelium.
4. PTH stimulates intestinal calcium absorption by promoting formation of 1, 25-dihydroxycholecalciferol in kidney.

On kidney: It acts synergistically with PTH to **increase calcium reabsorption** from kidney.

1. It increases **number of calcium pumps** in the epithelial cells of proximal and distal tubules.
2. Unlike PTH that causes phosphate excretion, vitamin D **increases phosphate reabsorption** from kidney.

On bone: It **acts on osteoblasts** that have receptors for vitamin D.

1. It increases **synthetic activity of osteoblasts.**
2. It is also necessary for normal **mineralization of bone.** Mineralization of newly formed osteoid depends on vitamin D.
3. It also **stimulates bone resorption**, not by directly ***increasing the osteoclastic activity***, but by stimulating various paracrine signals that originate from the osteoblasts. Activated osteoclasts produce a number of proteins including phosphatase and collagenase that **lyse bone matrix.**
4. It promotes development of osteoclasts from their precursor cells.
5. It also **increases osteocytic osteolysis.**
6. Thus, the direct effect of vitamin D on bone is to **mobilize calcium**, which is contrary to its overall effect of promoting mineralization.

In summary, vitamin D **increases calcium and phosphate absorption from intestine**, and their reabsorption **from kidney**. Thus, vitamin D increases plasma level of calcium and phosphate (Flowchart 62.4), that increases **bone mineralization**. This overshadows the direct action of vitamin to mobilize these minerals from bone.

Other actions: Receptors for vitamin D are also found in skeletal and cardiac muscles, breast, anterior pituitary, skin, lymphocytes and monocytes.

1. It **stimulates transport of calcium into skeletal and cardiac muscle**. It has been observed that deficiency of vitamin D results in muscle weakness and cardiac dysfunction.
2. It promotes **differentiation of immunological cells and keratinocytes** in the skin. Therefore, skin infection is high in vitamin D deficiency.
3. It **regulates growth of many tissues**. It also stimulates production of tissue growth factors.
4. Anti-aging protein exerts effects partly via 1,25-dihydroxycholecalciferol (Application Box 62.1).

Application Box 62.1

α-Klotho partly acts through Vit. D: The anti-aging protein α-Klotho that plays a major role in calcium and phosphate metabolism has been observed to act partly through 1,25-dihydroxycholecalciferol.

- α-Klotho facilitates membrane localization of proteins that are involved in calcium and phosphate reabsorption, such as TRPV5 and Na^+-K^+ ATPase.
- It enhances the activity of FGF-23 (fibroblast growth factor) by acting at the receptor level.
- FGF-23 ***decreases the renal NaPi-IIc activity*** and ***inhibits synthesis of 1α-hydroxylase*** that reduces the level of 1,25-dihydroxycholecalciferol.

Vitamin D Deficiency

(Rickets and Osteomalacia)

Deficiency of vitamin D causes **rickets in children** and **osteomalacia in adults.**

Causes

1. Inadequate intake
2. Lack of exposure to sunlight
3. Chronic liver disease (inadequate 25 hydroxylation)
4. Chronic renal disease (inadequate 1 hydroxylation)
5. Hypoparathyroidism
6. Anticonvulsant drugs like phenobarbital
7. Vit. D receptor deficiency
8. Vit. D dependent rickets (Hereditary deficiency of 1 α-hydroxylase, an autosomal recessive disorder).

Features

The disease is characterized by **inadequate mineralization of bone matrix**. Both trabecular and cortical bones are involved. In both adult and children, excess unmineralized osteoid accumulates in the bone. The concentration of calcium and phosphate is significantly low. **Bone strength is reduced**, and therefore, they distort in response to mechanical load.

In Children

Decreased mineralization diminishes bone rigidity that results in **bowing of the long bones** of lower limbs and ricketic chest. The **epiphyseal growth centers are affected** by defective mineralization of bone.

In Adults

As longitudinal growth of long bone is already completed in adults, bowing of bones does not occur. However, due to **increased unmineralized osteoid content**, bone pain, **vertebral collapse, and fractures** are common.

Treatment

Vitamin D supplement should start at the earliest.

Vitamin D Excess

Vitamin D excess usually occurs due to **excess intake** of the vitamin.

1. It causes hypercalcemia, hypercalciuria, and kidney stones.
2. Increased bone resorption is not uncommon.
3. Hyperphosphatemia is also present.

Other Hormones Affecting Calcium and Bone Metabolism

Glucocorticoids

Glucocorticoid decrease plasma calcium level by **inhibiting osteoclastic activity** and decreasing calcium absorption from intestine. Therefore, cortisol excess causes osteoporosis.

Growth Hormone

It increases calcium absorption from intestine, though it also promotes calcium excretion in urine. The net effect is mild increase in plasma calcium. Stimulates osteoblastic activity and bone formation.

Growth Factors

Promote protein synthesis in bone. Bone formation is increased.

Insulin

Promotes bone formation. Bone loss occurs in chronic diabetes.

Thyroid Hormones

In excess, cause hypercalcemia and hypercalciuria. The net long-term effects are **demineralization of bone** and osteoporosis.

Estrogen

Inhibits osteoclastic activity and prevents osteoporosis.

Testosterone

Maintains normal bone mass and **promotes bone development**.

CHAPTER SUMMARY

Key Concepts

1. The primary action of PTH is to increase the level of calcium and decrease the level of phosphate in the plasma. Though PTH acts on both osteoblasts and osteoclasts and activates both bone synthesis and resorption, the net effect is increased bone resorption and excess mobilization of calcium into plasma.
2. Calcitonin decreases the plasma calcium level by acting mainly on bones and kidney. It decreases osteoclastic activity and inhibits the bone resorption. The number and size of osteoclasts decrease.
3. Therefore, for normal bone health (balance between osteoblastic and osteoclastic activity), the normal concentration of PTH and calcitonin should be maintained.
4. Vit. D is also necessary for normal **mineralization of bone**. Mineralization of newly formed osteoid depends on vitamin D. It also increases **synthetic activity of osteoblasts**.

Important to Know (Must Read)

1. In examination, 'Describe the hormones regulating calcium and bone metabolism', 'Describe the regulation of secretion and physiological actions of parathyroid hormone (PTH)' may be asked as **Long Questions**.
2. Hypoparathyroidism, Effects of Parathyroidectomy, Hypocalcemic tetany, Calcitonin, Physiological actions of vitamin D, Causes, features and treatment of rickets and osteomalacia are usual **Short Questions** in exam.
3. In **Viva**, examiner may ask— Name the three main hormones regulating calcium and bone metabolism, List the other hormones regulating calcium and bone metabolism, List the physiological actions of parathyroid hormone, List the physiological actions of calcitonin, List the physiological actions of vitamin D, Name the features of hypocalcemic tetany, What is treatment of hypocalcemic tetany, What are types and features of hyperparathyroidism, What is osteitis fibrosa, Why hypercalcemia occurs in malignancies, What is pseudohypoparathyroidism and what are the types, What are the causes, features and treatment of rickets and osteomalacia, How is the secretion of PTH regulated, Physiological anatomy and cell types of parathyroid gland, Name the PTH receptors, What is parathyroid hormone related protein (PTHrP) and what are its functions, What is the mechanism of action of PTH, What are the factors that stimulate calcitonin secretion, What is calcitonin escape, What are the physiological significances of calcitonin escape, What are the clinical uses of calcitonin, What are the causes, features and treatment of Paget's disease, What are the sources of vitamin D, What are the steps of synthesis of vitamin D, What is the mechanism of action of vitamin D, Wdat are the functions of Vit D, What is α- Klotho and what are its functions, What are the features of vitamin D excess, What is the difference between osteoporosis and osteomalacia, What is Gley's glands.

CHAPTER 63

Pineal Gland

Learning Objectives

On completion of study of this chapter, the student **MUST** be able to:

1. Understand the importance of pineal gland in regulation of body functions.
2. List the hormones secreted from Pineal gland.
3. Give the steps of melatonin synthesis.
4. List the functions of pineal gland.

The student **MAY** also be able to:

1. Describe the functions of pineal gland.

Pineal gland, also known as ***epiphysis*** was initially described as the main controlling center in the brain that influences many CNS functions. In fact, for centuries, it has attracted attention of many researchers in physiology and medicine for its role in integral control of the being. However, till date functions of pineal gland are not clearly understood except its role in **melatonin secretion** and **control of light-dark cycle**. It is known to act as photoreceptor in fish, amphibian and reptiles, a biological clock in birds, and has become an endocrine gland in mammals. However, more research needs to be done in human beings to reveal the role of pineal in the evolutionary progression of the mankind.

PHYSIOLOGICAL ANATOMY

Pineal is embryologically derived from an evagination of the roof of third ventricle between the habenular and posterior commissures. Along with habenular and posterior commissures it makes up the epithalamus.

1. It is connected by a stalk to the posterior and habenular commissures (Fig. 63.1).
2. The stroma of the pineal gland consists of **neuroglial cells, pinealocytes, and parenchymal tissue.** Pinealocytes possess secretory function (Fig. 63.2).
3. It is **larger in size during infancy and childhood**. It regresses at the time of puberty and is **small in size in adults.**

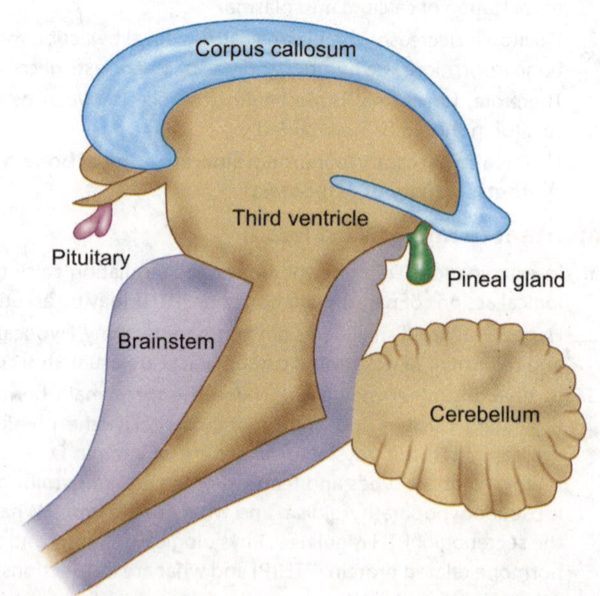

Fig. 63.1: Location of pineal in the brain.

4. The plasma level of melatonin, which is secreted from pineal gland, in children is about 250 pg/ml, which is much higher than the level in adults, i.e. about 70 pg/ml.

Hormones of the Pineal Gland

Pineal gland secretes the hormone **melatonin**. Recently, it has been detected that pineal gland secretes **many other**

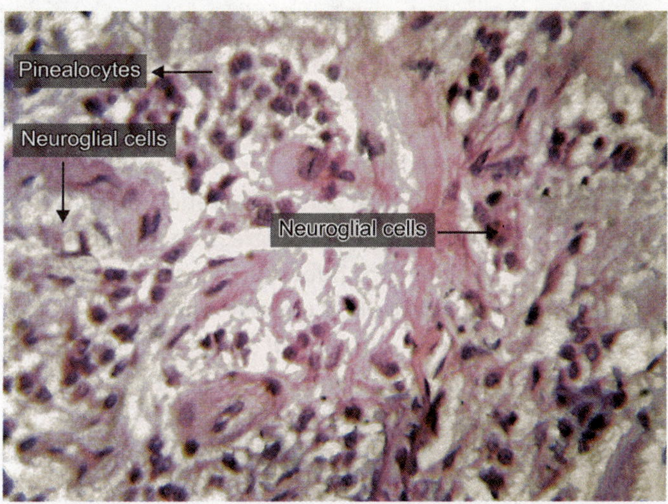

Fig. 63.2: Histology of pineal gland showing neuroglial cells and pinealocytes.
Courtesy: Figure 18.9B, Basic Histology, by V Subhadra Devi, 1st edition, 2016; Jaypee Brothers Medical Publishers (P) Ltd.

Flowchart 63.1: Synthesis of melatonin.

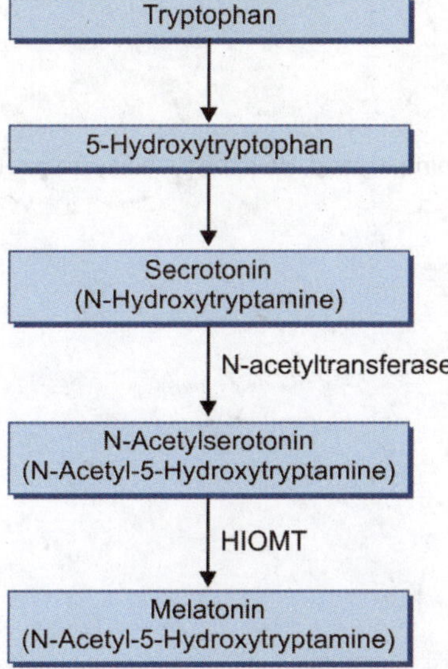

(HIOMT: Hydroxyindole-O-methyltransferase).

peptides that influence hypothalamic and other endocrine secretions. Peptides that have been identified in pineal gland in mammals are **arginine vasotocin, arginine vasopressin, oxytocin, pro-opiomelanocortin** derived peptides like *ACTH, α-MSH and β-endorphin*, **angiotensin II, renin like activity, and TRH and GnRH** like peptides. Thus, pineal gland might be involved in control of many endocrinal functions of the body.

Melatonin

Melatonin is N-acetyl-5-methoxytryptamine, which is synthesized from the amino acid tryptamine (Flowchart 63.1). It is synthesized by the parenchymal cells of the pineal gland and then released into circulation and CSF.

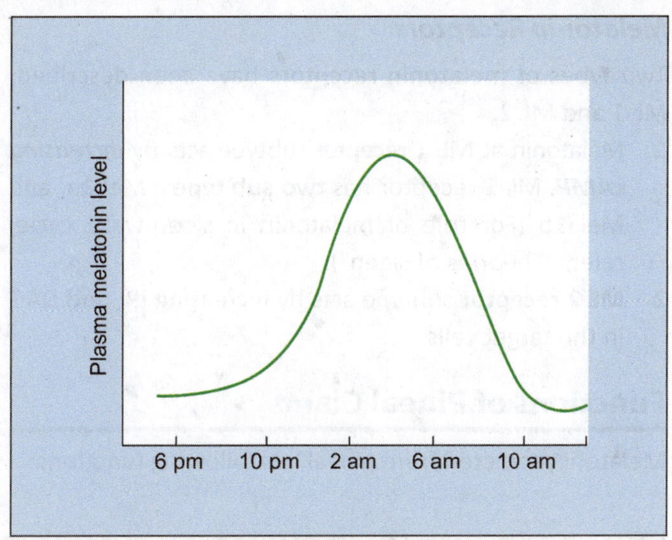

Fig. 63.3: Diurnal variation in melatonin secretion. Note, secretion is maximum between 11 PM and 7 AM.

Flowchart 63.2: Pathway from retina that causes melatonin secretion during night.

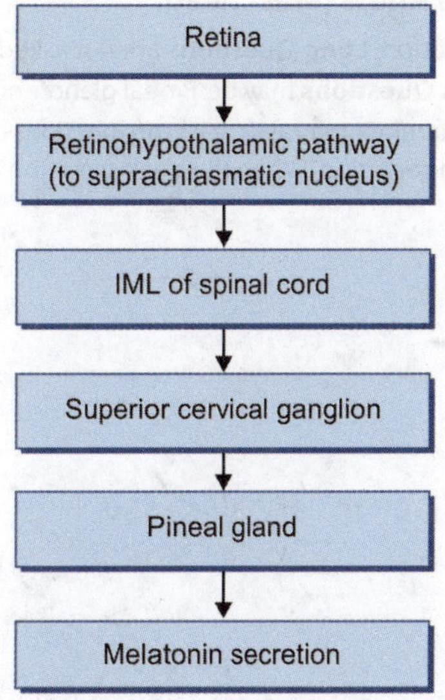

1. Melatonin secretion exhibits a remarkable **diurnal variation**. The secretion is maximum in the night, especially between 11 pm and 7 am (Fig. 63.3).
2. It is proposed that this **diurnal variation** is due to the alteration in sympathetic discharge to the pineal gland, mediated by norepinephrine via β receptors.
3. The **pineal sympathetic output** synchronized with light dark cycle is controlled by **inputs from retinohypothalamic pathway** that projects to suprachiasmatic nucleus.
4. Fibers from **suprachiasmatic nucleus** terminate in intermediolateral gray column of the thoracic spinal cord that in turn projects to *superior cervical ganglion* from where fibers originate to end in the pineal gland (Flowchart 63.2).

Melatonin Receptors

Two types of **melatonin receptors** have been described: ML 1 and ML 2.

1. Melatonin at **ML 1 receptor** subtype acts ***by increasing cAMP***. ML 1 receptor has **two sub types**: Mel 1a, and Mel 1b (For role of melatonin in sleep-wake cycle, refer, "Theories of sleep").
2. **ML 2 receptor** subtype acts by increasing IP_3 and DAG in the target cells.

Functions of Pineal Gland

Melatonin secreted from pineal has following functions:

1. Melatonin secreted from pineal has a definite **diurnal pattern**. This diurnal change in melatonin level is believed to coordinate the endocrinal responses of the body with the light-dark cycle in the environment.
2. Melatonin secreted from pineal **inhibits gonadal function**. It is believed that pineal secretion **inhibits the onset of puberty**. Therefore, regression of pineal stimulates the beginning of pubertal changes. It has been observed that ***precocious puberty and sexual precocity are associated with pineal abnormalities***.
3. In lower animals, melatonin influences the activity of melanophores and thereby controls **skin color**. However, such function in human appears to be uncertain.

CHAPTER SUMMARY

Key Concepts

1. Though pineal gland is known to secrete melatonin, and control circadian rhythm, it might have many more functions.
2. The size of pineal gland decreases with the maturation of sex organs. May be melatonin is meant of inhibition for basic instincts, especially functions related to mating.

Important to Know (Must Read)

1. In examination, **Long Questions** are not asked from this chapter.
2. The **Short Questions** may be 'Pineal gland' and 'Melatonin'.
3. In **Viva**, examiner may ask... List the functions of pineal gland, List the hormones of pineal gland, How the pathway from retina stimulates melatonin secretion, When the peak secretion of melatonin occurs.

CHAPTER 64

Local Hormones

Learning Objectives

On completion of study of this chapter, the student **MUST** be able to:

1. Name the local hormones.
2. Name the receptors and describe the functions of histamine and serotonin
3. Classify prostaglandins and describe their functions.
4. Give the functions of other local hormones.

The student **MAY** also be able to:

1. Describe the function of all local hormones.
2. Explain the role of local hormones in various functions and dysfunctions of the body.

DEFINITION AND TYPES

Definition: Local hormones are chemicals that are secreted locally from an endocrine tissue that are primarily involved in control of local tissue functions where they are secreted.

Types: The known local hormones are: renin, erythropoietin, ANP, melatonin, thymosin, histamine, serotonin, bradykinin, and prostaglandins.

Histamine

Source, Synthesis and Metabolism

Histamine is secreted from **mast cells and basophils**:

1. It is widely distributed in mammalian tissues.
2. It has highest concentration in the skin, gastric mucosa, pituitary and lungs.
3. Histamine is synthesized from the amino acid **histidine** by the action of enzyme *histidine decarboxylase*.
4. Histamine is converted to **methylhistamine** by *histamine-N-methyltransferase,* which is further converted to **methyl-imidazole-acetic acid** (Flowchart 64.1).

Flowchart 64.1: Synthesis and metabolism of histamine.

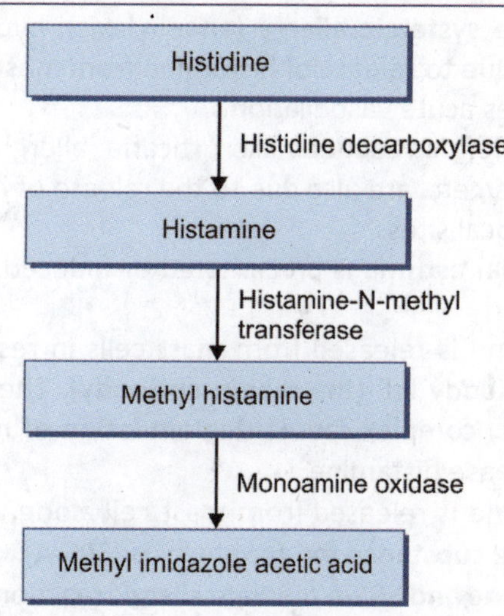

Histamine Receptors

Three types of histamine receptors have been described so far. They are: H_1, H_2 and H_3 receptors. All are found in brain and peripheral tissues.

H_1 receptors: They are attached to phospholipase C. On activation, they produce **IP_3 and DAG** in the cell. These receptors mediate inflammation and allergy.

H_2 receptors: Histamine at H_2 receptors acts by **increasing intracellular cAMP**. They are found in gastric mucosa and mediate gastric acid secretion.

H_3 receptors: They are found in CNS, especially in presynaptic membrane and are coupled to G proteins. They inhibit release of histamine and other neurotransmitters from presynaptic nerve terminals.

Physiological Actions

Histamine acts mainly on the cardiovascular system, smooth muscles, and exocrine secretions. It mediates inflammation and allergy.

On CVS

Histamine is a **potent vasodilator**. It decreases blood pressure (causes **hypotension**). It also **decreases the cardiac output**.

On Smooth Muscles

Histamine increases tone of most of the smooth muscles. It **increases intestinal motility** and causes **bronchoconstriction**.

On Exocrine Secretions

Histamine is a powerful **stimulator of HCl secretion** from parietal cells stomach. It also potentiates salivary, pancreatic, and intestinal secretions.

Role in Inflammation

It is an important mediator of inflammation. Histamine, by causing **local vasodilation** increases blood flow at the site of inflammation and by **increasing capillary permeability** causes local swelling. It mediates responses (triple response) to local injury.

Role in Allergy

Allergic reactions are mostly mediated via histamine:
1. **In acute systemic allergy** (anaphylaxis), hypotension occurs due to release of histamine from mast cell that produces acute vasodilation.
2. **Local allergic reactions** like urticaria, allergic rhinitis, hay fever, etc. are also due to the release of histamine at the local sites.
3. **Bronchial asthma** is precipitated or induced by histamine.
4. Histamine is released from mast cells in response to the antibody IgE (the **reagin antibody**). The antigen-antibody complex causes **degranulation of mast cells** and release histamine.
5. Histamine is released from mast cell along with **slow reacting substance for anaphylaxis** (SRS-A).
6. **Histamine and SRS-A** mediate allergic reactions. Hence, **antihistaminics** are mainstay of treatment for allergies.

Relation with Itch

Histamine acts as a neurotransmitter for itch sensation. Experimentally, when histamine is injected into the skin, it produces sever itch. Itching associated with skin allergy (urticaria) is cured by antihistaminics.

On CNS

Histamine is a neurotransmitter in many areas of the CNS. Histaminergic neurons project from tuberomamillary nucleus to all parts of the brain. These histaminergic fibers are involved in the control of blood pressure, sexual and ingestive behaviors, arousal and alertness, pain and secretion of anterior pituitary hormones.

Clinical Correlation

Antihistaminic Drugs

Antihistaminics are used frequently in clinical practice for the treatment of allergy and inflammations.

H_1 receptor antagonists: H_1 antagonists like **mepyramine and promethazine** are used to prevent histamine induced contractions of smooth muscles of intestine and bronchi. They are also used frequently in the treatment of allergies.

H_2 receptor antagonists: H_2 antagonists like **cimetidine, ranitidine, and famotidine** are used to inhibit histamine induced HCl secretion in the stomach. These drugs are frequently used in the treatment of peptic ulcer.

Serotonin

Source

Serotonin is 5-hydroxytryptamine (5-HT). It is distributed in various tissues. It is present in high concentration in GI tract, CNS, especially in the hypothalamus and brainstem, and skin. Due to its higher concentration in the intestine, it is also known as **enteramine**. It is also present in platelets and basophils.

Synthesis and Metabolism

Synthesis

Serotonin is synthesized from the amino acid **tryptophan**. Tryptophan is converted to **5-hydroxytryptophan** by the action of enzyme tryptophan hydroxylase. 5-hydroxytryptophan is then decarboxylated to form 5-hydroxytryptamine (serotonin) catalyzed by the enzyme 5-hydroxytryptophan decarboxylase (Flowchart 64.2).

Metabolism

Serotonin is metabolized by the enzyme monoamine oxidase to form 5-hydroxyindole acetic acid (5-HIAA), which is excreted in urine. 5-HIAA is physiologically inactive. However, the level of it in urine is **an index of serotonin secretion in the body**.

Serotonin Receptors

Till date, **seven types of serotonin receptors** have been identified. They are 5-HT_1, 5-HT_2, 5-HT_3, 5-HT_4, 5-HT_5, 5-HT_6, 5-HT_7. The 5-HT_1 is further subdivided into 5-HT_{1A}, 5-HT_{1B}, 5-HT_{1D}, 5-HT_{1E}, and 5-HT_{1F}. Also, 5-HT_2 is further subdivided into 5-HT_{2A}, 5-HT_{2B} and 5-HT_{2C}. The 5-HT_5 has two subtypes: 5-HT_{5A} and 5-HT_{5B}.

Flowchart 64.2: Synthesis and metabolism of serotonin.

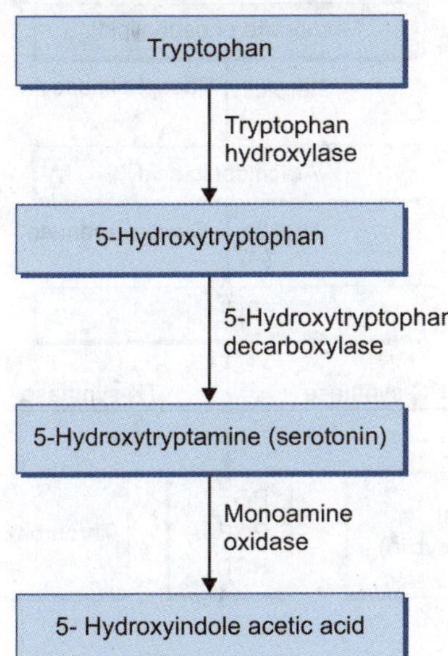

Physiological Actions

Serotonin mainly acts on cardiovascular system, respiratory system, kidney, smooth muscle, and nervous system.

Cardiovascular System

Serotonin, acting locally **produces vasoconstriction**. It facilitates **platelet aggregation**. These two functions of platelets are mediated via 5-HT_{2A} receptors, and are essential for temporary hemostasis. Serotonin also produces tachycardia.

Respiratory System

Serotonin increases bronchial tone (causes **bronchoconstriction**), which is mediated via 5-HT_{2A} receptors. In asthmatic patients, it induces the acute attack of asthma. It also stimulates rate of respiration.

Kidney

Serotonin has mild **antidiuretic effect**. It prevents diuresis by decreasing GFR, which occurs due to afferent glomerular arteriolar constriction. It also causes ureteric spasm and temporarily stops urination.

GI Tract

Serotonin **stimulates GI secretions and motility**. It promotes peristalsis and produce diarrhea. These effects are mediated by 5-HT_4 receptors.

Central Nervous System

It is released as a neurotransmitter in different parts of the brain. The most important serotonergic pathway in the brain is the **raphespinal system** that on stimulation produces analgesia. 5-HT_3 receptors are present in area postrema that on activation induces vomiting. 5-HT_6 and 5-HT_7 receptors are distributed throughout the limbic system, neocortex, cerebellum and spinal cord. It has following central functions:

1. Inhibits transmission of pain impulses in dorsal horn of spinal cord, and thus, it is an important component of **endogenous analgesia system.**
2. Stimulates **prolactin secretion** from anterior pituitary.
3. Regulates **circadian rhythm** (suprachiasmatic nucleus receives heavy serotonergic innervation). Serotonin is a strong **antidepressant**. Hallucinogens produce euphoria by releasing serotonin in the brain. Antidepressant drugs such as fluoxetine act by inhibiting serotonin reuptake in the brain.
4. Serotonin is a strong **anorectic agent**. It inhibits feeding by acting on hypothalamic and other feeding areas in the brain.
5. Serotonin **suppresses sleep** and serotonin antagonists enhance slow wave sleep.

Clinical Correlation

Increased serotonin activity is seen in some endocrine tumors, which is detected by estimation of urinary 5-HIAA. This is usually observed in **carcinoid syndrome**.

Bradykinin

Bradykinin is a peptide containing 9 amino acids (nonapeptide). It is synthesized in tissue and plasma.

Synthesis

Bradykinin is synthesized from high molecular weight kininogen (HMWK) by the action of plasma kallikrein in plasma and tissue kallikrein in tissue. Plasma kallikrein is formed from prekallikrein by activated clotting factor XII.

Physiological Actions

Bradykinin **resembles histamine in its physiological functions**:

1. It produces **vasodilation and increases local blood flow.**
2. It causes **contraction of visceral smooth muscle.**
3. It **increases capillary permeability,** attracts leucocytes to the site of injury and produces pain when injected into the skin.
4. It increases secretion from exocrine pancreas and salivary gland.
5. It also increases sweat secretion.

Clinical Importance

Bradykinin is secreted from **abnormal endocrine tumors** as seen ***in carcinoid syndrome***.

Prostaglandins

Prostaglandin was first described by Von Euler in 1937. It was named prostaglandin for its enumeration in the secretion from prostate gland. Afterwards, prostaglandins were found to be synthesized in various tissues of the body. They are **20-carbon unsaturated fatty acids** containing a cyclopentane ring. They act as local hormone in kidney, lungs, GI tract, uterus, skin and other tissues.

Scientist contributed

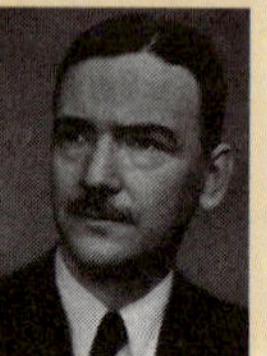

Ulf S von Euler (1905–1983)

Ulf Svante von Euler (1905-1983) was a Swedish physiologist and pharmacologist. He shared the **Nobel Prize in Physiology or Medicine in 1970** for his work on neurotransmitters. His short stay as a postdoctoral student in Dale's laboratory was very fruitful, where in 1931 he worked with John H Gaddum and discovered **substance P**. After returning to Stockholm, he pursued his research, and discovered four other important endogenous active substances, **prostaglandins,** vesiglandin (1935), piperidine (1942) and **noradrenaline** (1946).

Types

There are different types of prostaglandins. The commonest prostaglandins are PGE, PGF, PGI, PFH and PGA. Further, each has subcategories like are PGA_1, PGA_2, PGE_1, PGE_2, $PGF_{1\alpha}$, and $PGF_{2\alpha}$, etc.

Synthesis

Prostaglandins are synthesized from **arachidonic acid,** which is formed from membrane phospholipid by the enzyme **phospholipase A_2**:

1. Arachidonic acid is then converted to cyclic endoperoxides (PGH_2) by the action of enzyme **cyclooxygenase** (prostaglandin synthase).
2. PGH_2 is then converted to prostacyclin by the enzyme prostacyclin synthase or thromboxane A_2 by the enzyme thromboxane synthase (Flowchart 64.3).
3. PGH_2 is also converted to PGE_2, $PGF_{2\alpha}$, etc. by various isomerases.

Flowchart 64.3: Prostaglandin synthesis.

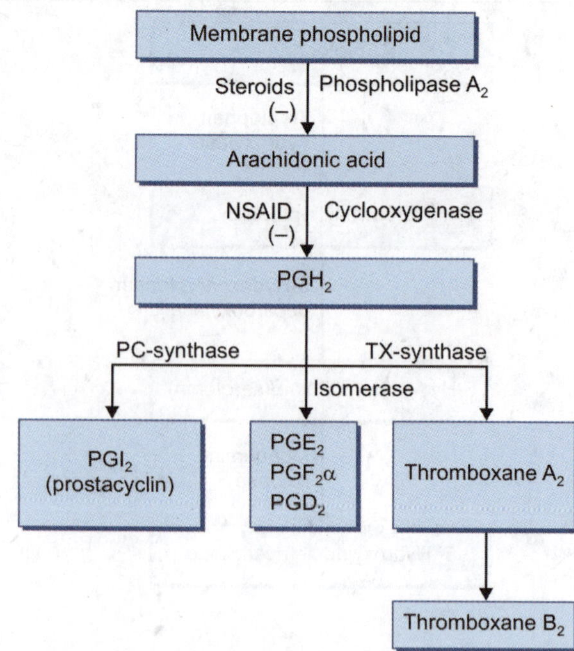

[NSAID: Nonsteroidal anti-inflammatory drugs; PC: Prostacyclin; TX: Thromboxane; (–): Indicates inhibition].

Physiological Actions

Prostaglandins are present in almost all the tissues of the body. They are mainly involved in the control of functions of various organ systems, hemostasis, and metabolisms and play an important role in inflammation.

Cardiovascular System

PGA_1 and PGA_2 cause peripheral arteriolar dilation. Prostacyclin produces vasodilation and thromboxane A_2 causes vasoconstriction.

Reproductive System

1. $PGF_{2\alpha}$ produces **contraction of gravid uterus**. The concentration of this chemical increases in the maternal blood during parturition. It is suggested that the increase in $PGF_{2\alpha}$ initiates labor in the presence of high concentration of oxytocin.
2. Prostaglandins facilitate **luteolysis** (regression of corpus luteum).
3. They decrease the secretion of progesterone.
4. Prostaglandins **increase in uterine fluid** and cause necrosis of blood vessels of the uterus just before the bleeding starts during menstrual cycle. It is proposed that prostaglandins **initiate the process of bleeding**.
5. It increases **secretion of GnRH** from hypothalamus.

Hemostasis

Prostacyclin *inhibits platelet aggregation and produces vasodilation* whereas **thromboxane A_2 and endoperoxides** *promote platelet aggregation and cause vasoconstriction*:

1. The balance between the prostacyclin and thromboxane A_2 determines the degree of **platelet plug** formation (refer to Fig. 20.9, Chapter 20).
2. Thus, prostaglandins greatly influence temporary hemostasis.

Respiratory System

Prostaglandin E causes *bronchodilation* whereas **$PGF_{2\alpha}$** produces *bronchoconstriction*. $PGF_{2\alpha}$ is implicated in the genesis of bronchial asthma.

GI System

Prostaglandins E and $F_{2\alpha}$ *inhibit absorption of sodium and water*:

1. The **watery diarrhea** produced in cholera is mediated by prostaglandins.
2. They also stimulate **intestinal motility**.

Central Nervous System

Prostaglandins act as neurotransmitters in various parts of the brain. PGE inhibits release of norepinephrine from the nerve endings.

Inflammation

Prostaglandin E and A increase capillary permeability during inflammation. PGE sensitizes the nerve endings to bradykinin and produces pain.

Metabolism

PGE_1 inhibits lipolysis, induced by ACTH, GH, glucagons, and epinephrine.

Clinical Correlation

Prostaglandin preparations are used in the treatment of different diseases.

1. **Steroidal anti-inflammatory drugs** such as cortisol inhibit prostaglandin production by inhibiting the enzyme phospholipase A_2.
2. **Nonsteroidal anti-inflammatory drugs** (NSAID) such as ibuprofen inhibit prostaglandin synthesis by inhibiting the enzyme cyclooxygenase (*see* Flowchart 64.3).

Carcinoid Syndrome

These are tumors of **enterochromaffin cells** of the GI tract or bronchus or pancreas:

1. A characteristic feature of carcinoid syndrome is the **episodic flushing** of the skin, associated with hypertension, abdominal pain, diarrhea, and bronchoconstriction.
2. These episodic attacks occur due to secretion of various chemicals from the tumor enterochromaffin cells.
3. Usually, these tumors secrete **excess of serotonin and histamine**.
4. Therefore, the disease is diagnosed by the **excretion of increased amount of 5-HIAA** in the urine.

Other Local Hormones

Renin

Renin is the hormone **secreted from JG cells of kidney** in response to hypovolemia and hypotension. It **converts angiotensinogen to angiotensin I**, which is further converted to angiotensin II by ACE (for details, refer renin-angiotensin system in Kidney).

Erythropoietin

Erythropoietin is the glycoprotein hormone containing 165 amino acids secreted mainly from **interstitial cells in the peritubular capillary bed of kidney**. It is the major regulator of erythropoiesis (for details, refer erythropoiesis in Section II "Blood").

ANP

Atrial natriuretic peptide (ANP) is a peptide hormone synthesized by the **atrial myocytes**. It has profound natriuretic and diuretic effect. Therefore, it is known as a natriuretic peptide. ANP contains 28 amino acids. A similar peptide is isolated in the brain, called as **brain natriuretic peptide** (BNP), which contains 32 amino acids. A third natriuretic peptide is also described, the **C type natriuretic peptide** (CNP), which contains 22 amino acids. The CNP is present in the brain, kidney, and vascular endothelial cells. Actions of natriuretic peptides are almost similar (for details, *see* ANP in 'cardiovascular system').

The **major functions of ANP** are:

1. ANP increases sodium excretion (**natriuresis**). This is occurs due to increased GFR, which is produced by dilation of afferent arteriole and relaxation of mesangial cells in the glomerulus of kidney. Also, ANP acts on kidney tubule to inhibit sodium reabsorption.
2. It increases water excretion (**diuresis**). This occurs, secondary to natriuresis.
3. It causes **vasodilation**, leading to decrease in blood pressure.
4. It also increases capillary permeability that causes extravasation of fluid into interstitial tissue space. This decreases blood volume and pressure.
5. It **decreases the sensitivity of blood vessels to constrictors** like catecholamines and angiotensin II.
6. It decreases heart rate and cardiac output.

Melatonin

Melatonin is secreted from the pineal gland. The secretion is more in children and less in adults. It inhibits gonadal function (for details, refer previous chapter).

Thymosin

Thymosin is the hormone secreted from thymus. Thymus is present in the mediastinum posterior to sternum. At birth it weighs about 10 g, which increases in size to about 30 g during adolescence. Thereafter, it decreases to about 5 g in adults and 2 g in elderly:

1. Thymosin controls the **development of lymphocytes** and plays an important role in immunity. It is secreted by the reticular epithelial cells of thymus (for details, refer Chapter 18).
2. **Development of the T cells** occurs in thymus during childhood and **thymosin plays a crucial role** in this process.
3. Hence, thymus has the central position in the development of **cellular immunity**. For details of T cell development, refer 'Immunity'.

CHAPTER SUMMARY

Key Concepts

1. Though local hormones act locally in the tissue where they are produced, some of them have systemic effects.
2. Many local hormones play important role in many physiological functions such as platelet aggregation, hemostasis, GI secretion and motility, menstrual bleeding, CV functions, neurotransmission in brain, glomerular filtration, bronchial activity, respiratory functions. Therefore, they play key role in many dysfunctions and diseases.

Important to Know (Must Read)

1. In examination, **Long Questions** are not asked from this chapter.
2. Physiological actions of histamine, Physiological actions of serotonin, Physiological actions of prostaglandins, Bradykinin, ANP, Carcinoid syndrome may be asked as **Short Questions** in exam.
3. In **Viva**, examiner may ask… List the physiological actions of histamine, List the physiological actions of serotonin, List the physiological actions of prostaglandins, List the physiological actions of bradykinin, List the physiological actions of ANP, What are the histamine receptors and where are they found, List some antihistaminic drugs and mention their uses, What is carcinoid syndrome and what are its features, What is the mechanism of action of anti-inflammatory drugs (both steroidal and nonsteroidal), List the local hormones, What is ANP and from where is it secreted, I list the steps of synthesis and metabolism of histamine, List the steps of synthesis and metabolism of serotonin, List the steps of synthesis of prostaglandins, List the serotonin receptors and their subtypes, What is thymosin and what are its functions.

SECTION–7

Reproductive System

PART A: GENERAL REPRODUCTIVE PHYSIOLOGY

65. Sex Differentiation and Development, Puberty and Menopause
66. Physiology of Puberty and Menopause

PART B: MALE REPRODUCTIVE PHYSIOLOGY

67. Male Reproductive System

PART C: FEMALE REPRODUCTIVE PHYSIOLOGY

68. Female Reproductive System: Functional Anatomy, Oogenesis and Follicular Development
69. Menstrual Cycle and Ovulation
70. Ovarian Hormones and Control of Ovarian Functions

PART D: PHYSIOLOGY OF CONCEPTION, PREGNANCY, LACTATION AND CONTRACEPTION

71. Physiology of Copulation
72. Pregnancy and Parturition
73. Physiology of Breast Development and Lactation
74. Physiology of Contraception

"To live, to love are signs of infinite things,
Love is glory from eternity's spheres.
Abased, disfigured, mocked by baser mights
That steal his name and shape and ecstasy,
He is still the Godhead by which all can change."

Sri Aurobindo (in 'SAVITRI')

CHAPTER 65

Sex Differentiation and Development, Puberty and Menopause

Learning Objectives

On completion of study of this chapter, the student **MUST** be able to:

1. Understand the physiology of sex determination and differentiation.
2. Describe the mechanism of sex differentiation and development in males and females.
3. List the abnormalities of sex differentiation and understand the physiological basis of their causation.
4. Apply the knowledge of sex determination and differentiation in understanding the physiology of reproductive system.

The student **MAY** also be able to:

1. Describe the mechanisms of dysfunctions of sex differentiation.

Reproduction serves a primary goal of the nature in preservation and perpetuation of the species. The creation of two sexually complete and different individuals in same species, known as **sexual dimorphism** is the central scheme of the nature to achieve its principal intention of continuation of species through reproduction. The complete sexual dimorphism is obtained through the attainment of **puberty**. The sexually matured adults then reproduce to maintain their progeny. Therefore, to appreciate the physiology of reproduction one should study the process of sex differentiation, development of gonads, gonadal functions, physiology of puberty and sexual maturation, the principles of functioning of the female and male reproductive systems, and the physiology of pregnancy, parturition and lactation.

SEX DIFFERENTIATION

Sex Determination

Normal Chromosomal Pattern

In a normal human being, there are 46 (23 pairs) chromosomes: 22 pairs are autosomes and one pair is sex chromosome (Fig. 65.1).

In Males

The pattern is 22 pairs of autosomes, and one X and one Y sex chromosomes (44 XY).

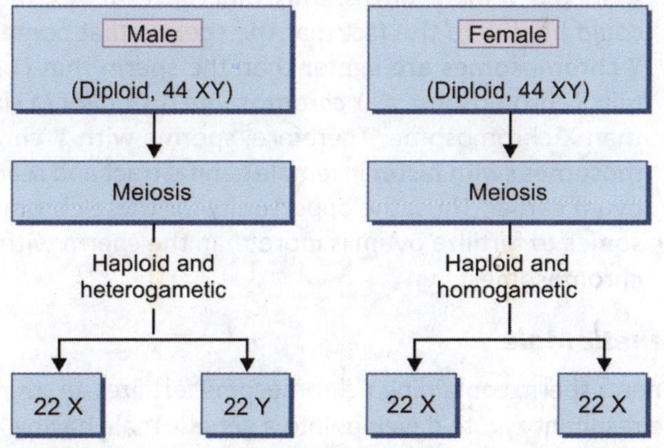

Fig. 65.1: Chromosomal pattern in males (44 XY) and females (44 XX).

In Females

The pattern is 22 pairs of autosomes and two X chromosomes (44 XX).

Sex Chromosomes

Gender is determined by the genetic inheritance of two chromosomes, called sex chromosomes. The two sex chromosomes are the **X chromosome**, the larger one, and the **Y chromosome**, the smaller one.

1. Females possess two X chromosomes and males have one X and one Y chromosome. Thus, ovum always contributes only one X chromosome, whereas half of the sperms contribute X and another half Y.

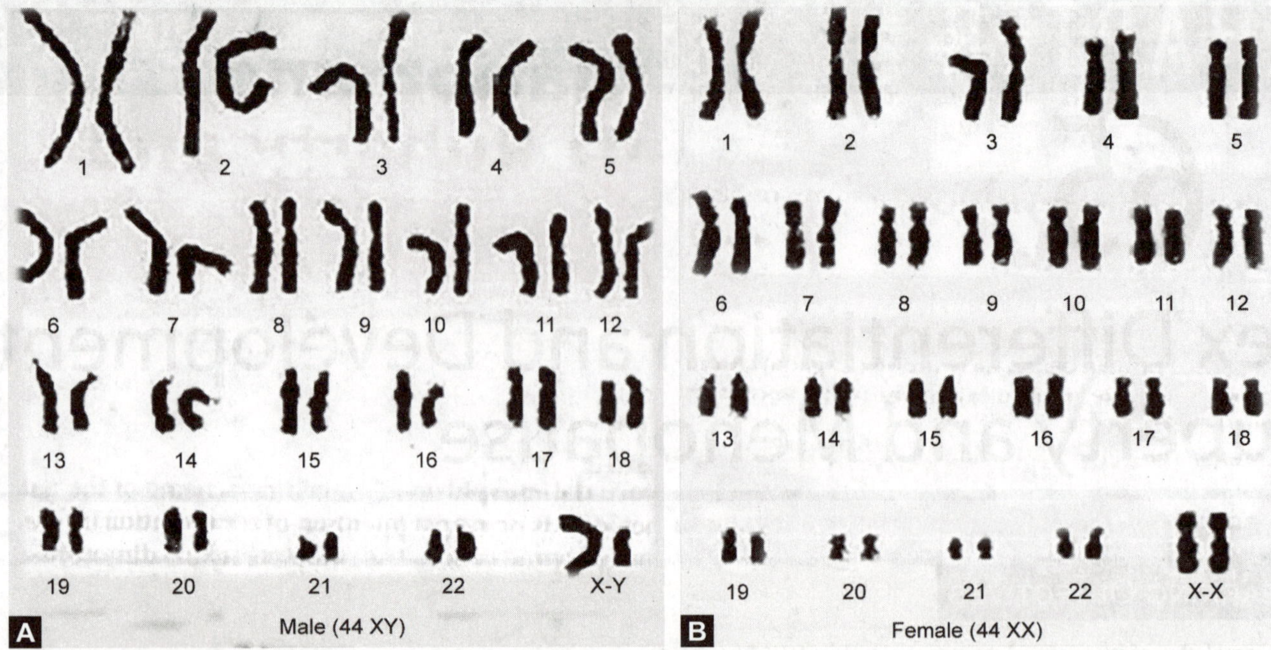

Figs. 65.2A and B: Chromosomal pattern (karyotyping) in males and females. Note, X chromosome is larger than Y chromosome.

2. Therefore, union of sperm and ovum (fertilization) usually results in half XX and half XY. Hence, ideally, births of male and female children should have been in equal proportion.
3. However, generally the **male births are slightly more than the female births**. This difference in sex ratio could be due to the fact that the sperms that contain **Y chromosomes are lighter** than the sperm that contain X chromosome as ***Y chromosome is smaller in size*** than X chromosome. Therefore, **sperms with Y chromosomes swim faster** in female genital tract and reach ovum earlier. Thus, the opportunity for these chromosomes to fertilize ovum is more than the sperm with X chromosomes.

Genetic Male

When a sperm containing Y chromosome fertilizes an ovum, the resultant zygote develops into a **genetic male** having XY pattern of sex chromosomes. The karyotype is **44 XY.**

Genetic Female

When a sperm containing X chromosome fertilizes an ovum, the resultant zygote develops into a **genetic female** having XX pattern of sex chromosomes. The karyotype is **44 XX.**

Sex Determination

Karyotyping

Sex determination is usually done by **karyotyping**, a technique used for determining sex chromosome composition by employing tissue culture visualization of all chromosomes. The differences in shape and size of chromosomes in males and females help in concrete determination of sex (Figs. 65.2A and B)

Demonstration of Sex Chromatin

This is a relatively easy method to demonstrate sex chromatin **(Barr body)** in leucocytes or mucosal cells of the oral cavity (refer to Fig. 5.7, Chapter 5).

1. Barr bodies are usually formed in females as they have two X chromosomes.
2. When two X chromosomes are present, one X chromosome is functional and other X chromosome which is nonfunctional condenses to form sex chromatin.
3. Thus, presence of **Barr body generally indicates female sex.**

Sex Differentiation

The process of sex differentiation includes the pattern of development of the gonads, genital ducts, and the external genitalia.

1. During pregnancy, no differences in the gonads of male and female fetuses occur during the first five weeks of gestation. This is called the **stage of indifferent gonads.**
2. The differentiation of gender starts from sixth week of intrauterine life and continues even after birth till the complete maturation of the gonad of either gender is achieved.
3. The process of development from the indifferent gonad to complete mature gonad of either gender is called the **sex differentiation.**

Cell Lines of Development: Following fertilization, two different cell lines develop in the indifferent gonad.

1. The **one cell line** forms the ***granulosa cells*** of the ovarian follicle and the ***Sertoli cells*** of the testicular seminiferous tubules. The cells of this cell line **nurse the germ cells** and promote their maturation, and finally guide their development into the ***genital duct system***. These cells in females **produce estrogen.**

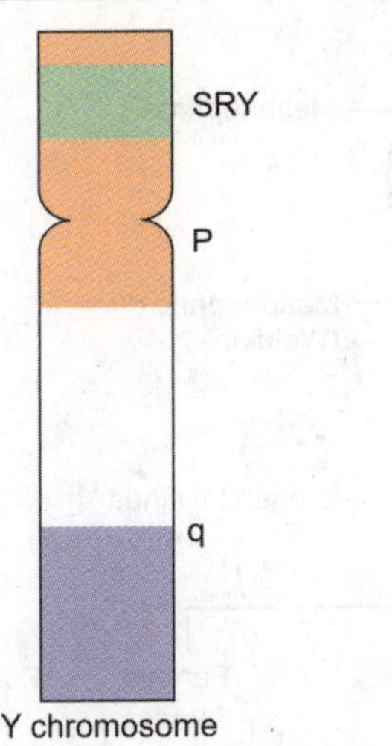

Fig. 65.3: Sex-determining region of Y (SRY) chromosome.

2. The **other cell line** of the indifferent gonad (the interstitial cells) forms ***theca cells*** in the ovary and ***Leydig cells*** in the testis. These cells mainly **secrete androgen**, which is essential for the development of ***male sexual characteristics*** and spermatogenesis. In females, they form the precursors for estrogen synthesis.

Differentiation of the Genetic Sex, Gonadal Sex and Phenotypic Sex

Genetic Sex

Male Genetic Sex

The male chromosomal pattern is 44 autosomes and a pair of sex chromosomes. The sex chromosomes in a normal male is X and Y. The presence of Y chromosomes determines the maleness of the individual, without which neither testis nor the male genital pattern develop.

1. The Y chromosome contains the **SRY gene** (sex-determining region of the Y) which is located on the distal part of its short arm (Fig. 65.3).
2. This gene encodes the **testis determining factor** (TDF). The TDF is a ***transcription factor*** that binds to DNA molecules.
3. A gene identical to SRY gene encodes a histocompatibility antigen known as **H-Y antigen**. These are glycoprotein antigens present on the surface of all male cells. Both these antigens are ***involved in rejection of male tissue*** by the female recipients. This H-Y antigen helps in **development of male gonads**, and masculinization.
4. Though SRY gene is essential for masculinization, *it is not adequate* for the complete maleness.
5. Virilization of the genital duct and external genitalia requires the presence of an **androgen hormone receptor**. This receptor is encoded by the gene present on the X chromosomes. Therefore, *X chromosomal gene also contributes to the development of maleness.*

Female Genetic Sex

The normal female chromosomal pattern consists of 44 autosomes and a pair of X chromosomes (XX).

1. In the absence of a Y chromosome, SRY gene is absent.
2. Therefore, TDF and H-Y antigen do not develop.
3. Hence, instead of male gonads ovaries develop when both the sex chromosomes are X.

Gonadal Sex

Male Gonadal Sex

In a normal genetic male, the seminiferous tubule starts to form at 6–7 weeks of gestation.

1. The Sertoli cells enclose the germ cells.
2. The **Leydig cells appear at 8–9 weeks**. The testis starts **secreting testosterone** during this period. This helps in development of male sex.
3. The SRY gene prevents the synthesis of estrogen and inhibits the enzyme aromatase, which inhibits the development of female systems.

Female Gonadal Sex

In a normal genetic female, the differentiation of indifferent gonad into the female gonads (ovaries) starts after nine weeks of gestation.

1. Both the X chromosomes in the **germ cells are activated**.
2. The germ cells then undergo divisions to **form oogonia** that continue to proliferate.
3. Immediately after the start of meiosis, oogonia are surrounded by granulosa cells.
4. Stroma appears inside it, which gives rise to interstitial cells. Now the germ cells are known as **primary oocytes**.
5. The female gonad remains in this stage (***primary oocyte stage***), i.e. in the stage of diplotene or late prophase of meiosis **for many years** until ovulation occurs.
6. Estrogen secreted from the granulosa cells help in the female development.

Phenotypic (Genital) Sex

The differentiation of genital duct and external genitalia requires hormones. The **basic principle** is that under the direction of a positive hormonal influence, the male gonadal system develops, and in the absence of any hormonal control, female genitals develop (Figs. 65.4 and 65.5). The development of brain is also linked to the phenotypic sex (Application Box 65.1).

In Males

In males, at about 9–10 weeks **Wolffian** or **mesonephric ducts** develop which gives rise to epididymis, vas deferens, seminal vesicles, and ejaculatory ducts.

1. Development of this system is presided by the appearance of Leydig cells in the testis that secrete testosterone.
2. Testosterone stimulates growth and differentiation of Wolffian duct into the male genital system (Flowchart 65.1).

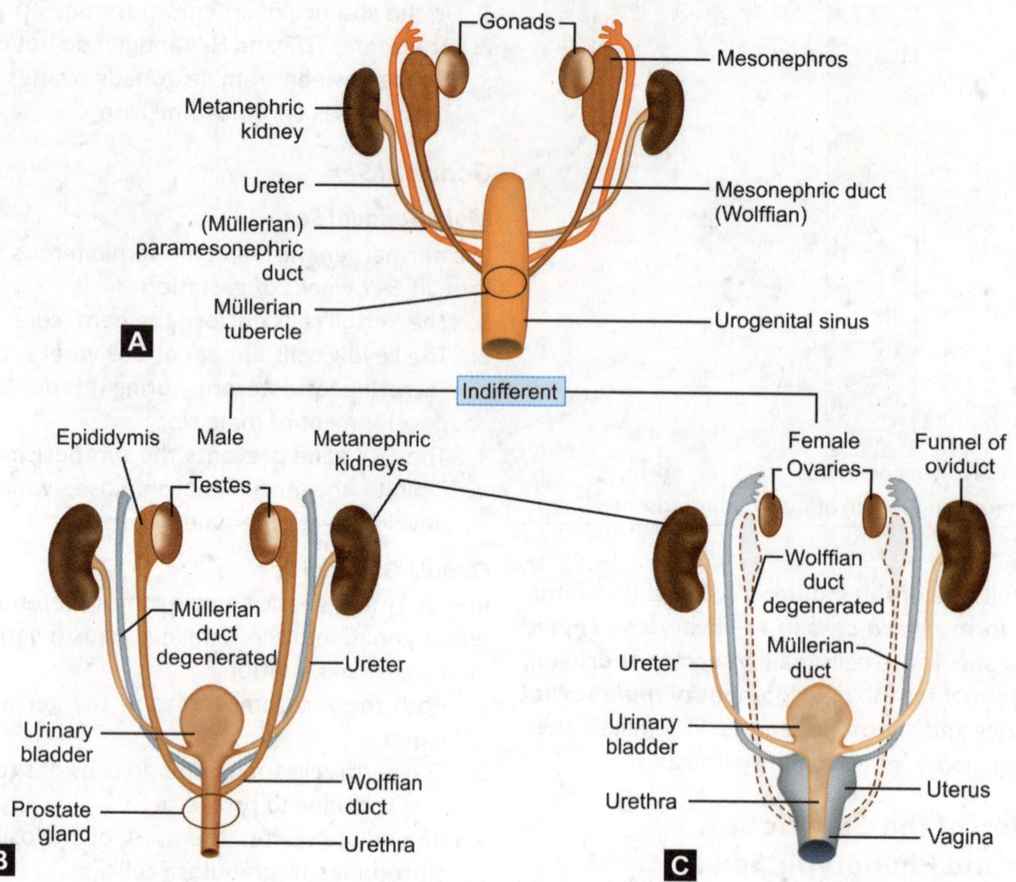

Figs. 65.4A to C: Differentiation of the male and female internal genitalia. (A) Indifferent stage; (B) Male internal genitalia; (C) Female internal genitalia. Note, in male, Müllerian duct degenerates, and in female, Wolffian duct degenerates.

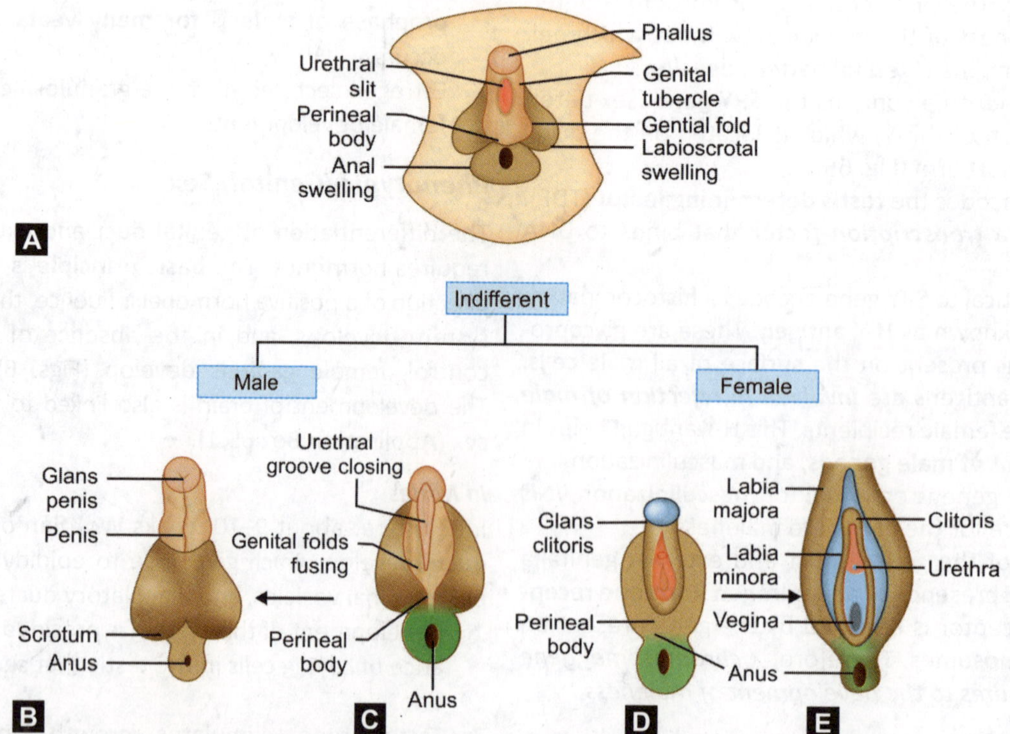

Figs. 65.5A to E: Differentiation of the male and female external genitalia. (A) Indifferent stage; (B) Male genitalia (7th to 8th week); (C) Male genitalia (at about 12th week); (D) Female genitalia (7th to 8th week); (E) Female genitalia (at about 12th week).

Flowchart 65.1: Mechanism of sex differentiation in male.

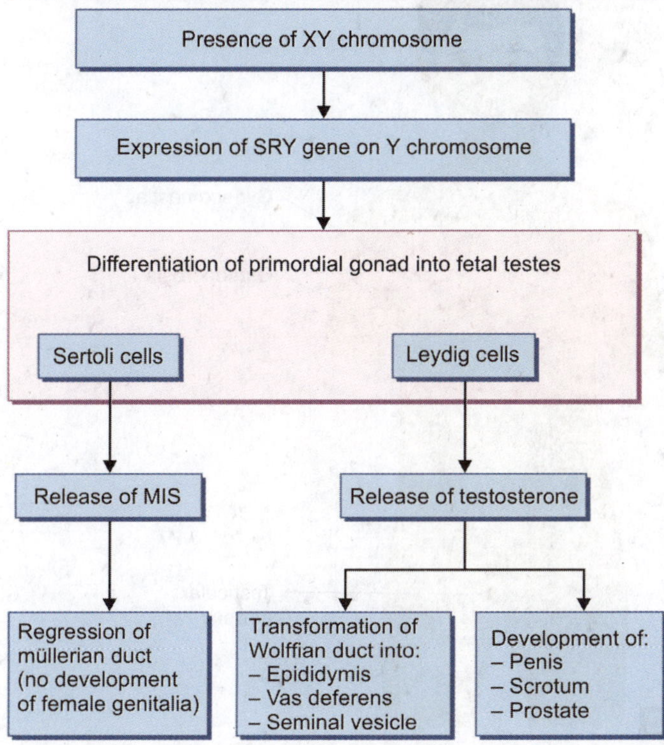

Flowchart 65.2: Mechanism of sex differentiation in female.

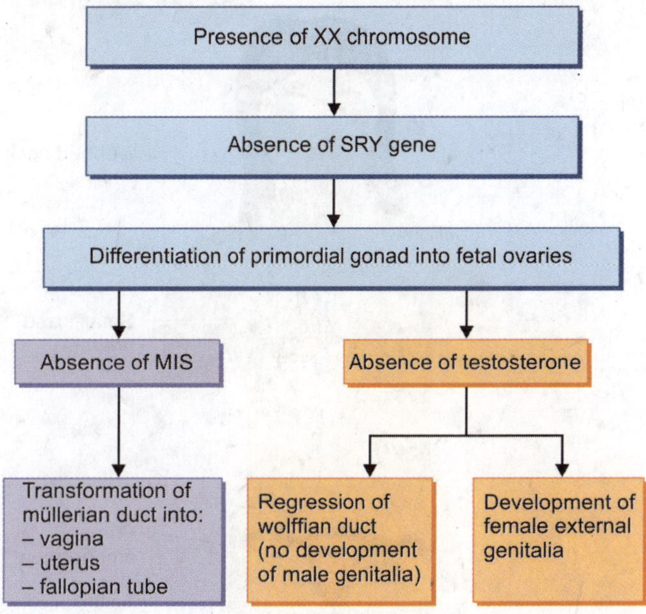

In Females

In females, the Wolffian duct degenerates at about 10–11 weeks as ovary does not secrete testosterone. From Wolffian ducts on each side, the **Müllerian ducts** arise, which develops into fallopian tubes and uterus.

Role of MIS: In males, müllerian ducts regress at about 8 weeks of gestation, the time during which Sertoli cells appear in the testis. The Sertoli cells produce a hormone called **müllerian inhibiting substance** (MIS). This is also known as *antimüllerian hormone* or *müllerian regression factor*.

1. MIS causes degeneration of müllerian duct by facilitating its apoptosis.
2. The SRY gene promotes the synthesis of MIS.
3. In females who **lack MIS**, ***müllerian duct continues to grow*** and form fallopian tubes, uterus, cervix, and vagina (Flowchart 65.2). This differentiation is completed by 18–20 weeks of gestation.

Müllerian Inhibiting Substance (MIS)

Also known as **antimüllerian hormone** or **müllerian regression factor**, MIS is a polypeptide hormone containing 536 amino acids **secreted by the Sertoli cells** of testis. It belongs to the **TGF β superfamily** of growth factors that includes activin and inhibin.

1. **In males**, though the secretion of MIS starts at 8–10 weeks of gestation, the level in plasma reaches its peak, i.e., about 50 ng/mL at 1 to 2 years of age. The concentration then declines gradually to a low level during puberty and a lower concentration of about 2–5 ng/mL is maintained through rest of life.
2. **In females**, granulosa cells of some ovarian follicles start secreting MIS at a low rate during puberty and continue in a similar fashion thereafter. Therefore, the adult female plasma level of MIS is same as that of males.
3. However, the exact role of MIS in adults, especially in females is not known.

Functions of MIS

1. **During early embryonic life**, MIS ***inhibits development of female gonads*** by promoting regression of müllerian duct. Therefore, it helps in male gonadal development.
2. Later **during fetal life** in males, it helps in ***testicular descent***.
3. In both sexes, it helps in maturation of germ cells.

Application Box 65. 1

Phenotypic sex development influences brain development: Development of brain is linked to the development of the external genitalia in the early part of life, which is influenced by exposures to androgens. It is proposed that the pattern of hypothalamic control of gonadotropin release that starts with the onset of puberty is determined earlier by the exposure to androgen in first few days of life. In the absence of androgen exposure, female pattern develops.

Abnormalities of Sex Differentiation

The abnormalities of sex differentiation can be broadly divided into two categories: chromosomal and developmental abnormalities.

Chromosomal Abnormalities

The common chromosomal abnormalities are Turner's syndrome, Klinefelter's syndrome, testicular feminization syndrome, superfemales and true hermaphroditism.

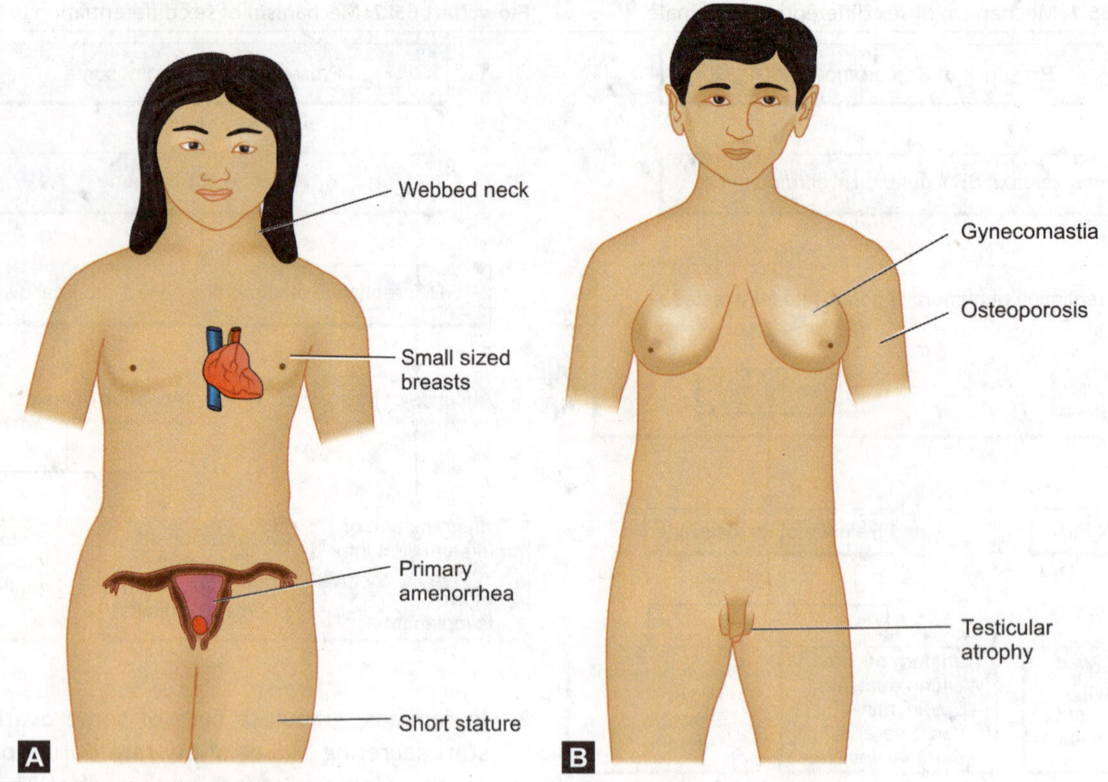

Figs. 65.6A and B: (A) Turner syndrome. Note the small breast, webbed neck and short stature in a female with this syndrome; (B) Klinefelter syndrome. Note the gynecomastia and small testis in a male with this syndrome.

Turner's Syndrome

This is otherwise known as **gonadal or ovarian dysgenesis**.

1. It is characterized by diminished sexual development, dwarfism, and webbing of the neck in patients with no gonadal tissue or rudimentary gonads (Fig. 65.6 A).
2. The chromosomal **pattern of sex chromosomes is XO**, which means there are 44 autosomes and one X chromosomes (total 45 chromosomes).
3. It results from nondisjunction of one of the X chromosomes during oogenesis.
4. Usually, it presents with *primary amenorrhea*. No sexual maturation occurs at puberty.

Klinefelter's Syndrome

This is the most common sex chromosome abnormality. The syndrome is otherwise called **seminiferous tubule dysgenesis**.

1. Typically, it is characterized by presence of feminine features in an apparent male with small testes (Figs. 65.6B).
2. The patient is genetically female, but the presence of an extra Y chromosome causes development of the testis. Therefore, the **karyotype is 47 XXY** (44 autosomes + XX sex chromosomes + one extra Y chromosomes).
3. They have male genitalia and at puberty male characteristics develop due to adequate testosterone.
4. But, seminiferous tubules are not properly developed and therefore, infertility results.
5. Thus, the syndrome usually presents with ***primary hypogonadism and infertility*** in male. Mental retardation is common.

Superfemales

This is a common aberration of sexual differentiation. Usually, it is **not associated with any characteristic abnormalities** and therefore remains undetected. The abnormality is commonly diagnosed while performing chromosomal analysis for some other causes. The **karyotype is XXX**.

Testicular Feminization Syndrome

The patients appear **normal females externally**. At puberty though breasts develop normally, the growth of pubic and axillary hairs is scanty. It causes ***primary amenorrhea***.

1. Though the external genitalia are of female type, there is *no development of uterus*. The vagina ends in a blind pouch.
2. The **gonads are testis**, with immature seminiferous tubules.
3. Therefore, it is called testicular feminization syndrome. Though testes are present, **spermatogenesis does not occur**. The patients are **genetic males** (XY karyotype).

True Hermaphroditism

This is a rare condition in which both testes and ovaries are present. Sometimes, ovary is present on one side and the testis on the opposite side. Both male and female sex differentiations occur with the development of combined female and male external and internal genitalia. Usually, the karyotype pattern is 46 XX-XY.

Other Chromosomal Abnormalities

Though other chromosomal abnormalities are not common, they do occur.

Transposition of Chromosome

Transposition of a part of one chromosome to other chromosome is possible. For example, genetic males may have XX chromosome pattern due to transposition of short arm of their father's Y chromosome into the father's X chromosome during meiosis. They receive X chromosome from their mother and transpositioned X chromosome from father.

Deletion of a part of Chromosome

Deletion of small portion of Y chromosome containing SRY gene occurs during meiosis. This results in females with XY karyotype.

Nondisjunction of Chromosome

Nondisjunction of chromosome 21 (an autosome) is not uncommon. This is called **trisomy 21**, which is associated with **Down's syndrome or mongolism**. It is not an aberration of sex chromosome, rather an autosomal abnormality.

Developmental Abnormalities

The developmental abnormalities are mainly hormonal disorders. However, nonhormonal abnormalities are also encountered. The hormonal abnormalities are broadly divided into **pseudohermaphroditisms** (both female and male patterns) and **enzyme deficiencies**.

Pseudohermaphroditisms

A **pseudohermaphrodite** is an individual with **genetic constitution and gonad of one sex**, but the **external genitalia of the other sex**. There are male and female pseudohermaphroditisms. In these conditions, the patients have normal gonadal development in accordance with their chromosomal sex, but afterward they develop heterosexual characteristics due to opposite hormonal excess.

Female Pseudohermaphroditisms

Male external genital development occurs in **genetic females** exposed to androgen during 8th to 13th week of gestation.

1. Source of androgen is usually **congenital virilizing adrenal hyperplasia** of fetus or **virilizing ovarian tumor** of the mother.
2. Sometimes it may be ***iatrogenically-induced*** following treatment of mother with androgens or progestational drugs.
3. In a typical female pseudohermaphrodite, the individual possesses ovaries, oviducts, but there is varying degrees of **masculine differentiation of external genitalia**.
4. The **chromosomal sex is female**.

Male Pseudohermaphroditisms

Development of female external genitalia in a **genetic male** is called male pseudohermaphroditism.

1. It is usually due to **defective testicular development**.
2. As MIS secreted from testis during early embryonic life prevents development of female gonads, in defective testicular development the internal genitalia are also of female pattern.
3. Male pseudohermaphroditism could also be due to **androgen resistance** that usually occurs in deficiency of 5α-reductase, the enzyme that forms dehydroepiandrosterone or due to defects in androgen receptors.
4. In **complete androgen resistance syndrome** (testicular feminizing syndrome), MIS is secreted as testes are normal; therefore, vagina ends blindly due to absence of internal genitalia.

Enzyme Deficiencies

Congenital **17α-hydroxylase deficiency** causes **male pseudohermaphroditism**. This also occurs in congenital adrenal hyperplasia in which enzyme defects block the formation of pregnenolone (for details, refer to Chapter 59, 'The Adrenal Cortex')

CHAPTER SUMMARY

Key Concepts

1. In males, The Y chromosome contains the **SRY gene** (sex-determining region of the Y), which encodes the **testis determining factor** (TDF). Another gene identical to SRY gene encodes a histocompatibility antigen known as **H-Y antigen**. Both these antigens are ***involved in rejection of male tissue*** by the female recipients. This H-Y antigen helps in **development of male gonads**, and masculinization.
2. Virilization of the genital duct and external genitalia requires the presence of an **androgen hormone receptor**. This receptor is encoded by the gene present on the X chromosomes. Therefore, X chromosomal gene also contributes to the development of maleness.
3. In the absence of a Y chromosome, SRY gene is absent. Therefore, TDF and H-Y antigen do not develop. Hence, instead of male gonads ovaries develop when both the sex chromosomes are X.

Important to Know (Must Read)

1. In examination, **Long Questions** are usually not asked from this chapter.
2. Mullerian inhibiting substance (MIS), Turner's syndrome, Klinefelter's syndrome, Pseudohermaphroditism, Testicular feminizing syndrome, Mechanism of sex differentiation in male, Mechanism of sex differentiation in female may be asked as **Short Questions** in exam.
3. In **Viva**, examiner may ask... How the genetic sex is determined in males and females, How the gonadal sex is determined in males and females, How the phenotypic (genital) sex is determined in males and females, What is called a genetic male and a genetic female? What are the methods for sex determination, What is MIS and what are its functions, What is the role of MIS in sex differentiation, What is SRY gene and what is its role, What is H-Y antigen and what is its role, List the chromosomal abnormalities, What are the features of Turner's syndrome, What are the features of Klinefelter's syndrome, What are the features of testicular feminizing syndrome, What is true hermaphroditism, What is pseudohermaphroditism and what are the types and features, What is superfemale, How the phenotypic sex development influences brain development.

CHAPTER 66

Physiology of Puberty and Menopause

Learning Objectives

On completion of study of this chapter, the student **MUST** be able to:

1. Understand the physiology of puberty in boys and girls.
2. Name the stages of puberty and the special features in each stage.
3. Understand the mechanism of onset of puberty.
4. Appreciate the physiological basis of causation of precocious puberty and delayed puberty.
5. Understand the mechanism of onset of menopause.

The student **MAY** also be able to:

1. Describe the mechanism of onset of puberty, and physiological basis of changes at puberty.
2. Explain the physiological basis of puberty abnormalities.

Puberty is the physiological phenomenon of attainment of sexual maturity. The ability to reproduce is attained with puberty and ceased with menopause. In females, reproducibility totally stops at menopause, whereas in males reproducibility continues.

PUBERTY

Definition

The period of **transition from the non-reproductive state to the state of reproductive functions that allows procreation** is defined as puberty. During this period, the hypothalamic-pituitary-gonadal axis is activated to bring the gametogenic functions of the gonads to their threshold of reproductive maturation.

1. Normally, gonads of both genders remain quiescent until the onset of puberty. Under the influence of gonadotropins secreted from pituitary, maturation of gonads occurs that in turn helps in maturation of the reproductive system.
2. This period of maturation is known as puberty or **adolescence**. During this period, the endocrine and gametogenic functions of the gonads first develop to the point where the reproduction becomes possible.

Age and Initiating Stimulus

Age of Onset of Puberty

The age of onset of puberty varies depending on various factors like socioeconomic and environmental conditions and genetic constitutions. In general, in developed countries, puberty occurs earlier than in the developing countries. In advanced nations, it occurs between the age of 8–13 in girls and 9–14 in boys. In developing nations, the age of onset of puberty is **11–16 years in girls** and **13–18 years in boys**.

Initiating Stimulus

The increased secretion of adrenal androgen, called **adrenarche**, occurs about 1 to 2 years before the onset of puberty.

1. This **increased adrenal androgen** is believed to stimulate the production of gonadal hormones that cause maturation of reproductive organs. As increase in adrenal androgen at this stage occurs without any alteration in ACTH or cortisol secretion, it is proposed that this is the primary and sole stimulus that heralds puberty.
2. One hypothesis suggests that increased secretion of adrenal androgen before puberty occurs due to secretion of **adrenal androgen stimulating hormone** (AASH) from pituitary. But actual nature and mechanism of it are not known.

Stages of Puberty

In Boys

The pubertal development in males occurs in five stages (by **Tanner method**, modified). Usually it is completed within 2 to 4 years from its onset.

Stage 1

This is the **preadolescent stage**. There is no enlargement of external genitalia (penis, scrotum and testes). No pubic hair is present. However, secretion of adrenal androgen is increased (**adrenarche**).

Stage 2

Testes enlarge to more than 2.5 cm, which occurs due to growth of seminiferous tubules.

1. Though this occurs due to the secretion of adrenal androgen (adrenarche), testicular androgen also contributes.
2. Testicular testosterone secretion increases significantly.
3. **Pubic hairs appear** in scanty at the root of the penis.

Stage 3

Penis enlarges in length. Scrotum and testes are further enlarged. ***Pubic hairs become darker and coarser*** above the pubis. **Sperm first appears** in the morning sample urine (**spermarchy**).

Stage 4

Penis enlarges in width and further in length. Scrotal and testicular enlargement continues. Pubic hair becomes adult type. **Ejaculation of sperm** occurs either in dreams, or on masturbation or by sexual act.

Stage 5

Full adult pattern of sexual features develops.

In Girls

The pubertal development in females also described in five stages (by **Tanner method**, modified). Usually, it is completed within 2 to 5 years from its onset.

Stage 1

This is **the preadolescent stage**. There is no breast development. No pubic hair is present. However, secretion of adrenal androgen is increased (**adrenarche**).

Stage 2

Breast development starts (**thelarche**). **Breast paillae is elevated** and the diameter of areola is increased. Secretion of estrogen from ovary increases significantly. Sparse hairs appear along the labia majora.

Stage 3

Breast enlarges with enlargement of areola. **Pubic hairs develop**, grow and become dark (**pubarche**). Hairs appear in axilla.

Stage 4

Breast further enlarges with areola and papillae projecting out of it. Pubic hair becomes adult type, but covers smaller area. **Menstrual cycle starts** (**menarche**), but irregular at the beginning.

Stage 5

Full adult pattern of breasts and pubic hairs develop. Menstrual cycle occurs regularly.

Mechanism of Onset of Puberty

The **hypothalamic neurons** gradually mature to ***secrete more GnRH***. This maturational process is genetically preprogrammed.

1. Dehydroepiandrosterone secreted from adrenal gland plays some role in the **maturation of hypothalamic neurons.**
2. The adipose tissue via secretion of **leptin** also plays some role in the determination of the time of onset of puberty (*see* below).
3. Normally, the secretion of GnRH, LH and FSH is not pulsatile before the onset of puberty. It is clear that **until puberty the release of GnRH is non-pulsatile**, which prevents puberty to occur.
4. It is not known what mechanism inhibits the **GnRH pulse generator** till puberty. However, before puberty, the GnRH is secreted in a **pulsatile pattern** that stimulates **pulsatile secretion of LH and FSH.**
5. It is proposed that this **pulsatile secretion of GnRH** brings about the onset of puberty. This theory is supported by the fact that experimental pulsatile injection of GnRH in immature monkeys produces normal menstrual cycle and the cycles continue till the pulsatile injection continues.

Role of Leptin

It has been observed that **body weight increases to a critical level** before the onset of puberty, especially in females. It is also observed that the onset of puberty is **delayed in girls with lower body weight**.

1. Leptin, the hormone secreted from adipose tissue cell is believed to help in the **maturation of hypothalamo-gonadal axis.**
2. This is supported by the experimental evidence that injection of leptin in female mice results in precocious puberty.
3. But, the exact role of leptin in the control of puberty is not known.

Abnormalities of Puberty

Abnormalities of puberty can be broadly classified into precocious puberty and delayed puberty.

Precocious Puberty

Precocious puberty may be of **two types**: true precocious puberty and precocious pseudopuberty.

True Precocious Puberty

Early development of **secondary sexual characteristics,** may be associated *with premature development of gonads* is known as true precocious puberty. Precocious puberty can occur in both girls and boys. This occurs due to early pubertal pattern of secretion of gonadotropin from pituitary.

True precocious puberty occurs due to following causes:

1. **Hypothalamic precocity:** Usually occurs due to tumor or infection of hypothalamus that causes premature increased secretion of GnRH.
2. **Gonadotropin independent precocity:** Precocious gametogenesis without increase in gonadotropin secretion. Usually, it occurs due to increased sensitivity of LH receptors to gonadotropins.
3. **Constitutional precocity:** When the actual cause of precocity can not be ascertained.
4. Tumor of pineal gland.

Precocious Pseudopuberty

The development of secondary sexual characteristics **without gametogenesis** is called as precocious pseudopuberty. This occurs due to exposure of immature males to abnormal quantity of androgen, and in immature females the abnormal exposure to estrogen.

Precocious pseudopuberty occurs due to following causes:

1. **Adrenal causes: Congenital virilizing adrenal hyperplasia** can lead to precocious pseudopuberty. **Androgen secreting or estrogen secreting tumors** of adrenal gland resulting in precocious pseudopuberty are not uncommon.
2. **Gonadal causes: Leydig cell tumor** of testis in male or **granulosa cell tumor** of ovary in females can cause precocious pseudopuberty.

Delayed Puberty

When onset of puberty is **delayed beyond the age of 17 in girls** and **20 in boys**, the condition is called delayed puberty.

1. It occurs usually due to **panhypopituitarism** that causes failure of maturation of gonads.
2. It is also associated with chromosomal abnormality of **XO pattern** or **gonadal dysgenesis**.
3. Puberty may be delayed in spite of presence of normal gonads, which is called **eunuchoidism** in males and **primary amenorrhea** in girls.

MENOPAUSE

With advancement of age, gonadal functions gradually decrease. In females, **ovaries become unresponsive** to the gonadotropins. The functions of gonads slowly decrease finally resulting in complete cessation of menstrual cycle. This is called menopause or **climacteric**.

Mechanism and Features

Mechanism of Menopause

The mechanism and purpose of menopause are not clear. The **female gonads progressively become unresponsive to gonadotropins** with advancing age. The mechanism by which ovarian responsiveness decreases is not known. Ovaries stop secreting progesterone and estrogen in appreciable amount. The *negative feedback effect* of ovarian hormones causes **increased secretion of luteinizing hormone (LH) and FSH**. The uterus and vagina become atrophic.

Age at Menopause

1. **In women**, onset of menopause occurs between the age of 45–55 years. In recent years, the age at menopause has gradually increased.
2. **In males**, though there is some decline in reproductive capacity from 5th decade of life, **climacteric does not occur**. Testicular functions and potency persist till 8th decade. Thus, in males, there is no **andropause** (male menopause).

Features of Menopause

Hot flushes (sensation of warmth spreading from trunk to the face) occur frequently. Night sweating, tachycardia, mental symptoms are also observed.

1. The mechanism of hot flushes is not exactly known but it coincides with the **surges of LH secretion.**
2. With the onset of menopause, **LH secretion is increased**, which occurs in episodes of 30–60 minutes. This is called **circhoral secretion of LH**.
3. Each hot flush **coincides with an episode of LH surge.** However, experimental evidences indicate that hot flushes are not due to episodic secretion of LH per se.
4. The decreased secretion of estrogen triggering some **hypothalamic mechanism** is proposed to cause both episodic secretion of LH and hot flushes.

Management of Menopause

The fear that the women will lose her womanhood may cause **psychological depression**.

1. It needs proper **care, counseling and assurance** of the spouse to make her understand and adjust to this physiological phenomenon of the nature.
2. In some cases, hot flushes and psychological symptoms become more problematic. In such women, **hormonal supplementation** of estrogen is usually helpful.
3. However, metabolic and other complications of estrogen should be kept in mind while continuing estrogen therapy for a longer period.

CHAPTER SUMMARY

Key Concepts

1. Increased secretion of adrenal androgens (adrenarche) sensitizes hypothalamo-pituitary-gonadal axis for pubertal changes. Dehydroepiandrosterone secreted from adrenal gland plays some role in the maturation of hypothalamic neurons, and GnRH secretion becomes pulsatile. **Pulsatile secretion of GnRH** brings about the onset of puberty.
2. Reproducibility totally stops at menopause, whereas in males reproducibility continues. Therefore, the male menopause is not definitive.

Important to Know (Must Read)

1. In examination, **Long Questions** are usually not asked from this chapter.
2. Precocious puberty, Stages of puberty in boys and girls, Mechanism of onset of puberty, Mechanism, features and management of menopause may be asked as **Short Questions** in exam.
3. In **Viva**, examiner may ask… Define puberty, What is the age of onset of puberty in boys and girls, What are the stages of puberty in boys, What are the stages of puberty in girls, Explain the mechanism of onset of puberty, What is true precocious puberty and what are its causes, What is precocious pseudopuberty and what are its causes, What is delayed puberty, What is menopause, What is the mechanism of menopause, What is the age of menopause, What are the features of menopause, How menopause can be managed.

CHAPTER 67

Male Reproductive System

LEARNING OBJECTIVES

On completion of study of this chapter, the student **MUST** be able to:

1. Name the different parts of male reproductive system, and give the functions of each.
2. List the functions of Sertoli cells and Leydig cells.
3. Understand the importance of blood-testis barrier in testicular functions.
4. Name the steps of spermatogenesis and describe the mechanism and regulation of spermatogenesis.
5. Understand the importance of semen analysis.
6. List the testicular hormones and describe the functions of testosterone.
7. List the secondary sex characteristics in males.
8. Understand the regulation of testicular functions.
9. Understand the physiological basis of testicular abnormalities.

The student **MAY** also be able to:

1. Describe the regulation of testicular functions and hypothalamo-pituitary-gonadal axis in males.
2. Describe the stages and mechanisms of spermatogenesis.
3. Explain the physiological basis of reproductive abnormalities in males.

The primary objective of the male reproductive system is to produce healthy sperms capable of fertilizing the ovum. The main specialty of male reproduction is that the male gametes are produced in millions and after puberty the process of production is a continuous phenomenon.

Scientist contributed

Enrico Sertoli (1842–1910) an Italian physiologist and histologist was a professor of anatomy and physiology at the Royal School of veterinary medicine in Milan, and after 1907, he worked only as a professor of physiology there. In Milan, he founded the **laboratory of experimental physiology**. He worked extensively on reproductive physiology. He is remembered for his 1865 discovery of the eponymous **Sertoli cell** that provide nourishment and support for developing sperm.

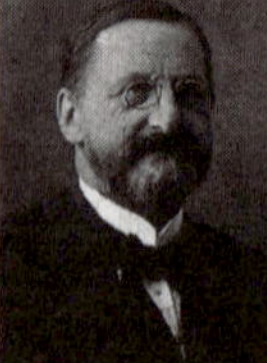

Enrico Sertoli
(1842–1910)

FUNCTIONAL ANATOMY

The male reproductive system consists of testes, epididymis, vas deferens, ejaculatory ducts, prostate, urethra, and penis. They have ***two important functions***, **spermatogenesis** (formation of spermatozoa) and **steroidogenesis** (synthesis of testosterone). Spermatozoa produced by testes enter the epididymis from where they pass into the vas deferens (Fig. 67.1). Epididymis and proximal part of vas deferens store sperms. At the time of ejaculation, sperms enter into the urethra in the body of prostate through the ejaculatory duct and via urethra they come out of the genital tract.

The Testes

In human beings, testes are located in scrotum. During intrauterine life, testes are placed in the abdominal cavity beneath the posterior abdominal wall. Gradually they **descend down to the inguinal canal** during mid-pregnancy. During two months before term, they descend further through the inguinal canal into the scrotum (Application Box 67.1).

Application Box 67.1

Separate domicile for male gonad: Testes are the male gonads that are placed in separate sacs almost hanging away from the body. In female, the gonads (ovaries) are well preserved in the abdominal cavity. Then, why has the nature provided separate external compartments for male gonads? Scrotum is the sac, which keeps testis at about 2– 3°C below the core body temperature and this cooler environment is highly favorable for spermatogenesis.

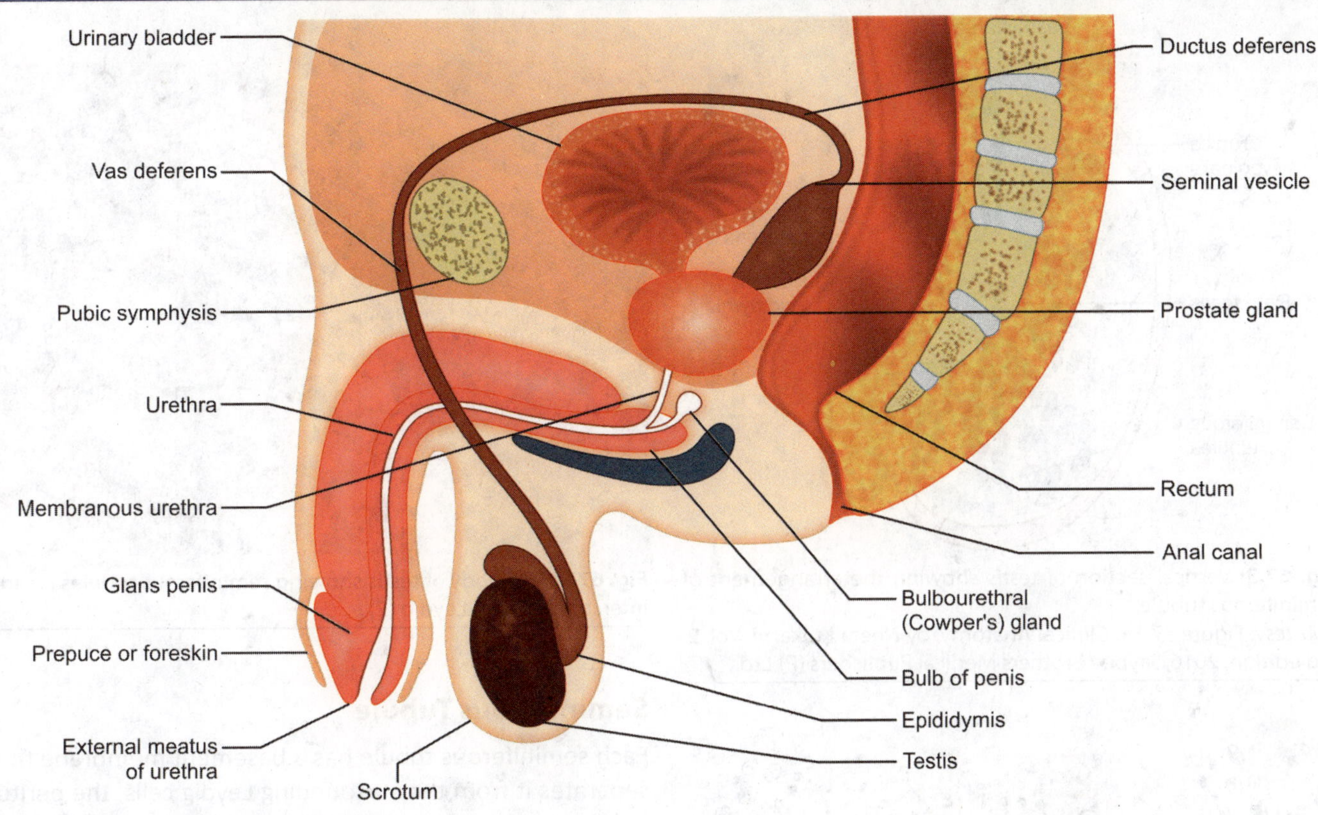

Fig. 67.1: Structures of male genital tract.

The **scrotal temperature is cooler** than core body temperature **for following reasons**:

1. **Anatomical location:** Scrotum forms sacs that are like **outpouching from the body**, which has **less direct transmission of the inner body temperature** into it. Testes being placed in the scrotum avails scrotal temperature.
2. **Pampiniform plexus of the blood vessels:** These plexuses of blood vessels **serve as counter-current exchanger** between warm arterial blood entering the testes and cooler venous blood leaving the testes (Fig. 67.2).
3. **Role of cremasteric & dartos muscles:** Cremaster muscle is a small band of skeletal muscle present in the spermatic cord that contracts or relaxes in response to change in environmental temperature.
   - It **contracts on exposure to sever cold** and elevates the testis and **relaxes in warm environment** and lowers the testis.
   - Also, a flap of smooth muscle is present in the fascial layer of scrotum, called **dartos muscle**, which contracts on exposure to cold. This increases **wrinkling of scrotal skin** and facilitates lifting of the testis.
   - Thus, cremasteric and dartos muscles on exposure to cold push testes close to the pelvic cavity where they can absorb body heat, and pull them away from the body in hot environment. Therefore, these muscles **prevent temporary sterility** in extreme weathers.

Weight of each testis is about 10–15 grams, length 5 cm and width 2.5 cm in adults. Testes receive blood supply from the spermatic arteries that originate directly from the aorta.

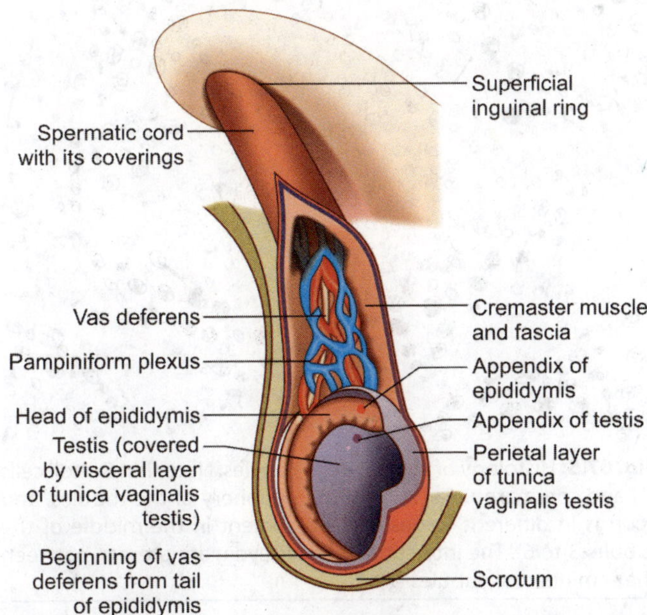

Fig. 67.2: Pampiniform plexus and cremaster muscle of the scrotum. *Courtesy*: Figure 57.12, Clinical Anatomy, Vol.2, 3rd Edition, by Neeta Kulkarni, 2016; Jaypee Brothers Medical Publishers (P) Ltd.

Functional Histology of Testis

Testes are covered by thick connective tissue membrane called **tunica albuginea**. Each testis is made up of seminiferous tubules. Hundreds of tubules are tightly packed to from a mass of coiled loops (Fig. 67.3).

1. Each loop begins and ends in a single duct called ***tubulus rectus***, which in turn drains into the epididymis.

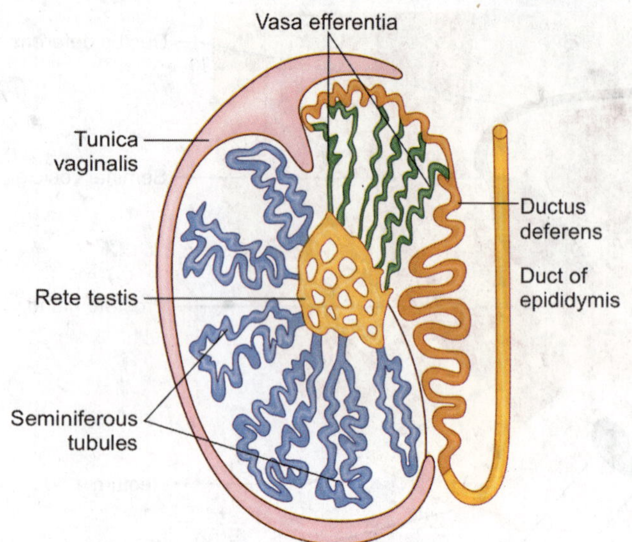

Fig. 67.3: Vertical section of testis showing the arrangement of seminiferous tubule.
Courtesy: Figure 57.14, Clinical Anatomy, by Neeta Kulkarni, Vol. 2, 3rd edition, 2016; Jaypee Brothers Medical Publishers (P) Ltd.

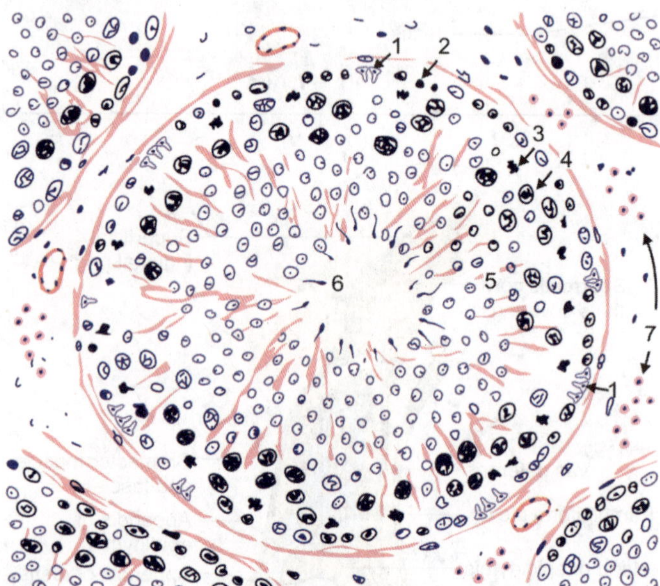

Fig. 67.5: Histology of seminiferous tubules. Note that Sertoli cells (1) and spermatoginia (2) lie in the periphery of the tubules, and sperms in different stages of development in the middle of the tubule (3 to 6). The interstitial cells of Leydig are present between the seminiferous tubules (7).

2. Tubules are arranged in lobules separated by septa formed by extensions of tunica albuginea. Each tubule is about 50 cm long and 250 μm in diameter.
3. **Myoid cells** are present surrounding the basal lamina of the seminiferous tubules and **interstitial cells of Leydig** are present in the space between the seminiferous tubules (Fig. 67.4).
4. Thus, testis consists of seminiferous tubules and interstitium that mainly contains Leydig cells, connective tissues and capillaries, and few myoid cells and fibroblasts.

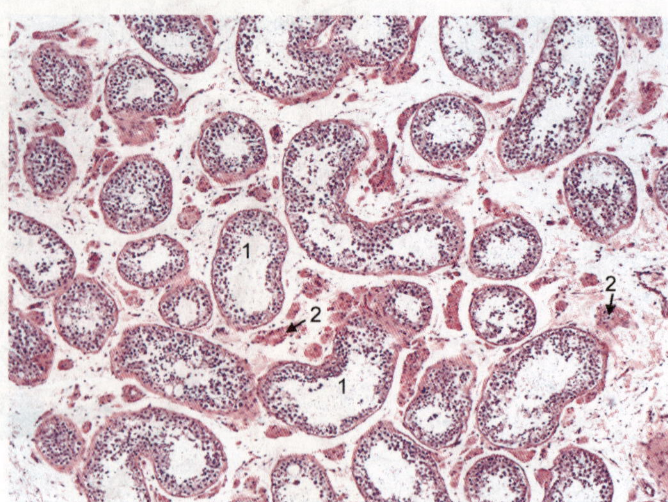

Fig. 67.4: Histology of testis showing seminiferous tubules (1) and interstitial cells of Leydig (2).

Seminiferous Tubule

Each seminiferous tubule has a basement membrane that separates it from the surrounding Leydig cells, the peritubular cells (myoid cells) and the connective tissue.

1. Spermatogonia and Sertoli cells are located in the wall of the tubule just beneath the basement membrane (Fig. 67.5).
2. There are **two principal cell types** in seminiferous tubules: somatic cells (**Sertoli cells**) and **germ cells** (Fig. 67.6).

Sertoli Cells

Sertoli cells are the sustentacular cells in seminiferous tubules, which form the major cell mass in them.

Structure of Sertoli cells

They are irregularly shaped cells that are extended from the basement membrane into the lumen of seminiferous tubule. Sperms are attached to the apical membrane of

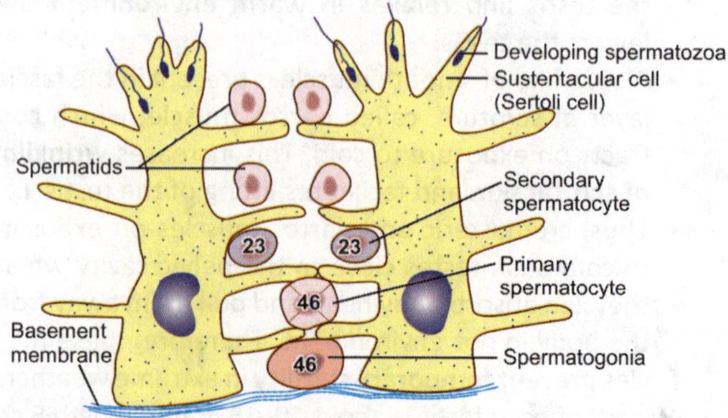

Fig. 67.6: Arrangement of Sertoli cells and germ cells in seminiferous tubule.

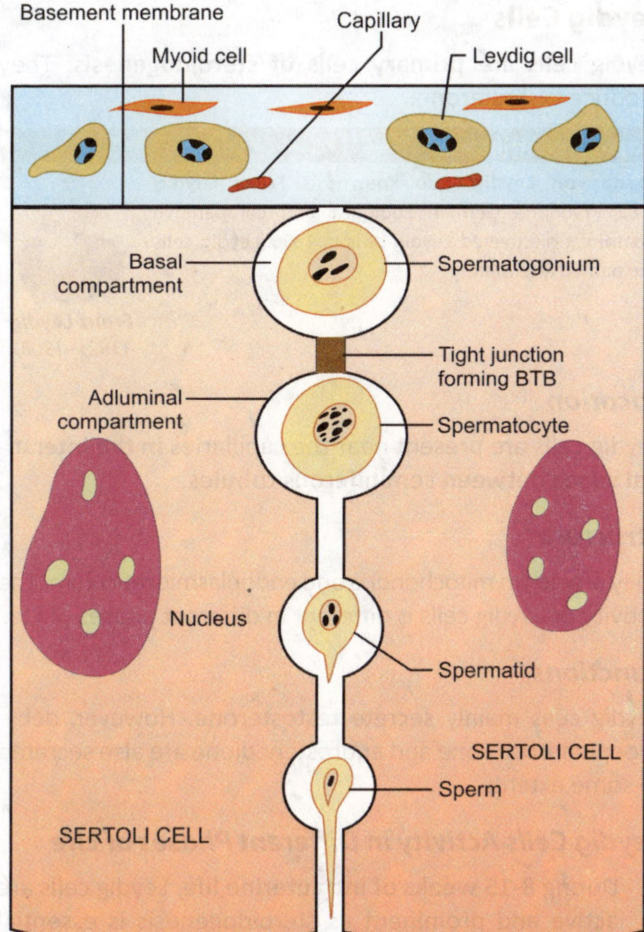

Fig. 67.7: Relationship (arrangement) of Sertoli cells with Leydig cells and germ cells. Note, tight junction between Sertoli cells that forms the blood-testis barrier (BTB) separates basal compartment containing spermatogonium from adluminal compartment containing spermatocytes, spermatid and sperm.

the Sertoli cells. At their bases, Sertoli cells are attached to each other by tight junctions. Tight junctions divide tubules into **two compartments:** basal compartment and adluminal compartment (Fig. 67.7).

Basal Compartment

The basal compartment is the *outer compartment* that mainly consists of **spermatogonium.** It is *exposed to circulating substances* as the capillaries are in close contact with it and substances from blood can easily be exchanged.

Adluminal Compartment

Adluminal compartment is the *inner compartment* that consists of **primary and secondary spermatocytes and spermatids.** It is *separated from blood-borne agents* by the tight junctions between the Sertoli cells close to basal lamina.

Blood-Testis Barrier

Because, the tight junctions between Sertoli cells are too tight (Fig. 67.7), they do not allow substances from interstitial space and blood to pass through them except steroids and few proteins. Thus, ***tight junction between Sertoli cells near the basal lamina*** forms the **blood-testis barrier** (BTB).

1. The BTB prevents the large molecules to be transported from interstitial tissue and basal compartment to the interior of the tubule (adluminal compartment).
2. However, **maturing germ cells pass through BTB** to enter into adluminal compartment. If maturing spermatocytes can pass through the BTB one could easily doubt the veracity of the barrier.
3. The **proposed explanation** is that when spermatocytes attempt to penetrate the barrier, the tight junction in front of them dislocate and give way for them, and immediately after the spermatocytes pass through the tight junctions the new tight junctions are concomitantly formed behind them.
4. Thus, physiologically, maturing germ cells pass through BTB without actually disrupting it.

Functions of BTB:

1. BTB **protects germ cells** in the seminiferous tubules from harmful elements in blood.
2. Antigenic elements are produced by germ cells during their growth and multiplication, which are capable of inducing immunological reactions in the body. BTB **prevents these antigenic products to escape into circulation** from tubule and thus prevents autoimmune reactions.
3. BTB maintains the composition of the fluid in the lumen of seminiferous tubules. The tubular luminal fluid contains less protein and glucose as they do not pass from blood through the BTB. However, it is rich in androgens, estrogens, K^+, inositol, glutamic and aspartic acids.
4. BTB maintains higher osmolality of luminal content of the seminiferous tubules, which favors the osmotic movement of fluid into the tubular lumen.

Functions of Sertoli Cells

Sertoli cells have multiple functions. Important among them are:

1. **Germ cell development:** Sertoli cells are critical to germ cell development. They provide structural support and nutrition to germ cells. Sertoli cells are rich in glycoproteins that nourish the germ cells.
2. **Phagocytosis:** Sertoli cells phagocytose residual bodies and damaged germ cells from the seminiferous tubules. *Residual bodies* are cytoplasmic fragments formed by excess cytoplasm resulting from transformation of spermatids to spermatozoa.
3. **Nourishment and growth of spermatids:** They nourish the developing spermatids. About 10 to 12 spermatids are attached to each Sertoli cells. Sertoli cells synthesize transferrin, an iron-transport protein that helps in development of sperms.
4. **Formation of tubular fluid:** They secrete fluid into the lumen of seminiferous tubule. This fluid later forms the major components of seminal fluid.

5. **Support spermiation:** This is the process of detachment of mature sperms from Sertoli cells into the lumen. In this process, *plasmin*, the proteolytic enzyme assists in release of sperms from Sertoli cells. Sertoli cells produce plasminogen activator that causes formation of plasmin.
6. **FSH and testosterone sensitivity:** Sertoli cells have receptors for FSH and testosterone. FSH receptors are present on the cell membrane and testosterone receptors are present within the nucleus. During puberty, receptors for these hormones on Sertoli cell increase. FSH increases cAMP in Sertoli cells and induces production of androgen-binding protein (*see* below) and plasminogen activator in Sertoli cells. These chemicals help in sperm development.
7. **Endocrine functions of Sertoli cells:** Sertoli cells secrete many hormones. These are:
   i. **Inhibin:** Inhibin suppresses FSH release from pituitary.
   ii. **Activin:** Activin stimulates release of FSH.
   iii. **Follistatin:** It decreases FSH secretion stimulated by activin.
   iv. **Müllerian regression substance:** During 8th week of gestation MIS is secreted from fetal Sertoli cells. MIS causes regression of müllerian duct in fetuses destined to become males.
   v. **Estrogens:** Sertoli cells contain the enzyme aromatase that converts androgen into estrogen.
8. **Secretory functions:** Sertoli cells secrete *androgen binding proteins* (ABP) and *H-Y antigen*. ABP maintains concentration of androgen in Sertoli cells, which is essential for maturation of spermatozoa. H-Y antigen is secreted by Sertoli cells during fetal life that controls development of testis.

   Androgen binding proteins (ABP): Sertoli cells secrete and synthesize ABP, a protein having molecular weight 90,000 into the luminal fluid. ABP has *high affinity for binding dihydrotestosterone* and *testosterone*. It is present in high concentration in luminal fluid. A high concentration of androgen in luminal fluid is essential for production and maturation of spermatozoa. ABP maintains this concentration of androgen in luminal fluid. It helps in *storage of androgen* in seminiferous tubule and facilitates transport of testosterone from testis to epididymis.
9. **Blood-testis barrier:** Sertoli cells provide the blood-testis barrier (BTB) for the seminiferous tubules. Thus, they protect the developing sperms from harmful effects of blood-borne toxins. Other functions of BTB are discussed above.

Germ Cells

Germ cells are **germinal epithelial cells** of seminiferous tubules. Each germ cell is a spermatogonium that forms spermatocytes and spermatozoa in the process of its development, i.e., spermatogenesis (*see* below).

Leydig Cells

Leydig cells are **primary cells of steroidogenesis**. They produce testosterone.

Scientist contributed

Franz von Leydig, also known as **Franz Leydig** (1821–1908), a German zoologist and comparative anatomist discovered Leydig cells in 1850. Leydig cells are named after him.

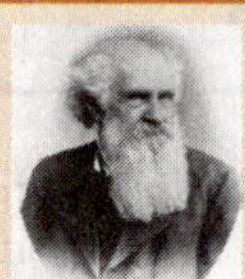

Franz Leydig
(1821–1908)

Location

Leydig cells are present near the capillaries **in the interstitial space between seminiferous tubules.**

Structure

They are rich in mitochondria and endoplasmic reticulum. The activity of Leydig cells is different in different phases of life.

Functions

Leydig cells mainly **secrete testosterone**. However, dehydroepiandrosterone and androstenedione are also secreted to some extent.

Leydig Cells Activity in Different Phases of Life

1. During **8-15 weeks of intrauterine life**, Leydig cells are active and prominent as steroidogenesis is essential for differentiation of male genital ducts. During this period, as hypothalamo-pituitary gonadal axis is not fully formed, steroidogenesis is controlled by hCG, not by LH.
2. Thereafter, Leydig cell activity decreases. **In male infants**, during 3–5 months of postnatal life, Leydig cell activity increases significantly that results in increased testosterone secretion. The physiological significance of this infantile testosterone surge is not known.
3. Leydig cells then remain dormant till puberty. At the **onset of puberty**, activity of Leydig cells in males attains maximum.
4. **After puberty**, Leydig cell activity decreases, but maintains at a basal rate till senescence.

Regulation of Leydig Cell Activity

Leydig cells have **receptors for LH.**

1. LH controls Leydig cell steroidogenesis by **cAMP-dependent mechanism**.
2. Leydig cells do not have receptors for FSH. However, FSH indirectly controls Leydig cells activity. FSH stimulates Sertoli cells to produce growth factors, which in turn promote the growth of Leydig cells.
3. Leydig cell activity is **stimulated by androgen and inhibited by estrogen.**

Interaction of Leydig cells with Sertoli cells

Sertoli cells do not produce testosterone, but have receptors for it. **Testosterone secreted from Leydig cell enters**

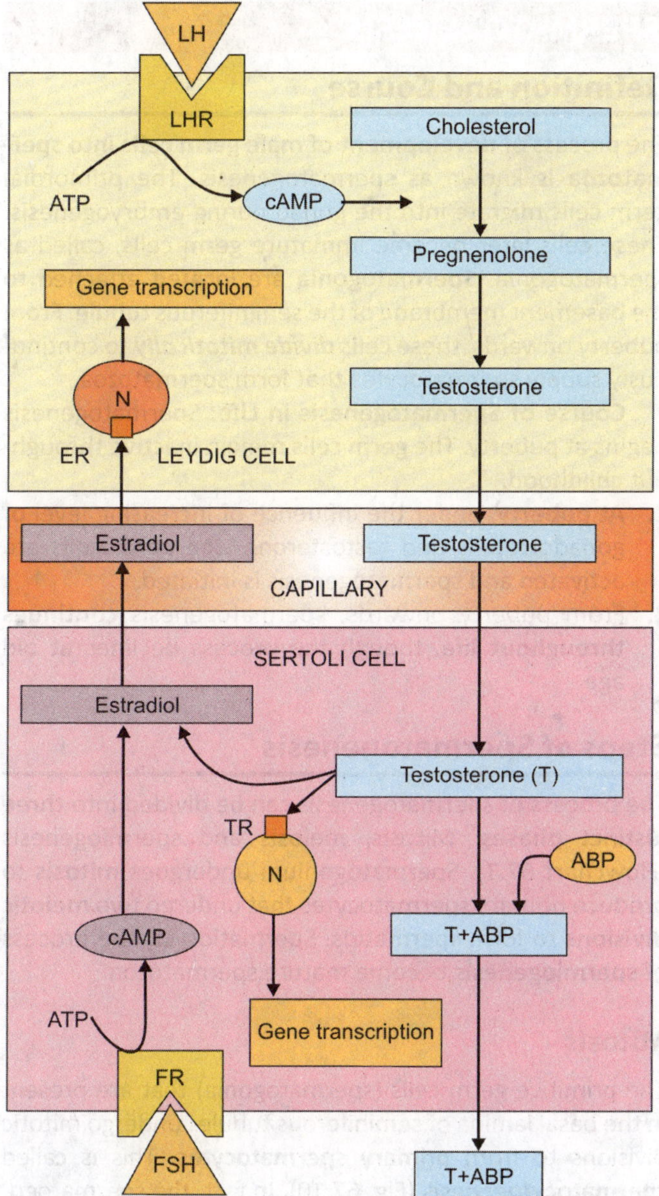

Fig. 67.8: Interaction between Leydig and Sertoli cells. Note, testosterone secreted from Leydig cells enters Sertoli cell and influences Sertoli cell functions. Similarly, estradiol produced in Sertoli cells enters Leydig cell and control Leydig cell functions. (LH: Luteinizing hormone; LHR: LH receptors; ABP: Androgen binding protein; FSH: follicle stimulating hormone; FR: FSH receptor; TR: Testosterone receptor; ER: Estrogen receptor; N: Nucleus).

Sertoli cells where it binds with the ABP. This testosterone is essential for three important functions:

1. Spermatogenesis
2. Functioning of Sertoli cells
3. Estrogen production in Sertoli cells.

Estrogen produced in Sertoli cells ***diffuses back into the Leydig*** cells and regulates Leydig cell function (Fig. 67.8).

Functions of Testis

Testis serves **three important functions.**

1. **Spermatogenesis**, i.e., production of sperms (*see* below)
2. **Steroidogenesis**, i.e. synthesis of steroid hormones, mainly testosterone, which is later, converted to dihydrotestosterone and estradiol (*see* below).
3. Testis **secretes other hormones** like activin, inhibin and follistatin that influence many other reproductive functions.

Epididymis

Seminiferous tubules open into a network of tubules, called **rete testis**. Rete testis opens into epididymis via *efferent ductules*.

Structure

Epididymis is located on the posterior aspect of the testis. It contains a **highly convoluted long duct**, which is about 5 meter in length. Epididymis is divided into **three parts**: head (the part close to testis), body and tail (Fig. 67.9).

Function

The function of epididymis is the **storage and maturation of spermatozoa** (Application Box 67.2).

1. About 99% of testicular fluid is reabsorbed in the epididymis and rete testis. Spermatozoa from tubular fluid and rete testis are transferred to epididymis almost passively as they are essentially immotile.
2. In epididymis, they **acquire the capacity for progressive forward movement** and the ability to attach to zona pellucida of ovum and penetrate into it.
3. Thus, the sperms obtained directly from testis are functionally immature, whereas **sperms obtained from body of the epididymis or further down in the male genital tract are fertile.**

Application Box 67.2

Fate of stored spermatozoa: Spermatozoa are carried from epididymis via vas deferens and ejaculatory duct into the urethra in penis to be removed out of it at the time of ejaculation. The fate of sperms that are not voided through ejaculation is not clearly known. It has been suggested that these sperms are ultimately phagocytosed by macrophages in the epididymis or voided slowly in urine. However, in Indian spiritual scriptures, it has been noted that sperms in the body are converted into vital energy, which can be further transformed into spiritual energy if properly utilized with the help of higher spiritual forces. Therefore, in practice of yoga, it has been advised to conserve and properly utilize the energy of the semen.

Vas Deferens

Epididymis empties its content into the vas deferens (Fig. 67.9), which *transfers sperms* further down in the duct.

1. Proximal part of vas deferens like epididymis ***stores the sperms***.
2. Vas deferens joins with the duct arising from seminal vesicle to from the ejaculatory duct.
3. The movement of sperm in vas deferens is active as they are capable of motility.
4. However, **contraction of muscle in the wall of vas deferens** facilitates the process of sperm movement.

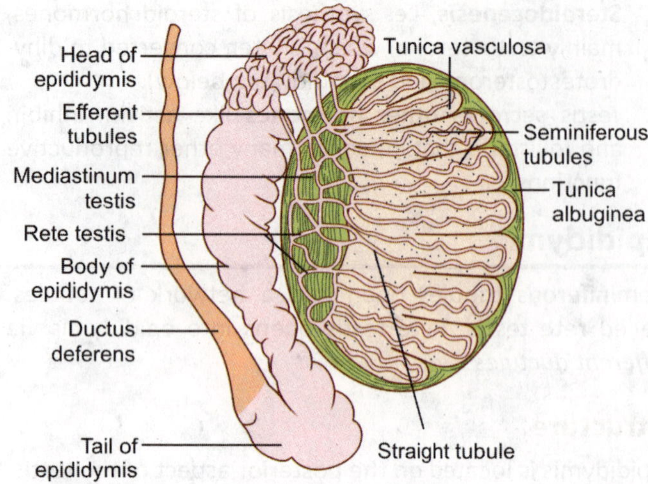

Fig. 67.9: Structure of epididymis. Note the head, body and tail of epididymis. The tail continues as ductus deferens.

Seminal Vesicle

There are two seminal vesicles located close to the prostate. They secrete a viscid and alkaline fluid called **seminal vesicular fluid**.

1. Seminal vesicular fluid contributes to **70% of the total volume** of the semen.
2. Rest 20% of the volume is contributed by epididymal fluid and fluid secreted from accessory sex glands, and 10% is contributed by sperms.
3. The seminal vesicles **secrete vitamin C and fructose**. The fluid appears yellowish as it contains flavins.
4. Most of the prostaglandins found in semen are contributed by seminal vesicle.

Accessory Sex Glands

Accessory male sex glands are prostate gland and bulbourethral glands of Cowper.

The Prostate Gland

The ejaculatory duct enters the prostatic portion of the urethra after passing through the prostate.

1. Prostate gland consists of 30–50 **branched tubuloalveolar glands** whose secretions empty into prostatic urethra.
2. The prostatic fluid contains **fibrinolysin, fibrinogenase** and large quantity of **acid phosphatase**. Fibrinolysin prevents sperm heads to clump.
3. Prostate gland also releases **a factor**, which contains sugar, sulfate and vitamin E derivative that also prevents sperm head to cluster.

Bulbourethral Glands

They secrete mucus and alkaline fluid. They also secrete the enzyme **hyaluronidase** that *facilitates penetrability of oocytes by sperms.*

SPERMATOGENESIS

Definition and Course

The process of **development of male germ cells into spermatozoa** is known as spermatogenesis. The primordial germ cells migrate into the gonad during embryogenesis. These cells later become immature germ cells, called as spermatogonia. **Spermatogonia** are located attached to the basement membrane of the seminiferous tubule. From puberty onwards, these cells ***divide mitotically*** to continuously supply spermatocytes that form spermatozoa.

Course of Spermatogenesis in Life: Spermatogenesis begins at puberty. The germ cells remain inactive throughout childhood.

1. **At puberty**, under the influence of increasing level of gonadotropins and testosterone, the germ cells are activated and spermatogenesis is initiated.
2. From puberty onwards, spermatogenesis **continues throughout life**, though the process declines at old age.

Steps of Spermatogenesis

The process of spermatogenesis can be divided into **three distinct phases**: Mitosis, meiosis and spermiogenesis (Flowchart 67.1). Spermatogonium undergoes **mitosis** to produce primary spermatocytes that undergo two **meiotic divisions** to form spermatids. Spermatids, by the process of **spermiogenesis** become mature spermatozoa.

Mitosis

The primitive germ cells (spermatogonia) that are present in the basal lamina of seminiferous tubules undergo mitotic divisions to from **primary spermatocytes**. This is called **spermatocytogenesis** (Fig. 67.10). In fact, the spermatogonia undergo many mitotic divisions to produce two types of spermatogonia: spermatogonia A and spermatogonia B.

Spermatogonia A: Spermatogonia A formed by mitotic divisions resemble the original spermatogonia and are the source of subsequent spermatogonia in the testis. Thus, they form the **spermatogonia reserve pool** in the testis.

Spermatogonia B: Spermatogonia B grow and enter adluminal compartment where they develop into primary spermatocytes.

Meiosis

The primary spermatocytes (diploid 4N DNA) undergo **two meiotic divisions**.

1. The first meiotic division forms **secondary spermatocytes** (haploid 2N DNA)) and the second meiotic division forms **spermatids** (haploid 1N DNA).
2. Spermatids contain half of the number of chromosomes (23 chromosomes, i.e., 22 autosomes and 1 sex chromosome, which is either an X or a Y chromosome).

Flowchart 67.1: Steps of spermatogenesis. Note, till the stage of primary spermatocyte, each cell contains 46 chromosomes and from secondary spermatocyte to spermatozoa, each cell contains 23 chromosomes (number indicated against each category of cells as 46 chromosomes and 23 chromosomes in bracket).

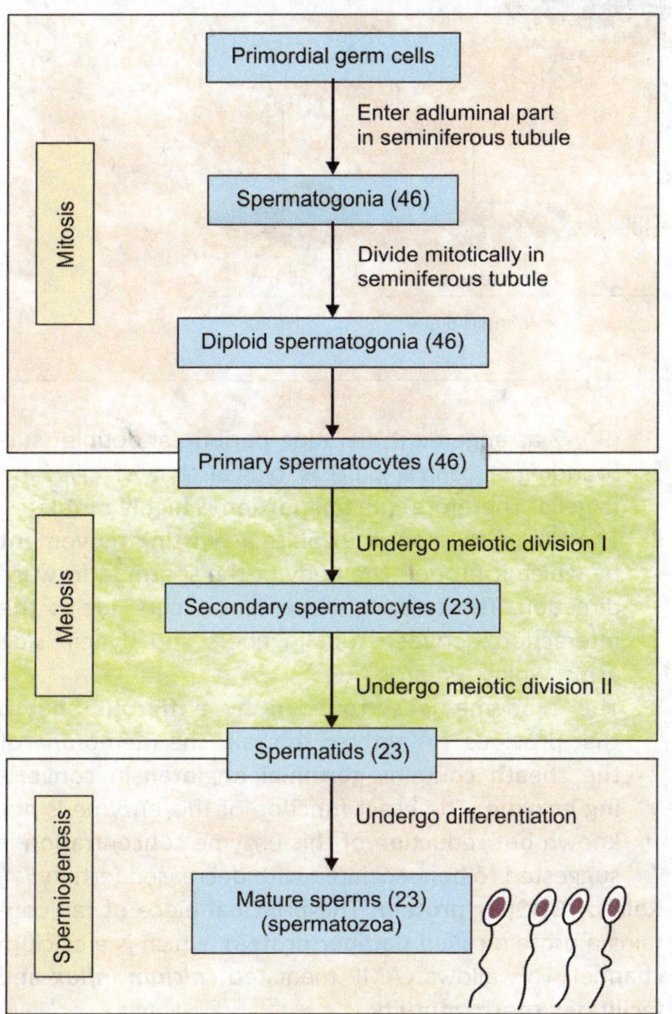

3. Of every four spermatids formed from primary spermatocytes, two of them contain X chromosome and two Y chromosomes.
4. Normally after undergoing several mitotic and two meiotic divisions in the process of spermatogenesis, *each spermatogonium yields 512 spermatids*.

Spermiogenesis

The process of development of spermatids into matured spermatozoa is called spermiogenesis. Spermatids are small, round and less characteristic cells. They undergo many structural changes to form spermatozoa (Fig. 67.10). The major changes are:

1. **Massive reduction in cytoplasm.** Cytoplasmic fragments are discarded as residual bodies.
2. **Elongation of the nucleus** to become head of spermatozoa.
3. Acquirement of an upper covering for the head called **acrosomal cap**.
4. Formation of a **middle piece and a tail piece** with the ability to move efficiently and swiftly.

All these changes occur in mature sperms to enable them to survive in a foreign and even hostile environment (**acidic vaginal pH**) in the female genital tract and to recognize and fertilize the ovum. These changes mainly help the sperm to move forward towards the ovum in the female genital tract, the movement known as **progressive motility** of the sperm.

Spermiation

Spermatozoa, after they are formed, remain in the lumen of the seminiferous tubule sticking to the apical membrane of the Sertoli cells. They **adhere tightly to the Sertoli cells**. The process of **detachment of head of spermatozoa and their free release** into the luminal fluid is called spermiation.

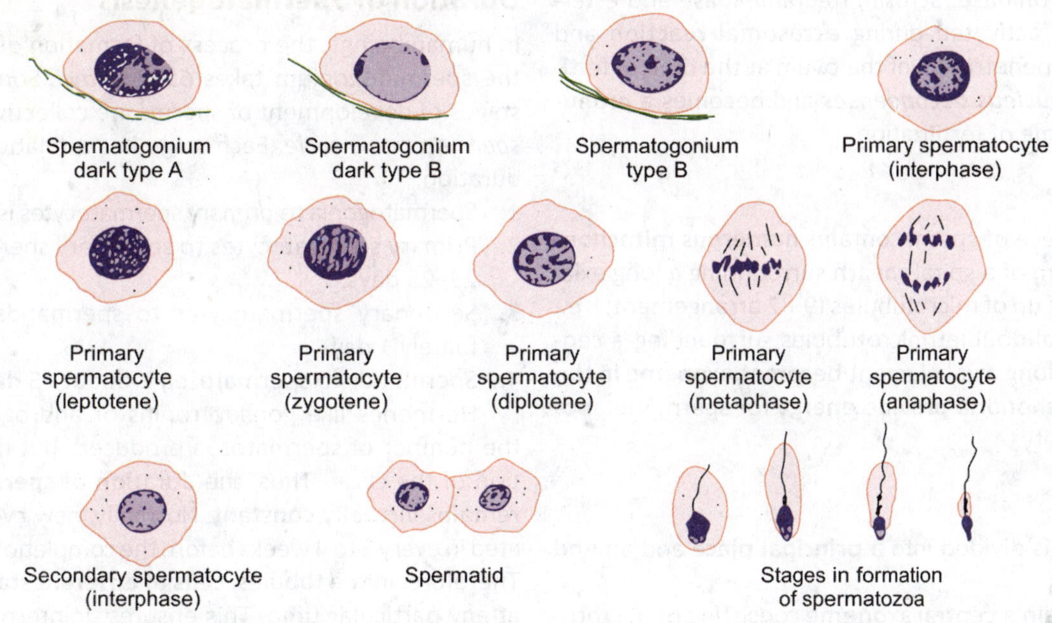

Fig. 67.10: Stages of spermatogenesis.

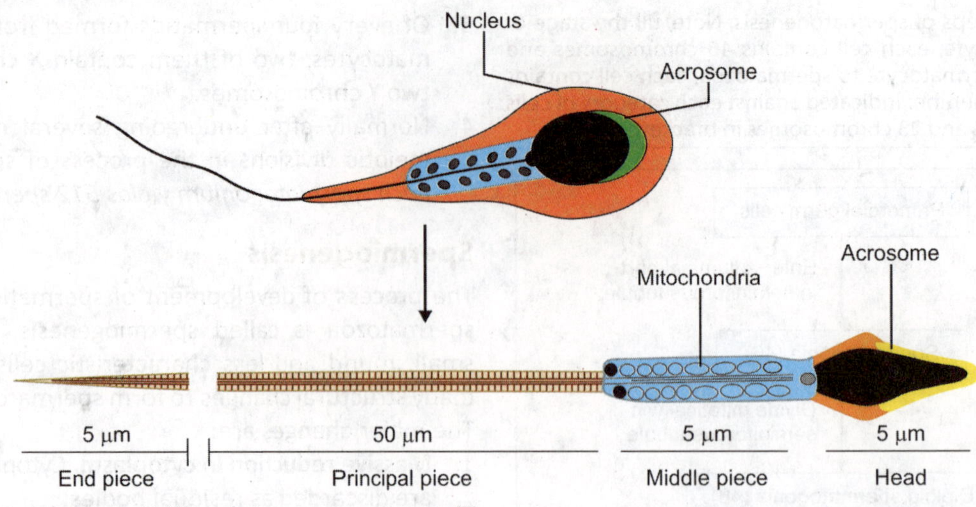

Fig. 67.11: Structure of immature (A) and mature spermatozoa (B).

Capacitation

When spermatozoa are ejaculated into the female genital tract, they undergo further maturation called capacitation. This includes **increase in further motility of sperms** and **preparation for acrosomal reaction**. However, capacitation is not so much essential for fertilization as fertilization can also occur in vitro.

Structure of Spermatozoa

A matured sperm is a motile cell rich in DNA, consisting of head, middle peace and tail (Fig. 67.11). A human sperm is about 65 μm long with average diameter of 2 μm.

Head

Head contains **a prominent nucleus** at the center, which is condensed with chromatin. The head is covered by a cap called **acrosome**, which is formed from Golgi apparatus. Acrosome is like a lysosome **rich in proteolytic enzymes** such as hyaluronidase, acrosin, neuraminidase and esterases that are activated during **acrosomal reaction** and help in sperm penetration of the ovum at the time of fertilization. The ***nucleus decondenses*** and becomes **a pronucleus** at the time of fertilization.

Middle Piece

The middle piece of sperm contains **numerous mitochondria** in the form of a spiral sheath surrounding a long axial filament made up of microtubules (9 + 2 arrangement; i. e., nine peripheral doublet microtubules surrounding a central pair). The long axial filament **becomes axoneme in the tail**. The mitochondria **provide energy** for sperm metabolism and motility.

Tail Piece

The tail piece is divided into a **principal piece** and an **end piece**.

1. They contain a central **axoneme** consisting of microtubules. The axial filament arrangement in microtubules (9 + 2 arrangement; i.e. nine peripheral doublet surrounding a central pair) is typical that of cilia and flagella. Therefore, the **tail portion is highly motile**.
2. The tail of the sperm exhibits **a twisting movement** by which it propels the body of the sperm in forward direction. The twisting movement occurs due to the interaction between tubulin fibers and dynein side arms, which requires ATP.
3. The axoneme is surrounded by a **fibrous sheath** that provides strength to the tail. The membrane of the sheath contains **germinal angiotensin converting enzyme**. The exact function of this enzyme is not known but reduction of this enzyme concentration is suggested to be associated with decreased fertility.

Role of CatSper protein: The principal piece of tail contains a protein called **CatSper protein**, which is a calcium channel. This allows cAMP mediated ***calcium influx*** and **facilitates sperm motility**.

Duration of Spermatogenesis

In human beings, the process of formation of sperm from the spermatogonium takes ***65–74 days***. Sometimes, the stages of development of sperms are collectively called as *spermatogenic cycle*. Each stage has a relatively constant duration:

1. Spermatogonia to primary spermatocytes is 16–20 days.
2. Primary spermatocytes to secondary spermatocytes is 23–25 days.
3. Secondary spermatocytes to spermatids is approximately 1 day.
4. Spermatids to spermatozoa is about 25 days.

Hormones like gonadotropins or androgen influence the number of spermatozoa produced, but not the duration of the cycle. Thus, the **duration of spermatogenesis remains virtually constant**. Normally, new cycles are initiated in every 2 to 4 weeks before the completion of old cycle. Therefore, in the tubules, **cells of different stages** are seen at any particular time. This ensures uninterrupted supply of spermatozoa throughout life.

Rate of Production of Sperms

A single spermatogonium **forms 512 spermatids**, if all of them remain alive.

1. Approximately, 200 millions of sperms are produced daily in an adult testis in humans. This is roughly same as the number of sperms in an ejaculate in a normal healthy adult. Expressed per unit weight of testicular tissue, about **6–7 million sperms are produced per gram per day**.
2. The rate of production of sperms falls progressively in old age. After the age of 50, the rate of sperm production is 3.5–4 million per gram of tissue.
3. The decrease in production in elderly is due to degeneration of germ cells during meiotic prophase. However, appreciable spermatogenesis continues even at the age of 90.

Differences between Spermatogenesis and Oogenesis

There are few basic differences in the process of gametogenesis in females and males. These are:

1. In females, mitotic proliferation of germ cells completes before birth, whereas in males, spermatogonia grow only at the time of puberty and then continue to proliferate throughout life.
2. In female, the meiotic division of primary oocyte produces only one ovum, whereas in males one primary spermatocyte produces four spermatozoa.
3. In female, second meiotic division is completed only upon fertilization, whereas in males second meiotic division is completed during spermatogenesis.

Factors Controlling Spermatogenesis

Factors controlling spermatogenesis can be broadly divided into ***two categories***: hormonal and environmental.

Hormonal Factors

Androgen, estrogen and gonadotropins mainly control spermatogenesis.

1. **Androgen:** Androgens **stimulate spermatogenesis**. LH creates an elevated local concentration of androgen in the testis by stimulating Leydig cells to secrete testosterone, and this **high intertesticular testosterone is essential for spermatogenesis.**
   - Testosterone secreted from Leydig cells diffuse into the seminiferous tubule. In tubule, only the Sertoli cells (not spermatogenic cells), have receptors for testosterone.
   - **Testosterone binds with ABP in the Sertoli cells** (Fig. 67.8), which maintains a high concentration of testosterone in the cell. However, it is not clearly known how testosterone promotes spermatogenesis.
   - It appears that, till the formation of spermatid does not depend on androgen, rather **spermiogenesis** (spermatids developing to spermatozoa) **is androgen dependent**.
2. **Estrogen:** Estrogen content of the fluid in the rete testis is high and there are **estrogen receptors in the rete testis**. Rete testis reabsorbs fluid and makes the spermatozoa concentrated, which is required for sperm maturation. The diluted volume of large fluid that enters rete testis and epididymis unless absorbed adequately results in infertility. **Estrogen concentrates the fluid** by facilitating fluid reabsorption.
3. **LH and FSH:** LH helps in spermatogenesis by **producing a high local concentration of androgen**. FSH maintains gametogenic functions of testis. It appears that FSH is required for initiation of spermatogenesis at the time of puberty, and then LH maintains it.

Environmental Factors

It is mainly the **temperature** that influences spermatogenesis. Lower environmental temperature facilitates spermatogenesis. Spermatogenesis **best occurs at 30 to 35**°C. However, very low temperature inhibits it. Conversely, **increased temperature inhibits spermatogenesis**. Therefore, in persons taking repeated hot bath or those who regularly use insulated athletic support for the scrotum, sperm count is invariably less. Generally, sperm count is more in comfortable winter and less in intense summer.

Semen Analysis

Semen analysis is one of the important tests **for assessment of male fertility**. It is performed to know if the sterility is related to sperm production. It is also performed after vasectomy, to check its completeness. It reflects the activity of the testes and accessory sex organs in males.

Analysis of freshly collected sample of semen gives the knowledge about the male fertility which is detected by examining the sample under microscope. Usually, the sample is collected after a period of sexual abstinence for 2 days.

Composition of Normal Semen

Volume	: 2 to 5 mL
Color	: White, opalescent
Specific gravity	: 1.028
Motility	: > 60% should be actively motile within 3 h of collection
Count	: > 40 millions/ml is considered normal (usually, 100 millions/ml is seen normally)
Liquefaction	: Should liquefy within half-an-hour
Morphology	:> 80% should have normal morphology
pH	: 7.3 to 7.5
Fructose content	: Fructose concentration is 2–7 mg/mL
Other biochemical constituents:	1. Prostaglandins 2. Ascorbic acid 3. Flavins 4. Phosphorylcholine

5. Ergothioneine
6. Fibrinolysin, fibrinogenase
7. Acid phosphatase
8. Zinc
9. Phospholipids
10. Cholesterol
11. Spermin
12. Citric acid
13. Phosphate
14. Bicarbonate
15. Hyaluronidase

Fructose and other biochemical compositions as noted above from serial No. 1 to 5 are synthesized and secreted from seminal vesicles. The secretion from seminal vesicle constitutes 60% of the semen volume. Other biochemical compositions from serial No. 6 to 11 are released from prostate. Secretion from prostate contributes to 20% of the total semen volume. Bicarbonate and phosphates are buffers in the seminal fluid. Normally, sperm motility is facilitated by **prostate specific antigen** (PSA) (Application Box 67. 3).

Application Box 67.3

PSA is a marker of prostate cancer: Prostate specific antigen (PSA) is 30 kDa serine protease formed and secreted from the prostate into the seminal fluid. **Semenogelin**, the sperm motility inhibitor is hydrolyzed by PSA. Thus, PSA facilitates sperm motility. The PSA gene has two androgen response elements. Though PSA is elevated in BHP (benign hyperplasia of prostate) and prostatitis, it is markedly increased in malignancy of prostate. Hence, elevated plasma PSA is used as a screening test for detection of prostate cancer.

Abnormalities

Volume

A low volume might suggest an anatomical or functional defect or an inflammatory condition of the genital tract. Volume decreases with advancing age.

Motility

In a normal sample, **at least 60% of the sperms should exhibit forward motility** within the first 3 hours of collection of the specimen. Motility less than 40% is associated with sterility. The speed of normal human sperm in female genital tract is 3 mm/min. Within one hour of ejaculation in the vagina, the sperms reach fallopian tube where they fertilize the ovum.

Count

Sperm count **below 20 millions/ml results in sterility**. A count between 20 to 40 millions/ml indicates borderline infertility.

Liquefaction

Delayed liquefaction of more than 2 hours suggests inflammation of accessory glands or enzyme defects in the secretory products of the glands.

Morphology

Normally **70% of the sperms should have normal morphology**. Abnormalities more than 30% indicate serious pathology. The abnormalities include abnormal shapes, and poorly formed head or tail. The abnormal sperms may have bifurcated tail, bifid head, spirally coiled tail, or absence of head (Figs. 67.12A to D).

pH

pH below 7.0 indicates semen content is mainly prostatic fluid, which may be due to congenital absence of seminal vesicle.

Fructose Content

The normal fructose content of semen is 2–7 mg/mL. Its absence indicates obstruction or absence of the ejaculatory ducts or seminal vesicle.

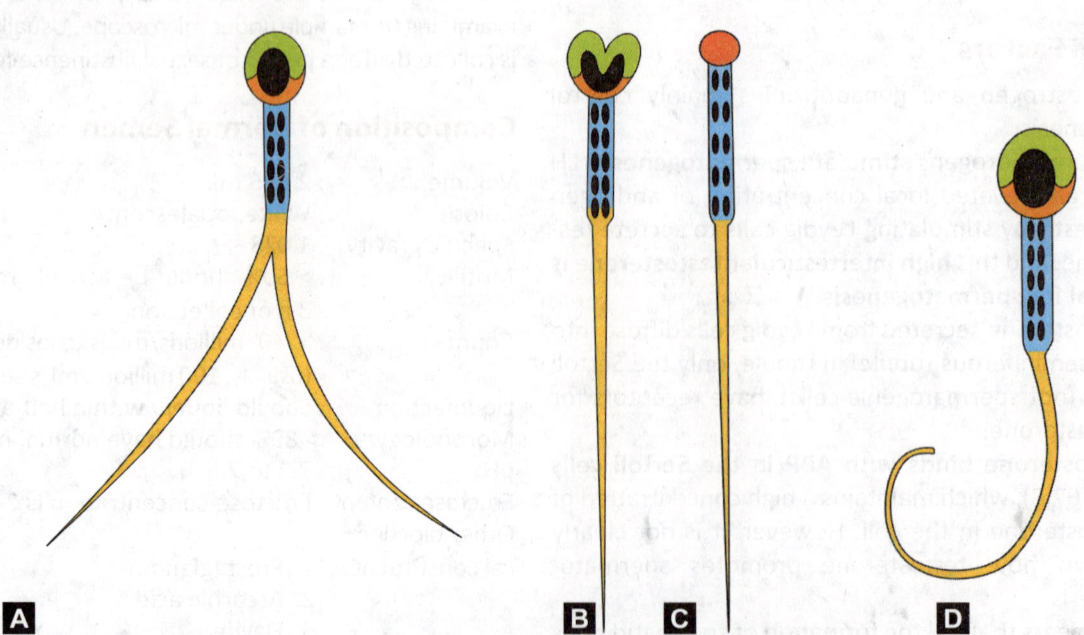

Figs. 67.12A to D: Abnormal sperms. (A) Bifid tail; (B) Bifid head; (C) No head; (D) Curved tail.

Effects of Vasectomy

Vasectomy is the bilateral ligation of vas deferens. This is the permanent contraceptive procedure for males. This is a safe and convenient contraceptive procedure.

1. About 50% of vasectomized males **develop antibodies against sperms**. However, the incidence is more following restoration of patency of the vas deferens in males those who wish to restore their fertility.
2. As such, restoration of patency of the vas (**recanalization**) is a difficult procedure. The anti-sperm antibodies further reduce the fertility.

TESTICULAR HORMONES

Testosterone

The principal steroid secreted from testis is testosterone. It is the essential hormone for male reproduction and its absence or decreased production leads to sterility. Primarily, it allows the development of male reproductive organs during fetal life, controls spermatogenesis, guides development of secondary sex characteristics and maintains male vigor.

Source

Testosterone is synthesized by the **Leydig cells of testis**. Testosterone is also secreted from **adrenal cortex, ovaries and placenta**. Thus, a small amount of testosterone is secreted in females.

Structure, Synthesis and Secretion

It is a C_{19} steroid hormone with an OH group at 17 position.

1. It is **synthesized from cholesterol** in Leydig cells of the testis. It is also formed from **androstenedione secreted from adrenal cortex**. Though, the biosynthetic pathways in the endocrine tissue that form steroid hormones are similar, minor differences exist among the enzymes that are involved in the process. For example, the 17α-hydroxylase is found in testis, whereas 11– and 21–β hydroxylases are found in adrenal cortex.
2. Therefore, in testis, pregnenolone is hydroxylated at 17 position.
3. Pregnenolone is converted to testosterone in two pathways: **delta 5** and **delta 4 pathways**. Major steps of **these pathways are** summarized in Figure 67.13.
4. Pregnenolone also forms progesterone, which forms 17α-hydroxyprogesterone, which in turn forms androstenedione and testosterone by **delta-4-pathway**.

The normal secretion rate of testosterone from testes is 4–10 mg per day. The normal plasma concentration of testosterone is **300–1000 ng/dL in adult males** and *30–70 ng/dL in females*.

Metabolism

About 98% of testosterone binds with plasma proteins and only 2% is free in plasma. The free testosterone

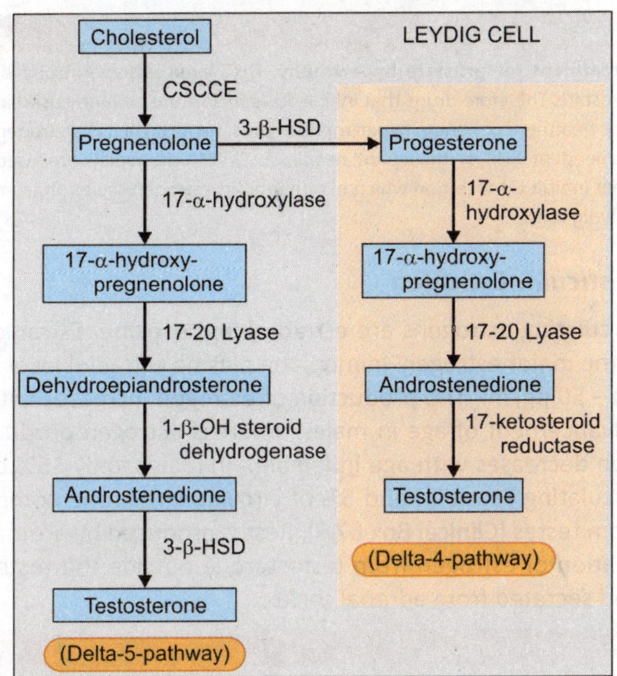

Fig. 67.13: Steps of testosterone synthesis. (CSCCE: Cholesterol side chain cleavage enzyme HSD: Hydroxy steroid dehydrogenase).

enters the target tissues in which it is converted to its active form **dihydrotestosterone** (DHT) by 5α-reductase and **estradiol** (17β-estradiol) by *aromatase*. Thus testosterone acts as prohormone and DHT is the biologically active hormone. DHT has 2–3 times more affinity than testosterone for binding with androgen receptors (Clinical Box 67.1). DHT causes hypertrophy of prostate (Clinical Box 67.2)

Clinical Box 67.1

Penis-at-14 syndrome: Normally, DHT which is formed from testosterone by the enzyme *5α-reductase* is essential for the development of male genitalia during early embryonic life. Therefore, deficiency of 5α-reductase in males results in confusing genitalia containing internal male and external female characters. In the absence of DHT, female genitalia predominate in genetic male (*male pseudohermaphroditism*) at birth. Undescended testis is a common feature in this condition and they are born as female children. At the time of puberty, testosterone secretion increases and they develop male figure with enlargement of clitoris to become a penis like structure. At this point in their life, they become boys and change their name and sex. They may even develop full male libido and do intercourse with women. As it occurs around the age of 14, syndrome is called penis-at-14-syndrome. It is common in Dominican Republic.

17–ketosteroids: About 65% binding of testosterone in plasma occurs with *gonadal steroid binding globulin* (GBG) and 33% with *sex steroid binding globulin* (SBG). Most of the circulating testosterone is converted into **17–ketosteroids** by the enzyme 17β-dehydrogenase and a small amount into **estrogen**. 17–ketosteroids possess about 20% of androgen activity. The **principal ketosteroids are androsterone and etiocholanolone**. Ketosteroids are excreted in urine. However, two-thirds of urinary ketosteroid is of adrenal origin and one-third of testicular origin.

Clinical Box 67.2

Treatment for prostate hypertrophy: DHT induces hypertrophy of prostate. Therefore drugs that inhibit *5α-reductase* are currently used in the treatment of benign hypertrophy of prostate (BHP). If it is androgen dependent BHP or malignant neoplasia, GnRH antagonists are used that inhibit LH secretion which in turn inhibits estrogen secretion from Leydig cells.

Testicular Estrogen

Circulating estrogens are **estradiol and estrone**. Estradiol is the major estrogen. In men, the plasma estradiol level is 20 – 50 pg/ml. The production of estrogen increases with advancement of age in males, whereas estrogen production decreases with age in female. In males, only 15% of circulating estradiol and 5% of circulating estrone comes from testes (Clinical Box 67.3). Rest is produced by aromatization of estrogen from testosterone outside the testes and secreted from adrenal cortex.

Clinical Box 67.3

Gynecomastia in males: In adipose tissues, skin, liver and brain, testosterone is aromatized to estrogen, which is then released into circulation. Therefore in men, circulating level of estrogen (estradiol and estrone) is almost close to the level of estrogen in follicular phase in females. However, men are protected from feminization due to high level of androgens and high responsiveness of tissues to androgens. Therefore, use of anabolic steroids or testosterone analogues (as athletes use), decreased testosterone secretion, estrogen producing testicular tumors, and tissue insensitivity to androgens result in gynecomastia.

Mechanism of Action

Testosterone like other steroid hormones acts by binding with the cytoplasmic nuclear receptors. In the cell, two pathways are activated: DHT pathway, and testosterone pathway (Fig. 67.14).

DHT pathway

This pathway is mainly active in **prostate, scrotum, penis, skin and bones**. The testosterone is converted to DHT by **5α-reductase**. DHT then binds with androgen receptors in the nucleus and induces RNA transcription to form various proteins. This causes **sexual maturation at puberty and external virilization**. Thus, DHT is mainly responsible for development of facial hair, skin changes, recession of hair line, and enlargement of prostate, scrotum, penis and bone.

Testosterone Pathway

Testosterone directly binds with testosterone receptors in the nucleus that induces m RNA activity. This pathway **mainly regulates gonadotropin secretion**, causes muscle development, **controls spermatogenesis**, and influences male **sex drive and libido**.

Physiological Actions

Testosterone is an **anabolic hormone**. It promotes growth of male reproductive system and causes development of secondary sex characters. Among various androgens, the potency in order of sequence is as follows:

- DHT > testosterone > androstenedione > DHEA
- DHEA is dehydroepiandrosterone.

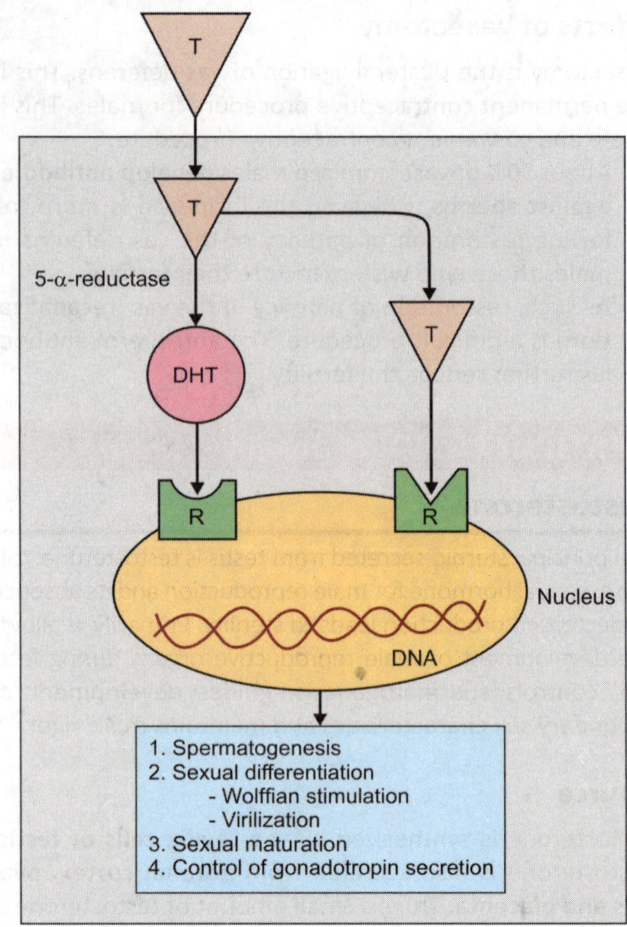

Fig. 67.14: Mechanisms of testosterone action. Note that testosterone (T) is converted to dihydrotestosterone (DHT) in the cell. There are separate receptors (R) for both testosterone and DHT in the nucleus. Therefore, two separate mechanisms exist in different cells for testosterone actions.

Development of Secondary Sex Characteristics

Testosterone is primarily responsible for changes in males that occur at puberty. It develops and maintains male secondary sex characteristics. These features mainly include changes in external and internal genitalia, distribution of body hair, skin changes, mental growth, voice change, change in body configuration and musculoskeletal changes.

1. **Changes in external genitalia:** Penis enlarges **in length and width**. The scrotum becomes more rugose and pigmented.
2. **Changes in internal genitalia:** Seminal vesicles increase in size and start secreting fructose. Prostate gland enlarges and secretion increases from prostate and bulbourethral gland.
3. **Growth and distribution of body hairs:** Hair growth is classified into **three groups** depending on their sensitivity to androgens: nonsexual, ambisexual and sexual. **Nonsexual hairs** are hairs of eyebrows and extremities.

Ambisexual hairs are the hairs in the axilla, and **sexual hairs** are the hairs in the face, chest and upper pubic triangle. Androgen stimulates growth of all types of hairs, though the effects are more on sexual and ambisexual hairs. It promotes hair growth in axilla, on the chest and pubic triangle, and around the anus. In the face, hairs grow in the form of moustache and beard. Pubic hairs grow with male pattern (in the shape of a triangle of which the apex is upward). The hair line on the scalp recedes in males. Therefore, it is believed that baldness is a sign of maleness.

4. **Skin changes:** In general, skin becomes tough. Secretion of sebaceous gland increases and becomes thick. This leads to **acne formation**. Sometimes acne vulgaris appears. Skin derived from urogenital sinus, i.e., the prepuce, clitoris, labia majora and scrotum becomes more sensitive. Skin in and around genitalia becomes more pigmented.
5. **Mental changes:** The individual becomes more **active and aggressive**. He takes more **interest in opposite sex**.
6. **Voice change:** Enlargement of larynx and thickening of vocal cord occur. Therefore, **voice becomes thick and deep**.
7. **Body configuration:** General increase in body height and girth occurs (growth spurt). Especially, **Broadening of the shoulder** occurs with general increase in size of skeletal muscles. These changes impart masculine phenotypic expression.
8. **Musculoskeletal changes:** Growth of long bones, pectoral girdle and vertebral bones occurs at puberty. Testosterone causes **closure of epiphysis** of long bone, ultimately limiting increase in height of the individual. It causes muscle hypertrophy, increases muscle protein synthesis and **increases muscle mass**.

Effects on Spermatogenesis

Testosterone **stimulates spermatogenesis**, the exact mechanism of which is not known. It is essential for sperm production and maturation.

1. It mainly **facilitates the process of spermiogenesis**.
2. It initiates spermatogenesis at puberty and then maintains it throughout adulthood and also in old age.

Effects during Embryonic Life

In male fetus, between 8th and 18th week testosterone causes the **differentiation of male genitalia**.

1. The **development of Wolffian duct** into epididymis, vas deferens and seminal vesicles depends directly on the effects of androgen.
2. Also, the **differentiation of urogenital sinus and genital tubercle** into penis, scrotum and testis is mediated by testosterone and DHT.
3. Further, **descent of testis** into scrotum is promoted by testosterone.

Anabolic Effects

Testosterone **increases the synthesis of proteins** and decreases its catabolism. This results in increased growth and development of bones and muscles.

1. It **causes sodium, potassium, calcium, phosphate, and water retention** from kidney.
2. It is used as an **anabolic drug** in patients suffering from wasting diseases. Athletes use it as anabolic steroids.

Effects on Brain

Many areas in the brain have androgen receptors. However, the receptors are **densely located in limbic areas**, especially in amygdala and septum, and in hypothalamus, pituitary and preoptic area.

1. In these areas, testosterone is **aromatized to estrogen** (Flowchart 67.2).
2. **Sexual dimorphism of neurons** in the brain with respect to their distribution, size, number and activity has been reported in preoptic area and amygdala.

Other Effects

Testosterone, by its negative feedback effects, **inhibits GnRH secretion** from hypothalamus and LH and FSH secretion from anterior pituitary. It **stimulates erythropoiesis**.

Flowchart 67.2: Fate of testosterone secreted from Leydig cells.

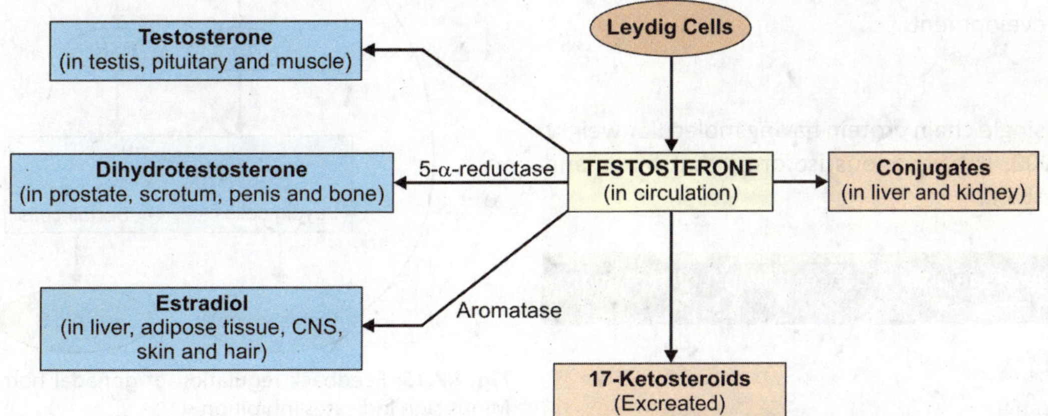

Other Testicular Hormones

Other testicular hormones are androgens other than testosterone, inhibin, activin and follistatin. Estrogen is also produced in testis by aromatization of androgen in Sertoli cells.

Androgens

Testis secretes androgens. Testicular androgens are testosterone (*see* above), **androstenedione** and **dihydrotestosterone**. Among them, testosterone is the major androgen (Table 67.1).

Inhibin

Source

Inhibin is secreted from **Sertoli cells of testes** in males and **granulosa cells** of ovaries in females.

Types and Structure

There are two types of inhibins: inhibin A and inhibin B. Inhibins are made up of **two subunits**: α and β. **The β subunit** is of two types βA and βB. The **inhibin A** is made up of αβA and **inhibin B** is made up of αβB. The α and β subunits are made up of polypeptides. Inhibin B is the FSH regulating peptide.

The homodimers and heterodimers of β subunits are formed. This results in formation of βAβB, βBβB, and βAβA. These are called **activins**. Activins and inhibins are found in the gonads, brain, and many other tissues. In bone marrow, activins stimulate leucopoiesis.

Functions

The main function of inhibin is to **provide feedback signal to inhibit FSH secretion** from anterior pituitary. Inhibin B mainly inhibits FSH secretion.

Activin

It is a polypeptide hormone with molecular weight of 30,000. Activin is **produced by Sertoli cells.**

1. It stimulates **secretion of FSH.**
2. Activin results from various combinations of βA and βB subunits of inhibin that forms βAβB, βBβB, and βAβA.
3. They stimulate WBC development in the bone marrow, formation of mesoderm during embryonic life and also gonadal development.

Follistatin

Follistatin is a single chain protein having molecular weight of about 40,000. It has various isoforms that binds and **inactivates activin.**

Table 67.1: Average plasma concentration (μg/lit) of androgens in adult male.

Testosterone	: 6.5
Androstenedione	: 1.5
Dihydrotestosterone	: 0.5

1. When activins bind with follistatin they loose their functions.
2. Thus, FSH secretion is reduced from pituitary cells.
3. Follistatin **influences developing spermatogenic cells** by a paracrine mechanism.

Regulation of Testicular Functions

The major function of testes is to secrete testicular hormones, especially testosterone that controls gametogenesis, sexual development and anabolic effects. Testicular functions are controlled by hypothalamic and pituitary inputs.

Hypothalamic Control

Hypothalamus secretes GnRH. **GnRH stimulates LH and FSH secretion** from anterior pituitary that in turn influences testicular steroidogenesis.

Pituitary Control

Anterior pituitary controls testicular functions by secreting LH and FSH. **FSH stimulates Sertoli cells to produce inhibin** that maintains the gametogenic functions of the testis. FSH also stimulates secretion of androgen binding protein. **LH stimulates Leydig cells to secrete testosterone,** which controls gametogenesis.

Steroid Feedback

Testosterone provides **negative feedback signal** to hypothalamus to inhibit the secretion of GnRH, and to gonadotrophs of anterior pituitary to inhibit secretion of LH (Fig. 67.15). Inhibin provides negative feedback effect on anterior pituitary to inhibit the secretion of FSH.

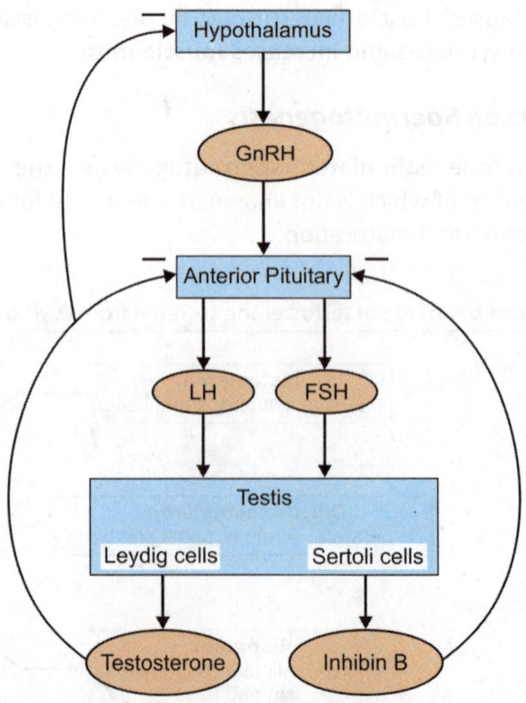

Fig. 67.15: Feedback regulation of gonadal hormone secretion. Minus sign indicates inhibition.

TESTICULAR ABNORMALITIES

Cryptorchidism

The failure of migration of testis from abdominal cavity into the scrotum during fetal development is called **undescended testis** or cryptorchidism. The usual site of undescended testis is inguinal rings.

1. From posterior wall of the abdomen testis first descends into the inguinal region and then from there into the scrotum.
2. The descent from abdomen into the inguinal region **depends on MIS**.
3. The descent from inguinal region to scrotum depends on testosterone and other factors.
4. Descent of testis normally completes **in few days before the birth**.

Treatment

Treatment with **gonadotropin hormones** facilitates the descent of testis. Surgical correction is required when the hormonal treatment fails.

Complications

Undescended testis **decreases sperm production**, as temperature is high in the abdomen. The **incidence of malignant tumors** is significantly more in undescended testis.

Male Hypogonadism

There are mainly **two types**: Hypergonadotropic hypogonadism and hypogonadotropic hypogonadism.

Hypergonadotropic Hypogonadism

If this occurs due to testicular dysfunctions, plasma level of gonadotropin is increased.

Hypogonadotropic Hypogonadism

This ocurs mainly due to tumor of hypothalamus or pituitary. Gonadotropin level in plasma is depressed.

1. If hypogonadism **occurs after puberty**, the secondary sex characteristics regress slowly as androgenic maintenance of these features is less essential. However, loss of libido is common.
2. If loss of Leydig cells **occurs from childhood**, ***eunuchoidism*** results.
   - Enuchoids are usually tall, with narrow shoulders and less muscular development.
   - The genitalia are small.
   - Though pubic hairs are present they are usually sparse and exhibit female pattern, i.e. triangle with base up.

Androgen Secreting Tumors

Hypersecretion of testis is usually due to a tumor in the testis. Leydig cell tumors secrete androgen and result in precocious puberty in prepubertal boys.

CHAPTER SUMMARY

Key Concepts

1. In males, gametogenesis is a continuous process. Gametes (sperms) are produced in millions every day, and the process continues throughout life starting from puberty, though the rate of production decreases in old age.
2. Sertoli cells provide support to the germ cells in the process of spermatogenesis. The tight junctions between Sertoli cells from the blood-testis barrier that provides protection to developing sperms from harmful blood born toxins.
3. Leydig cells secrete testosterone that provides hormonal stimulation for spermatogenesis.

Important to Know (Must Read)

1. In examination, 'Describe the steps of spermatogenesis and factors controlling spermatogenesis, may be asked as a **Long Question.**
2. Spermatogenesis, Factors controlling spermatogenesis, Functions of Sertoli cells, Leydig cells, Blood-testis barrier, Spermiogenesis, Semen analysis, Physiological actions of testosterone, Testicular abnormalities, are usual **Short Questions** in exam.
3. In **Viva**, examiner may ask... List the steps of spermatogenesis, List the factors controlling spermatogenesis, What is the duration of spermatogenesis, What is the rate of production of sperms, List the functions of testis, Why the scrotal temperature is lower than core body temperature, What is blood-testis barrier and what are its functions, What is the structure of a spermatozoa, What is the fate of stored spermatozoa, What is the composition of normal semen, How do you assess male infertility, What is the source of testosterone, List the physiological actions of testosterone, What are the secondary sex characteristics in male, List the functions of Sertoli cells, What are the functions of Leydig cells, What is the fate of testosterone secreted from Leydig cells, What is cryptorchidism and what is its treatment and complications, What is spermiogenesis and what are the changes that occur during this period, What is spermiation, What is capacitation, What is acrosomal reaction, What are the function of prostate glands, Why is the prostate specific antigen (PSA) a marker of prostate cancer, What is the use of 5α -reductase inhibitors in prostate hypertrophy, What is penis-at-14 syndrome, What is the source of estrogen in males, What are the causes of gynecomastia in males, What are the types and causes of male hypogonadism, What is eunuchoidism, What are the other testicular hormones and what are their functions, How is the testicular functions regulated, What is the mechanism of action of testosterone, What is CatSper protein and what is its function, , List the differences between spermatogenesis and oogenesis, What is the structure and function of epididymis, How do the Leydig cells and Sertoli cells interact, What are the function of vas deferens, What are the function of bulbourethral glands, What is the effect of androgen secreting tumors.

CHAPTER

68

Female Reproductive System: Functional Anatomy, Oogenesis and Follicular Development

Learning Objectives

On completion of study of this chapter, the student **MUST** be able to:

1. Correlate the functional organization of female reproductive tract with their functions.
2. Give the different parts of uterus and ovary, and list their functions.
3. Give the steps and regulation of oogenesis.
4. Understand the mechanism and regulation of different phases of ovarian follicle.
5. Describe the structure and function of corpus luteum.

The student **MAY** also be able to:

1. Describe the process of oogenesis.
2. Describe the ovarian follicular development.

The important event in female reproductive functions is the cyclical release of gamete during the reproductive cycles. The **ovarian changes** are mainly growth, maturation and release of ovum and secretion of hormones, and **uterine changes** are mainly endometrial alterations to nourish the implanted fertilized gamete, or shedding of endometrium associated with uterine bleeding in the absence of fertilization. The follicular development during each cycle is a detailed and organized process controlled by hypothalamo-pituitary-ovarian endocrine axis.

Scientist contributed

Regnier de Graaf (1641–1673), was a Dutch physician, anatomist and physiologist who made key discoveries in reproductive biology during his only 32 years of short life span. He was the first scientist who pioneered in the study of **physiology of reproductive system** in males and females. He had demonstrated ovulation in mammals. The ovarian follicles are named after him as **Graafian follicles** in recognition of his outstanding contribution in the field of reproductive physiology. He had also studied the pancreatic secretion.

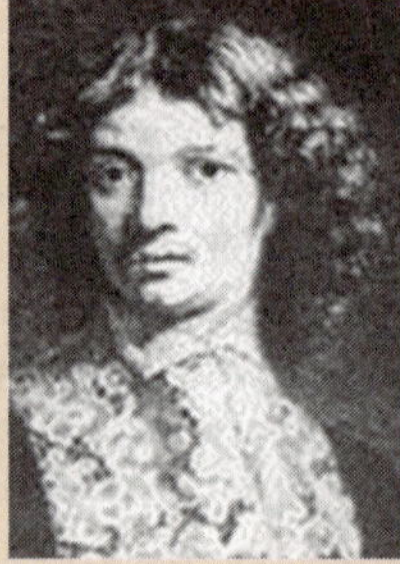

Regnier de Graaf
(1641–1673)

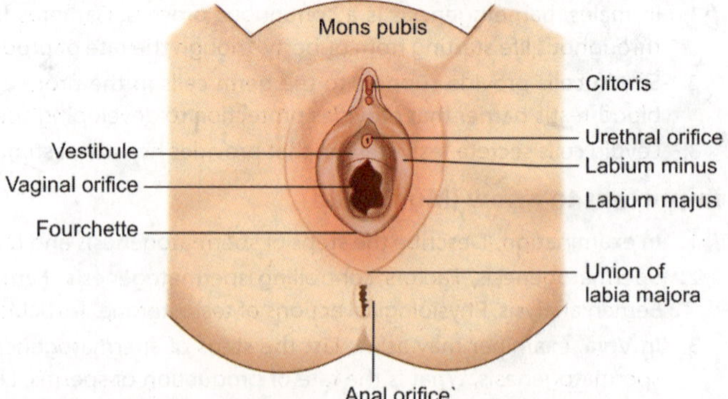

Fig. 68.1: Female external genitalia.
Courtesy: Figure 58.21, Clinical Anatomy, by Neeta Kulkarni, Vol. 2, 3rd edition, 2016; Jaypee Brothers Medical Publishers (P) Ltd.

FUNCTIONAL ANATOMY

External Genitalia

Female external genitalia include labia majora, labia minora, clitoris, vestibule of vagina and vestibular glands (Fig. 68.1). These structures are collectively called as vulva.

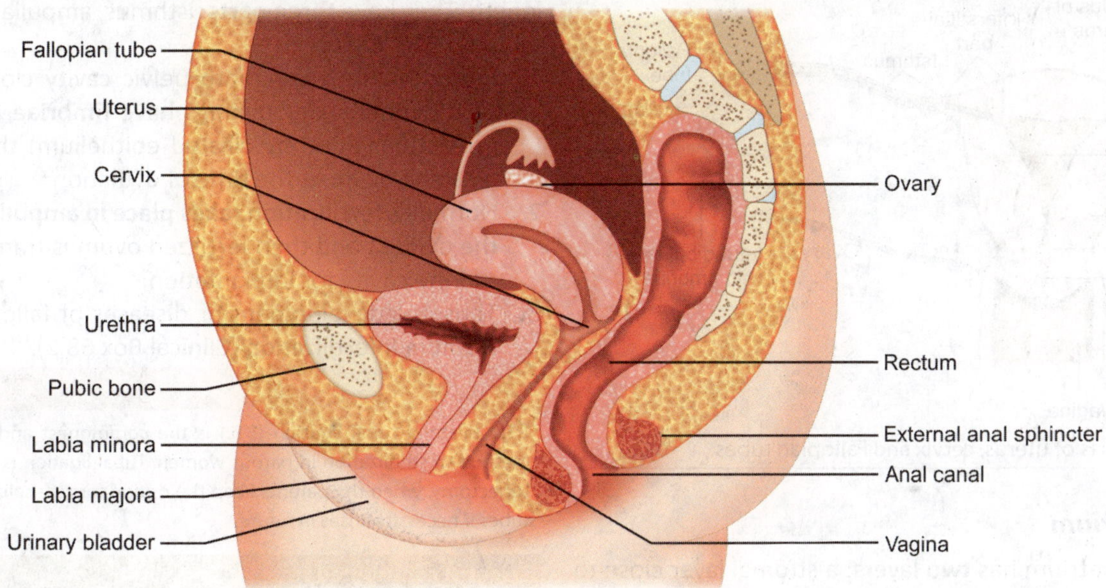

Fig. 68.2: Reproductive organs in female.

Labia Majora

Labia majora are **analogous to scrotum in males.** These are two major skin folds that form the outer lips of vaginal vestibule, which include vaginal and urethral openings.

Labia Minora

Labia minora are two minor skin folds present between labia majora and form inner lips of vaginal and urethral openings.

Clitoris

Clitoris is located at the anterior pole of vaginal vestibule. This is the ***female analogue of penis***. It consists of erectile tissue. The tip of the clitoris is the ***glans clitoris*** similar to glans penis.

Vaginal Vestibule

Vaginal vestibule contains two openings: vaginal and urethral openings. **Vaginal opening** lies below and posterior to **urethral opening**. In virgins, vaginal opening is partially closed by **hymen**, a thin fold of mucous membrane. **Vestibular glands** empty their secretion into the vaginal vestibule.

Internal Genitalia

The female internal reproductive organs are present in the pelvis and consist of vagina, uterus, fallopian tubes and ovaries (Fig. 68.2).

Vagina

This is a tubular canal which is present anterior to rectum and posterior to the urethra and bladder. It connects vaginal opening in the vestibule to the uterine cervix.

1. The length of vagina in adult is about 8 cm, but it is highly stretchable as its wall is folded normally. It can ***elongate to about double of its length*** during sexual act.
2. Under the action of relaxin, it **widens and stretches further during parturition.**
3. **Vaginal wall** contains muscle and contraction of vagina during sexual act facilitates the transportation of sperm into the uterus.
4. **Vaginal epithelium** changes during different ***phases of menstrual cycle***.
   - **In proliferative phase**, under the influence of estrogen, **cornification** (keratinization) of vaginal epithelium occurs that secretes thin mucus.
   - **In the luteal phase**, under the influence of progesterone, cornification of epithelium is reduced; rather, polymorphonuclear leucocytes infiltrate and epithelium proliferates to ***secrete thick mucus.***
5. **After menopause**, vaginal epithelium becomes thin and secretion is scanty. Therefore, post-menopausal vagina is dry and susceptible to infections.

Uterus

This is hollow organ having **thick muscular wall.** It is placed between bladder anteriorly and rectum posteriorly. It has **two parts**: the corpus (or the body) and the cervix (Fig. 68.3).

Body of Uterus

Uterus consists mainly of **two layers** (myometrium and endometrium) and uterine cavity.

Myometrium

The myometrium consists of multiple layers of smooth muscle.

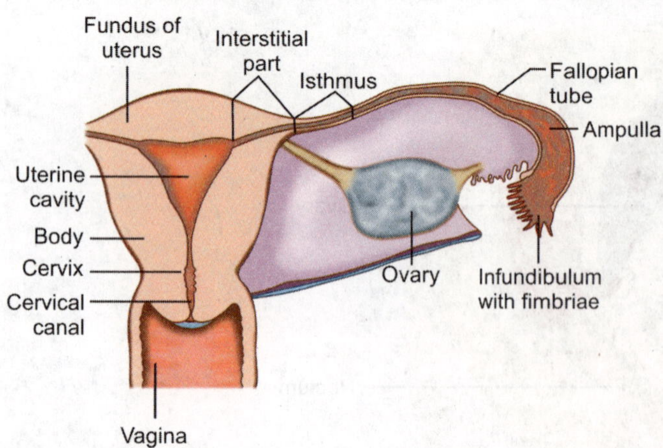

Fig. 68.3: Parts of uterus, cervix and Fallopian tubes.

Endometrium

The endometrium has **two layers**: a stromal layer close to myometrium and an epithelium.

1. **The stroma** is penetrated by spiral arteries and contains adequate connective tissue.
2. **The epithelium** contains uterine glands that are lined by columnar secretory cells. The glands also infiltrate into stroma. The ***arterial and glandular changes*** occur in different phases of menstrual cycle (*see* below).
3. **Shedding of endometrial tissue** at the end of luteal phase results in menstrual bleeding. Uterus enlarges during pregnancy to accommodate the growing fetus and expels the fetus at the time of parturition.

Uterine Cervix

The cervix is a **narrow muscular tube** that connects vagina with body of the uterus (Fig. 68.3). It has internal os, cervical canal and external os.

1. Cervical mucus changes from thick and viscous liquid to profuse, watery and highly elastic liquid, which forms the physiological basis of '**spinnbarkeit test**' for ovulation (spinnbarkeit refers to a highly elastic substance).
2. Under the influence of estrogen, cervical mucous forms typical '**fern pattern**', which disappears following ovulation.
3. **Cervical dilation** is done for uterine investigations (Clinical Box 68.1). Cervical dilation is the initial event in the initiation of parturition.

Clinical Box 68.1

D and C: Dilation of cervix is performed routinely in gynecological practice to obtain endometrial tissue from cervix or body of the uterus for diagnosis of various uterine pathologies. This is called dilatation and curettage (D and C). D and C are also performed therapeutically for treatment of few uterine diseases. Cervical dilation is done to evacuate the uterine content (conceptus) for abortion.

Fallopian Tubes

Two fallopian tubes (also called **oviducts**) arise from both sides of upper poles of uterus. Oviducts are 10–15 cm in length. They have **three parts**: isthmus, ampulla and infundibulum (Fig. 68.3).

1. **Infundibulum** opens into pelvic cavity close to ovaries. Infundibular openings have **fimbriae** (finger like projections lined by ciliated epithelium) that help in grasping ovum at the time of ovulation.
2. Normally, **fertilization takes place in ampullary part** of the oviduct and then fertilized ovum is transported to uterine cavity for implantation.
3. Thus, maldevelopment or diseases of fallopian tubes result in infertilization (Clinical Box 68.2).

Clinical Box 68.2

BTL: Bilateral tubal ligation (BTL) is the commonest and permanent method of sterilization in parous women. Tubal ligation is preferred to tubectomy, when the parents keep the option for recanalization of the tubes if necessity arises in future.

Scientist contributed

Gabriele Falloppio (1523–1562) was Italian physician and anatomist of 15th century who pioneered in studying the structure and functions of the reproductive organs. He demonstrated the seminal vesicle, the uterine tubes and the details of the mammalian reproductive systems. For his immense contribution in the field of reproductive system during his life span of less than 40 years, the uterine tubes of female reproductive system are named after him as **Fallopian tubes.**

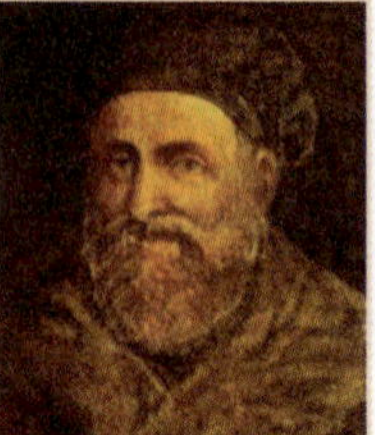

G Falloppio
(1523–1562)

The Ovaries

There are two ovaries each weighing about 10 g in adults. Each one present on both sides of uterus and are attached by ovarian ligaments. Ovary consists of **two zones**: the cortex, and medulla.

Cortex of Ovary

The cortex is the outer and the major zone lined by the germinal epithelium. It is surrounded by a layer of fibrous tissue called **tunica albuginea**.

1. Cortex contains oocytes. Each oocyte is enclosed within a follicle, the **ovarian follicle.** Ovarian follicles are present in their various stages of development (Fig. 68.4).
2. The matured ovarian follicle is called **Graafian follicle.**
3. The **stroma** of the ovary is present in between the follicles, which consists of supporting connective tissue and interstitial cells.

Medulla of Ovary

The inner zone of the ovary forms the medulla that contains different types of interstitial and connective tissue cells. Blood vessels and lymphatics enter the ovary through its hilum.

Functions of Ovary:

Ovary like testis performs many functions:

1. Oogenesis during fetal life.
2. Maturation of oocyte.

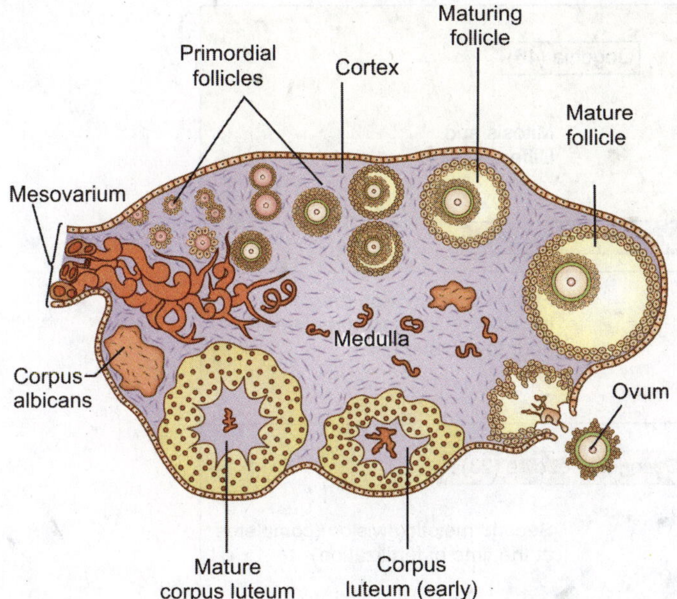

Fig. 68.4: Structure of ovary. The stroma of ovary has two parts: cortex and medulla. Note that the cortex contains ovarian follicle in different stages of development.

3. Ovulation
4. Secretion of female sex hormones and peptide hormones.

The primary function of ovary is to **develop ovarian follicles** and **release ovum at the time of ovulation**, and to **secrete steroid hormones** that control various reproductive and metabolic functions.

OOGENESIS

Unlike spermatogenesis that starts at puberty and continues throughout life, the **process of oogenesis starts in fetal life and ceases at menopause**. Also, the process of development of each spermatocyte is completed in few days, whereas **development of each oocyte that begins in intrauterine life is completed with ovulation** that occurs during menstrual cycle.

Thus, many sperms are produced in few days whereas single ovum is produced during each cycle, the development of which occurs at different stages of life till ovulation. The stages of **development of oocytes occur in three stages**: Oogonium becoming primary oocyte, primary oocyte converted to secondary oocyte, and finally secondary oocyte developing to mature ovum.

Oogonia Becoming Primary Oocyte

Oogonia

The primordial germ cells (oogonia) migrate from the ***yolk sac of embryo*** to the genital ridge at about 6th week of gestation. The, oogonia undergo ***many mitotic divisions*** and the number of oogonia reaches to about 7 millions. When mitosis cease, the oogonia are called ***oocytes***.

Primary Oocytes

The oocytes undergo **two meiotic divisions** (the meiotic cycle) at different stages of development to produce a haploid ovum. Oocytes in their preliminary stage of development are called primary oocytes.

First Meiotic Division

The first meiotic division starts in primary oocytes during fetal life, which occurs at about 8th week of pregnancy is **arrested in prophase**. The oocytes then grow in size.

1. However, the first meiotic division is not completed in fetal life, not even till puberty; in fact, it is completed just prior to ovulation.
2. Therefore, the **life span of a primary oocyte** can be up to 50 years, as ovulation can continue up to this age.
3. The suspension of oocyte division in prophase for such a long period depends on the internal hormonal environment provided by the surrounding supporting cells.

Oocyte Degeneration

The oocyte degeneration however, **starts from the intrauterine life** so that only about 1 million primary oocytes remain at the time of birth. By the time of puberty about 200,000 and by the age of 30 only about 26,000 oocytes remain in the ovary. At menopause, ovaries are virtually devoid of oocytes.

1. During a woman's life, only **about 400 oocytes are ovulated** and the other oocytes degenerate. The process of degeneration of oocyte is called **atresia**.
2. A **major difference in male and female gametogenesis** is that the process of spermatogenesis is a continuous phenomenon and the production of sperm is unlimited, whereas primary oocytes degenerate with age (Application Box 68.1).
3. As new oogonia cannot be manufactured in ovary, the **oocytes totally disappear at the time of menopause**.

Application Box 68.1

Age of oocyte contribute to health of children: Because of the peculiar pattern of development of oocyte in females, the life span of an oocyte may be as old as 50 years. The oocyte that ovulates at about 40 years of age is about 25 years older than the oocyte that ovulates at the age of 15. This one of the important factors that contribute to the anomalies in children born to older woman as the aged-eggs oocyte have degenerative changes and therefore their fertilization may result in defective embryo.

Primary Oocyte Converted to Secondary Oocyte

In fetus, oogonia develop into primary oocyte, which undergo first meiotic division. However, the first meiotic division is not completed in fetus. This is called as **meiotic arrest**. Thus, all eggs present at birth are **primary oocytes**

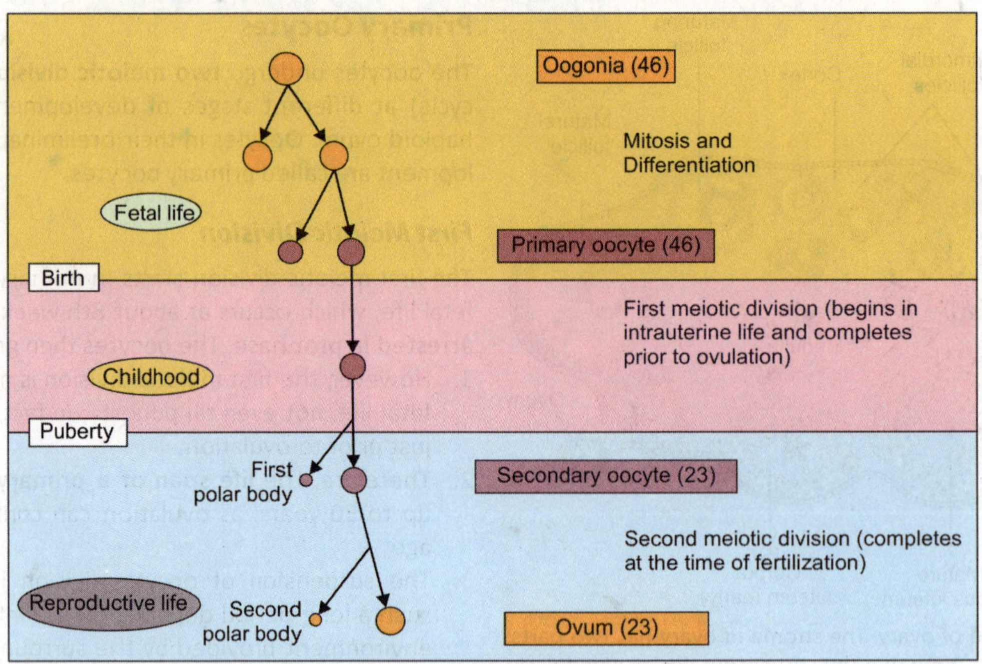

Fig. 68.5: Stages of oogenesis. Note, first meiotic division of oocyte begins during fetal life and completes prior to ovulation, whereas second meiotic division completes at the time of fertilization.

in meiotic arrest containing 46 chromosomes. This state continues until puberty.

1. The primary oocyte that is destined for ovulation **completes the first meiotic division just before the ovulation.**
2. This division results in production of two structures: one is the daughter cell, called **secondary oocyte** containing 23 chromosomes, and the other is the **first polar body** (Fig. 68.5).
3. However, the **cytoplasmic division is grossly unequal** in this process in which the secondary oocyte retains nearly all the cytoplasm with polar body containing very little of it. Thus, the polar body becomes completely nonfunctional.

Secondary Oocyte Forming Ovum

Second Meiotic Division

The second meiotic division **occurs in the secondary oocyte** after ovulation, and is **arrested in metaphase.**

1. The second meiotic division is **completed when the egg is penetrated by a sperm.** Thus, **meiotic cycle is completed only on fertilization.**
2. As a result of this meiotic division, **the ovum** containing 23 chromosomes and the **second polar body** are formed (Fig. 68.5). The polar body is extruded.
3. Thus, in the process of oogenesis, **each primary oocyte produces only one ovum.**

DEVELOPMENT OF OVARIAN FOLLICLE

The oocyte grows throughout their life in the ovarian follicle till ovulation when the ovum is released from the follicle (from the ovary). Along with development of oocyte in ovarian follicle, follicles also grow in different phases. This is called follicular growth or **folliculogenesis.**

1. It **starts during intrauterine life** and **continues till ovulation** that occurs during each menstrual cycle. Thus, a single ovarian follicle may develop **from fetal life till menopause.**
2. At the beginning of menstrual cycle, a number of follicles start growing. However, only the one **dominant follicle** finally matures and releases ovum, whereas rest **others undergo degeneration** (atresia).
3. About 99.9% of follicles present at birth undergo atresia during the reproductive life of a woman.

Stages of Follicular Development

Folliculogenesis occurs in four stages: Stages 1– 4 (Figs. 68.6A to D).

Stage 1 (Primordial Follicular Stage)

The ovarian follicle, also called **Graafian follicle** begins as a **primordial follicle** (Fig. 68.6A).

1. The primordial follicle consists of a **primary oocyte** at the center surrounded by a **layer of spindle cells** (flattened **pregranulosa cells**) that form granulosa cells later. A basal lamina is formed outside the spindle cells. The size of oocyte in primordial follicle is about 25 µm.
2. Primordial follicles form the **resting pool of follicles** in the ovary.
3. However, they *degenerate progressively from fetal life to menopause.*

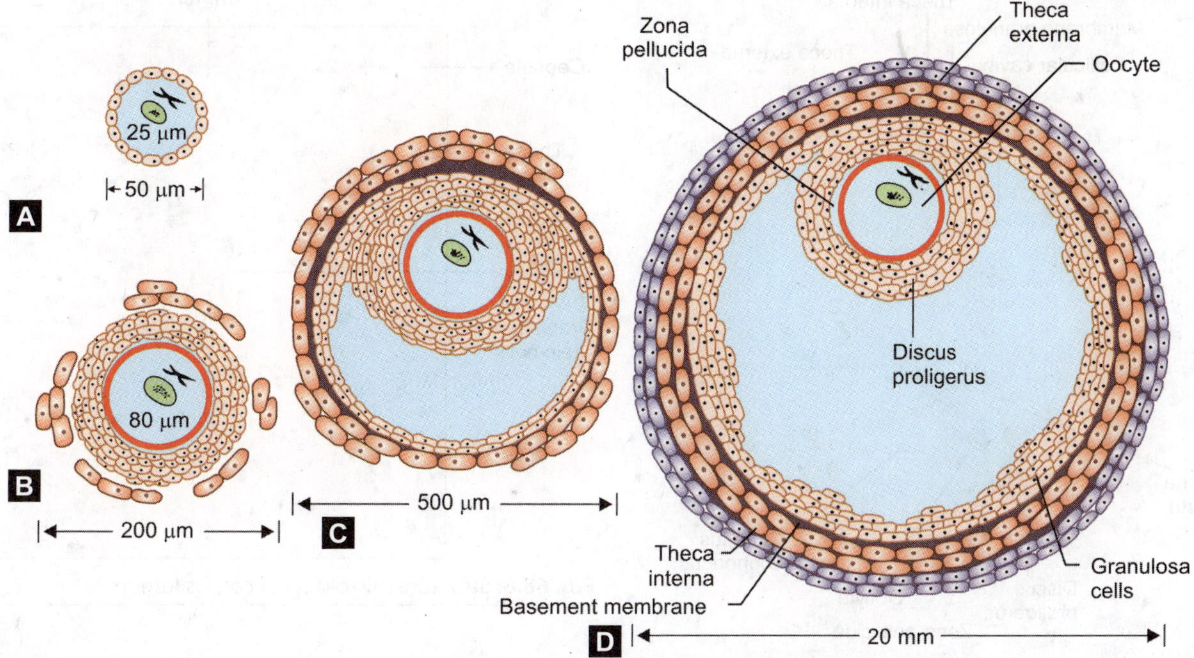

Figs. 68.6A to D: Stages of development of ovarian follicle. (A) Primordial follicular stage (Stage 1); (B) Primary follicular stage (Stage 2); (C) Secondary follicular stage (Stage 3); (D) Tertiary follicular stage (Stage 4, or Matured follicle).

4. The oocyte enters into **first meiotic division** and the division is **arrested in prophase**. This prophase of oocyte is maintained till just prior to ovulation.

Stage 2 (Primary Follicular Stage)

The primordial follicles grow into the **primary follicles**.

1. During this process the flattened pregranulosa cells (spindle cells) become **cuboidal granulosa cells** that further proliferate to form a continuous cell layer surrounding the oocyte (Fig. 68.6B). The size of oocyte increases to about 80-140 µm.
2. A type of ***glassy material*** consisting of mucopolysaccharide is secreted from granulosa cells, which forms a thick layer between the oocyte and the granulosa cell layer, called as **zona pellucida**.
3. The primordial follicle becomes primary follicle at about 28th weeks of gestation.
4. The prophase of first meiotic division of oocyte is maintained.

Stage 3 (Secondary Follicular Stage)

The primary follicle becomes **secondary follicle** in this stage during which the granulosa cells divide and form several layers of cells around the oocyte. Thus, the size of follicle increases enormously in this stage to about 500 µm.

1. At this, stage, follicle is called **preantral follicle.** However, small antrum may develop (Fig. 68.6C).
2. A layer of spindle cells (**pre or early theca cells**) is formed at the periphery of the basal lamina, which forms the theca cell layer in the next stage.
3. All these development occur slowly in the prepubertal ovary.
4. The oocyte is maintained in prophase of its first meiotic division.

Stage 4 (Tertiary Follicular Stage)

This is the final stage of follicular development. It occurs in **two sub-stages**: the early tertiary stage and the Graafian follicular stage.

Early Tertiary or Antral Follicular Stage

In this stage, the spindle cell layer surrounding the basement membrane proliferates and differentiates into inner **theca interna** and outer **theca externa.**

1. **Theca interna cells** multiply to form multiple cell layers and become steroidogenic.
2. **Theca externa cell** lie in a single layer and provide mechanical support to the follicle from outside.
3. Theca cells receive blood, lymphatic and nerve supply whereas **granulosa cells remain avascular** as blood vessel cannot penetrate the basement membrane.
4. A long with the expansion of theca cell layer, a fluid-filled space is created in the midst of granulosa cells, called as **antrum** (Fig. 68.6C). Therefore, the follicle in this stage is also called **early antral follicle** and the stage also as early ***antral follicular stage***.
5. The granulosa cells increase in number and **acquire receptors for FSH** and start secreting estrogen. In fact, the progression of early tertiary stage to the next stage of follicular development is **FSH dependent.**

Late Tertiary or Graafian Follicular Stage

This is the **most rapid stage** of development. It occurs only in the post-pubertal ovary.

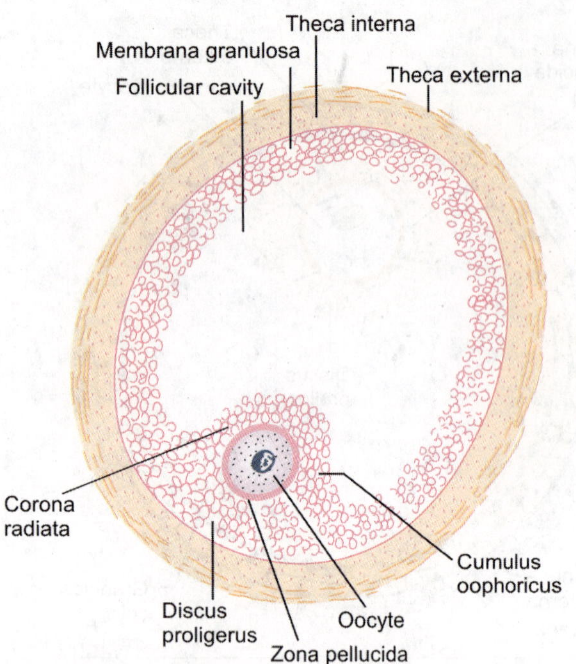

Fig. 68.7: Mature ovarian follicle showing 3 layers of granulosa cells.

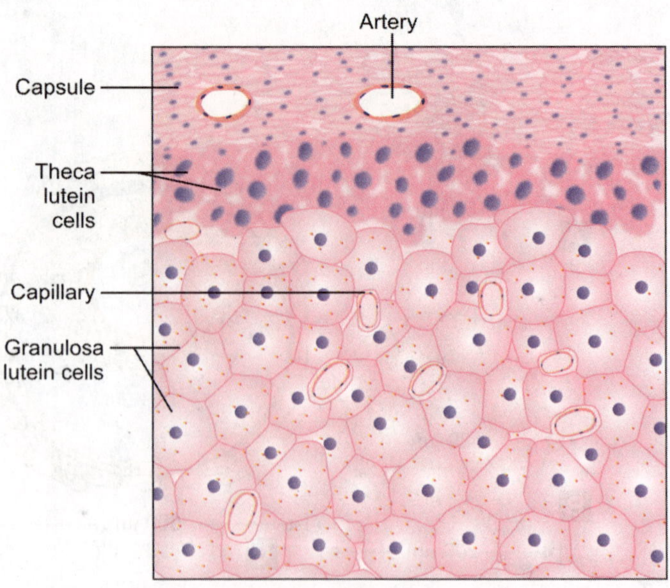

Fig. 68.8: Structure (histology) of corpus luteum.

1. After 5–7 days of onset of menses, a single follicle becomes **dominant follicle** for that cycle. The follicle in this stage is called **Graafian follicle** (Fig. 68.6D) and the stage is called *Graafian follicular stage*. It occurs in one ovary during each cycle.
2. The size of the antrum and the amount of antral fluid are increased significantly. This ***pushes the oocyte to the periphery*** of the follicle.
3. The mucopolysaccharide, which is present in the antral fluid, is depolymerized to increase the osmotic pressure of the fluid. However, the total *intrafollicular pressure* remains within 20 mm Hg.
4. The antral fluid **contains many hormones** such as estrogen, progesterone, FSH, LH, prolactin, androstenedione and growth factors, inhibin, activin, GnRH, CRH, opioid peptides and oxytocin.
5. It also contains plasminogen activator, mucopolysaccharide, proteins, electrolytes, glycosaminoglycans and proteoglycans.
6. The vascularity of theca increases.
7. The **granulosa cells in this stage** are anatomically divided into **three compartments**: antral, cumulus and mural granulosa cells (Fig. 68.7).
   Antral granulosa cells: Granulosa cells lining the antral cavity are called antral granulosa cells (Discus proligerous). Antral granulosa cells are **highly steroidogenic**.
   Cumulus granulosa cells: Granulosa cells surrounding the oocyte are cumulus granulosa cells (cumulus oophoricus).
   - Therefore, the granulosa cells that project into the antrum like a mound are collectively called as **cumulus oophorus**.
   - Cumulus granulosa cells are **less steroidogenic**.

   Mural granulosa cells: Granulosa cells that are attached to the basement membrane are called mural granulosa cells (Membrana granulosa). Mural granulosa cells are **highly steroidogenic**.
8. The diameter of the follicle in this stage is about 2.5 cm. The follicle is called **pre-ovulatory follicle** as it is ready for ovulation at this stage. The ***basement membrane*** close to the surface of the ovary undergoes **proteolysis** that slowly *leads to rupture of the follicle* resulting in release of oocyte from the follicle, the process called **ovulation**.
9. Just prior to ovulation, **the first meiotic division is completed.**
10. The oocyte is taken up by the fallopian tube.
11. **If fertilization occurs,** the penetration of ovum by the sperm **completes the second meiotic division**, which results in **functional ovum** (fertilized egg).
12. If fertilization does not occur, the oocyte begins to degenerate in 24 to 48 hours.

Corpus Luteum Formation

Luteinization

After ovulation, the ruptured follicle is quickly filled with blood, and at this time, the follicle is called **corpus hemorrhagicum**. However, the cells lining the follicle rapidly proliferate to replace blood with luteal cells that are rich in lipid. Now, the follicle is called **corpus luteum** and its appearance heralds the beginning of luteal phase of the cycle.

1. The corpus luteum is a yellow body made up of **endocrine tissue** that consists of **granulosa luteal cells, theca luteal cells and fibroblasts** (Fig. 68.8). The number of mitochondria, lipid droplets and the endoplasmic reticulum increase in the granulosa cells of corpus luteum. These morphological changes are collectively known as **luteinization**, which is ***essential for synthesis of more steroid hormones***.

2. The granulosa and theca cells of matured corpus luteum are respectively called as **granulosa lutein cells** and **theca lutein cells**.
3. Luteal granulosa cells are vascular unlike the follicular granulosa cells that are nonvascular.
4. Vascularity of luteal cells **facilitates the synthesis of steroid hormones** by promoting the supply of cholesterol from plasma to these cells.

Regulation of Luteinization

Progesterone, estrogen and androgen are formed in corpus luteum.

1. **Progesterone secretion** reaches its peak in menstrual cycle at about 7 days after ovulation, which correlates with the full maturity of corpus luteum. These hormones (Progesterone, estrogen and androgen) may be playing some role in luteinization.
2. However, **LH is the major stimulator of luteinization**. LH maintains the functions of corpus luteum by promoting luteinization of its cells, and therefore, LH is referred to as luteinizing hormone.
3. FSH increases the number of LH receptors on the cells.

Luteal Regression

If **fertilization does not occur**, corpus luteum degenerates in about 13 days after ovulation.

1. The endocrine cells of corpus luteum become necrotic, and are invaded by leucocytes and fibroblasts. This process is called **luteolysis** or luteal regression.
2. The exact mechanism of luteolysis is not known. However, it is proposed to be due to the action of **luteolysins** that are produced locally in the ovary. The proposed luteolysins are **oxytocin, prostaglandins and GnRH**.
3. Luteolysins promote luteal regression by preventing the action of LH on corpus luteum.
4. The degenerated corpus luteum is replaced by avascular and nonfunctional fibrous tissue, known as **corpus albicans**.

If **fertilization occurs**, the implanted fertilized ovum secretes hCG from its embryonic trophoblast, which has LH-like activity. Therefore, **hCG maintains luteinization** and promotes the functions of the **corpus luteum of pregnancy**.

Functions of Corpus Luteum:

1. The corpus luteum **secretes hormones**. During luteal phase, increased secretion of progesterone, estrogen and inhibin A occurs from corpus luteum. It also secretes androgen.
2. It provides endocrinal **environment for implantation of fertilized ovum**.
3. It **maintains the early part of pregnancy** by secreting progesterone in adequate concentration till the placenta becomes functional.

Infertility occurs due to luteal deficiency (Clinical Box 68.3)

Clinical Box 68.3

Luteal deficiency: One of the common causes of infertility is the luteal deficiency, also called **luteal insufficiency**, in which either luteinization of granulosa cells of corpus luteum is deficient due to less number LH receptors on luteal cells, or due to ovulation of prematurely developed follicle that contains less number of luteinized granulosa cells. FSH also promotes expression of LH receptors in the follicular cells. Therefore, FSH deficiency can also cause luteal insufficiency. Due to **inadequate secretion of progesterone** from malfunctioning corpus luteum, pregnancy is terminated very early. Luteal insufficiency is diagnosed by demonstrating a **low progesterone level in the midluteal phase in successive cycles**. The condition is treated by administration of progesterone that maintain follicular phase and early part of pregnancy, or clomiphene citrate that induces follicular development, or hCG that facilitates luteinization of granulosa cells of corpus luteum.

Atresia of Follicle

During the entire reproductive period of a woman, about 400 oocytes grow to culminate in ovulation. The follicles that do not become dominant undergo a ***process of degeneration*** called atresia. Atresia starts in fetal ovary soon after the appearance of primordial follicles. It occurs due to **apoptosis**, a process of programmed cell death.

Regulation of Follicular Development

Factors affecting development of follicles are different in different phases of follicular growth.

Primordial Follicular Stage

The growth of primordial follicle is not affected by gonadotropins. It is purely a local phenomenon.

Primary Follicular Stage

The **chemical substances secreted by oocyte** stimulate the transformation of pregranulosa cells to granulosa cells. The **products of granulosa cells** stimulate the formation of spindle (pre-theca) cells. **FSH and LH** stimulate the development of follicle toward the later part of gestation. During early childhood, though LH and FSH are secreted in low concentration, they are essential to maintain follicular growth. Follicular growth is impaired without gonadotropins.

Secondary Follicular Stage

At the time of puberty, secondary follicles start developing. The granulosa cells of secondary follicles **acquire FSH receptors** and secrete estrogen in less concentration. This **follicular estrogen** promotes further follicular development.

Early Tertiary Stage

Immediately after menarche (the first menstrual bleeding), in the early luteal phase of the same first cycle, usually the secondary follicles enter the tertiary follicular stage of development. The granulosa cells respond to FSH in the follicular phase of the next cycle.

1. The **FSH stimulates the granulosa cell** and increases the aromatase activity, which increases the synthesis of estrogen from androgen. The follicular concentration of estrogen increases.
2. **Estrogen** along with FSH induces expression of LH receptors on granulosa cells. Estrogen also conditions hypothalamo-anterior pituitary axis that maintains LH activity in the plasma.
3. **LH synthesis is increased** by estrogen at this point of time, which is essential for **pre-ovulatory surge of LH.**
4. **Estrogen** also *increases the number and sensitivity of LH receptors in the theca cells*. Therefore, **LH stimulates androgen synthesis** in theca cells that becomes substrate for estrogen production in the granulosa cells (Fig. 68.9).
5. LH also stimulates granulosa cells to produce progesterone. Therefore, progesterone concentration also increases.

Late Tertiary Stage

Between 5th to 7th days of follicular phase, only one follicle grows sufficiently to become the **dominant follicle.**

1. The aromatase activity and number of FSH receptors increase in the granulosa cells of dominant follicle. This increases the **synthesis of estrogen**, and more concentration of estrogen allows the dominant follicles to prime the hypothalamo-pituitary axis to generate LH surge just prior to ovulation. Under normal conditions, estrogen inhibits LH secretion.
2. But, when the plasma concentration of estrogen reaches about 200 pg/ml and maintains that high concentration for about 36 hours, estrogen stimulates LH secretion. Thus, the **positive feedback effect on LH** increases more secretion of LH. This leads to **LH surge**, which causes ovulation (see below). This positive feedback on LH secretion is due to the effect of estrogen both at the levels of hypothalamus and pituitary.
3. LH **increases progesterone secretion**, which increases the **proteolytic enzyme activity** and causes the distention of follicle due to rapid **increase in follicular fluid volume.**
4. LH also stimulates the activity of endoperoxide synthase that increases **synthesis of prostaglandins** and leukotrienes.
5. **Prostaglandins cause lysis of follicular wall** leading to rupture of follicle.

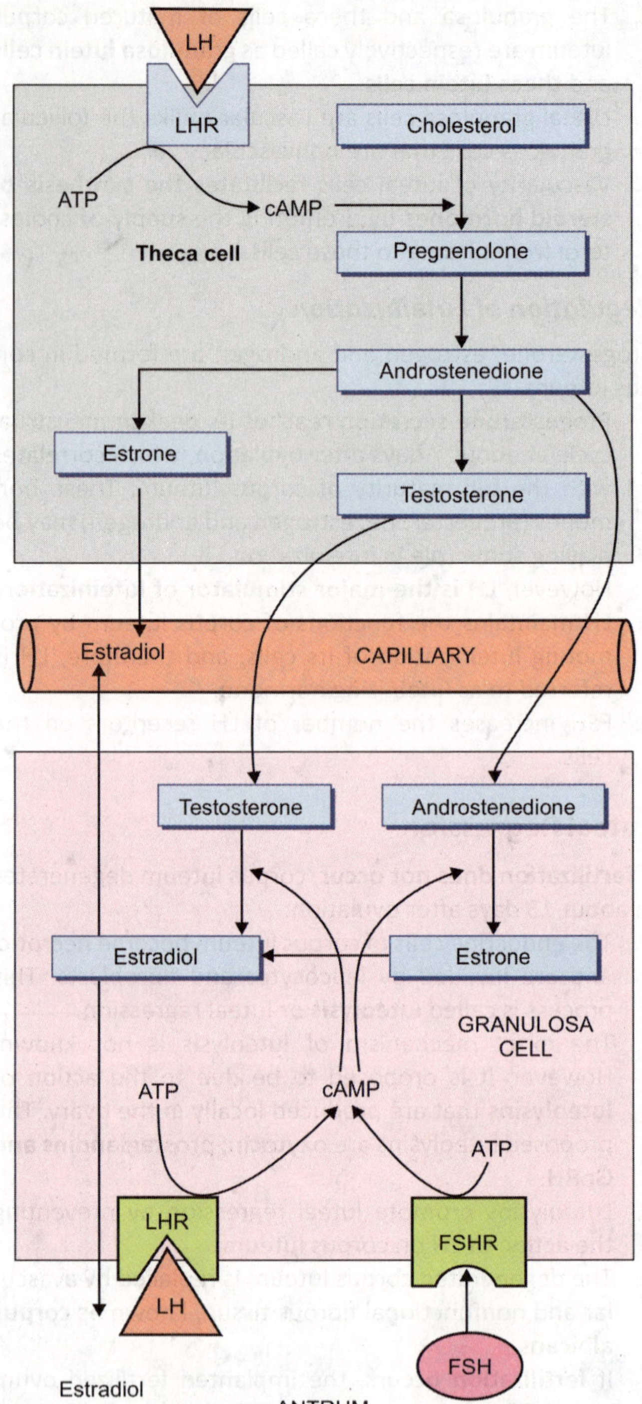

Fig. 68.9: Interaction of theca cell with granulosa cells. (LHR: LH receptor; FSHR: FSH receptor).

6. Breaking down of follicular wall is facilitated by the proteolytic enzyme **plasmin**. FSH, by stimulating the **activity of plasminogen activator** facilitates the formation of plasmin.
7. **Oxytocin causes contraction of follicular wall** and extrudes the oocyte. This is called **ovulation.** Immediately after LH surge, the number of LH receptors decreases. This desensitizes granulosa and theca cells to LH.

CHAPTER SUMMARY

Key Concepts

1. In females, the period of gametogenesis is restricted from puberty to menopause, which is less than for 40 years. Gametes (sperms).
2. The process of oogenesis starts in fetal life. The development of each oocyte that begins in intrauterine life is completed with ovulation that occurs during menstrual cycle.
3. If fertilization occurs, corpus luteum provides hormonal support for implantation of fertilized egg and maintenance of early part of pregnancy.

Important to Know (Must Read)

1. In examination, Long questions are usually not asked from this chapter. However, 'Describe the stages and regulation of ovarian follicle' may come as a **Long Question**.
2. Oogenesis, Corpus luteum, Graafian follicle, Stages of follicular development, Regulation of follicular development, may be asked as **Short Questions** in exam.
3. In **Viva**, examiner may ask…… How the corpus luteum is formed, What are the functions of corpus luteum, How is the lutenization regulated, What is luteal regression, What is luteal deficiency and what are its features, What is D and C, What are the functions of ovary, What are the stages of oogenesis, How the age of oocyte contributes to the health of children, List the stages of follicular development, How the early tertiary stage is regulated, How is the late tertiary stage regulated, What are the changes that occur in primordial follicular stage, What are the changes that occur in primary follicular stage, What are the changes that occur in secondary follicular stage, What are the changes that occur in tertiary follicular stage.

CHAPTER

69

Menstrual Cycle and Ovulation

Learning Objectives

On completion of study of this chapter, the student **MUST** be able to:

1. Name the phases of menstrual cycle.
3. Describe (with the help of a schematic diagram) the uterine, ovarian, and hormonal changes in menstrual cycle.
4. Define and understand the mechanism of ovulation.
5. List the indicators of ovulation and give the importance of ovulation.
6. Classify amenorrhea and name the common causes of different types of amenorrhea.
7. Give the physiological causes of anovulation.
8. Give the physiological basis of premenstrual syndrome.
9. Understand anorexia nervosa.

The student **MAY** also be able to:

1. Explain the mechanisms of ovulation.
2. Describe the physiological basis of different types of menstrual irregularities.

The fundamental difference in female and male reproductive functions is the cyclical release of gametes in females during their reproductive life. The structural and functional changes of female reproductive system during each cycle are synchronized with the changes in hypothalamo-pituitary-ovarian axis. The **ovarian changes** are mainly growth, maturation and release of gamete and secretion of hormones, and **uterine changes** are mainly endometrial alterations to nourish the implanted fertilized gamete, or shedding of endometrium associated with uterine bleeding in the absence of fertilization. These cyclical changes in human beings are called **menstrual cycles** and the uterine bleeding is called **menstruation**.

Menstrual cycles start at puberty, temporarily stop during pregnancy and lactation, and finally cease at menopause. During different stages of menstrual cycle, ovarian hormones, especially estrogen and progesterone provide feedback effects on hypothalamo-pituitary secretions generating typical cyclic release of gonadotropins from anterior pituitary. As hypothalamo-pituitary axis is subjected to various influences, menstrual cycle can easily be affected by stress and psychosocial and environmental factors.

MENSTRUAL CYCLE

The reproductive functions in women exhibit cyclical changes that occur regularly over a period of about one month. This is called menstrual cycle, which is the **periodic preparation of the reproductive system for fertilization and implantation of the fertilized ovum**. In human beings and primates, the reproductive cycle externally manifests by periodic vaginal bleeding, called as **menstruation**. Therefore, the cycle is called menstrual cycle. The first menstrual cycle is called **menarche**. The usual age for menarche is 12–14 years.

Duration and Phases of Menstrual Cycle

Duration of Menstrual Cycle

The length of menstrual cycle usually averages at about 28 days. However, the duration of cycles is never fixed in all women. Also, the duration of all cycles is not same in one woman. This is because menstrual cycle is frequently influenced by psychological, environmental, nutritional, and social factors.

1. Normally, it ranges from 21 to 35 days.
2. The cycle is described by number of days, the **first day** being the ***day of beginning of menstrual bleeding***.
3. The cycle becomes irregular toward menopause.
4. Nevertheless, irregularity in cycle length or in duration and quantity of bleeding in an apparently normal woman indicates dysfunctions of reproductive system, especially in the uterus or in the ovary.
5. Physiologically, menstrual cycle temporarily ceases during pregnancy and lactation.

Phases of Menstrual Cycle

Characteristically, the menstrual cycle is divided into two phases: **follicular phase and luteal phase**, separated by **ovulation** that occurs between these two phases.

Follicular Phase

This is the period **from the onset of bleeding to the day of ovulation**. This is called **follicular phase** as the dominant follicle in ovary matures in this phase to terminate in ovulation at the end of the phase.

1. This phase has two parts: the ***menstrual phase*** (the phase of menstrual bleeding), and the ***proliferative phase*** (phase of proliferation of the uterine endometrium).
2. Follicular phase is also called **preovulatory phase**.

Luteal Phase

This is the part of menstrual cycle **between ovulation and the onset of the next menstrual bleeding**.

1. This is called **luteal phase** as corpus luteum is formed in the ovary, which mainly controls activities of this phase.
2. This is also called the **secretory phase** as uterine endometrium is highly secretory during this phase.
3. Luteal phase is also called **postovulatory phase**

Length of Each Phase of Cycle

In a 28 days cycle, the follicular phase is of 14 days (1–14 days) and the luteal phase is of 14 days (15–28 days).

1. However, alteration of the length of menstrual cycle occurs due to alteration in the duration of follicular phase. Once ovulation occurs, menstrual bleeding starts after 14 days of ovulation.
2. Thus, the **length of the luteal phase remains constant** irrespective of the cycle length.

Menstrual bleeding occurs in the early part of follicular phase, and usually, ovulation occurs in the mid-cycle or more appropriately, at the end of the proliferative phase and just prior to the beginning of the luteal phase. Therefore, menstrual cycle is sometimes loosely divided into ***four phases***: bleeding phase, follicular phase, ovulatory phase, and luteal phase. However, it should be remembered that *bleeding phase is part of the follicular phase* and ovulation is not a separate phase, but an event that occurs at the junction between proliferative and secretory phases of the cycle.

Changes in Reproductive Organs in Menstrual Cycle

Changes in the Follicular Phase (Menstrual and Proliferative Phase)

Ovarian Changes

In the follicular phase, one follicle is selected to become the **dominant follicle** by 4th day. The mechanism of selection of a follicle to grow is not known.

1. The dominant follicle **develops into mature follicle** (for details of follicular development, *see* above).
2. The **granulosa and theca interna cells proliferate** and secrete estrogen.
3. The **antrum increases in size** and **stromal fluid increases in volume**.
4. The distended follicle ruptures at about 14th day resulting in ovulation.

Uterine Changes

In the early part of the follicular phase, along with the menstrual bleeding, layers of the uterine endometrium are sloughed. Under the influence of estrogen secreted from the developing follicle, **thickness of endometrium rapidly increases** from 5th to 14th day of the cycle. During this process, following uterine changes occur (Fig. 69.1C):

1. The uterine **endometrium undergoes hyperplasia and hypertrophy** and increases in size and thickness.
2. The **endometrial glands lengthen and glands are drawn out**. The glands are lined with columnar epithelium.
3. The endometrium is vascularized with **formation of more number of spiral arteries** that increase blood supply to the deeper layers. Increased blood supply further promotes growth of uterine mucosa.
4. Endometrial veins also grow in size.
5. **Myometrial excitability increases** due to the effect of estrogen.

As proliferation of endometrium is the major feature in this phase of the cycle, this is called proliferative phase. This is also called **preovulatory phase** as the changes occur before ovulation.

Change in Uterine Cervix

Under the effects of estrogen, **volume of cervical mucous increases.**

1. The **alkalinity and elasticity** of cervical mucous also increase.
2. This forms the physiological basis for **spinnbarkeit.**
3. The cervical epithelium becomes more **secretory**. Sperm easily passes through the estrogen-dependent cervical mucous.

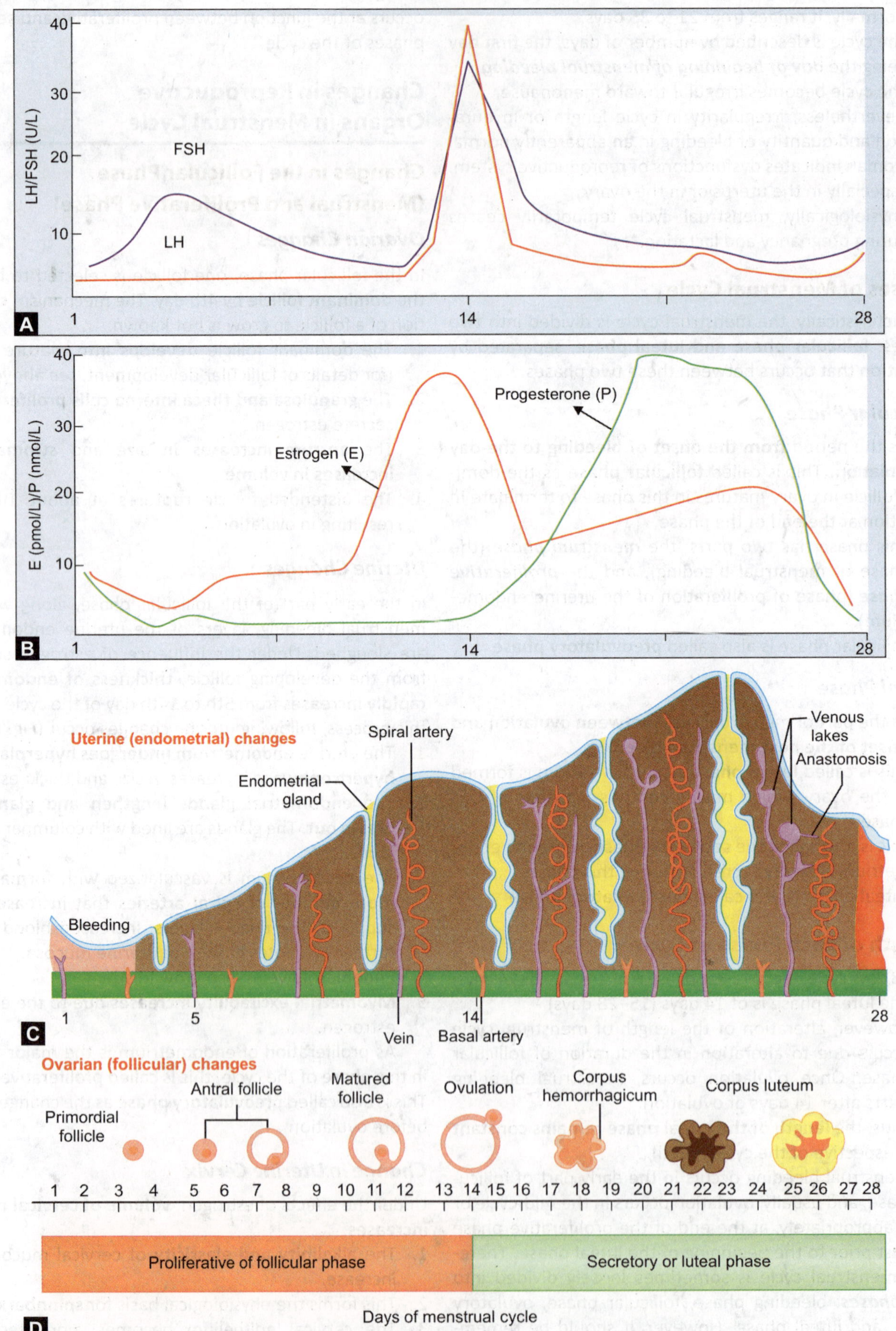

Figs. 69.1A to D: Changes in reproductive organs and secretion of hormones in menstrual cycle. (A) Changes in LH and FSH level; (B) Changes in estrogen and progesterone level; (C) Endometrial changes; (D) Follicular changes.

Vaginal Changes

During this phase, under the influence of estrogen, vaginal **epithelial cells become cornified** (keratinized). The **cornification index increases** from almost zero on day 1 to about 100 on 14th day.

Changes in the Luteal Phase (Secretory Phase)

Ovarian Changes

Luteal phase starts after ovulation. Following ovulation, follicle is **rapidly filled with blood**. Therefore, the follicle is called **corpus hemorrhagicum**. The blood clot inside the follicle is replaced by proliferation of granulosa cells. The granulosa and theca cells of the follicle undergo **luteinization** to become granulosa lutein cells and theca lutein cells. Thus, the follicle develops into **corpus luteum** (Fig. 69.1D). The luteal cells secrete progesterone and estrogen. If pregnancy occurs, corpus luteum persists; otherwise it degenerates between 26th to 28th days, and forms **corpus albicans**.

Uterine Changes

During the luteal phase, progesterone secretion increases significantly. Estrogen secretion also increases to some extent. Therefore, following uterine changes occur under the combined effects of estrogen and progesterone. However, major changes are due to the effects of progesterone.

1. The uterine glands become **coiled and tortuous**.
2. The glandular cells store glycogen and secrete **large quantity of carbohydrate-rich mucous and fluid.** Therefore, this phase is called **secretory phase**.
3. The **vascularity of endometrium increases further** due to combined effects of estrogen and progesterone secreted from corpus luteum. **Spiral arteries become tortuous** (Fig. 69.1C).
4. Due to increased blood supply and increased secretion, the endometrium becomes edematous and thick.
5. Endometrial veins form **venous lakes and anastomoses** (Fig. 69.2).
6. **Myometrial excitability decreases** due to the effects of progesterone.
7. Toward later part, due to regression of corpus luteum, progesterone and estrogen secretions decrease. Coiled arteries constrict that reduces blood supply to endometrium. The **foci of necrosis** appear in the endometrium at many places.
8. **Necrotic areas coalesce** and endometrium starts sloughing at the end of secretory phase that heralds the onset of bleeding.

Change in Cervical Mucous

Under the effects of progesterone, the **cervical mucous becomes thick and its elasticity decreases.** Sperm cannot easily enter through the progesterone-dominated cervical mucous.

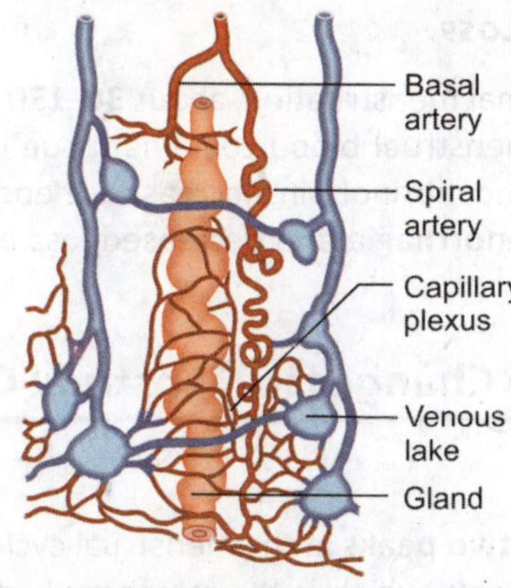

Fig. 69.2: Showing the pattern of venous lake and anastomosis formation in the endometrium in late secretory pahse. Also, note the basal and spiral arteries becoming more tortuous.

Vaginal Changes

Under the influence of progesterone, **vaginal epithelium proliferates** and secretes a **thick mucous**. The epithelium is infiltrated with leucocytes and **cornification decreases**.

Mechanism of Menstrual Bleeding

When **corpus luteum degenerates**, hormonal support of endometrium is withdrawn. This causes the ***endometrium to become necrotic***.

1. The **coiled arteries constrict** and reduce blood supply to endometrium.
2. The **foci of necrosis coalesce** leading to confluent hemorrhage, which occurs along with sloughing of endometrium.
3. This results in menstrual bleeding.

Mechanism

The mechanism is **initiated by decreased secretion of steroid hormones**.

1. Reduction in steroids causes **destabilization of lysosomal membranes** in the endometrial cells, which leads to release of **proteolytic enzymes** and **production of prostaglandins**, especially **PGF2α**.
2. The proteolytic enzymes cause **lysis of the endometrial tissue** and **PGF2α** causes vasospasm producing **endometrial ischemia** (Application Box 69.1). The ischemic changes result in **areas of local necrosis**, which is facilitated by proteolytic damage.
3. The foci of necrosis join with each other that result in sloughing of the uterine endometrium.

Application Box 69.1

Prostaglandins cause menstrual cramps: Vasoconstriction and uterine contractions are mediated by prostaglandins formed in the endometrium in response to the decrease in plasma estrogen and progesterone. The main mechanism of **dysmenorrhea** (menstrual cramps) is **overproduction of prostaglandins** causing excessive uterine contractions. Prostaglandins also cause smooth muscle contraction in other parts of body that accounts for nausea, vomiting, and headache associated with dysmenorrhea.

Amount of Loss

During a normal menstruation, about **30–130 mL of blood** is lost. The menstrual blood contains tissue debris, prostaglandins, and fibrinolysin. Increased menstrual loss is known as **menorrhagia** and decreased loss as **hypomenorrhea**.

Hormonal Changes in Menstrual Cycle

Estrogen

Estrogen has **two peaks** in the menstrual cycle.

1. **The fist peak**, which is the major peak, occurs about 48 hours before ovulation and **the second peak**, which the minor peak, occurs in the post-midluteal phase (Fig. 69.1B).
2. With the growth of ovarian follicle, estrogen concentration slowly increases in the early part of follicular phase. The concentration rises rapidly from 8th day of cycle to **reach the peak about one or two days before ovulation**. The concentration decreases thereafter and decreases further after ovulation.
3. About two days after ovulation (after the formation of corpus luteum), again estrogen concentration increases slowly to reach a **smaller peak** that occurs just after the midsecretory phase.

Progesterone

Progesterone concentration is minimal in the proliferative phase.

1. It starts rising following ovulation and reaches peak in 4 to 5 days after ovulation.
2. The **peak is maintained till corpus luteum is active.**
3. With regression of corpus luteum, progesterone concentration decreases toward the end of luteal phase.

LH

The concentration of Luteiuizing hormone (LH) remains low almost throughout the proliferative phase. However, about a day before ovulation, the **secretion of LH increases sharply** to reach the peak about 8–10 hours before ovulation. This is called **LH surge** (*see* below). Then, it declines fast in 24–48 hours and remains low in rest of the secretory phase (Fig. 69.1A).

FSH

Follicle-stimulating hormone (FSH) secretion **increases in the early part of the follicular phase** (during menstrual bleeding), and then declines slowly. Synchronous with the rise in LH, secretion of FSH **rises toward ovulation** and thereafter the pattern of change in FSH is similar with LH pattern.

Inhibins

The pattern of change in concentration of **inhibin B coincides with the change in concentration of FSH**, whereas the concentration of **inhibin A coincides with the pattern of progesterone**.

OVULATION

Ovulation is the **process of release of ovum** (oocyte) from the ovary that results from rupture of Graafian follicle at the end of the follicular phase of the menstrual cycle. Usually, ovulation **occurs on 14th day** in a 28 days cycle. However, if the cycle length is altered, ovulation occurs 14 days before the onset of menstrual bleeding as the **duration of luteal phase (which is 14 days) always remains constant.**

Mechanism of Ovulation

Ovulation occurs due to midcycle **LH surge.**

1. LH surge occurs due to high rise in estrogen concentration toward the later part of follicular phase that provides a **positive feedback effects on LH secretion** from pituitary.
2. Normally, a mild to moderate increase in estrogen for a brief period is inhibitory on LH secretion.
3. **Two-days prior to ovulation, *estrogen concentration increases*** to a higher level and when this high concentration is maintained for about 36 hours, the process of ovulation is initiated.
4. A series of biochemical and morphological changes occur in ovarian follicle that culminates in **follicular rupture**.
5. **Three chemical substances** are involved in rupture of ovarian follicle: **prostaglandins, cyclin D2** (a protein that regulates cell cycle), and **C-EBP** (CCAAT-enhancer binding protein). Decreased formation of these chemicals in ovary has been demonstrated to prevent ovulation in mice.

Steps of Follicular Rupture

1. LH surge increases release of **prostaglandins and bradykinin** that increase the ovarian blood flow. Thus, follicular blood flow increases.
2. The dominant follicle becomes **highly vascularized** and edematous. This increases the size of the follicle to about 25 mm.
3. Follicular blood flow also increases antral fluid volume, which in turn exerts pressure on the surrounding granulosa cells. The **cumulus-oophorus complex gets detached** from the follicular wall.
4. The **basement membrane** that separates granulosa cells and theca cells **disintegrates** due to intrafollicular pressure and the effects of proteolytic enzymes.

5. LH promotes **synthesis of plasminogen activator** by granulosa and theca cells, which causes conversion of plasminogen to plasmin. Plasmin causes **proteolysis of follicular wall**. Plasmin also activates the **synthesis of collagenase** that causes destruction of connective tissue matrix of the follicular wall and adjacent ovarian capsule.
6. Increased intrafollicular pressure and degeneration of the follicular wall facilitate the rupture of the follicle, which results in expulsion of oocyte from the follicle and the ovary.
7. FSH surge is not essential for ovulation (Application Box 69. 2)

Application Box 69.2

FSH surge occurs simultaneously: It should be noted that though midcycle FSH surge also occurs almost simultaneously along with LH surge, FSH surge is not essential for ovulation. However, FSH primes the follicular cells to express adequate number of LH receptors.

Indicators of Ovulation

It is important to know the day of ovulation for its physiological and clinical significance. The indicators of ovulation are as follows:

1. **Rise in of basal body temperature:** The basal body temperature (BBT) increases during ovulation by about 0.5°C. Accurate charting of this temperature can exactly detect the day of ovulation.
   a. It is recorded orally, early in the morning before getting up of the bed, and before taking any drink or washing the mouth.
   b. The increase in body temperature is due to the **influence of progesterone** that starts increasing with the beginning of secretory phase. Progesterone is thermogenic.
2. **Fleeting lower abdominal pain (mittelschmerz):** With ovulation, bleeding occurs into the antrum of the follicle.
   a. Small amount of **blood also escapes into the abdominal cavity**, which causes peritoneal irritation and produces fleeting (short-lived) lower abdominal pain.
   b. This is called as **mittelschmerz**.
3. **Vaginal discharge (spotting):** There may be **transitory increase in vaginal discharge** during ovulation.
   a. When rise in BBT is associated with mittelschmerz and spotting, they are collectively called as **ovulation cascade**.
   b. If all the three features are present, occurrence of ovulation is almost confirmed.
4. **Spinnbarkeit:** In the proliferative phase, estrogen makes the cervical mucous thin and alkaline.
   a. With the beginning of secretory phase, progesterone secreted from corpus luteum makes the cervical mucous thick and tenacious. Thus, **uterine mucous is thinnest at the time of ovulation and its elasticity is maximal.**
   b. Therefore, a drop of cervical mucous collected at the time of ovulation can be **stretched to as long as 10 cm or more** like a thread. This elastic nature of the mucous is called **spinnbarkeit.**
   c. **Decreased elasticity indicates ovulation** has already taken place.
5. **Fern test:** Under the effect of estrogen, the cervical mucous **before ovulation forms an arborizing fern like pattern**, when the mucous is spread on a slide.
   a. This is confirmed by microscopic examination of the mucous smear.
   b. Following ovulation, due to progesterone effect, the mucous become thick and fern pattern is not observed in smear of the mucous.
6. **Laparoscopic observation:** Demonstrating ovum in the abdominal cavity by laparoscopy confirms ovulation.
7. **Demonstration of LH peak:** LH surge occurs just prior to ovulation. Therefore, daily estimation of plasma LH in the periovulatory period will accurately detect the day of ovulation.

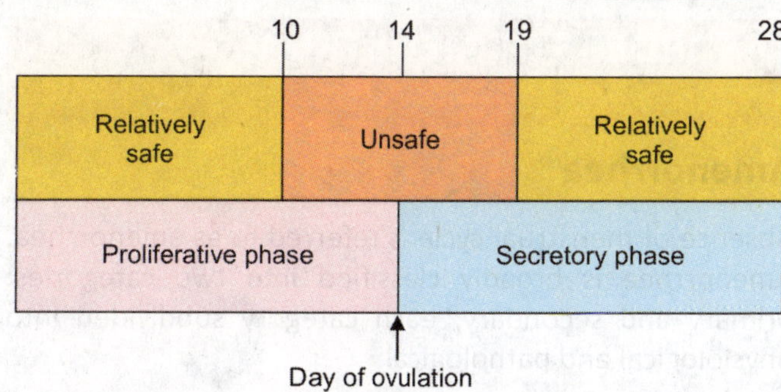

Fig. 69.3: Unsafe and safe periods in menstrual cycle. In regular cycles of 28 days, ovulation occurs on 14th day. Four days before and after ovulation (10th to 19th day of the cycle) is called unsafe period as unprotected sex leads to conception. Rest of the period is considered relatively safe, as chance of conception is minimal during these days.

Physiological Importance

Determination of day of ovulation **helps in family planning.**

1. The life span of ovum is about 72 hours.
2. Therefore, those who are **desirous of a child**, should have regular sexual act in the periovulatory period (day of ovulation, and two days before and after the ovulation).
3. **Those who want to avoid pregnancy**, should not have unprotected sexual act during the unsafe period (day of ovulation, four days before and after ovulation) of the cycle (Fig. 69.3).
4. Thus, it helps in **planning both conception and contraception** (for details, *see* "Female Contraceptives").

DISORDERS OF MENSTRUAL CYCLE AND OVULATION

Amenorrhea

Absence of menstrual cycle is referred to as amenorrhea. Amenorrhea is broadly classified into two categories: primary and secondary; each category subdivided into physiological and pathological.

Primary Amenorrhea

When menstruation has never occurred, the condition is called primary amenorrhea. There are physiological and pathological causes of primary amenorrhea.

Physiological Primary Amenorrhea

Amenorrhea occurs in many physiological conditions. Physiological amenorrhea is more common than pathological amenorrhea. The causes of physiological amenorrhea are:

1. **Before puberty:** Amenorrhea is normal in childhood and prepubertal age. Usually, menstruation starts at the age of 12–14 years.
2. **Constitutional amenorrhea:** Though menstrual cycle starts normally by the age of 16 years, sometimes it may not occur even at the age of 18 years or more, without there being any abnormality. This is called *constitutional amenorrhea*.

Pathological Primary Amenorrhea

When menstrual cycle *does not start till the age of 18 years due to some prevailing disease*, the condition is called pathological primary amenorrhea.

1. It usually occurs due to **congenital and genetic defects**. Examples are Turner syndrome, Kallman syndrome, etc.
2. **Congenital malformations** of reproductive tract like absence of uterus can also cause primary amenorrhea.

Secondary Amenorrhea

When menstrual cycle stops in a woman ***who had normal cycles before***, the condition is called secondary amenorrhea. There are physiological and secondary causes.

Physiological Secondary Amenorrhea

Physiological causes of secondary amenorrhea are more common than pathological causes.

1. **Peri-pubertal amenorrhea:** In first one to two years of onset of menarche, menstrual cycles are often anovulatory and therefore irregular. Menstruation does not occur even for 2–4 consecutive cycles. This is called peripubertal amenorrhea. This very common till the full pubertal and reproductive developments occur and is regarded as normal.
2. **Pregnancy:** Pregnancy is the ***commonest cause of secondary amenorrhea***. It is so common amongst all forms of amenorrhea that before investigating for the causes of amenorrhea, first, pregnancy should be ruled out.
3. **Lactation:** The prolactin concentration is high in the plasma of a lactating mother. Prolactin inhibits the secretion of gonadotropin-releasing hormone (GnRH), and therefore, ovulation is prevented. This is called **lactational amenorrhea**. This is the physiological basis of contraception in a lactating woman.
4. **Emotional disturbance:** Psychological trauma frequently causes amenorrhea by disrupting hypothalamic release of GnRH via limbic-hypothalamic connections.
5. **Change in environment:** Sudden change of place, especially exposure to extremes of climates is known to produce amenorrhea during the acclimatization period.
6. **Menopause:** Menstrual cycle ceases at menopause. This occurs due to failure of the ovary, to respond to gonadotropic stimuli. It occurs usually between the ages of 45–50 years. Menstrual cycles become initially irregular for 2–6 months before completely stopping at menopause.

Pathological Secondary Amenorrhea

Pathological secondary amenorrhea occurs due to a defect in hypothalamus, pituitary, ovary and uterus or due to a systemic disease or chronic use of some drugs.

1. **Hypothalamic disorders:** Hypothalamic diseases resulting in ***decreased secretion of GnRH*** leads to amenorrhea. The reduction in frequency of GnRH pulses rather than the absolute decrease in concentration of GnRH is the cause of hypothalamic amenorrhea. Recently, it has been observed that this occurs due to increased opioid activity and treatment with opioid blockers like naltrexone cures hypothalamic amenorrhea.
2. **Pituitary disorders:** Tumors and other diseases of pituitary (***hypopituitarism***) resulting in decreased secretion of gonadotropins leads to amenorrhea. Examples are **Sheehan's syndrome** (post-partum ischemic necrosis of anterior pituitary due to severe hemorrhage during childbirth) and **Simmond's syndrome** (complete destruction of anterior pituitary) etc.
3. **Ovarian diseases:** Diseases that ***decrease the production of estrogen and progesterone***, frequently lead to amenorrhea. In **Stein-Leventhal syndrome** (polycystic ovarian disease), amenorrhea occurs due to abnormal production of hormone leading to high LH-FSH ratio and high androgen level.
4. **Uterine pathology:** Congenital absence of uterus, underdeveloped uterus and severe infective or non-infective endometritis produce amenorrhea.
5. **Systemic illness:** Amenorrhea occurs in chronic illnesses like chronic hypothyroidism, chronic renal failure and cirrhosis of liver. Any systemic illness that leads to cachexia may also cause amenorrhea.
6. **Drugs:** Phenothiazine derivatives, reserpine, ganglion blocking agents and estrogen-progesterone preparations (pill contraceptives) are common drugs that prevent menstrual cycles. They mainly act by inhibiting hypothalamic release of GnRH.

Anovulation

Absence of ovulation during a menstrual cycle is called anovulatory cycle.

1. **Following menarche**, menstrual cycles may be anovulatory for first 1 to 2 years.
2. Few cycles may also be anovulatory in **lactating woman**, and about six months **before menopause**.
3. Anovulation also occurs in severe strenuous exercise or severer job related stress.
4. Except these physiological situations, anovulation is abnormal and occurs mainly due to **hormonal deficiencies.**

Treatment of Amenorrhea and Anovulation

If amenorrhea is due to hypothalamo-pituitary defects, **pulsatile administration of GnRH** gives successful result. In hypopituitarism, **sequential administration of FSH and hCG** is useful. If amenorrhea is due to pituitary tumor, their **surgical removal** should be considered. **Clomiphene**, that binds with estrogen receptors and blocks estrogen action, induces ovulation. Clomiphene increases LH and FSH secretion by *reducing the negative effects of estrogen*. For uterine pathologies, corrective surgeries should be performed.

Hypomenorrhea and Oligomenorrhea

Decreased menstrual bleeding in duration or amount or both is called **hypomenorrhea**. It may be constitutional, or due to uterine pathology or due to hormonal disorders.

Decreased frequency (cycle more than 35 days) of menstrual cycle is called **oligomenorrhea**. Usually, oligomenorrhea occurs in ***ovarian diseases*** in which menstruation is irregular and infrequent.

Dysmenorrhea

Dysmenorrhea means painful menstrual bleeding. It is classified into two categories:

1. **Primary dysmenorrhea** in which there is no visible pelvic pathology, and
2. **Secondary dysmenorrhea** in which a uterine or pelvic pathology is associated with it. Usually, it occurs due to passage of clots in flow.

Dysmenorrhea occurs due to accumulation of prostaglandins in the uterine fluid. Therefore, use of prostaglandin inhibitors usually gives relief from dysmenorrhea.

Menorrhagia, Metrorrhagia, and Polymenorrhea

Menorrhagia

Increased menstrual bleeding in amount, duration or both is called menorrhagia.

1. It is generally caused by conditions that affect **uterus and its vascular apparatus** rather than any ovarian dysfunction.
2. Or, sometimes it may be a manifestation of **coagulation disorder**.

Metrorrhagia

Bleeding occurring **between the periods** (acyclical and irregular) is called metrorrhagia. It usually indicates a *surface lesion in the genital tract*, which may be benign or malignant.

Polymenorrhea

When menstrual cycle **occurs frequently** (less than 21 days), it is called polymenorrhea. Usually, the amount and duration of bleeding remain normal.

Premenstrual Syndrome

Few women develop some nonspecific features about a week before the onset of menstrual bleeding that are combinely called as premenstrual syndrome (PMS) or **premenstrual dysphoric disorder** (PMDD).

Features: The usual features are edema, painful or swollen breasts, depression, loss of concentration, irritability, headache, behavioral changes, and emotional disturbances. These features disappear within 1–3 days after the start of menstruation.

Etiology: Though the salt and water retention has mainly been attributed to PMS, the exact cause of it is not known. Recently, it has been proposed that PMS occurs due to an excess and complex interplay between the sex steroids and brain neurotransmitters.

Treatment: Treatment with drugs that prematurely terminate luteal phase of the cycle does not give any substantial relieve, which indicates that the PMS is **not due to hormonal imbalance**. Also, the plasma concentrations of hormones usually found to be normal in these patients. However, treatment with alprazolam (**minor tranquilizer**), prozac (**serotonin uptake inhibitor**) and **GnRH agonist** give some relief. This proves the hypothesis that PMS is due to the complex interplay between the gonadal steroids and neurotransmitters in the brain.

Anorexia Nervosa

It is a complex behavioral disorder in women which manifests as severe anorexia (loss of food intake) associated with functional abnormalities.

1. **Amenorrhea** is seen in 30–40% of cases.
2. Patient is grossly **emaciated.**
3. Emaciation (low body fat) and stress **inhibit LH secretion** through endorphins.
4. Pubic hair development and breast development usually remain unaffected.

CHAPTER SUMMARY

Key Concepts

1. The duration of menstrual cycle is not constant even in a healthy woman, as it affected by many psychosocial factors that alter hormones related to hypothalamo-pituitary-gonadal axis. The luteal phase remains constant and alteration in cycle occurs due to change in proliferative phase.
2. BBT is a good sign of ovulation. But BBT should be recorded properly to note the exact change in temperature.
3. LH surge is an example of positive feedback mechanism.

Important to Know (Must Read)

1. In examination, "With the help of a suitable diagram, describe the uterine and ovarian changes during different phases of menstrual cycle" is usually asked as a **Long Question.**
2. Indicators of ovulation, Uterine changes during different phases of menstrual cycle, Ovarian changes during different phases of menstrual cycle, Hormonal changes during different phases of menstrual cycle, Amenorrhea, Premenstrual syndrome (PMS), Mechanism of ovulation, Mechanism of menstrual bleeding, are asked as **Short Questions** in exam.
3. In **Viva**, examiner may ask… List the indicators of ovulation, What is mittelschmerz, What is spinnbarkeit, What is spotting, What is ovulation cascade, What is fern test, What are the phases of menstrual cycle, What are the uterine changes during different phases of menstrual cycle, What are the ovarian changes during different phases of menstrual cycle, What are the hormonal changes during different phases of menstrual cycle, What are the vaginal changes during different phases of menstrual cycle, What is the duration of menstrual cycle, How do you calculate the day of ovulation, How does the determination of the day of ovulation help in family planning, List the steps of follicular rupture, What is the mechanism of menstrual bleeding, What is the role of prostaglandins in menstruation,

   What is amenorrhea and what are its types, What is primary amenorrhea and what are its types, What is physiological primary amenorrhea and what are its causes, What is pathological primary amenorrhea and what are its causes, What is secondary amenorrhea and what are its types, What is physiological secondary amenorrhea and what are its causes, What is pathological secondary amenorrhea and what are its causes, What is the treatment of amenorrhea, What is anovulation and what is its treatment, What is hypomenorrhea and what are its causes, What is oligomenorrhea and what are its causes, What is dysmenorrhea and what are its causes, What is menorrhagia and what are its causes, What is metrorrhagia and what are its causes, What is polymenorrhea and what are its causes, What is premenstrual syndrome (PMS), What are the causes , features and treatment of PMS, What is anorexia nervosa and what are its features.

CHAPTER 70

Ovarian Hormones and Control of Ovarian Functions

Learning Objectives

On completion of study of this chapter, the student **MUST** be able to:

1. List the ovarian hormones.
2. Describe the functions of ovarian hormones.
3. List the secondary sexual characteristics in females.
4. Understand the mechanisms of control of ovarian functions.
5. Apply the knowledge of ovarian functions to understand the abnormalities of female reproduction.

The student **MAY** also be able to:

1. Describe the control of ovarian functions.

OVARIAN HORMONES

Ovary secretes estrogens, progesterone, Inhibins and relaxin.

Estrogens

The naturally synthesized estrogens are **17β-estradiol, estrone, and estriol** (Fig. 70.1). Estradiol is 15 and 80 times more potent than estrone and estriol respectively.

Source

Estrogen is secreted from **granulosa cells of ovarian follicles, corpus luteum, and placenta**. Estrogen is not directly secreted from **adrenal gland**, but adrenal androgen is converted to estrogen by the enzyme aromatase.

Synthesis

Estrogen is a steroid hormone, synthesized from cholesterol (Flowchart 70.1). LH, acting on LH receptors located on **theca interna cells** converts cholesterol to androstenedione.

1. In theca cells, some androstenedione is converted into estradiol, but **most of it is supplied to granulosa cells to be converted into estrogen** in those cells.
2. FSH acting on the FSH receptors on the granulosa cells facilitates the conversion of androgen to estrogen by activating the activity of the enzyme aromatase.

A. 17-β-Estradiol

OH

HO

B. Estrone

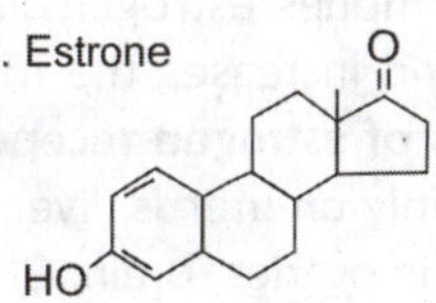

C. Estriol

OH

OH

HO

Fig. 70.1: Structure of estrogens.

3. However, mature granulosa cells also acquire LH receptors and directly form estrogen.

Secretion

Estrogen secretion occurs in **two peaks** during the menstrual cycle. A larger peak occurs during proliferative phase just before ovulation and a smaller peak in the midsecretory phase. The rate of secretion of estradiol is about 35 μg per day in the early follicular phase, **400 μg per day**

Flowchart 70.1: Synthesis of estrogens.

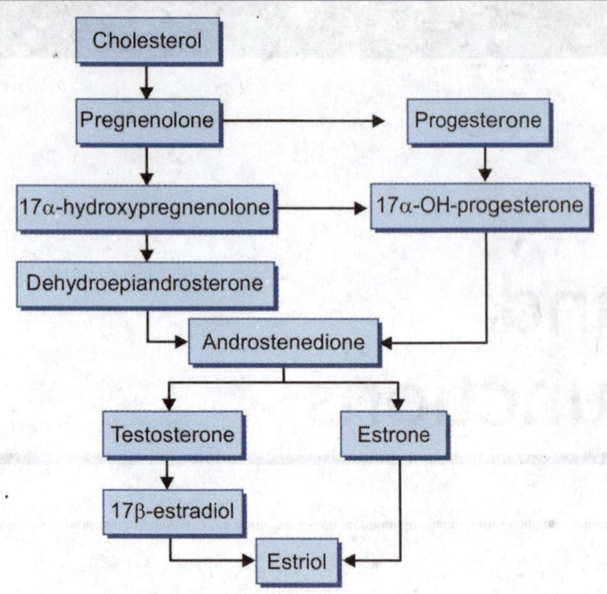

just before ovulation and 250 µg per day in the midluteal phase. Secretion of estrone is similar to the secretion of estradiol. The secretion is very low after menopause.

Metabolism

Like other steroid hormones, about **98% of circulating estrogen is bound to proteins**. 60% of the estrogen is bound to albumin and 38% to steroid-binding globulin. In liver, estrogens are metabolized through oxidation or are converted to their **glucuronide and sulfate derivatives** that are excreted in urine.

Mechanism of Action

Like other steroid hormones, estrogen binds with the receptor in the nucleus and increases the formation of mRNA. There are **two types of estrogen receptors**: ERα and ERβ. **ERα** are present mainly on uterus, liver, kidney and heart, and **ERβ** are present in ovaries, brain, GI tract, hemopoietic tissues, lungs and prostate. Estrogens have both **genomic and nongenomic actions**. Most of the actions are genomic that are mediated via production of mRNA. However, some of the effects are nongenomic that occur rapidly and are mediated via intracellular second messengers.

Physiological Actions

Effects on Female Reproductive System

Estrogen promotes growth of all components of female reproductive system. In general, it causes growth of smooth muscle and proliferation of epithelial lining of reproductive tract.

On ovary

Estrogen stimulates **growth of ovary and ovarian follicles**. Role of estrogen on follicular growth has been described in Chapter 70 'Follicular development'.

On Fallopian Tubes

Estrogen stimulates smooth muscle contraction of fallopian tubes and therefore increases fallopian tube motility. It also increases ciliary activity of the tubes.

On Uterus

Estrogen has wide ranging effects on uterus.

1. It **increases uterine size**. Therefore, in prepubertal girls or castrated females the uterus is small with thin myometrium.
2. During the follicular phase of menstrual cycle, estrogen causes **proliferation of uterine endometrium**.
3. During luteal phase, along with progesterone, it **increases uterine fluid secretion**. It also increases progesterone receptor on uterine endometrium. Thus estrogen prepares endometrium for progesterone action.
4. It **increases uterine blood flow**. Therefore, it increases myometrial size (Application Box 70.1).
5. It increases the **content of contractile proteins** in uterine smooth muscles. It increases the activity and **excitability of uterine muscle**. It also increases the **sensitivity of uterus to oxytocin.** Estrogen secretion increases towards term and all these uterine changes prepare the uterus for parturition.

Effects on Cervical Mucous

Under the influence of estrogen, cervical mucus becomes **abundant, clear, and watery**. These characteristics become more pronounced at the time of ovulation to allow sperm to easily pass through the cervical mucus barrier on their way to the uterus and fallopian tubes.

Application Box 70.1

Withdrawal bleeding: Chronic estrogen treatment causes excessive endometrial hypertrophy. In such patients, discontinuation of therapy causes sloughing of the uterine endometrium that produces bleeding. This is called withdrawal bleeding. Sometimes, bleeding also occurs during the course of treatment of estrogen over a longer period. This is called **breakthrough bleeding**.

Effects on Breast

Estrogen causes **breast enlargement during puberty**. Therefore, it is known as **"growth hormone of the breast"**. It causes **growth of ducts** of the mammary gland. It also causes **pigmentation of the areola**.

Effects on Secondary Sexual Characteristics

At the time of puberty, secondary sexual characteristics develop in girls due to the effects of estrogen. Following are the secondary sexual characteristics in females:

1. **Female body configuration:** Narrow shoulders and broad hips.
2. **Wide carrying angle:** Thighs that converge and arms that diverge.
3. **Female distribution of fat:** Fat deposition in the hips and breast (breast enlargement).
4. Voice remains **high pitched**, as no change in larynx occurs.

5. Less hair on the body and more hair on the scalp.
6. **Pubic Hair:** Female escutcheon of pubic hair. Pubic hair distribution in females forms a triangle with ***base upward and apex downward***.
7. **Internal Genitalia:** Vagina, uterus, ovary, fallopian tube grow in size and functions (as described above).

It is believed that growth of pubic and axillary hairs occurs due to androgen in females rather than estrogen.

Effects on Endocrine Organs

Estrogen has wide ranging endocrine effects.

1. Estrogen **inhibits LH secretion** by its negative feedback effects directly on pituitary and by indirectly inhibiting GnRH secretion from hypothalamus. However, before ovulation, the feedback becomes positive that results in LH surge.
2. Estrogen **inhibits FSH secretion**.
3. It **stimulates prolactin secretion**. However, it inhibits the milk producing action of prolactin on breast.
4. It **promotes the synthesis of angiotensinogen** from liver. Thus, it **activates renin-angiotensin system**. By increasing the formation of angiotensin II, it **increases blood pressure**, especially when estrogen is taken for a longer period; for example as contraceptive pill.
5. Estrogen **increases the formation of thyroxine-binding globulin**. Therefore, the free thyroxine concentration decreases in estrogen therapy and also in later part of pregnancy when estrogen concentration is high.
6. It **stimulates androgen secretion** from adrenal cortex (Application Box 70.2).

Application Box 70.2

Estrogen stimulates growth of animals: In farm animals, commercially available estrogen injections are given to increase the body weight of the animal. This occurs due to the **protein anabolic effect** of estrogen, which is **induced by increased androgen secretion** from adrenal cortex. Estrogen injection is known to promote growth of chickens and cattle.

Effects on CNS

By **activating neurons in the limbic system**, estrogen stimulates **libido**. Especially, acting on the suprachiasmatic area of hypothalamus, it produces **sexual behaviors**. Conversely, estrogen implantation into arcuate nucleus-ventral hypothalamus complex in experimental animals has been observed to produce ovarian atrophy.

Effects on Musculoskeletal System

Estrogen **stimulates bone growth.**

1. It prevents osteoclastic activity. Therefore, estrogen **prevents osteoporotic activity**.
2. Estrogen causes **epiphyseal closure**. Hence, it causes cessation of longitudinal growth of bone and therefore, **determines the height** of the female.
3. Estrogen has no direct effect on growth of skeletal muscle. However, by stimulating androgen secretion, it facilitates skeletal muscle development.

Effects on Water and Electrolyte Metabolisms

Estrogen promotes **salt and water retention** to some extent by directly acting on kidney tubules. This contributes to **ECF expansion and hypertension** in chronic estrogen therapy, in addition to its activation of renin-angiotensin system.

Effects on Lipid Profile

Estrogen is a strong **cholesterol lowering agent**, and therefore, it **prevents atherosclerosis**. Hence, coronary artery disease, especially myocardial infarction is less common in females during their reproductive life. Possibly, estrogen also increases HDL concentration in plasma.

Effects on Sebaceous Secretion & Skin

From sebaceous gland, estrogen promotes more fluid secretions. This antagonizes the thick sebaceous secretion of androgen. Thus, estrogen **inhibits the formation of acne**. Chronic high estrogen levels may produce cutaneous angiomas (Clinical Box 70.1)

Clinical Box 70.1

Hyperestrogenemia in liver diseases: Androstenedione is metabolized in liver. Therefore, in advanced liver diseases, circulating androstenedione concentration increases, that facilitates their conversion into estrogen. Hence, spider angiomas and breast enlargement are features of advanced stage of liver diseases.

Estrogen Preparations

Naturally occurring estrogens as extracted from plants have adverse effects when injected into farm animals. They may promote uterine and breast cancer. Therefore, **synthetic estrogens** that have no effects on uterine and breast tissue but have bone preserving and anabolic effects are used in humans and animals. This becomes possible due to the activation of selective estrogen receptor modulators in specific tissues. Examples of such estrogens are tamoxifen and raloxifene.

Progesterone

Source, Synthesis and Metabolism

Progesterone is secreted from **corpus luteum, placenta and ovarian follicle**. It is also an intermediate product in many steroid biosynthesis.

1. It is formed from pregnenolone. The plasma concentration of progesterone in follicular phase is about 0.9 ng/mL, and in luteal phase at its peak is 18 ng/mL.
2. Like other steroid hormones, progesterone is mainly bound to plasma proteins. Only 2% circulates freely in plasma, whereas 80% is bound to albumin and 18% is bound to corticosteroid-binding globulin.
3. In the liver, it is converted to **pregnanediol**, which forms **glucuronide conjugates** and excreted in urine (Flowchart 70.2).

Flowchart 70.2: Synthesis and metabolism of progesterone.

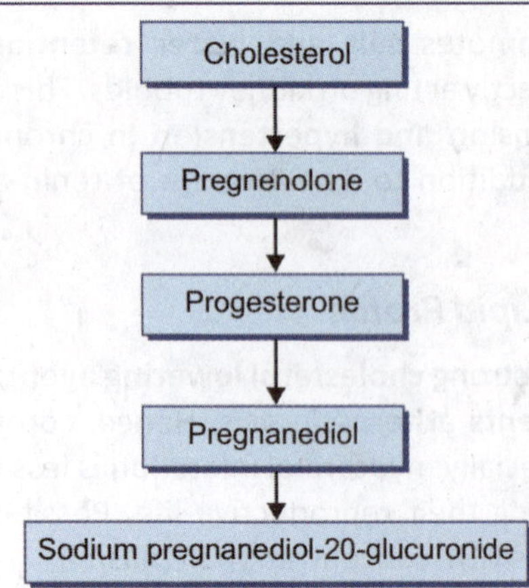

Mechanism of Action

Like other steroid hormones, progesterone acts on the receptors located in the nucleus, and the biochemical mechanism of action is through increased **gene transcription.**

Physiological Actions

Effects on Reproductive Organs

Progesterone **inhibits uterine myometrial contractions,** by following mechanisms:

1. It **opposes the stimulatory actions of estrogen** and locally generated prostaglandins. This is very *important for implantation of fertilized egg* and *continuation of pregnancy*.
2. It increases the rate of conversion of 17β-estradiol to less active estrogens.
3. Progesterone also directly **causes relaxation of uterine smooth muscles.**
4. It also **decreases excitability of myometrium** and the sensitivity of myometrium to oxytocin. Progesterone increases the membrane potential and decreases the spontaneous electrical activity of myometrial cells.

 Uterine quiescence is maintained throughout pregnancy by progesterone, which is crucial to **prevent premature expulsion of the fetus** (abortion).

Progesterone also has important effects on the secretion of mucus from the cervix. It causes the **cervical mucus to become thick and sticky**; in essence, this acts as a plug that prevents infective organisms from vagina to enter the uterus. This antibacterial blockage **protects the growing embryo** if conception has occurred.

Progesterone acts on estrogen-primed endometrium and **increases secretions from endometrial glands**. It inhibits proliferation of the cells lining the vagina.

Effects on Breast

It promotes growth of the breast, especially the **growth of the glandular tissue** (lobules and alveoli). It supports the differentiation of estrogen-prime ductal tissue. It also supports the secretory functions of breast during lactation.

Effects on Body Temperature

Immediately after ovulation, there is a small increase (approximately 0.5°C) in body temperature that occurs due to an action of progesterone on temperature regulatory centers in the brain. **Progesterone is thermogenic.**

Effects on Hypothalamo-Pituitary Axis

Progesterone has **negative feedback effects** on hypothalamo-pituitary axis. It **decreases LH secretion.** In large doses, it also potentiates the inhibitory effects of estrogen. Therefore, **it prevents ovulation.** Hence, it is used as a contraceptive agent.

Effects on Respiration

Progesterone **stimulates respiration and produces tachypnea**. Therefore, the PCO_2 decreases in pregnancy.

Effects on Blood Pressure

Progesterone **causes vasodilation** (relaxation of vascular smooth muscle). Therefore, **diastolic pressure decreases in pregnancy**. Thus, hypertension is never a feature of normal pregnancy. This also contributes to **wide pulse pressure in pregnancy** as systolic pressure increases due to ECF expansion.

On Electrolyte and Water Metabolisms

In large doses, progesterone produces **natriuresis and diuresis** by blocking the effects of aldosterone on kidney tubules.

Other Ovarian Hormones

Relaxin

Relaxin is a **polypeptide hormone.** Structurally it is similar to insulin and insulin like growth factors. The gene for relaxin is located on chromosome 9.

Source

Relaxin is secreted from **corpus luteum, placenta, uterus and breast tissue** in females, and **prostate glands** in males. The secretion of relaxin increases towards later part of pregnancy reaching a peak just before term.

Functions

1. It **relaxes pubic symphysis** and **pelvic joints and ligaments.**
2. It causes **softening and dilation of uterine cervix.** Thus it facilitates parturition.
3. It **inhibits uterine contraction.**
4. It promotes development of mammary gland.
5. In nonpregnant woman, it is secreted from corpus luteum in the secretory phase of menstrual cycle. However, its physiological significance is not known.
6. In males, it is secreted from prostate. It **facilitates sperm motility** and penetration of ovum by sperm.

Inhibins

Inhibins are secreted from granulosa cells of ovary. Inhibin **inhibits the secretion of FSH** from anterior pituitary (for details, refer 'Male Reproductive System').

Androgens

Androgens are secreted in women from **adrenal glands and ovaries**.

1. These androgens play some role in the female reproductive functions.
2. They **stimulate the growth of pubic and axillary hairs** and possibly they also promote **growth of skeletal muscle**.
3. They also help **maintain sexual desire (libido)**.
4. However, excess production leads to male body hair distribution, abnormal skeletal muscle growth, enlargement of clitoris and reduction in breast size.

CONTROL OF OVARIAN FUNCTIONS

Ovaries have the following major functions:

1. Synthesis and **secretion of gonadal hormones**.
2. Release of oocyte (**ovulation**) at the end of proliferative phase of the menstrual cycle.
3. Nourishment and **development of resident oocytes**.
4. Preparation of fallopian tube to **facilitate fertilization**.
5. Preparation of uterus for **implantation** of fertilized ovum.
6. Providing **hormonal support** to the embryo till placenta starts functioning.

The ovarian functions are controlled by hormones secreted from **hypothalamus, anterior pituitary and ovary**. They are GnRH, FSH and LH, and gonadal sex hormones. The major factor determining ovarian function is the **pulsatile secretion of GnRH** from hypothalamic neuroendocrine cells. The pattern of frequency and amplitude of GnRH pulses during a 24-hour period is different over the course of the menstrual cycle. Also, responsiveness of the pituitary to GnRH and of the ovaries to gonadotropins varies in different phases of the cycle.

Hypothalamic Control

Hypothalamus plays an important role in regulating ovarian functions by controlling the secretion of gonadotropins from anterior pituitary.

1. Hypothalamus secretes GnRH, which is released in **episodic bursts**. This **episodic secretion of GnRH** determines circhoral peaks of LH secretion. It has been experimentally observed that maintaining a constant and steady release of GnRH inhibits (Clinical Box 70.2), whereas episodic and pulsatile injection of GnRH stimulates LH secretion.
2. Episodic secretion of GnRH not only stimulates LH secretion, but also regulates secretion of other hormones that **control menstrual cycle**.
3. The **frequency of GnRH burst** is important in bringing the LH surge.
4. Also, the sensitivity of gonadotrophs of anterior pituitary to the GnRH burst is important in bringing **LH surge**, which increases towards ovulation.
5. The higher concentration of **estrogen stimulates this frequency towards the later part of follicular phase** that finally culminates in LH surge.
6. However, the exact site of **GnRH pulse generator** in the hypothalamus is not known.
7. Progesterone, androgen, catecholamines, enkephalins and endorphins inhibit frequency of GnRH pulses.

Clinical Box 70.2

Long-acting GnRH analogs: As described above, a constantly elevated GnRH level in plasma inhibits LH secretion by down-regulating receptors on gonadotrophs. Therefore, long-acting GnRH analogs are used in **treatment of precocious puberty** as it inhibits LH secretion by chronically maintaining a GnRH level. It is also used in **therapy of prostate cancer**.

Pituitary Control

The anterior pituitary secretes LH and FSH. The major target organs of these hormones are gonads. Therefore they are called **gonadotropins**. Primarily, they control ovarian functions in both the phases of menstrual cycle. Ovarian control by gonadotropins has a similar analogy with testicular control (Clinical Box 70.3).

Clinical Box 70.3

Analogy with testis: The granulosa and theca cells of ovarian follicle are similar to the Sertoli and Leydig cells of testis. Sertoli cells provide microenvironment in testis in which the germ cells develop and mature, and Sertoli are stimulated by FSH. **Granulosa cells resemble Sertoli cells** in their function by providing environment for development of oocyte, and for their control by FSH. Like Sertoli cells granulosa cells also secrete inhibin-B that controls FSH secretion from pituitary. The **theca cells are similar to the Leydig cells** in that they produce androgens and are stimulated mainly by LH.

The Pattern of Secretion of Gonadotropins

The **FSH level** in plasma slowly increases in the early part of the follicular phase and then steadily decreases in the remainder of the phase and then increases rapidly towards the end of the phase to attain a mid-cycle peak (refer to Fig. 69.1, Chapter 69).

1. The **LH in level plasma** is low in most part of the cycle except in the periovulatory period. It starts increasing rapidly about a day before ovulation to reach a very **large mid-cycle peak**, called LH surge.
2. This is followed by a rapid decline of LH in the luteal phase.

Regulation by FSH

A number of primary and early antral follicles are always present in the ovary between puberty and menopause. Further development of these follicles beyond these stages requires stimulation by FSH.

1. **Before puberty,** the concentration of FSH in the plasma is too low to bring such development.
2. **After puberty**, during first half of each menstrual cycle, increase in FSH secretion stimulates follicular growth. FSH stimulates **proliferation of granulosa** cells to produce estrogen, and stimulates **enlargement of the antrum.**
3. FSH also primes the granulosa and theca cells to the effect of LH.

Regulation by LH

LH acts on the theca and granulosa cells. These cells are converted to luteal cells as follicle becomes corpus luteum after ovulation. LH **causes luteinization** of these cells. LH surge is responsible for ovulation to occur (for details, refer "Mechanism of Ovulation" in previous chapter).

The Ovarian Control

Ovary controls its own functions by secreting hormones that directly influence granulosa cell function or indirectly influence hypothalamic-pituitary-ovarian axis (feedback control).

The Pattern of Secretion of Gonadal Hormones

Estrogen

After remaining low in the first week, estrogen first increases slowly and then rapidly in the second week as the dominant ovarian follicle grows and secretes more estrogen.

1. **Estrogen peak occurs about two days before ovulation** and then decreases rapidly in next two days.
2. The second but **slow and small peak** of estrogen occurs in luteal phase due to its secretion from corpus luteum.

Progesterone

Progesterone release is low during the follicular phase.

1. But, soon after ovulation, progesterone concentration **increases rapidly in luteal phase** due to its release in large amount from corpus luteum.
2. Inhibin-B secretion resembles the secretory pattern of FSH.

Direct Regulation

Theca cells secrete androgen, which facilitates secretion of estrogen by the granulosa cells.

Feedback Regulation

The dominant follicle secretes estrogen that inhibits gonadotropins (the **negative feedback effect**) from pituitary and GnRH secretion from hypothalamus (Fig. 70.2).

1. When plasma concentration of estrogen is very high the secretion of gonadotropin increases (the **positive feedback effect**).

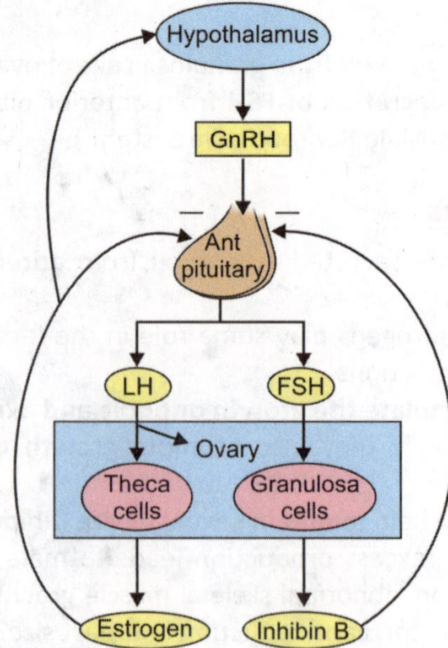

Fig. 70.2: Feedback regulation of ovarian functions.

2. But, how exactly low concentration of estrogen exerts negative feedback inhibition and high concentration provides positive feedback effect on the secretion of gonadotropins is not clearly known.
3. However, the effect is partly mediated via hypothalamus. Large dose of **progesterone inhibits LH secretion** and **potentiates the usual inhibitory effect of estrogen**. Therefore, **combination of estrogen and progesterone** is used in the prevention of ovulation.

The increase in plasma inhibin concentration in the luteal phase also contributes to the suppression of FSH secretion. Therefore, in the luteal phase, plasma concentrations of the gonadotropins are very low.

Thus, ovarian events via hormonal feedback mechanisms control the hypothalamus and anterior pituitary secretions. Therefore, it should be remembered that, though the hypothalamus and anterior pituitary are fundamental regulator of ovarian functions, the **real controller is the ovary itself**, as its own hormones (ovarian hormones) profoundly influence hypothalamo-pituitary axis via their feedback regulations.

APPLIED ASPECTS

Reproductive abnormalities that either lead to or occur due to ovarian dysfunctions can broadly be classified into two categories: genetic and hormonal abnormalities.

Genetic and Hormonal Abnormalities

Following genetic abnormalities are common in women, and are associated with hormonal dysfunctions:

GnRH Resistance

This occurs due to **decreased number and sensitivity of GnRH receptors** on gonadotrophs of pituitary.

FSH Resistance

This occurs due to **decreased number and sensitivity of FSH receptors** on granulosa cells of pituitary.

LH Resistance

This occurs due to **decreased number and sensitivity of LH receptors on granulosa and theca cells** of ovarian follicles.

Aromatase Deficiency

The enzyme aromatase is required for synthesis of gonadal hormones. Aromatase (CYP 19) **converts testosterone to estradiol and androstenedione to estrone**. Therefore, its deficiency leads to **estrogen deficiency and amenorrhea**.

McCune-Albright Syndrome

This is an example of **receptor protein (G protein) abnormality** in which G_{sa} is active in some cells and defective in others. It causes endocrine dysfunctions associated with **precocious puberty, amenorrhea and galactorrhea**. Lina Medina of Peru was the commonly quoted example of Albright syndrome.

Kallmann's Syndrome

This is a **hypogonadal form of deficiency of LH and FSH neurons** that occurs due to failure of migration of these neurons from the olfactory bulb. The GnRH secretion from hypothalamus is less and therefore deficiency occurs in secretion of LH and FSH. Pubertal maturation of testes in males and ovaries in females fail to occur (**hypogonadotropic hypogonadism**).

CHAPTER SUMMARY

Key Concepts

1. The major function of estrogen is development secondary sexual characters in women including the development of breast and reproductive structures. It causes proliferation of endometrium and follicular development in preovulatory phase of menstrual cycle. It protects from atherosclerosis and cardiovascular risks.
2. The major function of progesterone is relaxation of uterine smooth muscle and decreases excitability of the myometrium in early part of pregnancy. This favors implantation and prevents abortion. It causes uterine changes in the secretory phase of the cycle. It decreases BP.
3. Ovarian functions are controlled mainly by feedback regulation of hypothalamo-pituitary-gonadal axis driven by the circulating ovarian hormones.

Important to Know (Must Read)

1. In examination, 'Describe the physiological actions and regulation of secretion of estrogen and progesterone' may be asked as a **Long Question.**
2. Physiological actions of estrogen on female reproductive system, Secondary sexual characteristics in females, Physiological actions of progesterone, Hypothalamic control of ovarian function, Pituitary control of ovarian function, Ovarian control of ovarian function may be asked as **Short Questions** in exam.
3. In **Viva**, examiner may ask... Name the hormones secreted from ovary, What are the functions of estrogen, Name the secondary sexual characteristics in women, What are the physiological actions of estrogen on female reproductive system, on breast, on secondary sexual characteristics, on endocrine organs, on CNS on musculoskeletal system, on water and electrolyte metabolism, on lipid profile, Why is estrogen used in animal farms, Why does hyperestrogenemia occur in liver diseases, What are the estrogen preparations, List the functions of progesterone, What is the mechanism of action of estrogen and progesterone, What are the functions of relaxin, What is the function of inhibin released from ovary, What are the functions of androgens in women, List the functions of ovary, How does the hypothalamus control the ovarian function, What is the use of long-acting GnRH analogs, How does the pituitary control the ovarian function, How does the ovary regulate its own function, List the genetic and hormonal abnormalities in women, What is McCune-Albright syndrome, What is Kallmann's syndrome.

CHAPTER

71

Physiology of Copulation

LEARNING OBJECTIVES

On completion of study of this chapter, the student **MUST** be able to:

1. Understand the blood supply and innervation of the erectile tissues of the penis.
2. Learn the mechanism of erection of penis.
3. Understand the process of emission and ejaculation.
4. Describe the sexual responses in females.
5. Appreciate the mechanism of orgasm.
6. Define impotence and give its physiological basis.

The student **MAY** also be able to:

1. Describe the processes and mechanisms involved in male and female sexual act.

Copulation is the process of **mating** that occurs in human being by coitus, or the sexual act. Though the physiology of mating is similar in primates, the **sexual responses of male and female** are different in human being. It is important to understand the physiology of copulation to learn the pathophysiology of impotency, which is quite common in the present society.

MALE SEXUAL ACT

In sexual intercourse, male is the active partner. The major events of male sexual act include:

- Erection of penis,
- Penetration of penis into the vagina, and
- Ejaculation.

These are the **series of reflexes that are integrated in the spinal cord** and mediated via ***autonomic and somatic nerves***.

1. Male genital tract receives both **sympathetic and parasympathetic** innervation, and in addition, penis receives the **somatic innervation**.
2. Though the sexual act per se is *mainly a neural process*, its overall integration is a **behavioral phenomenon** that includes hormonal, biochemical and psychological interactions.

Erection

Blood supply: Penis is supplied by **internal pudendal arteries** that enter the organ as **dorsal artery of penis** from its dorsal surface. Dorsal artery penetrates deeply into the erectile tissues of penis as **deep artery** (Fig. 71.1). **Venous drainage** from penis occurs by ***dorsal vein***.

Mechanism

Erection occurs due to dilatation of **the penile arterioles filling the erectile tissues** of the penis by blood. The erectile tissues of penis are **three in numbers: two corpora cavernosa** and **a corpus spongiosum** (Fig. 71.2).

1. In normal state, penis is flaccid due to paucity of blood in the spaces of these erectile tissues.
2. **Upon arousal**, mainly the spaces in **cavernous erectile tissue fill with blood** and penis becomes **turgid** (Fig. 71.3).
3. Relaxation of the ***smooth muscles of corpora*** allows increased flow of blood into corporal interstices (cavernous spaces) that increases the volume and rigidity of the penis.
4. As **veins are compressed** by the erectile tissues filled with blood, engorgement of penis **inhibits venous return** and keeps the interstices filled with blood, which maintains erection.

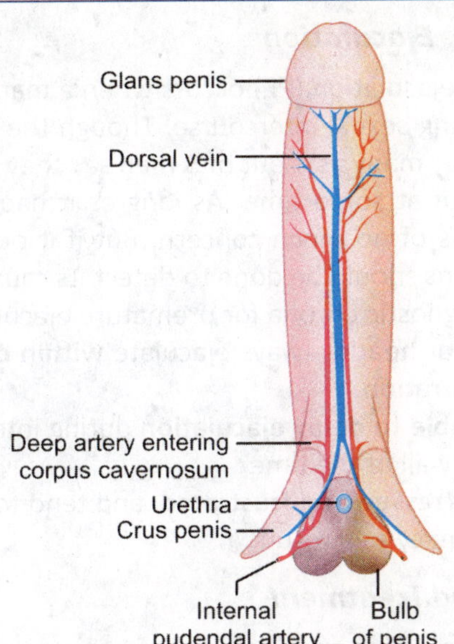

Fig. 71.1: Blood supply of penis. Blood supply to penis is from internal pudendal artery that enters penis from its dorsal surface as dorsal artery and penetrate deep into the organ as deep artery.

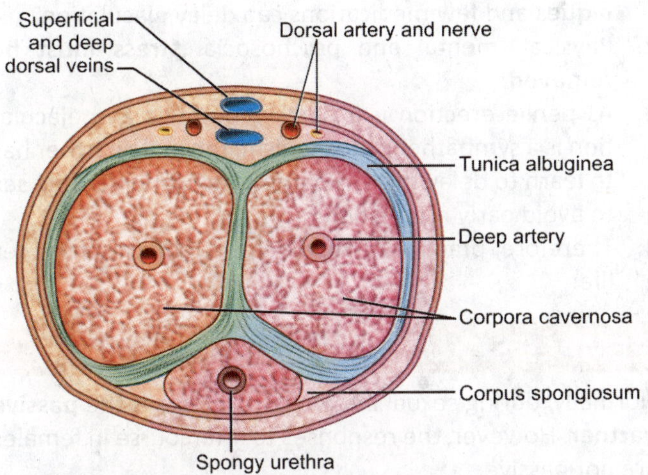

Fig. 71.3: Transverse section of penis. Note, the major erectile tissues are two corpora cavernosa (CC) that are separated by median septum and penetrated by deep artery (DeA) of penis at their center. Increased blood flow into the cavernous spaces (CS) in these erectile tissues makes the penis turgid. (DA: Dorsal artery, U: Urethra; CSp: Corpus spongiosum).
Courtesy: Figure 58.32, Clinical Anatomy, Vol. 2, 3rd edition, by Neeta Kulkarni, 2016; Jaypee Brothers Medical Publishers (P) Ltd.

Parasympathetic Control

Penile erection is mainly achieved by **parasympathetic activity** that relaxes smooth muscles of corpora, causes vasodilation and increases blood flow to the corporal interstices.

1. The effects are mediated via parasympathetic fibers in **nervi erigentes** (pelvic splanchnic nerves) that release acetylcholine, VIP and nitric oxide (NO) (Flowchart 71.1).
2. Nonadrenergic noncholinergic fibers are present nervi erigentes that are rich in NO. NO plays an important role in causing erection of the penis.

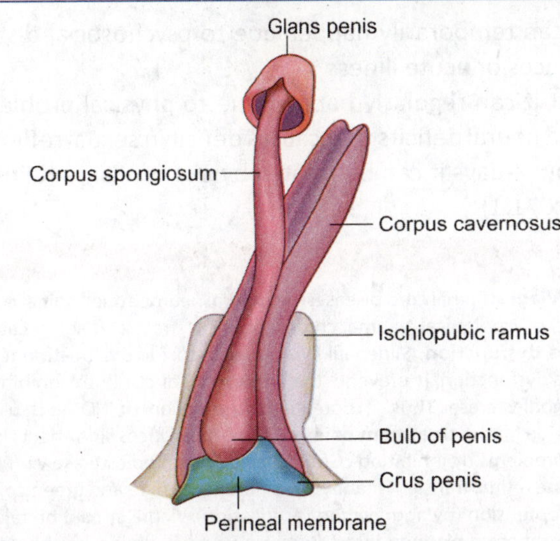

Fig. 71.2: Muscles of penis.
Courtesy: Figure 58.30, Clinical Anatomy, by Neeta Kulkarni, Vol. 2, 3rd edition, 2016; Jaypee Brothers Medical Publishers (P) Ltd.

Flowchart 71.1: Mechanism of penile erection.

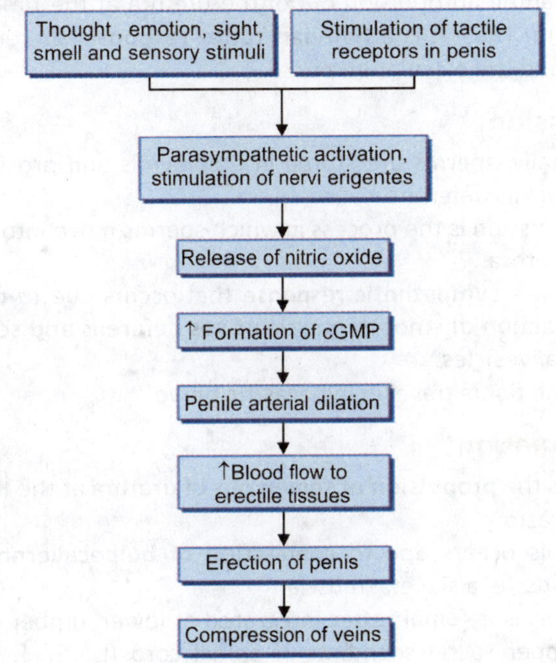

3. **NO activates guanylyl cyclase that increases the production of cGMP**, which is a potent vasodilator. The drugs that inhibit the breakdown of cGMP such as tadalafil, vardenafil and sildenafil are very useful in the treatment of erectile dysfunctions.

Impotency

Impotency is the erectile dysfunction in males. It is the inability to keep the penis adequately erected to be penetrated into the female genital tract.

1. **Erectile dysfunction** (ED) or impotence is sexual dysfunction characterized by the inability to develop or maintain an erection of the penis during sexual activity in humans.

2. It can temporarily happen due to psychosocial disturbances or acute illness.
3. But it can regularly happen due to physical problems and neural deficits that causes deficit in sexual reflexes.
4. Now-a-days it can be treated by use of Viagra (Clinical Box 71.1)

Clinical Box 71.1

Use of Viagra: Spinal cord diseases, peripheral neuropathies, spinal cord injuries, psychological trauma, chronic physical stress and aging cause **erectile dysfunction**. Sildenafil (Viagra) is used for the treatment of erectile dysfunction. It prevents the breakdown of cGMP by inhibiting phosphodiesterase. Thus, it potentiates the action of NO. It is used worldwide for the **treatment of impotence**. It produces side effects like visual problems by inhibiting cGMP specific phosphodiesterase V1 (PDE V1) in the retina, transient inability to differentiate blue and green color, and hypotension (by aggravating vasodilation). Viagra should be taken one hour before planned intercourse. However, it should not be used regularly for its known side effects.

Ejaculation

Ejaculation is the emission of semen from the male genital tract and its propulsion out of the urethra at the time of orgasm. Thus, it is a **two-part reflex response**: the emission and the ejaculation *per se*.

Emission

Normally, sperms are stored in epididymis and proximal part of vas deferens.

1. Emission is the process in which sperms move into the urethra.
2. It is a **sympathetic response** that occurs due to **contraction of smooth muscle of vas deferens and seminal vesicles**.
3. The fibers travel in hypogastric nerve.

Ejaculation

This is the **propulsion of semen out of urethra** at the time of orgasm.

1. This occurs due to **contraction of bulbocavernosus muscle**, a skeletal muscle.
2. This is a **spinal reflex** integrated at lower lumbar and upper sacral segments of spinal cord (L_5, $S_{1\text{-}3}$). The efferent fibers traverse in pudendal nerve.
3. It is proposed that the **carbon monoxide (CO) is the transmitter** in the neural circuit of ejaculation as evidenced from the fact that the ejaculatory performance is diminished when the gene responsible for the enzyme **HO_2 (heme oxygenase)** is knocked out. HO_2 normally catalyzes the formation of CO. Retrograde ejaculation occurs in diabetes (Application Box 71.1).

Application Box 71.1

Retrograde ejaculation: The internal urethral sphincter constricts at the time of emission. When this sphincter fails to constrict, the sperms instead of passing down the urethra enter the urinary bladder. The quantity of ejaculate decreases and sperms appear in urine (more than 15 sperms per high power field). Usually it occurs in diabetic neuropathy, multiple sclerosis and use of sympatholytic drugs.

Premature Ejaculation

Premature ejaculation (PE) occurs when a man ejaculates sooner during sexual intercourse. Though the prevalence of PE vary, as many as 1 out of 3 men say they experience this problem at some time. As long as it happens infrequently, it is of no much concern. But if it occurs often, investigations should be done to detect its cause.

The diagnostic criteria for premature ejaculation are:

1. Always or nearly always ejaculate **within one minute of penetration.**
2. Are **unable to delay ejaculation** during intercourse all or nearly all of the time.
3. Feel **distressed and frustrated**, and tend to avoid sexual intimacy as a result.

Causes and Treatment

Both **psychological and biological factors** can play a role in premature ejaculation. Although many men feel embarrassed to talk about it, premature ejaculation is a common and treatable condition.

1. **Regular counseling, learning the proper sexual techniques** and few medications can delay ejaculation.
2. Physical, mental and psychosocial **stress must be removed.**
3. As penile erection is a parasympathetic and ejaculation is a sympathetic mechanism, the male partner has to learn to delay the sympathetic activation during sex to avoid early ejaculation.
4. Therefore, practice of **Yoga** helps a lot to improve sex life.

FEMALE SEXUAL ACT

Normally, during sexual intercourse, female is the **passive partner**. However, the responses to intercourse in females are not passive.

1. The female responses are characterized by **marked increase in blood flow and muscular activities** in many parts of the body.
2. Increased sexual excitement is accompanied by **engorgement of the breasts** and **erection of the nipples, increased diameter and length of clitoris** due to increased blood flow into these structures.
3. Nipple and clitoris have rich sensory innervation. Therefore, clitorial and nipple stimulations during sexual act add to sexual excitement.
4. Blood flow also increases to vagina due to release of VIP from vaginal nerves and **increased fluid secretion from vagina** lubricates vaginal epithelium.
5. Mucous secretion is also increased from vestibular glands.

Sexual desire in women is possibly ***dependent on androgens***, because sex drive is maintained long after the menopause, when estrogen level in plasma is very low. Therefore, it is believed that androgens secreted by the adrenal glands maintain sexual appetite in females.

Vaginal Changes

Vaginal secretion increases during sexual excitation and intercourse.

1. This occurs mostly due to **release of VIP** from vaginal nerves.
2. **Vestibular glands** secrete mucus that also helps in lubrication.
3. The **stimuli** for vaginal secretion are tactile stimulation of clitoris, labia minora, breast and sexual excitement. Visual, olfactory and auditory stimuli aid to the excitement.
4. The sexual gratification in females culminates in **orgasm** that manifests as ***rhythmic vaginal contractions*** mediated by autonomic influences (Application Box 71.2).

> **Application Box 71.2**
>
> **Male orgasm should coincide with female orgasm:** For the best conjugal life and to derive maximal pleasure of sexual act, orgasms of male and female should appear concurrently during the sexual act. As female is the passive partner in the sexual act, orgasm in females comes usually later. Therefore, the male partner should learn to stimulate the female partner appropriately and adequately even before the initiation of intercourse so that orgasms in both arrive together. In males, orgasm occurs with ejaculation, following which the penis becomes flaccid. Unless female orgasm is attained along with the male orgasm, the female does not derive actual pleasure from the act, and repeated failure to attain orgasm in females is harmful both physically and mentally. Therefore, gradually the male should know the time of orgasm of his partner and should learn to maintain penile erection till then. Usually, after marriage it takes at least a year or more for both the partners to adjust to eachothers' physical and emotional needs to bring at once their orgasms. Thus, sexual act is more an art than science.

ORGASM

It is the climax of sexual excitement and pleasure that occurs with satisfactory intercourse. The natural sexual act culminates with orgasm.

Orgasm (climax) in female is associated with a **pleasurable feeling** accompanied by sudden increase in skeletal muscle activity, increased heart rate and blood pressure, and ***rhythmic contraction of the vaginal wall***. Though, **vaginal contraction** during orgasm facilitates sperm transport, it is **not essential for fertilization** since conception can occur in the absence of orgasm.

Orgasm results in following psychological, physical and reflex responses.

1. Increase in heart rate, may be up to 150 beats/min
2. Increase in systemic arterial BP
3. Rapid breathing
4. Flushing of face
5. Sweating
6. Increased skeletal muscle activity

All these changes are due to increased epinephrine secretion into the circulation. There may be associated stimulation of the anterior pituitary, adrenal cortex and the thyroid gland.

Fate of Sperms in Female Genital Tract

Normally 10^8 to 5×10^8 motile sperms are released into the female vagina on ejaculation. The sperms move at the rate of **1–3 mm/min** and only about **100 sperms reach the oviduct within 30 minutes**. Vaginal contraction during mating facilitates sperm movement.

1. The fluid medium in the uterus is favorable for sperms. **Uterine muscular movements** and ciliary activity may aid in migration of sperms within the uterus.
2. Some **spermatozoa can survive** in a viable state within the slightly alkaline medium of the cervical mucus for up to **48 hours**.
3. Finally, only one sperm fertilizes the ovum.
   - The initial process is called **capacitation** which makes the sperm (spermatozoon) able to adhere to the ovum.
   - It is followed by the **acrosomal reaction** in which one spermatozoon releases enough lytic enzymes locally to penetrate the cumulus cells and the zona pellucida that surrounds the ovum.
4. The remaining sperms disintegrate and liquefy in the female genital tract.

CHAPTER SUMMARY

Key Concepts

1. Penile erection is a parasympathetic and ejaculation is a sympathetic mechanism. Therefore, to one must learn to delay the sympathetic activation to avoid early ejaculation.
2. The orgasms of male and female partner should occur simultaneously in an effective sex.
3. Yoga is helpful for healthier sex life.

Important to Know (Must Read)

1. In examination, there will be no **Long Question** from this chapter.
2. Male sexual responses, Female sexual responses, and Orgasm, may be asked as **Short Questions** in exam.
3. In **Viva**, examiner may ask… Speak the mechanism of male sexual responses, Mechanism of erection, emission, ejaculation, What is the role of NO, What is nerve erigentis, What is the role of parasympathetic and sympathetic nerves in male sexual act, Mechanism of male sexual responses, Mechanism of female sexual responses, Definition and mechanism of orgasm, Definition and causes of impotency, Definition and causes of premature ejaculation, Mechanism of action of Viagra, Fate of sperm in female genital tract.

CHAPTER 72

Pregnancy and Parturition

Learning Objectives

On completion of study of this chapter, the student **MUST** be able to:

1. Understand the importance of learning the physiology of pregnancy.
2. Understand the physiology at different steps of pregnancy starting from fertilization to fetal maturation.
3. List the placental hormones and mention their functions.
4. List the causes of female infertility.
5. Understand the concept, indication and steps of in-vitro fertilization.
6. Describe various systemic maternal changes in pregnancy.
7. Understand the mechanism of parturition.

The student **MAY** also be able to:

1. Describe the physiology of fertilization and fetal development.
2. Explain the feto-maternal changes in pregnancy.
3. Describe the physiological changes in different stages of labor.

Pregnancy is the most precious event in the life of a married woman as it proves her fertile capability, and brings completeness to her womanhood. Pregnancy occurs when a **mature oocyte is fertilized by a sperm**. The introduction of sperm into the female genital tract should ideally occur in the period of two days before and one day after ovulation. This is because the sperms following their ejaculation into the vagina remain capable of fertilizing **an egg usually for 24 to 48 hours** (though they may survive for 3 to 5 days in the female genital tract) and the fertilizable life of the ovulated egg is about 24 hours. Thus, if ovulation occurs on 14th day of the cycle, for conception to occur the coitus should take place on 12th, 13th, 14th, and 15th days (the ***fertile period***) of the menstrual cycle).

PHYSIOLOGY OF PREGNANCY

Transport of Gametes

Transport of Egg

Following ovulation, the oocyte is extruded onto the surface of the ovary or into the abdominal cavity. The fimbriae located at the end of the fallopian tube **actively pick up** the oocyte.

1. The fimbriae contain smooth muscle and are lined with ciliated epithelium. Immediately after ovulation, **smooth muscle of the fimbriae contract**, which make the fimbrial end of the tube migrate close to the oocyte. The cilia of fimbriae beat in waves toward the interior of the duct.
2. These **ciliary motions** sweep the egg into the fallopian tube as the egg emerges from follicle to the ovarian surface. Inside the fallopian tube, egg movement is driven by fallopian-tube cilia, which is a normally a slow process.
3. Therefore, the egg takes **about four days to reach the uterus**. Hence, for fertilization to occur, it must naturally happen **in the distal portion of fallopian tube** (within a day of ovulation) because of the short viability of the unfertilized egg (Fig. 72.1).

Transport of Sperm

During the act of intercourse, some sperms are propelled from the vagina to the cervix, and **many enter cervical canal after the sexual act**. Though usual **transit time** of sperm to reach fallopian tube is 4–6 hours, within few minutes of ejaculation, sperms have been detected in the

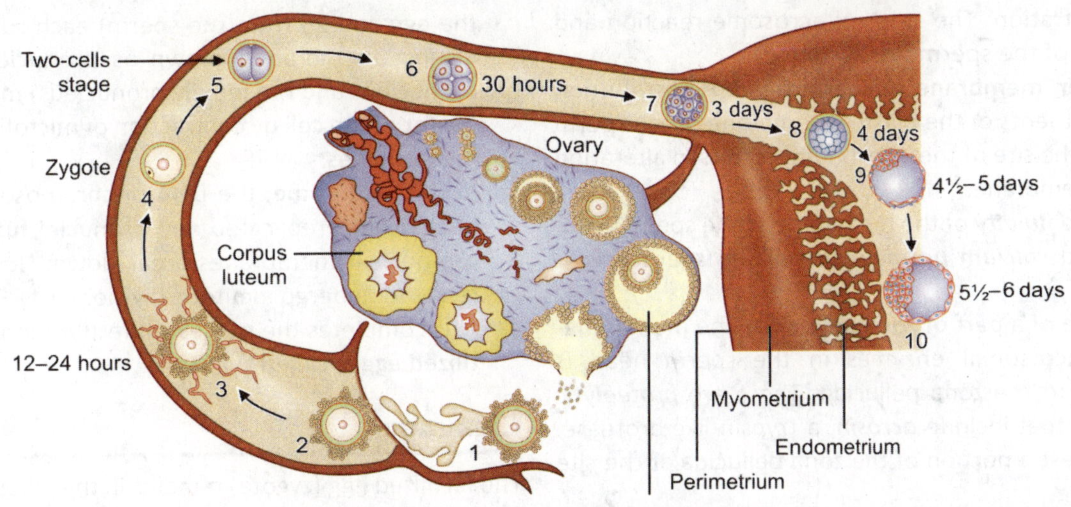

Fig. 72.1: Events in fertilization and implantation of fertilized egg. 1: Ovulation; 2: Tube picking up the oocyte; 3: Fertilization with extrusion of 2nd polar body; 4: Zygote formation; 5: Two-cell stage; 6: Four-cell stage; 7: Early morula (Day 17); 8: Late morula (Day 18); 9: Early blastocyst stage; 10: Early implantation.

uterus and tubes. However, many *sperms die in the vagina due its acidic environment* (vaginal pH is 5.5–6).

Transport of Sperm in the Cervix

Passage of sperms through cervix is favored by:

1. **Nature of cervical mucous:** Sperm transport is **favored by estrogen-induced changes** in consistency and orientation of the mucous. Estrogen makes the mucous **thin and elastic**.
2. **Orientation of the mucous:** Also, under the influence of estrogen, **cervical mucous is oriented in parallel** that favors the transport of sperm. Thus, sperms can easily swim through estrogen-dependent cervical mucous.

Transport of Sperm in the Uterus

Transport of the sperm through the entire length of the uterus and then into the fallopian tubes occurs due to sperm's own motility and uterine contractions.

Transport of Sperm in the Fallopian Tube

In the fallopian tube, sperm motility is facilitated by three factors:

1. Ciliary movement in the tube
2. Peristaltic activity of the tube
3. Flow of fluid in the tube.

Though several millions of sperms are deposited in the vagina, only about 50–100 reach the fallopian tube. This is the major reasons that **there must be many millions of motile sperms** in the seminal fluid for fertilization to occur. Thus, decreased count and motility of sperms lead to infertility in males.

Changes in Sperm in Female Genital Tract

Sperms undergo changes in the female genital tract that make them able to fertilize the egg. These changes are collectively called **capacitation**, which occurs after sperms spend one to several hours in female genital tract. Capacitation includes **two major changes** in sperms:

1. The wavelike beating of the tail of the sperms is replaced by **whip-like movements** that propel the sperm forward in strong lurches.
2. **Alteration in the plasma membrane** (modification of surface proteins) of sperms that makes them capable of fusing with the surface of the egg.

Freshly ejaculated sperm cannot immediately penetrate the ovum; only a capacitated sperm is capable of doing so.

Fertilization

Fertilization is the process of union of sperm with egg that **results in zygote formation**. Normally, fertilization occurs in the **ampullary portion of the fallopian tube**. Fertilization takes place in **four steps**: Fusion of sperm with egg, acrosome reaction and sperm penetration, polyspermy block, and formation of zygote.

Fusion of Sperm with Egg

It begins with the fusion of a sperm and egg. Many sperms move between the cumulus cells (granulosa cells still surrounding the egg) to bind to the *zona pellucida* of the egg.

1. The **zona pellucida contains glycoproteins** that serve as receptors for sperm surface proteins.
2. The sperm contains many such proteins and therefore **bind simultaneously to many receptors** on the zona pellucida.

Acrosome Reaction

The binding sperm to the zona pellucida triggers *acrosome reaction* in the bound sperm, which is required for sperm penetration: The steps of acrosome reaction and penetration of the sperm are as follows:

1. **Change in membrane of sperm head:** Redistribution of constituents of the plasma membrane of the sperm head at the site of the attachment results in alteration in the membrane.
2. ***Increased fluidity*** of the membrane of the sperm head.
3. Increased ***calcium permeability*** of the sperm membrane.
4. **Digestion of a part of zona pellucida:** The membrane-bound acrosomal enzymes in the sperm head is exposed to the zona pellucida. These are *proteolytic enzymes* that include ***acrosin***, a trypsin-like protease. They digest a portion of the zona pellucida at the site of binding.
5. **Penetration of sperm through perivitalline space:** As the zona pellucida gives way, sperm advances through this coating using its propulsive force of the tail. Then, sperm penetrates the ***perivitalline space*** (the space surrounding the egg membrane) to reach the egg's plasma membrane.
6. **Fusion of sperm head with egg membrane:** The sperm head fuses with the egg's membrane, which is facilitated by sperm surface protein, called ***fertilin***. Then, sperm slowly enters the egg's cytoplasm (ooplasm).

Polyspermy Block

Only one sperm penetrates the egg. This is because, as soon as the sperm penetration starts, immediately **a series of changes** occur in the egg that prevent the entry of additional sperms. This is called *polyspermy block*. There are **two mechanisms** of polyspermy block:

1. The initial fusion of the sperm with egg plasma membranes triggers a reaction that **changes the membrane potential** of the egg. The change in egg membrane potential prevents additional sperm binding.
2. The secretory vesicles that are located in the peripheral part of the egg cytoplasm release their contents into perivitalline space (the narrow space between the egg plasma membrane and the zona pellucida) by exocytosis. These vesicular content contains enzymes that enter the zona pellucida and cause **inactivation of sperm-binding sites** on zona pellucida and **hardening of the entire zona pellucida**. Thus, binding of additional sperms to the zona pellucida is prevented.

Zygote Formation

The sperm penetration of egg is called fertilization. The fertilized egg **completes its second meiotic division in next few hours**.

1. As a result of the second meiotic division, the second polar body is formed, which is extruded from ooplasm.
2. The remaining haploid nucleus containing 23 chromosomes is transformed into **female pronucleus** in two to three hours. The two sets of chromosomes (23 from the egg and 23 from the sperm) each surrounded by distinct membranes known as **pronuclei** (the male pronucleus and the female pronucleus) **migrate to the center** of the cell by contraction of microfilaments and microtubules.
3. In the mean-time, the DNA of chromosomes in both pro-nuclei is replicated and **pronuclei fuse**. Then the pro-nuclear membranes break down. Now, the cell is ready to undergo a mitotic division.
4. This completes the process of fertilization and the **fertilized egg is called zygote**.

Cleavage

The fertilized egg (zygote) remains in the fallopian tube for three to four days. While in the fallopian tube, a **number of mitotic cell divisions** take place. This process of mitotic cell divisions is known as **cleavage**. The cell divisions are unusual in that no cell growth takes place before each division. Therefore, the 16 to 32 cell conceptus that enters the uterus is essentially the same size as that of original fertilized egg.

The first cell division takes place in 24 hours to produce two unequal sized cells, the structure called **blastomere**. Then each cell divides to form a four cell conceptus, eight cell conceptus and **morula** (16 to 32 cell conceptus) in 48, 72, and 96 hours, respectively. Twin is formed if dividing cells grow into two independent cell masses (Application Box 72. 1).

Application Box 72.1

Development of twins: Each of the cells of blastomere is a totipotent cell. They have the capacity to develop into an entire individual. Therefore, **identical (monozygotic) twins** result when, at the time of cleavage, the dividing cells are completely separated into two independently growing cell masses. And, fraternal or **dizygotic twins** result when, two eggs being ovulated and fertilized simultaneously.

After fertilization, the conceptus slowly moves from the ampulla of the fallopian tube into the uterus (Fig. 56.1). Till the morula stage, the conceptus is in the fallopian tube. Until implantation in the uterus, the conceptus is enclosed in the zona pellucida. The **intact zona pellucida has three functions**:

1. It prevents the adhesion of the conceptus to the inner wall of the fallopian tube.
2. It protects the conceptus from mechanical damage while being transported from ampulla of the tube into the uterus.
3. It also prevents the early immunological rejection of the conceptus.

Blastocyst Formation and Implantation

The morula enters uterus about four days of fertilization. After reaching the uterus, the conceptus floats free in the intrauterine fluid for approximately three days, during

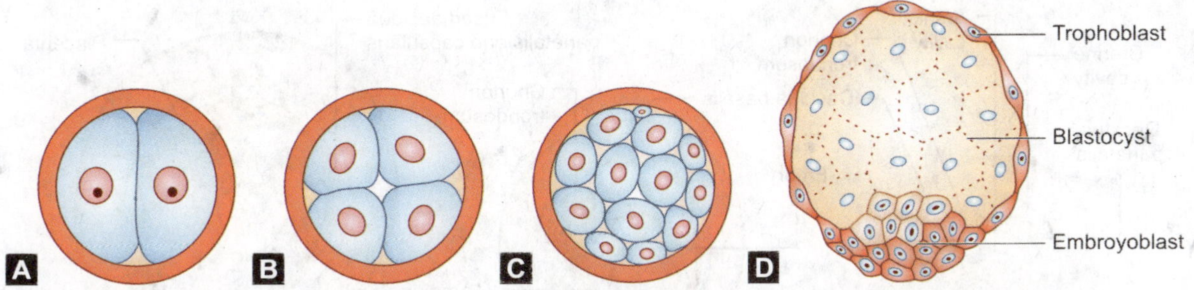

Figs. 72.2A to D: Stages in formation of blastocyst. (A) Two-cell stage; (B) Four-cell stage; (C) Morula; (D) Blastocyst stage.

which it further undergoes cell divisions. Now, the conceptus is known as a **blastocyst**, the stage which the cells have lost their totipotentiality and have begun to differentiate. Blastocyst derives nourishment from the uterine fluid. The blastocyst consists of **three components** (Figs. 72.2A to D):

1. **Trophoblast:** An outer layer of cells of blastocyst is called **trophoblast**. The trophoblast consists of extraembryonic ectodermal cells present on embryonic membrane. It helps in implantation of the conceptus and contributes to placenta formation. Trophoblast and its membrane secrete human chorionic gonadotropin (hCG).
2. **Embryoblast:** An inner cell mass called **embryoblast** that gives rise to fetus.
3. **Balstocele:** A central fluid-filled cavity of blastocyst is called **blastocele**. It forms amniotic cavity.

In subsequent development, the inner cell mass gives rise to the fetus. The trophoblast surrounds the embryo or fetus throughout its development and is involved in its nutrition as well as in the secretion of several important hormones.

Implantation and Early Development

Implantation is the **attachment of the blastocyst to the endometrial surface** of the uterine wall.

1. It occurs about 7–8 days after fertilization. Implantation occurs in estrogen and progesterone primed uterus.
2. By the time the zygote develops into the blastocyst, the menstrual cycle reaches about day 21 of the normal menstrual cycle or 7th post-ovulatory day, during which the **endometrium is being prepared by progesterone** secreted from corpus luteum.
3. During this period, embedding of the blastocyst into the endometrium (implantation) begins. Progesterone prepares the endometrium for implantation of blastocyst.
4. The **trophoblast cells are very sticky**, especially at the **region that overlie the inner cell mass** and this part of blastocyst adheres to the uterine wall for implantation. Implantation outside uterus leads to ectopic pregnancy (Clinical Box 72.1).

Mechanism of Implantation

Implantation occurs due to almost simultaneous changes in blastocyst that is to be implanted and the endometrium

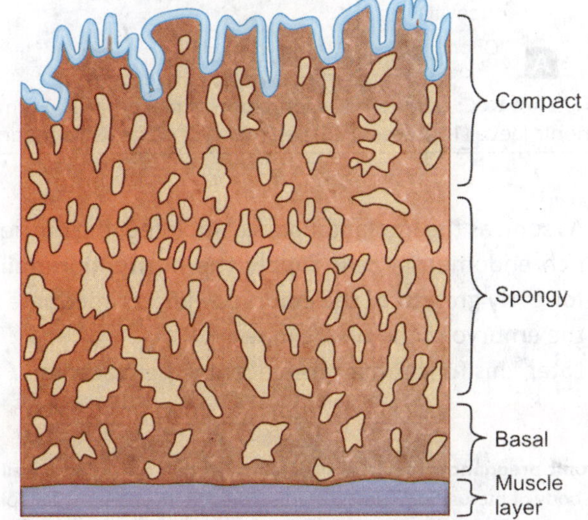

Fig. 72.3: Structure of decidua.

that allows implantation to occur, and interaction of blastocyst with the endometrium.

Changes in Blastocyst

Enlargement of blastocyst (before implantation) results in **rupture of zona pellucida**. The trophoblast cells are denuded and become **negatively charged**. This facilitates the **blastocyst attachment** to endometrium via surface glycoprotein. The initial contact between blastocyst and endometrium induces **rapid proliferation of the trophoblast**.

Interaction of Blastocyst with Endometrium

The proteolytic enzymes secreted by the trophoblast allow the **blastocyst to bury in the endometrium**. Microvilli of trophoblast cells interdigitate with endometrial cells and **form junctional complexes**.

Changes in Endometrium

At the site of contact, endometrium also undergoes changes. By the influence of progesterone, endometrium undergoes **decidualization**. In this process, the endometrial cells are hypertrophied and their glycogen and lipid content increase. The endometrium at the site of implantation is called **decidua** (Fig. 72.3).

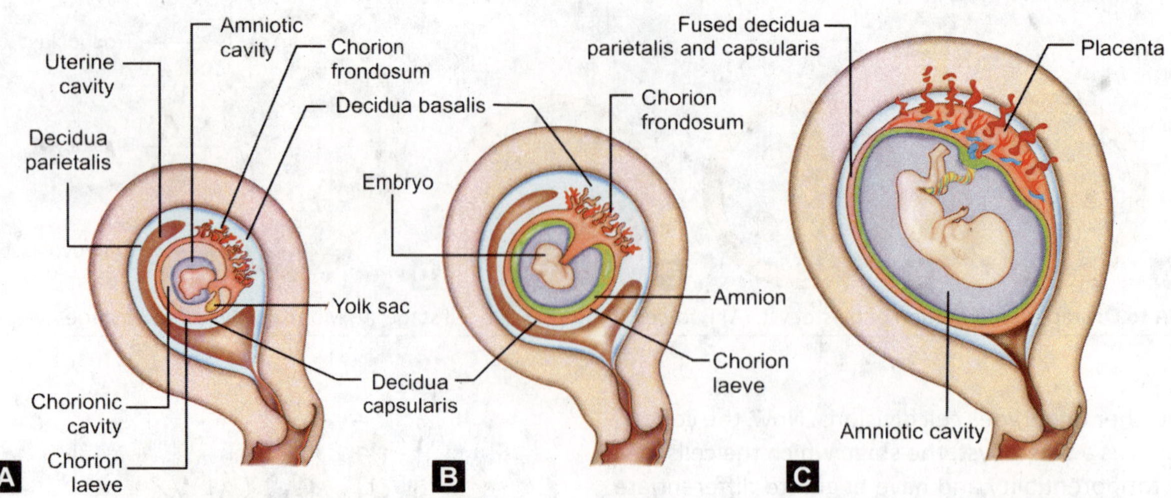

Figs. 72.4A to C: Stages in the formation of placenta. (A) Formation of amniotic cavity (end of 8th week); (B) Formation of amnion and chorionic laeve (10th week); (C) Beginning of placenta formation (12th week).

1. As soon as the implantation is completed, the nutrient-rich endometrial cells **supply the nutrients required for early growth of the embryo**, which is adequate for the embryo in the first few weeks.
2. Later, this function is taken over by the placenta.

Clinical Box 72.1

Ectopic pregnancy: The usual site of implantation is the dorsal wall in the body of uterus. Sometimes, a fertilized egg remains in the fallopian tube and gets implanted in the wall of the tube. This is called **tubal ectopic pregnancy**. Rarely, a fertilized egg may go backward from the fallopian tube into the abdominal cavity, where implantation may occur. Very rarely, fertilization may take place in the abdominal cavity. In both the cases, **abdominal ectopic pregnancy** occurs. Ectopic pregnancies usually do not continue for long as there is **no uterine support** for the developing embryo. However, early surgery should be performed to terminate ectopic pregnancy as there is risk of rupture and maternal hemorrhage.

Placentation and Amnion Formation

Placenta Formation

Implantation is completed in about 10–12 days after ovulation. The trophoblast cells become **cytotrophoblasts** (large polyhedral cells) that are surrounded by **syncytiotrobhobalsts** (cells with no boundaries). The blood vessels in the endometrium dilate and form lacunae. **Chorionic villi**, the functional units of placenta begins to form at about 12th day from fertilization (Figs. 72.4A to C).

Placenta is the combination of interdigitating fetal and maternal tissues that serves as the organ of exchange between mother and fetus during pregnancy. The **fetal part of the placenta** is formed by the outermost layers of trophoblast cells, **the chorion**, and the **maternal part** is formed by the endometrium underlying the chorion.

Chorionic villi (fingerlike projections) originate from trophoblast cells and extend from the chorion into the endometrium. The chorionic villi contain a rich network of capillaries. Each villus is surrounded by a pool of maternal blood called **placental sinus**, supplied by maternal arterioles.

Arrangement of Placental Circulation

The maternal blood flows into placental sinuses via the uterine artery and come out via the uterine veins. Simultaneously, blood flows from the fetus into the capillaries of the chorionic villi via the umbilical arteries and come out of the villi back to the fetus via the umbilical vein. All these umbilical vessels are contained in the umbilical cord, a long, rope-like structure that connects the fetus to the placenta.

Formation of Amnion

Once placenta is well formed, the **fetal heart begins to pump blood at about 5th week of gestation**. A layer of epithelial cells in the villi and a layer of endothelial cells in the fetal capillaries separate the maternal and fetal blood. Exchange of materials between maternal and fetal blood occurs between these layers. A space is formed between the inner cell mass and the chorion, called the **amniotic cavity** (Fig. 72.5A).

1. The cavity enlarges and is slowly lined by epithelial cells layer derived from the inner cell mass called the **amnion**, or **amniotic sac**.
2. Amnion finally fuses with the chorion to form a single combined membrane that surrounds the fetus (Fig. 72.5B). The fluid in the amniotic cavity is the **amniotic fluid** (Clinical Box 72.2) that buffers mechanical stress and temperature variations. The fetus floats in the amniotic cavity. Fetus is attached to the placenta by the umbilical cord. Eventually, it is only the amniotic sac that separates the fetus from the uterine lumen.

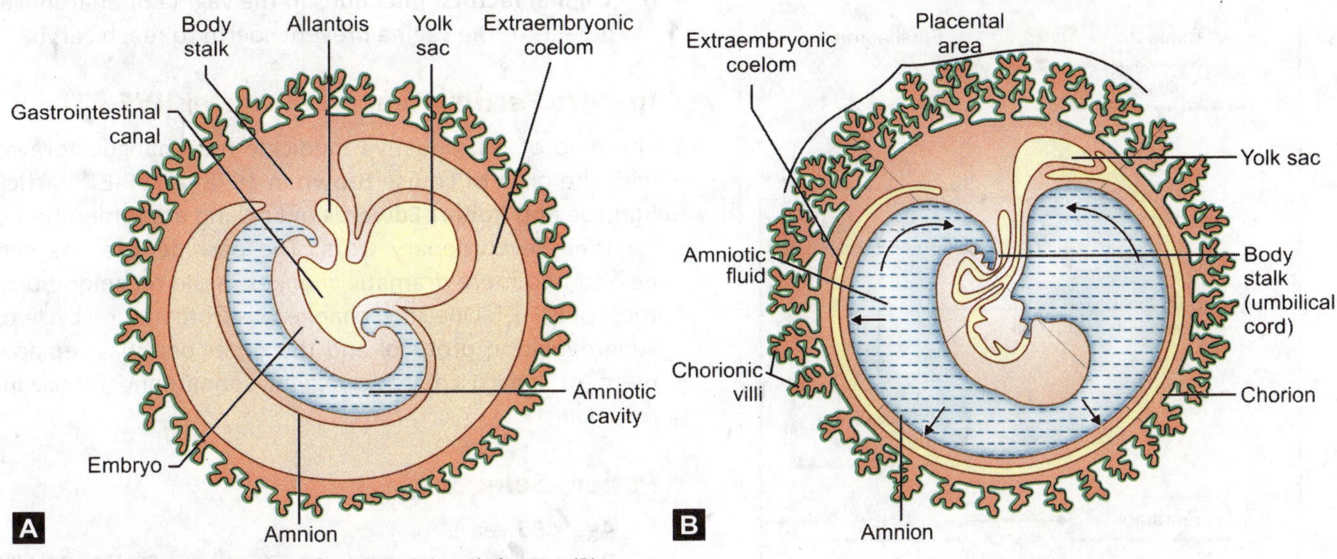

Figs. 72.5A and B: Formation of amnion (A) and chorion (B).

> **Clinical Box 72.2**
>
> **Amniocentesis:** Aspiration of fluid from the amniotic sac is called amniocentesis. Amniocentesis can be done as early as the 16th week of pregnancy by inserting a needle into the amniotic cavity. Few genetic diseases can be diagnosed by the demonstrating certain chemicals in the amniotic fluid or in sloughed fetal cells in the fluid. The chromosomes of these fetal cells can also be examined for diagnosis of certain disorders and determination of fetal sex. However, amniocentesis for diagnosis of fetal sex has been banned in India.

Techniques for Fetal Sex Diagnosis

In addition to amniocentesis, there are two other techniques of fetal diagnosis: chorionic villus sampling, and ultrasound.

Chorionic villus sampling: It involves obtaining tissue from chorionic villi of the placenta. The advantage is that it can be performed **as early as 10th weeks of pregnancy**. However, it carries higher risks including miscarriage.

Ultrasound: Ultrasound, especially with the help of 4D (four-dimensional) machine, that provides details of the picture of the fetus from all angles, fetal sex can be diagnosed as early 12th week.

Organogenesis and Fetal Nutrition

Once placenta is formed, fetus derives nutrition directly from the mother's blood. Therefore, **maternal nutrition is crucial** for the fetal development. Malnutrition in mother causes fetal growth retardation.

1. Organogenesis starts as early as 5th to 8th weeks of pregnancy. Therefore, deficiency of specific nutrients from first-trimester onwards results in specific fetal organ deficiency. For example, deficiency of folic acid leads to fetal neural defects.
2. The developing fetus is also subjected to influences by many **non-nutritional factors** like noise, radiation, chemicals and infections to which the mother is exposed. Especially, drugs (like aspirin etc.), alcohol and cigarette smoke consumed by the mother can cause birth defects in the fetus. These chemicals are known **teratogens**.

Fetus as a Graft

Half of the fetal genes that are from the father differ from the genes that originate from the mother. Therefore, fetus and mother are **two genetically different individuals**. Hence, the fetus is in essence a graft (foreign transplant) in the mother. However, the fetal graft is not rejected by the mother, due to three mechanisms:

1. Trophoblast of placenta that separates mother and fetal tissues expresses **HLA-G**, a nonpolymorphic gene, instead of expressing HLA-I and II, the polymorphic genes. As antibodies are formed only against polymorphic genes, they do not develop against fetal tissues.
2. T cells that are activated against fetal proteins are destroyed (**undergo apoptosis**) by Fas, a placental surface ligand.
3. Placenta that forms barrier between fetal and maternal blood protects fetus from immunological insults by the mother, by **preventing transfer of immunological materials**.

Fetoplacental Unit

For steroidogenesis, fetus and placenta interact closely. This is called fetoplacental unit. Placenta forms pregnenolone from cholesterol, which in turn forms progesterone.

1. **Placental pregnenolone** enters fetal circulation and become substrate for synthesis of **dehydroepiandrosterone** (DHEA) and **16-hydroxydehydroepiandrosterone** (16-OHDHEA) in fetal adrenal.

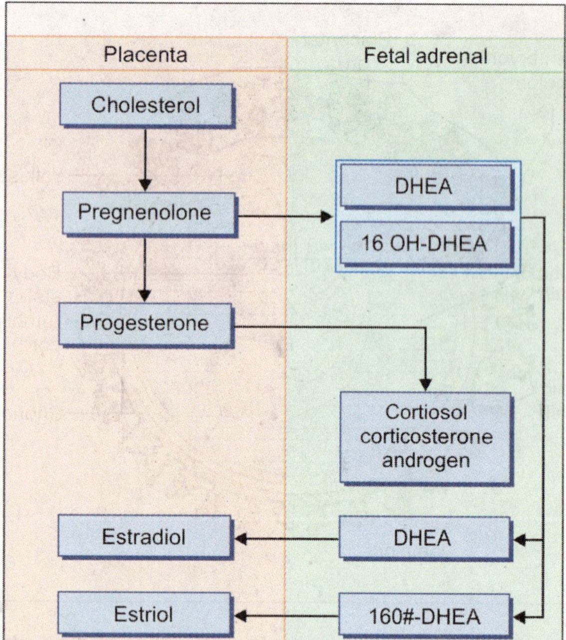

Fig. 72.6: Interaction between placenta and fetal adrenal gland for steroidogenesis.

2. Formation of 16-OHDHEA also occurs in the fetal liver. DHEA and 16-OHDHEA formed in fetus are taken back into the placenta, where DHEA forms estradiol and 16-OHDHEA forms estriol.
3. **The placental progesterone** also enters fetal adrenal and forms cortisol, corticosterone and androgen in adrenal cortex of fetus (Fig. 72.6).

Clinical Significance

The major estrogen formed by placenta is estriol for which the substrate is fetal adrenal 16-OHDHEA. Therefore, **excretion of estriol in maternal urine is a good index of health of the fetus.**

Female Infertility

Infertility is defined as the inability of a couple to achieve conception after one year of unprotected sexual intercourse. In females, infertility may be due to following causes;

1. **Ovarian factors:** Anovulation (absence of release of ovum from the ovary) causes infertility. For details of anovulation, refer previous chapter.
2. **Peritoneal factor:** Pelvic adhesion or pelvic peritonitis prevents fallopian tube to pick up the ovum from pelvic cavity.
3. **Tubal factors:** Partial or complete bilateral tubal obstruction resulting from infective or noninfective salpingitis prevents fertilization to occur.
4. **Uterine factors:** Endometritis, intrauterine adhesions, or anatomical defects can prevent implantation of the fertilized ovum.
5. **Cervical factors:** Thick cervical mucus or presence of sperm antibodies in the mucus makes the sperm impenetrable.
6. **Vaginal factors:** Infections in the vagina or anatomical defects in the vagina prevent sperm to reach cervix.

In-Vitro Fertilization and Transfer (IVF-ET)

The field of reproductive medicine has changed forever with the birth of **Louise Brown** in 1978 by IVF-ET. **Patrick Steptoe and Robert Edwards** of England are remembered for their revolutionary work. The past decade has witnessed two more dramatic changes in the technique protocol of IVF-ET. One such change was from natural cycle to superovulation protocol and the other one was replacement of laparoscopy by vaginal sonography for ovum retrieval.

Patient Selection

- Age < 35 years
- Presence of ovarian reserve (D-3, seum FSH < 10 IU/L)
- Husband-normal seminogram
- Couple must be screened negative for HIV and hepatitis
- Normal uterine cavity as evaluated by hysteroscopy/sonohysterography.

Principal steps of an ART cycle

- Down regulation using GnRH agonist
- Controlled ovarian stimulation
- Monitoring of follicle growth
- Oocyte retrieval
- Fertilization in vitro
- Transfer of gametes of embryos
- Luteal support with progesterone.

Oocyte Retrieval

Oocyte retrieval is done aseptically through **vaginal route** under ultrasound guidance.

1. With the development of vaginal transducers, **vaginal needle aspiration** is done about **36 hours after hCG administration** but before ovulation occurs. Intravenous analgesia and sedation (propofol) is adequate in most of the cases.
2. The oocyte is easily recognizable as a single cell surrounded by a mass cumulus cell. After recovery, the oocytes are maintained in culture in vitro for 4–6 hours.

Fertilization in Vitro

The sperm used for insemination in vitro is prepared by the wash and swim up or density gradient centrifugation (preferred) technique.

1. Approximately 50,000 to 100,000 capacitated sperm are placed in the culture media containing the oocyte within 4–6 hours of retrieval. The eggs may demonstrate signs of fertilization when examined 16–18 hours after insemination (presence of two pronuclei in the presence of a second polar body).

Table 72.1: Hormones secreted from placenta.

A. Steroid hormones
1. Estriol
2. 17-β estradiol
3. Estrone
4. Progesterone
B. Protein hormones
1. hCG
2. hCS
3. Relaxin
4. Prolactin
5. CRH
6. GnRH
7. β-endorphin
8. α-MSH
9. Dynorphin-A
10. Insulin like growth factors
11. ACTH

2. Sperm density and motility are two most important criteria for successful IVF. The semen is collected just prior to ovum retrieval.

Embryo Transfer

The fertilized ova at the 6–8 blastomere stage are placed into the uterine cavity close to the fundus about 3 days after fertilization through a fine flexible soft catheter transcervically. Not more than three embryo are transferred per cycle to minimize multiple pregnancy.

PLACENTAL HORMONES

Placenta is an endocrine organ as it secretes many hormones (Table 72.1). When fertilization takes place, corpus luteum fails to regress. Corpus luteum secretes hormones that support pregnancy in its early part. Once placenta is fully formed and starts secreting hormones (usually after sixth weeks of pregnancy), functions of corpus luteum slowly decline. Corpus luteum remains vestigial after eighth week. Therefore, **ovariectomy after eighth week** of pregnancy does not result in abortion.

hCG

The **human chorionic gonadotropin** (hCG) is the gonadotropin secreted from syncytiotrophoblast of placenta. The **syncytiotrophoblast cells** start producing hCG between 6–8 days after fertilization.

Structure

It is a **glycoprotein hormone** containing galactose and hexosamine. It is made up of **two subunits**: α and β. The α **subunit** contains 92 amino acids and has molecular weight

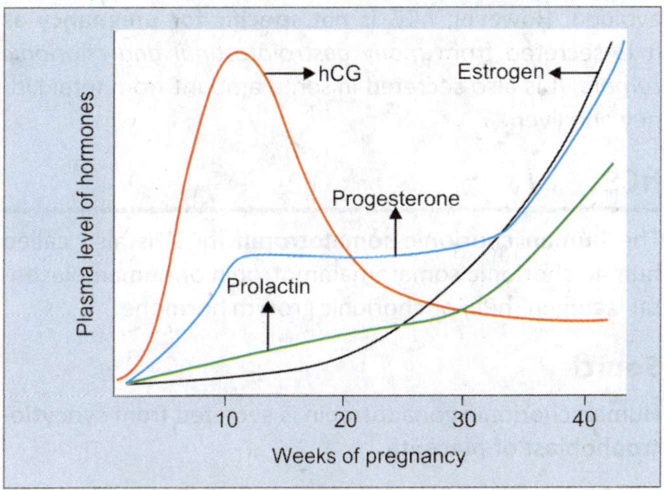

Fig. 72.7: Level of various hormones in maternal plasma throughout pregnancy.

18,000 whereas as the β **subunit** contains 145 amino acids and has molecular weight 28,000. The α subunit of hCG is similar to the α subunit of LH, FSH and TSH.

Secretion

Human chorionic gonadotropin secretion is more in the early pregnancy. It appears in maternal plasma as early as **sixth day after fertilization.** Its concentration increases rapidly to reach a **peak in about 10–12 weeks** of gestation, when the concentration is about 5 mg/mL. Then, the concentration decreases to 75% at about 25th weeks and remains at that level till term (Fig. 72.7). Associated with the decline of hCG secretion, the *placenta begins to secrete estrogen and progesterone in large amount*.

Functions

Human chorionic gonadotropin binds to **LH receptors in corpus luteum.** Therefore, it has mainly luteinizing and luteotropic activities. It has very less FSH activity.

1. It **stimulates progesterone production** from corpus luteum.
2. hCG plays a critical role in **placental steroidogenesis**.
3. hCG also helps in **sexual differentiation** in male fetus.
4. hCG **stimulates vomiting centers** in the brain. Therefore, morning sickness (sense of nausea and vomiting in the morning) is an early feature of pregnancy. Morning sickness is common in the first pregnancy, and usually disappears after first trimester.

Clinical Significance

Human chorionic gonadotropin is detected in plasma as early as 6 days after conception. Therefore, demonstrating hCG in plasma by RIA is a **pregnancy diagnostic test.** hCG appears **in urine from 14th day** of conception onwards. Detection of hCG in urine is easier, as blood collection is avoided. However, hCG is **not specific for pregnancy** as it is secreted from *many gastrointestinal and chorionic tumors*. It is also secreted in some amount from fetal kidney and liver.

hCS

The **human chorionic somatotropin** (hCS) is also called human chorionic somatomammotropin or human placental lactogen (hPL) or chorionic growth hormone.

Source

Human chorionic gonadotropin is secreted from **syncytiotrophoblast of placenta**.

Structure and Secretion

Structurally, it is **similar to human growth hormone**. hCS, GH and prolactin are formed from common precursor hormone. It contains 191 amino acids and has molecular weight 22,000. Secretion of hCS starts from **third week of pregnancy** and slowly rises till term. The peak concentration in plasma is achieved at term when it is about 15 mg/ml.

Functions

Human chorionic gonadotropin has functions similar to growth hormone and prolactin.

1. It promotes growth of mammary gland and **stimulates production of milk**. Therefore, it is also called **human placental lactogen**. However, hCS is less potent in milk production than prolactin secreted from anterior pituitary.
2. It **stimulates somatic growth of the fetus**. Therefore, it is also called growth hormone of pregnancy.
3. It causes **maternal lipolysis** and releases FFA from fat tissues.
4. It **decreases glucose utilization** in mother. It induces maternal insulin resistance and glucose intolerance.
5. It alters fuel availability for the fetus by antagonizing maternal glucose consumption and enhancing fat mobilization. This ensures **adequate supply of fuel for the fetus.**

Clinical Significance

The quantity of hCS secreted is proportional to size of the placenta. Therefore, a **low hCS level in third trimester indicates placental insufficiency**.

Other Hormones

1. **Relaxin** secreted from placenta causes ***uterine relaxation*** in the early part of pregnancy like progesterone to facilitate implantation and prevent expulsion of fetus. Its concentration in plasma is highest (1 ng/mL) in first trimester of pregnancy. Toward term, it causes relaxation of pubic symphysis and pelvic ligaments to facilitate delivery of fetus.

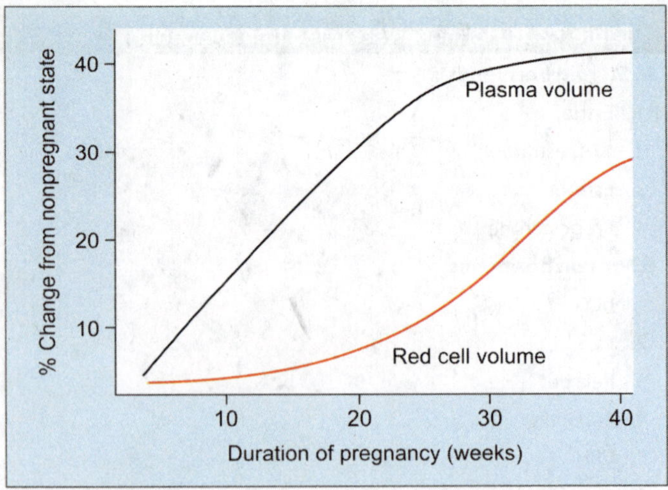

Fig. 72.8: Changes in plasma volume and red cell volume in pregnancy. Note, plasma volume increases early and attains about 40% increase, whereas, red cell volume increases gradually attains about 30% increase.

2. **Progesterone** causes myometrial quiescence and promotes continuation of pregnancy (*see* Fig. 72.7).
3. **Estrogen** secretion increases slowly in third trimester and reaches peak at term. The major estrogen secreted in pregnancy is **estriol**, which normally secreted in very less amount from the ovary of a nonpregnant woman. Estrogen facilitates parturition (discussed below).

MATERNAL CHANGES DURING PREGNANCY

Pregnancy is a state of altered physiology. Remarkable physiological changes occur in maternal systems during pregnancy. These changes are primarily meant to supply adequate oxygen and nutrients to fetus for its growth and development, and remove CO_2 and waste products from the fetal circulation. The major maternal changes are increase in blood volume and cardiac output, hyperventilation, increased renal blood flow and glomerular filtration, and considerable weight gain.

Changes in Blood Volume

There is rapid and significant increase in total blood volume in pregnancy. The increase is about 40% of the prepregnant stage, which occurs due to increase in both plasma and cell components (Fig. 72.8).

1. The **increase in plasma volume** is primarily due to the **expansion of ECF volume**. ECF volume increases by about 7 liters (about 40% above the prepregnant state), which accounts for about 70% increase in blood volume. The increase in ECF volume is due to *sodium and water retention*. The increase in plasma volume occurs at the earliest, as early as first month of gestation. The increase occurs by 400 mL at 8 weeks and 1 liter by 16 weeks of gestation.

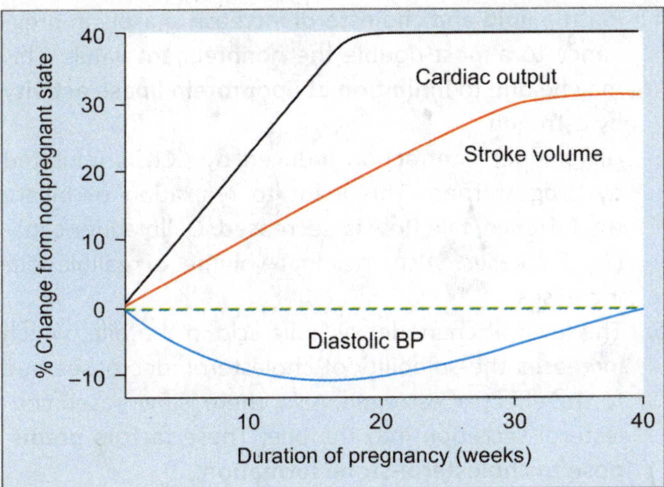

Fig. 72.9: Changes in cardiac output, stroke volume, and diastolic pressure in pregnancy. Cardiac output increases by about 40%, and stroke volume increases by about 30%, whereas diastolic pressure decreases by about 10%.

2. **Increase in red cell mass** occurs slowly after 16 weeks of gestation and the increase is usually about 20–30%. Erythropoiesis is stimulated in pregnancy due to **increased erythropoietin production**.

As increase in red cell mass is slower and lesser than the increase in plasma volume, there is a relative decrease in the red cell count **due to hemodilution**, though actually the red cell production is more. This is called **physiological anemia of pregnancy**.

Hematological Changes

Hematological changes are primarily designed to increase oxygen supply to the fetus and protect the fetus against infections.

1. **Red cell count increases** to about 20–30%, which is slower than the increase in plasma volume (as described above).
2. There is **moderate leucocytosis**. Leucocytosis occurs mainly due to **neutrophilia**. Moreover, **shift occurs to left in Arneth count**.
3. *Platelet count remains almost normal* in normal pregnancy.
4. The **increase in procoagulant activity** is among the striking hematological changes in third trimester of pregnancy. This occurs due to increased **hepatic synthesis of clotting factors by estrogen**. Fibrinogen concentration increases 2–4 times. Also, significant increase occurs in the level of factor VII, VIII, IX, and X.

In abnormal pregnancies, DIC (disseminated intravascular coagulation) occurs due to excess and unusual acceleration of procoagulant activities.

Changes in Cardiovascular System

Cardiac Output

The major hemodynamic change in pregnancy is the ***increase in cardiac output***. Cardiac output starts increasing in the early phase of pregnancy and is significantly high by the end of first trimester (Fig. 72.9). The increase in cardiac output reaches its maximum, i.e. about 40% increase from nonpregnant state, in mid-pregnancy and then remains elevated at that level till term. The increase in cardiac output is due to the increase in both stroke volume and heart rate.

Stroke Volume

Stroke volume **increases by about 30%**, which peaks at about 24 weeks of pregnancy. Increase in stroke volume is mainly due to increased end-diastolic volume (EDV), which occurs due to increased venous return as a consequence of increased blood volume.

Heart Rate

Heart rate **increases by about 10–15%**, reaching its peak at term.

Systolic BP

Systolic pressure **increases in pregnancy**, which is mainly due to increased cardiac output. The increase occurs more in the second and third trimester.

Diastolic BP

Diastolic pressure **falls slowly**, reaching a nadir at about 20th week, which then slowly increases to normal by term. Fall in diastolic pressure is due to the **vasodilation effect of progesterone**. **Pulse pressure** is wide due to increase in systolic and decrease in diastolic pressures.

LVET and PEP

Pre-ejection period (PEP) and left-ventricular ejection time (LVET) are reduced. However, cardiac output is high due to tachycardia and increased EDV.

Regional Blood Flow

In consequence to increased cardiac output and improved hemodynamics, blood flow increases in uterine, renal, mammary and cutaneous vascular bed.

Changes in Respiratory System

Respiratory changes aim to improve supply of oxygen to the fetus and removal of carbon dioxide from the fetus.

1. The most striking effect is the **increase in minute ventilation**. This increase begins in the early part of pregnancy. The increase is about 30% at the end of 8th week, which continues to increase to reach the peak of more than 50% of the nonpregnant value. The increase in ventilation is due to the **stimulation of respiratory centers by estrogen**.
2. Respiratory rate does not increase significantly. The increase in ventilation is mainly due to the **increase in tidal volume** (TV).

3. Residual volume **(RV) decreases by 20%**.
4. Expiratory reserve volume (ERV) decreases by 15%. Due to decrease in RV and ERV, **functional residual capacity decreases**.
5. Inspiratory reserve volume (IRV) increases. Increase in TV and ERV **increases inspiratory capacity**.
6. Diffusing capacity of alveolar membrane does not change significantly.

In third trimester, inspite of elevation of diaphragm due to increase in size of uterus, ventilation is not impaired significantly.

Changes in Kidney Functions

1. **Renal blood flow increases** by 35% that parallels the increase in blood volume and cardiac output. **Renal vasodilation** occurs due to increased local production of prostaglandins that facilitates increased renal plasma flow.
2. There is remarkable **increase in glomerular filtration rate** (GFR). Significant increase in GFR occurs as early as 2nd week, which reaches to about 40% by midpregnancy and continues at that level till term.
3. The **load of filtered glucose increases** without increase in tubular capacity to reabsorb glucose. Therefore, **glycosuria** is common in pregnant woman. Aminoaciduria also occurs.
4. Inspite of increased GFR and sodium load, **ability to excrete sodium and water remain normal** in normal pregnancy. However, ECF expansion occurs due to increased reabsorption of water and sodium.

Changes in GI System

GI **motility is decreased**. As a result, gastric emptying time is increased.

1. Due to increased transit time for chyme to pass though intestinal lumen, more water is absorbed that leads to **constipation**.
2. Toward term, enlarged uterus presses on the stomach, which increases intragastric pressure.
3. This results in propulsion of acid-gastric content into the esophagus leading to **reflux esophagitis**.

Changes in Hepatobiliary System

1. Hepatic blood flow remains unchanged despite marked increase in cardiac output.
2. Total serum protein decreases due to decrease in serum albumin. This is due to expansion of plasma that occurs without increase in synthesis of plasma proteins by the liver, which causes **dilutional hypoalbuminemia**. The γ-globulin concentration decreases. However, hepatic synthesis of fibrinogen increases.
3. Though SGPT and SGOT do not change much, **alkaline phosphatase** concentration increases 2–4 times.
4. Plasma **lipid and cholesterol increase** sharply in pregnancy to almost double the nonpregnant value. This may be due to **inhibition of lipoprotein lipase activity** by estrogen.
5. Gallbladder contraction induced by CCK is inhibited by progesterone. This leads to relaxation of biliary tract. Hence, **bile flow is decreased**. Gallbladder capacity increases. Also, residual volume of gallbladder increases.
6. The level of chenodeoxycholic acid in the bile, which increases the solubility of cholesterol, decreases due to the effect of estrogen. Also, there is increased cholesterol secretion into the bile. These factors **predispose to cholesterol-stone formation**.

Changes in Endocrine System

Pituitary Secretions

The **size of anterior lobe increases** two to three times during gestation, which is mainly due to increase in size and number of **prolactin secreting cells**.

1. **Prolactin** secretion starts increasing from end of first trimester and at term it is almost 10 times more than the pre-pregnant level.
2. However, due to negative feedback effects of estrogen, **gonadotrophs decrease in size**. The **hypothalamo-pituitary-ovarian axis is suppressed** by high level of sex steroids. This **decreases LH and FSH secretion**, and therefore **ovulation does not occur** during pregnancy.
3. **Growth hormone** secretion decreases and ***TSH secretion remains normal*** in pregnancy.
4. ACTH secretion is usually **suppressed**. However, ACTH secretion increases toward term due to its secretion from placenta.

Thyroid Secretion

Increase in GFR increases the renal clearance of iodine.

1. **Depletion of iodine pool** occurs due to increased renal excretion of iodine. This leads to moderate **increase in size of the thyroid gland,** unless dietary intake of iodine increases in pregnancy.
2. High level of circulating estrogen in the later part of pregnancy **increases TBG** (thyroxine binding globulin) production. Therefore, though secretion of T_3 and T_4 is increased, **euthyroid state is maintained in pregnancy**.

Adrenocortical Secretion

Secretion of **glucocorticoid and mineralocorticoid is increased** in pregnancy. The plasma free cortisol concentration increases due to its displacement from CBG (cortisol binding globulin). However, clinical hypercortisolism is not encountered.

Calcium Metabolism

The demand for calcium increases in pregnancy to facilitate fetal bone formation. This is achieved partly by **increased absorption of calcium** from GI tract by vitamin D and partly by the **increase in parathyroid hormone secretion**. However, total serum calcium decreases in the third trimester as fetal skeletal development is accelerated toward term. Therefore, calcium supplementation is invariably given in the later part of pregnancy.

Body Weight Gain

A major external change in the pregnant woman is the increase in body weight. In the first and second trimesters, it occurs mainly due to **fat deposition** induced by progesterone that stimulates food intake and diverts glucose for fat formation. In the third trimester, it is mainly due to increase in **size of fetus and uterus**. However, **fluid retention** significantly contributes to it. Body weight gain is usually more in eclampsia (Clinical Box 72.3).

Clinical Box 72.3

Toxemia of Pregnancy: About 5–10% of pregnant women develop edema, proteinuria and hypertension, known as **pregnancy-induced hypertension** (PIH). When all these features are present, the condition is called **pre-eclampsia**. If convulsion is associated, the condition is termed **eclampsia**. These two syndromes are collectively called toxemia of pregnancy. The maternal and fetal mortality is high in eclampsia. Exact mechanism of toxemia of pregnancy is not known. It is possibly due to the abnormal vasoconstriction of the maternal blood vessels and inadequate invasion of the endometrium by trophoblast cells that lead to poor blood perfusion of the placenta.

PARTURITION

Pregnancy terminates either in abortion or in parturition. When pregnancy terminates at or before 28th weeks of gestation (as per the Indian standard), the condition is called **abortion**; and termination after 28th week is called **parturition**. Normally, pregnancy terminates in parturition at term.

The **duration of normal pregnancy** in human is approximately **40 weeks from the first day of last menstrual cycle**, or 38 weeks from the day of ovulation. When pregnancy completes its full duration, is called **"term pregnancy"**. Delivery of the fetus at term through vaginal route is called parturition (as fetus can also be delivered by cesarean section). When fetus is delivered after 28th week and before 37th complete week of gestation, is called **premature infant**.

1. The smooth muscle (myometrium) of **uterus remains relaxed in most part of the pregnancy** due to the effect of **progesterone**.
2. In last few weeks of pregnancy, due to **increased level of estrogen**, uterine muscle cells **synthesize more connexin**, the protein that form gap junctions. This facilitates coordinated **contractions of myometrium**.

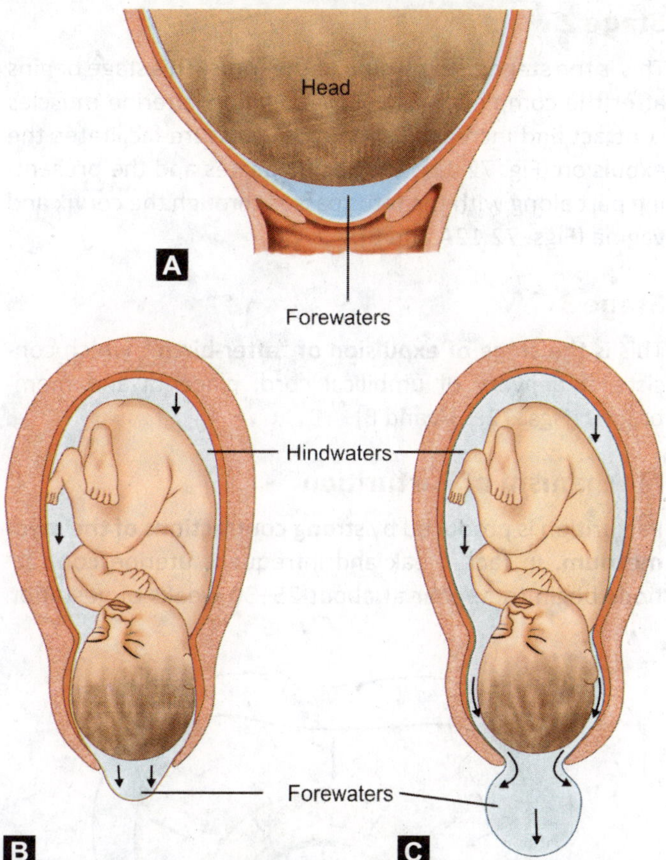

Figs. 72.10A to C: First stage of labor. Note the dilatation of cervix followed by formation of bag of membrane and forewaters.

3. However, the cervix of the uterus becomes soft due to enzymatic lysis of its collagen fibers.
4. **Relaxin** secreted from placenta and ovaries **facilitate cervical softening and dilation.**
5. Estrogen induces the synthesis of **oxytocin receptors**, which enhances uterine smooth muscle contraction.

Stages of Labor

Presence of following signs indicates the **onset of labor**:

1. Painful uterine contractions (***labor pain***).
2. Slight blood-stained mucus discharge from vagina, called as "**show**". This occurs due to minor hemorrhage from lower uterine segment and mucus secreted from cervix.
3. Commencement of **dilatation of internal os**.
4. Formation of **bag of water** (protrusion of amniotic sac).

Normal labor is divided into **three stages**:

Sage 1

This is the **stage of dilatation of cervix**. This is the preparatory stage during which cervix dilates to allow the expulsion of the fetus. First the formation of bag of membrane and forewaters occurs and then the membrane ruptures (Figs. 72.10A to C).

Stage 2

This is the **stage of expulsion of the fetus**. This stage begins after the completion of cervical dilation. Uterine muscles contract and increased abdominal pressure facilitates the expulsion (Fig. 72.11). The vagina dilates and the presenting part along with the fetus passes through the cervix and vagina (Figs. 72.12A and B).

Stage 3

This is the **stage of expulsion of "after-birth"**, which consists of delivery of umbilical cord, placenta and membranes (Figs. 72.13A and B).

Mechanism of Parturition

Parturition is produced by **strong contractions of the myometrium**. In fact, weak and infrequent uterine contractions begin to appear at about 25–30 weeks of gestation that gradually increase in magnitude and frequency as pregnancy advances. However, these are not the labor contractions. Labor contractions start with the onset of parturition. In the last month, the presenting part of the fetus, which is head in 90% of pregnancies (**cephalic presentation**) (Figs. 72.10A to C), descends toward cervix along entire uterine contents. At the **onset of parturition**, the **amniotic sac ruptures**, and the amniotic fluid flows through the vagina.

1. The **uterine contractions** become strong and appear every 10–15 min. Contraction waves originate in the upper part of the uterus and move downward toward cervix. Gradually, contractions increase in intensity and frequency.
2. The **cervix progressively dilates** to attain a maximum diameter of about 10–12 cm. Once cervical dilation is complete (Figs. 72.10A to C), every new contraction moves the fetus downward in the birth canal.
3. Finally, very strong uterine contractions push the fetus through the cervix and vagina (Fig. 72.11).
4. At this stage, the mother, by **bearing down** to increase abdominal pressure, adds to push the baby in the birth canal (Figs. 72.12A and B).
5. Within minutes of delivery of the baby, both the **umbilical cord and the placenta are delivered** (Figs. 72.13A and B). Placenta, which remains tightly adhered to uterine wall throughout pregnancy, is separated from it by a series of waves of uterine contractions and delivered after the delivery of the baby (hence, called *after birth*).

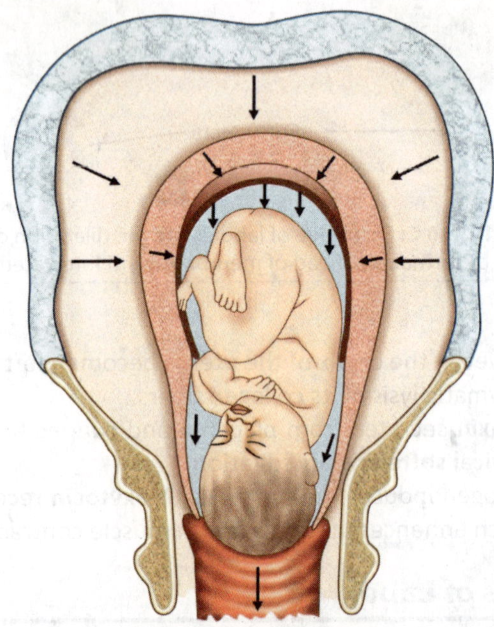

Fig. 72.11: Second stage of labor. Note the expulsion of the fetus by uterine contraction, of fetus facilitated by increased abdominal pressure.

Parturition Reflex

Parturition is a reflex phenomenon. The inherent rhythmic contractions of smooth muscle cells of the myometrium are facilitated by **stretch** imparted by the growing fetus.

1. Toward term, the pregnant uterus synthesizes and secretes **prostaglandins** (PGE_2 and $PGF_{2\alpha}$) that area potent stimulators of uterine muscle contraction (Fig. 72.14).
2. **Oxytocin** causes stronger uterine muscle contraction and also stimulates uterus to synthesize more prostaglandins.

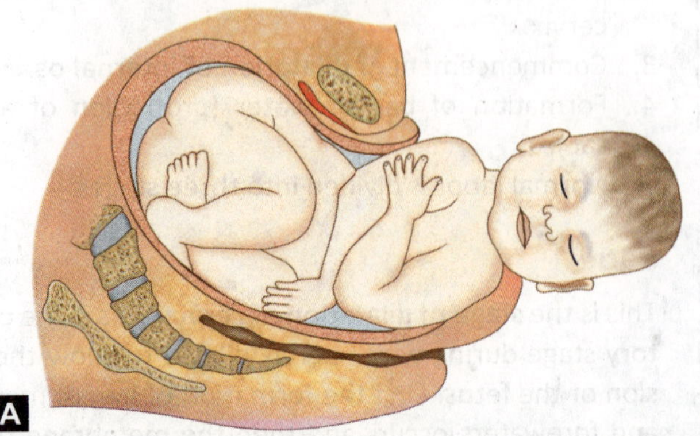

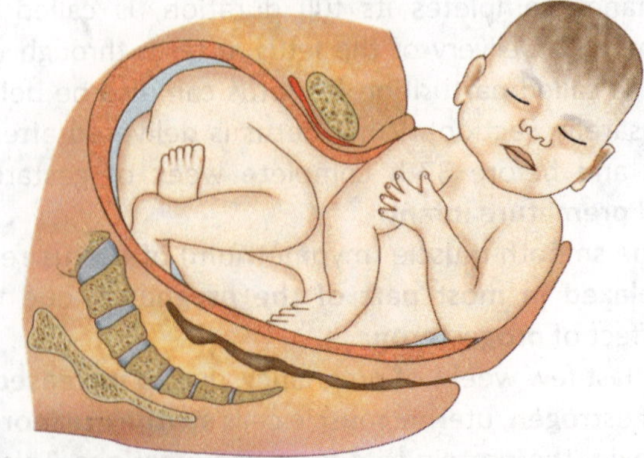

Figs. 72.12A and B: Second stage of labor. Note the dilatation of vagina and delivery of the head of fetus (A) followed by the body (B).

3. **Estrogen** increases uterine muscle excitability and contractility. Under the effect of estrogen, the **number and sensitivity of oxytocin receptors in uterine muscle cells increase** during the last few weeks of pregnancy.

Role of Oxytocin

Oxytocin is reflexly **secreted from posterior pituitary** in response to inputs originating in hypothalamus.

1. When descending part of the fetus (which is usually head) presses on the lower part of the uterus and cervix, **stimulation of stretch receptors** increases impulses via ascending sensory fibers through spinal cord to thalamus.
2. These fibers from their pathway in brainstem give **collaterals to hypothalamus** which in turn activates posterior pituitary.

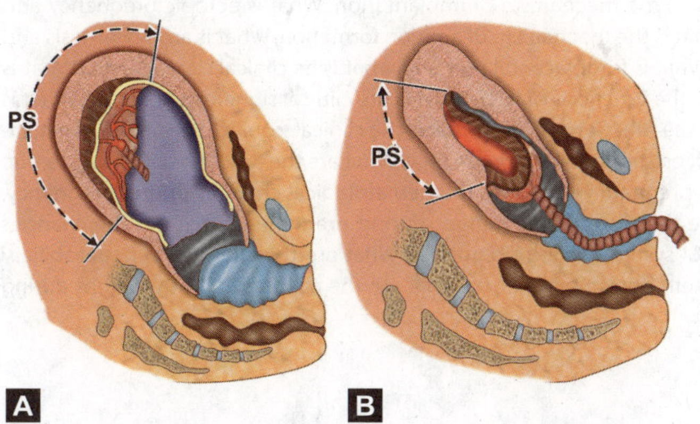

Figs. 72.13A and B: Third stage of labor. Note the separation of placenta (A), followed by expulsion of it (B). (PS: Placental surface).

3. Oxytocin is released from posterior pituitary that increases uterine contractions. The uterine contractions exert **positive feedback effect** on oxytocin secretion (Flowchart 72.1).
4. As part of the efferent limb of the reflex pathway is hormonal as in milk ejection reflex, parturition is another example of **neurohumoral reflex**.

Flowchart 72.1: Changes in cardiac output, stroke volume, and diastolic pressure in pregnancy. Cardiac output increases by about 40%, and stroke volume increases by about 30%, whereas diastolic pressure decreases by about 10%.

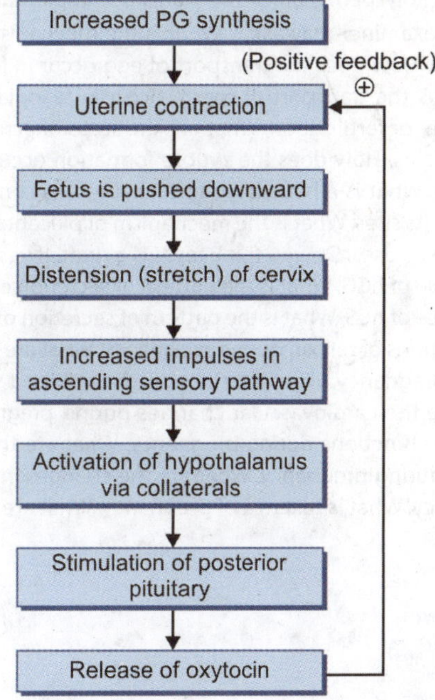

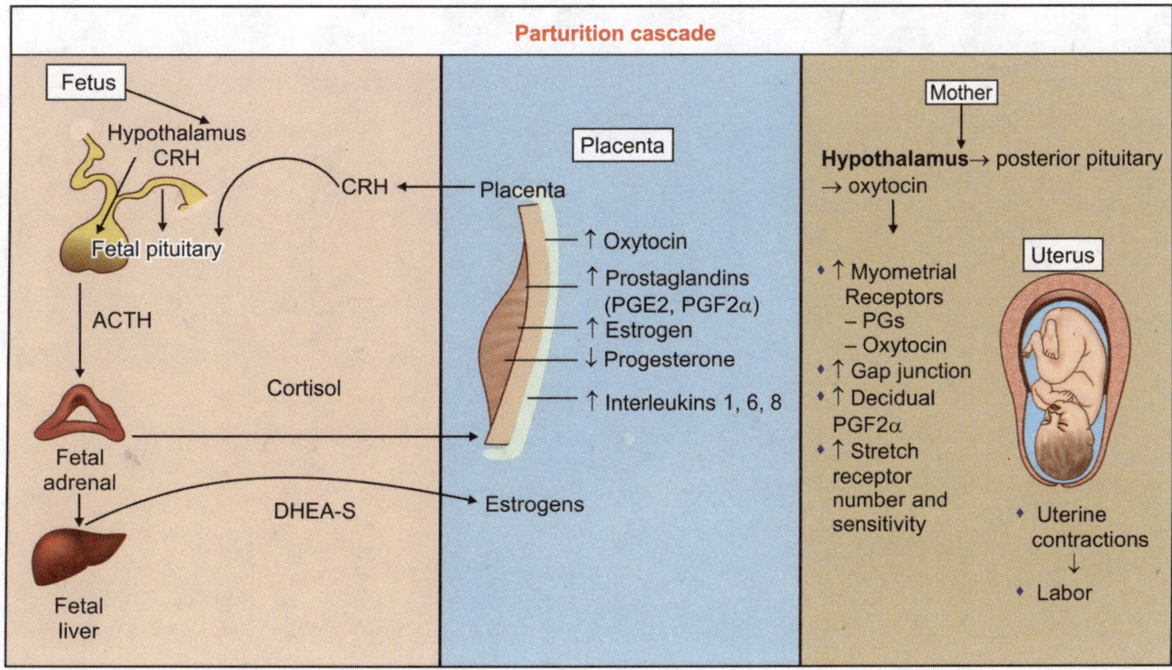

Fig. 72.14: Initiation of parturition.

CHAPTER SUMMARY

Key Concepts

1. Pregnancy starts with implantation of fertilized egg.
2. Placental hormones support fetal growth and continuation of pregnancy.
3. Pregnancy is an altered state of physiology, in which blood volume increases, C.O. and systolic BP increase, but diastolic BP decreases. All these changes facilitate blood and nutrition supply to fetus.
4. Parturition reflex is a neurohumoral reflex.

Important to Know (Must Read)

1. In examination, "Describe the maternal changes during pregnancy" may be asked as a **Long Question**.
2. Parturition reflex, Human chorionic gonadotropin (hCG), Human chorionic somatotropin (hCS), Cardiovascular changes during pregnancy, Respiratory changes during pregnancy, Hematological changes and changes in blood volume during pregnancy, Acrosome reaction, Polyspermy block, Mechanism of implantation, Fetoplacental unit, Female infertility may be asked as **Short Questions** in exam.
3. In **Viva**, examiner may ask… What is the mechanism of parturition reflex, List the placental hormones, What are the causes of female infertility, How does the transport of egg occur in female after ovulation, How does the transport of sperm occur in the cervix, uterus, How does the transport of sperm occur in fallopian tube, What are the changes occur in sperm in female genital tract, What is the usual site for fertilization, What are the steps of acrosome reaction and sperm penetration, What is polyspermy block and what are its mechanisms, How does the zygote formation occur, What is the mechanism of twin formation, What are the functions of intact zona pelucida, What is a blastocyst and what are its components, What is the mechanism of implantation, What is ectopic pregnancy and what are its sites, What is the mechanism of placenta formation, What is the mechanism of amnion formation, What is amniocentesis and what are its uses, Do you think fetus is a graft, if yes explain why, What is fetoplacental unit and what is its clinical significance, What is the source of hCG, What is the pattern of secretion of hCG, What are the functions of hCG, What is the clinical significance of hCG, What is the source of hCS, What is the pattern of secretion of hCS, What are the functions of hCS, What is the clinical significance of hCS, What are the functions of relaxin during pregnancy, What are the functions of estrogen during pregnancy, What are the functions of progesterone during pregnancy, What are the changes in blood volume during pregnancy, What are the hematological changes during pregnancy, What are the cardiovascular changes during pregnancy, What are the respiratory changes during pregnancy, What are the changes in kidney functions during pregnancy, What are the changes in GI system during pregnancy, What are the changes in hepatobiliary system during pregnancy, What are the changes in endocrine system during pregnancy, What are the changes in body weight during pregnancy, What is toxemia of pregnancy, What are stages of labor.

CHAPTER

73

Physiology of Breast Development and Lactation

Learning Objectives

On completion of study of this chapter, the student **MUST** be able to:

1. Understand the development of breast in different phases of life of women.
2. Understand the mechanism of lactogenesis.
3. List the composition of human milk.
4. Correlates the physiology of breast development and lactation with abnormalities of breast development and lactation.

The student **MAY** also be able to:

1. Describe the mechanisms and regulation of breast development.
2. Describe the mechanisms of lactogenesis and lactation.

BREAST DEVELOPMENT

The primary function of female breast is **synthesis and secretion of milk**. In mammals, especially in humans, milk secreted from breast (for breastfeeding) is the chief source of nutrition for the offspring. As breast milk contains all the ingredients necessary for complete development of the infant, deficient breastfeeding, especially in first six months during infancy results in retardation of growth. Therefore, in females, nature has designed the development of breast with the attainment of reproducibility and preparation of breast for lactogenesis and lactation during pregnancy, so that as soon as the baby is born, breast milk, the natural and the best nutrition for the newborn is available.

Structure of Breast

Breast is a mass of fibrofatty tissue containing **alveoli and ducts.**

1. Ducts in breast branch all through the mammary tissue and converge at the nipples.
2. Ducts begin in saclike glands called **alveoli.** Alveoli are the sites of milk secretion and they look like bunches of grapes with stems terminating in the ducts (Figs. 73.1A and B).
3. **Ductules** originate from alveoli. Ductules open to ducts that in turn drain to **lactiferous ducts.**
4. Lactiferous duct terminates in dilated **lactiferous sinus.**
5. Sinuses open to nipple through **nipple-pores.**
6. The alveoli and ducts are surrounded by specialized contractile cells called **myoepithelial cells.** ***Contraction of myoepithelial cells*** causes **milk ejection** into the lactiferous sinuses.

Breast Development in Different Phases of Life

Full development of breast requires many hormones.

1. The major hormones controlling development of mammary gland are estrogen, progesterone, prolactin, growth hormone (GH), thyroxine and cortisol.
2. Generally, **estrogen stimulates the development of duct system** and **progesterone promotes growth of lobulo-alveolar system.**
3. GH, prolactin and cortisol synergize the estrogen and progesterone effects.
4. **During pregnancy and lactation**, breast development and lactogenesis are dependent on prolactin and adrenal steroids.

During Intrauterine Life

Breast develops from **ectoderm**. When embryo is 7 mm in length, mammary tissue appears as a ridge called **mammary**

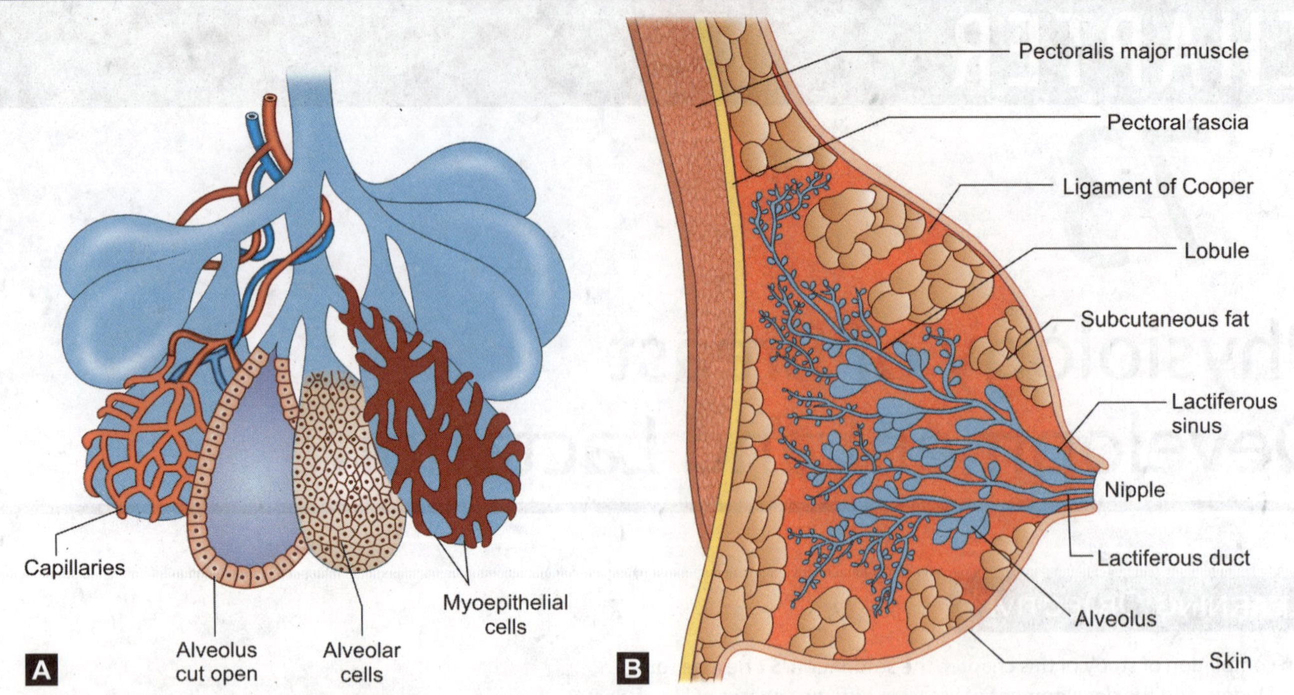

Figs. 73.1A and B: Structure of basic unit of mammary gland (A); Structure of adult breast (B).

crest, one on each side, extending along the ventrolateral body wall from axillary to the inguinal region.

1. The caudal part of the ridge regresses and the thoracic region condenses to form **primordial mammary bud** when the embryo is about 12 mm in length.
2. After 5th month of gestation, the primitive mammary bud forms about 20 **secondary buds** that form ductal system in the mature gland.
3. These ducts undergo proliferation in third trimester of pregnancy in response to various hormones.
4. **At birth**, mammary gland is rudimentary.
5. In some newborns, small quantity of milk is secreted due to high prolactin concentration in them at that time. This is called ***'witch milk'***.

During Childhood

After birth, breast **regresses due to lack of hormonal support** and remains in a quiescent stage. The growth of breast occurs with the general growth of the body till puberty, which is proportionate to the somatic growth.

During Puberty

Before puberty, the breasts are small with less glandular structure. With the onset of puberty in girls, marked enlargement of breast occurs due to the **effects of estrogen**.

1. The breast development is mainly due to **enhancement of duct growth and branching of ducts** with relatively little growth of the alveoli.
2. The breast enlargement is significantly contributed by **fat deposition**.
3. When menstrual cycle starts at puberty, **progesterone** secretion commences in the luteal phase of each cycle, which contributes to breast enlargement by stimulating the **growth of alveoli.**
4. The areola enlarges and becomes more pigmented.

During Each Menstrual Cycle

During each menstrual cycle, temporary changes in breasts occur in different phases of cycle due to proliferation and regression of ductal and alveolar tissue in response to fluctuations in plasma level of estrogen and progesterone. Especially, **in the late luteal phase, breast size increases due to alveolar growth** in response to progesterone and **ductal growth in response to estrogen.**

During Pregnancy

Prominent changes occur in breast during pregnancy. Breast enlargement occurs due to the stimulatory effects of high plasma concentrations of **estrogen, progesterone, prolactin, and hCS.**

1. Appreciable breast enlargement occurs after second month of gestation.
2. The **areola and nipple increase in size and become more pigmented.**
3. **Montgomery tubercles** appear in the areola (Figs. 73.2A and B).
4. Alveoli, ducts and glands gradually increase in size.
5. In the last trimester, acini differentiate into **secretory glands.**
6. Parenchymal cells of **alveoli undergo hypertrophy** increasing the size of the breast. All these changes are meant to prepare breasts for lactogenesis and lactation.

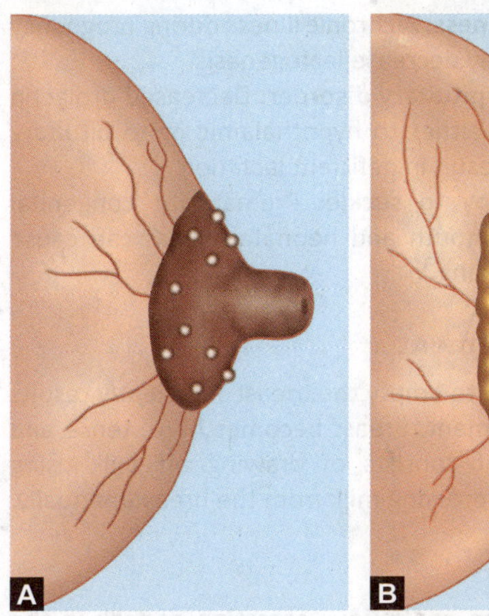

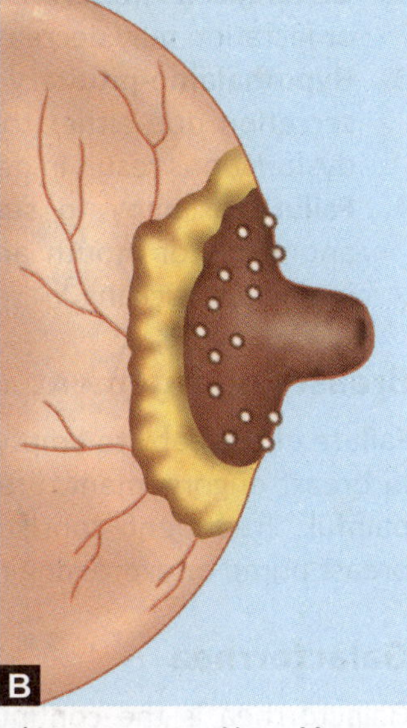

Figs. 73.2A and B: Mammary gland in pregnancy. Note, Montgomery tubercles in areola and size and vascularity of breast increases from 2nd trimester (A) to 3rd trimester (B).

During Lactation

A lactating breast is large in size with nipple projecting about 2 cm beyond the areola. Breast changes during lactation occur mainly due to the **action of prolactin** secreted from anterior pituitary. Prolactin also stimulates the production of milk.

LACTOGENESIS AND LACTATION

Though prolactin level is high in later part of pregnancy, milk production does not occur due to the **inhibitory effects of estrogen and progesterone** at their high concentrations on lactogenesis.

1. **Estrogen increases secretion of prolactin** and along with prolactin promotes breast growth and differentiation. But, along with progesterone, it **antagonizes prolactin action on milk production** and secretion.
2. **Following parturition**, estrogen and progesterone concentration in plasma falls appreciably as placenta, which was secreting large amount of these hormones is no more present. Decreased level of these hormones facilitates **unopposed milk production by prolactin**.
3. The role of prolactin in lactogenesis has been described in the Chapter "Anterior Pituitary".

Role of hypothalamus: The immediate fall in estrogen level following parturition decreases **prolactin secretion** from its peak pre-parturition level to new **post-partum basal level**. However, prolactin level **still remains very high** till the mother continues to nurse the breast milk.

1. Superimposed upon this high basal level, **large secretory bursts of prolactin** occur during each nursing period. This **episodic burst of prolactin** signals the breasts for maintenance of milk production. These **prolactin pulses** continue for several days after the mother completely stops nursing her infant.
2. The mechanism mediating prolactin pulses is initiated by **stimulation of nipple receptors by suckling** that sends afferent input to the hypothalamus.
3. This input **inhibits hypothalamic release of dopamine**. As normally dopamine inhibits prolactin secretion, decreased dopamine release stimulates prolactin secretion.
4. **Prolactin also inhibits GnRH secretion** from hypothalamus that **prevents ovulation**. Therefore, till mother continues to nurse the baby, normally ***pregnancy does not occur***.
5. This is the natural procedure of **contraception**, which aims at spacing the subsequent pregnancies.

Suckling also initiates **milk-ejection reflex** (for details, refer Chapter "Posterior Pituitary") that transfers milk from breast into the mouth of the baby.

Table: 73.1: Composition of human milk.

Component	Average Quantity
Water	87%
Solids	13%
Proteins (gm%)	2.5
Carbohydrate (gm%)	6
Fats (gm%)	5
Calcium (mg%)	40
Phosphorous (mg%)	30
Magnesium (mg%)	5
Sodium (mg%)	15
Potassium (mg%)	60
Vitamin C (mg%)	4.5
Vitamin A (µg%)	5
Vitamin D (IU)	5
Vitamin B1 (µg%)	15
Riboflavin (µg%)	45
Niacin (µg%)	180
Vitamin B6 (µg%)	10
Pantothenic acid (µg%)	200
Calories/100 g	67

Breast Milk

Immediately after delivery, a watery fluid is secreted from breasts called **colostrum**, which is rich in protein. Colostrum secretion is replaced by milk in about 24 to 48 hours.

1. **Mother's milk contains all nutrients in adequate quantity**: carbohydrate in the form of lactose (milk sugar), protein (casein), fat, minerals, vitamins and water (Table 73.1).
2. Milk contains **antibodies** meant for protecting the newborn from various infections.
3. Milk also contains **growth factors and hormones** that help in physical development and maturation, and large number of **neuropeptides and endogenous opioids** that facilitate the development of brain and behavior of infant.

4. Some of these substances are synthesized by the breast tissue itself, not just transported from blood to milk. It is virtually impossible to produce mother's milk in a commercial formula.
5. The milk proteins are not destroyed in the GI tract as low gastric acidity in newborn fails to denature them.
6. Also, the intestinal epithelium in infant is **more permeable to proteins** than in the adult, which facilitates their absorption. Thus, mother's **milk proteins easily enter into blood of the infant**. However, infectious agents like AIDS virus and various drugs can easily be transmitted through breast milk.

Abnormalities of Breast Development and Lactation

Small Breasts

Small breast due to poor breast development is common. This may be constitutional, genetic and familial. However, during pregnancy small breast becomes bigger and usually mils secretion becomes adequate.

Polythelia

Polythelia is more number of breasts. More number of breasts can develop in the milk line starting from axilla to the groin. Usually these multiple breasts are small in size. These are small and flat breast, and the nipples may be inverted or small that impede suckling and breast feeding.

Deficient Lactation

Deficiency of lactation can occur due to following causes.

1. **Poor breast development**, which may be constitutional, genetic and familial. A small, flat or inverted nipple may impede suckling.
2. **Generalized illness:** A chronic illness during pregnancy or lactation may decrease lactogenesis.
3. **Hypothalamo-pituitary disorder:** Decreased prolactin secretion due either to hypothalamic or to pituitary dysfunctions result in deficient lactation
4. **Failure of baby to suckle:** Prematurity, congenital anomalies of mouth and neonatal illness can cause inefficient suckling.

Breast Engorgement

Failure of the baby to empty the breast sufficiently results in breast engorgement. Breast becomes hard, tense and painful. Treatment consists of drawing off milk using breast pump or expressing milk from the breast manually.

Galactorrhea

Galactorrhea is the continuous secretion of milk in the absence of recent pregnancy. Though it is common in woman, it can also occur in man.

1. In women, when it is associated with amenorrhea, the condition is called **galactorrhea-amenorrhea syndrome**. The tumor of pituitary gland causing excess secretion of prolactin can cause this syndrome (**hyperprolactinemia-galactorrhea syndrome**).
2. It is also seen in **Chiari-Frommel syndrome**, which is characterized by excess lactation, amenorrhea, and superinvolution of uterus dating from pregnancy.
3. It occurs due to persistent prolactin secretion without secretion of FSH and LH.
4. Galactorrhea may occur **due to some drugs** such as reserpine, phenothiazine derivatives, α-methyldopa and tricyclic antidepressants.
5. Galactorrhea may be seen **in hypothyroidism** in which increased TRH secretion (feedback effects of low thyroxine) stimulates prolactin secretion.

CHAPTER SUMMARY

Key Concepts

1. Estrogen stimulates the development of duct system and progesterone promotes growth of lobulo-alveolar system.
2. During pregnancy breast size increases under the influence of estrogen, progesterone, prolactin, and hCS. Prolactin increases synthesis and secretion of milk after delivery.
3. Brest milk is the best nutrition for the infant as it contains all the ingredients including minerals, vitamins and antibodies.

Important to Know (Must Read)

1. In examination, **Long Questions** are usually not asked from this chapter.
2. Development of breast, Breast milk, Mechanism of lactation, may be asked as **Short Questions** in exam.
3. In **Viva**, examiner may ask... What is the composition of breast milk, What are the abnormalities of lactation, What is Galactorrhea, what are its causes and features, When does breast engorgement occur, What is Polythelia, How does the breast develop during intrauterine life, What changes do occur in the breast during childhood, How does the breast develop during puberty, What changes do occur in the breast during each menstrual cycle, What changes do occur in the breast during pregnancy, What changes do occur in the breast during lactation, What is the mechanism of lactogenesis and lactation.

CHAPTER 74

Physiology of Contraception

Learning Objectives

On completion of study of this chapter, the student **MUST** be able to:

1. Classify contraceptives for males and females.
2. Name the temporary and permanent methods of contraception.
3. Give the mechanism of action of contraceptives.
4. Say which contraceptive will be better for which type of couple.

The student **MAY** also be able to:

1. Describe the mechanisms, merits and demerits of different types of contraceptives.

India is a highly populous nation. One of the major problems India facing in recent years is birth control. In April, 1976, India formulated its first 'National Population Policy', and 'National Population Policy–2000' is the latest in the series. All these policies primarily aim at reducing the birth rate.

When birth control procedures work prior to implantation of the fertilized egg, they are called **contraceptives**, and when work after implantation (cause death of the embryo), they are termed as **abortifacients**.

CLASSIFICATION

Contraceptive methods are classified into following categories:

1. Barrier methods
   - Physical methods
   - Chemical methods
2. Intrauterine devices
3. Hormonal methods
4. Post-conceptional methods
5. Permanent methods

They may also be classified as **temporary** and **permanent methods.**

Methods of contraception
- Temporary
  - Barrier methods
  - Natural contraception
  - Intrauterine contraceptive devices (IUCDs)
  - Steroidal contraception
- Permanent
  - Female
    - Tubal occlusion
  - Male
    - Vasectomy

Physical Methods

In Males

Condom is the most widely used barrier device in male. It prevents sperm to be deposited in the vagina. The biggest advantage is that it provides **protection against sexually transmitted diseases.**

In Females

Diaphragm is the most commonly used vaginal barrier. A **spermicidal jelly** is usually used along with the diaphragm. Another female barrier device is **vaginal sponge.**

Chemical Methods

Various spermicidal agents like foams, creams and suppositories are inserted manually into vagina before intercourse. These act as 'surface active agents' that attach themselves to sperms and decrease their oxygen uptake and kill them. They are not usually used due to their high failure rate.

Intrauterine Devices

Intrauterine devices (IUDs) are most effective contraceptive devices for a parous lady (who has borne at least one child).

Types

The IUDs are of **three generations** (Figs. 74.1A to D):

1. **First generation IUD**

   Lippes Loop

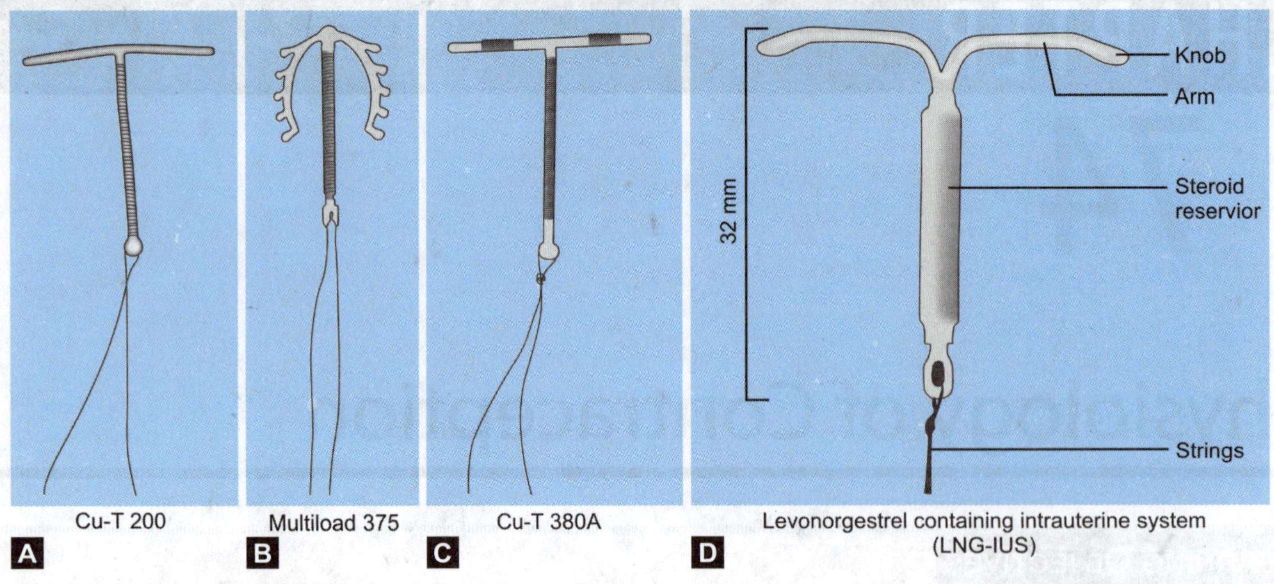

Figs. 74.1A to D: Commonly used IUDs.

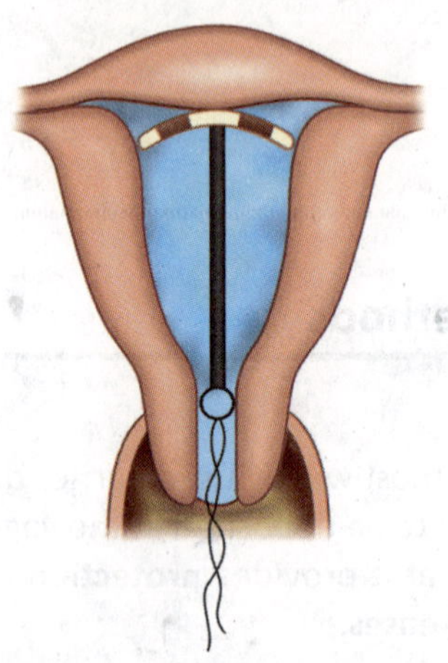

Fig. 74.2: Cupper in the uterus, T implanted as a foreign body.

2. **Second generation IUD**
   Earlier devices: Copper–7; Copper T–200
   Newer devices: Copper T variants (T–Cu 220C; T–Cu 380A; T–Cu 380Ag)
3. **Third generation IUD** (with hormonal preparation)
   Progestasert: A T-shaped device filled with 38 mg of progesterone.
   Levonorgestrel–20 (LNG-20): A T-shaped IUD releasing 20 mcg of leveonorgestrel, a synthetic steroid.

Mechanism of Action

IUD works by several mechanisms.

1. Usually, they work after fertilization has occurred but before implantation is completed. The presence of these small objects in the uterus brings about uterine changes that **interfere with the endometrial preparation** for acceptance of the blastocyst. Thus, implantation is prevented.
2. They also act as **foreign body** in the uterine cavity (Fig. 74.2) causing cellular and biochemical changes in the endometrium and the uterine fluid that impair the viability of the gamete. Therefore, the chance of fertilization is reduced.
3. **Copper facilitates cellular reaction** in endometrium, composition of cervical mucus, impairs sperm motility and impairs capacitation of sperm.
4. Hormone releasing devices increase the viscosity of cervical mucus by releasing progesterone. They **make mucous thick**, so that sperm cannot enter uterus. They also make the endometrium unfavorable for implantation.

Merits and Demerits

Merits and demerits of IUDs are summarized in Table 74.1.

Hormonal Contraceptives

1. **Oral contraceptive pills**
   - Combined pill
   - Progestogen only pill
   - Post-coital pill
   - Once-a-month pill
   - Male pill
2. **Depots** (slow releasing formulations)
   - Injectable preparations
   - Subcutaneous implants
   - Vaginal rings

Oral Contraceptive Pills (OCPs)

Presently, OCPs contain 30–35 mcg of estrogen and 0.5 to 1 mg of progesterone. The pill is given for 21 days from 5th day of the cycle. Oral contraceptives are based on the principle that estrogen and progesterone **inhibit pituitary**

Table 74.1: Merits and demerits of IUDs (Cu devices and hormone releasing IUDs).

Advantages	Disadvantages
• Inexpensive: Cu-T distributed free of cost through government channels	• Require motivation
• Simplicity in techniques of insertion and most cost effective of all methods	• Limitation in its use
• Prolonged contraceptive protection after insertion (5–10) years and suitable for rural population of developing countries effects	• Adverse local reactions manifested by menstrual abnormalities, PID, pelvic the pain and heavy periods. Beside are less with third generation of IUDs
• Systemic side effects are nil. Suitable for hypertensives, Breastfeeding women, and epileptics	• Risk of ectopic pregnancy
• Reversibility to fertility is prompt after removal	

gonadotropin release, thereby *preventing ovulation*. Progesterone only pill affects the composition of the cervical mucus, reducing the ability of the sperm to pass through the cervix, and inhibit the estrogen-induced proliferation of the endometrium, making it inhospitable for implantation.

Side Effects of OCP

Though OCPs are 100% effective in preventing pregnancy, there are risks of few side effects, especially when consumed for many years.

Cardiovascular Side Effects

Myocardial infarction, cerebral thrombosis, venous thrombosis and hypertension have been reported. These side effects are more seen in aged (more than 35 years) woman and in smokers. *Hypertension* occurs due to fluid retention and increased angiotensin level. Estrogen *increases renin-angiotensin activity* and thereby increases angiotensin II production which is a potent vasoconstrictor.

Carcinogenesis

Increased risks of cervical cancer and breast neoplasia have been reported. Hepatic tumors occurs rarely.

Metabolic side Effects

OCPs decrease HDL and alter blood coagulability. These two factors *facilitate atherosclerosis* and proneness to myocardial infarction and stroke. They also cause *glucose intolerance* and insulin resistance.

Miscellaneous

Other side effects include cholestatic jaundice, breast tenderness, weight gain and migraine.

Depots

Subcutaneous implants are contraceptive (progestogen) capsules (Norplant) implanted beneath the skin that releases hormone slowly and last for five years. Injectable forms (intra-muscular injection of progestogen substance like Depo-Provera every three months) are also available. Vaginal ring containing levonorgestrel has been found to be effective.

Post-Conceptional Pills

Contraceptives can be used **within 72 h** after intercourse (post-coital contraception).

1. These pills interfere with ovulation, transport of the conceptus to the uterus, or implantation.
2. Usually, high dose of estrogen, or two large doses (12 h apart) of a combined estrogen-progestin oral preparations are prescribed.
3. Most effective with fewer side effects is the **pill RU 486** (mifepristone), which antagonizes progesterone activity by binding competitively with progesterone receptors in the uterus.
4. This causes the endometrium to erode and the contractions of the fallopian tubes and myometrium to increase.

Other Methods

The Rhythm (Safe Period) Method

The rhythm method is the **abstinence from sexual intercourse during the fertile period** of the cycle (near the time of ovulation).

1. In 28 days regular cycles, normally ovulation occurs between 12th and 16th day (usually on 14th day). Functionally sperm can survive for two days and ovum for 3 days.
2. Therefore, unprotected intercourse should be avoided during the **fertile period** of the cycle, which will fall between 2 days before and 3 days after ovulation i. e. from 10th day to 19th day of the cycle (refer Fig. 69.4; Chapter 69). Rest of the period in the cycle is considered to be **safe period**.
3. However, the day of ovulation is not always fixed even in regular cycles and cycle length is also not always regular. Moreover, only the **length of luteal phase is constant**, which is 14 days from the day of ovulation, and practically it is difficult and tedious to know the day of ovulation.
4. Therefore, in practice, **shortest cycle minus 18 days gives** the first day of fertile period and **longest cycle minus 10 days** gives the last day of fertile period. For example, if the duration of shortest cycle is 25 days (25 – 18 = 7th day) and duration of longest cycle is 32 days (32 – 10 = 22nd day), the unprotected intercourse should be **avoided between 7th and 22nd day** of any cycle.

Table 74.2: Failure rate of contraceptive methods in first 12 months of use.

Methods	Pregnancy rate per 100 women years (approx.)
No method	85
Natural (calendar, temperature, mucus)	25
Withdrawal	27
Lactation amenorrhea	2
Condom (male)	15
Condom (female)	21
Diaphragm	16
IUCD:	
Cu-T 380 A	0.8
LNG 20	0.1
Combined oral pill	0.1
Progestin only pill	1
DMPA and NET injectables	0.3
Norplant	0.05
Implanon	0.01
Vasectomy	0.15
Tubectomy	0.15

Failure rate is further less when methods are used correctly and consistently.
(IUCD: Intrauterine contraceptive devices; Cu-T: Copper-T; LNG: Levonorgestrel; DMPA: Depot medroxyprogesterone acetate; NET: Norethisterone).

5. However, pregnancy has been documented due to intercourse on any day of the cycle. Therefore, it is believed that no period in any cycle, even during the bleeding phase is absolutely safe.

Coitus Interruptus

In this method, during fertile period, the male partner withdraws penis from vagina before ejaculation. Thus, sperm is not deposited in the female genital tract in the fertile period.

Breast-feeding

Till the mother continues to nurse the baby with breast feeding, ovulation does not occur. This is because prolactin secreted during lactation produces **lactational amenorrhea** by inhibiting GnRH secretion.

Table 74.3: Effectiveness of contraceptive methods.

Contraceptive effectiveness chart (WHO 2007)	Pregnancy/100wy
• **Most effective methods** Implants, IUDs, sterilization (male and female)	< 2
• **Very effective methods** Injectables, LAM, COCs, POPs, patch, vaginal rings	3–9
• **Effective methods** Male condom, diaphragm, female condom Fertility awareness methods	10–20
• **Least effective methods** Spermicides	21–30

Family Planning Operations

Government of India encourages people of India with different incentives to opt for family planning operation after a couple are blessed with a child ('we two-ours one' policy). It is done either by male or female sterilization.

Male Sterilization

Male sterilization is performed by **vasectomy**. In vasectomy, bilateral ligation of vas deferens is performed instead of sectioning the vas as recanalization can be taken up in future whenever needed. However, antibodies developed against spermatozoa following vasectomy causes infertility following restoration of patency of the vas.

Female Sterilization

Female sterilization is performed by **bilateral tubal ligation**. Tubal recanalization can also be performed later whenever needed.

Failure Rates of Contraceptive Methods

Failure rates of various contraceptive methods are summarizes in Table 74.2.

Effectiveness of contraceptive methods: Summarized in Table 74.3.

CHAPTER SUMMARY

Key Concepts

1. The best method in nulliparous woman is OCP and parous women are IUDs. However, there are failures in all methods.
2. The only dependable methods are sterilizations.

Important to Know (Must Read)

1. In examination, 'Classify contraceptives, describe the mechanism, merits and demerits of various contraceptive methods used in females and males' may be asked as **Long Questions**.
2. Intrauterine devices (IUDs), Oral contraceptive pills (OCPs) may be asked as **Short Questions** in exam.
3. In **Viva**, examiner may ask... List the contraceptive methods in female, List the contraceptive methods in male, What are the different types of IUDs, What is the mechanism of action of IUDs, List the hormonal contraceptives, What is the mechanism of action of OCPs, What are the side effects of OCPs, What is a post-conceptional pill, What is a Depot, How is the safe period calculated in the rhythm method, What is coitus interruptus, How does breast-feeding prevent conception, What is male sterilization, What is female sterilization, What is the physical contraceptive method in male, What is the physical contraceptive method in female, What is the chemical contraceptive method in male, What is the chemical contraceptive method in female.

SECTION–8

Renal System

75. General Introduction and Functional Anatomy of Kidney
76. Renal Blood Flow
77. Glomerular Filtration
78. Tubular Functions
79. Mechanisms of Urine Concentration and Dilution
80. Water Excretion, Diuresis, and Diuretics
81. Acidification of Urine
82. Kidney Function Tests and Pathophysiology of Renal Failure
83. Physiology of Micturition and Bladder Dysfunctions

"He is the godhead growing in human lives
And in the body of earth-being's forms:
He is the soul of man climbing to God
In Nature's surge out of earth's ignorance."

Sri Aurobindo (in 'SAVITRI')

CHAPTER 75

General Introduction and Functional Anatomy of Kidney

LEARNING OBJECTIVES

On completion of study of this chapter, the student **MUST** be able to:

1. List the functions of kidney.
2. Name the parts of the nephron and give their main functions.
3. Correlate histological modification at different segments of nephron with their specific functions.
4. List the differences between cortical and juxtamedullary nephrons.
5. Give the detail ultrastructure of glomerulo-capsular filtration barrier.
6. Describe the details of structure and functions of JG apparatus.
7. Explain the functions of renin-angiotensin system.

The student **MAY** also be able to:

1. Describe the structural and functional organization of different parts of the nephron.
2. Describe the role of JG apparatus in health and disease.

KIDNEY PLAYS HOMEOSTATIC ROLE

The kidneys play a vital role in homeostatic functions of the body. Therefore, impairment of kidney functions leads to many homeostatic abnormalities. Extracellular fluid (ECF) compartment is the interface between the external and the internal (cellular) milieus of living creatures. Water, minerals, nutrients and gases pass through the ECF before entering the cellular compartment, and cellular waste products pass through the ECF before being excreted from the body. Hence, **maintenance of ECF volume and composition**, the aim of many homeostatic mechanisms, is vital for organ functions. Kidneys play principal role in this homeostasis.

In clinical practice, biochemical investigations are important weapons of clinician's diagnostic armamentarium. These routine and special investigations from medical or surgical wards and clinics are generally meant to reveal kidney functions and dysfunctions, directly or indirectly. Medical students, interns, residents and consultants need to learn more of kidney physiology to understand and interpret the reports of these investigations. Moreover, understanding renal physiology helps physicians learn the pathophysiology of renal diseases and plan the management strategies of these disorders.

Functions of Kidney

1. **Urine formation and excretion of waste products:** The primary function of the kidneys is to **excrete waste products of metabolisms** from the body such as urea, creatinine, uric acid, etc. dissolved in urine. Kidneys form urine and excrete many toxic waste products from the body dissolved in urine. Thus, kidneys prevent their accumulation to a dangerous level in the body.
2. **Regulation of ECF volume:** Kidneys play an important role in regulation of ECF volume of the body. Many hormones such as aldosterone, ADH, ANP, angiotensin etc. involved in regulation of ECF volume act on kidney tubules to achieve this function. These hormones modify **reabsorption of sodium and water from kidneys** to control ECF volume.
3. **Regulation of blood pressure (BP):** Kidneys contribute mainly to **long-term regulation of arterial volume and pressure**. Renin secreted from kidney activates renin-angiotensin-aldosterone axis that plays an important role in regulation of BP. Many hormones act on kidney to regulate blood volume and pressure. Kidneys have also their intrinsic mechanisms to alter sodium and water excretion to regulate BP.

4. **Regulation of electrolyte composition of body fluids:** Composition of electrolytes in ECF is mainly the function of kidney. **Excretion and reabsorption of electrolytes** from kidneys directly influence their concentration in ECF. Kidneys also contribute to vitamin D synthesis that controls plasma calcium concentration.
5. **Acid-base balance:** Kidneys contribute significantly to acid-base balance by controlling **bicarbonate excretion and H^+ secretion**. Thus, it controls blood pH and pH of other body fluids. Therefore, kidney abnormalities may cause metabolic acidosis or alkalosis.
6. **Regulation of plasma osmolality:** By controlling **NaCl and water reabsorption**, kidneys control plasma osmolality. Change in plasma osmolality provides feedback signal for secretion of ADH that acts on kidney to regulate the osmolality.
7. **Regulation of erythropoiesis: Erythropoietin**, the major regulator of erythropoiesis is secreted from interstitial cells in the peritubular capillary bed of kidney. Therefore, kidney diseases result in anemia.
8. **Endocrine functions:** Kidney secretes **thromboxane A_2** and **prostaglandins**, in addition to the secretion of erythropoietin. Kidneys secrete **renin** that activates renin-angiotensin system. Kidneys also form **calcitriol** (1,25-dihydroxycholecalciferol), the active form of vitamin D_3 from 25-hydroxycholecalciferol.
9. **Gluconeogenesis:** Though kidneys are not the primary site of gluconeogenesis, in starvations, synthesis of glucose from noncarbohydrate sources, especially from glutamine occurs in these organs.

FUNCTIONAL ANATOMY

Kidneys are primary organs of the urinary system that also includes ureters, urinary bladder, and urethra. Kidneys form urine from the blood, which is excreted through the ureters and stored in the bladder. Once volume of urine in the bladder attains a critical level, micturition reflex is activated that expels urine through the urethra.

Gross Anatomy

Kidneys are bean shaped paired **retroperitoneal organs** present in the posterior part of the abdomen just above the waist between the **last thoracic and third lumbar vertebrae.** The right kidney is slightly lower in position due to the presence of liver on the right side.

1. Size of each kidney in adult is roughly about the size of one's fist (11 cm in length and 6 cm in width), and the weight is about 150 g.
2. Kidneys are covered by a thick capsule called **renal capsule**.
3. The medial border of kidney is concaved and the center of the concavity is called **renal hilus**, from which the ureter comes out of the organ (Fig. 75.1).

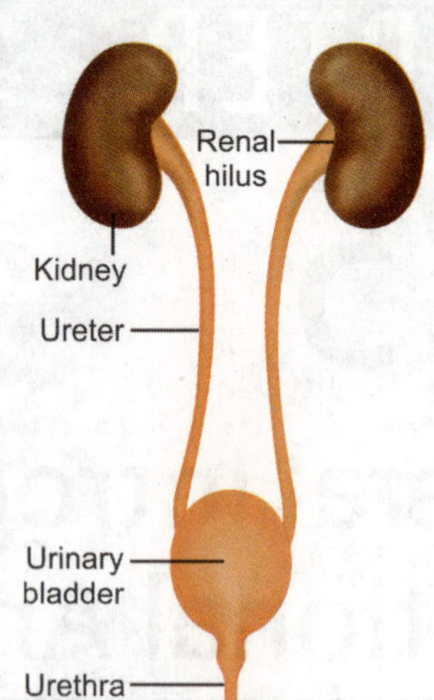

Fig. 75.1: Components of urinary system.

Internal Structures of Kidney

When the kidney is cut vertically into two halves, two distinct regions are seen: The outer cortex and the inner medulla.

Cortex

The cortex is **granular in appearance** and contains all glomeruli, convoluted tubules and cortical portion of collecting ducts.

Medulla

The medulla is **striated in appearance** due to presence of loop of Henle, medullary portion of collecting duct and blood vessels that are arranged in parallel.

The medulla is divided into 8–12 conical masses, called the **renal pyramids** that appear in a radiating pattern. Medullary pyramids originate at the corticomedullary junctions and terminate into a **papilla**, which is present within the **minor calyx**. Minor calyces unite to form **major calyx**. The major calyces open into **renal pelvis**, which is the upper expanded portion of the ureter (Fig. 75.2).

Parts of the Nephron

Nephron is the **basic structural and functional unit** of the kidney. There are about 1.2 millions of nephrons in each kidney in human beings. The nephrons are hollow tubes through which the blood is filtered and modified to finally form urine. A nephron consists of renal corpuscle, proximal convoluted tubule (PCT), loop of Henle, distal convoluted tubule (DCT), and collecting duct system (Fig. 75.3). Each segment of the nephron consists of a single layer of epithelial cells placed on the basement membrane that are modified to perform specific transport functions suitable for that segment. The total length of the nephron ranges from 45 to 65 mm.

The Renal Corpuscle

The renal corpuscle, also called Bowman's capsule, contains the **glomerulus**, a tuft of capillaries. **Bowman's capsule** filters blood from glomerular capillaries to form the **ultrafiltrate**, which is delivered into proximal tubule (details of renal corpuscle is described below).

The Proximal Tubule

This is the **initial segment** of the nephron, hence called proximal tubule (PT). As most part of it is coiled, proximal tubule is also called **proximal convoluted tubule** (PCT). It ends in a small straight segment that continues to form loop of Henle. The PT is about 15 mm long and 40 µm in diameter. PT **recovers most of the filtrate** for its considerable capacity of reabsorption. Hence the tubular cells of PT exhibit features that correlate with their functions (Fig. 75.4A).

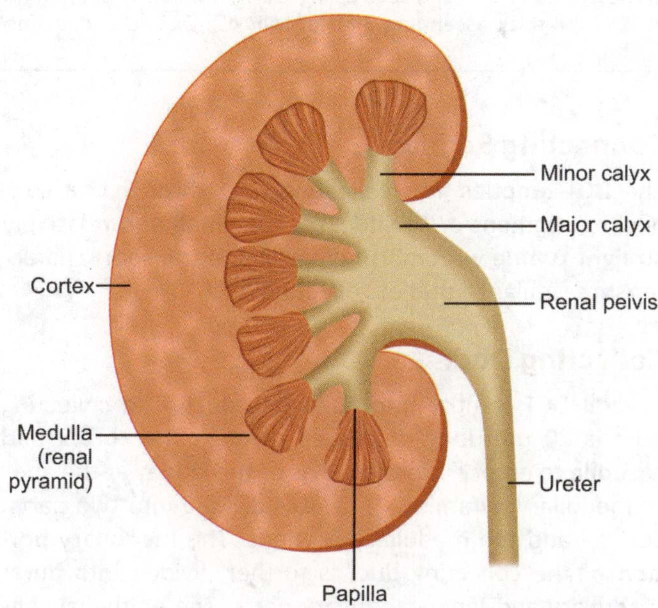

Fig. 75.2: Gross histological structure of kidney in sagittal section.

1. The proximal tubular epithelial cells have **extensive folding of the apical membrane**. Also, apical membrane contains **microvilli (brush border)** that further increase the luminal surface area for transport of ions and water.
2. The basolateral membrane of epithelial cells has multiple infoldings.
3. The epithelial cells **contain many mitochondria** that are present toward the basal part of the cells.
4. The adjoining epithelial cells are **bound to each other by tight junctions** at their luminal ends creating **paracellular and basolateral spaces** that help in transport of solutes and water.

The PT is divided into **two parts**: The initial major convoluted portion (**pars convoluta**) and the distal smaller straight portion (**pars recta**) that opens into loop of Henle. Pars convoluta constitutes about 70% of the PT. The number of infoldings of luminal border and the number of mitochondria in pars recta are less than in pars convoluta.

Loop of Henle

Loop of Henle (LOH) is the continuation of pars recta of PT. It consists of descending and ascending limbs. The **descending limb** is thin throughout in all nephrons, whereas the **ascending limb** has thin and thick portions in a typical juxtamedullary nephron.

1. Thus LOH ***in juxtamedullary nephrons*** has **three parts**: thin descending, thin ascending and thick ascending limbs.
2. In a ***cortical nephron***, thin ascending part of LOH is almost absent.
3. The total length of LOH varies from 14 to 26 mm depending on the type of nephrons (*see* below). The thin limb is about 2 to 14 mm long and the thick limb is about 12 mm long.
4. About **15% of filtrate is reabsorbed in LOH**. The LOH of juxtamedullary nephrons plays an important role in **counter-current mechanism of urine concentration**.

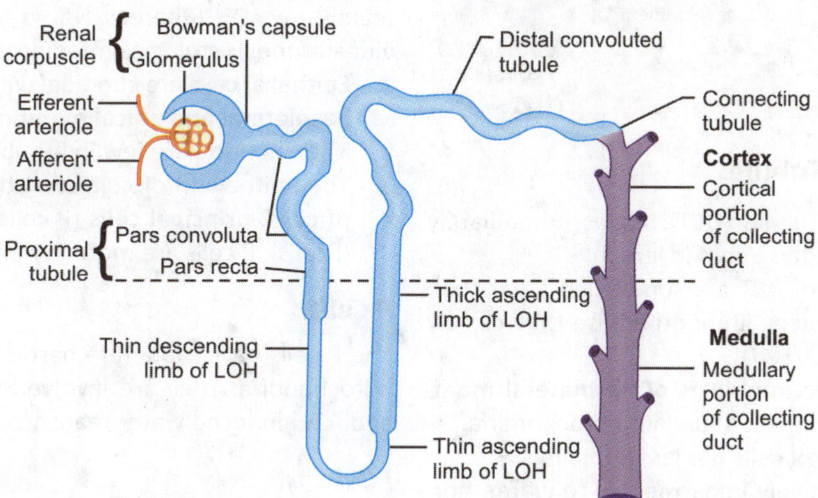

Fig. 75.3: Parts of a nephron. Parts of nephron in this picture are drawn wide apart from each other and length of PCT has been shortened to show their distinctness.

Thin Limb of LOH

The length of hairpin loop depends mainly on the length of thin part, which varies from 2 mm in superficial or cortical nephrons to 14 mm in juxtamedullary nephrons (*see* Fig. 75.3). **In cortical nephrons**, thin segment is very short and has no ascending portion and barely penetrates medulla. **In juxtamedullary nephrons**, the thin segment is long, has an ascending portion and penetrates deep into the medulla. The diameter of thin limb of LOH is about 15 μm. The structure of thin segment of LOH is simple suggesting the passive nature of exchange of solutes and water in this part.

1. The **epithelial cells are flat** with relatively **smooth apical and basolateral membranes.**
2. Cells contain few mitochondria (Fig. 75.4B).

Thick Limb of LOH

The transition between thin and thick parts of ascending limb is abrupt. The tubular diameter increases from 15 μm to 30 μm. Changes also occur in histology that suits for active transport of solutes and water.

1. Epithelial cells are small and cuboidal.
2. The basolateral membrane of cells has **extensive infoldings.**
3. The luminal surface of cells has less infoldings.
4. Cells contain **numerous mitochondria** that are mainly located toward basal part (Fig. 75.4C).

The thick ascending limb of LOH terminates in DCT. The junction between the thick ascending limb and DCT comes in contact with the afferent or efferent arteriole **to form JG apparatus** (described below). The tubular epithelial cells at this junction are histologically modified **to form macula densa**.

Scientist Contributed

Friedrich Gustav Jacob Henle (1809–1885) was a German physician, pathologist, and anatomist who had described the details of kidney structure. He is credited with the discovery of the **loop of Henle in the kidney**. He was an important figure in the development of modern medicine.

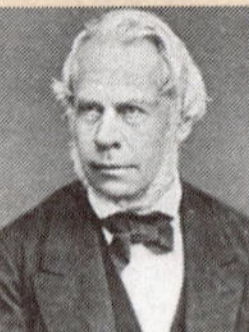

FGJ Henle
(1809–1885)

Distal Convoluted Tubule

The distal convoluted tubule (DCT) begins immediately after the macula densa. It is 5 mm in length.

1. The epithelial cells of DCT are somewhat larger than those of thick ascending limb; otherwise they closely resemble them (Fig. 75.4D).
2. They have **extensive infoldings of basolateral membrane** of cells that contain abundant mitochondria.
3. The luminal surface of cells has less infoldings.

Though, DCT is **relatively impermeable to water**, hormones like aldosterone and ADH facilitate its absorption in this segment.

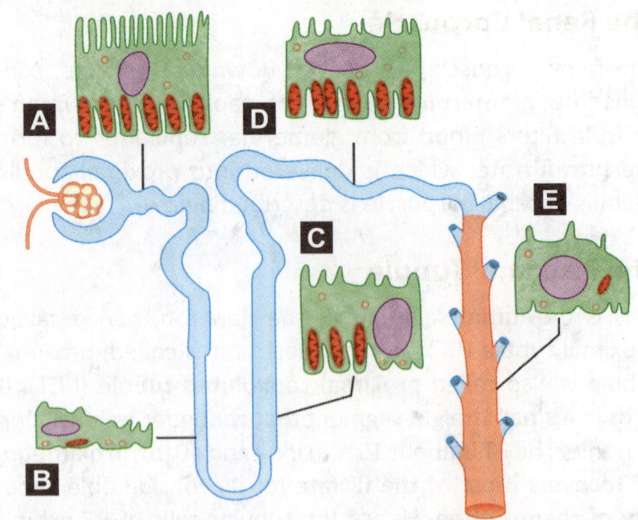

Figs. 75.4A to E: Histological specialties of different parts of nephron. Note the structural differences in epithelial cells of different parts (as described in the text) such as in PCT (A); thin descending limb of LOH (B); thick ascending limb of LOH (C); DCT (D); collecting duct (E).

Connecting Segment

The DCT empties into collecting duct through the connecting segment or tubule. This is a **small and relatively straight tubule** with morphological and transport characteristics similar to that of collecting duct.

Collecting Duct

Several DCTs empty into collecting duct. The collecting duct is 20 mm long. It **passes through the cortex and medulla** to empty into the pelvis of the kidney at the apex of medullary pyramids. Thus, it is divided into two parts: cortical and the medullary portions. The **medullary portion** of the collecting duct is further divided into outer medullary and inner medullary parts. The epithelial cells of collecting duct are modified to participate in transport of ions and water. The water permeability is controlled mainly by ADH whereas Na^+ transport is controlled by aldosterone. Histological modifications are as follows:

1. Epithelial cells are cuboidal with **minimal infoldings of basolateral and apical membrane.**
2. Mitochondria are few in number (Fig. 75.4E).
3. The epithelium of collecting duct contains **two types of cells**: **principal cells** (P cells) and **intercalated cells** (I cells). P cells are more in number than I cells.

P Cells

The P cells have moderate basolateral infoldings and few mitochondria. They are involved in sodium reabsorption and ADH-induced water reabsorption.

I Cells

The I cells contain more microvilli, more basolateral infoldings and more mitochondria. They are involved in acid secretion and bicarbonate transport. Few I cells are also present in DCT.

Secretory Cells of Kidney

The secretory or **endocrine cells** in kidney are mainly two types:

1. **Juxtaglomerular (JG cells) cells:** JG cells **secrete renin** that activates renin-angiotensin system.
2. **Interstitial cells (IS cells):** Three are two types of interstitial cells: cortical and medullary.

Cortical interstitial cells are of two types: Phagocytic and fibroblast-like cells. **Fibroblast-like cells** (peritubular interstitial cells) secrete erythropoietin. **Medullary interstitial cells** are of two types: type-I and type-II. **Type-I medullary interstitial cells** secrete prostaglandins, especially PGE_2.

Types of Nephron

Anatomically, there are **three types of nephrons**:

1. Superficial nephrons
2. Mid-cortical nephrons
3. Juxtamedullary nephrons

Glomerular capsules of superficial nephrons are located in the superficial layer of the cortex, hence called superficial nephrons. Similarly, the renal corpuscles of mid-cortical nephrons are located in middle of the cortex. However, physiologically, superficial and mid-cortical nephrons are considered as **cortical nephrons** due to their similarity in histological morphologies and functions.

Cortical Nephrons

The renal corpuscle of cortical nephrons is located in superficial region of the cortex. The glomerulus is usually smaller. LOH of these nephrons is short. LOH **does not have a thin ascending limb** (Fig. 75.5).

1. However, the total length of the nephron is almost same as the juxtamedullary nephron, as the DCT is longer.
2. Efferent arteriole supplying cortical nephron **branches into peritubular capillaries** that surround the segments of the nephron of its own and of adjacent ones (Table 75.1).

Juxtamedullary Nephrons

The renal corpuscle of juxtamedullary nephrons is located in the juxtamedullary region of the cortex, i.e. the inner region of the cortex close to medulla.

1. The glomerulus is usually larger.
2. They **have long loop of Henle** that extends deep into the medulla. They also have a thin ascending part of LOH.
3. The efferent arterioles form peritubular capillaries and a series of vascular loops called **vasa recta** (for details, *see* next chapter).

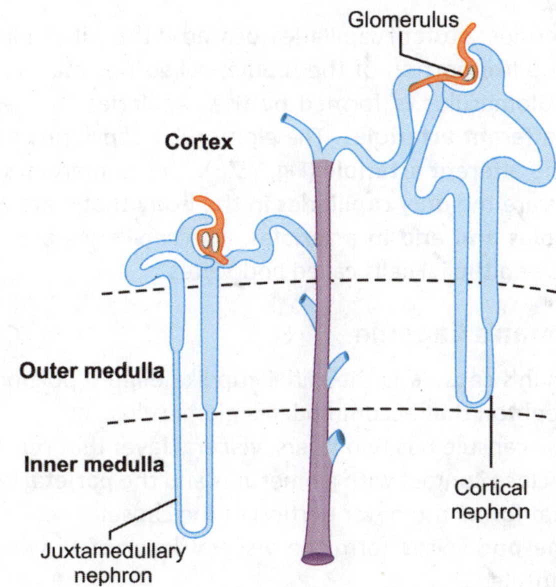

Fig. 75.5: Differences between cortical and juxtamedullary nephrons. Note that the renal corpuscle is located in superficial layers of cortex in cortical nephron and close to corticomedullary junction in juxtamedullary nephron. Also note the size of glomerulus which is small in cortical nephron and large in juxtamedullary nephron. In cortical nephron, the loop of Henle is small, does not have a thin ascending limb and does not extend into the inner medulla. In juxtamedullary nephron, the loop of Henle is long, has a thin ascending limb and extends deep into the inner medulla.

Table 75.1: Differences between cortical and juxtamedullary nephrons.

	Cortical nephrons	Juxtamedullary nephrons
1. Location of renal corpuscle	In the superficial region of cortex	In the juxtamedullary region of the cortex
2. Number	85% of total	15% of total
3. Length of LOH	Shorter	Longer
4. Length of thin limb of LOH	Shorter, and thin ascending is almost absent	Longer, and thin limb has ascending & descending parts
5. Size of glomerulus	Usually small	Usually large
6. Rate of filtration	Slow	High
7. Efferent arteriole	Forms peritubular capillaries.	Forms peritubular capillaries and vasa recta.
8. Efficiency in concentrating urine	Less	More
9. Renin content	More	Less
10. Main function	Urine formation &excretion of waste products	Urine concentration

Ultrastructure of Renal Corpuscle

Renal corpuscle consists of **Bowman's capsule** that contains **glomerulus** and **mesangium**. This executes the first step in urine formation. The formation of urine involves **three major steps:** Ultrafiltration, tubular reabsorption, and tubular secretion. **Ultrafiltration, the first step in urine formation** occurs in the renal corpuscle in which plasma is differentially filtered to form the tubular fluid. This is the initial and important step of urine formation as it considerably contributes to the volumes and composition of urine.

Glomerulus

Glomerulus, a tuft of capillaries located in the initial dilated and cup like portion of the tubule, called Bowman's capsule. Glomerulus is formed by the capillaries that arise from **afferent arterioles**. The glomerular capillaries drain into the **efferent arteriole** (Fig. 75.6). The glomerular capillaries are the **only capillaries in the body that start with arterioles and end in arterioles**. The capillaries are covered by epithelial cells called podocytes.

Bowman's Capsule

Bowman's capsule is the initial cup like dilated portion of the nephron that accommodates glomerulus.

1. The capsule has two layers: **visceral layer** that remains in close contact with glomerulus and the **parietal layer** that forms the outer portion of the capsule.
2. The **podocytes** form the visceral layer of Bowman's capsule.
3. The parietal layer of the Bowman's capsule is formed by **parietal epithelial cells** (Fig. 75.7A). The space between visceral and parietal layers is called **Bowman's space**.

Scientist contributed

Sir William Bowman (1816–1892) was an English surgeon, histologist and anatomist. He is best known for his research using microscopes to study various human organs. was the first scientist to propose the theory of kidney secretion and glomerular filtration. He gave the classical account of striated muscle, lens and ciliary muscle. The renal capsule that contains glomerulus is known after him as **Bowman's capsule**.

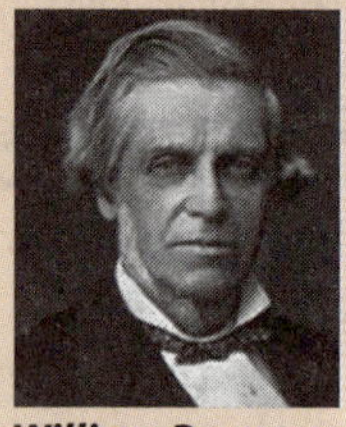

William Bowman *(1816–1892)*

Filtration Barrier

The endothelial cells of glomerular capillaries are covered by basement membrane. Podocytes surround this basement membrane. The capillary endothelial cells, basement membrane, and foot process of podocytes form the filtration barrier (Fig. 75.7B) through which blood from glomerular capillaries is filtered to form the tubular fluid.

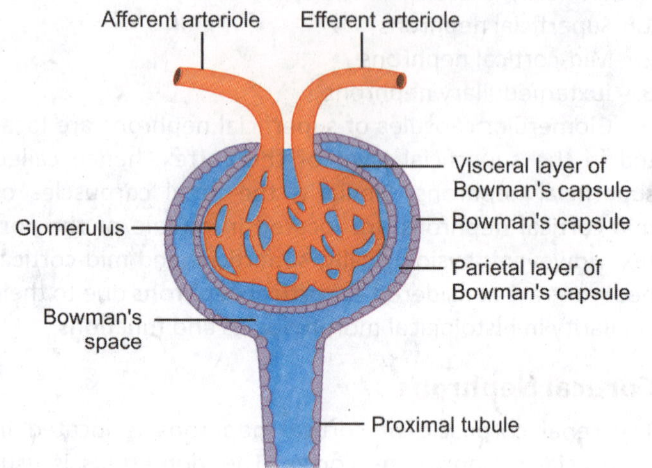

Fig. 75.6: Structure of renal corpuscle.

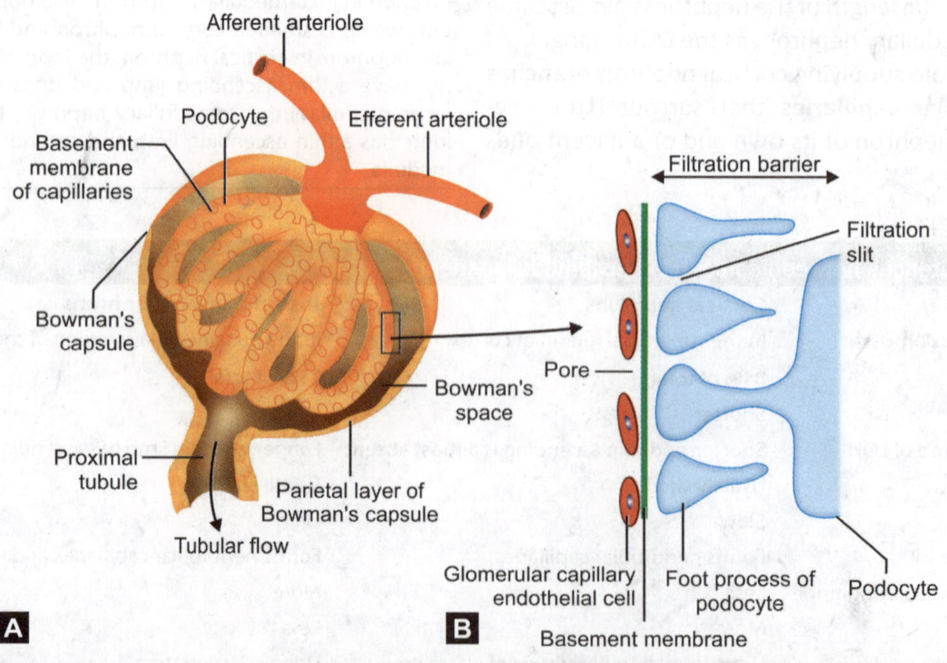

Figs. 75.7A and B: (A) Ultrastructure of renal corpuscle; (B) Structure of glomerulo-capsular filtering membrane.

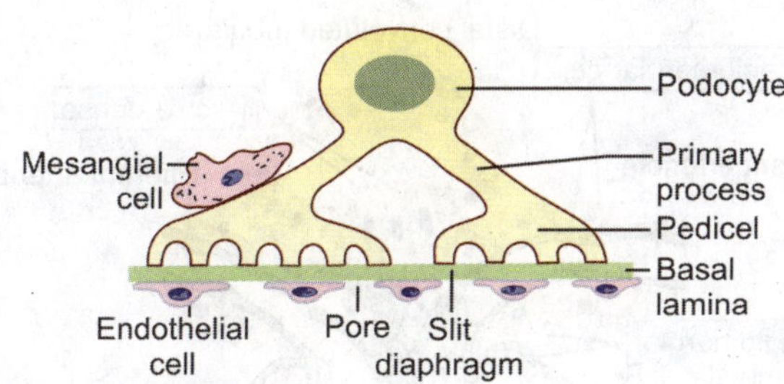

Fig. 75.8: The filtration slit.

Capillary Endothelium

The endothelium of glomerular capillaries is of **fenestrated type** as it contains fenestra (**pores** or windows).

1. These pores are large in diameter (50 to 100 nm in diameter) and therefore, they freely allow passage of large molecules through them. This allows water and small solutes like sodium, urea, and glucose to pass through the capillary endothelium.
2. The endothelial cells are **negatively charged** due to presence of anionic glycoproteins on their surface. The proteins in plasma are also anionic.
3. Therefore, **protein molecules are not easily filtered** through the filtration barrier. Hence, normally protein is absent in urine.

Basement Membrane

The basement membrane is made up of a **meshwork of fine fibrils** entrenched in a gel like matrix. It is an important **barrier for the proteins** as the matrix contains collagen, laminin, fibronectin, and other negatively charged proteins.

Foot Processes of Podocytes

The podocytes (**foot cells**) form the third or the **inner layer of the filtration barrier.**

1. Podocytes constitute the **visceral layer of Bowman's capsule**. They are the **epithelial cells**.
2. Their extensions terminate as foot processes that lie on the outer layer of the basement membrane (*see* Fig. 75.7B). The foot processes of podocytes interdigitate to cover the basement membrane. The interdigitating processes are separated by gaps (the space between adjacent foot processes) called **slit pores** or **filtration slits**, having width of 20 nm (Fig. 75.8).
3. The filtration slits are bridged by a thin diaphragm called **filtration slit diaphragm** that contains small rectangular pores, which do not allow free passage of molecules.
4. The filtration slit diaphragm is made up of a key molecule called **nephrin**. The nephrin molecules form a zipper-like structure. Minute rectangular pores with dimensions of 40 x 140 Å are formed between the prongs of the zipper.
5. Thus, filtration, especially of protein molecules is **greatly restricted by nephrins**.

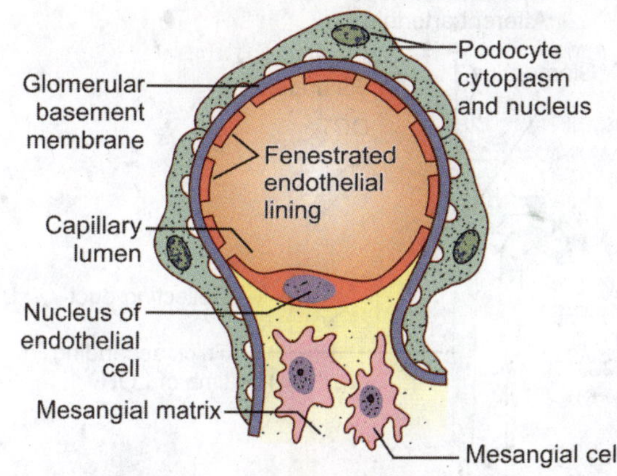

Fig. 75.9: Location of mesangial cells in the glomerulus. Note the relation of podocytes to glomerular capillary.

6. Filtration slit diaphragm also contains negatively charged particles that prevent passage of proteins.

As we understand from the anatomy of filtration barrier, filtration through glomerulo-capsular filtration barrier occurs **mostly through extracellular route** that consists of pores in the capillary endothelial cell layer, basement membrane and slit pores in the foot processes of podocytes of Bowman's capsule epithelium. The molecules with effective molecular radius 20 to 45 Å and cationic molecules are easily filtered through the filtration barrier. In diseases like nephrotic syndrome, the permeability of the glomerular capillaries to proteins increases that leads to proteinuria (Application Box 75.1).

Application Box 75.1

Nephrin mutation causes proteinuria: Nephrin, the key component of filtration slit diaphragm is mutated in **congenital nephrotic syndrome**. Abnormality of nephrin molecules allows free filtration of protein molecules resulting in massive proteinuria, the outstanding feature of the disease.

Mesangium

This is an important component of renal corpuscle. It consists of **mesangial cells** and **mesangial matrix.**

Mesangial Cells

Mesangial cells are derived from blood monocytes and are the components of **mononuclear phagocyte system**. Mesangial cells are present in the mesangium, close to the glomerular capillaries (Fig. 75.9). The function of mesangial cells are:

1. They provide **structural support** for the glomerular capillaries.
2. They **secrete extracellular matrix** (the glomerular or **mesangial matrix**).
3. They secrete **prostaglandins and cytokines**.
4. They are **phagocytic** in nature. They kill and remove the foreign organisms and debris in the kidney by phagocytosis.

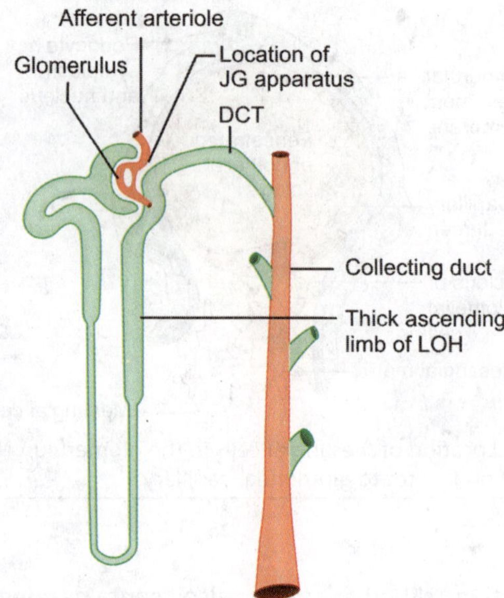

Fig. 75.10: Location of JG apparatus. When terminal part of thick ascending limb of LOH comes in contact with glomerulus and afferent and efferent arterioles, modifications in vascular and tubular cells form JG apparatus.

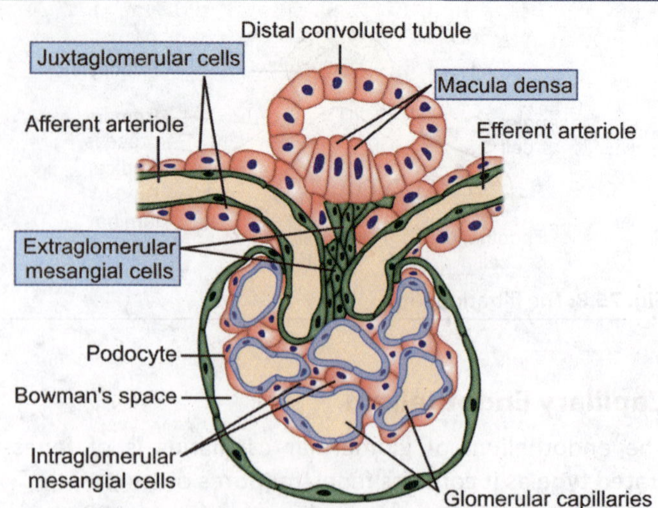

Fig. 75.11: Components of JG apparatus. JG apparatus is formed by modified smooth muscle cells mainly of afferent arteriole (JG cell), modifi ed epithelial cells of ascending limb of LOH (macula densa) and extraglomerular mesangial cell (Lacis cell). *Courtesy*: Figure 54.12, Clinical Anatomy, by Neeta Kulkarni, Vol. 2, 3rd edition, 2016; Jaypee Brothers Medical Publishers (P) Ltd.

5. The mesangial cells contain **contractile units** that are present in close contact with glomerular capillaries. Therefore, contraction or relaxation of mesangial cells influences alteration in GFR by changing blood flow through glomerular capillaries or by **changing capillary surface area.**
6. Mesangial cells that are present outside the glomerulus are called **extraglomerular mesangial cells**. They are also called **lacis cells** or **Goormaghtigh cells.** They are mainly located between the afferent and efferent arterioles. They secrete some quantity of renin and erythropoietin, and also possess phagocytic activity.
7. Mesangial cells are involved in the development of **immune complex-mediated glomerular disease.**

JUXTAGLOMERULAR APPARATUS

Structure

The thick ascending limb of loop of Henle when comes in contact with the glomerulus of the same renal corpuscle, structural modifications occur in the tubule and afferent and efferent arterioles (Fig. 75.10). The entire modified structure (tubular and vascular components and the cells between them) is called juxtaglomerular apparatus (JGA), which includes:

1. Macula densa of the thick ascending limb of LOH,
2. Juxtaglomerular cells (the modified muscle cells mainly of afferent arterioles), and
3. Lacis cells (extraglomerular mesangial cells).

Macula Densa

Macula densa cells are **modified epithelial cells** of the thick ascending limb of LOH when it comes in contact with the afferent and efferent arterioles.

1. The terminal portion of the thick ascending limb of LOH that passes through the angle formed by afferent and efferent arterioles of the same nephron possesses this tubular epithelial modification. This appears as a **dense area** (hence, called macula densa) in the tubule as epithelial cells are densely packed in this region (Fig. 75.11).
2. Macula densa **acts as the sensor** that monitors the **change in ionic composition** and **rate of flow of the tubular fluid** in the lumen of the tubule.
3. It provides appropriate **feedback signal to renal corpuscle** to change the rate of filtration so as to meet the need of the kidney functions.
4. Therefore, this is an important component in the tubuloglomerular feedback circuit (*see* below).

Juxtaglomerular Cells

Juxtaglomerular (JG) cells are the granular **epitheloid cells** present mainly in the tunica media of the afferent arteriole (few are also present in efferent arteriole) that come in contact with the terminal part of thick ascending limb of LOH.

1. In fact, these granular cells are **modified vascular smooth muscle cells** with an epithelioid appearance.
2. The cells are highly granular as they **contain many secretory granules.**
3. They are also called **Polkissen cells.**
4. JG cells **secrete renin** that activates renin-angiotensin system.

Lacis Cells

Lacis cells are present in the triangular space formed by efferent and afferent arterioles and the macula densa. Lacis cells are the **mesangial cells present outside the**

glomerulus; hence called **extraglomerular mesangial cells.** These are agranular cells that secrete some quantity of renin and erythropoietin.

Functions of JG Apparatus

1. JG cells secrete renin that activates **renin-angiotensin system**, which is involved primarily in the **regulation of blood volume and pressure**.
2. Macula densa cells act as sensor that detects the change in rate of flow and volume of flow in the tubule, and composition of tubular fluid. This provides feedback signal to the glomerulus to change the rate of filtration, which forms the physiological basis of **tubuloglomerular feedback**. Thus, they **control glomerular filtration.**
3. Lacis cells **secrete renin and erythropoietin**.

RENIN-ANGIOTENSIN SYSTEM

Renin secreted from JG cells of kidney activates angiotensinogen to angiotensin I, which on further enzymatic action gets converted into angiotensin II and III. Hence, this system is called renin-angiotensin system (RAS). RAS is primarily involved in the control of blood volume and blood pressure.

Scientist Contributed

Robert Adolf Armand Tigerstedt (1853–1923) Finnish-born medical scientist and physiologist who, with his student Per Bergman, discovered **renin** at the Karolinska Institute, Stockholm in 1898. He studied the nerve response to various kinds of mechanical stimulation. His important contribution was the discovery of **a pressor substance (renin) formed in the kidney,** which is discharged into circulation from renal veins, & regulates blood pressure, salt and water homeostasis and is an important therapeutic target.

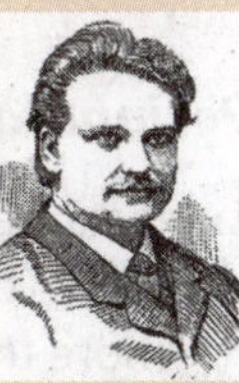

RAA Tigerstedt *(1853–1923)*

Renin

Renin is an **acid protease** secreted from JG cells of kidney. This is a glycoprotein having the molecular weight of 37,326. Like other peptide hormones, it is synthesized as **preprorenin** (406 amino acids), **prorenin** (383 amino acids), that finally becomes **renin** (340 amino acids). Renin acts as an enzyme to **convert angiotensinogen to angiotensin I.**

Regulation of Renin Secretion

Renin activates the renin-angiotensin system, which is essential for regulation of ECF volume, blood volume and blood pressure. Control of ECF volume is closely related to control of plasma electrolyte concentration, especially Na^+, Cl^- and K^+. Therefore, change in plasma concentration of these solutes affects renin secretion. Blood volume and pressure are also affected by sympathetic activity, circulating catecholamine and ADH. Therefore, alteration in these factors alters renin-secretion.

Factors that increase renin secretion:

1. Decreased blood volume and/or pressure
2. Decreased plasma Na^+ concentration, increased K^+ concentration
3. Increased sympathetic activity (stimulation of JG cells via renal nerve)
4. Increased circulating catecholamines
5. Prostaglandins

Factors that decrease renin secretion:

1. Increased plasma Na^+ concentration (increased sodium reabsorption via macula densa)
2. Increased blood pressure (increased afferent arteriolar pressure)
3. ADH
4. Angiotensin II

Conditions in which secretion of renin is high:

1. Hypotension
2. Hyponatremia
3. Hyperkalemia
4. Hypovolemia (like hemorrhage)
5. Dehydration
6. Constriction of renal artery (renal artery stenosis)
7. Cardiac failure
8. Standing
9. Cirrhosis of liver
10. Psychological depression

Role of Sodium in Renin Secretion

Sodium is an important electrolyte that controls renin secretion. Decreased plasma sodium **decreases the filtration of sodium** through the renal corpuscle (glomerular filtering membrane). This **decreases Na^+ concentration in the tubular fluid**. The decreased Na^+ load is **sensed by the cells of macula densa**, which immediately provides feedback information to the JG cells to secrete renin. Renin activates RAS that results in angiotensin II formation. **Angiotensin II increases sodium and water reabsorption** that restores ECF volume. The opposite mechanism operates when sodium concentration increases in plasma.

Angiotensinogen

This is a **glycoprotein synthesized in liver**. It contains 453 amino acids. The concentration of angiotensinogen in the plasma increases by following hormones:

1. Glucocorticoids
2. Thyroid hormones
3. Estrogen
4. Cytokines
5. Angiotensin II

Angiotensin II provides a positive feedback for further synthesis of angiotensinogen. Angiotensinogen is *physiologically inactive*. It **acts as precursor for the formation of angiotensin I**. Angiotensin I is converted to angiotensin II by angiotensin converting enzyme.

Flowchart 75.1: Renin-angiotensin system. (ACE: Angiotensin converting enzyme).

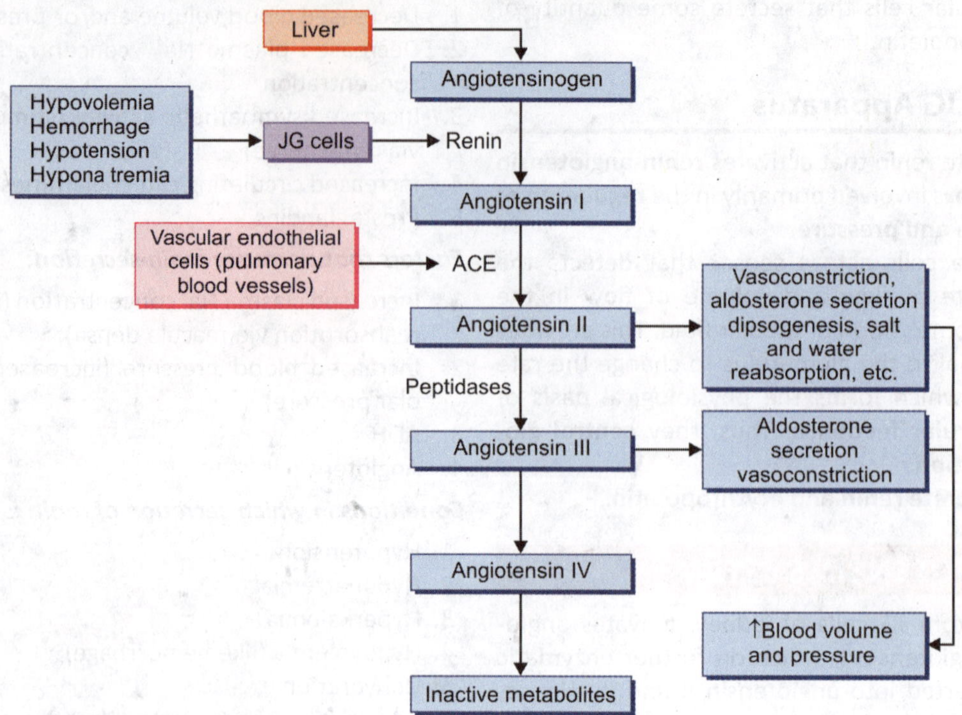

Angiotensin Converting Enzyme

Angiotensin converting enzyme (ACE) is a **carboxypeptidase** that acts on angiotensin I to **convert it to angiotensin II**. Though ACE is synthesized and secreted by the endothelial cells of blood vessels throughout the body, it is more formed in **blood vessels of lungs**. Hence, major conversion of angiotensin I to angiotensin II occurs in the lungs. ACE exists in **two forms**: somatic form and general form. However, physiological significance of existence in two forms is not known. ACE also **inactivates bradykinin**.

Angiotensin II, III and IV

Angiotensin II is formed from angiotensin I by the action of ACE. Angiotensin II has short plasma half-life of 1–2 min as it is rapidly metabolized by various peptidases and is rapidly converted to form **angiotensin III** (Flowchart 75.1). Angiotensin III is converted to **angiotensin IV**. Physiologically, ***angiotensin II is the most active angiotensin***. Angiotensin III and IV are also physiologically active. Plasma renin concentration is measured to determine the angiotensin activity in the body.

Physiological Actions of Angiotensins

Angiotensin I

It acts as **precursor for angiotensin II**. Otherwise, it is physiologically inactive.

Angiotensin II

This is the most important among all angiotensins. All of its actions are aimed at **increasing the blood volume and pressure**. The functions of angiotensin II can be divided into central and peripheral functions.

Peripheral Actions

1. It is one of the **most potent angiotensin I vasoconstrictors**. The vasoconstriction potency of is about 8 times more than that of norepinephrine. Thus, when injected, it increases blood pressure drastically. However, the vasoconstrictor activity of angiotensin II ***decreases in cirrhosis of liver and in patients with hyponatremia***. A chronic increase in angiotensin II level in plasma in these conditions ***decreases the angiotensin II receptors*** on the smooth muscle of blood vessels. Therefore, the vasopressor activity of angiotensin II is less in hepatic cirrhosis and hyponatremic conditions.
2. It **increases the synthesis and secretion of aldosterone** from adrenal cortex. In fact, angiotensin II is the major regulator of aldosterone secretion. Therefore, the RAS is also called ***renin-angiotensin-aldosterone axis***. Aldosterone increases sodium and water reabsorption from kidney that *increases ECF volume*.
3. Angiotensin II directly increases the **release of norepinephrine (NE)** *from the post-ganglionic sympathetic neurons*. Thus, it also potentiates vasoconstriction through NE release.
4. Angiotensin II causes **contraction of mesangial cells** that decreases the glomerular filtration. Therefore, angiotensin II ***decreases GFR***.
5. Angiotensin II increases **sodium, and water reabsorption** from proximal convoluted tubules of kidney.

Central Actions

1. Angiotensin II acts on the **brain centers to decrease the sensitivity of the baroreflex**. This potentiates the pressure effect of angiotensin II.
2. It **stimulates the thirst centers** in the brain to increase water intake. It does not penetrate the blood brain barrier. However, it acts on the **circumventricular organs** (the structures present outside the blood brain barrier) that include subfornical organ (SFO), organum vasculosum of lamina terminalis (OVLT), area postrema (AP) and the posterior pituitary. SFO and OVLT are amongst the thirst centers in the brain.
3. Angiotensin II **increases the secretion of ADH** from posterior pituitary.
4. It **increases the secretion of ACTH** from anterior pituitary.
5. It **acts as neurotransmitters** in some areas of the brain.

Angiotensin III

Angiotensin III possesses about **40% vasopressor activity of angiotensin II**. However, it has **100% aldosterone secreting activity** of angiotensin II. Thus, angiotensin II and III are involved in aldosterone secretion, whereas angiotensin II in primarily involved in the regulation of blood volume and pressure.

Angiotensin IV

This is the recently discovered angiotensin. It has some biological activities in the brain. Probably, it stimulates vasomotor center.

Angiotensin II Receptors

There are ***two types of angiotensin II receptors***: Angiotensin 1 (AT_1), and angiotensin 2 (AT_2).

AT_1 Receptors

These receptors are present in the **arteries and adrenal cortex**. Acting on AT_1 receptors, angiotensin increases intracellular calcium level via phospholipase C that forms **diacylglycerol and IP_3**. There are **two sub-types of AT_1 receptors**, AT_{1A}, and AT_{1B}. **AT_{1A} receptors** are present in blood vessels, and brain, and **AT_{1B} receptors** are present in adrenal cortex and anterior pituitary.

AT_2 Receptors

These receptors are attached to G proteins that **increase the intracellular cGMP**. These receptors are mainly present in fetuses and neonates. However, they are also present in brains in adults.

Clinical Importance of RAS

RAS is implicated in the **genesis of hypertension**. Renin increases angiotensin formation that causes intense vasoconstriction, which in turn increases blood pressure. Therefore, the conditions in which renin secretion is high, blood pressure is invariably high. This is the important physiological basis of **renal hypertension**.

1. In experimental animals, hypertension is produced by constricting the renal artery (producing renal ischemia). This is called **Goldblatt hypertension**.
2. Etiologically, hypertension is classified into three categories depending on the concentration of renin in the plasma: **hyper-renin hypertension, normo-renin hypertension, and hypo-renin hypertension**.
3. In the treatment of hypertension, the drugs that inhibit ACE (**ACE blockers**) are very effective in controlling blood pressure than other group of drugs.
4. The commonly administered ACE blockers are **captopril** and **enalapril**. Angiotensin II receptor blockers like **losartan** have been recently tried.

Tissue RAS

In many tissues, there is renin-angiotensin system (RAS) that generates A II independent of plasma A II. They are found in blood vessels, uterus, placenta, exocrine pancreas, heart, adipose tissue, anterior pituitary, pineal and brain. The exact function of tissue RAS is not known.

INNERVATION OF KIDNEY

Renal nerve controls renal blood flow, glomerular filtration rate, and electrolyte and water reabsorption from the kidney.

1. Renal nerve contains **sympathetic noradrenergic fibers**.
2. There is **no parasympathetic innervation of kidney**.
3. Sympathetic fibers also secrete **dopamine**.
4. Stimulation of sympathetic fibers causes constriction of both afferent and efferent arterioles. However, afferent arteriolar constriction is more. This **decreases renal blood flow and glomerular filtration rate**.
5. The JG cells are innervated by sympathetic fibers. Activation of sympathetic fibers results in **increased renin secretion**.

CHAPTER SUMMARY

Key Concepts

1. Kidney is an important structure for homeostasis of ECF volume and composition.
2. The structural medications of tubular epithelial cells in different parts of the nephrons are primarily meant for their participation in specific functions.
3. The loop of Henle of Juxtamedullary nephron is longer to facilitate its role in urine concentration.
4. JG apparatus is placed at a vital location in the tubule to sense and regulate blood volume and pressure through renin secretion.

Important to Know (Must Read)

1. In examination, Long questions are usually not asked from this chapter. However, 'Describe the functional importance of structural modification of tubular epithelial cells in different parts of the kidney tubules', and 'Describe the structure and functions of JG apparatus in heath and disease', can come as **Long Questions**.
2. Juxtaglomerular (JG) apparatus, rennin, Angiotensin II (AT-II), Differences between cortical and juxtamedullary nephrons, Structure and functions of glomerulus, Functions of podocytes, Renal filtration barrier, are asked as **Short Questions** in exam.
3. In **Viva**, examiner may ask… List the functions of kidney, What is the structure of JG apparatus, What are the macula densa cells and what are their functions, What are the JG cells and what are their functions, What are the Lacis cells and what are their functions, Functions of different parts of nephron, How are epithelial cells modified in different parts of nephrons, Structure of the filtration barrier, How are filtration slits formed, What are the functions of podocytes, How is the renin secretion regulated, What are the factors that increase renin secretion, What are the factors that decrease renin secretion, What are the conditions in which renin secretion is high, How the AT-II is synthesized, List the central functions of AT-II, List the peripheral functions of AT-II, What is the clinical importance of renin-angiotensin system.

CHAPTER

76

Renal Blood Flow

Learning Objectives

On completion of study of this chapter, the student **MUST** be able to:

1. Appreciate the arrangement of arterial supply and venous drainage in renal circulation.
2. Understand why kidney is susceptible to early hypoxic damage in shock.
3. Understand the principles of measurement of renal blood flow (RBF).
4. Describe the mechanisms of regulation of RBF.
5. List the hormones that cause renal vasoconstriction and vasodilation.

The student **MAY** also be able to:

1. Describe the measurement and explain the regulation of RBF.

RENAL CIRCULATION

Kidneys receive about 23.5% of the cardiac output though they constitute less than 0.5% of the total body weight. The blood flow to kidneys is about 1260 mL/min or 420 mL/100 g of tissue/min. Thus, blood flow per unit weight of the kidney tissue is much more in comparison to other organs:

1. However, there is a difference in the regional distribution of renal blood flow, with flow being maximum in cortex and minimum in medulla. Average blood flow **in the cortex is about 5 mL/min/g** of tissue and **in medulla, about 0.5 mL/min/g** of tissue (Fig. 76.1).
2. The low blood flow in medulla **helps to maintain hyperosmolality in the medullary interstitium** that plays an important role in counter-current mechanism of urine concentration.

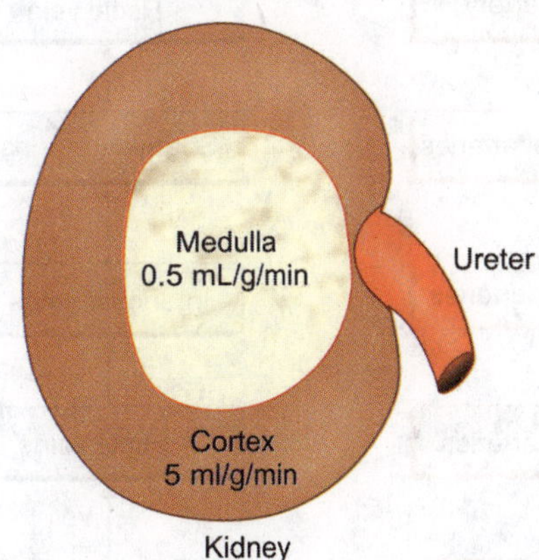

Fig. 76.1: Difference in cortical and medullary blood flows in kidney.

Functional Anatomy

Arterial Supply

Each kidney is supplied by a single **renal artery** that originates from aorta:

1. Renal artery branches to form **anterior and posterior divisions** that form total five **segmental arteries**.
2. Each segmental artery branches into **interlobar artery**, which in successive divisions forms **arcuate artery, interlobular artery** (cortical radial artery) and **afferent arteriole**.
3. Afferent arteriole gives rise to **glomerular capillary** network (glomerulus) that finally drains to **efferent arteriole**.
4. Efferent arterioles lead to a second capillary network, which is formed around the renal tubules (hence called **peritubular capillaries**) (Fig. 76.2).

Venous Drainage

The venous system of kidney parallels the arterial system:

1. Efferent arterioles form peritubular capillaries or vasa recta which drain into interlobular veins. The subsequent sequence of drainage is arcuate veins, interlobar veins, segmental veins and finally the renal vein (Flowchart 76.1).

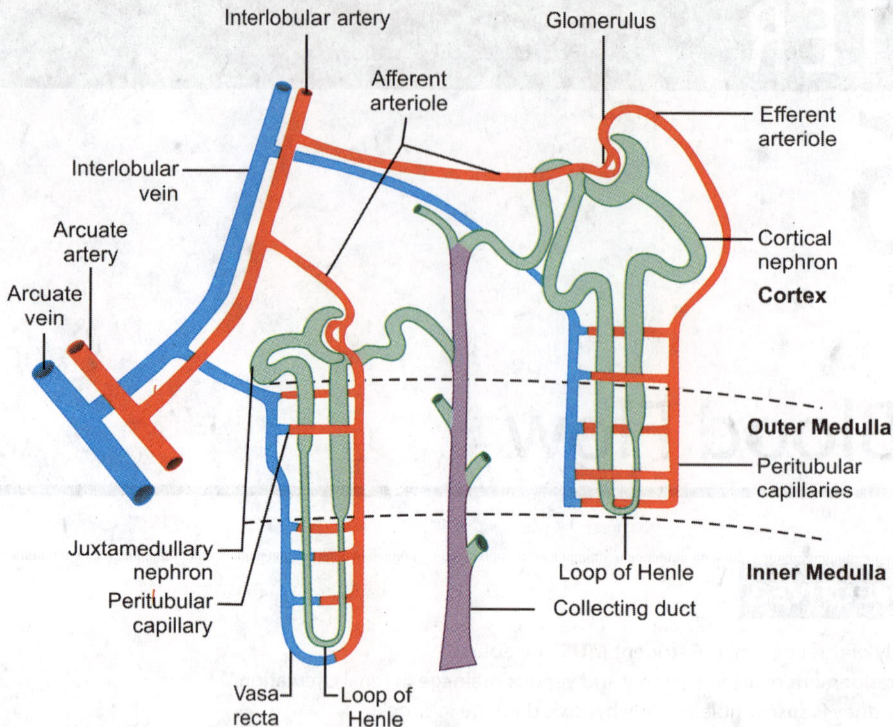

Fig. 76.2: Blood supply to kidney. Note the arrangement of peritubular capillaries in cortical nephron, and peritubular capillaries and vasa recta in juxtamedullary nephrons.

Flowchart 76.1: Sequence of arterial supply and venous drainage in kidney.

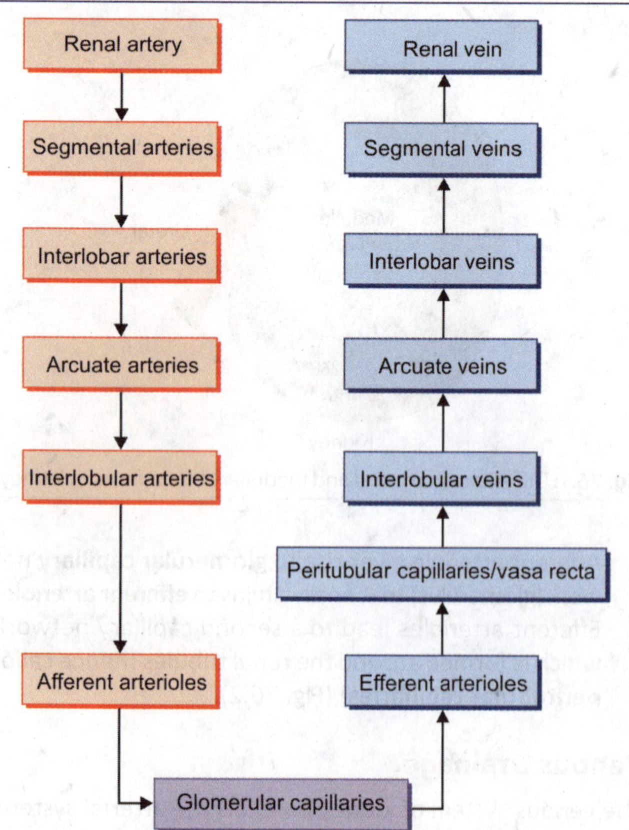

2. In the medulla of kidney, blood supply is derived from efferent arteriole of juxtamedullary glomeruli. These efferent arterioles in juxtaglomerular nephrons, in addition to formation of **peritubular capillaries**, form an extra set of capillaries called **vasa recta** (Fig. 76.2).
3. Vasa recta are straight and long capillaries that run deep into the medulla. Thus, there are **descending and ascending limbs** of vasa recta that remain in close contact with each other.
4. This arrangement of vasa recta helps it to function as the **counter exchanger** in urine concentrating mechanism by exchanging substances between blood flowing into and out of medulla. The blood from the inner medulla returns to the cortex in the ascending limb of vasa recta.

Functions of Vasa Recta

1. It provides oxygen and nutrients to the nephron segments.
2. It delivers substances to the nephron for secretion into the tubular lumen.
3. It serves as a pathway for the return of reabsorbed water and solutes to the circulatory system.
4. It participates in concentration (as counter current exchange) and dilution of urine.

Importance of Renal Blood Flow (RBF)

The flow of blood through kidneys serves following important functions:

1. Supplies oxygen, nutrients, and hormones that control kidney functions.
2. Delivers metabolites and waste products to the kidney for their excretion in the urine.
3. Controls concentration and dilution of urine.
4. Influences solute and water reabsorption from kidney.
5. Determines GFR (RBF is the main determinant of GFR).

As kidneys maintain blood volume, blood pressure and ionic composition of body fluids, alteration in RBF leads to serious consequences. Adequate renal blood flow is essential for these homeostatic functions. Therefore, in hemorrhagic shock, one of the primary objectives of treatment is to maintain renal blood flow so that azotemia does not develop and excretion of waste materials in urine continues to occur.

Oxygen Consumption of Kidneys

Kidneys are metabolically active organs. Therefore, the oxygen consumption by kidneys per unit tissue (6 mL per 100 g of tissue per min) is **more than other metabolically active organs** like liver (2 mL per 100 g of tissue per min) and brain (3.3 mL per 100 g of tissue per min). A greater blood flow to kidneys (**23.5% of the cardiac output**) ensures a higher oxygen supply to the organs.

1. However, oxygen supply to kidneys is more than they normally need. The oxygen consumption by kidneys as a whole is much less, which is about 18 mL per min, in comparison to 52 mL per min for liver, 50 mL per min for skeletal muscles, 45 mL per min for brain and 30 mL per min for heart.
2. Therefore, the **arteriovenous oxygen difference across the kidney is considerably less** than the other organs (Application Box 76.1). This ensures **adequate oxygen reserve** for kidneys in various physiological conditions.
3. Nevertheless, inspite of adequate oxygen supply to kidneys, damage to renal tissues occurs in hypoxic conditions as in shock (*see* below, in physiological significance).

Physiological Significance

The vascular arrangement in most part of kidney tissue permits shunting of a greater fraction of oxygen in the arterial blood to the venous blood before blood passes through the capillaries. Therefore, inspite of adequate oxygen supply to kidneys, the oxygenation of renal tissue is not as high as expected. Hence, kidney is **susceptible to hypoxic damage in shock**.

Application Box 76.1

Venous blood of kidney is bright red: The venous blood of kidney has a bright red color as the red cells in it have high oxyhemoglobin content. This is due to the low renal extraction of oxygen, because kidneys receive much more oxygen than they utilize. Thus, oxygen reserve for kidney is adequate in physiological conditions. Therefore, normally, venous content of oxygen is high (oxyhemoglobin content is more), which makes it bright red.

MEASUREMENT OF RBF

Principle of Measurement

RBF can be measured by **Fick principle**. Also, electromagnetic flow-meter and other flow-meters measure RBF. With the application of Fick principle, RBF is detected by measuring the amount of a given substance taken up by the organ per unit time and dividing this value with the arterio-venous (AV) difference of the substance across the organ (kidney).

Kidney filters blood to form urine. Therefore, renal blood flow equals the amount of a substance excreted per unit time divided by its renal AV difference. The substance used for measurement of RBF should have **following properties**:

1. The substance used should be measurable in the arterial and venous blood
2. Should not be metabolized
3. Should not be stored
4. Should not be produced by the kidney, and
5. By itself, should not affect the blood flow.

Usually the substance used for RBF measurement is **para-aminohippuric acid** (PAH), as it possesses all the above-mentioned properties. RBF is measured by using the appropriate formula that uses renal plasma flow (RPF) and hematocrit (*see* below). Renal blood flow is renal plasma flow (RPF) divided by 1 minus hematocrit (Hct).

$$\text{Renal blood flow} = \text{RPF} \times \frac{1}{1 - \text{Hct}}$$

Thus, first RPF and hematocrit are estimated. Hematocrit is determined by centrifuging a blood sample. RPF is measured by clearance of PAH infused intravenously.

Measurement of Renal Plasma Flow

RPF is measured by **injecting PAH** and then determining the concentration of PAH in urine and plasma. The **extraction ratio** (i.e. arterial concentration minus renal venous concentration divided by arterial concentration) for PAH is high, because PAH is filtered from the glomerulus and secreted by tubular cells:

1. Following its injection, 90% of PAH from the arterial blood is removed in the kidney through its single circulation.
2. Therefore, usually renal plasma flow is calculated by **dividing the amount of PAH in urine by the plasma level of PAH** (concentration of PAH in renal venous blood is ignored). Peripheral venous plasma is used as the concentration of PAH in peripheral plasma is essentially identical to that in the arterial plasma reaching the kidney.
3. The value obtained is called **effective renal plasma flow** (ERPF) to emphasize that the level in the renal venous plasma is not measured. In human being, ERPF is about 625 mL/min in average.

$$\text{ERPF} = \frac{U_{PAH} \times V}{P_{PAH}} = \text{Clearance of PAH } (C_{PAH})$$

For example, when concentration of PAH in urine (U_{PAH}) is 12.4 mg/mL, urine flow (V) is 1 mL/min, and concentration of PAH in plasma (P_{PAH}) is 0.02 mg/mL, ERPF is calculated as follows:

$$ERPF = \frac{12.4 \times 1}{0.02} = 620 \text{ mL/min}$$

ERPF is converted to actual renal plasma flow by the following method:

As the average PAH extraction ratio is 0.9,

$$\text{Actual RPF} = \frac{\text{ERPF}}{\text{Extraction ratio}} = \frac{620}{0.9} = 689 \text{ mL/min}$$

If hematocrit (Hct) is 47%, then RBF will be:

$$RBF = RPF \times \frac{1}{1-Hct} = 689 \times \frac{1}{1-0.47}$$

$$= 689 \times \frac{1}{0.53} = 1300 \text{ mL/min}$$

Thus, renal blood flow, as calculated from the above equations is 1300 mL/min.

Regulation of RBF

Renal blood flow is regulated by neural, hormonal, and local factors, and by autoregulatory mechanisms.

Neural Factors

Sympathetic Control

Stimulation of renal **sympathetic fibers** causes ***vasoconstriction that decreases renal blood flow***:

1. Therefore, conditions that activate renal sympathetic fibers such as hemorrhage, cold, pain, exercise, anesthesia, etc. decrease blood flow to kidney. Though sympathetic stimulation in these stressful situations aim at diverting blood from splanchnic circulation to vital organs, stimulation for a longer duration as occurs in hypovolemic shock causes *renal shutdown and azotemia*.
2. Sympathetic stimulation also **increases renin secretion** from JG cells that **activates renin-angiotensin system**. Formation of **angiotensin II** causes renal vasoconstriction and further decreases blood flow.
3. Fortunately, angiotensin II and sympathetic stimulation to kidneys stimulate the production of **local prostaglandins** (PG E_2 and I_2) that produce vasodilation and oppose the vasoconstriction effects. Therefore, sympathetic stimulation unless intense and longstanding, can not ordinarily compromise renal functions.

Table 76.1: Hormones affecting renal blood flow.

A. Vasoconstrictors	B. Vasodilators
Epinephrine	ANF
Norepinephrine	Dopamine
Angiotensin II	Histamine
Adenosine (A_1 receptor)	Kinins
Endothelin	EDRF
Vasopressin	PG E_2
Thromboxane A_2	PG I_2
	Acetylcholine
	Adenosine (A_2 receptor)

Hormonal Factors

Circulating catecholamines and other vasoactive peptides like angiotensin II cause renal vasoconstriction (Table 76.1). However, dopamine in high dose causes renal vasodilation. Therefore, **dopamine is preferred for the treatment of cardiogenic shock**, as its systemic effect increases blood pressure and its renal vasodilation effect maintains renal perfusion.

Local Factors

Locally produced **metabolites and chemicals** like ***CO_2 and prostaglandins*** cause renal vasodilation and maintain renal blood flow. Though **adenosine** is a potent vasodilator in coronary and cerebral circulations, it causes constriction in renal vascular bed.

Autoregulation

Blood flow to kidney is maintained at a relatively constant level despite the change in systemic pressure range between 80 to 180 mm Hg. This is called autoregulation of renal blood flow (Fig. 76.3).

Myogenic Mechanism of Autoregulation

1. The renal autoregulatory mechanism is an **intrinsic phenomenon** as it is also observed in isolated and denervated kidney.
2. However, it is absent when renal vascular smooth muscle is paralyzed by drug administration. This indicates that the autoregulation is mainly due to direct contractile response of renal smooth muscle

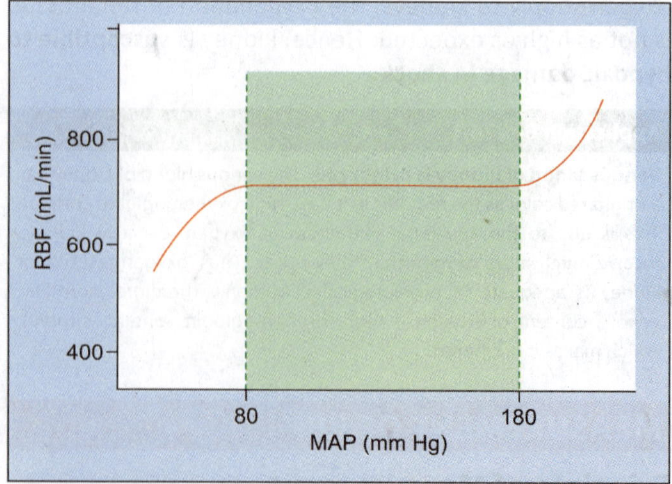

Fig. 76.3: Autoregulation of renal blood flow (RBF). Note, within the mean arterial pressure (MAP) range of 80 –180 mm Hg, renal blood flow almost remains constant.

(of afferent arteriole) to stretch. This is called the **myogenic mechanism of autoregulation.**

3. In this process, increased pressure in the blood vessel causes stretch of the vessel wall that **opens cation channels resulting in depolarization**. This leads to **voltage-dependent opening of calcium channel** causing calcium influx. **Increased intracellular calcium** causes vasoconstriction.
4. Opposite changes occur when blood pressure decreases.

Metabolic Mechanism

Local **metabolic mechanism** also contributes to autoregulation of blood flow, in which NO, prostaglandins, adenosine and other metabolites produced in the tissue influence blood flow.

Glomerulotubular Feedback Mechanism

Glomerulotubular feedback mechanism also plays role in autoregulation of blood flow, in which composition and flow of tubular fluid determine RBF and glomerular filtration.

CHAPTER SUMMARY

Key Concepts

1. RBF is 23.5% of cardiac output, which is much more compared to other organs. This adequate blood supply maintains RBF in conditions of hypovolemia and protects kidney functions.
2. The peritubular capillaries and vasa recta are in close contact with the tubules to facilitate the exchange between tubules and ECF.
3. RBF has well developed autoregulatory mechanisms that adjust blood flow to it despite sudden change in blood volume and pressure in systemic circulation.

Important to Know (Must Read)

1. In examination, **Long Questions** are usually not asked from this chapter.
2. Regulation of renal blood flow, Measurement of renal plasma flow, are asked as **Short Questions** in exam.
3. In **Viva**, examiner may ask....... How much is the RBF, How are vasa recta and peritubular capillary formed, List the sequence of arterial supply and venous drainage in kidney, What are the principles of measurement of renal blood flow, What is the method of measurement of renal plasma flow, What is effective renal plasma flow, List the factors regulating renal blood flow, List the neural factors affecting renal blood flow, List the hormones affecting renal blood flow , What is the autoregulation of renal blood flow, List the functions of vasa recta, What is the importance of renal blood flow, Why is kidney susceptible to hypoxia in shock, Why is the venous blood of kidney bright red.

CHAPTER 77

Glomerular Filtration

LEARNING OBJECTIVES

On completion of study of this chapter, the student **MUST** be able to:

1. Define GFR and give its normal value.
2. Explain the mechanism of glomerular filtration.
3. List the factors that affect GFR.
4. List the chemicals that cause contraction, and chemicals that cause relaxation of mesangial cells of kidney.
5. Give the principles of measurement of GFR.
6. List the conditions that alter GFR.
7. Understand the mechanisms of regulation of GFR.

The student **MAY** also be able to:

1. Describe and explain the mechanisms regulation of glomerular filtration.

The glomerular filtration is the first step in urine formation. This involves **ultrafiltration of plasma** that takes place through the *glomerulocapsular filtering membrane*. The product of filtration is called **filtrate** (the ultrafiltrate of plasma) that flows down the tubular lumen. The composition of the filtrate is altered as it passes through different parts of the tubule to finally become the urine. As the rate of filtration is the major determinant of tubular load, the final output from tubule (the volume of urine) depends on glomerular filtration. In general, factors that impair filtration decrease urine formation, and the factors that facilitate filtration increase urine formation. Therefore, determination of glomerular filtration is an important test in the assessment of kidney functions.

MECHANISM OF GLOMERULAR FILTRATION

Glomerular filtration occurs through the ***glomerulocapsular filtration barrier*** that consists of fenestrated capillary endothelium, the basement membrane and podocytes of capsular epithelium (for details, refer "Filtration Barrier" in Chapter 75) This is governed by ***two major factors***: **pressure gradients** or starling forces (hydrostatic and osmotic pressure gradients) across the glomerular capillary wall and **filtration coefficient** (size of the capillary bed and permeability of the capillaries).

Glomerular filtration = $K_f\,[(P_{GC} - P_T) - (\Pi_{GC} - \Pi_T)]$

When, K_f is filtration coefficient (the product of glomerular capillary wall permeability and the effective filtration surface area), P_{GC} is the mean hydrostatic pressure in glomerular capillaries, P_T is mean hydrostatic pressure in tubule, Π_{GC} is glomerular capillary oncotic pressure, and Π_T is osmotic pressure of the filtrate in the tubule.

Pressure Gradients

The pressure gradients across glomerular capillary wall are different from the pressure gradients along the capillaries of other vascular beds. Therefore, quality and degree of filtration are different through the filtration barrier. Like other capillary beds, the pressure gradients are due to operation of **Starling forces** that are **hydrostatic and oncotic pressures**.

Hydrostatic Pressure Gradient

The hydrostatic pressure in glomerular capillary is **considerably higher** than the capillary pressure in other parts of the body. This is because the afferent arterioles directly arise from interlobular arteries and they are short and straight:

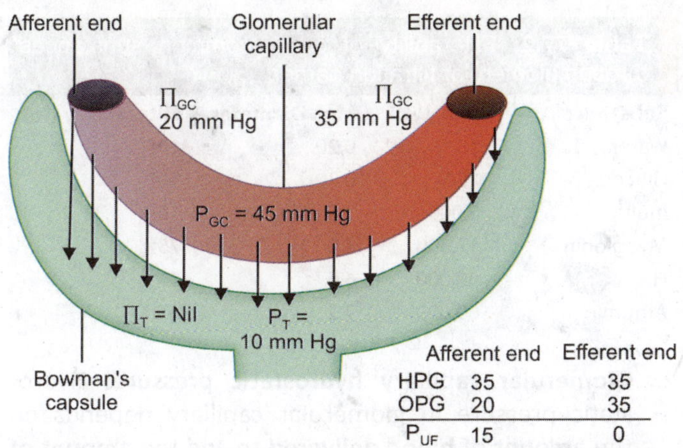

Fig. 77.1: Mechanism of filtration along the glomerular capillary membrane. Note, filtration occurs almost along the entire length of capillary membrane. However, the degree of filtration is maximum at afferent arteriolar end, which gradually decreases to almost zero at the extreme efferent end of the capillary. The magnitude of arrow indicates the degree of filtration. (P_{GC}: Mean hydrostatic pressure in glomerular capillaries; P_T: Mean hydrostatic pressure in tubule; Π_{GC}: Glomerular capillary oncotic pressure; Π_T: Osmotic pressure of the filtrate in the tubule. HPG: Hydrostatic pressure gradient; OPG: Osmotic pressure gradient).

1. The glomerular capillary pressure at the afferent arteriolar end is same as **at efferent arteriolar end**, i.e. 45 mm Hg.
2. This pressure is *opposed by* the hydrostatic pressure **in Bowman's capsule**, which is 10 mm Hg.
3. Therefore, the hydrostatic pressure gradient across the filtering membrane is 35 mm Hg (45–10 mm Hg) towards the capsule.
4. Thus, hydrostatic pressure **strongly favors filtration** across the entire glomerular capillary membrane from its afferent end to efferent end (Fig. 77.1).

Osmotic Pressure Gradient

The hydrostatic pressure gradient is opposed by the osmotic pressure gradient. Osmotic pressure gradient depends on the glomerular capillary **oncotic pressure** and the **osmotic pressure of the filtrate in the tubular fluid**:

1. Oncotic pressure at the afferent arteriolar end is 20 mm Hg and at the efferent arteriolar end is 35 mm Hg.
2. This pressure is **opposed by tubular fluid osmotic pressure**. However, the osmotic pressure of the tubular fluid is negligible.
3. Therefore, the **osmotic pressure gradient is towards capillary lumen** and the magnitude is more at efferent end than at afferent end.

The Net Filtration Pressure: The net filtration pressure (P_{UF}) across the glomerular membrane depends on the **difference between the hydrostatic pressure gradient and the glomerular capillary oncotic pressure** (as the oncotic pressure of tubular fluid is negligible).

$$P_{UF} = (P_{GC} - P_T) - \Pi_{GC}$$

At the afferent end of glomerular capillary, the net filtration pressure is:

Afferent P_{UF} = 35 mm Hg – 20 mm Hg
= 15 mm Hg outward

At efferent end of glomerular capillary, the net filtration pressure is:

Efferent P_{UF} = 35 mm Hg – 35 mm Hg
= 0 mm Hg

Thus, the net filtration gradient is **always from glomerular capillaries towards the tubule**, which is high at afferent arteriolar end that slowly declines to almost nil at efferent arteriolar end.

Filtration Coefficient

Filtration coefficient (K_f) is the product of **glomerular capillary wall permeability** and the **effective filtration surface area** (size of the capillary bed).

Capillary Permeability

Glomerular capillaries are **highly permeable**, i.e. about 50 times that of capillaries in skeletal muscle. However, **filtration depends on** the size and shape of the molecules and the electrostatic charge they carry.

Molecular Size

Molecular size is an important determining factor of filterability of the substance. Neutral substances with molecular diameter of less than 4 nm are freely filtered and substances with **diameter of more than 8 nm are not filtered**.

Shape

The elongated particle with large molecular weight can pass easily, whereas globular particle of same molecular weight cannot pass through.

Electrostatic Charge

The particles with **positive charge can easily pass** through the glomerular filtering membrane than the negatively charged particles:

1. This is because the glomerular capillary wall is negatively charged due to the presence of **sialoproteins**.
2. Therefore, permeability of cationic molecules is more than neutral and anionic molecules.
3. The effective diameter of circulating albumin is less than 8 nm, but albumin is anionic. Therefore, normally **albumin is not filtered** through the glomerular capillaries.
4. However, in **diseases in which the charge of glomerular capillaries is lost** as occurs in glomerular nephritis, albumin appears in urine.

Clinical Significance

Normally, about less than 100 mg of protein is excreted in urine per day. This is not due to the filtration of proteins by the glomerular membrane, rather **due to secretion** by the tubular cells.

Table 77.1: Factors that alter mesangial cell activity.

A. Factors that produce contraction of mesangial cells
- Angiotensin II
- Norepinephrine
- Endothelins
- ADH
- PDGF (platelet derived growth factor)
- PAF (platelet activating factor)
- Histamine
- Thromboxane A_2
- PGF_2
- Leukotrienes

B. Factors that produce relaxation of mesangial cells
- Dopamine
- ANP (atrial natriuretic peptide)
- cAMP
- PGE_2
- Nitric oxide
- Bradykinin

1. In fact, protein is not secreted, but it appears in tubular fluid due to **shedding of tubular epithelial cells.**
2. **Albuminuria**, which refers to excretion of significant amount of albumin in urine, is normally absent.
3. However, albuminuria is seen in diseases in which:
   - There is increase in the size of the pores in the glomerular membrane, or,
   - There is disruption of electrostatic force of glomerular membrane proteins.

Size of the Capillary Bed

The surface area for filtration of the capillary bed depends on the size of **mesangial cells**. The *contraction of mesangial cells decreases the area* available for filtration and *relaxation of mesangial cells increases the area* for filtration. Thus, **mesangial cell contraction impairs and relaxation facilitates GFR**. The factors that alter mesangial cell activity are listed in Table 77.1.

GLOMERULAR FILTRATION RATE

Definition and Normal Value: Glomerular filtration rate (GFR) is defined as the amount of filtrate formed by glomerular filtering membrane of both the kidneys in a unit time. Normally, it is **125 mL/min** (7.5 L/h or 180 L/day.

Factors Affecting GFR

The GFR is influenced by factors that alter renal blood flow, pressure gradients, glomerular capillary permeability and surface area for filtration:

1. **Change in renal blood flow:** Increased blood flow to kidney increases the delivery of blood to glomerulus that promotes filtration and conversely decreased flow decreases filtration. Thus, renal vasodilation maintains GFR.

Table 77.2: Filterability of some common substances through glomerular filtration barrier.

Substance	Mol. Wt.	Mol. Diameter	Filterability (%)
Water	18	0.20	100
Glucose	180	0.70	100
Inulin	5,000	2.8	100
Myoglobin	17,000	4.0	75
Hb	68,000	6.6	3
Albumin	69,000	7.2	0.01

2. **Glomerular capillary hydrostatic pressure:** Hydrostatic pressure in glomerular capillary depends on the **amount of blood delivered** to and the **amount of blood drained** from the glomerulus:
   a. Afferent arteriolar dilation or efferent arteriolar constriction increases capillary hydrostatic pressure and therefore, increases GFR.
   b. Conversely, afferent arteriolar constriction or efferent arteriolar dilation decreases GFR.
3. **Change in capsular hydrostatic pressure:** Hydrostatic pressure in the Bowman's capsule and tubule opposes filtration. **Tubular obstruction increases tubular hydrostatic pressure** and therefore decreases GFR.
4. **Oncotic pressure:** Osmotic pressure in glomerular capillaries due to plasma proteins opposes filtration. Therefore, **hypoproteinemia results in more GFR**. Conversely, dehydration decreases GFR and urine formation.
5. **Glomerular capillary permeability:** Integrity of glomerular capillary is an important determinant of GFR. Increased capillary permeability increases GFR as occurs in glomerulonephritis.
6. **Effective filtration surface area:** Size of filtration area depends on mesangial cells:
   a. Mesangial cell contraction distorts the capillary lumen and decreases the area available for filtration.
   b. Conversely, relaxation of mesangial cells increases filtration.
   c. Many hormones and chemicals control GFR by altering mesangial cell activity.
7. **Size, shape and electrical charge of the macromolecules Molecular size** determines the filterability of the substance:
   a. Any substance having molecular weight less than 10,000 can be freely filtered by the glomerular filtration barrier and molecules with weight more than 10,000 have restricted filterability (Table 77.2).
   b. Most of the proteins in plasma are larger molecules and therefore can not be filtered. Also, the molecular shape influences filterability.
   c. **Slender and supple molecules can easily pass through** than the spherical and rigid molecules.
   d. Due to the presence of negatively charged particles in all the three layers of glomerular filtration barrier, **molecules with negative charges can not easily be filtered**, whereas neutral and cationic substances can do so.

Filtration Fraction

Filtration fraction (FF) is the **ratio of the GFR to renal plasma flow**:

1. Normal FF ranges between **0.16 to 0.20**. This is a better **index of glomerular activity**. For example, decreased blood pressure increases FF without much change in GFR.
2. **In hypotension**, renal plasma flow decreases. However, GFR decrease is less than the decrease in renal plasma flow as efferent arteriolar constriction maintains GFR. Thus, *FF remains elevated*.

Measurement of GFR

Concept of Renal Clearance

Measurement of GFR and RBF is based on the principle of renal clearance. **Renal clearance of a substance is defined** *as the volume of plasma from which that substance is completely cleared (removed) per unit time*. When a substance is removed in urine, a certain volume of plasma is cleared (freed) of that substance. Therefore, clearance assesses an important aspect of kidney function as normally kidney is capable of clearing the substance from the plasma. The clearance of a substance can easily be assessed by determining the concentrations of the substance in plasma and urine, and by estimating the urine flow rate. The formula is as follows:

$$C_X = \frac{U_X \times V}{P_X}$$

When, C_X is the clearance of the substance, U_X is the concentration of substance in urine, V is the urine flow in unit time, and P_X is the concentration of substance in the arterial plasma.

Inulin Clearance Test

Inulin clearance test is commonly used for the assessment of glomerular filtration. It can be measured by measuring the concentration of the substance in urine and the plasma concentration of the substance. The substance **should be freely filtered through the glomeruli and should neither be secreted nor be reabsorbed** by the tubules.

GFR is equal to the concentration of the substance (x) in urine times the urine flow per unit time divided by the arterial plasma concentration of the substance.

$$GFR = \frac{U_X \times V}{P_X}$$

When, U_X is the concentration of substance in urine, V is the urine flow in unit time, and P_X is the concentration of substance in the arterial plasma. As the substance is not metabolized in the body the concentration in the venous plasma can be taken for the concentration in arterial plasma. This value of GFR is called the *clearance of the substance* (C_X).

Criteria of the substance used:

1. It should be freely filtered by the glomeruli.
2. It should be neither reabsorbed from nor secreted in the renal tubules.
3. It should not be synthesized or stored or altered in the kidney.
4. It should not be metabolized in the body.
5. It should be non-toxic to the body.
6. Its concentration in plasma and urine should be easily measured.

The substance usually used is **inulin**, a polymer of fructose, as it meets all the criteria of an ideal substance for measuring GFR.

It is injected intravenously initially as a bolus dose and then through the continuous infusion to maintain a constant concentration in the arterial plasma. Once, inulin equilibrates with body fluids, the urine and plasma sample are collected for its estimation.

For example, if urine concentration is 40 mg/mL, plasma concentration is 0.25 mg/mL and rate of urine flow is 0.8 mL/min. Then:

$$C_{IN} = \frac{U_{IN} \times V}{P_{IN}} = \frac{40 \times 0.8}{0.25}$$

$$C_{IN} = 128 \text{ mL/min}$$

As inulin is neither reabsorbed nor formed, altered and stored in kidney, the *filtered load of inulin equals the rate of inulin excretion*. Therefore, **inulin clearance equals the GFR.**

Creatinine Clearance Test

Endogenous creatinine clearance is used clinically to estimate GFR. Creatinine is the **end product of creatine phosphate**, a skeletal muscle derivative. It is produced continuously in the body and excreted continuously in urine. Therefore, the concentration of creatinine in plasma and urine are normally stable. Its concentrations are measured in plasma and urine and the urine flow rate is (volume of urine formed per unit time) determined. Then, creatinine clearance is calculated as:

$$C_{Creatinine} = \frac{U_{Creatinine} \times V}{P_{Creatinine}}$$

The **advantages** are that no infusion of creatinine is required.

Conditions that Alter GFR

GFR changes in different physiological and non-physiological conditions. The changes are due to the change in renal blood flow, glomerular oncotic pressure, glomerular hydrostatic pressure, change in plasma protein concentration, etc.

Exercise: GFR decreases in exercise ***due to sympathetic stimulation*** that causes more afferent arteriolar constriction than constriction of efferent arteriole.

Pregnancy: In pregnancy, RBF and **GFR increase**. RBF increases due to increase in blood volume, cardiac output and decreased renal vascular resistance. GFR increases mostly secondary to increase in RBF. However, hormonal changes also a play a role. About 40–50% increase of GFR occurs in second and third trimesters of pregnancy.

Posture: Maintaining body in ***standing position for a longer duration decreases GFR*** due to sympathetic stimulation and decreased effective blood volume (pooling of blood in veins of lower limbs and abdomen). Conversely, **supine posture increases GFR.**

Sleep: GFR is usually less during sleep due to decresed circulatory activity. However, supine position maintains GFR.

Weather: GFR is ***more in rainy season and less in summer***. In summer, decreased ECF volume decreases GFR. In winter and rainy season, GFR is more due to decreased loss of water from the body and less humidity.

Gender: GFR is ***less in females*** than in males.

Age: GFR decreases in geriatric age group due to ***functional loss of nephrons***. GFR is also less in children.

Food Intake: Diet rich in proteins increases GFR.

Regulation of GFR

Usually, factors that affect RBF also affect GFR. Thus, regulation of glomerular filtration involves neural mechanisms, hormonal mechanisms, myogenic mechanism and tubuloglomerular feedback.

Neural Mechanism

Both the afferent and efferent arterioles are innervated by sympathetic fibers:

1. The sympathetic activity in the renal nerve is less when the blood volume is normal. When blood volume decreases, increased renal sympathetic activity and increased circulating catecholamines cause renal vasoconstriction that in turn decreases RBF and GFR.
2. ***Activation of sympathetic fibers causes constriction of afferent arteriole*** that decreases blood flow to glomerulus and therefore, decreases GFR.
3. Thus, sympathetic stimulation as occurs in emotion, fear, pain, etc. decreases GFR.

Hormonal Mechanism

Various hormones affect GFR. These include angiotensin, histamine, dopamine, ANP, endothelin, bradykinin, nitric oxide, adenosine, glucocorticoids and prostaglandins.

Angiotensin

ngiotensin II causes constriction of afferent and efferent arterioles. However, the ***effect on* afferent arteriole is more** than that on the efferent arteriole. Therefore, it decreases GFR.

Histamine

The release of histamine locally plays an important role in the control of GFR. Though, histamine causes arterial dilation and increases renal blood flow. However, by causing **contraction of mesangial cells** it decreases GFR.

Dopamine

Dopamine causes **renal vasodilation**:

1. Thus, it increases renal blood flow and GFR.
2. Dopamine also **relaxes mesangial cells** and therefore, increases GFR.
3. Dopamine is produced by proximal tubular cells. Acting locally, it **inhibits renin secretion** from JG cells that decreases angiotensin II production.
4. This also contributes to increase in GFR.

ANP

Increased blood volume increases ANP secretion:

1. ANP causes **dilation of the afferent arteriole** and constriction of the efferent arteriole.
2. Therefore, it **considerably increases GFR.**
3. This contributes to decrease in blood volume by increasing urine formation (diuresis).

Endothelin

Endothelin is a **potent vasoconstrictor**:

1. It is secreted from the endothelial cells of the renal blood vessels, mesangial cells, and cells of the distal tubules.
2. It produces significant **vasoconstriction of both afferent and efferent arterioles.**
3. Therefore, it appreciably decreases GFR.

Nitric Oxide

The endothelial derived relaxing factor **(EDRF)** is the nitric oxide:

1. EDRF causes significant renal **vasodilation** and **dilation of both afferent and efferent arterioles.**
2. This also opposes the vasoconstriction effect of angiotensin II and catecholamines.
3. Thus, EDRF causes **profound increase in GFR.**

Bradykinin

Bradykinin is synthesized from kininogen:

1. It is a **potent vasodilator.**
2. It stimulates release of NO and prostaglandins.
3. Thus, it **increases GFR.**

Adenosine

Adenosine is produced by the kidney tissue:

1. It causes **constriction of the afferent arteriole** and therefore **decreases GFR.**
2. It also plays a role in tubuloglomerular feedback.

Glucocorticoids

Glucocorticoids increase RBF and GFR. But, the mechanism of alteration of GFR by glucocorticoids is not clearly known.

Prostaglandins

Prostaglandins are formed and secreted by kidney:

1. They increase RBF by **decreasing the vasoconstrictor effects of catecholamines and angiotensin II**.
2. PGE_2 causes **relaxation of mesangial cells** that contributes to increases in GFR.
3. In conditions like hypotension and shock, prostaglandins play important role in regulation of GFR.
4. **In hypovolemic shock**, sympathetic activation causes renal vasoconstriction, which deteriorates kidney functions.
5. However, renal vasodilation effect of prostaglandins in shock *protects kidney by opposing the sympathetic constrictor activity* and maintaining renal blood flow.

Autoregulatory Mechanisms

Similar to autoregulation of RBF, GFR is also autoregulated. The autoregulation of GFR maintains a constant rate of glomerular filtration despite change in systemic arterial pressure within the **range of 80–180 mm Hg** (Fig. 77.2). This is mainly due to the myogenic theory and theory of tubuloglomerular feedback.

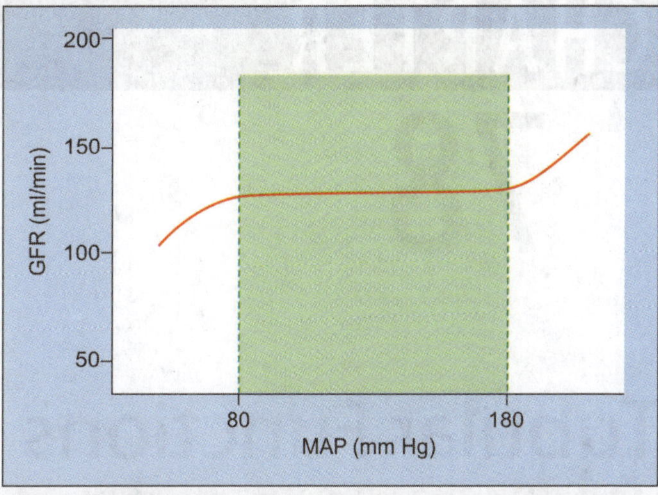

Fig. 77.2: Autoregulation of glomerular filtration rate (GFR). Note, within the mean arterial pressure (MAP) range of 80–180 mm Hg, GFR almost remains constant.

Myogenic Theory

Myogenic mechanism controls renal blood flow and GFR. When arterial pressure increases, the afferent arteriole is stretched and **stretch-induced contraction** of the smooth muscles of afferent arteriole decreases GFR. Opposite mechanism operates in hypotension.

Tubuloglomerular Feedback

Increased renal arterial pressure increases pressure in the glomerular capillaries:

1. This increases GFR and flow of fluid in the tubule, which is **sensed by macula densa cells.**
2. Tubular cells provide **signal to the glomerular apparatus** that causes **afferent arteriolar constriction** to decrease GFR and bring it back to normal and maintain the constancy of load delivered to the tubule. This is called *tubuloglomerular feedback*.
3. The exact mechanism of macula densa cells sensing and then signaling the JGA is not clearly known. However, it is now clear that **macula densa senses the flow dependent changes in NaCl reabsorption.**
4. The likely mediators are **adenosine and NO.**
5. Though adenosine produces vasodilation in most of the vascular beds, it causes **constriction of afferent arteriole.**
6. The macula densa cells synthesize both vasoconstrictor (adenosine), and vasodilator (NO) metabolites. Thus, the change in afferent arteriolar activity is brought about depending on the need by alteration in the secretion of these vasoconstrictor and dilator agents.

CHAPTER SUMMARY

Key Concepts

1. Though GFR depends on hydrostatic and osmotic pressure gradients, normally hydrostatic pressure gradients plays a bigger role. However, integrity of filtering membrane is the most important.
2. Inulin clearance test is the best method to measure GFT.
3. Sympathetic regulation and tubuloglomerular feedback are major systems for regulating GFR.

Important to Know (Must Read)

1. In examination, 'Describe the mechanism, measurement and factors affecting glomerular filtration rate (GFR)' is usually asked as a **Long Question.**
2. Mechanism of GFR, Measurement of GFR, Regulation of GFR, Tubuloglomerular feedback, Filtration fraction, may be asked as **Short Questions** in exam.
3. In **Viva**, examiner may ask...... Define GFR, give its normal value, List the factors affecting GFR, How do the Starling forces (hydrostatic and osmotic pressure gradient) affect GFR, What is filtration coefficient, What are the factors that affect glomerular capillary permeability, List the factors that affect mesangial cell activity, Define filtration fraction, give its normal value, Define renal clearance, give its formula, List the criteria of the substance used to measure GFR, List the conditions that alter GFR, List the neural mechanisms regulating GFR, List the hormonal mechanisms regulating GFR, Explain the autoregulation of GFR, What is tubuloglomerular feedback and how it works.

CHAPTER 78

Tubular Functions

Learning Objectives

On completion of study of this chapter, the student **MUST** be able to:

1. Understand the importance of tubular functions in urine formation.
2. Appreciate the basic transport mechanisms that function across the tubular epithelium.
3. Understand the transport mechanisms of various solutes and water in different parts of renal tubule.
4. Describe the reabsorption of sodium and glucose from kidney tubules.
5. Define and explain transport maximum and renal splay.
6. Correlate tubular functions with its dysfunctions.
7. Understand the mechanisms of regulation of ions and water from kidney tubules.
8. Learn the importance of tubuloglomerular feedback and glomerulotubular balance.

The student **MAY** also be able to:

1. Explain the role of proximal tubule, loop of Henle, and distal tubule in urine formation.
2. Explain the mechanisms of sodium and water reabsorption from kidney tubules.
3. Explain the mechanism of tubuloglomerular feedback and glomerulotubular balance.

STEPS OF URINE FORMATION

Formation of urine occurs in **three steps**: Ultrafiltration of plasma through renal corpuscle, reabsorption of water and solutes from the tubular fluid, and secretion of selected solutes into the tubular fluid (Fig. 78.1).

1. Thus, after glomerular filtration, **tubular handling of the filtrate is the most important step** in the process of urine formation. Glomerular filtration is a nonspecific process in the sense that mechanism of filtration is not different for water and different solutes; whereas **tubular transports are selective processes** as solvent and different solutes are either reabsorbed or secreted by mechanisms specific to their transport.
2. Tubular exchange of water and electrolytes **finally determines the volume and composition of urine**.
3. Thus, tubular mechanisms are most important processes in **determination in urine volume and composition**. By modulating the reabsorption and secretion of substances of its luminal fluid, renal tubule plays an important role in the **control of composition, osmolality, pH and volume of ECF**.

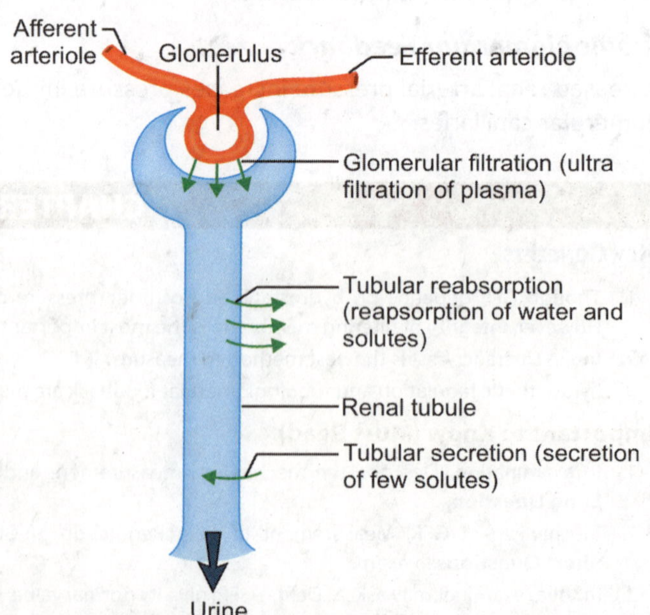

Fig. 78.1: Major steps of urine formation. Note, glomerular filtration, tubular reabsorption and tubular secretion are three main processes in formation of urine. Number of arrows indicates the magnitude of the process.

Scientist contributed

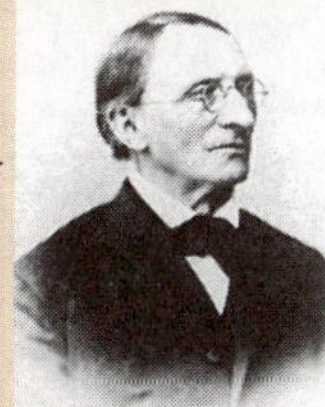

CFW Ludwig (1816–1895)

Carl Friedrich Wilhelm Ludwig (1816–1895) a German Physician and Physiologist, in 1865, at University of Leipzig developed the Physiological Institute, designated today after him as *Carl Ludwig Institute of Physiology*. Ludwig researched several topics, such as the physiology of blood pressure, urinary excretion, and anesthesia. He worked on renal tubular functions, in addition to his works on cardiovascular physiology. He was the first scientist to propose the **theory of renal secretion,** in relation to control of blood volume and BP.

The glomerular filtration rate (GFR) is 180 liters/day, whereas quantity of urine formed is about 1.5 liters/day, which is less than 1% of the glomerular filtrate. Thus, the renal tubules have **vast capacity to reabsorb water and solutes**. Usually, glucose and HCO_3^- are almost reabsorbed completely; water, Na^+ and Cl^- are reabsorbed more than 99%; K^+ is reabsorbed more than 90% and urea is reabsorbed about 50% of the filtrate in the renal tubules (Table 78.1).

COMMON PRINCIPLES OF TUBULAR FUNCTIONS

The major function of tubule is to **reabsorb water and solutes** from the tubular fluid, which is crucial for water and electrolyte homeostasis of the body. These transport mechanisms for various substances are different in different parts of the kidney tubule.

Transport Mechanisms

Processes of transport across tubular epithelium can be broadly divided into two categories: passive and active. Transport of solutes involves both passive and active processes, whereas water reabsorption is a passive phenomenon.

Passive Transport Mechanisms

The passive transport mechanisms include diffusion, facilitated diffusion, solvent drag and osmosis.

Diffusion

The solutes are transported by means of diffusion from their area of higher concentration to the area of lower concentration. This is the transport along the chemical gradient. Especially, uncharged solutes like glucose are transported by this mechanism. However, though charged solutes especially ions are also transported by diffusion, their electrical gradient greatly influences this passive transport.

Table 78.1: 24 hours filtration and reabsorption of various substances in nephrons (in order of % reabsorption).

Substance	Filtered	Reabsorbed	% Reabsorption
Glucose (mmol)	800	800	100
HCO_3^- (mEq)	4,500	4,500	100
Na^+ (mEq)	26,000	25,850	99.4
Cl^- (mEq)	18,000	17,850	99.2
Water (L)	180	178.5	99.2
*K^+ (mEq)	600	560	99.3
Urea (g)	56	29	51.7

*Among the solutes, K^+ is also secreted in the tubule

Facilitated Diffusion

In this transport mechanism, a **specific carrier protein** in the membrane facilitates the process of diffusion. *Reabsorption of glucose via glucose transporter* is an example of facilitated diffusion. Sodium and potassium ions are also reabsorbed from kidney tubule through the water, filled channels created by the carrier proteins. Transport of glucose, proteins and urea from the tubular fluid are other examples of facilitated diffusion.

Coupled transport, which is a form of facilitated diffusion, serves as major mechanism of transport of solutes in the tubules. There are **two mechanisms of coupled transports**: symport mechanism, and antiport mechanisms.

Symport Mechanism

The symport mechanism is the process of coupled transport of two or more solutes in same direction by a carrier protein. The examples are the transport of Na^+-glucose, Na^+-amino acid, etc.

Antiport Mechanism

Antiport mechanism is the process of coupled transport of two or more solutes in opposite direction by a carrier protein. An example is the **Na^+–H^+ exchange** in the proximal tubule that reabsorbs Na^+ from the tubular fluid in exchange for secretion of H^+ into it.

Solvent Drag

When bulk amount of water is reabsorbed, the **solutes dissolved in water are also transported** along with water across the tubular epithelium. This process is called solvent drag. This contributes to reabsorption of substantial amount of solutes in the proximal tubule.

Osmosis

When a considerable amount of osmotically active solute is transported, water is reabsorbed along with it **to maintain the osmotic balance**. This is the major mechanism for **reabsorption of water** from the tubular lumen. For example, water reabsorption follows reabsorption of Na^+ and Cl^- from the tubular fluid. Conversely, increased osmolality of tubular fluid increases water excretion, known as **osmotic diuresis** (Application Box 78.1).

Application Box 78.1

Glycosuria causes osmotic diuresis: Osmotic diuresis typically occurs in diabetes mellitus. In diabetes, when plasma glucose is more than renal threshold, glucose appears in urine (glycosuria). More glucose in tubular fluid causes water retention that leads to polyuria. This differentiates from water diuresis seen in diabetes insipidus that occurs due to ADH deficiency.

Table 78.2: Various transporters in apical membrane of epithelial cells in different segment of kidney tubule.

Site	Transporter	Function
PCT	Na^+-Glucose CT	Na^+ and glucose uptake
	Na^+-Pi CT	Na^+ and Pi uptake
	Na^+-AA CT	Na^+ and AA uptake
	Na^+-lactate CT	Na^+ and lactate uptake
	Na^+-H^+ exchanger	Na^+ uptake and H^+ secretion
Thick limb	Na^+-K^+- Cl^- CT	Na^+, K^+, and Cl^- uptake
of LOH	Na^+-H^+ exchanger	Na^+ uptake & H^+ secretion
	K^+ channel	K^+ secretion
DCT	NaCl CT	Na^+ and Cl^- uptake
CD	ENaC	Na^+ uptake

(CT: Cotransporter; Pi: Inorganic phosphate; AA: Amino acids PCT: Proximal tubule, DCT: Distal tubule; CD: Collecting duct.

Active Transport Mechanisms

Transport of solutes is considered to be active when **ATP is utilized in the process**. In this mechanism, solutes are transported from the area of lower concentration to the area of higher concentration. The best example of active transport mechanism is the **Na^+-K^+ pump**.

1. The Na^+-K^+ ATPase is mainly located in the basolateral membrane of the tubular epithelial cells. This pumps sodium out of the tubular epithelial cells and potassium into the cell.
2. The **other examples** include H^+-ATPase, H^+-K^+ ATPase, Ca^{++}-ATPase, etc. Various transporters in different segment of tubule are listed in Table 78.2

Secondary Active Transport

This is the major mechanism by which **Na^+, glucose and associated solutes are reabsorbed** from kidney tubules. The active transport mechanism, i.e. Na^+-K^+ ATPase located in the basolateral membrane of epithelial cells pumps Na^+ out of the cell. This creates a low concentration of Na^+ in the tubular cells. Therefore, Na^+ is reabsorbed from the tubular fluid along its concentration gradient into the tubular cells.

1. The carrier protein for Na^+ facilitates reabsorption of Na^+ into the tubular cells. Glucose is reabsorbed by the same carrier protein that reabsorbs Na^+.
2. Therefore, reabsorption of glucose by this mechanism is an example of secondary active transport (for details, *see* blow).
3. The similar mechanism operates in the epithelial cells of intestine.

Key Concepts in Transport Mechanisms

Paracellular Pathway of Transport

Close to apical membrane, tubular epithelial cells have **tight junctions** between them. Immediately after the tight junctions between the epithelial cells, the lateral intercellular space starts.

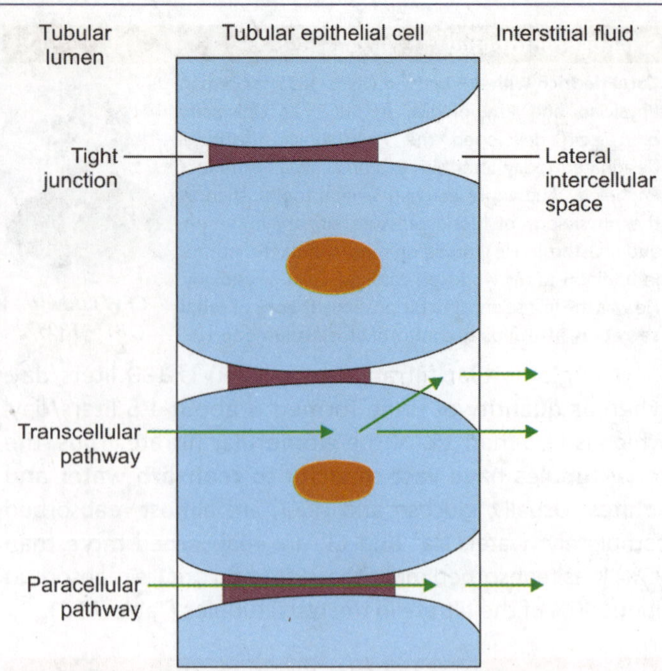

Fig. 78.2: Mechanisms of transcellular and paracellular transports across the renal tubular epithelium. Note that paracellular transport occurs through the tight junction between epithelial cells.

1. However, these tight junctions are not very tight and they have **leaky channels.** When transport of solutes and water occurs **between the cells through tight junctions and lateral intercellular space**, the process is called transport across the paracellular pathway.
2. A considerable quantity of **Ca^{++} and K^+ are reabsorbed** in proximal tubule via paracellular pathway.
3. Some amount of Na^+ and water is also reabsorbed via this route.
4. This is to differentiate from the **transcellular pathway** of transport in which transport occurs through the cell.
5. Transport of sodium and glucose from tubular fluid into the tubular cells and from there into the ECF is the example of transport via transcellular pathway (Fig. 78.2).

Transport Maximum

The transport systems in the renal tubule like transport systems in other parts of the body have their maximal rate, which is called as the **transport maximum (Tm).**

1. This is the rate at which the **tubule maximally transports a particular solute**. That means, the amount of a particular solute transported depends on the amount of the solute in tubular fluid present up to the Tm for the solute.
2. Tm is the amount of the substance **delivered to the tubule per minute**.
3. When the concentration of the solute in tubular fluid is more than the Tm concentration, the mechanism of transport is **said to be saturated**, and beyond this there will be no appreciable increase in transport of the solute. For example, the Tm for glucose is 375 mg/min. in males and 300 mg/min. in females.

Tubular Load

The quantity of a solute ***filtered by the glomerulo-capsular filtering barrier*** and presented to the tubular fluid is the tubular load.

1. Tubular load determines the amount of the substance to be reabsorbed from the tubule, as normally, a constant fraction of the load is reabsorbed by the kidney tubules, which is called ***glomerulotubular balance***. Tubular load also **determines the Tm for the substance.**
2. The amount of the substance delivered to the tubular fluid per unit time (tubular load of the substance) greatly contributes to the maximum quantity of the substance that can be reabsorbed.
3. However, Tm depends on **plasma concentration of the substance** and the **rate of filtration** of the substance, i. e. plasma concentration × GFR.
4. For example, **Tm for glucose is 375 mg/min**, which indicates that plasma concentration of glucose up to 300 gm%, tubule can transport glucose totally from the tubular fluid (300 mg/100 mL × 125 mL/min).
5. However, normally, glucose appears in urine above 200 mg% (more accurately, above 180 mg% of venous blood) of plasma level. This is because of the mechanism of renal splay for glucose (for details, *see* "Glucose Reabsorption" below).

Renal Threshold

This is the **concentration of the solute in the plasma at or above which the solute first appears in urine** or appears in more amount than its normal concentration.

1. For example, normally glucose is not present in urine and its renal threshold is 180 mg% in venous plasma (200 mg% in arterial plasma).
2. Therefore, glycosuria occurs when plasma concentration of glucose is above 180 mg%.

TUBULAR FUNCTIONS

Proximal Tubular Functions

The proximal tubule is the most important part of the nephron as it reabsorbs **about 67% of the filtered water, Na^+, Cl^-, K^+, and HCO_3^-** and **almost all the filtered glucose and amino acids.**

1. The proximal tubule has convoluted and straight portions. Though the convoluted part (PCT) comprises 70% of the tubule, **functionally both the parts are similar** with few minor differences.
2. The primary focus of reabsorption process in the proximal tubule is directed at the **Na^+ reabsorption**, which is usually **secondary to electrochemical gradient created by Na^+-K^+ pump** located on the basolateral membrane of the epithelial cells.
3. Reabsorption of water and most of the solutes is directly or indirectly linked with this pump. Therefore, abnormalities of this pump (i. e. Na^+ reabsorption process in the tubule) results in many renal dysfunctions.

Important Facts: The fluid in the early part of proximal tubule is almost **isosmotic to plasma.**

1. Na^+ and its two major anions Cl^- and **HCO_3^-** are the major solute in plasma and glomerular filtrate.
2. **HCO_3^- is reabsorbed** mainly in the convoluted portion of the proximal tubule leading to its drastic fall in rest of the tubule.
3. **Cl^- is reabsorbed** in the second half of the proximal tubule (later part of convoluted portion and straight portion) which creates a lumen positive transepithelial potential difference that favors passive reabsorption of Na^+.
4. About of 67% of filtered **K^+ is reabsorbed** along with 67% of water.
5. **Glucose and amino acids are almost completely reabsorbed** in proximal tubule resulting in their steep fall in rest of the tubule.
6. Thus, at the end of proximal tubule, only one-third of Na^+, Cl^- and K^+ remain with almost absence of glucose, amino acid and bicarbonate in the tubular fluid.
7. However, **urea concentration is increased** as it is not at all absorbed in this part of the tubule.

Na^+ Reabsorption

In proximal tubule, reabsorption of Na^+ is important among all transport processes as it generates the major driving force for reabsorption of water and other solutes. From tubular fluid, Na^+ enters the tubular epithelial cells along the electrochemical gradient. Inside the tubular cells, concentration of Na^+ is about 35 meq/L in comparison to about 140 meq/L in the tubular fluid.

1. The lower intracellular concentration of Na^+ is due to the activity of **Na^+-K^+ pump located on the basolateral surface of the cells.** Vigorous activity of Na^+-K^+ ATPase constantly removes three Na^+ out of the cell for bringing in two K^+ for each cycle of the pump. This active transport mechanism **constantly creates a low concentration of Na^+ in the cell.**
2. The Na^+ removed from the cell into the lateral intercellular space enters interstitial fluid, and the K^+ pumped into the cell diffuses out of it through basolateral membrane mostly via K^+ channels.
3. Thus, the **net effect** is the decreased Na^+ level in tubular cells. This causes Na^+ from tubular fluid to enter the tubular cells (Fig. 78.3).
4. As the Na^+ entry from the luminal surface into the cells utilizes the energy generated by Na^+-K^+ pump on the basolateral surface, the process of **Na^+ reabsorption is an active transport mechanism.** About 67% of filtered Na^+ is reabsorbed in proximal tubule (Application Box 78.2).

Cotransport and Antiport Mechanisms: From tubular fluid, entry of Na^+ into the tubular cells occurs via various *cotransport and antiport mechanisms* that are located on the apical cell membrane.

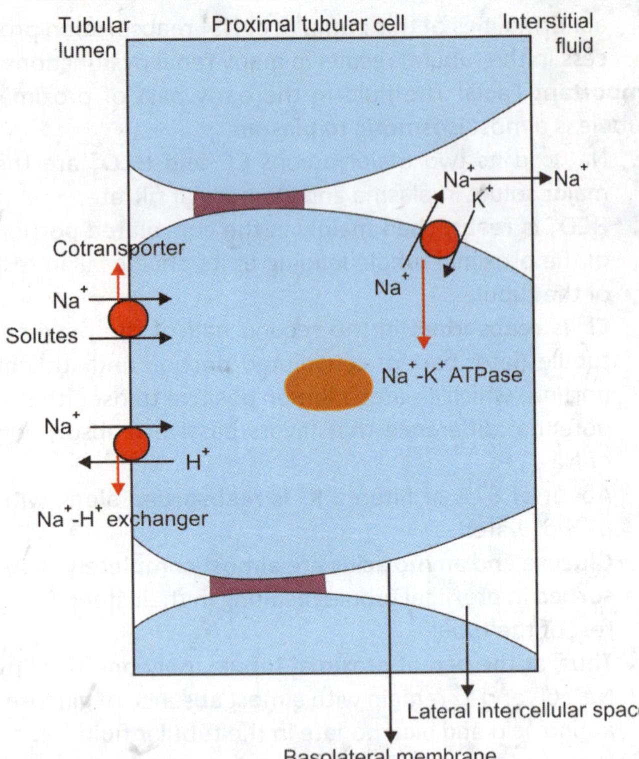

Fig. 78.3: Mechanism of Na^+ reabsorption in proximal tubule. Note that Na^+ pumped out of the cell by Na^+-K^+ ATPase located on the basolateral membrane creates the gradient for Na^+ transport from tubular fluid into the tubular cells. Na^+-K^+ antiport located on the apical membrane contributes considerably for transfer of Na^+ from tubular fluid into the cell.

1. The carrier protein that transports Na^+ also **cotransports glucose, amino acids, phosphates,** etc. Therefore, reabsorption of these solutes is considered as **secondary active transport** (for details, *see* below).
2. Na^+ is also transported from tubular fluid by antiport, especially by **Na^+-H^+ exchanger** which reabsorbs Na^+ into the cell in exchange for secretion of H^+ into the luminal fluid. Normally, Na^+-H^+ exchanger is the primary mechanism of entry of Na^+ into the epithelial cells, which accounts for about 60% of the total Na^+ entry.

Associated Anion Reabsorption: Na^+ reabsorption is accompanied by **reabsorption of anions,** such as HCO_3^- and Cl^- to maintain electroneutrality. However, process of anion absorption along with Na^+ is different in first and second half of proximal tubule.

Application Box 78.2

% of Na^+ reabsorption in different parts of tubule: Normally, 67% of filtered Na^+ is reabsorbed in proximal tubule which occurs mainly by Na^+-H^+ exchange. About 25% of Na^+ is reabsorbed in thick ascending limb of loop of Henle that occurs via Na^+-2Cl-K^+ cotransporter. In DCT, about 5% is reabsorbed by Na^+-Cl^- cotransport mechanism. Remaining of about 3% is reabsorbed in collecting duct via **ENaC (epithelial Na channels)**.

In First Half of Proximal Tubule

In first half of proximal tubule, Na^+ reabsorption is mainly **associated with HCO_3^- and organic solutes** like glucose, amino acids, phosphates, etc.

1. Thus, Na^+ and HCO_3^- reabsorption in the first part of PCT is **coupled to the transport of organic molecules.**
2. Therefore, simultaneous reabsorption of Na^+, bicarbonate, and organic solutes from the proximal tubular fluid **establishes an osmotic gradient** that results in reabsorption of water.

In Second Half of Proximal Tubule

In second half of proximal tubule, Na^+ reabsorption is mainly **associated with Cl^- reabsorption via transcellular and paracellular pathway**. In the later part of proximal tubule, Na^+ reabsorption is coupled with the Cl^- rather than bicarbonate or organic solutes because of **two reasons.**

1. In distal part of proximal tubule, concentration of Cl^- is very high, whereas the concentration of glucose and amino acid is less in this region as Na^+ and bicarbonate are preferentially reabsorbed in the first half of PCT.
2. Also, presence of more **chloride-anion antiporter** in the distal part of the proximal tubule facilitates transport of Cl^- into the cell. Na^+ that enters cell is pumped out of it to enter ECF via Na^+-K^+ pump located on the basolateral membrane. The Cl^- leaves the cell by means of K^+-Cl^- symporter located on the basolateral membrane. Thus, Na^+ and Cl^- are reabsorbed from tubular fluid into the interstitial fluid via tubular cells. This is called **transcellular pathway of reabsorption** of solutes. Increased concentration Na^+ in lateral-interstitial space creates an electrical gradient for Cl^- ions also to move through the paracellular pathway. This is because the *tight junctions between the tubular cells at their apical margin contain leaky channels* that transport Cl^- along its electrical concentration gradient from the tubular fluid into the interstitial space. This is called **paracellular pathway of reabsorption** solutes. This paracellular pathway of solute reabsorption constitutes about 25% of NaCl reabsorption in the proximal tubule.

Thus, Na^+ reabsorption helps in reabsorption of Cl^-, HCO_3^-, other cations and anions and various organic solutes. Transfer of organic and inorganic solutes from tubular fluid into the interstitial space **creates the osmotic gradient for the reabsorption of water** in the proximal tubule.

Water Reabsorption

Normally, 65% of the filtered water is reabsorbed in the PCT.

1. The driving force for water reabsorption is the **transcellular osmotic gradient**, which is established by absorption of Na^+ and accompanying solutes.
2. **Transcellular and paracellular reabsorption** of NaCl and other solutes from tubular fluid into the lateral intercellular and interstitial spaces increases the osmolality of fluid in these spaces.
3. Permeability of epithelium of proximal tubule to water is extremely high. Water passes through the epithelial cells **via water channels (aquaporin 1)** present in the cell membranes and also through the water channels present in the paracellular route (in tight junctions between the cells).

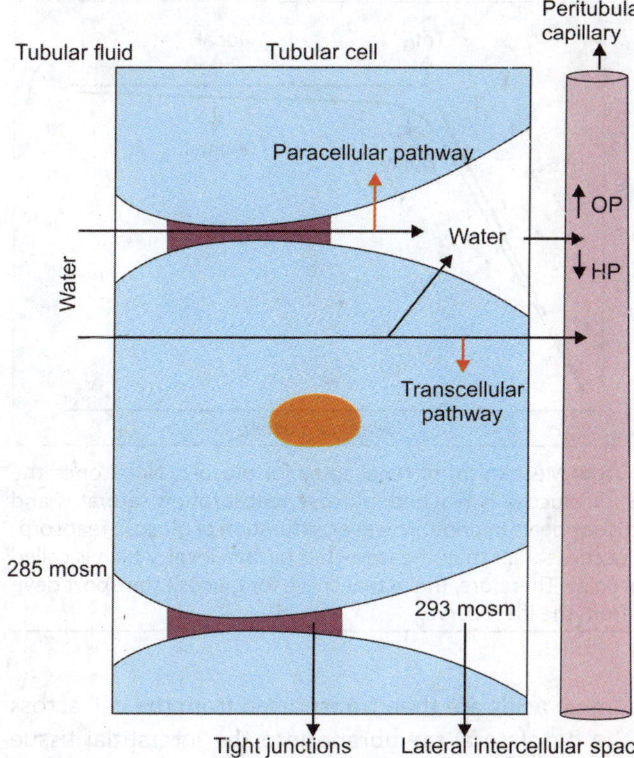

Fig. 78.4: Mechanism of water reabsorption in proximal tubule. Note, water reabsorption is efficient inspite of small difference between osmolality of tubular and interstitial fluids. Water is reabsorbed via both transcellular and paracellular pathways. High oncotic pressure (OP) and low hydrostatic pressure (HP) in peritubular capillary favor reabsorption of water.

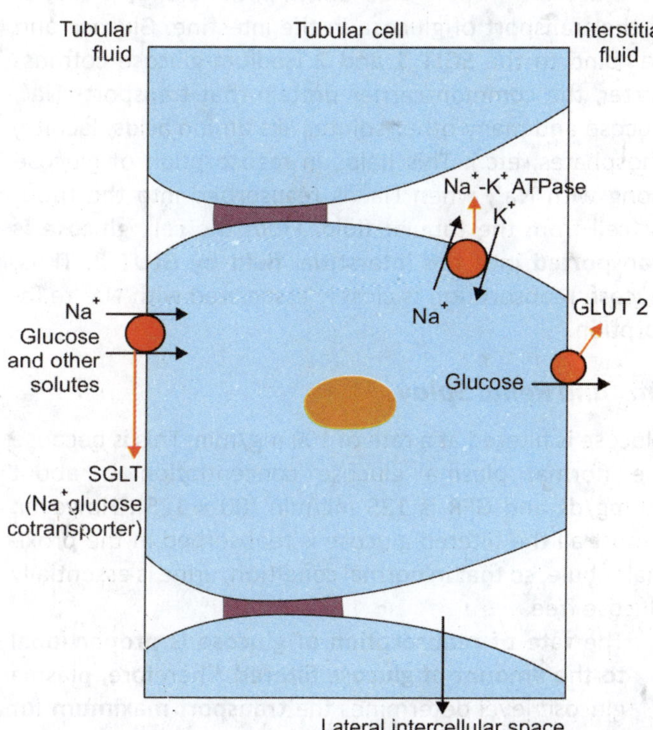

Fig. 78.5: Mechanism of glucose reabsorption in proximal tubule. From tubular fluid, glucose is reabsorbed into tubular cell along with Na^+ by SGLT (sodium-glucose cotransporter). Na^+-K^+ ATPase located on the basolateral membrane actively pumps Na^+ (primary active transport) out of the cell and creates the gradient for Na^+ transport from tubular fluid into the tubular cells. Glucose is cotransported into tubular cell by the same carrier protein (secondary active transport), and then from cell into interstitial fluid by GLUT 2.

4. Therefore, even a smaller osmotic gradient (osmolality of interstitial fluid of about 293 mosm/L against osmolality of tubular fluid of about 285 mosm/L) result in adequate movement of water. Thus, water flows along the osmotic gradient **via the transcellular and paracellular pathways** (Fig. 78.4).
5. Hence, reabsorption of water is coupled with the reabsorption of solutes, especially with that of Na^+ and Cl^- (as NaCl is osmotically most active).
6. The transfer of large amount (**bulk flow**) of water helps in transport of ions like K^+ and Ca^{++} that are carried along with water. This process is called **solvent drag**.
7. Accumulation of water in the interstitial space increases the hydrostatic pressure that favors transfer of water from there into the ECF.

Role of Peritubular Capillaries

The peritubular capillaries play and important role in absorption of solutes and water from the tubule. Peritubular capillaries are derived from efferent arteriole and therefore receive blood from the glomerulus.

1. As the blood draining from glomerulus has already been filtered in the glomerular capillary and protein has not been filtered through the filtration barrier in the renal corpuscle, **blood in peritubular capillary has high oncotic pressure**.
2. Moreover, the **hydrostatic pressure is also less in peritubular capillaries** as blood has passed through the upstream resistance vessels before entering these capillaries.
3. Thus, high oncotic and low hydrostatic pressures favor uptake of water from the interstitial tissue space surrounding tubules.
4. This transfer of water from peritubular space into peritubular capillaries maintains the gradient for water reabsorption from tubular lumen.

Glucose Reabsorption

Glucose is **reabsorbed completely from tubular fluid in the proximal tubule**.

1. It is reabsorbed **along with Na^+** in the tubule. Na^+ is pumped out of the tubular cells by Na^+-K^+ pump located on the basolateral membrane. This decreases intracellular Na^+ concentration and creates gradient for Na^+ entry into the cell from the tubular fluid.
2. The carrier protein that transports Na^+ also reabsorbs glucose (**sodium-glucose cotransporter**).
3. Thus, reabsorption of glucose from the luminal membrane is **secondary transport to the active process** located on the basolateral membrane of the cells and, therefore, is a typical example of **secondary active transport** (Fig. 78.5).

Glucose transport mechanism in the kidney is similar to the transport of glucose in the intestine. Glucose and Na^+ bind to the **SGLT 1 and 2** (sodium-glucose cotransporter, the common carrier protein that transports Na^+, glucose and many other solutes like amino acids, lactate, phosphates, etc.). This helps in reabsorption of glucose along with Na^+, when Na^+ is reabsorbed into the tubular cell from the tubular fluid. From the cell, **glucose is transported into the interstitial fluid by GLUT 2**. Thus, glucose reabsorption is closely associated with Na^+ reabsorption.

Tm_G and Renal Splay

Glucose is filtered at a rate of 100 mg/min. This is because the normal plasma glucose concentration is about 80 mg/dL and GFR is 125 mL/min (80 × 125). However, almost all the filtered glucose is reabsorbed in the proximal tubule, so that in normal condition, urine is essentially glucose free.

1. The **rate of reabsorption of glucose is proportional to the amount of glucose filtered**. Therefore, plasma glucose level determines the **transport maximum for glucose** (Tm_G).
2. The normal Tm_G is 375 mg/min in males and 300 mg/min in females. When Tm_G is exceeded, the glucose appears in urine. As the **renal threshold** is the Tm_G divided by GFR, the predicted value for renal threshold will be about 300 mg/dL, when Tm_G is 375 mg/min and the GFR is 125 mL/min (Tm_G divided by GFR should have been about 300 mg/dL).
3. However, the actual renal threshold is much below the predicted value, i.e. about 200 mg/dL in arterial plasma and 180 mg/dL in venous plasma.
4. Therefore, when the graph of Tm_G is plotted, the actual curve deviates from the ideal curve. This deviation is called **renal splay** (Fig. 78.6). The splay is due to **two reasons**:
   - Tm_G is not same in all the tubules, and
   - Amount of glucose removed from each tubule is not complete even when the amount filtered is below the Tm_G.

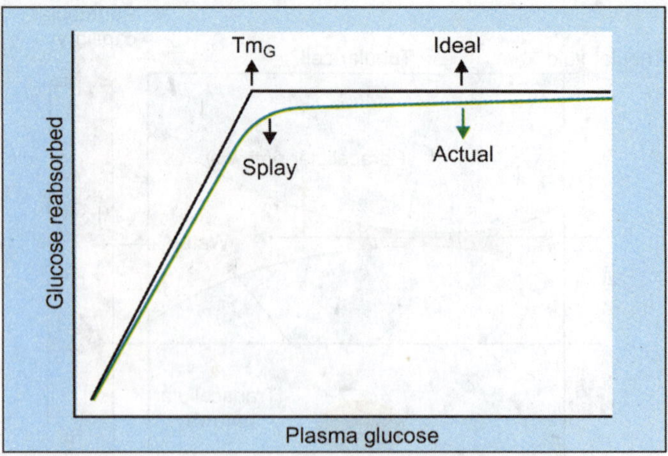

Fig. 78.6: Mechanism of renal splay for glucose. Note, once the TmG for glucose is reached, glucose reabsorption saturates and glucose appears in urine. However, saturation of glucose reabsorption occurs earlier than the expected plasma level, which is called renal splay. Therefore, the actual curve for glucose transport deviates from the ideal curve.

Protein Reabsorption

Normally proteins do not appear in the urine as they are almost **totally reabsorbed in the proximal tubule**. The glomerulus filters only a small quantity of proteins, which is about 7 g/day.

1. Amino acids from the tubular fluid are also *reabsorbed by means of the carrier proteins that reabsorb Na^+ and glucose* (**secondary active transport**).
2. Also, enzymes present on the apical membrane of the epithelial cells of PCT partially degrade the proteins and endocytose them.
3. The proteins in the cell are **degraded by the cellular enzymes** into their **respective amino acids**.
4. Amino acids are then transported from the cell across the basolateral membrane into the interstitial tissue space and from there into the blood.
5. By these mechanisms almost all the filtered proteins and amino acids are reabsorbed in proximal tubule. Therefore, urine is practically **protein free**.
6. But, when amount of protein filtered is more or protein reabsorption is less, proteinuria occurs (Clinical Box 78.1). Usually proteinuria occurs due to the disruption of the glomerular filtering membrane as occurs in glomerulonephritis that increases the tubular load of proteins.

Clinical Box 78.1

Proteinuria: The protein that appears in urine comes from two sources. The primary source of protein in the urine is the **excess filtration** by the glomerular membrane or **less reabsorption** in the proximal tubule. The other source may be the **protein synthesized by the cells** of thick ascending limb of loop of Henle, which is called **Tamm-Horsfall protein**. This protein is usually excreted in urine as the mechanism for protein reabsorption is primarily located in the proximal tubule.

Transport of Organic Solutes

The proximal tubule **secretes various organic cations and anions**. Many of these ions are produced by metabolism, such as uric acid.

1. Many exogenous organic substances like PAH, drugs, etc. are also secreted by the proximal tubule. Usually, these organic compounds are bound to plasma proteins that prevent filtration of the substances via the glomerular membrane. However, the substances are **transported from the peritubular capillaries into the tubular cells** from where they are secreted into the tubular fluid.
2. Therefore, the excretion of this organic compound in urine via their secretion by the tubular cells (rather than through filtration), constitutes an *important mechanism for their elimination* from the body.

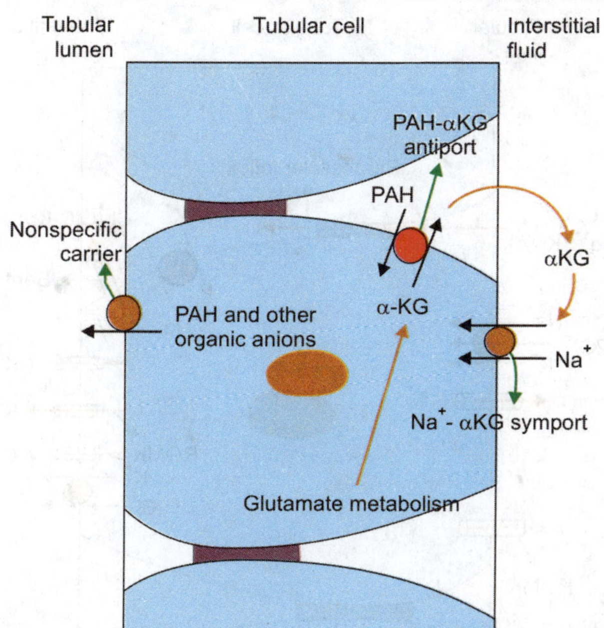

Fig. 78.7: Mechanism of PAH secretion. Note, PAH-αKG antiport located on the basolateral membrane exchanges PAH from interstitial fluid with αKG produced in the cell. PAH is then secreted into the tubular lumen by a less specific carrier protein that also transfers other organic anions. Therefore, presence of other organic anions impairs PAH secretion and vice versa.

Physiological Significance

Interference in renal transport of organic compounds help in treatment of many metabolic diseases. For example, **gout** occurs due to accumulation of uric acid in plasma. Therefore, aim of treatment of gout is **to decrease the plasma uric acid level**. Uric acid is both secreted and reabsorbed in proximal tubule. Thus, one mechanism to decrease uric acid level in gout is to promote its excretion by decreasing absorption in PCT.

PAH Transport

PAH is an **organic anion secreted across the proximal tubular cells**. The pathway for this secretion **has low specificity**, which means many other organic anions like bile salts, oxalates, urates, etc. are also secreted by this mechanism.

1. PAH enters the proximal tubular cells via basolateral membrane in exchange for α-ketoglutarate (αKG), i.e. via PAH-αKG antiport mechanism. Normally, αKG is produced in the cell by glutamate metabolism (Fig. 78.7).
2. The αKG that comes out of the cell into the interstitial tissue space is taken back in to the cells by **Na^+-α KG symport**.
3. PAH is then taken into the tubular fluid along its concentration gradient. The mechanism that transports PAH into the tubular cell is **non-specific**.
4. Therefore, increased plasma concentration of one anion decreases the secretion of the other. For example, urinary excretion of PAH decreases in individual receiving penicillin, and, similarly, excretion of penicillin decreases in individual receiving PAH.
5. Therefore, **during the World War II**, when the availability of the penicillin was less, the **penicillin was administered along with hippuric acid**, which resulted in prolonged action of penicillin by decreasing its secretion through the tubular cells. Thus, penicillin in low dose could achieve the desirable therapeutic effects.

Defects in proximal tubular reabsorption causes Fanconi syndrome (Clinical Box 78.2).

Clinical Box 78.2

Fanconi syndrome: This is a **generalized defect in proximal tubular reabsorption** involving amino acids, glucose, phosphate, uric acid, sodium, potassium, bicarbonate and proteins. This renal disease occurs due to **mutation of the carrier or transporter proteins** that may be either inherited as autosomal or X-linked trait or acquired in diseases like multiple myeloma, amyloidosis, heavy metal toxicity and from chemotherapeutic drugs. Thus, impaired ability of the PCT to reabsorb these organic and inorganic compounds results in glucosuria with normal plasma glucose, hypophosphatemia, hypouricemia, hypokalemia, aminoaciduria, low molecular weight proteinuria and proximal renal tubular acidosis. **Rickets and osteomalacia** commonly occurs secondary to hypophosphatemia. **Salt wasting and polyuria** are also common.

Chloride Reabsorption

Chloride is mainly ***reabsorbed secondary to Na^+ reabsorption*** in the proximal tubule to maintain electroneutrality. Recently, ***separate chloride channels*** have been identified in the kidney tubules. It has been observed that these Cl^- channels are ***linked with Ca^{++} channels***. But, how these two channels interact and operate is not clearly known. Defect in Cl^- channels causes Dent's disease (Clinical Box 78.3).

Clinical Box 78.3

Dent's disease: This is a disease of childhood that results from ***mutation of gene for chloride channels***. Number of Cl^- channels decreases in kidney tubules in this dysfunction. As Cl^- channels are linked with Ca^{++} channels, abnormality also occurs in calcium excretion. Therefore, hypercalciuria and kidney stones occur in this disease. The disorder presents with hypercalciuria, low molecular weight proteinuria, calcium nephrolithiasis and nephrocalcinosis in male children (female children are usually asymptomatic).

Functions of Loop of Henle

The loop of Henle (LOH) has descending and ascending limbs. **LOH of juxtamedullary nephrons** are longer than cortical nephrons and dip deep into the medullary pyramid.

1. In **juxtamedullary nephrons**, descending limb of LOH is totally thin, whereas ascending limb has thin and thick portions.
2. All the segments (thin descending, thin ascending and thick ascending segments) have different transport properties and permeability. Fluid from proximal tubule that enters LOH **is almost isotonic**, whereas **fluid leaving LOH is considerably hypotonic** having osmolality of 100 msom/kg of H_2O (in comparison to 285 msom/kg of H_2O of plasma and proximal tubular fluid).

3. This is because solutes are reabsorbed in ascending limb of LOH without reabsorption of water that makes the fluid more dilute.
4. Reabsorption of solutes into the interstitium from LOH plays a **critical role in counter current mechanism** of urine concentration.
5. **Cortical nephrons** are more in number and LOH of these nephrons help in urine formation, whereas juxtamedullary nephrons are less in number and LOH of these nephrons help in urine concentration.

Transport of Solutes

LOH reabsorbs about 25% of the filtered NaCl and K^+, 30% of filtered Ca^{++}, and 65% of filtered Mg^{++}. The **descending limb of LOH is permeable to water but not to the solutes,** whereas the **ascending limb is impermeable to water.** Na^+, K^+, and Cl^- are cotransported out of the thick segments of the ascending limb.

Descending Limb

Descending limb is permeable to water, but not to solutes. Therefore, fluid in terminal part of descending limb becomes hypertonic as water moves out of the tubule to enter the interstitial space.

Thin Ascending Limb

In the thin part of ascending limb of LOH, transport mechanism is predominantly a passive phenomenon, and permeability to water is less. Though passive transport of NaCl occurs to some extent, active transport of Na^+ is almost nil.

Thick Ascending Limb

In the thick ascending limb of LOH, the fluid becomes more dilute (hypotonic) as Na^+ and Cl^- are taken out of the tubular fluid.

1. The active transport system for Na^+ is well developed in this segment of LOH. Reabsorption of Na^+ from tubular fluid is dependant on a carrier protein on the apical membrane that transports **1 Na^+, 1 K^+, and 2Cl^-** from the lumen into the cell. 1Na^+-1K^+-2Cl^- cotransporter membrane protein is also present in airways, epithelial cells of GI tract and salivary gland.
2. From tubular cells, Na^+ is transported into the interstitial fluid by Na^+-K^+ pump, which is quite efficient in thick ascending limb of LOH (Fig. 78.8).
3. K^+ from cells diffuses back into the tubular fluid and also into the interstitium passively through **ROMK and other membrane K^+ channels.**
4. Cl– that enters the cell is **co-transported with K^+** into the interstitial fluid.
5. Transepithelial transfer of these solutes creates a potential difference between tubular and interstitial fluid space, which drives transfer of solutes, especially **transport of Na^+, K^+, Mg^{++} and Ca^{++} via paracellular pathway**.
6. Thus, transport of solute occurs by both transcellular and paracellular routes.

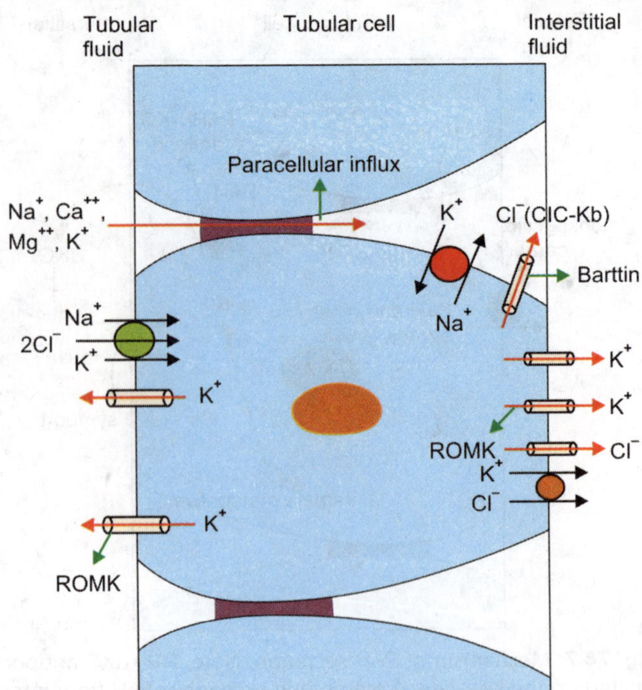

Fig. 78.8: Mechanism of solute transport in thick portion of ascending limb of LOH. Na^+-K^+ ATPase located on the basolateral membrane actively pumps Na^+ out of the cell and creates the gradient for Na^+ transport from tubular fl uid into the tubular cells. However, in this part of nephron, Na^+ transport is coupled with K^+ and Cl^- via Na^+-K^+-2Cl^- channel (1 Na^+-K^+-2Cl^- cotransporter, which is blocked by furosemide group of diuretics). K^+ from the cell is taken out by K^+ and ROMK channels located on both basal and apical membranes. Cl^- from the cell is taken out by Cl^- channel and ClC-Kb channel formed by Barttin, a membrane protein located on basolateral membrane. K^+-Cl^- symport on basal membrane also transfers Na^+ and Cl^- from the cell.

7. However, the tubular epithelium of thick ascending limb of LOH **is almost impermeable to water**; therefore, solute transfer in this part of the tubule is **not associated with transfer of water.**
8. Defect in thick ascending limb transport process causes Batter syndrome (Clinical Box 78.4).

Clinical Box 78.4

Bartter syndrome: This is a rare syndrome that occurs due to defective transport of solutes in thick ascending limb of LOH. It occurs due to mutation of gene for **Barttin**, an integral membrane protein essential for function of Cl^- channels (ClC-Kb Cl^- channels). Also, mutation of gene that causes synthesis of transporter proteins, such as 1Na^+-1K^+-2Cl^- cotransporter and ROMK K^+ channel occurs in this syndrome. The disease is characterized by chronic hyponatremia and hypovolemia that causes activation of renin-angiotensin system. The resultant increase in aldosterone secretion causes hyperkalemia and alkalosis. **Hypertension does not occur**. Patients of Bartter syndrome with mutated Barttin are **deaf** because the defect in stria vascularis in inner ear, which maintains high concentration of K^+ in scala media contains ClC-Kb Cl^- channels.

Reabsorption of Water

The loop of Henle reabsorbs approximately **15% of the filtered water, which occurs exclusively in the descending limb**, the ascending limb being impermeable to it.

1. The descending limb except at its terminal portion is highly permeable to water. Inspite of active transport of solutes in thick ascending limb of LOH, **water is not reabsorbed**.
2. Both thin and thick portions of ascending limb of LOH are **almost impermeable to water**. Furosemide is a loop diuretic (Clinical Box 78.5).

Clinical Box 78.5

Loop Diuretics: The loop diuretics like furosemide **inhibit the 1Na^+-1K^+-2Cl^- symporter**. This inhibits NaCl reabsorption from the thick ascending limb of loop of Henle. Thus, loop diuretics cause **natriuresis and kaliuresis and increase osmolality of tubular fluid** that lead to increase water excretion. However, K^+ depletion may result from long use of loop diuretics. Hence, K^+ supplement is usually given to patients under chronic furosemide therapy.

Functions of Distal Convoluted Tubule

Reabsorption of Solutes and Water

Distal convoluted tubule (DCT) is essentially the extension of the thick ascending limb of LOH. Hence, physiologically, it is close to thick ascending limb of LOH.

1. Therefore, DCT is **relatively impermeable to water** whereas solutes are transported. As solute is removed in excess of solvent, **further dilution of the tubular fluid occurs** in this part of the nephron.
2. In the initial segment of distal tubule, Na^+ and Cl^- are reabsorbed from tubular fluid into the tubular cells by Na^+-Cl^- symporter (Fig. 78.9).
3. Na^+ is removed from tubular cells to interstitial space by Na^+-K^+ pump located on the basolateral membrane, and Cl^- is removed by Cl^- channels.
4. However, *inspite of osmotic gradient* across the tubular epithelium, *water reabsorption is poor*. Only about 5% of the filtered water is removed in DCT.
5. Thus, dilution of the tubular fluid that begins in the thick ascending limb of LOH continues in the DCT. Thiazide diuretics act on DCT (Clinical Box 78. 6).

Clinical Box 78.6

Thiazide diuretics: Thiazide diuretics such, as chlorthiazide, and metolazone diuretics, act by inhibiting Na^+-Cl^- cotransporter in the early part of DCT. This causes natriuresis and diuresis.

Functions of Collecting Duct

Though collecting duct is considered as distal part of nephrons, strictly speaking, it is not the part of an individual nephron. However, as solute and water reabsorption continues in collecting duct system, physiologically, it is an essential component of a nephron.

1. As collecting duct is the terminal part of the nephron, its ability to alter transport of solutes and water contributes considerably to final osmolality, composition and volume of urine.
2. Most of the ***excreted K^+* in urine comes from collecting duct** as it secretes a significant quantity of this cation.

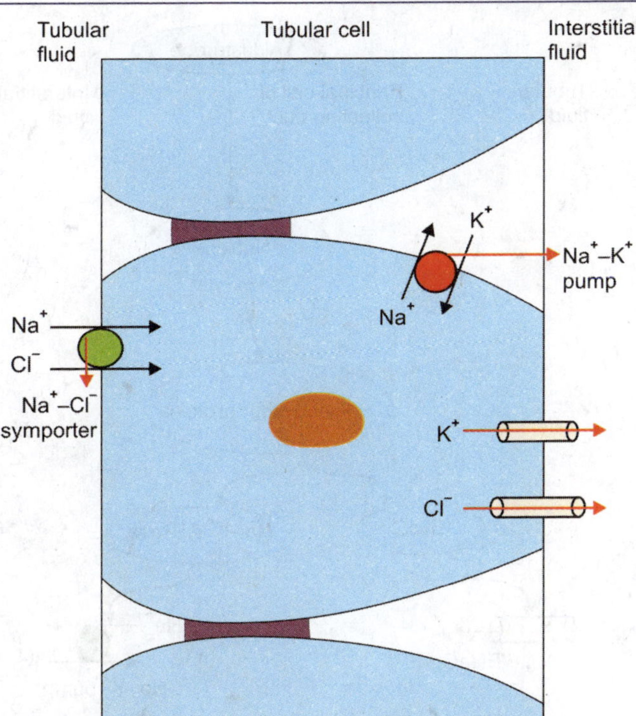

Fig. 78.9: Mechanism of solute reabsorption in distal convoluted tubule. Na^+-K^+ ATPase located on the basolateral membrane actively pumps Na^+ out of the cell and creates the gradient for Na^+ transport from tubular fluid into the tubular cells. However, in this part of nephron, Na^+ transport is coupled with Cl^- via Na^+-Cl^- cotransporter, which is blocked by thiazide group of diuretics. K^+ and Cl^- from cell are taken out by K^+ and Cl^- channels located on basal membrane.

3. Transport processes in collecting duct are influenced and fine-tuned by **hormones, such as aldosterone and ADH**.

Reabsorption of Solutes

Epithelium of collecting duct contains **two types of cells**: principal cells and intercalated cells.

1. The **principal cells** reabsorb Na^+ and secrete K^+, whereas **intercalated cells** secrete either H^+ or HCO_3^-.
2. Thus, principal cells contribute to K^+ metabolism and intercalated cells play an important role in acidification of urine.
3. Intercalated cells also reabsorb HCO_3^- and K^+.

Principal Cells

Principal cells are present abundantly in the epithelium of collecting duct.

1. The **reabsorption of Na^+ and secretion of K^+** in the principal cells depends on Na^+-K^+ pump in the basolateral membrane (Fig. 78.10). This pump provides chemical gradient for the movement of Na^+ from the distal tubular fluid into the cells. K^+ is secreted from blood via principal cells into the tubular fluid.
2. K^+ secretion in the collecting duct mainly occurs **in the cortical part**.

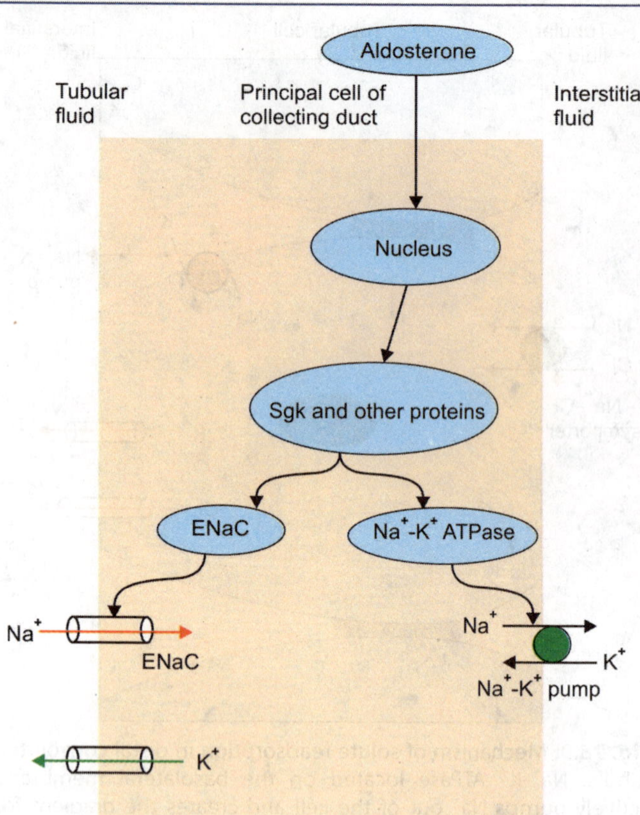

Fig. 78.10: Mechanism of Na^+ reabsorption and K^+ secretion in principal cells of collecting duct. Note, aldosterone increases activity of epithelial Na^+ channels (ENaC) that increases Na^+ reabsorption, and also stimulates activity of Na^+-K^+ ATPase that helps in generating gradient for Na^+ absorption and K^+ secretion.

3. In physiological conditions, most of K^+ in urine comes from collecting duct secretion.
4. Though, in conditions of K^+ excess like high K^+ diet, collecting duct secretes more K^+, in K^+ depletion it reabsorbs K^+.
5. **K^+ secretion is facilitated by aldosterone.**

Role of Aldosterone

Na^+ is reabsorbed from tubular fluid by principal cells by diffusion through Na^+ channels in the apical membrane of epithelial cells. These Na^+ channels are known as **epithelial sodium (Na) channels** or **ENaC**.

1. **Aldosterone facilitates genomic activity** to produce **sgk and other proteins** that form ENaC in the cells and their insertion into the luminal membrane (Fig. 78.10).
2. Thus, aldosterone increases the activity of ENaC and increases reabsorption of Na^+. Na^+ that enters cell is pumped out into interstitial space by **Na^+-K^+ pump**, the activity of which is **also promoted by aldosterone.**
3. Thus, aldosterone, acting on collecting duct (mainly cortical part), increases Na^+ absorption and facilitates K^+ excretion.
4. Therefore, **hypernatremia** (and expansion of ECF) and **hypokalemia are features of hyperaldosteronism.**
5. K^+-sparing diuretics inhibit Na^+ reabsorption in collecting duct (Clinical Box 78.7).

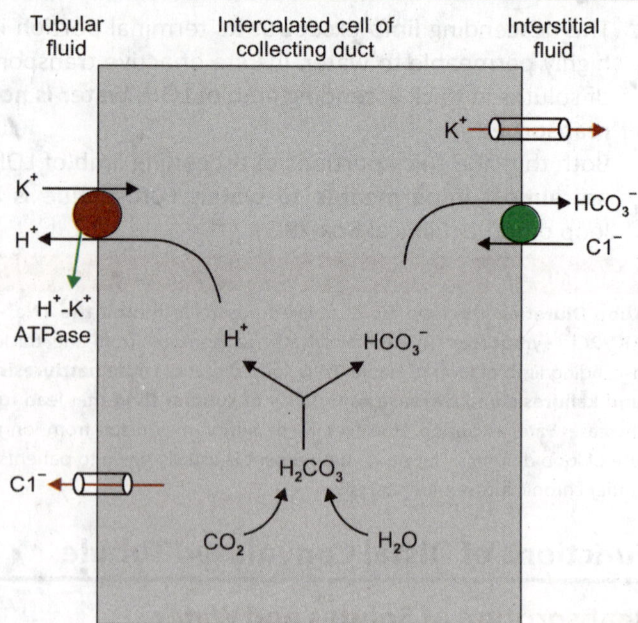

Fig. 78.11: Mechanism of H^+ secretion by intercalated cells of collecting duct. Note, H^+ is secreted by activation of K^+-H^+ pump activity.

Clinical Box 78.7

K^+-sparing diuretics: K^+-sparing diuretics like amiloride and spironolactone **inhibit Na^+ reabsorption from collecting duct** by antagonizing the effect of aldosterone. Amiloride directly inhibits the Na^+ channels (ENaC) on the luminal membrane and spironolactone inhibits Na^+-K^+ pump on the basolateral membrane. Inhibition of Na^+ reabsorption decreases the magnitude of negative charge in the lumen. This facilitates Cl^- reabsorption by paracellular pathway. Because it decreases the negative charge in the lumen, it also decreases K^+ secretion into the tubular fluid. Thus, it **decreases K^+ excretion in the urine.** Therefore, they are called K^+-sparing diuretics. This is usually used in patients with increased K^+ excretion in the urine.

Intercalated Cells

These cells are scattered among the major cells in the collecting duct.

1. On the luminal side, the membrane contains **H^+-K^+ ATPase that pumps H^+ into the cell and K^+ into the tubular fluid** (Fig. 78.11).
2. In the cell, H^+ and HCO_3^- are formed from dissociation of H_2CO_3. H^+ is secreted into the tubular lumen and HCO_3^- is reabsorbed into the interstitial space.
3. Thus, intercalated cells contribute **to acidification of urine** and conservation of K^+.

Reabsorption of Water

Collecting duct has two parts: the cortical part and the medullary part. The reabsorption of solute and water from the collecting duct mainly **depends on the efficacy of ADH acting on it.**

Cortical Part

In the cortical part, ADH increases the permeability of collecting duct to water by inserting **aquaporin-2** water channels, especially on the luminal membrane of the principal cells.

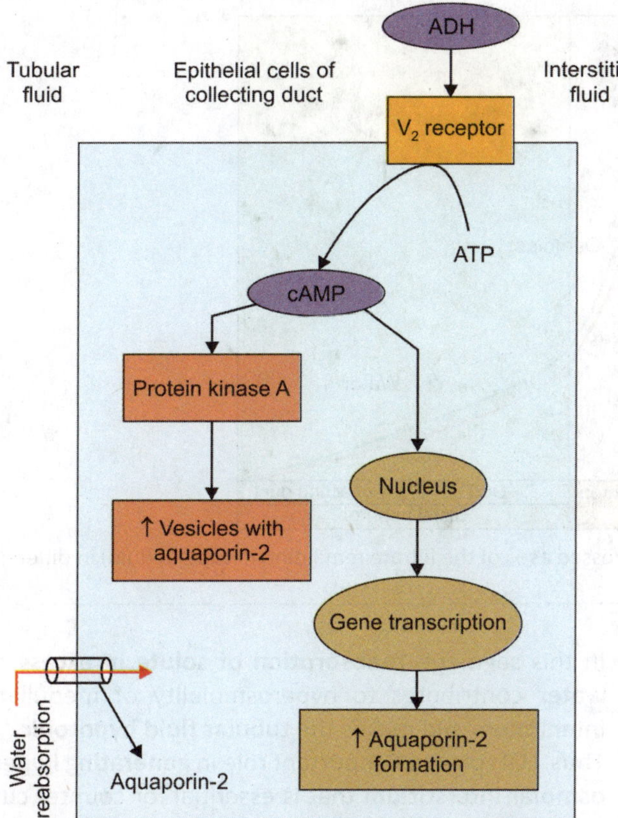

Fig. 78.12: Mechanism of water reabsorption by epithelial cells of collecting duct. ADH increases cAMP formation in the cell by acting on V2 receptors. cAMP stimulates protein kinase A activity that promotes insertion of vesicles containing aquaporin 2 on cell membrane. cAMP also stimulates gene transcription that promotes formation of new aquaporin 2 in the cell.

1. ADH binds with V_2 receptor on the basolateral cell membrane, where it activates adenylate cyclase to **increase the production of cAMP**.
2. cAMP activates protein-kinase A, which promotes the **insertion of vesicle containing aquaporin-2** on the luminal surface of the epithelial cells (Fig. 78.12) that increases the water permeability.
3. cAMP also **increases gene transcription** that increases **formation of aquaporin-2.**
4. In the presence of ADH, water moves out of the hypotonic tubular fluid into the cells of the cortical collecting duct and then from there into the interstitium of the cortex. This helps in **reabsorption of about 10% filtered water** and the tubular fluid becomes isotonic.
5. The isotonic fluid then enters the medullary portion of the collecting duct.

In Medullary Part

In this portion of the collecting duct **osmolality of interstitium is very high**.

1. Water is reabsorbed from the tubular fluid into the hypertonic medullary interstitium by osmotic effect, which **accounts for about 5% of water reabsorption**.
2. This plays an important role in **counter-current mechanism** and makes the urine concentrated.

In human beings, **in the presence of adequate ADH**, osmolality of urine may reach 1400 mosm/kg of H_2O (99.7% of filtered water is reabsorbed). **In the absence of ADH**, the cells of collecting duct are relatively impermeable to water. Therefore, urine becomes hypotonic (osmolality as low as 30 mosm/kg. of H_2O) in the absence of ADH (Clinical Box 78.8). However, collecting duct is not totally impermeable to water and, therefore, even in complete absence of ADH, about 2% filtered water is reabsorbed.

Clinical Box 78.8

Diabetes Insipidus: This is a condition of excess urine formation (polyuria) that occurs due to ADH deficiency (**neurogenic DI**) or failure of collecting duct to respond to the hormone (**nephrogenic DI**). The nephrogenic form, which is an X-linked recessive type, occurs due to **mutation of the gene for V2 receptors.**

Other Tubular Dysfunctions

Liddle's Syndrome

This is a rare **autosomal dominant disorder** characterized by clinical **features similar to hyperaldosteronism** consisting of increase in ECF volume, hypertension, hypokalemia, and metabolic alkalosis. However, **aldosterone and renin level in plasma are less.**

1. In this disease, the **amiloride-sensitive Na^+ channels become hyperactive**, which results in reabsorption of inappropriately large quantity of Na^+ and increased K^+ excretion from the tubular fluid.
2. This is accompanied by reabsorption of large quantity of water. Thus, ECF expansion occurs that causes hypertension.

Pseudohypoaldosteronism

There are **two forms** of pseudohypoaldosterinism: Type I and type II.

Pseudohypoaldosteronism Type 1

This is a rare autosomal disease, which is just opposite to that of Liddle's syndrome. The **dominant form** is due to the *mutation of mineralocorticoid receptor gene* and the **recessive form** is due to the *mutation of amiloride-sensitive epithelial Na^+ channels*. The disease is characterized by significant **reduction in ECF volume** and, therefore, the condition is **associated with hypotension**. The decreased Na^+ channels and decreased aldosterone activity in the tubule impair Na^+ reabsorption. Consequently, increased Na^+ excretion is accompanied by excretion of large amount of water. This causes contraction of ECF compartment and hypotension.

Pseudohypoaldosteronism Type II

In type II pseudohypoaldosteronism, (also called as **Gordon syndrome**), an autosomal dominant disease, hyperkalemia, hypertension and metabolic acidosis occur secondary to **overactivity of thiazide-sensitive Na^+-Cl^- cotransporter** in DCT.

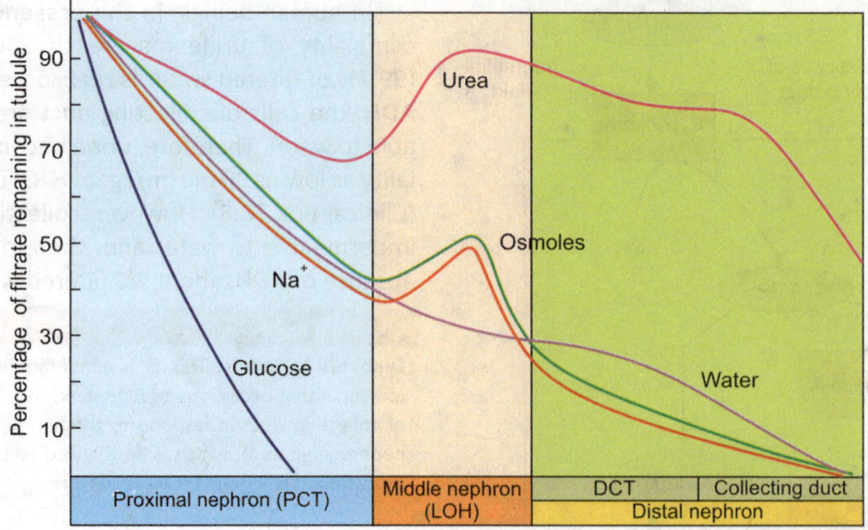

Fig. 78.13: Magnitude of reabsorption of water and various solutes (expressed as % of the filtrate remaining in tubular fluid) in different parts of nephron.

Gitelman's Syndrome

This is an autosomal recessive disorder that has similarity with features of Bartter syndrome like hypokalemia, metabolic alkalosis, salt wasting, elevated renin and aldosterone level, and normal BP. However, hypomagnesemia and hypocalciuria differentiates it from Bartter syndrome.

1. The disease occurs due to **mutation of thiazide-sensitive Na^+-Cl^- transporter**.
2. Decreased Na^+ reabsorption in DCT leads to volume depletion and hypokalemia.
3. Loss of activity of thiazide-sensitive transporter increases calcium reabsorption causing hypocalciuria.

Summary of Tubular Functions

From the above discussion on tubular functions, we learn that nephron is **functionally divided into three parts**: proximal segment, middle segment and distal segment.

Proximal Nephron

The proximal nephron **is the proximal tubule** that absorbs about **67% of the solutes and water** (Fig. 78.13). Proximal nephron is nonselective and reabsorbs solute and solvent maximally. Thus, it greatly **contributes to electrolyte and volume homeostasis.**

1. In proximal nephron, Na^+ and water reabsorption are closely coupled as the epithelial water permeability is very high and **paracellular pathway** of absorption of solute and water **is well developed** (as the *tight junctions between the cells are leaky*).
2. Inspite of a small osmotic gradient across tubular epithelium, the quantity of water reabsorbed is large due to greater permeability of PCT to water.
3. However, the tubular fluid is isosmotic.

Middle Nephron

Loop of Henle constitutes the middle segment of the nephron.

1. In this segment, **reabsorption of solute in excess of water** contributes to hyperosmolality of medullary interstitium and makes the **tubular fluid hypotonic.**
2. Thus, LOH plays an important role in **generating hyperosmolar interstitium** that is essential for counter current mechanism of **urine concentration.**

Distal Nephron

DCT and collecting duct form the distal nephron. Distal nephron **is selective in reabsorption** and absorbs smaller quantity of water and solutes. About **8% of Na^+ and 18–20% of water is reabsorbed** in this part of the tubule (Fig. 78.14).

1. **Na^+ and water reabsorption are not coupled as water permeability is very poor** in distal nephron.
2. The tubular fluid is hypotonic.
3. Inspite of a steep osmotic gradient across the epithelium, reabsorption of water is extremely poor in the absence of aldosterone and ADH.
4. The **paracellular route of transport is not well developed** as the junctions between epithelial cells are really very tight.
5. Distal nephron **contributes to concentration and acidification of urine.**

REGULATION OF IONS AND WATER REABSORPTION

Regulation of NaCl and Water Reabsorption

Normally, of the total Na^+ is filtered (26,000 meq) of in the glomerulus per day, 99.4% (25,850 meq/day) is reabsorbed in the tubule. Of the filtered Na^+, about 67% is reabsorbed in the PCT, 25% in LOH, 5% in DCT and 3% in collecting duct (Fig. 78.15).

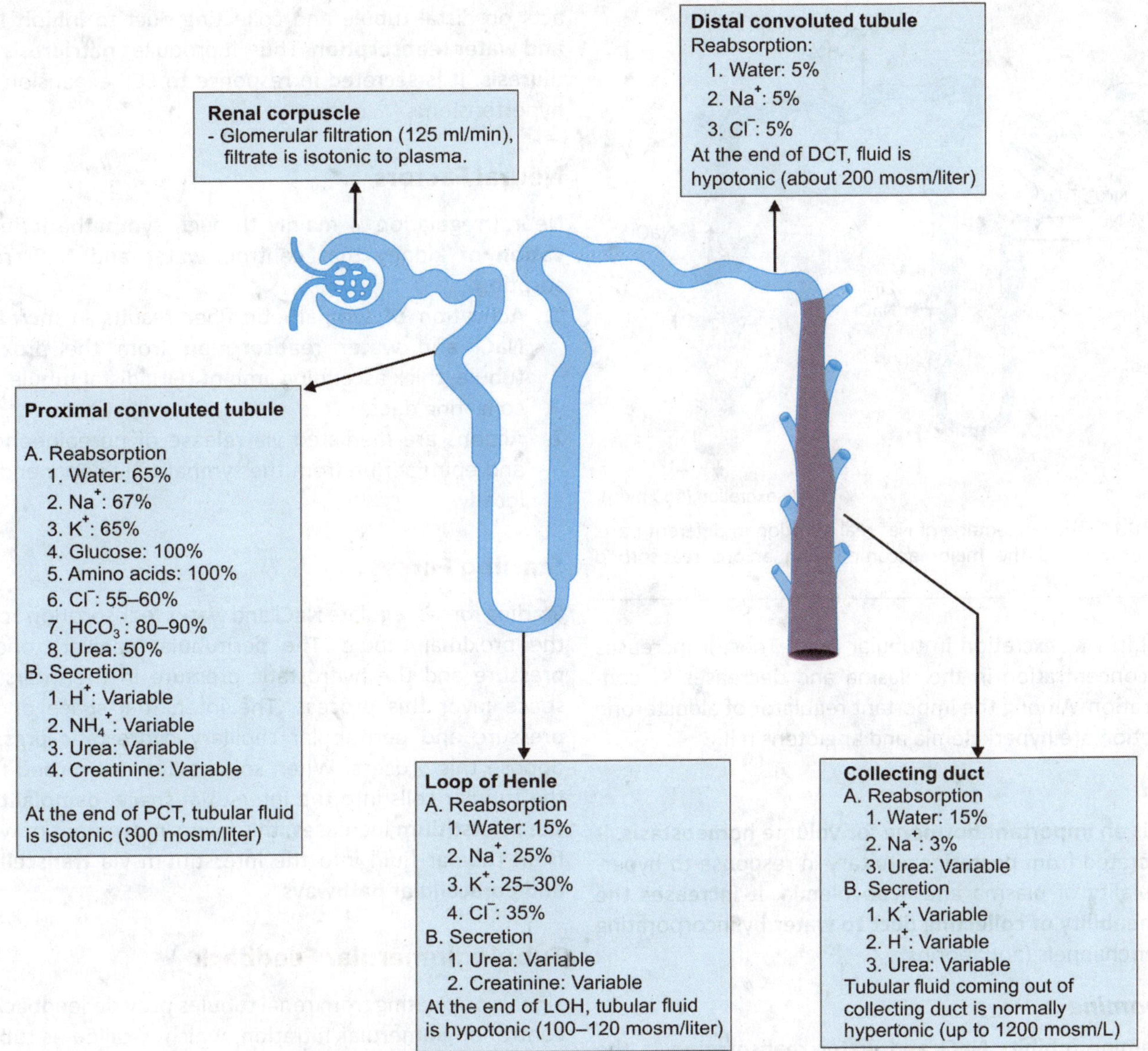

Fig. 78.14: Summary of functions of nephron. Note, the change in composition and osmolality of the filtrate as it passes through different parts of nephron, starting from the glomerular filtration to urine (fluid coming out of collecting duct) formation.

1. Reabsorption of Na^+ **facilitates the reabsorption of many other solutes** and establishes **osmotic gradient for reabsorption of water.**
2. The total urinary Na^+ output ranges between 1 meq and 400 meq (average about 150 meq) per day, depending on the dietary salt intake of the person.
3. Regulation of NaCl and water reabsorption is primarily the function of various **hormones acting on kidneys.**
4. Neural factors, starling forces, tubuloglomerular feedback and glomerulotubular balance also play role in Na^+ regulatory mechanisms.

Hormonal Factors

The major hormones that influence NaCl and water reabsorption form kidney are angiotensin II, aldosterone, ADH, dopamine, glucocorticoid, urodilatin and ANP.

Angiotensin II

Angiotensin II acts mainly on proximal tubule of the kidney. It increases **NaCl and water reabsorption** and causes expansion of ECF volume. It is secreted in conditions of hypovolemia and hypotension.

Clinical Correlation: Captopril that inhibits angiotensin converting enzyme (**ACE inhibitor**) decreases ECF volume and blood pressure. This prevents formation of angiotensin I to angiotensin II. Therefore, decreased concentration of angiotensin II decreases NaCl and water reabsorption from proximal tubule, and decreases vasoconstriction. This is used for the **treatment of hypertension and in conditions of ECF volume expansion.**

Aldosterone

Aldosterone stimulates reabsorption of NaCl and water from collecting duct. It **acts on Na^+-K^+ pump and ENaC.** It

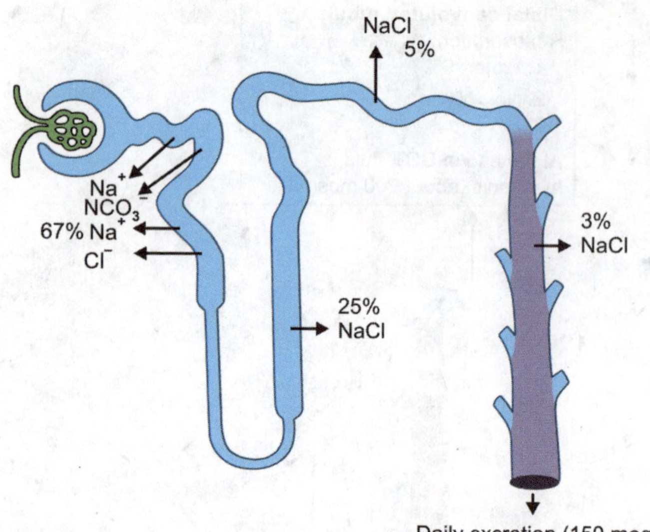

Fig. 78.15: The percentage of Na^+ reabsorption in different parts of nephron and the major accompanying anions reabsorbed with Na^+.

facilitates K^+ excretion in tubular fluid. Thus, it increases Na^+ concentration in the plasma and decreases K^+ concentration. Among the important regulator of aldosterone secretion are hyperkalemia and angiotensin II.

ADH

This is an **important hormone for volume homeostasis**. It is secreted from posterior pituitary in response to hyperosmolality of plasma and hypovolemia. It **increases the permeability of collecting duct to water** by incorporating water channels (aquaporins).

Dopamine

Dopamine **inhibits NaCl and water reabsorption** in the proximal tubule. Thus, it causes **natriuresis and diuresis**. Dopamine secretion increases in expansion of ECF volume.

Glucocorticoids

Glucocorticoids have **mild mineralocorticoid (aldosterone) activity**. They increase water and NaCl reabsorption.

Urodilatin

This is a polypeptide hormone containing 32 amino acids **secreted by the distal tubule and collecting duct.** It acts on the kidney tubule locally. It acts exclusively on collecting duct to **inhibit NaCl and water reabsorption** from the medullary part of the collecting duct. It is a potent natriuretic and diuretic hormone like that of ANP. However, recently the validity of this hormone has been questioned.

ANP

This is a polypeptide hormone containing 28 amino acids, secreted from myocytes of atria of the heart. It acts on distal tubule and collecting duct to **inhibit NaCl and water reabsorption.** Thus, it produces **natriuresis and diuresis**. It is secreted in response to ECF expansion and hypertension.

Neural Factors

Neural regulation is mainly through **sympathetic innervation** of kidney that controls water and NaCl reabsorption.

1. Activation of sympathetic fiber results in **increased NaCl and water reabsorption** from the proximal tubule, thick ascending limb of LOH, distal tubule, and collecting duct.
2. Actions are mediated via release of norepinephrine, and epinephrine from the sympathetic nerve endings locally.

Starling Forces

Starling forces regulate NaCl and water reabsorption across the proximal tubule. The peritubular capillary oncotic pressure and the hydrostatic pressure in the interstitial space favor this process. The interstitial space oncotic pressure and peritubular capillary hydrostatic pressure oppose this process. When solutes are reabsorbed from the tubular cells into the interstitial space, **osmolality of the interstitium** increases, this favors movement of water from tubular fluid into the interstitium via **transcellular and paracellular pathways.**

Tubuloglomerular Feedback

Signals originating from renal tubules provide feedback for control of glomerular filtration, which is called as tubuloglomerular feedback.

1. In this process, the **rate of flow of and the concentration of NaCl** in the tubular fluid of thick ascending limb of LOH and initial part of distal tubule provides feedback information to the glomerulus to control the rate of filtration.
2. When the rate of flow through the tubule increases, rate of filtration decreases and when the rate of tubular flow decreases, rate of filtration increases in the same nephron.
3. Thus, the change in glomerular filtration maintains a **constancy of tubular load,** i. e. a constant volume of fluid delivered to the tubule.

Role of Macula Densa

The **macula densa** in the terminal part of thick ascending limb of LOH act as **sensor** that detects the rate of flow of fluid through it.

1. Macula densa cells provide signal to the afferent arteriole. When tubular flow is high, concentration of Na^+ and Cl^- in tubular fluid becomes high.

2. More quantity of **Na^+ and Cl^- enters the macula densa cells** via $1Na^+$-$1K^+$-$2Cl^-$ cotransporter located in their apical membrane. Increased Na^+ in the cell **increases Na^+-K^+ ATPase activity**.
3. Increased ATP hydrolysis results in formation of more **adenosine**. Adenosine acts on the A_1 adenosine receptors to increase the **release of Ca^{++}** from macula densa cells that causes **constriction of afferent arteriole** (Flowchart 78.1).
4. Thus, **glomerular filtration is decreased**. Opposite mechanism operates when tubular flow decreases.

It is also believed that a similar mechanism operates to **control renin secretion** from JG cells that influence glomerular function through angiotensin II. Also, change in diameter of the afferent arteriole is mediated by secretion of chemicals like **thromboxane A_2 and prostaglandins** locally. Alteration in glomerular filtration is also achieved by changing the surface area for filtration, which is brought about by constriction or relaxation of the **mesangial cells**.

Flowchart 78.1: Mechanism of tubuloglomerular feedback (FB).

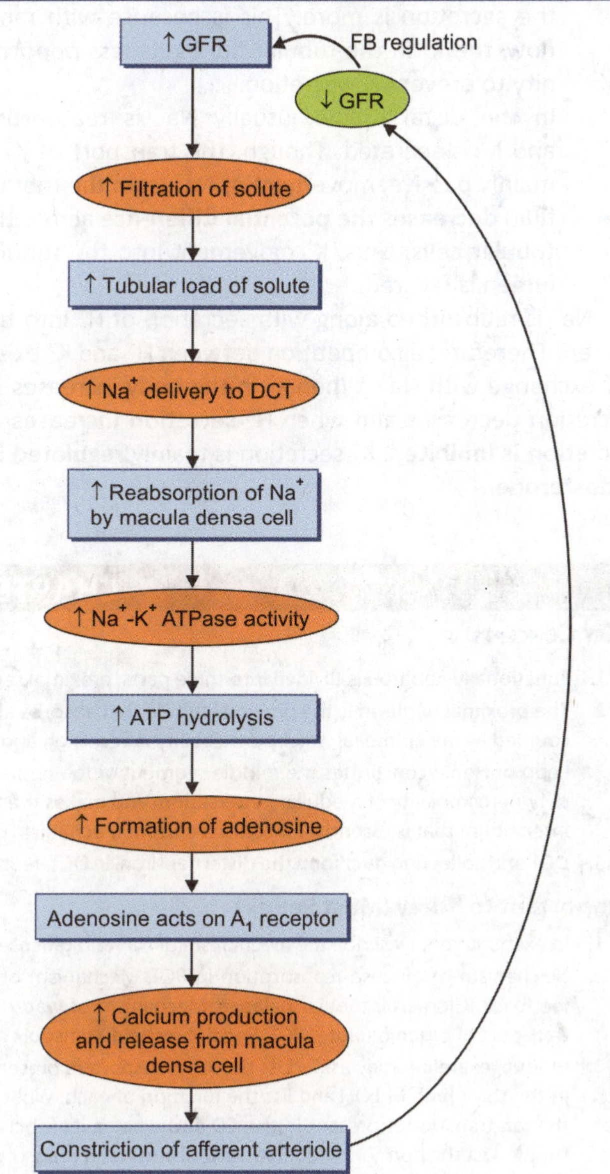

Glomerulotubular Balance

Increase in GFR increases the load of solutes, especially of Na^+ in the tubular fluid. This increases reabsorption of Na^+ from the proximal tubule. Normally, a constant fraction of filtered solute is reabsorbed. That means, a constant percentage of the tubular load is reabsorbed by the proximal tubule. This is called glomerulotubular balance.

There are **two possible mechanisms** for glomerulotubular balance:

1. **Change in oncotic and hydrostatic pressures between peritubular capillaries and lateral intercellular space:** This mechanism is more effective for Na^+. Increase in GFR increases protein concentration in the blood that leaves glomerular capillary, i.e. protein content becomes more in efferent arteriole. Efferent arteriolar blood enters the peritubular capillaries. Therefore, **oncotic pressure in the peritubular capillaries increases**, which causes increased Na^+ reabsorption from tubular fluid. This is also accompanied by increased fluid movement into the interstitial space (lateral intercellular space) and then from there into the blood.
2. **Increased load on the tubule:** With increased GFR, filtered load of Na^+, glucose and amino acids on the tubule increases. Increased Na^+ reabsorption is associated with increase in glucose and amino acid reabsorption through the same carrier proteins. Thus, more solutes are reabsorbed.

Regulation of K^+ Excretion

K^+ is the primary intracellular cation. Its gradient across the cell membrane is mainly determined by the electrical potential across the membrane. As excitability of nerves and muscles depends on this electrical potential, precise control of K^+ level in plasma is very essential, in which kidneys play an important role.

1. Normally 600 meq of K^+ is filtered in 24 hours of which **99.3% (560 meq) is reabsorbed.**
   - The major reabsorption of K^+ takes place in the proximal tubule, which removes about 65% of its filtered load.
   - In thick ascending portion of LOH, about 25–30% of K^+ reabsorption takes place.
   - However, about 50 meq of **K^+ is secreted from the distal tubule**. Thus, the net excretion of K^+ in urine is about 90 meq/day.
   - Minor reabsorption and secretion of K^+ also take place in collecting duct, especially by the intercalated cell (Fig. 78.16).
2. The rate of secretion of K^+ by distal tubular cells is **proportionate to the rate of flow of fluid** through it.

- When the flow of fluid in the distal tubule is rapid, the secretion is more. This is because with rapid flow, the K^+ in the tubular fluid gets less opportunity to prevent K^+ secretion.
- In the distal tubule, usually Na^+ is reabsorbed and K^+ is secreted. Though, the transport of K^+ is mainly passive, movement of Na^+ from the tubular fluid **decreases the potential difference** across the tubular cells; thus, K^+ movement into the tubular lumen is favored.

Na^+ is reabsorbed along with secretion of H^+ into the lumen. Therefore, a competition between H^+ and K^+ exists for exchange with Na^+. When K^+ in the body increases H^+ secretion decreases and when **H^+ secretion increases K^+ secretion is inhibited**. K^+ secretion is mainly **regulated by aldosterone**.

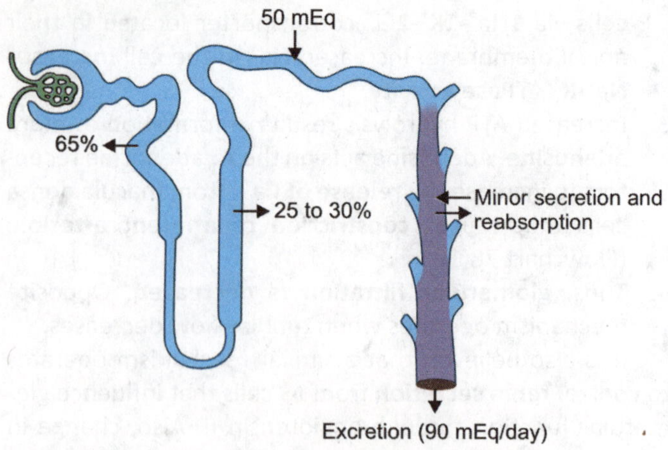

Fig. 78.16: Transport of K^+ in different parts of the nephron.

CHAPTER SUMMARY

KEY CONCEPTS

1. Functionally nephron is divided into three parts: proximal segment, middle segment and distal segment..
2. The proximal nephron is the proximal tubule that absorbs about 67% of the solutes and water. Na^+ and water reabsorption are closely coupled as the epithelial water permeability is very high and paracellular pathway of absorption of solute and water is well developed.
3. Loop of Henle constitutes the middle segment of the nephron. In this segment, reabsorption of solute in excess of water contributes to hyperosmolality of medullary interstitium and makes the tubular fluid hypotonic. It plays important role in generating hyperosmolar interstitium that is essential for counter current mechanism of urine concentration.
4. DCT and collecting duct form the distal nephron. In DCT, reabsorption of water is extremely poor in the absence of aldosterone and ADH.

Important to Know (Must Read)

1. In examination, 'Describe the mechanism of Na^+ and glucose reabsorption in proximal renal tubule' may be asked as a **Long Question.**
2. Mechanism of glucose reabsorption in PCT, Mechanism of Na^+ reabsorption in PCT, Functions of Loop of henle, Tubuloglomerular feedback, Glomerulotubular balance, Mechanism of water reabsorption in CD, Mechanism of solute transport in CD, Mechanism of transport of organic solutes PCT, Renal threshold, transport maximum, Renal splay, may be asked as **Short Questions** in exam.
3. In **Viva**, examiner may ask… List the ion transporters present in the PCT and list the function of each, List the ion transporters present in the thick limb of LOH and list the function of each, What is the ion transporter present in the DCT and what is its function, What is the ion transporter present in the CD and what is its function, What is the percentage of Na^+ reabsorption in different parts of renal tubule, List the hormones regulating NaCl and water reabsorption from kidney tubule, What is tubuloglomerular feedback and what is its mechanism, What is glomerulotubular balance and what is its mechanism, What is the mechanism of glucose reabsorption in PCT, What is T_{MG} and what is its value, What is renal threshold for glucose and what is its value, What is renal splay and what are the reasons for it, List the cell types present in the collecting duct and give their functions, What is the mechanism of water reabsorption in CD, What is the mechanism of action of K^+ sparing diuretics, give example, What is the mechanism of action of loop diuretics, give example, What is the mechanism of action of thiazide diuretics, give example, What is the mechanism of chloride reabsorption in PCT, What is the mechanism of K^+ excretion from kidney tubule, What is the mechanism of protein reabsorption in PCT, What are the sources of protein that appears in urine in proteinuria, What are the mechanisms of reabsorption of organic solutes in PCT, What is Fanconi syndrome and what are its causes and features, What is Dent's disease and what are its causes and features, What is Bartter syndrome and what are its causes and features, What is Liddle's syndrome and what are its features, What is pseudohypoaldosteronism and what are its types and features, What is Gitelman's syndrome and what are its features.

CHAPTER

79

Mechanisms of Urine Concentration and Dilution

LEARNING OBJECTIVES

On completion of study of this chapter, the student **MUST** be able to:

1. Acquire the concept of a counter current system.
2. Understand and describe the countercurrent mechanism of urine concentration.
3. Appreciate the importance of urine concentration.

Student **MAY** also be able to:

1. Explain the application of counter current mechanism in different situations.

GENERAL CONCEPT

In human beings, urine can be formed with an osmolality of as high as 1400 mosm/kg of H_2O and as low as 30 mosm/kg of H_2O. Such a capability of kidneys to pass urine with extremes of osmolality is a fundamental necessity for volume and electrolyte homeostasis. Though glomerular filtrate is about 180 liters a day, only about 1.5 liters of urine is excreted daily. Therefore, normally, kidney excretes a concentrated urine to prevent volume depletion from the body, in which **osmolality of urine is an index of its concentrating and diluting capacity**.

1. **Under physiological conditions**, urine osmolality is a **function of solvent (water) excretion**. That means, when kidney excretes osmotically concentrated urine, in effect, water output is reduced considerably, and when kidney excretes osmotically dilute urine, water excretion is increased significantly.
   - Thus, when kidney takes the responsibility of regulating the ECF volume of the body by changing its solvent output, the solute concentration automatically changes, which changes the urine osmolality.
   - For example, when the individual is exposed to a desert like condition or to a high environmental temperature, **kidney maintains effective blood volume by reducing the urine output**, and in the process it excretes concentrated urine. In fact, for excreting urine with osmolality of 1400 mosm/kg of H_2O, kidney excretes about 0.5 L of urine in a day. Thus, it prevents dehydration and hypovolemia by saving about 1 L of effective blood volume (as normal urine output is about 1.5 L per day).
   - By executing this regulatory process, kidney decreases the amount of water that we are obliged to drink (as water may not be available) in such extreme conditions. Hence, in a true sense, kidney is the best friend of human beings as it reduces the obligatory task of drinking water in adverse situations. Conversely, kidney also has the **task of excreting a water load** from the body by forming a large quantity of dilute urine.
2. **In pathological conditions**, increased urine osmolality is due to change in solute output, and **excretion of water is secondary to the change in osmolality** of tubular fluid.
   - For example, in diabetes mellitus, glycosuria results in osmotic diuresis. In such a condition, increased excretion of solute in urine is accompanied by increased volume output that results in dehydration.
   - Thus, in disease conditions, water loss in urine is a forced phenomenon in response to solute load in the urine, in which kidney fails to regulate the volume loss, and therefore dehydration sets in.
   - Thus, mechanisms and the consequences of increased urine osmolality in physiological and pathological situations are in effect, have different perspectives.

Diluting and Concentrating Ability of Kidney

Normally, the change in urine osmolality is brought about **mainly by the action of ADH** on collecting duct of kidney. **In the presence of ADH**, urine osmolality may be as high as 1400 mosm/kg of H_2O with volume of urine at about 0.5 liter per day (0.27% of glomerular filtrate) and **in the absence of ADH**, urine osmolality may fall to as low as 30 mosm/kg of H_2O with urine volume at about 23 liters per day (more than 12.7% of glomerular filtrate). **In diabetes insipidus**, which occurs due to ADH deficiency, urine output is **more than 20 liters per day**.

1. Thus, ADH, which is an external factor for kidney plays an important role in urine concentration and dilution. However, also kidney has its own **intrinsic mechanism** to concentrate and dilute urine.
2. To produce diluted urine to excrete a volume overload is a rare physiological phenomenon.
3. But, to form concentrated urine to prevent volume loss, which is encountered frequently in life, is a challenge to and responsibility of the kidneys.
4. As such, normally kidneys excrete concentrated urine, which is less than 1% of glomerular filtrate. Kidneys further concentrate urine in the presence of volume contraction.

Thus, kidney is well equipped with an inherent and well developed mechanism to concentrate urine in normal as well as abnormal conditions, the mechanism which is known for more than 50 years as **countercurrent mechanism** of urine concentration.

Requirements of a Counter Current Mechanism

The mechanism by which urine is concentrated is known as countercurrent mechanism. In medulla of the kidney, there is **an increasing gradient of osmolality from outer region to inner region of medulla** with highest osmolality at the tip of the renal papillae. This osmolality gradient, which is produced and maintained by the counter current mechanisms, is essential for urine concentration. Countercurrent means **flow of fluid in opposite direction in adjacent structures.** For any countercurrent mechanism to operate, it **requires three conditions**:

1. There should be two tubes (inflow and outflow tubes) that should run parallel to each other.
2. The movement of fluid in one tube should be in opposite direction to the other.
3. The tubes should be in close proximity to each other and should be selectively permeable.

The best example is the **maintenance of air temperature in a furnace**, in which the input duct carries cool air from outside into the furnace and output duct carries hot air from the inner furnace to outside. The temperature of the hot air in the output duct is exchanged with the cool air of the input duct as both of them are in close thermal contact with each other (Fig. 79.1). Thus, temperature of fresh air of the input pathway increases as it passes deep into the furnace and becomes maximum at the tip (deepest part) and the temperature in the output pathway decreases as air comes out of the furnace. As a result, *inner temperature of the furnace circulates in the furnace without much loss to the environment*. Consequently, **a high temperature is maintained** inside the furnace. Similar mechanism is also applied for preserving heat in heating the air of a building. Heat preservation of such systems becomes more effective when the passive diffusion of heat from the ascending limb is replaced by or **added with active pumps** that push heat forcefully out of the ascending pathway into the descending pathway.

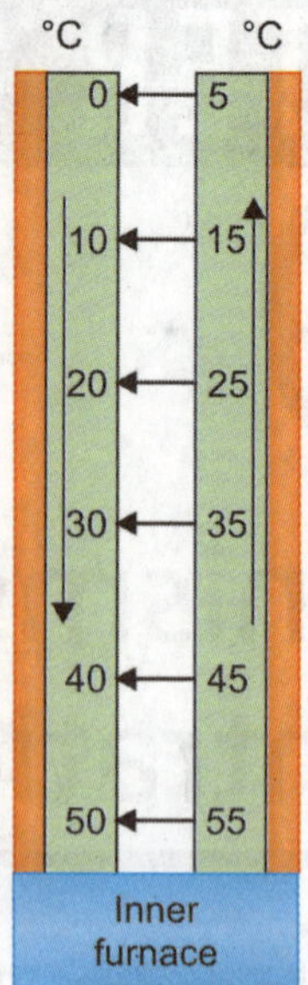

Fig. 79.1: Mechanism of counter-current heat exchange between inflow (downward arrow) and outflow (upward arrow) tubes of a furnace. Note, cooler air of inflow tube exchanges heat with hot air of outflow tube, so that the heat is maintained in the inner furnace. Thick outer wall of inflow and outflow tubes are meant to insulate the tubes.

In kidney, countercurrent mechanisms of similar nature operate. **Two countercurrent processes** work in the medulla of the kidney: countercurrent multiplication system and countercurrent exchange system. Loop of Henle (LOH) acts as **countercurrent multiplier** and vasa recta as **countercurrent exchanger**.

1. **In LOH,** fluid flows deep into the medulla along the descending limb and from medulla into the cortex along the ascending limb. The descending and ascending limbs for their selective permeabilities for water and solutes, **establish an osmotic gradient** in the medulla.
2. **In vasa recta**, blood flows in opposite direction in descending and ascending vessels during which **water and solutes are exchanged passively** between capillary blood vessels. This passive exchange in vasa recta **maintains the osmotic gradient**.
3. Collecting duct is juxtaposed to LOH and vasa recta (Fig. 79.2), and acts as an **osmotic equilibrating device**.

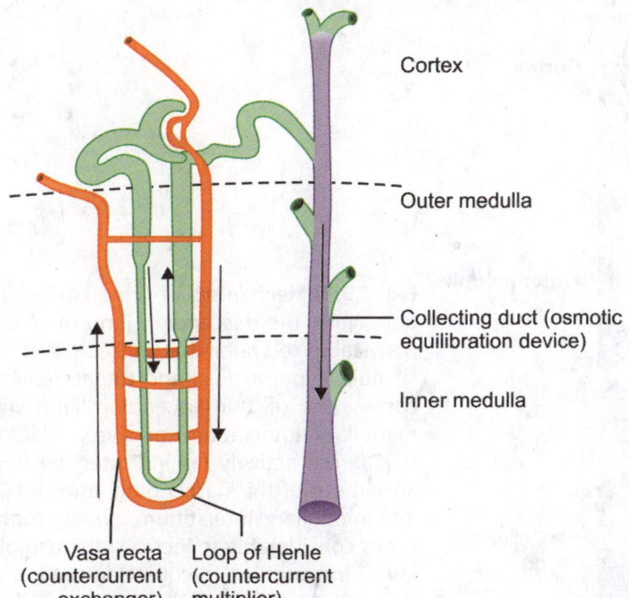

Fig. 79.2: Components of counter-current mechanism in kidney for concentration of urine. Note that the flow is in opposite direction in descending and ascending limbs of loop of Henle (as indicated by arrows inside), and vasa recta (as indicated by arrows outside vasa recta). This close proximity of descending and ascending limbs in a parallel arrangement and the opposite direction of flow in limbs are essential components of a counter-current mechanism to be effectively operative. Also, note the direction of flow in collecting duct (as indicated by arrow within the collecting duct).

Counter current mechanism also operate in other vascular beds (Application Box 79.1).

Application Box 79.1

Countercurrent mechanism helps penguin to stand on ice for a long: Ability of the kidney to concentrate urine is a critical adaptation of life on land. Countercurrent mechanisms not only operate in medulla of kidney, but also in **many vascular beds** where the blood vessels lie close to each other and allow exchange of solute, solvent and temperature between them. For example, exchange of heat between the inflowing and outflowing vessels of the feet of penguin helps penguin to maintain its body temperature when it stands on ice for a long.

Countercurrent Multiplication System

This is the process in which a small osmotic gradient established at any level of LOH is multiplied into a larger gradient. The osmotic gradient created at any level of LOH is called **single effect**, which is due to *movement of solute out of the water impermeable ascending limb of LOH*. Solute deposition in medulla is accompanied by removal of water from the descending limb.

As tubular fluid in the loop enters the deeper layers of medulla, it is more concentrated that creates increasing gradient of osmolality along the axis of the loop, called **axial gradient**. Magnitude of the axial gradient depends on three main factors:

1. The rate of fluid flow
2. Strength of single effect
3. The length of LOH.

Slower the fluid flow, larger the single effect and greater the loop length, the bigger is the axial gradient. Conversely, faster the fluid flow, smaller the single effect and shorter LOH reduces the axial gradient.

When the rate of flow is slower, time taken for transport of solutes in the ascending limb of LOH is more, and therefore, the **strength of single effect** and consequently the magnitude of axial gradient is enhanced. **When LOH is longer**, a greater axial gradient is generated as the chance for multiplication becomes higher.

Countercurrent Exchange System

The solute gradient created in the medulla by LOH is **maintained by vasa recta**.

1. The exchange of solutes and water takes place purely passively between descending and ascending limbs of vasa recta and this process of exchange **decreases the dissipation of the solute gradient** from medullary interstitium.
2. Water is removed from descending limb of vasa recta into the hyperosmolal interstitium, which is taken back by ascending limb of vasa recta (Fig. 79.3).
3. Thus, vasa recta **prevents dilution of osmolality of interstitium**.
4. Moreover, solutes come out of ascending limb and enter the descending limb of LOH, which ensures trapping of solutes in the medulla.
5. Thus, the process of exchange of water and solutes between descending and ascending limbs of vasa recta **maintains the gradient of osmolality established by LOH**.

COUNTERCURRENT MECHANISM

The countercurrent mechanism for urine concentration depends on **generation and maintenance of an increasing osmolality gradient** along the medullary pyramid from its outer layer to its deepest part. As discussed above, two systems operate to generate and maintain the high osmolality gradient in the medullary interstitium.

1. The osmolality gradient is **generated by the loop of Henle**, which acts as countercurrent multiplier, and **maintained by vasa recta**, which acts as countercurrent exchanger.
2. However, **collecting duct contributes in this process by equilibrating the gradient** (acts as equilibrating device). Thus, renal countercurrent mechanism depends on integrated functioning of loop of Henle, vasa recta and collecting duct.

Role of Loop of Henle: The Counter-Current Multiplier

The loop of Henle acts as counter current multiplier. About 30% of the volume originally filtered by the renal corpuscle enters LOH, which is isosmotic. In LOH, selective reabsorption of solutes and water occurs in its different segments that contribute to generate higher osmolality in medullary interstitium.

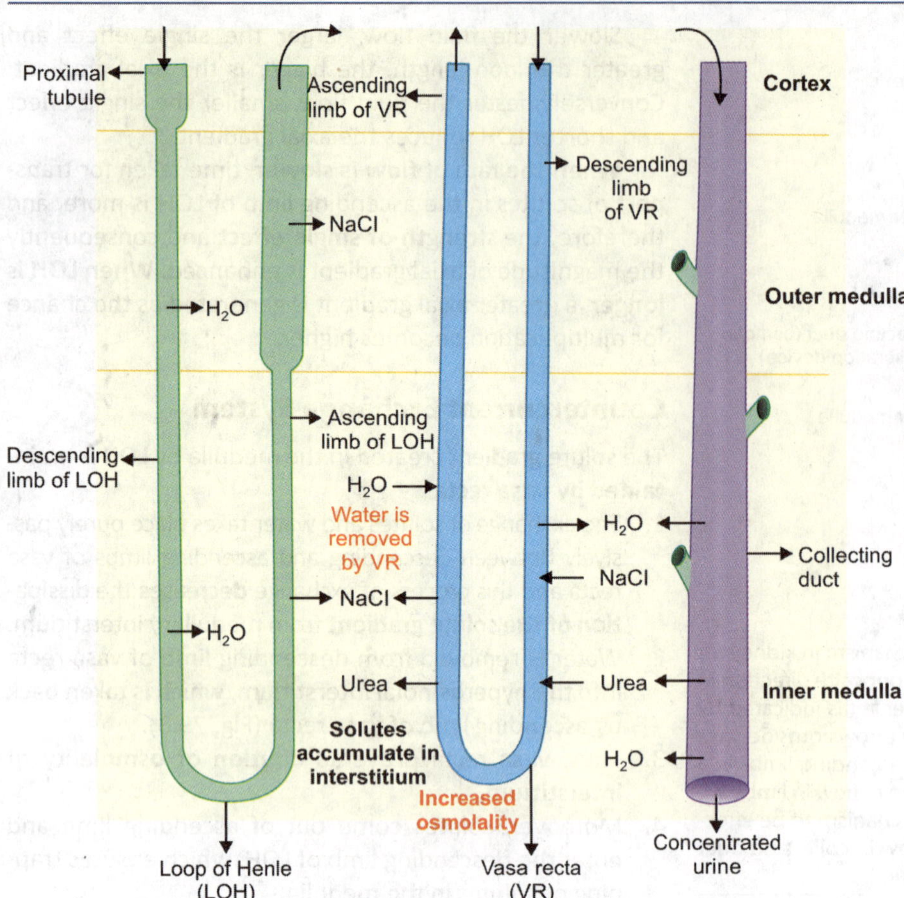

Fig. 79.3: Mechanism of urine concentration. Note, the descending limb of LOH is permeable to water that makes the tubular fluid hyperosmolal and therefore, NaCl comes out of thin ascending limb into medullary interstitium passively. NaCl is transferred actively (as indicated by thick arrow) out of thick ascending limb of LOH into medullary interstitium, which contributes considerably to increase the osmolality of interstitium. In collecting duct, urea diffuses out of the tubular fluid that aids to increase the interstitial osmolality. Water that comes out of collecting duct (and also from descending limb of LOH) is removed from medullary interstitium by vasa recta, which helps to maintain higher osmolality in the interstitium. This higher interstitial osmolality transfers water from tubular fluid leaving collecting duct and makes the urine concentrated. Arrows indicate direction of flow.

1. **Descending limb of LOH is highly permeable to water**, but **impermeable to solutes**. Therefore, fluid that flows down in the descending limb **becomes increasingly hypertonic** as water is selectively removed. Thus, fluid in the tip of the loop is highly concentrated and its osmolality is more than the interstitial osmolality.
2. **Thin ascending limb of LOH** is passively permeable to solutes. Due to high osmolality of fluid at the tip of the hairpin loop and in thin ascending limb of LOH, and the permeability of thin ascending limb to solutes, **solutes are passively transported from the hypertonic tubular fluid in to the interstitium.** However, the thin ascending limb of LOH is **relatively impermeable to water**. Therefore, every time the tubular fluid passes through the thin ascending limb of LOH, extra solutes enter the interstitium. This helps in multiplication of the interstitial osmolality.
3. Moreover, in **thick ascending limb of LOH**, Na^+ and Cl^- are **actively transported** from the tubular fluid due to vigorous activity of Na^+-K^+ ATPase in this part of the loop (Fig. 79.3). This actively removes solutes from the tubular fluid into the interstitium and **considerably aids in building up of a higher interstitial osmolality**. This makes the tubular fluid entering the distal tubule hypotonic.

The countercurrent multiplier role of LOH **depends on its length.** LOH of medullary nephrons are much longer than that of cortical nephrons. Therefore, though cortical nephrons are considerably more than medullary nephrons, higher osmolality is built only in the medullary interstitium. This is because **more Na^+ and Cl^- move down their concentration gradient along a longer thin ascending limb** into the interstitium and also **more are actively transported** along a greater length of thick ascending limb of LOH

Role of Collecting Duct

Collecting duct acts as osmotic equilibrating device. It contributes to urinary concentration by ***two ways***: first by its permeability to water and second for its permeability to urea.

1. **Collecting duct is permeable to water**. Therefore, *water moves out of tubular fluid* in the collecting duct into the hyperosmolal interstitium both in the cortical and medullary part. This *makes the tubular urine hypertonic*.
2. **Urea transported in collecting duct** also greatly *helps in generating osmotic gradient* in the medullary pyramid. In renal tubule, some quantity of urea is reabsorbed in PCT. However, *except in the inner medullary portion of the collecting duct, the rest of tubular epithelium is relatively impermeable to urea*. Some amount of urea is secreted into tubular fluid in the descending limb of LOH. Therefore, by the time tubular fluid reaches the medullary part of collecting duct, its urea concentration is very high. In the inner medulla, **urea moves from the tubular fluid into the interstitium passively**. When urea is removed from tubular fluid into the interstitium, *water moves out of tubular lumen* along with urea to maintain osmotic balance. Thus, **urine is**

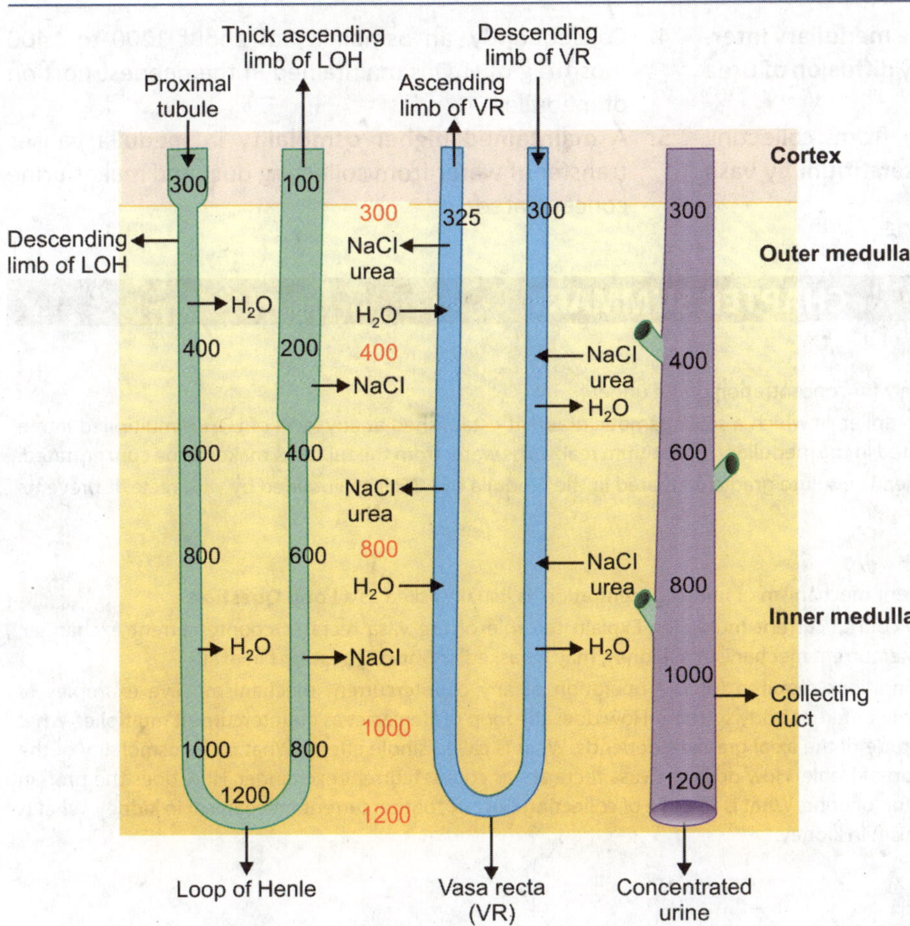

Fig. 79.4: Osmotic gradient across the medulla of kidney from its outer regions to the inner regions. Note, the tubular fluid and blood in vasa recta entering into medulla becomes gradually hyperosmolal and fluid and blood leaving medulla becomes gradually hypoosmolal. This occurs due to mechanisms as described in Figure 79.3. Thus, interstitial osmolality (mosm/kg of water) increases gradually from outer layers to inner layers of medulla reaching about 1200 mosm/kg of water in innermost part. This osmolal gradient transfers water from tubular fluid of collecting duct leaving the medulla that makes urine concentrated. Arrows indicate direction of movement. (VR: Vasa recta).

more concentrated. Water that enters the interstitium is taken up by vasa recta (*see* below) and consequently osmolal dilution of interstitium is prevented.

Urea Transporters: The movement of urea in collecting duct of kidney is facilitated by **urea transport protein A1** (UT-A1). There are **two types of urea transporters** that help urea transport by facilitated diffusion: urea transporter A (UT-A) and urea transporter B (UT-B). **UT-A** is found in kidney and **UT-B** in red cells. In kidney, **UT-A has four subtypes**: UT-A1 to UT-A1-4. The **UT-A1 is influenced by ADH**. Therefore, ADH facilitates urea reabsorption in kidney. The transport of urea and water in the collecting duct further helps in building up of hyperosmolality of the interstitium (Application Box 78.2).

Application Box 78.2

Protein content of diet controls concentration of urine: Urea content of tubular fluid depends mainly on the urea filtered in the glomerular filtering membrane, which depends on the **protein content of the diet**. Low-protein diet impairs the ability of kidney to maximally concentrate urine as this decreases the urea content in the medullary interstitium. Conversely, **high protein diet makes the urine concentrated**.

Role of Vasa Recta: The Counter-Current Exchanger

The concentration gradient generated by loop of Henle will not be long lasting if NaCl and urea accumulated in the interstitium are removed by circulation. However, the **osmolal gradient is maintained by the vasa recta**, which acts as counter current exchanger.

1. **In the descending limb** of vasa recta, **solutes diffuse into the vessels** (that carries blood into the medullary pyramid), and in the ascending limb **solutes diffuse out of the vessel** that carries blood toward the cortex.
2. Thus, solutes keep circulating in the interstitium. The movement of water is opposite to the movement of solutes.
3. **Water diffuses out of the descending limb and into the ascending limb** of the vasa recta (Fig. 79. 3). Thus, while solutes recirculate in the medulla, water is removed from it. Therefore, hypertonicity of the interstitium is maintained.
4. Water in the vasa recta enters general circulation and helps in maintaining ECF volume.

Net Effect

Every time tubular fluid passes through LOH, **water comes out of descending limb** into interstitium (which is removed by ascending limb of VR) and **solutes come out of ascending limb** (NaCl diffuses passively into interstitium in thin ascending portion and pumped actively into interstitium in thick ascending limb).

1. A longer LOH accumulates more solutes across its length from outer layers into deeper layers of medulla. Thus, **osmolality increases along LOH** as it dips into the medulla (Fig. 79.4).

2. This causes a **higher osmolality in the medullary interstitium**, which is further enhanced by **diffusion of urea from the collecting duct** into it.
3. Water also moves out passively from collecting duct, but **water is removed from interstitium by vasa recta**.
4. Consequently, an osmolality of about 1200 to 1400 mosm/kg of H_2O is maintained in the deepest portion of medulla.
5. A **maintained higher osmolality** in medulla causes transfer of water from collecting duct and makes urine concentrated.

CHAPTER SUMMARY

Key Concepts

1. The counter-current system is meant mainly for concentration of the urine.
2. Loop of Henle acts as counter current multiplier, in which a small osmotic gradient established at any level of LOH is multiplied into a larger gradient. The osmotic gradient created in the medullary interstitium reabsorbs water from the tubule & makes urine concentrated.
3. Vasa recta is the counter-current exchanger. The solute gradient created in the medulla by LOH is maintained by vasa recta. It prevents dilution of osmolality of interstitium.

Important to Know (Must Read)

1. In examination, "Describe the countercurrent mechanism of urine concentration" is usually asked as a **Long Question.**
2. Explain the role of the loop of Henle as countercurrent multiplier, Explain the role of the vasa recta as countercurrent exchanger, Explain the role of collecting duct in countercurrent mechanism in kidney, may be asked as **Short Questions** in exam.
3. In **Viva**, examiner may ask... List the conditions required for the operation of any countercurrent mechanism, Give examples of countercurrent mechanisms that operates in different body systems, How does the loop of Henle act as countercurrent multiplier, What are the three factors on which the magnitude of the axial gradient depends, What is called single effect , What is the osmolality of the filtrate in the PCT and at the tip of the loop of Henle, How does the vasa recta act as countercurrent exchanger, How does the protein content of the diet control the concentration of urine, What is the role of collecting duct in countercurrent mechanism in kidney, What is the role of urea in countercurrent mechanism in kidney.

CHAPTER

80

Water Excretion, Diuresis, and Diuretics

LEARNING OBJECTIVES

On completion of study of this chapter, the student **MUST** be able to:

1. Understand the mechanism of water reabsorption from kidney tubule.
2. Understand the concept of obligatory and facultative reabsorption of water.
3. List the difference between water and osmotic diuresis.
4. Describe the mechanism of water reabsorption in kidney tubules.
5. List the diuretics and give their mechanism of action.
6. Appreciate the functions of aquaporins

The student **MAY** also be able to:

1. Describe the physiological basis of use of diuretics.

WATER EXCRETION

Controlled excretion of urine from the body is an important function of kidney. The volume of urine is determined by the quantity of water reabsorbed from renal tubule. Normally, kidney reabsorbs more than 99% of the filtered water. Therefore, though the GFR is about 180 liters per day, only 1 to 1.5 liters of urine is formed in 24 hours. Even when, more than 23 liters of urine is formed per day as occurs in ADH deficiency, kidney absorbs about 87% of the filtered water. Thus, the capacity of kidney to reabsorb water is enormous. This is the major mechanism of volume homeostasis of the body.

Types of Water Reabsorption

Water reabsorption in renal tubules is of two types: obligatory and facultative.

Obligatory Reabsorption

Obligatory reabsorption of water is the water reabsorption that occurs secondary to reabsorption of solutes. This accounts for about **85% of the total water reabsorption** in tubules and most part of it occurs in proximal tubule.

Facultative Reabsorption

Facultative reabsorption of water is the water reabsorption that occurs secondary to the effects of hormone, especially ***ADH and aldosterone***. This accounts for about **15% of total water reabsorption** from kidney and occurs mostly in distal parts of nephron (in collecting duct and DCT).

Aquaporins

Transport of water across the membrane of epithelial cells depends on the presence of **aquaporins**, the water channels made up of proteins. **Thirteen aquaporins** have been identified till date. In human beings, **four types of aquaporins** have been characterized so far. These are aquaporin-1, aquaporin-2, aquaporin-5, and aquaporin-9. Aquaporins-1 and 2 are mainly involved in water reabsorption from kidney (Table 80.1).

Scientist contributed

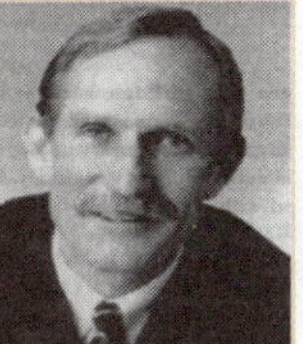

Peter Agre

Dr Peter Agre received **Nobel Prize in Chemistry** in 2003, for his unique discovery of **aquaporins (water channels)** that revolutionized the mechanism of water absorption from kidney tubules and other epithelia of the body. He worked at John Hopkins University, Baltimore, USA and shared the Nobel Prize with **Roderick MacKinnon**. Initially he was granted NIH funding for study of Rh blood group antigen. While isolating Rh antigen protein, Agre and colleagues found another protein of 28kDa from the red cells, the water pores (the aquaporins).

Aquaporins in Kidney

Most of the aquaporins are found in kidney. **Aquaporin-1** is found mainly in proximal tubule and loop of Henle, and

Table 80.1: Distribution and functions of main 9 types of aquaporins.

Types	Distribution	Functions	Expression in other tissues
A. Renal aquaporins			
Aquaporin 1	Apical and basolateral membrane of PCT and thin descending limb of LOH	67% of water reabsorption in PCT is due to AQP-1 Imparts free water permeability in thin descending limb of LOH	Multiple organs
Aquaporin 2	Apical membrane of late DCT and vesicles of principal cells of cortical part of CD	Mediate ADH effects	Testis
Aquaporin 3	Basolateral membrane of late DCT and cortical CD	Mediate ADH effects	Multiple organs
Aquaporin 4	Basolateral membrane of late DCT and cortical CD	Mediate ADH effects	Brain, other organs
Aquaporin 6	Vesicles of intercalated cells of CD	Acts as an internal ion channel of I cells	
Aquaporin 7	Apical membrane of PCT	Water absorption in PCT	Testis and adipocytes
Aquaporin 8	Intracellular vesicles in cortex and medulla; in PCT	Exact function not known	Testis, epididymis, pancreas, liver, colon, heart, placenta
B. Extrarenal aquaporins			
Aquaporin 5	Salivary glands, lungs, eye		
Aquaporin 9	Liver, leucocyte, brain, spleen, lungs, epididymis, testis		

aquaporin-2 in the collecting duct. These aquaporins (aquaporins-1 and 2) control water reabsorption in renal tubules. Knock out of aquaporin 1 in PCT in experimental animals decreases water reabsorption by about 70%. These animals fail to maintain water balance in dehydration. This signifies the importance of aquaporin 1 in proximal tubule in water reabsorption (for details of aquaporins, refer page 594).

Aquaporins in Extrarenal Tissues

In addition, **aquaporin-5** is found in lacrimal gland and **aquaporin-9** is present in liver, spleen, lungs, and leucocytes. The role of aquaporins in extrarenal tissues is not clearly known.

Structure and Functions of Aquaporins

Aquaporins were discovered by Peter Agre and his team. Aquaporins have **six membrane spanning regions,** with intracellular membrane spanning both amino and carboxy terminals (Fig. 80.1). They form tetramers in the cell membrane, with **each monomer acting as a water channel.**

The distribution and function of main 9 types of aquaporins are listed in Table 80.1.

Applied Aspects

1. Nephrogenic diabetes insipidus is characterized by **decreased expression of aquaporin 2** in CD and DCT.
2. In chronic heart failure, there is increased expression of aquaporin-2.

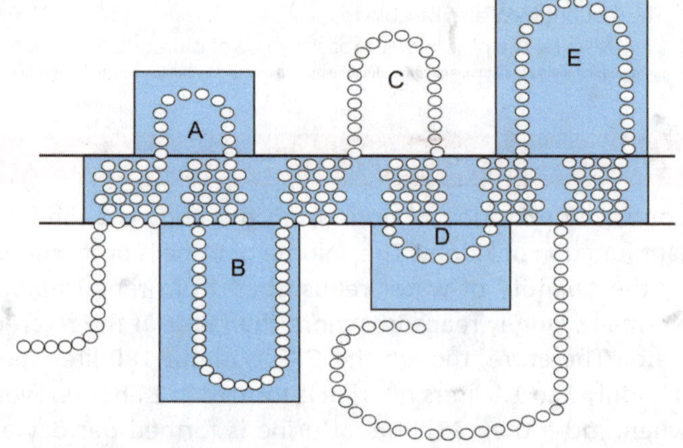

Fig. 80.1: Structure of Aquaporin-1.

Mechanism of Water Reabsorption

In Proximal Tubule

Normally, **65% of the filtered water** is reabsorbed in the proximal tubule.

1. The driving force for water reabsorption is the **transcellular osmotic gradient**, which is established by absorption of Na^+ and accompanying solutes.
2. Permeability of epithelium of proximal tubule to water is extremely high, due to the presence of aquaporin-1 in the cell membranes.
3. Water also passes through the **water channels present in the paracellular route** (through tight junctions present between epithelial cells). Therefore, even a smaller osmotic gradient across the tubular cells results in adequate movement of water.

In LOH

The loop of Henle reabsorbs approximately **15% of the filtered water**.

1. The ascending limb of LOH is impermeable to water and water reabsorption **occurs mainly in the descending limb**.
2. The water reabsorption in descending limb of LOH **is a passive process** that occurs secondary to higher osmolality of medullary interstitium.

In DCT

DCT is **relatively impermeable to water**. Inspite of osmotic gradient across the tubular epithelium, water reabsorption is poor. Only about **5% of the filtered water** is removed in DCT, which is influenced by aldosterone and ADH. However, solute is removed actively in excess of solvent in this part of nephron.

In Collecting Duct

Collecting duct (CD) has two parts: cortical and medullary. Reabsorption of solute and water from the collecting duct mainly depends on the concentration of ADH acting on it. About 12–15% of water is reabsorbed in collecting duct.

Cortical CD

In the cortical part, **ADH increases permeability** of collecting duct to water by inserting **aquaporin-2** water channels. ADH binds with **V_2 receptor** on the basolateral membrane of tubular cell, where it **activates adenylate cyclase** to increase the production of cAMP. cAMP activates proteinkinase A, which promotes the formation and insertion of vesicle containing aquaporin-2 on luminal surface of the epithelial cells that increases water permeability. Therefore, in the presence of ADH, water moves out of relatively hypotonic tubular fluid into interstitium of the cortex, which accounts for a substantial reabsorption of water in CD in the presence of the hormone.

Medullary CD

In the medullary portion of the collecting duct, water is reabsorbed from the tubular fluid into the hypertonic medullary interstitium **along the osmotic gradient**, which accounts for 5–10% of water reabsorption. This **plays an important role counter-current mechanism** and makes the urine concentrated.

DIURESIS AND DIURETICS

Diuresis is the **excess excretion of water** in the urine. **Physiologically**, it occurs due to failure of mechanisms that concentrates urine. **In diseases**, it occurs due either to absence of ADH that results in **water diuresis** or to excretion of osmotically active solutes that leads to **osmotic diuresis**.

Diuresis

Diuresis is of broadly **two categories**: water diuresis and osmotic diuresis. Generally, diuresis occurs when **osmolality of the tubular fluid is more** or the **reabsorptive capacity of the tubule for water is less**. The former is called osmotic diuresis and the later is called water diuresis.

Water Diuresis

Water diuresis is the excretion of large volume of water without loss of excess of solute. This occurs when the capacity of the kidney tubule to reabsorb water is impaired.

1. Normally, the level of *ADH determines the amount of water to be reabsorbed* from the kidney.
2. Therefore, ADH deficiency, results in water diuresis. For example, in diabetes insipidus, urine is dilute and more in volume.
3. Water diuresis can be physiologically demonstrated by drinking a large amount of hypotonic fluid like water, in which polyuria occurs in 15 to 40 minutes of water ingestion.

Osmotic Diuresis

Increased concentration of **osmotically active particles in the tubular fluid** increases the excretion of water. This is called as osmotic diuresis.

1. This is typically seen in diabetes mellitus in which increased filtration of glucose (increased tubular glucose load) causes glycosuria, this causes osmotic diuresis. By osmotic effect, solutes hold water in the tubule (prevents reabsorption of water) that causes diuresis.
2. Osmotic diuresis is also produced by **administration of mannitol**. Mannitol is filtered in kidney but not reabsorbed and therefore, produces diuresis by its osmotic effect.
3. Osmotic diuresis can also be produced by infusion of large amount of NaCl or urea.

Diuretics

Diuretics are substances that promote diuresis (increased excretion of water in urine). In medical practice, diuretics are usually used to decrease the ECF volume. Frequently, administered diuretics are loop diuretics, aldosterone antagonists, thiazide diuretics, carbonic anhydrase inhibitors, xanthines, large quantities of osmotically active substances, ethanol, acidifying salts, vasopressin antagonists, and water.

Loop Diuretics

Furosemide (lasix) and ethacrynic acid are loop diuretics.

1. They act by ***inhibiting Na^+-K^+-$2Cl^-$ cotransporter in the thick ascending limb*** of loop of Henle.
2. This inhibits Na^+, K^+, and Cl^- reabsorption causing diuresis with loss of these electrolytes.

Aldosterone Antagonists

Spironolactone is the commonly administered aldosterone antagonist.

1. It *inhibits the action of aldosterone* on the kidney tubule. Thus, it ***inhibits*** Na^+***-***K^+ ***exchange*** that leads to natriuresis and diuresis with retention of K^+ in the body. Hence, it is called K^+ ***sparing diuretic***.
2. **Amiloride and triamterene**, other K^+ sparring diuretics compete with sodium for a site in the ENaC (epithelial Na channel) and block sodium reabsorption and potassium secretion.
3. Thus, they produce diuresis with retention of K^+.

Thiazide Diuretics

Usually administered thiazide diuretic is **chlorothiazide**. It **inhibits** Na^+**-**Cl^- **cotransporter in the early part of distal tubule**. Thus, increased excretion of NaCl produces diuresis.

Carbonic Anhydrase Inhibitors

The usually administered diuretic is **acetazolamide** (diamox). As the name suggests, it inhibits carbonic anhydrase activity in renal tubular cells.

1. It decreases H^+ secretion into tubular fluid.
2. Normally, H^+ is exchanged with Na^+ in luminal membrane of tubular epithelial cells by Na^+**-**H^+ **antiport.**
3. Therefore, decreased H^+ secretion results in increase in Na^+ (and also K^+) excretion that leads to diuresis.

Xanthines

Xanthines such as caffeine and theophylline act as diuretics. They inhibit tubular reabsorption of Na^+. They also increase GFR.

Osmotically Active Substances

Administration of large quantities of osmotically active substances like mannitol and glucose produce osmotic diuresis by increasing their concentration in tubular fluid.

Ethanol

Ethyl alcohol produces diuresis by **inhibiting ADH secretion.**

Acidifying Salts

Acidifying salts like calcium and ammonium chloride act as diuretic by **increasing the tubular acid load**. The H^+ is buffered, but an anion is excreted with Na^+ when the ability of kidney to replace Na^+ with H^+ is exceeded.

Vasopressin Antagonists

ADH antagonists inhibit the action of ADH on kidney tubules.

Water: Increased water consumption (hypervolemia) *inhibits ADH secretion*.

CHAPTER SUMMARY

Key Concepts

1. Diuresis is mainly for excreting excess water from the body when there is volume overload or ECF expansion.
2. In diabetes, osmotic diuresis occurs due to glycosuria.
3. Loop diuretics such as furosemide are commonly used in clinical practice.

Important to Know (Must Read)

1. In examination, no **Long Question** will be asked from this chapter.
2. Mechanism of water reabsorption in kidney, Types and mechanisms of diuresis, Aquaporins, may asked as **Short Questions** in exam.
3. In **Viva**, examiner may ask... What is obligatory reabsorption of water, What is facultative reabsorption of water, What is the mechanism of action of aquaporins, What is osmotic diuresis, give example, What is water diuresis, give example, List the important diuretics and give their mechanism of action.

CHAPTER

81

Acidification of Urine

Learning Objectives

On completion of study of this chapter, the student **MUST** be able to:

1. Appreciate the purpose of acidification of urine.
2. Mention the factors that contribute to acidification of urine.
3. Learn the mechanisms of acidification of urine.
4. Understand the responses of kidney in acid-base disorders.

The student **MAY** also be able to:

1. Explain the mechanisms of acidification of urine.

GENERAL CONCEPTS

Normally, pH of plasma is maintained within a narrow range of 7.35 to 7.45. To maintain this slender plasma pH range, major systems that work continuously and effectively are **buffer systems, respiratory system and renal system**. These three mechanisms work in concurrence. However, **kidney plays an important role in long-term control of pH** as most of the acid load from plasma is removed through renal system.

1. According to the increase or decrease of plasma pH, **body excretes or retains acids and bicarbonates and urine becomes acidic or alkaline** respectively.
2. **Alkalization of urine** is rare, which occurs mostly in pathological conditions.
3. However, during daily normal metabolism, **acids are produced continuously**. Therefore, unless acids are excreted, they accumulate in the body and produce acidosis.
4. In order **to prevent acidosis,** body excretes excess acids through kidney into urine, the process that leads to acidification of urine, which is a normal physiological phenomenon.

Excretion of acids through urine **serves three important functions**:

1. **Eliminates extra acids** that are harmful to our body. This prevents development of acidosis.
2. Contributes to **normal acid-base balance** of body.
3. **Protects from urinary tract infection** by preventing entry of pathogens by virtue of acidic pH of urine, which is especially important in females.

Factors Influencing Acidification of Urine

Four important factors contribute to acidification of urine:

1. Renal acid excretion
2. Renal bicarbonate reabsorption
3. Acid-base status of the body
4. Other factors (mainly hormonal).

Renal Acid Excretion

Kidney contributes to acid-base balance **by excreting acid,** which is proportionate to the production of non-volatile acids in the body. Kidney also **prevents bicarbonate loss** to achieve this purpose.

1. The major contribution to acid-base balance is by renal bicarbonate loss or gain as filtered load of HCO_3^- (about 4300 meq/day) is much higher than the filtered load of non-volatile acid, which is about 80 meq/day.
2. Most of the filtered HCO_3^- is reabsorbed. The reabsorption of filtered HCO_3^- and excretion of acid are achieved through the **process of H^+ secretion.**
3. Most of the H^+ secreted into the tubular fluid, which is about 4400 meq/day, *serves to reabsorb the filtered HCO_3^-*, and only about 100 meq/day is excreted in urine. Therefore, normally urine is mildly acidic.

Ammonium (NH_4^+) synthesis and excretion by kidney plays an important role in maintenance of acid-base balance. For each NH_4^+ excreted in urine, one HCO_3^- is added to the systemic circulation. This replenishes the HCO_3^- lost during titration of non-volatile acid (Application Box 81.1). For acid-base balance, the net acid excretion should be equal to the net non-volatile acid production. In general, the process is designated as **net acid excretion**.

Application Box 81.1

Titratable Acids: Kidney excretes non-volatile acids and replenishes HCO_3^- lost, during titration. However, kidney cannot excrete the free acids; instead excretes the salts of free acids while excreting H^+ with other anions, the **urinary buffers**. The main buffer in the urine is phosphate buffer. Other buffers are bicarbonate and ammonia buffers. The **different urinary buffers are collectively known as titratable acids.** The term titratable acid refers to the method of estimation of an acid. In a laboratory, to estimate urine acid, alkali is added to urine sample to titrate its pH to that of plasma. The quantity of alkali added is equal to the H^+ titrated by these urine buffers. Therefore, this is called the titratable acid.

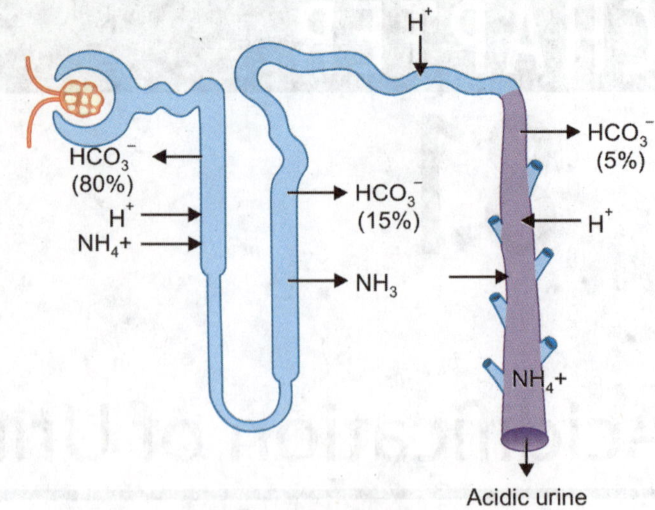

Fig. 81.1: Renal tubular handling of HCO_3^-, H^+ and NH_4^+. Arrows indicate the direction of movement.

Renal Bicarbonate Reabsorption

Normally, the amount of bicarbonate reabsorbed from tubular fluid equals the amount filtered. Therefore, under normal conditions, **HCO_3^- is not excreted in urine**.

1. About 80% of the total filtered bicarbonate is reabsorbed in PCT and 15% in thick ascending limb of LOH and 5% in the collecting duct (Fig. 81.1).
2. The mechanism of **bicarbonate reabsorption in PCT** involves **Na^+-H^+ antiporter** in the apical surface of the epithelial cells (for details, *see* below).
3. In the thick part of ascending limb of LOH, mechanism is similar to that in the PCT.
4. **In DCT and collecting duct**, reabsorption does not require Na^+-H^+ antiporter.
5. In *intercalated cells* in these parts of nephron, H^+ and HCO_3^- are produced by hydration of CO_2, which is catalyzed by carbonic anhydrase. From the cell, H^+ is secreted into the tubular fluid **by H^+-ATPase or K^+-H^+ ATPase** and HCO_3^- is added to interstitium by Cl^--HCO_3^- antiporter present in the basolateral membrane.

In PCT, permeability to H^+ and HCO_3^- is more. Therefore, the pH of tubular fluid in the PCT is about 6.5. In collecting duct, permeability to H^+ is low. Therefore, *tubular fluid in this part of the tubule is more acidic*, having pH about 4.5. This ability of the collecting duct to reduce the tubular fluid pH is **physiologically important for excretion of urinary buffers.**

Formation of New Bicarbonate (Role of Ammonia)

Urinary ammonium excretion is intimately associated with acid-base balance.

1. Ammonium is **important in HCO_3^- formation.** In the kidney, ammonium is produced by **metabolism of glutamine.**
2. Glutamine and Na^+ salts are the non-volatile acids. Kidney metabolizes glutamine, excrete NH_4^+ with acid-salts and add $NaHCO_3$ to the body.
3. In this process, **new HCO_3^- is formed** which is dependent on the ability of the kidney to excrete the NH_4^+ in the urine (for details, *see* below).

Acid-Base Status of the Body

Systemic acid-base balance affects acid secretion and HCO_3^- reabsorption and hence, acidification of urine. Therefore, acidification of urine cannot be addressed without mentioning acid-base balance.

1. **In metabolic acidosis**, acidification of intracellular fluid increases H^+ gradient between tubular cell and lumen. This results **in increased H^+ secretion.**
   - Acidification of intracellular fluid also increases the insertion of transporters into the apical membrane of the cells that **increases the net H^+ ATPase activity.**
   - Therefore, H^+ secretion is more, which in turn increases HCO_3^- reabsorption, especially in PCT.
   - HCO_3^- reabsorption is increased from the kidney to nullify the increased acidity of body fluids.
2. **In metabolic alkalosis**, HCO_3^- reabsorption as well as acid secretion from kidney is decreased thereby causing a **decrease in urine acidification rate.**
   - In metabolic alkalosis, when plasma bicarbonate level goes beyond 28 mmol/L, renal threshold for bicarbonate reabsorption crosses its limits and the bicarbonate ions start appearing in the urine.
   - Hence, urine acidification drops down.
3. **In respiratory acidosis,** when pCO_2 increases, the H^+ formation increases by the action of carbonic anhydrase. This causes **increased reabsorption of bicarbonate and acidification of urine.**
4. The reverse happens in case of **respiratory alkalosis.**

Other Factors

Aldosterone, parathormone, angiotensin II and plasma K^+ contribute to acidification of urine.

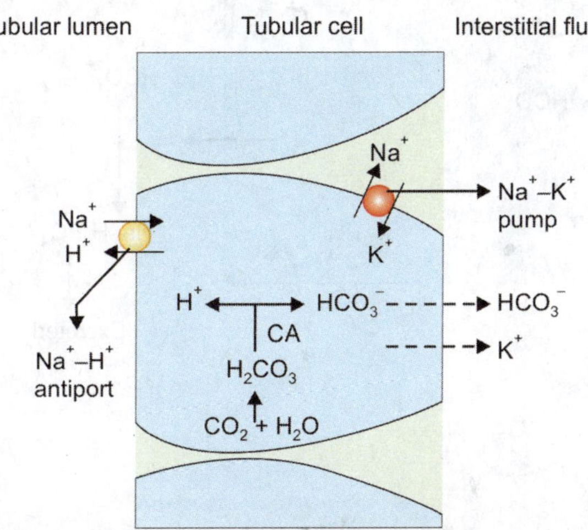

Fig. 81.2: Mechanism of acid secretion in PCT. H^+ formed from dissociation of $H_2CO_3^-$ is transferred into tubular fluid by Na^+–H^+ antiport located on apical membrane of tubular epithelial cell and HCO_3^- diffuses into interstitial fluid. Thus, H^+ secretion in PCT is Na^+-dependent.

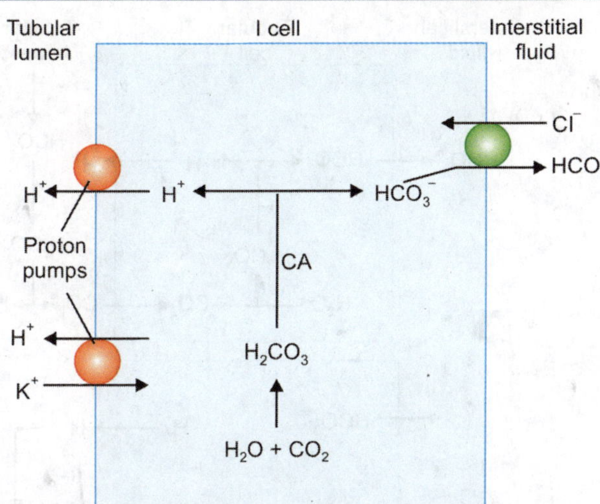

Fig. 81.3: Mechanism of acid secretion in distal tubular cells (by intercalated (I) cells in DCT and CD). H^+ formed from dissociation of $H_2CO_3^-$ is transferred into tubular fluid by proton pumps (H^+ ATPase or K^+-H^+ ATPase) located on apical membrane of tubular epithelial cell and HCO_3^- diffuses into interstitial fluid by HCO_3^--Cl^- antiport located on basolateral membrane. Thus, H^+ secretion in DCT and CD is mostly Na^+-independent.

1. **Aldosterone** increases H^+ secretion from the tubular cells into the tubular fluid. Therefore, it contributes to urine acidification and alkali reabsorption in the kidney.
2. **Angiotensin II** secondarily affects Na^+ concentration and Na^+-H^+ exchange, hence affects urine acidification.

MECHANISM OF URINE ACIDIFICATION

Acidification of urine is due to various mechanisms operating in different parts of the nephron, especially in PCT, DCT and collecting duct.

Acidification in Proximal Tubule

Increased CO_2 in the body represents increased acidity in systemic circulation.

1. In proximal tubular cells, CO_2 binds with H_2O to form carbonic acid. Dissociation of carbonic acid produces H^+ and HCO_3. Both the formation and dissociation of carbonic acid is catalyzed by the enzyme **carbonic anhydrase** at the brush border. This **serves two purposes.**
   - First, it helps to trap the acid in the form of CO_2 which cannot be removed from kidney fully even after diffusion through tubular walls.
   - Second, it cleaves and extracts the acid and helps in its active secretion into the lumen while retaining the alkaline bicarbonate inside the cell.
2. **Secretion of H^+ into tubular fluid** occurs via Na^+-H^+ antiporter (Fig. 81.2).
3. The **bicarbonate ion diffuses into the interstitium** as K^+ ion does.
4. The Na^+ ion from tubular cells enters interstitium in exchange of a K^+ by Na^+-K^+ ATPase.
5. Thus, cellular K^+ concentration remains unaffected, while Na^+ concentration decreases. The decreased Na^+ concentration initiates entry of Na^+ ions from luminal side into cell, which is coupled with secretion of H^+. Thus, urine **acidification at PCT is dependent on Na^+ concentration.**

Parathormone inhibits Na^+-H^+ exchanger in apical cell membrane of PCT and therefore, affects urine pH. It should be noted that as the carbonic anhydrase plays a vital role in PCT, drugs that inhibit its action (**carbonic anhydrase inhibitors**) decrease the process of acidification of urine.

Acidification in Distal Tubules and Collecting Duct

Unlike in PCT, the distal tubular cells acidify urine independent of their Na^+ concentration. In DCT, secretion of H^+ occurs by **active (ATP-driven) proton pumps.**

1. Aldosterone increases distal tubular acid secretion by acting on these pumps directly.
2. The **I cells of DCT** are equivalent to the parietal cells of stomach as they actively secrete acid. These cells are rich in carbonic anhydrase. The number of H^+ pumps employed at the membrane increases for increased acid secretion.
3. **Band 3 protein**, an anion exchanger protein located at the basolateral membrane acts as **chloride-bicarbonate exchanger** (Fig. 81.3). It transports bicarbonate ion into interstitium, thereby it retains bicarbonate ion and acidifies urine.
4. Apart from this, **H^+-K^+ ATPase** to some extent secretes H^+ and absorbs K^+ in the collecting tubules. pH changes of tubular fluid in DCT may be acute (Application Box 81.2)

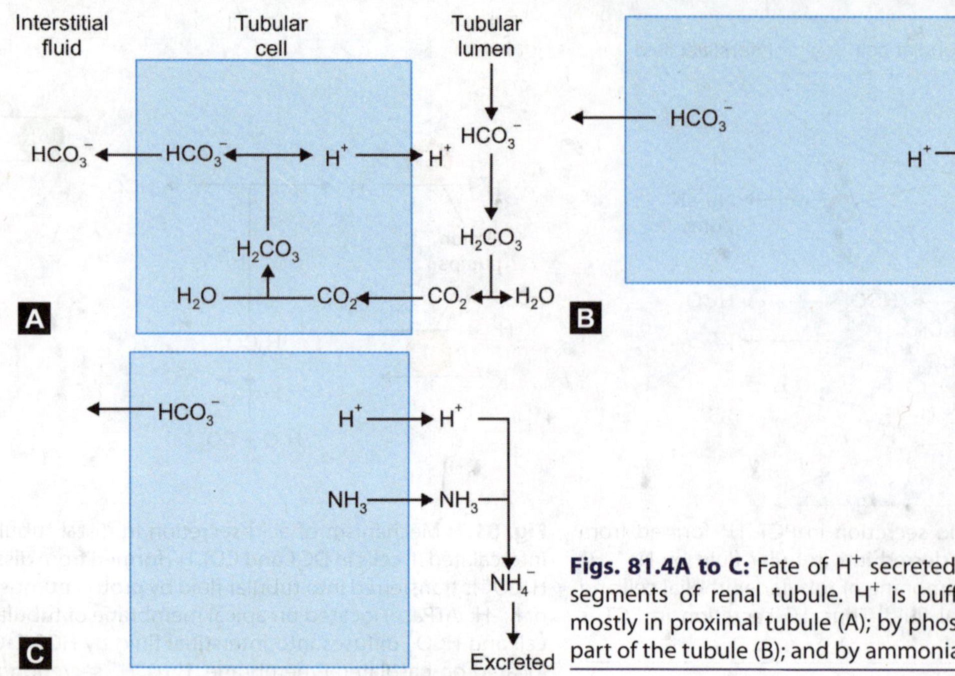

Figs. 81.4A to C: Fate of H^+ secreted by tubular cells in different segments of renal tubule. H^+ is buffered by bicarbonate buffer mostly in proximal tubule (A); by phosphate buffer mostly in distal part of the tubule (B); and by ammonia buffer in PCT and DCT (C).

Application Box 81.2

Maximum acidification: The minimum urinary pH at which maximal acidification can be achieved is 4.5. At this pH, H^+ concentration of urine is 1000 times more than that in plasma. This pH of tubular fluid is usually attained in the collecting ducts. Though acid secretion is more in PCT, it contributes to moderate change in urinary pH as the carbonic acid breaks down into carbon dioxide and water. On the other hand, urinary pH changes are acute in DCT though its acid secreting capacity is less.

Further Modifications in Acidification

After saturation of acid secreting mechanisms, there would be no further urine acidification. However, constant removal of H^+ by the action of urinary buffers from the tubules makes it possible for further acid secretion. It occurs via three different **buffering mechanisms** at different regions of tubules (Figs. 81.4A to C).

In PCT

Reaction with **bicarbonate buffers** occurs in the tubular fluid in PCT. Bicarbonate ion after filtration into tubular fluid reaches a concentration of about 24 millimoles. At this concentration, it is an effective buffer for the tubular acids. It forms carbonic acid that breaks down into carbon dioxide and water at the brush border of PCT by the action of carbonic anhydrase. The carbon dioxide diffuses into tubule cell and reacts with water molecule to resecrete acid into tubule and reclaim bicarbonate ion into interstitium (Fig. 81.4A).

In DCT and Collecting Duct

Secreted acid reacts with dibasic **phosphate buffer** whose pK value is closer to urinary pH (Fig. 81.4B). The relative concentration of phosphate buffer here is more and effective, as it is not reabsorbed in PCT. The reaction is:

$$Na_2HPO_4 + H^+ \rightarrow Na^+ + NaH_2PO_4$$

The monobasic phosphate gets excreted while sodium gets reabsorbed. In DCT and collecting tubules, phosphate gets concentrated due to increased absorption of water. Hence, phosphate buffer is more active in these parts of nephron.

In PCT and DCT

In PCT and DCT, **ammonia buffer** also woks. Soluble ammonia diffuses through cell membrane down its concentration gradient into tubular fluid. Here it reacts with acid to form ammonium ion, which subsequently gets excreted. Hence, it maintains the ammonia gradient for further ammonia diffusion. This is called **nonionic diffusion.** In case of acidosis, amount of ammonia diffusion into urine increases and hence the excretion of ammonium ion increases (Fig. 81.4C). The mechanism that increases ammonia diffusion into urine in acidosis is still not clear. However, the probable mechanism may be as follows.

In PCT

In proximal tubular cells, ammonium is produced from glutamine. Each **glutamine molecule produces two molecules of NH_4^+** and a **divalent anion.**

1. Each anion is metabolized to produce two molecules of HCO_3^- that enter the blood as new HCO_3^- and NH_4^+ enters the tubular fluid.
2. Glutamine becomes glutamate by glutaminase, which in turn forms α-ketoglutarate (α-KG) by glutamic dehydrogenase.
3. α-KG is converted to glucose by gluconeogenesis that enters interstitial fluid and from there into blood. NH_4^+ formed during this process is secreted into tubular fluid.
4. The mechanism of NH_4^+ secretion involves **Na^+-H^+ antiporter** that substitutes NH_4^+ for H^+ (Fig. 81.5). A

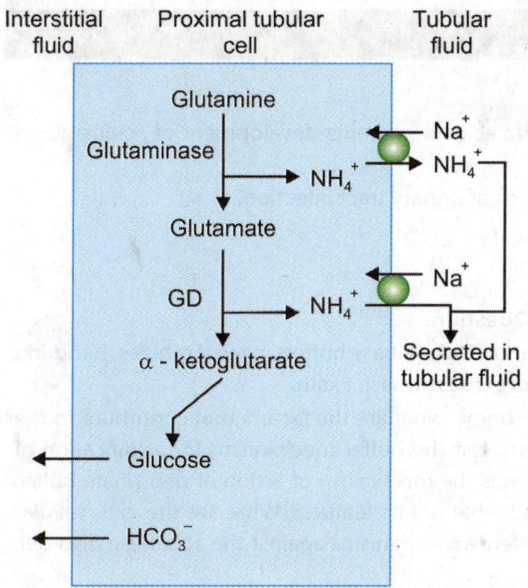

Fig. 81.5: Mechanism of NH_4^+ secretion that occurs mostly in proximal tubule. Note, NH_4^+ is formed during glutamine metabolism and its secretion involves Na^+-H^+ antiporter that substitutes NH_4^+ for H^+. GD: glutamic dehydrogenase.

substantial amount of this NH_4^+ is reabsorbed in thick ascending limb of loop of Henle, which accumulates in the medullary interstitium.

In Collecting Duct

In the collecting duct, the tubular cells are **not permeable to NH_4^+** but permeable to NH_3.

1. NH_3 diffuses from the interstitium into the tubular fluid.
2. H^+ is also secreted by the intercalated cells into the tubular fluid, and combines with NH_3 to form NH_4^+, which is excreted in the urine.
3. Thus, *H^+ secreted in the collecting duct is essential for the excretion of NH_4^+.*
4. Therefore, when H^+ secretion in collecting duct is decreased, net acid excretion is decreased (Clinical Box 81.3). This in turn decreases the transfer of new HCO_3^- to the blood to replenish the amount utilized by buffering of non-volatile acid.

Clinical Box 81.3

Fanconi Syndrome: Renal tubular acidosis (RTA) is the condition in which acidification of urine is decreased. In such a situation, kidneys are incapable of excreting a large amount of acid to balance the production of non-volatile acid. This results in **metabolic acidosis**. An example of RTA is Fanconi syndrome. When the defect is in the proximal tubule, the condition is called **proximal RTA** and when the defect is in distal part of the tubule, the condition is called **distal RTA**. Failure to produce and excrete NH_4^+ decreases the amount of net acid excreted by kidneys that results in metabolic acidosis.

RESPONSE OF KIDNEY TO ACID-BASE DISORDER

The pH of blood is maintained within a narrow range of 7.35 to 7.45. When pH falls acidosis occurs and when pH increases alkalosis occurs. When this imbalance occurs *primarily due to alteration in HCO_3^-*, the condition is called **metabolic acidosis or alkalosis**, and when it occurs primarily due to *alteration in blood PCO_2* the condition is called **respiratory acidosis or alkalosis**.

The body has three general mechanisms to maintain pH produced by the acid-base disorder:

1. Extracellular and intracellular buffering.
2. Adjustment in blood PCO_2 by mainly changing the rate of ventilation
3. By adjusting the renal acid secretion.

Accordingly, the mechanisms are called extracellular and intracellular defenses, respiratory defense and renal defense.

Extracellular and Intracellular Defenses

The extracellular buffering occurs immediately whereas intracellular buffering occurs slowly. **Extracellular buffering** includes **bicarbonate, phosphate, and protein buffers**. The **intracellular buffers** are mainly **phosphate, protein and hemoglobin buffers**.

Respiratory Defense

This defense mechanism against acid-base disorder operates within few minutes, which is mainly mediated by the **rate of ventilation** that determines the level of pCO_2 in blood. Increased ventilation decreases pCO_2 and decreased ventilation increases pCO_2 (for details, refer chapter "Acid-Base Balance" in Section XIII). For example, in metabolic acidosis, increase in concentration of H^+ increases ventilation by stimulating central chemoreceptors. The typical example is **Kussmaul respiration** seen in diabetic ketoacidosis.

Renal Defense

The renal defense mechanism takes several days to be effectively operative. This is because kidney takes hours to days to synthesis the enzymes that are involved in NH_4^+ synthesize. *Ammonium ion is the major urinary acid*. When the pH of urine falls below 6, excretion of ammonium ions increases.

1. **In acidosis**, secretion of H^+ by the kidney is increased, and filtered bicarbonate is totally reabsorbed.
   - Synthesis and excretion of NH_4^+ are also increased. This **increases total acid excreted by the kidney**.
   - New HCO_3^- generated during the acid excretion returns to blood that increases plasma bicarbonate.
   - In case of chronic acidosis like **diabetic ketoacidosis**, excretion of NH_4^+ can be increased 10 folds.
2. Conversely, **in alkalosis** secretion of H^+ by the kidney is inhibited. This **decreases bicarbonate reabsorption** and therefore, urine becomes alkaline (for details, refer chapter "Acid-Base Balance" in Section XIII).

CHAPTER SUMMARY

Key Concepts

1. Acids are continuously produced in the body by metabolism. Kidney eliminates extra acids & prevents development of acidosis, and therefore normally urine becomes acidic.
2. Acidic urine also prevents growth of bacteria in urinary tract and prevents the incidence of urinary tract infection.
3. Bicarbonate buffer and ammonia buffers are important buffers in the renal tubules.

Important to Know (Must Read)

1. In examination, 'Describe the mechanism of acidification of urine' is asked as a **Long Question.**
2. Mechanism of acidification of urine in PCT, Mechanism of acidification of urine in DCT and CD, Acid-base buffers in renal tubules, Handling of acid load by kidney, Response of kidney to acid base disorder, may be asked as **Short Questions** in exam.
3. In **Viva**, examiner may ask....... How is excretion of acids through urine helpful for our body, what are the factors that contribute to the acidification of urine, What do you mean by titratable acids, what are its components, List the buffer mechanisms for acidification of urine in PCT, DCT and CD, What is the mechanism of action of bicarbonate buffer, What is the mechanism of action of phosphate buffer, What is the mechanism of action of ammonia buffer, What is Fanconi syndrome and what are its features, What are the extracellular and intracellular defenses against the acid-base disorder, What are the respiratory defense mechanisms against the acid-base disorder, What are the renal defense mechanisms against the acid-base disorder.

CHAPTER

82

Kidney Function Tests and Pathophysiology of Renal Failure

Learning Objectives

On completion of study of this chapter, the student **MUST** be able to:

1. Classify kidney function tests (KFTs).
2. Understand the physiological basis of each KFT.
3. Learn the concept of clearance tests.
4. Understand the physiological basis of genesis and management of acute and chronic renal failures.

The student **MAY** also be able to:

1. Describe the procedure, application, merits and demerits of kidney function tests.

KIDNEY FUNCTION TESTS

As urine formation, the primary function of kidney is achieved by **two principal mechanisms**, the glomerular ultrafiltration, and tubular reabsorption & secretion, kidney function tests are physiologically grouped into two broad categories:

1. Tests that assess glomerular functions (**glomerular function tests**)
2. Tests that assess tubular functions (**tubular function tests**).

A. Glomerular function tests:

1. Blood urea determination
2. Blood creatinine estimation
3. Inulin clearance test
4. Creatinine clearance test
5. Urea clearance test
6. PAH clearance test
7. Estimation of proteins in the urine

B. Tubular function tests:

1. Urine concentration test
2. Urine dilution test
3. Detection of uric acid excretion
4. Test for acidification of urine
5. Test for alkalinisation of urine
6. Test for amino acids in urine

However, **clinically**, kidney function tests are divided into **four categories**:

1. **Routine tests:** Complete urine analysis, measurement of BUN in blood, and measurement of serum electrolytes.
2. **Tests for further assessments:** Clearance test, determination of urine and plasma osmolality, and concentration and dilution tests.
3. **Specific tests:** Tests to assess renal acidification, tests to assess renal handling of sodium, measurement of renal plasma flow, and excretion of exogenous compound like PSP.
4. **Special tests:** Ultrasonography, CT scan, MRI, etc.

Routine Urine Analysis

In clinical laboratories, urine analysis is performed routinely for assessing the degree of kidney dysfunctions in kidney diseases and other diseases that affect kidney functions. Routine urine analysis includes analysis of **physical and biochemical characteristics** of urine.

Physical Characteristics

Volume

The normal volume of urine excreted is about 1–1.5 liters per day. **Urine volume increases** in excess water intake, high protein diet, diuretic therapy, diabetes mellitus, diabetes insipidus, and sometimes in chronic renal diseases. **Urine volume decreases** in excessive sweating, hot climate, dehydration, hypotension, hypovolemia, kidney diseases, acute renal failure, antidiuretic therapy, edema due to variety of causes, and shock.

Oliguria and Anuria

A person on normal diet can excrete the solute load at maximum concentration when the urine volume is between 300 to 500 ml/day.

1. Volume below this is termed as **oliguria**.
2. When urine flow is totally absent or less than 50 ml/day, the situation is called as **anuria**.
3. Oliguria and anuria could be due to **decreased urine production** (as seen in renal failure, renal infarction, rapidly progressive glomerulonephritis etc.) or **due to obstruction to urine flow** (as seen in urinary calculi, prostatic enlargement, atonic bladder, pelvic or retroperitoneal tumors, urethral strictures, urethral infection, urethral valves etc.).

Polyuria

When urine volume is inappropriately high (> 3 liters per day), the situation is called polyuria. Polyuria could be due to **osmotic diuresis** (increased urinary solute excretion) or due to **water diuresis**. The common causes of polyuria are:

1. Excessive fluid intake
2. Osmotic diuresis (due to hyperglycemia and hypercalcemia)
3. Neurogenic diabetes insipidus (decreased ADH secretion)
4. Nephrogenic diabetes insipidus (due to tubular defects, interstitial renal disease, hypokalemia, hypercalcemia, drugs such as lithium)
5. Diuretics
6. Psychogenic polydipsia
7. Increased frequency of micturition (as occurs in urethritis, cystitis, prosatitis) may cause polyuria.

Nocturia

Waking up in the night to void urine is called nocturia. It may occur due to polyuria, but often it is due to more fluid intake before going to bed in the night or use of diuretic in the night. It can also occur in chronic kidney diseases and prostatic enlargement, or in sleep disturbances/disorders without functional abnormalities of urinary tract.

Appearance

Normally, urine is clear. It becomes turbid when kept in a container for a long time as urea is converted to ammonium carbonate by the action of bacteria, which makes the urine alkaline and results in precipitation of calcium and magnesium phosphates. Urine may also be turbid if it contains more **phosphates** (as in alkaline urine) or **pus** as seen in infection of urinary tract, or **chyle** as occurs in obstruction of lymphatics of the urinary tract (for example, in filariasis).

Odor

Normally, the odor of urine is **mildly aromatic** due to presence of volatile organic acids. However, if kept for a long time, urine gives unpleasant ammoniacal smell due to conversion of urea into ammonium carbonate. **Diabetic urine** gives acidotic-fruity odor due to the presence acetone in the urine. Excretion of different drugs in the urine also changes the smell of urine.

Color

Normal urine is **straw colored** or amber-yellow in color, which is due to the presence of the pigment **urochrome** in it.

1. Urine becomes **yellow in bilirubinuria**, as occurs in jaundice.
2. Urine becomes **dark** in alkaptonuria, melanuria (seen in malignant melanoma), and,
3. **Red** in hematuria, hemoglobinuria, myoglobinuria, porphyria or following intake of rifampicin (anti-tubercular antibiotic).

Specific Gravity

The normal specific gravity of urine is 1.005-1.030 (the theoretical range is 1.003 – 1.035). Specific gravity of urine of 1.010 normally corresponds to urine osmolality of 285 mosm/kg.

1. Specific gravity **decreases when urine is diluted** (as seen in diabetes insipidus) and **increases when urine is concentrated** (as occurs in dehydration).
2. Specific gravity also increases when urine contains glucose, protein and contrasts. In chronic renal failure, specific gravity is fixed at 1010.

Biochemical Characteristics

Reaction of Urine

Normally, urine is ***mildly acidic***; the average pH being 6 (ranging between 4.5–7.5).

1. ***After a normal meal***, urine becomes alkaline due to *alkaline tide* that occurs with secretion of acid in the stomach, which adds bicarbonate into the plasma.
2. However, ***if the meal is rich in protein***, urine becomes acidic due to formation of sulfates and phosphates of amino acids in tubular fluid.
3. ***If the meal is rich in vegetables***, then the urine becomes alkaline as organic acids like citric and tartaric acids extracted from vegetables are converted to bicarbonate in the body.
4. **Alkaline urine** is also feature of type II distal renal tubular acidosis, urinary tract infection by urease producing organisms, acetazolamide therapy and following ingestion of alkali.

Proteins in Urine

Normally, glomerulus is not permeable to substances with molecular weight more than 69000. Therefore, **normally proteins are absent in urine**.

1. Proteinuria occurs when glomerular filtering membrane is damaged in various glomerular diseases. **Albumin** being a smaller molecule passes easily through the damaged glomerulus than the heavier globulins.

Table 82.1: 24-hr urinary protein and protein-creatinine ratio in different conditions.

24 h urinary protein (g)	Protein/Creatinine ratio	Significance
< 0.03	<2.5 in males <3.5 in females	Normal
0.03–0.3	3.5–15	Microalbuminuria
0.3–0.5	15–50	Dipstick positive
> 2.5	> 250	Glomerular disease likely
> 4.0	> 400	Glomerular disease

2. Therefore, in proteinuria, albumin predominates in urine. The molecular weight of **hemoglobin** is 67000; therefore, hemoglobinuria occurs in hemolysis. Though, normally **proteins are not filtered** by glomerulus, a very less amount (less than 150 mg per day) of it is excreted in urine, which is **secreted by the tubular epithelial cells**.
3. However, this trace quantity of protein is not detected by routine urine analysis test. The normal protein content of 24 hour urine is < 0.03 g.

Protein-Creatinine Ratio

The normal protein-creatinine ratio in a random urine sample is < 2.5 in males and < 3.5 in females (Table 82.1). Ratio > 3.5 indicates microalbuminuria and > 15 indicates proteinuria.

Proteinuria

Proteinuria is seen in nephritis, nephrosis, urinary tract infections (UTIs), eclampsia, heart failure and later part of pregnancy. strenuous exercise, Normally, protein filtered is reabsorbed by the tubule. Therefore, either in increased filtration or in diseases of tubule, proteinuria occurs. Protein in urine is detected by **heat and acetic acid test, sulphosalicylic acid test**, or by using **Esbach's albuminometer.**

Bence-Jones Proteinuria

Bence-Jones protein is the B lymphocyte secreting immunoglobulin light chain protein. If it is present in blood it is freely secreted in urine. This occurs in multiple myeloma, amyloidosis and plasma cell dyscrasias. This is used as a marker in myeloma in which **myeloma protein** (*Bence-Jones proteins*) increases in plasma.

Microalbuminuria

Excretion of 24 hr urinary protein 30-300 mg (0.03 to 0.3 g) is described as microalbuminuria.

1. This is an early sign of glomerular dysfunction.
2. Patients with diabetes should be regularly screened for microalbuminuria to detect early development of diabetic nephropathy.
3. A persistent microalbuminuria has recently been found to be associated with increased risk of atherosclerosis and cardiovascular mortality.

Blood in Urine

Blood in urine is called **hematuria**. It may be microscopic hematuria or may be detected by patient (macroscopic hematuria). It indicates bleeding from anywhere in renal tract. Commonly, hematuria is seen in glomerulonephritis and injury to ureter, urinary bladder or urethra. It is detected by **Benzidine test.**

Hemoglobinuria and Myoglobinuria

Presence of hemoglobin (usually without red cells) in urine (hemoglobinuria) indicates intravascular hemolysis and presence of myoglobin in urine (myoglobunuria) indicates rhabdomyolysis.

Reducing Sugars in Urine

The presence of sugar in urine is called **glycosuria** (or more accurately, **glucosuria**). Normally, **glucose does not appear** in urine. Glucosuria occurs in conditions in which renal threshold (plasma glucose >180 mg%) for glucose is exceeded as in diabetes mellitus. Glucose in urine is detected by **Benedicts test.**

Glycosuria occurs due to:

1. Diabetes mellitus
2. Kidney diseases (**renal glycosuria**) due to decreased renal threshold
3. **Alimentary glycosuria** (lag storage glycosuria) in which transitory rise in blood glucose occurs following meals. It may be seen in normal people, after gastric surgery (rapid absorption of glucose into circulation due to rapid gastric emptying), hyperthyroidism, peptic ulcer and hepatic disease.
4. **Gestational glycosuria**: Glycosuria is common in normal pregnancy as renal threshold for glucose falls in pregnancy due to increased GFR. However, gestational diabetes should be ruled out.

Other Biochemical Tests

Ketone Bodies in Urine

The ketone bodies are acetoacetate, β-hydroxybutyrate and acetone. Excretion of ketone bodies in urine is called **ketonuria.** Normally, **ketone bodies are not present** in urine. Ketonuria occurs in severe diabetes mellitus, starvation, chronic vomiting, etc. Ketone bodies in urine are detected by **Rothera's test and Gerhardt's test.**

Bile Salts in Urine

Bile salts appear in urine in the **early phase of obstructive jaundice.** Bile salts are detected by **Hay's test and Petenkoffer's test.**

Bile Pigments in Urine

Bile pigments (bilirubin and biliverdin) appear in urine in obstructive jaundice. **Bilirubinuria** is detected by modified van den Berg reaction or Fouchet's test.

Urobilinogen in Urine

Normally, the main pigment in the urine is **urochrome.** However, small amounts of **urobilinogen** may also be present in urine. Urobilinogen excretion increases in persistent fevers, liver diseases, diseases of biliary tract and hemolysis. This is detected by **Ehrlich test and Schlesinger's test** for urobilinogen.

Measurement of (NPN) in Urine

The non-protein nitrogen (NPN) in urine includes **urea, creatinine and uric acid**. These compounds are excreted from the body mainly through urine. Their concentration in urine increases in different physiological and pathological conditions.

1. Determination of **creatinine** is an important test for renal function.
2. **Urea** level is altered in many conditions. Even, increased intake of protein increases urea in urine. Hence, urea estimation is a *non-specific kidney function test*. However, blood urea concentration is a good index of renal functions.
3. **Uric acid** is increased in urine in conditions that are associated with increased purine catabolism.

Clearance Tests

Clearance tests mainly determine the glomerular function. *GFR provides the most useful index* for assessment of severity of the renal disease.

Clearance is defined as the **quantity of blood or plasma cleared of a substance for unit time.** This is expressed as ml per minute. It is the ml of plasma, which contains the amount of that substance excreted by the kidney within a minute. Actually, it estimates the amount of plasma that passes through the glomeruli per minute with complete removal of that substance (to account for the substance actually appears in the urine).

$$\text{Clearance} = \frac{\text{mg of substance excreted per minute}}{\text{mg of substance per ml of plasma or serum}}$$

It is calculated by using the formula, $C = \frac{U \times V}{P}$

Where U = concentration of the substance in urine;
P = concentration of the substance in plasma or serum and V = the ml of urine excreted per minute. The value is expressed as ml/minute.

Measurement of the clearance is predominantly a test of glomerular filtration rate (GFR). The relation between clearance value and GFR may be depicted as shown in Table 82.2.

The clearance of a substance, which is completely filtered but neither reabsorbed nor secreted by the tubule is ideally used to measure GFR. Therefore, **inulin clearance test is the standard test for measurement of GFR.** The **PAH clearance** determines the substance filtered and secreted but not reabsorbed. Therefore, it is best used for measurement of **renal plasma flow**. Normally, the RPF is 700 mL per minute and GFR is 120 mL per minute. Therefore, it is obvious that one fifth of the plasma that passes through the glomerulus becomes glomerular filtrate which is known as **filtration fraction.**

In normal practice, creatinine clearance test, urea clearance test, and inulin clearance test are used for determination of kidney functions.

Table 82.2: Relationship between GFR and clearance value.

Mechanism	Result	Example
Substances filtered but neither reabsorbed nor excreted.	GFR = clearance	Inulin
Substances filtered, reabsorbed & excreted	GFR = clearance	Uric acid
Substances filtered & partially reabsorbed	Clearance < GFR	Urea, & creatinine
Substances filtered & secreted, but not reabsorbed	Clearance > GFR	Diodrast & PAH

Blood Investigations

Blood tests for assessing kidney functions are serum urea, creatinine, uric acid and electrolytes.

Serum Urea

Normal serum urea level is 15 – 40 mg%. Increased serum urea is seen in:

1. High intake (high protein diet, GI hemorrhage)
2. High production (trauma, burn, infections)
3. Reduced urinary excretion (renal failure, hypovolemia).

Serum Creatinine

Normal serum creatinine is 0.7–1.5 mg% in males and 0.5–1.2 mg% in females. It increases in:

1. High production (increased muscle mass, rhabdomyolysis)
2. Reduced excretion in urine (renal failure, drugs like trimethoprim, cimetidine).

Serum Electrolytes

Normal serum sodium value is 136 to 145 mM/L and normal serum potassium value is 3.5 to 5 mM/L.

Hyperkalemia is an important feature of renal dysfunctions.

Tubular Function Tests

The primary function of tubule is to reabsorb solutes and water from the tubular fluid. Therefore, **detecting concentration of solutes in urine** gives the knowledge of tubular functions. The simplest tubular function test is the **measurement of specific gravity** of the urine.

Determination of Specific Gravity

The **specific gravity depends on the concentration of solutes** whereas the osmolality detects the presence of osmotically active particles in the urine. For example, in proteinuria specific gravity is significantly increased whereas osmolality is mildly elevated.

Other Tests

Tubular functions are determined by **concentration** and **dilution tests.** The earliest manifestation of the renal disease is the inability to concentrate urine. This is detected by concentration test.

Concentration Test

The patient is advised to eat normal food at 6 PM but fluid intake is restricted to 200 mL. He is further advised not to take anything throughout night. Next morning, at 7 AM, the bladder is emptied and this first specimen is discarded. At 8 AM, urine collected and this second specimen is obtained for measuring specific gravity.

1. **If specific gravity is more than 1.022**, the renal function is normal.
2. **If specific gravity is below this value**, a third sample is collected at 9 AM.
3. If this sample gives **specific gravity less than 1.022**, then the concentrating ability of the kidney is considered to be impaired.

Determination of Urine Volume

The measurement of the volume of urine passed in 24 hours is a simple test of tubular function. The urine volume is measured separately during night time and during day time.

1. Normally, the **volume of urine in night is half the volume** of urine excreted during day time.
2. An **increased excretion of urine during night** is an early indication of tubular dysfunctions.

Measurement of Osmolality

Osmolality of urine varies widely between 60–1200 mosm/kg. Urine osmolality is usually an **index of plasma osmolality**, which normally ranges between 285–295 mosm/kg. Therefore, the plasma and urine osmolalities are detected and the **ratio of osmolality of urine to plasma** is recorded. The **normal ratio is 3–4.5**. Urine osmolality is detected by ADH test, dilution tests, and free water clearance.

ADH Test

Normally, ADH reabsorbs water from the kidney tubule. With tubular dysfunction, effectiveness of tubular water reabsorption by ADH decreases, as seen in nephrogenic diabetes insipidus. *Five units of ADH are injected* and urine samples are collected for 24 hours for estimation of specific gravity and osmolality. Normally, at least one sample should have the **specific gravity more than 1.020 and osmolality of 800 mosm/kg.**

Dilution Test

The patient is not allowed to drink water or fluid after 10 PM. The bladder is emptied at 7AM in the next morning and patient is allowed to take a water load of 1.2 liter in half an-hour. Hourly urine samples are collected for four hours for determination of volume, specific gravity, and osmolality of each sample. Normally, a person **excretes the total water load in four hours** and the specific gravity of at least one sample should fall to 1.003 and osmolality to 50 mosm/kg.

Osmolal Clearance or Free Water Clearance

It actually detects the concentrating and diluting ability of the kidney. Therefore, it is a better test for tubular function. Osmolal clearance is defined as the **volume of plasma water that is cleared of its solutes** to excrete urine with same specific gravity as that of plasma.

$$\text{Osmolar clearance (Cosm)} = \frac{\text{Uosm}}{\text{Posm}} \times V$$

Where, Uosm is the urine osmolality, Posm is the plasma osmolality, and V is the urine excreted per minute.

When **urine is hypotonic to plasma,** more water is excreted. This is expressed as free water clearance (C water). C water is equal to V – Cosm ml/minute.

Usually this is used to **differentiate polyuria** of diabetes insipidus, diabetes mellitus, and excess water drinking.

Specific Tests

Tests for Urine Acidification

Usually, *acid loading test* is performed to detect the ability of the kidney to acidify urine. **Ammonium chloride** is given to the subject as an enteric coated tablet (0.1 g/kg b.w.).

1. Urine is collected every hour for 4–8 hours for determination of pH of urine and ammonia excretion of each sample.
2. At least, **one sample should have pH of 5.3** or less and **ammonia excretion should be 30–90 mmol per hour.**

Tests for Renal Handling of Na^+

The subject is given a load of 100 mmole of sodium as sodium chloride. Normally, 60–80 mmole of sodium is excreted per day. Then, the patient is given **sodium free diet for 7 days** (daily intake less than 10 mmole). After a week, urinary sodium output is estimated.

1. A normal person **decreases Na^+ excretion to 10 mmole** per day after 7 days. When tubular function is impaired, ability to reabsorb sodium is lower.
2. In such conditions, natriuresis continues regardless of Na^+ intake.

PSP Test

The PSP or **phenolsulphthalein (phenol red) test** is used for determining the **secretory capacity of the tubule**. The subject is allowed to drink 600 mL of water following which PSP is given intravenously (6 mg in 1 mL solution). Bladder is emptied after 15 minutes, 30 minutes, 60 minutes and 120 minutes, and excretion of the phenol red is noted in each sample. Normally, the **phenol content is 35% in the first sample** and **70% of the dye should be eliminated in two hours**. In tubular dysfunctions, the dye excreted in first sample is less and also the total amount excreted in two hours will be less. This is a useful test for detection of **early stage of kidney disease.**

Special Tests

Special tests to assess kidney functions include **ultrasonography, intravenous pyelography, computed tomography** and **magnetic resonance imaging. Renal biopsy** (percutaneous needle biopsy) is useful in some selective diseases.

RENAL FAILURE

Renal failure is the condition of decreased urine output due to loss of renal function that develops over a period of days to years. This is of two types: acute renal failure and chronic renal failure.

Acute Renal Failure

Definition and Causes

Acute renal failure (ARF) refers to a sudden, but usually reversible loss of renal function that develops over a period of days or weeks and is usually accompanied by a reduction in urine volume. The causes of ARF are listed in Table 82.3. The commonest pre-renal cause of ARF is hypovolemic shock and commonest renal cause is acute tubular necrosis (ATN). ATN usually occurs due to ischemia or nephrotoxicity caused by chemicals or bacterial toxins or both.

Table 82.3: Causes of renal failure.
I. Causes of acute renal failure
A. Prerenal causes
1. Systemic causes
– Heart failure
– Blood or fluid loss
2. Local causes
– Renal artery stenosis
3. Under-perfusion of kidney
B. Renal causes
1. Acute tubular necrosis/toxic/septic renal failure
2. Glomerular diseases
3. Interstitial kidney diseases
C. Postrenal causes
1. Obstruction to urine outflow
– Kidney stones
– Kidney tumors
– Prostatic enlargement
II. Causes of chronic renal failure.
1. Diabetes mellitus
2. Hypertension
3. Glomerular diseases (e. g. IgA nephropathy)
4. Renal interstitial diseases
5. Renal artery stenosis
6. Congenital and inherited (e.g. polycystic kidney disease, Alport syndrome)
7. Systemic inflammatory diseases (e.g. SLE, vasculitis)

Features

Patient is usually **oliguric** (24 hr urine volume < 500 mL).

1. **Hyperkalemia** is common. **Dilutional hyponatremia** and metabolic acidosis may be present. **Hypocalcemia** is common due to decreased production of 1,25 dihydroxycholecalciferol.
2. **Uremic features** include anorexia, nausea, vomiting, apathy, confusion, muscle twitching, hiccoughs, fits and coma.
3. **Pulmonary edema** may be present due to increased pulmonary capillary permeability.
4. **Anemia** is common.
5. **Bleeding** may occur due to platelet dysfunctions or disturbances in coagulation cascade. Spontaneous GI hemorrhage is not uncommon.

Treatment

Emergency resuscitation and follow up treatment include:

1. **Hyerkalemia is treated immediately** to prevent development of life threatening cardiac arrhythmias. ***Calcium gluconate*** (10 mL of 10% solution) is given i.v. to stabilize membrane potential. ***Insulin and glucose solution*** (5 units of insulin + 50 mL of 50% glucose) is injected i.v. along with sodium bicarbonate. Insulin facilitates entry of K^+ into the cell and immediately decreases plasma K^+ level. Glucose is given to combat insulin-induced hypoglycemia. Sodibicarb prevents acidosis. Dialysis may be needed in extreme cases.
2. **Circulating blood volume should be optimized.** For pre-renal ARF, hypovolemia is treated with rapid infusion of blood or plasma or isotonic saline and CVP should be monitored regularly.
3. **Metabolic acidosis is corrected** by isotonic sodium bicarbonate infusion.
4. **Fluid and electrolyte balance** is monitored after initial resuscitation. Fluid intake should equal the urine output.
5. **Treatment of underlying cause** include treatment for ATN or surgical removal of obstruction in post-renal ARF.
6. **Infection should be controlled** promptly.
7. **Renal replacement therapy** (intermittent hemodialysis, hemofiltration, intermittent hemodiafiltration and peritoneal dialysis) is considered if there is severe uremia, hyperkalemia and metabolic acidosis.

Chronic Renal Failure (CRF)

Definition

Chronic renal failure (CRF) refers to an irreversible deterioration in renal function that develops over a period of years. Initially, it manifests only as biochemical abnormality, but eventually loss of endocrine, metabolic and excretory functions of kidney leads to the development of signs and symptoms of renal failure, which are referred to as uremia. When death is likely without renal replacement therapy, it is called **end-stage renal failure** (ESRF).

Etiopathogenesis

CRF is caused by any condition that destroys structure and functions of kidney. Presently, the commonest causes of CRF are diabetes mellitus and hypertension (Table 82.3). Disturbances in water, electrolyte and acid-base balance contribute to the clinical picture in CRF. Uremia is caused by accumulation of many intermediary products of metabolism, called as uremic toxins.

Features

CRF may be detected as raised blood urea and serum creatinine during routine investigation of patients of diabetes, hypertension, proteinuria and anemia. Unless GFR falls below 30 mL/min, patient remains asymptomatic. Nocturia occurs due to loss of concentric ability of kidney and increased osmotic load on nephron.

1. Tiredness and breathlessness are common.
2. ESRF patients appear ill and anemic and may show signs of sodium and water depletion. They present with anorexia, nausea, vomiting, hiccough, pruritus, muscular twitching, fits and drowsiness.
3. Features of metabolic acidosis such as *Kussmaul respiration* may be present.

Treatment

Consists of identifying the renal disease, identify the precipitating factors and preventing the further renal damage. Diabetes, hypertension and anemia are promptly treated. Fluid and electrolyte balance is maintained. Metabolic acidosis is corrected. Renal replacement therapy (dialysis/ renal transplantation) is instituted.

CHAPTER SUMMARY

Key Concepts

1. Physiologically, kidney function tests are done to assess glomerular filtration and tubular functions. Estimation of protein and glucose in urine, and pH of urine are routine tests.
2. Clearance test, ADH test and concentration/dilution tests are specific tubular function tests.
3. Hyperkalemia is an acute condition in ARF, and is immediately treated by IV insulin in glucose solution.

Important to Know (Must Read)

1. In examination, **Long Questions** are usually not asked from this chapter. However, 'Describe the physiological basis and application of kidney function tests' may come as a long question.
2. Tubular function tests, Glomerular function tests, Clearance tests, Urine analysis, Acute renal failure, Chronic renal failure may be asked as **Short Questions** in exam.
3. In **Viva**, examiner may ask....... List the glomerular function tests, List the tubular function tests, Physiologically, how do you classify kidney function tests, Clinically, how do you classify kidney function tests, What are the normal physical characteristics of urine, What is oliguria and anuria, What is polyuria and what are its causes, What is nocturia, What is protein-creatinine ratio in urine, What is proteinuria, What is Bence-Jones proteinuria, What is microalbuminuria, What is glycosuria and what are its causes, Define clearance, what is its formula and what area the substances used to calculate clearance, How does the urine concentration test is performed, What is ADH test, How does the urine dilution test is performed, What is osmolal clearance or free water clearance, What are the tests for urine acidification, What is PSP test and what is its use, What are the causes, features and treatment of acute renal failure, What are the causes, features and treatment of chronic renal failure.

CHAPTER 83

Physiology of Micturition and Bladder Dysfunctions

Learning Objectives

On completion of study of this chapter, the student **MUST** be able to:

1. Understand the relation of functional anatomy of urinary bladder with its functions.
2. Appreciate the innervation and arrangement of sphincters of urinary bladder.
3. Learn the mechanism and control of micturition reflex.
4. Explain the graph of cystometrogram.
5. Understand the physiological basis of bladder dysfunctions.

The student **MAY** also be able to:

1. Describe the abnormalities of bladder dysfunctions.

Urinary bladder stores urines. It accumulates urine without much rise in pressure in it and empties its content at appropriate time following suitable rise in pressure.

1. Urine from kidneys flows down to the bladder through ureters due to the **action of gravity**, which is **aided by peristaltic movements of ureter**.
2. Peristaltic waves in ureters originate by a **pacemaker tissue located close to the calyces** at a frequency of about one per minute.
3. Once in the bladder, **regurgitation of urine back into the ureter is prevented** passively by a **valvular flap** present at the entry point of the ureter at the base of the bladder. Ureteric pain occurs when ureters are distended by stones or by obstructions.

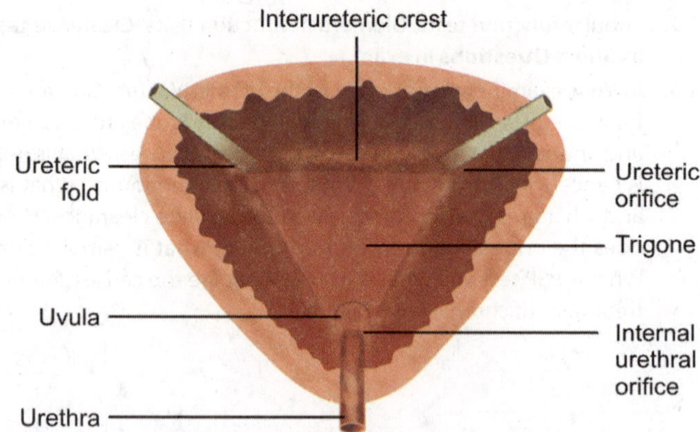

Fig. 83.1: Interior structure of the urinary bladder. Note, thick bladder wall is due to the thick detrusor muscle.

URINARY BLADDER

Functional Aspects

Bladder Wall

Urinary bladder is a sac like structure present in the pelvic cavity.

1. It is a **distensible organ** made up of smooth muscle, called **detrusor muscle** (Fig. 83.1), depicting the Latin word 'pushes down'.
2. Detrusor muscles are arranged in **three bundles**: spiral, longitudinal and circular.
3. Contraction of the detrusor causes emptying of the bladder.
4. The **epithelium of the bladder** is formed by a superficial layer of flat cells and a deep layer of cuboidal cells.

Innervation

Bladder is innervated by both sympathetic and parasympathetic fibers (Fig. 83.2).

1. **Parasympathetic fibers** originate from the **sacral 2, 3 and 4 segments** of the spinal cord and reach the bladder via pelvic nerves,

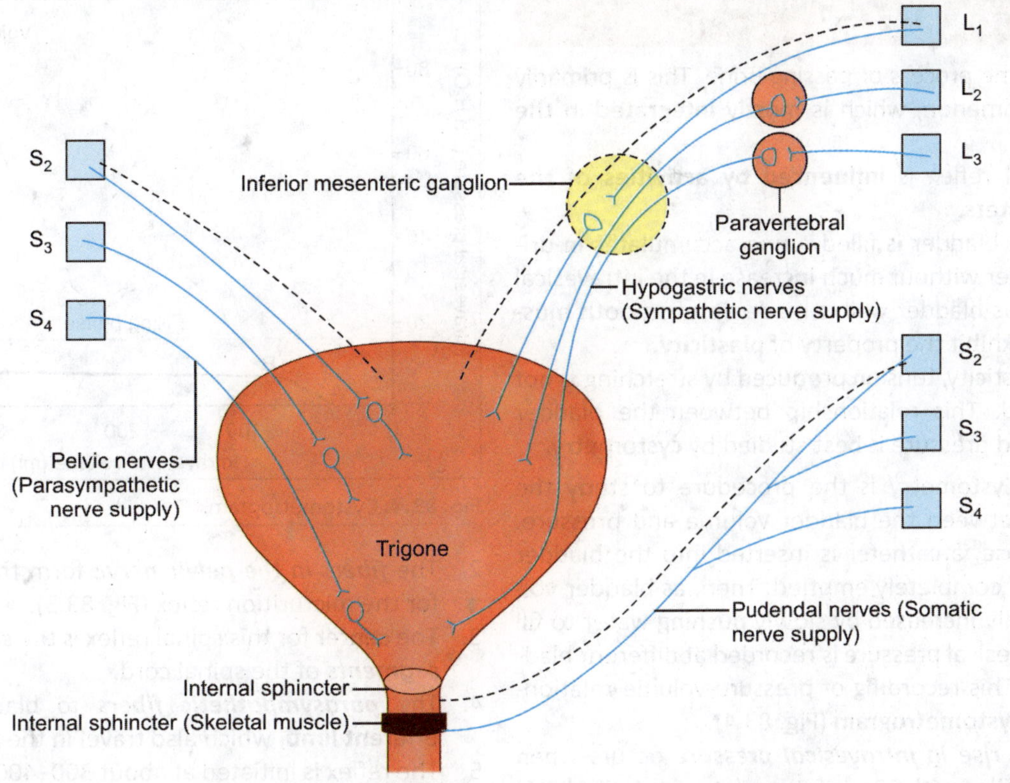

Fig. 83.2: Structure and innervation of urinary bladder. Dotted lines represent sensory innervation.

2. The **sympathetic fibers** originate from **lumbar 1, 2 and 3 segments** of the spinal cord and reach the bladder via hypogastric nerve (Fig. 83.2).
3. The **somatic fibers** originate from **S_2, S_3 and S_4** and innervate bladder and external sphincter via pudendal nerve.
4. Filling of bladder, desire to pass urine and painful distension, all these sensations of bladder are mediated by **afferents in the pelvic nerve.**

Urethral Sphincters

There are **two sphincters:** Internal and external (Fig. 83.3).

1. The **internal sphincter**, which is located at the neck of the bladder, is made up of a bundle of smooth muscle (***sphincter vesicae***), and innervated by **sympathetic (hypogastric) and parasympathetic (pelvic) nerves.** Therefore, the internal sphincter is **under autonomic control.**
2. The **external sphincter** is made up of a flap of skeletal muscle, which is present around the urethra in its proximal part (***sphincter urethrae***). The external sphincter is **innervated by somatic (pudendal) nerve** and therefore **under voluntary control.**

Functions of Urinary Bladder

Urinary bladder serves **two functions:**

1. **Storage of urine** up to a critical volume.

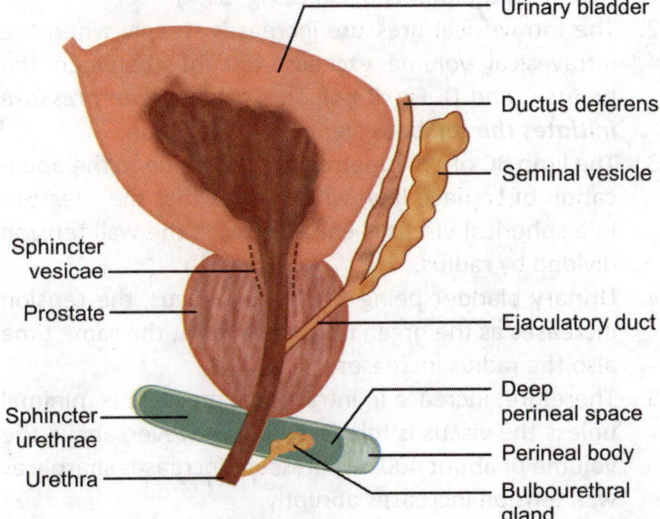

Fig. 83.3 : Sphincter vesicae (internal sphincter of bladder) and sphincter urethrae (external sphincter of bladder).

2. **Emptying urine** into urethra when the critical volume is attained.

The external sphincter is kept closed most of the time. The sensation of bladder filling is experienced at the bladder volume of about 150 mL and the **sensation to pass urine** is experienced at bladder volume of **150–250 mL. At volume of about 400 mL**, the sensation to pass urine becomes **uncomfortable** and at about 700 mL, it becomes very painful leading to loss of control.

MICTURITION REFLEX

Micturition is the process of passing urine. This is primarily a reflex phenomenon, which is mostly **integrated in the spinal cord**.

1. This spinal reflex is **influenced by activities of the higher centers**.
2. Unless the bladder is filled, urine accumulates in urinary bladder without much increase in the intravesical pressure, as bladder wall is made up of smooth muscles that exhibit the property of **plasticity**.
3. Due to plasticity, tension produced by stretching is not maintained. This relationship between the bladder volume and pressure is best studied by **cystometry.**

Cystometry: Cystometry is the procedure to study the relationship between the bladder volume and pressure. For this purpose, a catheter is inserted into the bladder and bladder is completely emptied. Then, as bladder volume is gradually increased by slowly pushing water to fill bladder, intravesical pressure is recorded at different bladder volumes. This recording of pressure-volume relationship is called **cystometrogram** (Fig. 83.4).

1. The ***initial rise in intravesical pressure*** occurs when bladder is filled with 50 ml of water (at point A, Fig. 83.4) and thereafter no significant increase in pressure occurs with increase in volume to about 400 ml (between the points B and C, Fig. 83.4).
2. The intravesical pressure increases steeply when the intravesical volume exceeds 400 mL (between the points C and D, Fig. 83.4). This ***sharp rise in pressure initiates the reflex*** triggering of micturition.
3. The limb BC of cystometrogram is flat due to the application of **Laplace law**, which states that the pressure in a spherical viscus is equal to twice the wall tension divided by radius.
4. Urinary bladder being a spherical viscus, the tension increases as the organ fills. However, at the same time also the radius increases.
5. Therefore, increase in intravesical pressure is minimal unless the viscus is relatively full. However, above the volume of about 400 mL, pressure increases sharply as wall tension increases abruptly.

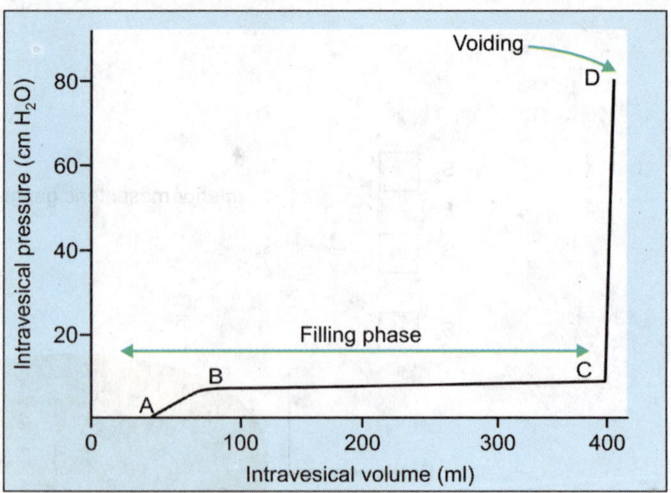

Fig. 83.4: Cystometrogram.

Mechanism of Micturition

The urge to pass urine is initiated with filling of the bladder, which is sensed by stretch receptors. The stretch receptors that are present in the wall of the bladder send impulses in the afferent nerve that initiate reflex contraction.

Stimulus and Reflex Arc

Filling of the bladder, causing stretch of bladder wall is the stimulus.

1. The **stretch receptors** that are present in the wall of the bladder send impulses in the afferent nerve that initiate reflex contraction.
2. The ***fibers in the pelvic nerve*** form the **afferent limb** for the micturition reflex (Fig. 83.5).
3. The **center** for this spinal reflex is the ***sacral 2, 3, and 4 segments*** of the spinal cord.
4. The ***parasympathetic fibers*** to bladder constitute **efferent limb**, which also travel in the pelvic nerve.
5. The reflex is initiated at about 300–400 ml of intravesical volume.
6. Normally, the **sympathetic fibers do not play role** in micturition. However, the sympathetic activation causes **contraction of bladder muscle** that prevents semen from entering the bladder during ejaculation.

Mechanism

Micturition is a **parasympathetic activity**.

1. Parasympathetic stimulation causes ***contraction of detrusor and relaxation of internal sphincter***, so that the urine passes forcefully into the urethra.
2. Contraction of abdominal muscle and descent of diaphragm ***increases intra-abdominal pressure***. During micturition, the ***pelvic, perineal and levator ani muscles relax***. This causes ***downward pull of detrusor muscle*** and aids to initiation of its contraction.
3. At this stage, *perineal muscles and external sphincter can be made to contract voluntarily* to prevent micturition to occur.
4. The **voluntary control** of micturition is influenced by ***cortical activities*** and by *learning to contract the external urethral sphincter*.
5. Once in the urethra, the urine is emptied **in females** by the effect of gravity and pressure from the pelvic floor, whereas **in males**, urine is emptied by *contractions of bulbocavernosus muscle*.
6. The voluntary contraction of abdominal muscles helps in expulsion of urine.

Control of Micturition

The micturition reflex is controlled by **centers in the brainstem**.

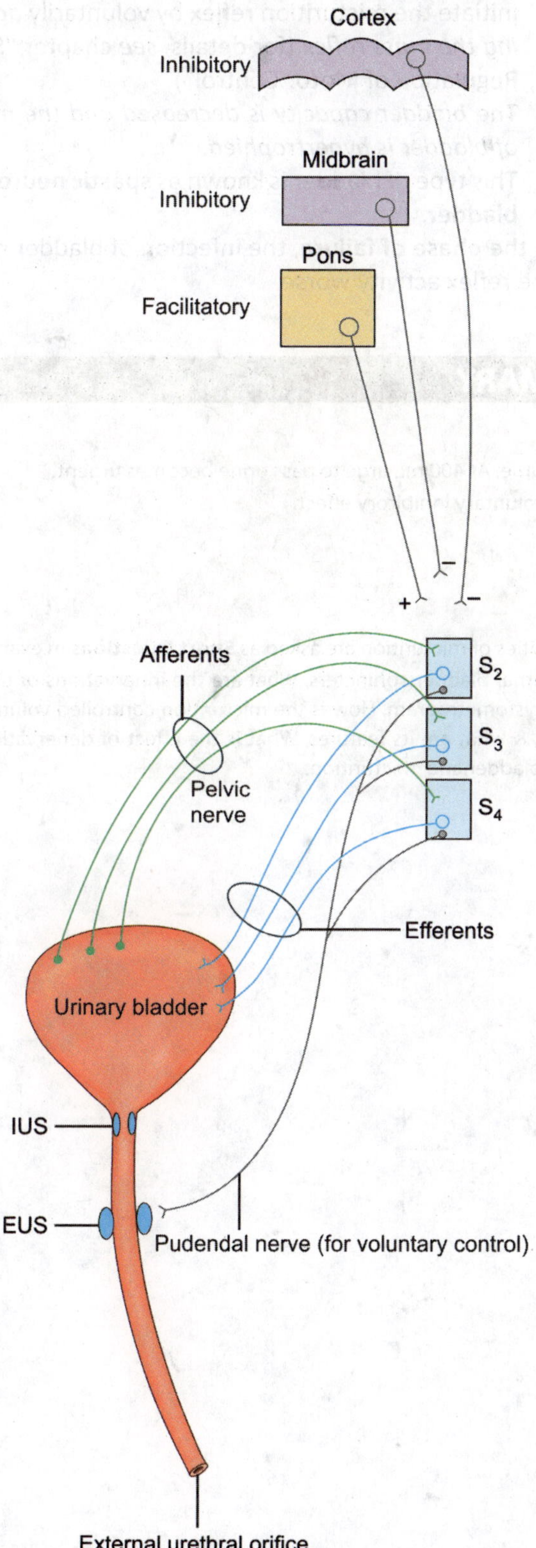

Fig. 83.5: Control of micturition reflex. Fullness of bladder is sensed by afferents in pelvic nerve and parasympathetic efferents also travel in pelvic nerve. Note, midbrain and cortex inhibit and pons facilitates reflex activity. Voluntary prevention of micturition is achieved by contracting external urethral sphincter (EUS), which is mediated through somatic efferents in pudendal nerve. (IUS: Internal urethral sphincter).

1. The **facilitatory area** is present in pons and the **inhibitory area** is present in midbrain (Fig. 83.5). Therefore, ***section of neuraxis above pons*** promotes activity of micturition reflex in which less filling of bladder triggers its reflex evacuation, and ***section above midbrain*** does not affect it.
2. **Posterior hypothalamus** also contains a *facilitatory area for micturition*.
3. **Cortex** has *voluntary inhibitory control* on micturition. In children, below three years of age, cortical inhibition is not well developed; hence they often pass urine without their knowledge.
4. Control on urination starts to **develop at about two years** of age and completes by three years.

BLADDER DYSFUNCTIONS

Abnormalities of Micturition

The **lesions at different segments of neuraxis** result in bladder dysfunctions. There are ***three major neural defects*** that produce bladder dysfunctions:

1. Interruption of afferent fibers (**deafferentation**).
2. Interruption of both afferent and efferent fibers (**denervation**).
3. Interruption of influences from the facilitatory and inhibitory areas in the brain (**spinal cord transection**).

   In these lesions, bladder may contact, but the contraction is not enough to empty the viscus. Therefore, **residual urine** is always left in the bladder.

Deafferentation

When, fibers originating from **the sacral roots** of the spinal cord are experimentally destroyed, **reflex contraction of bladder is abolished.**

1. The bladder is **distended, thin-walled and hypotonic**.
2. However, some contractions occur (due to intrinsic response of the smooth muscles to stretch).
3. Such type of bladder is seen in *tabes dorsalis*.

Denervation

When both the **afferent and efferent fibers are cut**, bladder becomes **flaccid and distended** at the beginning.

1. However, gradually the muscle of the bladder becomes active and the contraction of the bladder muscle removes urine in the form of dribbles.
2. Later, the bladder is **shrunken and bladder wall becomes hypertrophied**.
3. This is typically seen in the **tumors of cauda equina or filum terminale**.
4. The hyperactive bladder suggests ***denervation hypersensitivity*** of bladder muscles.

Spinal Cord Transection

When the spinal cord is transected, typically **three phases** are observed: phase of shock, phase of recovery (increased reflex activity), and phase of failure.

1. During **the phase of spinal shock**, the bladder becomes ***flaccid and unresponsive***. The *overflow incontinence* (urine dribbles through the sphincter when the bladder is overfilled) occurs.
2. In the **phase of recovery**, micturition reflex is the ***first reflex activity to return***. However, voluntary control or control by the higher centers is abolished after transection.
   - The spinal man (the human being following transection of the spinal cord) can train himself to initiate the micturition reflex by voluntarily *activating the mass reflex* (for details, *see* chapter "Spinal Regulation of Motor Control").
   - The *bladder capacity is decreased and the muscle of bladder is hypertrophied*.
   - This type of bladder is known as **spastic neurogenic bladder.**
3. In the **phase of failure**, the infection of bladder makes the reflex activity worse.

CHAPTER SUMMARY

Key Concepts

1. The initiation of micturition reflex occurs at 150 to 200 mL of bladder volume. At 400 mL urge to pass urine becomes urgent.
2. Micturition reflex is parasympathetic phenomenon. Cortical control has voluntary inhibitory effect.
3. Spastic neurogenic bladder is seen in spinal cord injury.

Important to Know (Must Read)

1. In examination, **Long Questions** are usually not asked from this chapter.
2. Micturition reflex, Cystometrogram, Mechanism of micturition, Abnormalities of micturition are asked as **Short Questions** in exam.
3. In **Viva**, examiner may ask... What are the functions of internal and external bladder sphincters, What are the innervations of urinary bladder, List the functions of urinary bladder, What are the phases of a cystometrogram, How is the micturition controlled voluntarily, How is the micturition controlled involuntarily, What is deafferentation, & what are its features, What is the effect of denervation on bladder and micturition, What is the effect of spinal cord transaction on bladder and micturition.

Index

Page numbers followed by *f* refer to figure, *fc* refer to flowchart and *t* refer to table

A

Abdomen 1019
ABO 124
  agglutinins 118
  antigen 120*f*
  blood groups 119
  phenotypes 120*t*
  system 117
Abscess 163
Absorption 342, 423, 425
Acanthocyte 85
Accommodation reflex 311, 1191, 1192*fc*
Acetazolamide 708
Acetic acid test 717
Acetylcholine 241, 242, 291, 332, 345, 352, 406, 437, 792, 990, 991, 1118
Achalasia cardia 402, 403*f*, 985
Achilles tendon reflex 490, 497
Achondroplasia 1281
Acid 408, 709
  arachidonic 448
  base balance 72, 660, 709, 1266, 1269
    regulation of 1268
  base disorder 713
    types of 1270*t*
  base homeostasis, principle of 1266
  base status 710
  excretion of 709
  hydrochloric 348, 426
  hypersecretion of 359
  lactic 1255
  nicotinic 1289
  nonvolatile 1266
  peptic disease 358
  phosphatase 594
  production, nonvolatile 1268
  protease 667
    enzyme 554
  secretion
    autoregulation of 353
    capacity 357
Acidic chyme 367, 405
Acidophil cells 461*f*
Acidosis 709, 713, 941, 942*fc*, 796, 940, 1256, 1269
  metabolic 710, 713, 720, 942, 1269
  respiratory 710, 713, 942, 958, 1269, 1270
Acinar cells 365
  pancreatic 366*f*
Acini, types of 343*f*
Acinus 343
Acne
  formation 625, 1235
Acquired immunodeficiency syndrome (AIDS) 180
Acrosome 596
  reaction 635
Acute hypotension, causes of 865
Adenine 30*f*
Adenohypophysis 460
Adenoleukodystrophy 20
Adenosine 282, 674, 680, 697, 855, 993, 1119
  metabolites 993
  triphosphate 270
Adenylate cyclase 447, 558, 561, 707
Adhesion 184, 189
Adie tonic pupil 310
Adipose tissue blood flow 1261
Adrenal
  androgen 584
    stimulating hormone 584
  cortex 433, 599, 669
  gland 623, 627
  medulla 297, 304, 991
    role of 298
Adrenaline test 315
Adrenarche 584, 585
Adrenergic receptor kinase 985
Adrenocorticotropic hormone 455, 460, 471
Ageusia 1228
Agglutinins 116, 119
Agglutinogens 116
Agnosia
  auditory 1011
  visual 1011
Agranulocytes 127
Agraphesthesia 1012
Agraphias 1146
Air
  conduction 1212, 1218
  embolism 126, 955
  pressure 1205
Airway
  branching of 881
  diameter of 902
  management 963
  obstruction 967, 969
  resistance 901, 902*f*, 967
  tree 881
Akinesia 1085
Albumin 74, 486, 677, 716
  bilirubin complex 374
  globulin ratio 74
Albuminuria 74, 678
Alcohol 862, 992
  intoxication 954
Alder-Reilly anomaly 134
Aldosterone 693, 695, 711
  antagonists 708
  role of 692
  secretion 668, 868, 1248
Alkaline
  bile secretion 337
  phosphatase 644
  urine 716
Alkalosis 713, 1269, 1270, 1271
  metabolic 710, 1269, 1270
  respiratory 710, 713, 958, 1269, 1271
Allergic reactions 126
  acute 142
  chronic 142
Allergy 139, 141, 178, 570
  systemic 179
Allodynia 1015, 1022
Alpha rhythm 1116
Alveolar
  arterial oxygen gradient 971
  capillary membrane 910, 911, 958
    layers of 910, 911*f*
  growth 650
  pressure 891, 917
  stability 901
  surface tension 918
  ventilation 907, 909, 910
    measurement of 909
Alveoli 649
  epithelium of 899*f*
  growth of 650
  lobules of 469

Alveolocapillary membrane 1259
Alzheimer's disease 1129, 1141
Amacrine cell 1170, 1182
Ambisexual hairs 601
Amenorrhea 469, 470, 582, 620, 621, 629
- lactational 620, 656
- treatment of 621

Amiloride 708
Amine 990
- and peptide hormones, transport of 437
- hormone 441, 445
  - synthesis 434
- production of 390

Amino acid 33, 409, 433, 465, 475, 557, 561, 685, 686, 688, 990, 1285, 1285*t*
- classification of 1285
- duodenal infusion of 368
- entry 465

Ammonia
- buffer 712
- role of 710

Ammonium
- chloride 719
- excretion of 1269

Amnesia 1140
- anterograde 1140
- retrograde 1135, 1140

Amniocentesis 639
Amnion, formation of 638, 639*f*
Amniotic cavity 638
- formation of 638*f*

Amniotic fluid 638
- embolism 211

Amniotic sac 638
- ruptures 646

Ampulla of Vater 363
Amygdala 309, 841
Anal sphincter 418, 418*f*
Analgesia 1022
- systems 1020

Anaphylaxis 142, 179
Androgen 94, 597, 602, 627
- binding proteins 592
- hormone receptor 579
- resistance 583
- secreting tumors 603
- secretion 625

Androstenedione 599, 602
Anemia 94, 105, 107, 109, 111, 121, 123, 147, 720, 1293
- aplastic 111
- causes of 109
- chronic 123
- classification of 110*t*
- degree of 1236
- dimorphic 349
- hemolytic 111
- iron deficiency 111
- macrocytic 110, 111*f*, 388
- megaloblastic 95*f*, 96, 135*f*, 1291
- microcytic hypochromic 110*f*, 1291
- pernicious 336, 425
- sickle cell 112

Anesthesia 885, 995, 1011, 1072
Angina pectoris 850, 1018
Angiotensin 667–669, 674, 680, 695, 711
- converting enzyme 668, 668*fc*, 864
- formation of 667

Angiotensinogen 667
Anhydrosis 309, 310
- facial 309

Anions 386, 493
Anisocytes 84
Ankle clonus 1057
Ankyrin 16, 86
Anorectal angle, acute 418
Anorexia 1246
- nervosa 621, 1111

Anovulation 621
Antacids 360
Anterolateral system 1008, 1009, 1009*f*, 1030
Antiadrenergic drugs 864
Antibacterial chemicals 138
Antibiotics 164, 175, 175*t*, 177, 179, 360, 651
Antibodies 1249
- dependent cell-mediated cytotoxicity 160
- functions of 176
- monoclonal 178
- production of 155
- structure of 176, 176*f*
- therapy 178
- types of 175

Anticoagulation therapy 206
Anti-D antibody 121
Antigen 169
- recognition 170
- ingestion of 170

Anti-inflammatory
- cytokines 387
- drugs 821

Antimüllerian hormone 581
Antioxidants 1296, 1298
Antral
- contraction 408, 409
- follicular stage 609
- granulosa cells 610

Antrectomy 353
Antrum, enlargement of 628
Anuria 716
Anxiety 1130
Aorta 860
- gonad mesonephros 79

Aortic arch, wall of 829
Aphasia 1144, 1145
- anomic 1146
- transcortical 1146
- types of 1145

Aphonia 1145
Aplastic anemia, causes of 111
Apnea 959
- abrupt onset of 959
- deglutition 399

Apocrine glands 1235
Apoptosis 37, 38, 611
- molecular mechanisms of 37
- regulation of 37
- steps of 38

Appetite 1247
- juice 354
- regulation 342
  - disorder of 1293

Apraxia 1035, 1151
APUD cell 335
- system 386

Aquaporins 477, 705, 706
Aqueous humor 1168
Arachidonic acid 572
- derivative 444

Arachnoid granulations 1156
Arcuate artery 671
Arcuate fasciculus 1144
Arcuate nucleus 456
Areflexia 1072
Argentaffin cells 386
Arginine vasopressin 476*f*, 567
Argyll Robertson pupil 310, 1192
Arneth count 133, 134
Arrhythmia 768, 770
- atrial 771
- cardiac 424, 770
- ventricular 772, 772*f*

Arterial pressure 476, 476*f*, 681*f*, 824, 824*f*, 832*f*, 837*f*, 1274
- pulmonary 860

Arterial pulse 797, 799
- abnormal 801*f*

Arterial system 733
Arteries 669, 733, 814*f*
- disease, coronary 850
- hepatic 370, 856
- hypophyseal 457, 460
- interlobular 671
- peripheral 789
- pudendal 630
- pulmonary 731
- renal 671
- spiral 615, 617
- systemic 731

Arteriolar arcade 852
Arteriovenous pressure gradient 917
Arthritis, rheumatoid 1248, 1299
Articulation, disorder of 1146

Artificial ventilation, method of 961
Arytenoids 881
Ascending pathways 1007
Ascites 874
Ascorbic acid 1288
Asphyxia 957
  stages of 957
Aspiration 1301
Astereognosis 1012
Asthma 903
  bronchial 570, 801
Astigmatism 1175
Astrocytes 977
  functions of 977
Ataxia 1095, 1096, 1250
Atherosclerosis 201, 733, 863, 1284, 1296, 1299
  coronary 850
Athetosis 1087
Atrioventricular valves 738
Atrium 730, 738
Atropine 304, 318
  sulphates 963
Auditory canal, external 1202
Auditory ossicles, destruction of 1217
Auer bodies 134
Autoantibodies 179, 246, 493
Autoimmune
  disease 179, 493
  hemolytic anemia 195
  pernicious anemia 425
Autolysis 19
Autonomic
  diseases 309
  dysfunctions 309, 324
  failure 309
  function
    tests 312
    control of 306
  ganglia 304
    role of 307
  imbalance 323
  nervous system 285, 287–289, 293*t*, 311, 976
  neuraxis 307
  neuropathy 409
  organization, part of 306
  reflexes 308, 1073
    spinal 308
  regulation 826, 840
Autonomous nervous system 295
Autophagosomes 19
Autosomal dominant disorder 112, 693
Axoaxonic synapse 982
Axodendritic synapse 981*f*, 982, 982*f*
Axon 216, 220, 238, 979
  cylinder 979
  hillock 216, 979
  reflex 307, 853, 853*f*
  types of 217
Axoneme 596
Axoplasm 979
Axoplasmic transport, types of 219
Axosomatic synapse 981*f*, 982
Axoxonic synapse 981*f*
Azathioprine 177
Azurophilic granules 134, 185

B

B cells 168, 170, 173
  development of 168, 168*f*
B lymphocytes 164
Babinski's sign 1065, 1068, 1073
Bachman's tract 742
Bachman's bundle 742
Bacteria
  colonic 390
  intestinal 119, 387
Bacterial growth 379
Bacteroides fragilis 387
Bainbridge reflex 771, 798, 835, 835*f*
Baker's muscular dystrophy 273
Balstocele 637
Barbiturates 992
Barometric pressure 954
Baroreceptor 829, 945
  information 304
  reflex 798, 829, 830*f*, 832
    pressure range of 831*f*
    sensitivity 313
Barr body 133, 578
Barrett's esophagus 402
Barrier methods 653
Bartter syndrome 690
Basal
  acid output 356
  blood pressure 824
  body temperature 619, 1239
  cells 1224
  compartment 591
  electrical rhythm 394
  firing rate 298
  ganglia 121, 1043, 1071, 1075, 1082, 1083, 1083*f*, 1084*f*
    dysfunctions of 1085
    functions of 1085
    nuclei of 1084*f*
    parts of 1082*f*
  heart rate 744, 1260
  heat production 1241
  lamina 24, 242
    anchoring junctions 25
  metabolic
    activity 1240
    rate 489
  metabolism 489
  sympathetic
    activity 298
    tone 298
Basement membrane 242, 610, 618, 665
Basilar membrane 1213
  depression of 1212
Basophil 141, 141*t*, 142
  cells 461*f*
  count 143*t*
  granules 142
  megakaryocyte 185
  structure of 142*f*
Basophilic erythroblast 92
Bazett's formula 769
Bell-Magendie law 1004
Benedicts test 717
Benzodiazepine drugs 992
Beriberi 1289
  infantile 1289
Bernard-Soulier syndrome 189
Bernoulli's principle 804
Beta rhythm 1116
Betazole test 356
Bezold-Jarisch reflex 835
Bicarbonate 713, 1269
  carbonic acid buffer system 1267
  deficit 1269
  excess 1270
  ions 929
  reabsorption 710, 713
    renal 710
  reclamation of 1269
Bickel pouch 355
Bigger Golgi apparatus 557
Bile
  acidification of 381
  acids 379, 380, 380*f*, 381
    fecal estimation of 380
    pool 380
    secretion 381
    source of 379
  canaliculi 371, 378
  concentration of 381
  duct 378
  flow 644
  pigments 380, 419, 717
  salt 379, 380, 717
    activated lipase 423
    functions of 379
  secretion 341, 370, 371, 379, 381
    regulation of 381
  stasis 382
  storage of 381
  supersaturation of 382
Biliary secretion 378
Bilirubin 101, 107, 121, 374, 375
  diglucuronide 101
  glucuronide 374, 376
  metabolism 101*f*, 374, 375*f*
  production of 375
Bilirubinuria 716, 717
Binocular vision 1189

Biochemical tests 717
Biot's respiration 959
Bipolar 760
  cell 1182
  chest leads 761
  lead 760
  limb leads 760
  neurons 221, 979, 1221
Bladder
  dysfunctions 725
  epithelium of 722
  function 315
  internal sphincter of 723*f*
  muscle, contraction of 724
  wall 722
Blast cells 129, 131
Blastocele 637
Blastocyst 637
  formation and implantation 636
Blastomere 636
Bleeding 194
  disorder 189, 208
  mucocutaneous 210
  tendency 209
  time 194, 208
Blind loop syndrome 388
Blood 8, 71, 1240
  brain barrier 25, 845, 845*f*, 1105, 1160
    structure of 1160*f*
  calcium 206
  cells 145
    white 127
  coagulation 184, 189, 190, 192, 196, 199, 200, 200*f*, 201, 209, 548
    regulation of 205
  collection 125, 205
  composition of 71
  disorders, study of 71
  flow 300, 345, 844*t*, 850*f*, 855, 856, 857, 912, 955, 1234, 1261, 1263
    aortic 780
    autoregulation of 842
    cerebral 845, 1261
    coronary 839, 1261
    dynamism of 205
    endothelium-mediated regulation of 842
    medullary 671
    pulmonary 916, 965, 970
    regional 643
    regulation of 857
    renal 644, 669, 671, 672, 674*t*, 678
    sluggishness of 211
    types of 805
    visceral 1261
  functions of 72
  gas analysis 970
  group 116, 117
    A 119
    AB 119, 124
    antigens 116
    associated diseases 123, 123*t*
    B 119
    group O 119
    systems 117*t*, 122
    method of 120*f*
    use of 116
  hypercoagulability of 211
  indices 107
  loss
    anemia 110
    gastrointestinal 111
  oxygenation of 860
  peripheral 78, 147*f*, 148*f*
  physiology 71
  pressure 313, 338, 476, 625, 626, 823, 824, 829–831, 831*f*, 834, 836, 837
    diastolic 823
    pulmonary 965
    reflex regulation of 829
    regulation of 659, 667, 822, 826
    systemic 857
    systolic 490, 823, 1261
  smear, peripheral 114*f*
  storage of 125, 926
  stream 351
  testis barrier 591, 592
  thymic barrier 152
  transfusion 116, 123–125, 870
  venous 789
    pooling of 1250
  vessel 277, 457, 730–732, 825, 842, 847, 863, 1014, 1073
    cerebral 845
    coronary 848
    pampiniform plexus of 589
    radius of 806
    size of 191
    smooth muscle of 835
  viscosity of 73, 793, 806
  volume 63, 72, 73, 476, 642, 1262, 1273, 1274
    determination of 72
    peripheral 735
    regulation of 667
Body
  cavities 159
  color 72
  configuration 601
  fluid
    compartments 63
    ionic composition of 65
    osmolality 1275
    volumes 64, 1272
  protection 1236
  righting reflex 1077
  secretions 160
  size 1239
  systems 8
  temperature 89, 489, 626, 797, 1110
    regulation 11
    rhythm 1238
  weight gain 645
Bohr effect 930
Bone 465, 552, 561
  cells 552*f*
  composition of 551
  conduction 1212, 1218
  constituent of 551*t*
  demineralization of 551
  density 555
  formation 553, 554, 565
    stages of 553*f*
  growth 625
  marrow 76, 78, 164
    biopsy 78
    examination 77
    failure 123
    needle aspiration 78
    smear 195*f*
    study of 71
    transplantation 78
    types of 76
  matrix 564
    destruction of 554
  metastases 560
  mineralization of 547, 564
  morphogenic protein 1221
  parts of 551
  physiology 550
  resorption 553, 554, 559, 561, 562, 564
  strength 564
  structure of 551, 552*f*
  tissue 554
Bony cochlea 1205
Botulinum toxin 244, 402, 984, 985
Bowditch phenomenon 750
Bowel
  disease, inflammatory 420
  habits, abnormal 420
Bowman's capsule 661, 664, 665, 677
Bowman's glands 1220
Bowman's membrane 1166
Bowman's space 664
Boyle's apparatus 961
Bradycardia 767, 798, 829, 833–835, 841
  causes of 800
Bradykinesia 1085
Bradykinin 162, 345, 571, 680, 836, 853
Braggpaul method 961
Brain 601, 951, 975, 995, 1014, 1129*f*, 1140, 1143, 1156*f*
  abscess 1159
  arterial supply of 846*f*
  cells 489, 1158
    maturation of 489

diseases 959
injury 957, 960
lobes of 1147, 1150, 1152*f*
mechanisms 341
motor loop of 1030
natriuretic peptide 573
stem centers 1061
tumor 833, 1159, 1160
Brainstem 479, 724, 976, 1005, 1007, 1041
auditory evoked responses 1219
lesion 1039, 1219
motor nuclei 1043
nuclei 1034, 1070
organization 293
parasympathetic division 301
reticular system 300
role of 308
transection of 935
Breast 624, 626, 652, 1284
cancer of 560
development 469, 649, 652
and lactation, abnormalities of 652
engorgement 632, 652
enlarges 585
milk 651
structure of 649
tissue 621, 626
hyperplasia of 469
Breathing 889, 936, 959
abdominothoracic 892
chemical control of 937
control of 932
mechanics of 886, 965, 966
patterns 959*f*
types of 892
Broca's aphasia 1145
Broca's area 1144
Brodmann's area 1033, 1151*f*, 1210
Bronchopulmonary segments 884
Brown-Schilder's disease 20
Brown-Séquard syndrome 1037, 1038
Brunner's gland 384, 387
Brush border 331
intestine 421
peptidases 423
Bruxism 1122
Buccal mucosa 345
Buerger disease 310
Buffer systems 709
Buffy coat 72
preparation 72
Bulbocavernosus muscle, contraction of 632
Bulbospinal pathway 828
Bulbourethral glands 594
Bundle branch block 773, 773*f*
Bundle of His 744*f*
Bundle of Kent 773
Burn 123, 211
sepsis 211
shock 869
Burr cells 85
Bursa
development of 164
equivalents 164, 168

C

Cabot's ring 86
Caisson disease 955
Calbindin 451, 550, 563, 564
Calcitonin 550, 556, 561, 562
gene 561
protects bone loss 562
Calcium 197, 451, 547, 551, 559, 564, 1291
absorption of 426, 550, 645
accumulation 188
and phosphate, intestinal control of 550
bilirubinate stones 382
binding proteins 448, 450, 451
calmodulin
kinase 450
system 449, 451*f*
channel 564, 756
blockers 852, 864
closure of 754, 755
efflux 280
functions of 547
gluconate 720
induced calcium release 256
influx 242, 279, 756, 984
ions 748
influx of 755
mediated exocytosis 434, 547, 984
metabolism 547, 548*f*, 645
pumps 564
reabsorption of 550, 559, 564
role of 259, 279
sensing receptors 557
sparks 756
Calmodulin 277, 280, 451
dependent kinases 450
Caloric nystagmus 1102
Canalicular
flow 381
system 186, 188, 350
Canaliculi 552
Cancer 36, 1294
genetic basis of 36
Cannon wave 783, 784*f*
Capillaries
density 1264
endothelium 665
fragility test 208
hydrostatic pressure 918
microcirculation 817*f*
network, system of 733
plexus 457
tube method 208
types of 816
Capsular hydrostatic pressure 678
Captopril 669, 1228
Carbaminohemoglobin 106
Carbamylcholine 245
Carbohydrate 18, 364, 408, 899, 1282, 1283
absorption of 421, 422
digestion 364, 421
and absorption of 421
malabsorption syndromes 422
metabolism 465, 491, 1289
moiety 473
sources and functions of 1283, 1283*t*
types of 1283
Carbomonoxyhemoglobin 106
Carbon
chain, length of 1283, 1284
dioxide 106, 796, 925
dissociation curve 930*f*
transport 928
monoxide 632, 927
Carbonic anhydrase 351, 711
inhibitors 708
Carboxyhemoglobin 106
Carcinogenesis 655
Carcinoid syndrome 571, 573
Cardiac
cycle 778, 780*f*, 782
failure, congestive 959
index 787
massage, external 963
muscle 247, 249, 276, 282, 739, 740*f*, 746, 748, 1014, 1240
fiber, structure of 739*f*
output 787, 788, 790, 793, 813, 824, 958, 1072
autoregulation of 794
measurement of 788
regulation of 794
rhythm 768
tamponade 737, 792
tissues 753
valve 738, 739*f*
hemolysis 99
Cardiogenic shock, treatment of 674
Cardiovascular
autonomic functions 312
disorder, hypothalamic 1111
system 8, 571–573, 643, 729, 731*f*, 1289
Carnitine, synthesis of 1288
Carotid
arteries, internal 845
bodies 833, 937, 937*f*

sinus 829, 829*f*
nerve 830
wall of 829
tunnel syndrome 1003
Carpopedal spasm 560
carpal component of 561*f*
Cartilage, functions of 881
Catalase 138, 1298
Catecholamine 282, 298, 793, 831, 867, 991, 1241, 1255, 1263
secretion of 1246
Catechol-O-methyltransferase 992
Catsper protein 596
Cauda equina, tumor of 725
Cavity, abdominal 619
Cecum, distention of 415
Celiac disease 387
Celiac ganglion 297
Cell 553*f*, 557, 742, 938, 951, 1009
adhesion 24
molecules 25*f*, 26, 27, 27*f*
body 216, 220
dendritic 145, 151, 170
functions of 446
hemoglobin 107
membrane 13, 86, 187
functions of 16
structure of 13, 14*f*
nucleus of 441
organelles 16, 216
replication, role of 1296
shrinkage 38
structure of 13*f*
types of 77*f*, 386, 552, 557, 662
volume 51
measurement of 73
Cellular
enzymes 688
immunity 164, 170, 171*f*, 573
steps of 170
immunotherapy 178
organization 13
systems 188
Central
blood volume 735, 1236
hypoventilation 910
nervous system 571, 573, 975, 976*f*, 981
development of 489
neurons 289
reflexes 333, 334
venous pressure 735, 814
Centricular failure 801
Centroacinar cells 362
Centromedian 1026, 1028, 1030
Ceramide generation 38
Cerebellar cortex, layers of 1090*f*
Cerebellum 1031, 1043, 1071 1075, 1088, 1092, 1092*f*, 1093, 1093*f*
connection of 1089*f*
functions of 1089, 1089*f*, 1093
Cerebral
artery, posterior 1031
blood flow, autoregulation of 847*f*
hemorrhage, artery of 1064
Cerebrocerebellum 1090, 1092
Cerebrospinal
fluid 64, 847, 1155
tract 1068
Cervical
dilatation 479
ganglion 296, 344
lymph nodes 309
Cervix, dilatation of 645
Charcot's artery 1064
Charcot's triad 1096
Charcot-Bouchard aneurysm 863
Charcot-Leyden crystals 142
Chediac-Higashi syndrome 134
Chemical
thermogenesis 1246
vasodilation 1246
Chemoreceptor 997, 1224, 1226
peripheral 937
reflex 798, 833, 833*f*, 867
sensitivity of 938
structure of 937
Chemoreflex
coronary 835
pulmonary 835
Chemotaxis 137, 162
Cheyne-Stokes respiration 959
Chiari-Frommel syndrome 652
Chloride
ions, secretion of 339
reabsorption 689
Chlorothiazide 708
Chlorpromazine 410
Chlorpropamide 478
Cholecalciferol 550, 556, 563, 1287
Cholecystectomy 382
Cholecystitis
acute 382, 1019
chronic 382
Cholecystokinin 336, 366, 1109
secretion, regulation of 337*fc*
Cholelithiasis 382
Cholera 386, 425, 447
toxin 447
Cholesterol 433, 599, 1284
hydrolase 364
metabolism 390
stone 382
formation 644
synthesis of 491
Cholesteryl ester hydrolase 423
Cholinergic neurons, role of 396, 1140
Chondrocyte 490, 553, 554
proliferation of 561
size and number of 464
Chorda tendineae 738, 739*f*
Chorda tympani 1225
Chorea 1086, 1087
Chorionic villi 638
Choroid 1166
Christmas disease 210
Chrohn's disease 387
Chromaffin cells 298, 460
Chromophil 460
cells 460
types of 460
Chromophobe 460
cells 461, 461*f*
Chromosomal
disorders 31
sex 583
translocation 36
Chromosome 1, 24, 28, 120, 122, 123, 167, 198, 199, 368, 583
nondisjunction of 583
structure of 28, 29*f*
types of 29*f*
Chronic hypotension, causes of 864
Chvostek's sign 560
Chyle 716
Chyme 348, 354, 405
enters duodenum 342
Cilia 22, 159
functions of 881
movement of 1213
Ciliary
body 1166, 1167
parts of 1167
ganglion 303
motions 634
Circadian rhythm 43, 308, 436, 471, 571, 1107, 1120
Circle of Willis 845
Circulation, dynamism of 1259
Clasp-knife phenomenon 1057
Clathrin 53
mediated endocytosis 54
Clitoris 605
length of 632
Clofibrate 486
therapy 479
Clomiphene 621
Clonal deletion 176
Clonus 1057
Clot retraction 189, 190, 193, 202
functions of 202
time 194, 208, 209
proliferation of 202
Clotting time 208
Cluster region 1009
Coagulation of blood 196
abnormalities of 209

Coating proteins 53
Cobalophilin 425*f*
Cocaine test 315
Cochlea 1205, 1213
  role of 1213
Cochlear hair cell, structure of 1207*f*
Codeine 414
Coenzyme A 1290
Coitus
  interruptus 656
  reflex 1073
Cold 1246
  acclimatization 1248
  antibodies 119, 124
  induced vasodilation 1248
  pressure test 315
  receptor 997, 1002, 1023, 1243
  saline 790
Collagen 191, 553
  synthesis 559, 1288
Collecting duct, functions of 691
Colon 416
  distention of 419
  motility of 416
  physiology of 389
Colonic bacteria
  functions of 390
  migration of 414
Colony-stimulating factors 82, 131
Color blindness 1195, 1196
Color vision 1193
  theories of 1194
Colostomy 418
Colostrum 651
Columnar epithelial cells 349, 365
Complement system
  activation of 173, 175*f*
  classical pathway of 173
Complete androgen resistance syndrome 583
Cone pigments 1178
Constipation 309, 419, 644
Contraception 651
  physiology of 653
Contraceptive
  hormonal 654
  methods 656, 656*t*
  oral 473
  pills, oral 654
Contractile system 188
Convergence theory 1019, 1019*f*
Convulsion, stage of 957
Copper facilitates cellular reaction 654
Cordotomy, anterolateral 1022
Cords 154
Cornea 1166
  layers of 1166*f*
Corneal transplant 1166
Corona radiata 1063
Coronary blood flow
  measurement of 849
  regulation of 849
Corpora, smooth muscle of 630
Corpus albicans 611, 617
Corpus hemorrhagicum 610, 617
Corpus luteum 610, 617, 623, 625, 626, 641
  degeneration of 480
  formation 610
  functions of 611
  structure of 610
Corpus spongiosum 630
Cortex 150, 151*f*, 153, 725, 1005, 1035, 1043, 1071, 1075, 1077, 1147, 1148, 1235
  auditory 1209
  cerebellar 1090
  cerebral 1185*f*
  frontal 1222
  limbic 828, 841
  orbitofrontal 1225
  parietal 1062
  piriform 1222
  somatosensory 1033, 1043, 1062, 1079, 1080
  vocalization of 1079
Corticospinal tracts 1043, 1061–1063
Cough 963
Cranial
  nerve 303, 304, 1018
    nuclei 293
  pain fibers 1016
Craniosacral outflow 293, 301
Creatine kinase 851
Creatine phosphate 270
Creatinine 718
  clearance test 679
Crohn's disease 420
Cross-bridge 254
  cycle 260
    continues 280
  detachment 271
  formation 260
  theory 259
Crural monoplegia 1068
Cryptorchidism 603
Crypts of Lieberkühn 384, 389
Cubilin 425
Cuboidal epithelium 482*f*
Cumulus oophorus 610, 618
Cuneate fasciculus 1008
Cuneocerebellar tract 1091
Cushing's disease 834
Cushing's reflex 799, 833, 834, 834*f*, 847, 867
Cutaneous blood flow, regulation of 852
Cyanide poisoning 951
Cyanmethemoglobin 106
Cyanosis, degree of 1236
Cyclic guanosine monophosphate 448
Cyclosporine 177
Cystinuria 423
Cystometrogram 315, 724, 724*f*
Cytochrome oxidase activity 489
Cytokine 139, 140, 144, 179, 180, 667
  secretion of 472
  therapy 178
Cytolysis 172, 174
Cytoplasm 13, 441, 979
Cytosine 30*f*
Cytoskeletal
  proteins, proteolysis of 39
  structures 13
  system 186, 187
Cytoskeleton, cytoplasmic 187
Cytotoxic Drugs Act 22
Cytotoxic T cells 164, 166, 172
Cytotrophoblasts 638

D

Dacryocyte 85
Dale's phenomenon 984
Dantrolene sodium 1250
Dead space, measurement of 908, 909*f*
Deafness 1212, 1217–1219
  treatment of 1218
Decidua, structure of 637*f*
Decubitus ulcers 1074
Deep
  cerebellar nuclei 1090, 1091*f*
  pain 1015, 1018
  reflexes 1073
  tendon reflexes 1064
Defecation 160, 418
  reflex 308, 418*f*
Deglutition, disorder of 399
Degradation, metabolic 486
Dehydration 64, 1242
  hypernatremic 1246
  hyperosmotic 1276
  hypo-osmotic 1276
Dehydroepiandrosterone 639
Deiter's nucleus 1065
Delayed puberty 586
Delta rhythm 1116
Dementia 1086, 1141
Dendrites 216, 220, 979
Dense
  bodies 188, 278
  core granules 991
  granules 188
  lymphoid tissue 153
  tubular system 187*f*, 188, 424
Density 741, 818
Dent's disease 689
Deoxycorticosterone 992

Deoxyribonucleic acid 29
Dephosphorylate proteins 446
Depolarization, atrial 757, 761, 764
Depresses myocardium 796
Dermatomal theory 1019
Dermis 1234, 1235
Descemet's membrane 1166
Descending pathways 1061
Desmosomes 25
Detrusor muscle 722, 724
Deuterium oxide 65
Dextrose 125
Diabetes 309, 1003, 1284
  insipidus 478, 693, 700, 1111
  mellitus 1294
Diabetic ketoacidosis 713, 959
Diabetic urine 716
Diapedesis 137, 162
Diaphragm 653, 887
  contraction of 887*f*
Diarrhea 309, 338, 386, 390, 419, 573
  treatment of 387
Diastolic dysfunction 782
Dicrotic pulse 800
Dicrotic wave 799, 800
Diencephalon 975
Dietary
  fats 1284
  fibers 1283
  requirements 1282
Digestion and absorption 421
Digestive enzymes, activation of 11
Dihydropyridine receptor 255
Dihydrotestosterone 599, 602
Di-iodotyrosine 485
Dilution test 718, 719
Diphtheria 951
Diplegia 1069
Diplopia 246
Discomfort, abdominal 403
Disseminated intravascular
    coagulation 210, 211*f*
Distal
  convoluted tubule 662
  nephron 694
  stomach 404, 405
  tubule, part of 708
  tubules 711
Distant vision 1188
Distention, abdominal 419
Disuse atrophy 1064
Diuresis, osmotic 683, 707, 716
Diuretics 821, 836, 864, 875, 949
Döhle bodies 136
Dominant follicle 610, 612, 615
Donnan effect 49
Dopamine 451, 468, 558, 669, 680, 696,
    870, 991, 992, 1086, 1109
  receptors, types of 992
Dopaminergic systems 1127, 1127*f*
Dorsal column 1010
  nuclei 1009, 1025, 1030
  pathway 1008, 1008*f*, 1010, 1011
  sensations 1011
Dorsal horn laminae 1005*f*
  cells of 1005
Dorsal noradrenergic bundle 1105
Dorsal nuclei 1028
Dorsal respiratory group 932
Dorsal rhizotomy 1022, 1076
Dorsal root 1004, 1016
  fibers 237
  ganglia 1002
Dorsal spinocerebellar tract 1091
Dorsal vein 630
Double helix structure 30*f*
Douglas bag 970
Down's syndrome 31, 31*f*, 583
Drinker's method 961, 963
Drowning 918, 958
Dry beriberi 1289
Dubois formula 788
Duchenne muscular dystrophy 273
Ducts 649
  branching of 650
  cell 365
  cystic 378
  growth 650
  of Rivinus 343
  of Stensen 343
  of Wharton 343
  proliferation of 469
  system, development of 649
Ductular secretion 381
Ductus arteriosus 860
Ductus venosus, closure of 860
Duffy system 122
Duke method 208
Dumping syndrome 410
Duodenal ulcer 358, 364, 405
Duodenum 354, 408, 423, 424
  stretching of 409
Dwarfism, metabolic 1281
Dysarthria 1145
Dysbarism 955
Dysesthesia 1012
Dysgeusia 1229
Dysmenorrhea 617, 621
Dysmetria 1095
Dysosmia 1223
Dysphagia 400, 1144
Dyspnea 873, 969
Dysrrhythmia 770
Dystrophin 253

E

Ear, functions of 1202
Ebner's glands 1226, 1234
Echinocyte 85
Eclampsia 211
Ectoderm 649
Edema 820, 821, 874
  cerebral 949
  formation 74, 820
  pulmonary 720, 918
  treatment of 821
Edinger-Westphal nucleus 293, 303
Edridge-Green Lantern test 1196
Eicosanoids, synthesis of 1284
Einthoven's triangle 759, 760, 760*f*, 770
Ejaculation 632
  premature 309, 632
Ejection fraction 788
Elastic tissue 732
Elastin 375
Electrical rhythm 394
Electrocardiogram, mechanics of 759
Electroencephalogram 1115
Electrolyte 465, 1275
Electromagnetic flow meter 788, 849
Electronystagmography 1102
Electroretinogram, waves of 1200*f*
Embden-Mayerhoff pathway 86, 87
Embryo transfer 641
Embryoblast 637
Emotions, physiology of 1132
Encephalitis 1159
End diastolic volume 750, 800, 1260
End stage renal failure 721
Endocardium 737, 738
Endochondral maturation 490
Endochondral ossification 490, 553
Endocrine
  cells 350, 386, 460, 663
  communication 436
  gland 431, 432, 432*f*, 453
  neoplasia syndrome, multiple 559
  organs 432, 625
  system 8, 644
  tissue 610
  tumors, abnormal 571
Endocytic vesicle 54*f*, 55
Endocytosis 54, 138, 170, 425, 441, 471
  constitutive 54, 54*f*
  types of 54
Endogenous
  analgesia system 571, 993
  ceruloplasmin 1298
  neural analgesia system 1021*f*
  opioid systems 1021
  pain-inhibiting system 1067
  pyrogens 1249
  water gain 1273
Endolymph 1213
Endometrial glands 615, 626
Endometrium 637
Endomysium 250*f*

Endoneurium 222
Endoplasmic reticulum 17, 52, 188, 484*f*, 548
  structure of 18
Endorphin 1021, 1022, 1263
  receptors 1021
  system 271
Endoscopic retrograde cholangiopancreatography 369
Endothelial
  cells 371, 732, 818
  injury 211
Endothelin 282, 680, 836
Endothelium 1166, 1167
Energy
  restoration 301
  source 1254
  utilization 295
Enteric nervous system 288, 331, 332*f*, 333, 395
Enteritis 381
Enterobacter aerogens 387, 390
Enterochromaffin cells 329, 335, 339, 350, 385, 386, 573
Enterocytes 424
Enteroendocrine cells 335
Enterogastric reflex 355, 409
Enterogastrone 354
Enteroglucagon 338
Enterohepatic circulation 379, 380
Enterokinase 423
Enteropeptidase 364
Enzyme 144, 163, 345, 364, 386, 1285
  cascade hypothesis 11, 201
  component 364
  deficiencies 583
  intestinal 386*t*
  linked immunosorbent assay 439
Eosinophil
  cationic protein 140
  count 141
  derived chemicals 139*t*
  derived neurotoxin 140
  granular contents 139
  mediated inflammatory reactions 140
  peroxidase 140
  structure of 139
Eosinophilia, causes of 141*t*
Ependymal cells 978
Epidermis 159, 1233
  deepest layer of 1234
Epididymis 593
  structure of 594*f*
Epiglottis 881
Epilepsies, types of 1122
Epinephrine 870, 991
Epineurium 222
Epiphyseal
  cartilage, growth of 464
  closure 625
  plate 551
Epiphysis 466, 551, 566
  closure of 554, 1278
  fusion of 466
Epistaxis 194
Epithalamus 1031
Epithelial cell 150, 151, 151*f*, 165, 358, 386, 662, 665, 1225
  function 1286
  intestinal 24*f*
  parietal 664
Epitheliocytes 150
Epithelium 329, 605, 1166, 1168
  intestinal 387
  olfactory 1220
Epitheloid cells 666
Erectile
  dysfunction 309, 631, 632
  tissues 630, 999
Ergosterol 1287
Erlanger-Gasser classification 237
Erythroblast 92, 121
  orthochromatic 92
Erythroblastosis fetalis 121
Erythrocyte 83, 93
  sedimentation rate 88
Erythrocytosis 115*t*
Erythroid stem cells 92
Erythropoiesis 90, 93, 93*t*, 96, 491
  duration of 93
  medullary 90
  regulation of 93, 94, 660
  sites and stages of 90
  stages of 90, 91*f*
  steps of 91
Erythropoietin 82, 93, 573
  production 643
  synthesis of 868
Esbach's albuminometer 717
Escherchia coli 390
Esophageal
  leads 761
  motility 401
  peristalsis 402
  sphincter 349, 399, 401, 402, 410
Esophagus 328, 394, 399, 402
  parts of 401
  structure of 401*f*
  upper part of 401
Esthesia 995
Estradiol 600
Estriol 642
Estrogen 94, 451, 597, 599, 612, 618, 623, 625, 628, 642, 650, 667, 862, 1109
  functions of 624
  level of 645
  receptors, types of 624
  stimulates growth 625
  structure of 623*f*
  synthesis of 612, 624*fc*
Ethylenediamine tetra-acetic acid 206
Etidronate 562
Eustachian tube 1204
  dysfunctions 1204
  obstruction 1217
Evans blue dye 65
Exercise physiology 1252
Exocrine pancreas
  deficiency of 424
  structure of 362
Exocrine secretions 570
Exocytic vesicles, formation of 56*f*
Exocytosis 55, 171, 243
  constitutive 55, 56*f*
Exogenous pyrogens 1249
Exophthalmos 493*f*, 494
Expiratory muscles, strength of 967
External sphincter, contraction of 418
Extracellular
  fluid 1267
    compartment 63
  matrix 24
  organisms 164
Extracorpuscular defects 112
Extrafusal muscle fibers 1046
Extraglomerular mesangial cells 666, 667
Extralobular ducts 365
Extramedullary hemopoiesis 79, 121
Extraocular muscles 246, 1198, 1198*f*
Extraparenchymal
  dysfunction 968
  inspiratory dysfunction 968
Extrapyramidal
  structures 1071
  systems 1042, 1064, 1071
  tracts 1061
Extrarenal tissues 706
Extrasystole 748
Extrathyroidal tissue 492
Extravascular destruction 99, 101
Extrinsic
  neural
    control 333
    regulation 333
  proteins 15
  regulation 795, 842
  system of clotting 201
Eye 454
  intrinsic muscles of 1168
  movements of 1198, 1200
Eyeball movement 1095

F

Facial pain, acute 1025
Fallopian tube 624, 635
  ampullary portion of 635
  distal portion of 634
Family planning operations 656
Fanconi syndrome 689, 713
Farrell pouch 355
Fat
  absorption of 379
  deposition 645, 650
  digestion 367, 409
    disorder of 423
  emulsification of 379
  fecal estimation of 369
  metabolism 465, 491
  restriction of 863
  soluble vitamins, absorption of 379, 425
Fatigue 246, 874, 1254
Fatty acids 409, 423, 849, 1110, 1254, 1255, 1283, 1284
  unsaturated 160
Fear, emotions of 1130
Febrile reaction 125, 126
Fecal stercobilinogen 376
Female Sexual Act 632
Fern test 619
Ferric reductase 426
Ferricytochrome 1298
Ferritin, formation of 1288
Fertile period 655
Fertilization 627, 635
  in vitro 640
Festinant gait 1086, 1086f
Fetal
  adrenal gland 640f
  basal ganglia 1086
  circulation 859, 859f
  growth 466
  hemoglobin 104
  liver 164
  tissues 860
  tolerance 177
Fetus 562
  head of 646f
Fever 163, 958, 1248, 1249
  genesis of 1249fc
  pathogenesis of 1249
Fibers 297t, 363, 417, 674, 723, 724, 1018
  cholinergic 827, 1114
  corticohypothalamic 1105
  corticoreticular 1064
  corticospinal 1064
  corticothalamic 1026, 1028, 1031
  monoaminergic 1114
  noradrenergic 669
  parasympathetic 278, 304, 722, 724
  peripheral 1015
  somatic 723
Fibrillation, atrial 757, 772
Fibrin
  degradation products 203, 203f, 204
  monomer 201
    polymerization of 201, 202
  polymer, stabilization of 201, 202
  stabilization 202fc
  threads spread 202
Fibrinogen 74, 88, 89, 191, 197, 201
  concentration 209
Fibrinolysis 183, 202, 203
  activation of 203f
  inhibitor of 204
Fibrinolytic deficiency 204
Fibroblast 663, 1288
Fibrofatty plaques 1296
Fibrosis 1073
  cystic 37, 365, 368
  pulmonary 958
Fibrous pericardium 737
Fick method 789
Fick principle 789, 846, 849
Filaments, organization of 278
Filopodia 187
Filtration slit diaphragm 665
Fimbriae contract, smooth muscle of 634
Fine needle aspiration cytology 496
Flaccid paralysis 1068
Flavin 1289
Flexion reflex 1058t
  afferents 1057f
Flexor
  muscles 1073
  planter response 1068
  reflex 1057, 1073
  spasm 1073
  tone 1073
Flow volume curve 903, 903f
Fluid
  component 71
  retention 645
  tonicity of 1275
  volume 1110
    disorder of 1275
Focal adhesion complexes 22
Foliate papillae 1224
Folic acid 94, 852, 1288, 1290
  deficiency 1291
Follicle
  atresia of 611
  stimulating hormone 460, 618
Follicular
  Development
    regulation of 611
    stages of 608
  estrogen 611
  fluid volume 612
  rupture 618
    steps of 618
  wall, proteolysis of 619
Folliculogenesis 608
Folliculostellate cells 461
Follistatin 473, 602
Forced expiratory volume 967
Forced vital capacity 893, 966
Formiminoglutamic acid 1291
Fornix 1105
Fovea centralis 1170
Frank-Starling law 741, 750, 791, 794
Fresh frozen plasma 73, 210
Frey syndrome 310
Friedreich's ataxia 1096
Frontal lobe syndrome 1153
Fundus 1171
Fungemia 211
Fungiform papillae 1224
Furosemide 707, 864
Fusimotor fibers 1049
Fusimotor system 1046

G

G cells 335, 350
G protein 442
  couple receptors 443
  diseases 444
  gustducin 1227
  types of 443
Gait 1096
Galactorrhea 629, 652
Galactose 117, 422
Gallamine 245
Gallbladder 379, 379t, 381
Gallop rhythm 785
Gallstone 368, 382, 382f
  formation 379
Gametes, transport of 634
Gamma aminobutyric acid 992
Ganglia 293, 296–298
  cell bodies of 293t
  collateral 290, 297
  mesenteric 331
  parasympathetic 308
  paravertebral 291f, 296
    chain of 744
  sacral 297
  sympathetic chain of 294
Ganglion 296
  blockers 304
  cells 1183
  submandibular 303, 344
  trigeminal 1025
Gap junction 739, 987
  functions, regulation of 26
Gas
  analysis, respiratory 970
  exchange 884, 910, 915, 969, 970

molecular weight of 911
solubility of 911
partial pressure of 912t
Gastrectomy 360, 426
Gastric
acid 345, 424
secretion 337, 352, 353, 353t
stimulation of 336
atrophy 426
distension 342
emptying, regulation of 408
function tests 356
glands 349
inhibitory peptide 338, 340, 354
juice 350, 407, 408
composition of 350
lipase 423
motility 337, 404
electrophysiology of 406
types of 406
mucosa, growth of 336
oxyntic gland, parts of 350f
peristalsis 407
pits 349
rugae 349
secretion 338, 341, 348, 351, 356t, 1223
regulation of 336fc, 353f, 354
secretory products 357
slow waves 406
ulcer 358, 405
Gastrin 335, 352, 409
blockers 360
provocative tests 357
secretion, control of 336
trophic action of 336
types of 336
Gastrinoma 336
Gastritis 358
acute 358
chronic 358
classification of 358t
Gastrocolic reflex 417
Gastroduodenal
content 409
junction 405
mucosa 405
Gastroduodenostomy 360f
Gastroenteritis, acute 387
Gastroileal reflex 415
Gastrointestinal
system 8, 327, 572
tract 277, 328, 571
Gastrojejunostomy 360
Gastroparesis 409
Gastroscopy 358
Gene
amplification 33, 36
augmentation 37
correction 36
expression 32
rearrangement 33
replacement 36
therapy 34, 36
transcription 489, 626
Genetic sex
female 579
male 579
Geniculostriate pathway 1184f
Genital
duct system 578
stimulation 479
tract, diseases of 111
tubercle 601
Genitalia 600, 605, 625
external 580f, 583, 600, 604, 604f
Genitourinary diseases 111
Gentamycin 1217
Gerhardt's test 717
Germ cell 579, 590, 590f, 591, 591f, 592
development 591
Germinal angiotensin converting enzyme 596
Ghrelin 1109
Giant
cells 145
osteoclasts 559
Gibbs-Donnan effect 49
Gibbs-Donnan equilibrium 59, 59f
Gigantism 466
Gitelman's syndrome 694
Glands
cardiac 349
conserve sodium 1248
hormone 435
intestinal 384, 385f, 389
secretory 650
sublingual 343, 344
submandibular 343, 344
Glandular tissue, growth of 626
Glanzmann thrombasthenia 202
Glial cells 977, 978f
functions of 977
types of 977
Gliomas 978
Global hypothalamic syndrome 1110
Globulin 74, 88
Glomerular
apparatus 681
capillary 671, 677
endothelium 56
hydrostatic pressure 678
membrane 677f
oncotic pressure 677
permeability 678
filtration 676, 697
barrier 678t
rate 644, 669, 678
function tests 715
Glomeruli, olfactory 1221
Glomerulocapsular filtration barrier 676
Glomerulotubular feedback mechanism 675
Glomerulus 661, 664
Glomus cells, transplantation of 1086
Glossopharyngeal nerves 936f
Glottis 881
Glucagon 338, 793, 796, 1263
Glucocorticoid 565, 667, 681, 696
hormones 821900
therapy 177
Gluconeogenesis 491, 660, 1255
Glucose 491, 1255
absorption of 491
galactose malabsorption syndrome 422
hepatic release of 1255
intolerance 491
reabsorption 53, 687
solution 720
utilization 642
Glucuronide 624
conjugates 625
Glutamate 992, 1213, 1227
decarboxylase 992
Glutamine
metabolism of 710
molecule produces 712
Glutathione peroxidase 1292, 1298
Glycine 992
Glycocalyx, functions of 15
Glycocholic acid 379
Glycogen 1254, 1255
Glycogenolysis 300, 478
Glycolytic enzymes, inhibitor of 206
Glycopeptide 476f
Glycoprotein 187, 441
hormone 444, 641
receptors 187, 188f
Glycosaminoglycans 207
Glycosides, cardiac 741
Glycosuria 644, 683, 717
gestational 717
Glycosylation 470
Goblet cells 386, 389
Goiter 1291
multinodular 493
Goldblatt hypertension 669, 863
Goldman-Hodgkin-Katz equation 60
Golgi
apparatus 18, 216, 484f
bottle neuron 1055
complex 18
structure of 18f
tendon organ 1048, 1052, 1056
structure of 1052f
type 221, 222
Golgi-Mazzoni corpuscle 998

Goll and Burdach tract 1008
Gonadal
  dysgenesis 586, 1281
  function 568
  growth 465
    curve 1279
  hormone 433, 473, 1279
    secretion of 627, 628
  sex 579
  steroid binding globulin 599
Gonadotropin 460, 627
  hormones 603
  independent precocity 586
  releasing hormone 455
  secretion of 627
Goodpasture syndrome 179
Goormaghtigh cells 666
Gout 689
Graafian follicle 604, 608, 610
Gracile fasciculus 1008
Grand mal epilepsy 1122
Granular lymphocytes 160
Granule 134, 1234
  cell 1221
  secretory 134, 434
Granulocytes 127
  and mononuclear cells, role of 160
  development of 130f
Granulomatous diseases, chronic 123, 1299
Granulosa 629
  cells 578, 609–612, 612f, 623
  lutein cells 611
Grasp reflex 1078
Graves' disease 493
Gravid uterus, contraction of 572
Growth 464, 600, 1278
  and development, physiology of 1278
  cone 239
  curve 1278
  factors 144, 561, 565
  hormone 94, 455, 460, 461, 471, 490, 565, 644, 796, 1255, 1279
    insensitivity 1281
    receptor 463
  patterns of 1278
  periods of 1280
  regulation of 1279
  spurt 1278
    infantile 1278
    pubertal 1278, 1279f
Guanine 30f
  exchange factors 443
Guanylin 339
  receptors 339
Gustation 1224
  physiology of 1225
Gustatory
  pathway neurons 1229
  receptor cell 1224, 1225
  stimuli 1227
  transduction, mechanics of 1226
Gynecomastia 600

H

Haber's reaction 1298
Hageman's factor 198, 200
Hair 1235
  bulb 1235
  cells 1098, 1098f, 1100, 1206, 1213, 1215
    depolarize 1215
    repolarize 1215
    senile degeneration of 1217
    stimulation of 1100f
    structure of 1098f
    toxic degeneration of 1217
  follicle 999, 1235
  follicle, nonsinus 999
  parts of 1235, 1235f
  structure of 1235
  types of 1235
Haldane gas analyzer 970
Haldane-Priestley method 970
Haloperidol 410
Hamilton's dye dilution method 789
Haptoglobin 100
Hartnup disease 423
Hashimoto's thyroiditis 495
Hassall's corpuscle 151f
Haundice, hepatic 375, 376
Haustral contractions 417
Haversian canals 551
Hay's test 717
Headache 1250
Heart 304, 729, 730, 737, 739, 744, 745f, 747, 749, 763, 807, 863
  block 772, 773
  chambers 872
    wall of 737
  conducting system of 742, 742f
  denervation of 744
  disease, coronary 1284, 1294
  electrophysiology of 751
  failure 785, 872, 873f, 874f
    pathophysiology of 871
    types of 871
  functional anatomy of 736
  heterometric autoregulation of 794
  lung preparation 794, 794f
  muscle 490, 749f
  pacemaker of 746
  rate 304, 312, 313, 316, 317, 490, 643, 743, 744, 747, 756, 767, 782, 793, 795, 798, 825, 1247, 1260, 1262
    regulation of 798
  sound 784, 785
  tissues of 754f
Heartburn 402
Heat 271, 717, 1245
  acclimatization 1247, 1248
  balance 1240
  collapse 1250
  conductance 1248
  dissipation 1241, 1246
  exhaustion 1242, 1250
  flow 1240, 1246
  gain, mechanics of 1241
  generation 1239
    and transfer, principles of 1239
    rate of 1239
  loss 1245, 1247, 1254
    neurons 1244
    mechanics of 1242fc, 1242t
    pulmonary 1241, 1243
    radiant 1241
  metabolic 1240
  preservation 1240
  production 271, 1239, 1244, 1246
    neurons 1244
    mechanics of 1240, 1242fc
    rate of 1239
  shock protein 449
  stress 1249
  syncope 1250
  transfer 1239
Heatstroke 1250
Heidenhain's pouch 355
Heimlich maneuver 962
Heinz bodies 105
Helicobacter pylori infection 359
Helminthic infections 140
Helper cells 165
Hematemesis 359
Hematocrit 88, 806
Hematopoiesis 76
Hematopoietic stem cell 78
  abnormalities of 115
Hematuria 717
Heme 103, 374
  oxygenase 426
Hemianesthesia 1012
Hemiballismus 1032
Hemicholinium 245
Hemidesmosomes 25
Hemiglobin 106
Hemiglobincyanide 106
Hemineglect syndrome 1035
Hemiplegia 1064, 1069
Hemochromatosis 426
Hemodilution 105
Hemoglobin 103, 104, 717, 923
  A 104
  A2 104
  abnormal 105

buffer system 1268
catabolism 374
electrophoresis 112
estimation 107
fate of 104*f*
ligands 105
solution, viscosity of 99
synthesis, steps of 104*fc*
types of 104
Hemoglobinuria 107, 125, 717
Hemolysis
acute 179
intravascular 100*f*, 112
Hemolytic
anemia, causes of 112*t*
jaundice, causes of 101*t*
transfusion reactions, acute 125
Hemopexin 101
Hemophilia 209
A 209
B 210
types of 210
Hemopoiesis 76, 78, 551
hepatic stage of 155
regulation of 82
sites and stages of 79
steps of 80
types of 81
Hemorrhage
acute 110
cerebral 863, 1159
chronic 111
Hemosiderosis 426
Hemostasis 183, 184, 184*fc*, 185, 190, 193, 572
inhibitor of 193
steps of 183
Henderson-Hasselbalch equation 1267
Heparin 193, 206, 207
Hepatic
blood flow, regulation of 856
canaliculi, lumen of 381
duct 363, 370, 371, 378
glucose output 491
glycogenolysis 491
lobules 371*f*
neoglucogenesis 465
Hepatitis 381
Hepatobiliary system 378, 378*f*, 644
Hepatocytes 379
Hering-Breuer reflex 943
Heterochromatin clumps 92
Heterometric autoregulation 750, 791
Hexaxial reference system 766, 766*f*
Hexoses 1283
Hierarchial system 435
High-pressure
baroreceptors 829
nervous syndrome 954, 955
volume receptors 1274
Hinge region 176
Hip bones 555
Hirschsprung's disease 310, 419
His bundle 743
electrogram 776, 777*f*
His-Purkinje fibers 747
His-Purkinje system 757
Histalog test 356
Histamine 142, 162, 179, 352, 353, 390, 569, 570, 680, 837, 853, 993, 1023
receptors 569
test 356
Histaminergic system 1129
Histidine 569
Hodgkin's cycle 11, 229
Holger-Neilson method 961, 962, 963*f*
Hollander test 357
Holmgren's wool-matching test 1196
Homeostasis 9, 1158
Hormone 152, 282, 339, 396, 409, 433, 438, 439, 442, 446*f*, 468, 486, 642, 691, 819, 916, 926, 1102
action 51, 437–439, 441
anabolic 600
antidiuretic 475, 826, 1263
binding 437
domain 449
classification of 433*t*
concentration 438
degradation and disposal of 438
disposal of 438
functions of 431
gastrointestinal 335
half-life of 438
homeostasis 434
hypophysiotropic 457
hypothalamic 454, 456, 460
intrinsic 334
luteinizing 455, 460, 473
pancreatic 370
receptor complex 441, 444
secretion 460
ectopic 434
measurement of 438
regulation of 12, 434
synthesis of 34
testicular 599, 602
thymic 152
transport of 437
trophic 435
types of 433
Horn cells, Anterior 1045, 1046
Horner's syndrome 309, 311
Horse-radish peroxidase 219
Hot flushes 586
Howell Jolly bodies 86
Human
blood 119
chorionic gonadotropin 641, 642
growth hormone 642
milk, composition of 651*t*
placental lactogen 642
Humoral hypercalcemia 561
Humoral immunity 164, 172
steps of 172
Hunger contractions 406
Huntington's disease 1086
Hyaline mass 151
Hyaluronidase 594
Hybridoma 178
Hydrocephalus 342, 1159
Hydrochloric acid
action of 426
secretion of 348
Hydrops fetalis 121
Hydrostatic pressure 49, 687, 697, 820, 835
gradient 676, 677, 819, 918
Hydroxyapatite crystals 551, 553
Hydroxylation 559
Hydroxylysine 559
Hydroxyproline 554, 559
Hydroxyprolinuria 465, 554
Hyerkalemia 720
Hyperaldosteronism 692, 693
Hyperalgesia 1015, 1022
Hyperbaric oxygen therapy 952
Hypercalcemia 561, 562, 776
osteolytic 561
Hypercapnia 939, 940*f*, 941, 957, 958
Hypercomplex cells 1186
Hyperdefecation 491
Hyperemia 842, 854, 855
Hyperesthesia 1012, 1038
Hyperestrogenemia 625
Hypergonadotropic hypogonadism 603
Hyperkalemia 126, 720, 776, 776*f*
Hyperlipidemia 862, 1299
Hypermetropia 1175
Hypernatremia 692, 776
Hyperosmolar interstitium 694
Hyperoxaluria 20
Hyperparathyroidism 559, 560
Hyperpathia 1012, 1022
Hyperplasia 282, 465, 468
Hyperpnea
anticipatory 1257
spontaneous 959
Hyperprolactinemia 468, 470
galactorrhea syndrome 652
Hypersensitivity 240, 247, 247*f*, 442, 725
Hypersomnia 1123
Hypersympathetic state 491
Hypertension 282, 308, 625, 690, 861, 861*t*, 862, 863, 1284, 1294
degree of 861
endocrinal 862
genesis of 669

neurogenic 862
pathophysiology of 861
pulmonary 949
renal 669, 862
systolic 861
treatment of 695
types of 861
Hyperthermia 1240, 1244, 1249, 1250, 1254
malignant 1250
Hyperthyroidism 492, 493, 495, 496
Hypertonic
fluid 1275
solution 87, 409
use of 1161
Hypertrophy 282, 465, 1073
vascular 970
Hyperventilation 910, 959
voluntary 958
Hypervitaminosis D 1287
Hypesthesia 1011
Hypoalbuminemia 74, 644
Hypoalgesia 1022
Hypocalcemia 560, 720, 776
Hypocapnia 958
Hypochlorous acid 138
Hypochromia 84, 110
Hypochromic cells 84
Hypogeusia 1228
Hypoglycemia 410
Hypogonadism, male 603
Hypogonadotropic hypogonadism 603, 629
Hypokalemia 692, 776
Hypomenorrhea 618, 621
Hyponatremia 479, 668, 720, 776
Hypoparathyroidism 560
Hypophyseal artery, superior 457, 460
Hypoproteinemia 678
Hyposmia 1223
Hypotension 338, 570, 679, 693, 834, 835, 841, 864
acute 179, 865
chronic 864
orthostatic 309, 313
pathophysiology of 861
postural 865
Hypothalamic
centers, role of 1244
hypothyroidism, hypothalamic 494
integration, mechanics of 1245, 1245*fc*
neurochemicals, role of 1121
neurons, maturation of 585
syndrome 456, 1110
Hypothalamo-gonadal axis, maturation of 585
Hypothalamo-hypophyseal tract 456, 457, 457*f*, 1105
Hypothalamo-pituitary
adrenocortical axis 472, 453
axis 453, 456, 626, 457*f*
disorder 652
gonadal axis 453
ovarian axis 644
target endocrine gland axis 435
thyroid axis 453
Hypothalamo-sympatho-adrenal-axis 453
Hypothalamus 308, 453, 454*f*, 627, 840, 1029, 1104*f*, 1105–1107
anterior 829, 1244
arcuate nucleus of 455, 456, 993
connection of 454*f*
functions of 1104, 1106
integrates 292
modulates histamine 1122*fc*
nuclear groups of 1105*f*
paraventricular
cells of 479
nuclei of 457, 475
posterior 308, 725, 1244
posterolateral part of 829
role of 308, 651, 1107, 1110
suprachiasmatic nucleus of 471
thermosensitivity of 1244
Hypothermia 1242, 1244, 1251
Hypothesis, traveling wave 1214
Hypothyroidism 471, 494–496, 652, 1291
hypopituitary 471
treatment of 495
Hypotonia 1068
Hypotonic solutions 87
Hypoventilation 910, 950, 957, 971
peripheral 910
regional 971
Hypovolemia 48, 410, 477, 1242, 1250
Hypoxemia 969, 971
Hypoxia 96, 238, 845, 854, 920, 938, 939*f*, 940*f*, 941, 942, 945, 950, 951, 957
acute 951
chronic 952
histotoxic 951, 952
hypoperfusion 951
hypoxic 950, 952
subacute 951
types of 950
Hysteresis loop 895

I

Idiopathic thrombocytopenic purpura 194
Ileocecal sphincter, function of 415
Ileum, distention of 415
Iliac crest puncture 78
Immune complex disease 179
Immune system 432, 433
gastrointestinal 332
Immunity 72, 74, 155, 158, 372, 1236
types of 159*t*
Immunodeficiency syndromes, congenital 179
In vitro fertilization 640
Infarction
myocardial 191, 774, 835, 850
postmyocardial 323
Infertility, female 640
Inflammation
acute 163
chronic 163
steps of 161*f*
Ingestion 138, 1241
Inguinal canal 588
Inhibin 473, 602, 618, 627
A 602
B 602
Injury
pulmonary 970
severity of 240
spinal 311
Insomnia 1122
Inspiratory muscles, strength of 967
Insulin 86, 565, 793, 796, 900, 1279
growth factor binding proteins 466
secretion 410
test 357
Integral membrane proteins, functions of 15
Integration, hypothalamic 455*fc*
Intensity 996, 1000
discrimination 1228
Interleukins 82, 94, 131, 180, 186
Interstitial cells 417, 573, 590, 590*f*, 663
medullary 663
Interstitial fluid volume, measurement of 65
Interstitium, osmolality of 693, 696
Intestinal
circulation, regulation of 855
epithelium, integrity of 380
flora, functions of 387
mucosa, growth of 387
secretion, functions of 387
smooth muscles, electrophysiology of 413
Intestine
bacterial flora of 328
large 329, 390*f*, 416, 417, 424
length of 414
small 328, 385*f*, 397, 413*f*, 423, 426
Intra-abdominal pressure 410, 419, 724
Intracellular
binding 27
buffers 713
calcium 675
concentration 823
camp 299, 300

dehydration 1276
digestions 19
fluid 64, 1267
compartment 64
homeostasis 12
organisms 164, 170
receptor system 448
Intracorpuscular defects 112
Intracranial pressure 847
role of 847
Intrafusal fibers 1046, 1048
Intragastric pressure 406, 407
Intrahepatic obstruction 376
Intralaminar nuclei 1030
Intranasal tube 952
Intrapleural pressure 791, 889, 890
measurement of 889
Intrauterine
devices 653
fetal transfusion 122
Intrinsic mutagenesis theory 1296
Inulin 679
clearance test 679, 718
Iodide, high dose of 493
Iodine 1291
deficiency 483
metabolism of 484*f*
Iodotyrosine deiodinase 485
Ion channel 40, 42, 245
blockers 231
Ipsilateral limb, flexion of 1058
Iris 94, 104, 1167, 1291
Iron
absorption of 426
deficiency anemia 110, 111, 112*f*, 426
storage of 426
Irritable bowel syndrome 419
Ischemia 415, 1003
acute 1003
cerebral 958
chronic 1003
myocardial 769, 774, 850
Ischemic tissue death 212
Ishihara chart 1196, 1196*f*
Isotonic
contraction, concentric type of 1253
fluid diarrhea 447
Isotopic tests 495
Itch 1023
receptors 1023
Ivy pouch 355

J

Jak-stat pathway 449, 463
Jaundice 374, 376, 717
acholuric 101, 376
causes of 375
degree of 1236
hemolytic 101, 101*f*, 102, 107, 121, 375, 376
laboratory diagnosis of 376
neonatal 376
obstructive 375, 375*f*, 376, 382
pathophysiology of 370
types of 375, 376*t*
Jejunum, mucosa of 385*f*
Jendrassik's maneuver 1051, 1052
Joints, pelvic 626
Jugular venous pulse 783, 783*f*
Juvenile
neutrophil 131, 133
red cells 93, 96
Juxtacrine communication 437
Juxtaglomerular cells 666
Juxtamedullary nephrons 661–663, 689

K

Kallikrein-Kinin system 836
Kallmann's syndrome 629, 1223
Kanamycin 1217
Kaposi's sarcoma 180
Kasper Hauser syndrome 1281
Kell system 123
Keratin 1234
Keratinocytes 563
Keratocytes 85
Keratohyalin 1234
Keratomalacia 1287
Kernicterus 845, 1160
Ketogenesis 465
Ketone bodies 717
Ketonuria 717
Kety method 846
Kidd system 123
Kidney 478, 492, 562, 571, 659, 669, 863
disease 74, 719
function tests 715
internal structures of 660
oxygen consumption of 673
secretory cells of 663
tubular cells 477*fc*
tubule 684*t*
Killer cells 166
Klinefelter's syndrome 31, 31*f*, 582, 582*f*
Klüver-Bucy syndrome 1133, 1152
Korotkoff's sounds 805
Korsakoff's psychosis 1289
Krause's end-bulb 998, 99*f*
Kulchitsky cells 386
Kupffer cells 558
Kussmaul breathing 959
Kussmaul respiration 713
Kwashiorkor 1293

L

Labia majora 605
Labia minora 605
Labor
first stage of 645*f*
second stage of 646*f*
stages of 645
third stage of 647*f*
Labyrinthine righting reflex 1077, 1101
Lacrimal gland 291*f*, 1166
Lactate dehydrogenase 851
Lactation 469, 620, 651
Lactic acid 1254, 1256, 1258
Lactoferrin 138, 345
Lactogenesis 562, 651
Lactose intolerance 422, 1283
Lactotrophs
hyperplasia of 468
proliferation of 466
Lambert-Eaton myasthenic syndrome 246
Lamina 1005
propria 329
terminalis, organum vasculosum of 476, 1249
Laminar flow 805, 805*t*, 901
Landsteiner's law 119
Langerhans cells 1234
Language 1143
and speech, physiology of 1143
defects 1151
disorders 1146
functions 1148
Lanugo hairs 1235
Laplace law 724, 807, 807*f*, 898
Laron dwarfism 1281
Laryngopharynx 881
Laryngospasm 560
Larynx 881
Lee-White method 208
Lemniscal system 1008
Lens 1168
Leptin 1108
Lethargy 1246
Leucocytes 127
alkaline phosphatase score 134
apoptosis of 133
development of 128*f*
life span of 129*fc*
types of 128*t*
Leucocytosis 133, 643
Leucoerythroblastic reaction 97
Leucopoiesis 129*fc*
duration of 132
regulation of 131
stages of 128
Leukemia 146
acute 146
chronic 147

Leukocytes 132
Leukopoiesis 128
Leukotrienes 448
Lewis factor 1018
Lewis lead 761
Lewis system 122
Lewis-Hunting response 1248
Leydig cell 579, 591*f*, 592, 601*fc*, 627
Libido, inhibition of 469
Liddle's syndrome 693, 1271
Lidocaine 231
Ligandin 374
Limb muscles, proximal 1063
Limbic dysfunctions 1153
  types of 1131
Limbic lobe 1125, 1126*f*
Limbic system 841, 1030, 1125, 1131
  functions of 1129
  role of 1133
Lipid 1283
  bilayer, functions of 15
  digestion 364
    and absorption of 423
  soluble substances 15, 349
  types of 1283
Lipolysis 491
Lipoprotein lipase activity, inhibition of 644
Lipoxides 1298
Lissauer tract 1016
Liver 371, 470, 856, 1293
  cells 371
  cirrhosis of 668
  diseases 74, 625
  fibrosis of 856
  function tests 370, 372, 373*t*
  glycogens 1255
  lobule, structure of 371*f*
  physiology of 370
  role of 205
Lobules 150, 371
Locus ceruleus 308, 1034
  system 1128
Loop of Henle 559, 661, 663, 701
  functions of 689
  role of 701
Low pressure
  collecting system 734
  volume receptors 1274
Lower motor neuron 1045, 1064, 1068
  paralysis 1068
Lower respiratory tract 879, 881
Lown-Ganong-Levine syndrome 774
Lumbar puncture 1156, 1158
Lungs 883, 894
  blood vessels of 668
  capacities 893, 965, 966
  chest wall interaction 897
  collapse 900
  compliance 894, 896
    measurement of 894
  disease
    chronic 910
    obstructive 906
    restrictive 906
  expansion 944
  lobes of 884
  pancoast tumor of 309
  perfusion of 1259
  size 896
  stretching of 900
  tissues 968
  volume 892, 896, 902, 902*f*, 916, 965, 966
Luteinisation, regulation of 611
Luteolysis 572, 611
Lutheran system 123
Lymph node 153, 153, 164, 168*f*
  mesenteric 332
Lymphadenopathy 147, 148, 157
Lymphatic 153
  bulbs 155
  drainage system 156*f*
  nodules 389, 412
  role of 918
  tissue 152, 329
  types of 156
  vessels 152
Lymphoblast 81, 131, 147, 165, 173
Lymphoblastic leukemia, acute 147*f*
Lymphocytes 145, 160
  development of 573
Lymphocytopenia 145, 146*t*
Lymphocytosis 145
  causes of 144
Lymphoid
  follicles 168*f*
  growth curve 1279
  organ 153, 164
  stem cells 80, 128
  tissue 153, 331
    masses of 155
Lymphopoiesis 151
Lymphotoxin 172
Lyse bone matrix 564
Lysolecithin 367
Lysophospholipase 140
Lysosomal
  enzymes 19*t*, 485
  membranes 617
  storage diseases 20, 20*t*
Lysosome 18, 19
  functions of 19
  types of 19, 19*fc*
Lysozyme 138, 345

M

Macrocyte 84
Macrocytosis 84
Macrophages 99, 143, 144, 151, 160, 170
Macula densa 666, 696
  cells of 667
  role of 696
Magnesium, absorption of 564
Malabsorption syndrome 387
Male Sexual Act 630
Mammalian spinal motor neuron 60*t*
Mammary gland 650*f*, 651*f*, 1235
Mammillothalamic tract 1031, 1105
Mannose binding lectin pathway 175
Mantle cell 168
Marasmus 1292, 1293
Marey's law 832
Marrow, white 77
Mass
  peristaltic movement 418
  reflex 1073, 1074
Mast cells 141, 141*t*, 142, 569
  granules 142
  degranulation of 570
Mastocytosis 142
  systemic 142
Matrix 1085
May-Hegglin anomaly 134
McCune-Albright syndrome 444, 629
Meal stimulation test 368
Mean corpuscular hemoglobin 107
  concentration 107
Medulla 150, 151*f*, 1071
Megakaryoblast 81, 185
  formation of 185
Megakaryocytes 185, 195, 195*f*
  proliferation of 186
Megakaryopoiesis 185
Megalocolon 310
Meiosis 594
Meiotic division 608
Meissner's corpuscle 997, 998*f*
Meissner's plexus 333
Melanin, quantity of 1234
Melanocytes 1234, 1234*f*
Melanopsin 1178
Melatonin, synthesis of 567*fc*
Membrane
  carbohydrates 15
  cytoskeleton 187
  enzyme phospholipase C 447
  fluidity of 14
  glycoproteins 187
  lipid, amphipathic nature of 14*f*
  phospholipid-phospholipase system 447, 447*f*
  protein 15

defects 16
deficiency of 189
role of 189, 984
skeleton 86
toxins 231
Memory
B cells 168, 173
deficit 1152
intercortical transfer of 1139
T cells 166, 172
types of 1135
Menarche 585, 614, 621
Mendelian dominant 862
Meniere's disease 1218
Meningitis 1158
Menopause 577, 584, 586, 605, 620, 621
management of 586
Menorrhagia 618, 621
Menstrual bleeding 615, 617, 621
Menstrual cycle 436, 585, 614–616, 618, 619*f*, 627, 650
and ovulation, disorder of 620
duration and phases of 614
duration of 614
Menstrual phase 615
Mental
relaxation 864
retardation 490
Mepyramine 570
Merkel apparatus 998
Merkel cells 998
Merkel disk 998, 998*f*
Merocrine glands 1234
Mesangial cells 665, 665f, 666, 678, 680, 681, 697
contraction of 668, 680
Mesangial matrix 665
Mesangium 664, 665
Mesencephalic locomotion generator 1074, 1078
Mesencephalon 975
Mesenteric ganglion, superior 297
Mesolimbic dopaminergic system 1105
Mesonephric ducts 579
Metabolic theory 842
Metamyelocytes 131, 148
Metencephalon 976
Methemalbumin 101
Methemoglobin 106
Methyl-imidazole-acetic acid 569
Methyl-tetrahydrofolate 95
Metrorrhagia 621
Microcirculation 733, 816
Microcyte 84
Microcytosis 84, 110
Microelectrode 225
Microfilaments, structure of 21*f*
Microglia 978
Microtubules 22, 187
Microvilli 384
Micturition 724
abnormalities of 725
frequency of 309
reflex 308, 308*f*, 724, 1073
control of 725
Midbrain reflexes 1077
Middle ear 1202
cavity 1203*f*
Midline nucleus 1026
Migrating motor complex 396, 407
Milk
ejection reflex 436, 479, 480, 651
production of 642
synthesis 469
Minerals, absorption of 426
Minute ventilation 907, 1257*t*
Miosis 309, 310
Miraculin 1228
Missense mutation 36
Mitochondria 16, 216, 596, 661
structure of 17*f*
Mitochondrial
cytochromes, synthesis of 489
diseases 17
enzymes 17*t*, 1264
matrix 17
membrane 16, 17
Mitosis 594
Mitotic cell divisions 636
Mitral valve 730, 738
Mixed deafness 1217, 1218
Molecules, movement of 45*f*
Moles 48, 66
Monge's disease 949
Monoamine oxidase 992
Monoaminergic pathways 1067
Monoblast 81, 131
Monoclonal antibody, use of 178
Monocyte 143, 160
count 144
structure of 143*f*
Monoiodotyrosine 485
Mononuclear phagocyte 978
system 143, 144, 160, 665
cells of 552
Monoplegia 1068, 1069
Monosodium glutamate 1227
Monosynaptic reflex 1055
Monro-Kellie doctrine 847
Montgomery tubercles 650
Mossy fiber inputs 1091
Motion sickness 1102
Motor
aphasia 1145
cortex 1043, 1061, 1062, 1079
defect 1038, 1151, 1153
fibers 1049
functions 1030
homunculus 1079, 1080
lamina 1005
nerve system 1049
neurons 222, 233, 980, 1045, 1055, 1058, 1068
bombardment of 1072*f*
spinal 1070
nuclei 1029
signals 1041
system 1042*f*
organization of 1040, 1042
segmental organization of 1044
unit 1046, 1058, 1253
recruitment 1046, 1253
role of 1253
size of 272
structure of 272*f*
Mountain sickness
acute 949
chronic 949
Mouth-to-mouth breathing 961
Mouth-to-nose breathing 961
Mucosa 329
associated lymphoid tissue 153, 155
intestinal 385
Mucus membrane, olfactory 1220*f*, 1221
Müllerian duct 581
Müllerian inhibiting substance 581
Müllerian regression
factor 581
substance 592
Multiorgan dysfunctions 211
Multiprotein complex 984
Multiunit smooth muscle 276
Murmurs 786
Muscarinic receptors 291, 304
Muscle 1044, 1048, 1053, 1056, 1255
abdominal 410
antigravity 1056, 1075
atrial 752
atrophy 1064
bundle 249*f*, 250*f*
circular 405, 416, 417
contraction 262, 1052
functional unit of 1253
molecular mechanisms of 259
sliding-filament theory of 258
types of 1253
cramp 274, 492
fatigue 270
fiber 249*f*, 271*t*, 272
organization of 278
type of 1253
flaccidity of 1068
heart reflex 1260
ossicular 1204
pain 1018
proteins 251
relaxation 262

respiratory 1240
size of 1253
spindle 1046, 1048, 1049, 1056
functions of 1050
sensitivity of 1050
structure of 1048, 1049*f*
sprain 274
strength 273
stretch of 1050, 1055
tone 281, 1056, 1057, 1073, 1094
weakness 238, 246
white 272
Muscular dystrophy 253, 273
Muscularis externa 329, 405, 412, 413*f*
Muscularis mucosa 329, 384
contraction of 414
Musculoskeletal system 8, 625
Mutant gene, detection of 35
Mutation 35
theory 1295
Myasthenia gravis 152, 245, 246*f*
Myelencephalon 976
Myelin sheath 217*f*, 241
Myelination 233
Myelinogenesis 217
Myeloblast 81, 130, 131
Myeloblastic leukemia, acute 147
Myelocytes 148
Myeloid
leukemia, chronic 134, 147
stem cells 80, 92, 128, 128*f*
Myeloma cells 178
Myelopathy, anterior 1039
Myeloperoxidase 138
Myenteric plexus, deficiency of 402
Myocardial infarction
acute 769, 851*f*, 1019
anterior 775*f*
Myocarditis 775
Myocardium 737, 737*f*
Myocyte 250
atrial 573
Myoepithelial cells 818
contraction of 479
Myofilaments 278*f*
Myogenic theory 681, 842
Myoglobin 926
Myoglobinuria 717
Myometrium 605, 626, 646
contraction of 645
Myopathies
inflammatory 274
metabolic 274
Myopia 1175
Myosin 251, 1218
filament, structure of 251*f*
head 251
phosphorylation of 280
rotation of 260
heavy chain 490
hinge 251
light-chain
dephosphorylation of 280
kinase 280, 823
phosphatase 280
molecule, structure of 251*f*
polymers of 251
Myotatic reflex 1054, 1056
Myotonia 274

N

N-acetylgalactosamine 117
Naïve B cell 168
Naïve T cells 165
Narcolepsy 1122
Narcotic poisoning 957
Natriuresis 479, 573, 696
Natriuretic peptide, atrial 573, 826, 836
Natural killer cells 160
Nausea 409, 1250
Necrosis
foci of 617
intestinal 855
Neher and Sakmann model 43
Neonatal
autoimmune thrombocytopenia 195
oxygen radical diseases 1298
Neospinothalamic pathway 1016, 1017
Neostigmine 246
Nephrin 665
mutation 665
Nephron
cortical 661, 663
functions of 220, 695*f*
parts of 660, 661*f*
types of 663
functional loss of 680
Nerve 298, 1015
action potentials 1215
deafness 1219
fiber 232, 236, 237, 996
classification of 237, 237*t*
transection of 1003
gases 245
growth factor 221
transfer of 219
injury 238, 239, 247*f*
facial 311
grading of 238
occulomotor 311
lesions, multiple 1037
olfactory 1221
pelvic 417, 418, 723, 724
peripheral 1002
root
lesion 1038
trigeminal 1022
somatic 418, 976
trigeminal 1019
Nervous system 8, 223*fc*, 297, 432, 489, 491, 975, 1221
divisions of 975
functions of 976
parasympathetic 303*f*
peripheral 217, 976
somatic 289*f*
Neural reflexes, types of 333
Neuralgia 1022
trigeminal 1022, 1025
Neurexins, role of 983
Neuroendocrine cells 335
Neurogenic secretory diarrhea 395
Neuroglia 223, 977
types of 223*fc*
Neuroglial cells 566, 567*f*
Neurohumoral reflex 480, 647
Neurohypophysis 457, 460
Neuromuscular
disorders 910
dysfunctions 245
junction, structure of 241, 242
transmission 241, 242, 243*fc*, 246*f*, 550
blockade of 244
Neuron
cholinergic 396, 1129
growth of 220
higher order of 1008
hypothalamic 585
myelination of 489
postganglionic 290, 291, 296, 298
postsynaptic 982, 988
preganglionic 290, 294, 295
presynaptic 982
pseudounipolar 221, 979
retinal 1182, 1183
second order of 1007, 1009
serotonergic 1105, 1114
structure of 215, 215*f*, 978
types of 221, 221*fc*, 979
unipolar 221, 979
Neuropeptide 456, 993, 1109
Neurosis, colonic 419
Neurotransmitter 291, 292, 298, 304, 332, 432, 444
synthesis 489
vesicles 217
migration of 242
Neutrophil 131, 133, 134*f*, 135*f*, 148, 160, 162
count 136, 136*t*
phagocytosis 136
structure of 134*f*
Neutrophilia 643
Neutrophilic myelocytes 131
Neutrophilopoiesis 136

Niacin 1289
functions of 1289
Nicotinic receptors 291, 304, 991
Nifedipine 949
Night blindness 1286, 1287
Night terrors 1123
Nightmares 1123
Nipple
erection of 632
receptors, stimulation of 651
Nissl bodies 979
Nissl granules 216
Nitric oxide 105, 282, 396, 405, 680, 837, 994
Nitrogen
excretion 489
narcosis 954
washout method 969
Nitrous oxide 849
Nocturia 716
Nocturnal
dyspnea, paroxysmal 874
enuresis 1123
hemoglobinuria, paroxysmal 99
paroxysmal dystonia 1123
secretion 1107
Node of Ranvier 217, 218f
Non-isotopic tests 495
Nonsteroidal anti-inflammatory drugs 573
Noradrenaline 298, 299
Noradrenergic system 1128, 1128f
Norepinephrine 282, 292, 313, 991, 1118
inhibits 406
Normoblasts 92
Normochromic normocytic anemia 110
Normocytic cell 84f
Northern blotting 34, 35
Noxious stimulus 1073
Nuclear
chain fibers 1048, 1049
chromatin, fragmentation of 39
Nuclei 293
groups of 1026
hypothalamic 455fc, 475f, 1130
intrinsic 1030
nonspecific 1028, 1031
parasympathetic 293
Nucleoplasm 24
Nucleotide, composition of 30f
Nucleus 23, 979
accumbens 1130
ambiguous 304, 399
decondenses 596
emboliformis 1090
fastigius 1090
functions of 24
gigantocellularis 1066
globosus 1090
gracilis 1009
paragigantocellularis 1020
paraventricular 456, 457
raphe magnus 1020, 1067
reticularis pontis 1066
spinal 1024
structure of 23, 23f
suprachiasmatic 567, 1186
supraoptic 457
tractus solitarius 293, 308, 399, 409, 743, 829, 1225, 1226, 1226f, 1274
Nutrition
disorder of 1292
physiology of 1282
Nystagmus 1199, 1200
postrotatory 1102

O

Obesity 862, 1293, 1294, 1299
Oculomotor nerve 303
Odor 716
Odorant stimulus, type of 1223
Ohm's law 804
Olfaction
mechanics of 1222
physiology of 1222
Oligodendrocytes 217, 977
Oligomenorrhea 621
Oligopeptides 433
Oligosaccharides 117
Oliguria 716
Olivary complex, superior 1208
Olivocerebellar tract 1091
Oncotic pressure 48, 72, 74, 677, 678, 820
Oocyte 579, 608
Oogenesis 597
stages of 608f
Oogonia 579
Opsonins 137
Optic 1172
chiasm, lesion of 1190
disk 1171
nerve 1105
lesion of 1190
tract, lesion of 1190
Oral rehydration therapy 419, 424
Oral sugar tolerance test 422
Organ of Corti 1206, 1206f
Organelles, cytoplasmic 188
Organic molecules, transport of 686
Organogenesis 639
Organs
circumventricular 669, 1160, 1160f
contraction of 156
retroperitoneal 660
visceral 465
Orgasm 633
female 633
male 633
Oropharynx 880
Orthopnea 874
Osmolality, measurement of 719
Osmosis 47, 87, 683
Osmotic fragility test 87
Osmotic pressure 48, 74, 408
gradient 677, 820, 918
measurement of 49
Ossicles, immobility of 1217
Osteoarthritis, treatment of 1265
Osteoblasts 552, 559, 564, 1288
function of 553
Osteoclastic activity, stimulation of 559
Osteoclasts 552–554, 559
Osteocytes 552
Osteoid 490, 551–553
Osteolysis
osteocytic 553, 559, 564
stimulation of 559
Osteomalacia 689
Osteopetrosis 555
Osteoporosis 554, 1265
development of 549
postmenopausal 554
Osteoprogenitor cells 552
Otic ganglion 303, 344
Otoacoustic emissions 1219
Otolith organs 1065, 1066, 1076, 1077, 1098, 1100f
structure of 1099f
Otosclerosis 1217
Ovarian changes 604, 614, 615, 617
Ovarian control 628
Ovarian diseases 620, 621
Ovarian dysgenesis 582
Ovarian follicle 623, 625
development of 608, 609f
Ovarian functions 628f
control of 623, 627
Ovarian hormones 623, 626
Ovarian tumor 583
Ovaries 599
Ovulation 204, 469, 618, 619, 635
Oxidative decarboxylation 1289
Oxidative fibers 272
Oxidative phosphorylation 489, 1289
Oxidative stress 106, 1297
degree of 106
Oxygen 300, 491, 796
arterial content of 789
burst 1299
consumption 789, 1256t
content 927, 928
extraction 928
hemoglobin dissociation curve 924, 924f

saturation 927
measurement of 928
tension 916
therapy 949, 950, 952, 963
transport 922
utilization 491
Oxyhemoglobin 105
formation 923
Oxyntic cells 349
structure of 350
Oxyntic gland 349
Oxyphil granules 557
Oxytocin 479, 567, 611, 646
receptor 480, 645
role of 647

P

Pacemaker 742, 747
cells 742
Pacinian corpuscles 997, 1000*f*, 1010
Paget's disease 562
Pain 367, 828, 846, 1008, 1014, 1016, 1018, 1030
abdominal 359
acute 1015
autoinhibition of 1021
chronic 1015
fibers 834, 1016
gate control theory of 1021
inflammatory 1015, 1022
itch and temperature, physiology of 1014
modulating systems 1020
neuropathic 1015, 1022
pathways 1016
peripheral 1015
recognition 1020
sensation 406
somatic 1015
stimuli 1039
superficial 1015
syndromes 1022
types of 1015
visceral 1015, 1016, 1018, 1019
Paleospinothalamic pathway 1016
Pallanesthesia 1011
Pallidothalamic tract 1030
Pampiniform plexus 589*f*
Pancreas 363*f*
gastrin secreting tumor of 359
Pancreatic
acinus, structure of 363*f*
amylase 364, 421
deficiency 425
duct 362, 363
epithelial cells 365*f*
enzymes
activation of 379
functions of 364*t*
function tests 368
juice, secretion of 337
lipase 364, 379, 423, 424
secretion 328, 341, 362, 363, 365*f*, 366, 366*t*, 1223
functions of 364
regulation of 367*f*
stimulation of 368
tissue 364
Pancreatitis
acute 364, 367
chronic 368
hemorrhagic 367
Paneth cells 339, 385
Pantothenic acid 1290
Papez circuit 1031, 1127*f*
Papilla 660, 1234
Papillary muscle 762
Para-aminohippuric acid 673
Para-aortic splanchnopleura 79
Paracellular pathway 684, 686, 694
Paracrine signals 554
Paradoxical sleep 1119
Parafollicular cells 482, 483*f*, 561
Parageusia 1229
Paralysis 1068, 1069
oculosympathetic 309
patterns of 1068
Paralytic ileus 415
Paranasal sinuses 880
Paraplegia 1069, 1073
Parasites, killing of 140
Parasitic infections 122
Parasthesia 995
Parasympathetic nerve, stimulation of 345
Parasympathetic system 288, 290, 291, 301, 311, 333
stimulation of 436
Parathormone 547, 556, 711
Parathyroid glands 481, 556, 556*f*, 557*f*
Parathyroid hormone 556, 557
secretion 645
Parathyroidectomy 560
Parenchymal tissue 566
Paresis 1068
Paresthesia 1039
Parietal cell, structure of 350*f*, 351*f*
Parietal cortex, posterior 1080
Parietal lobe 1150
posterior 1033, 1080
Parkinson's disease 1085
Parosmia 1223
Parotid duct 343*f*
Parotid gland 343
innervation of 344*f*
Pars intermedia 459
Partial thromboplastin time 208, 209
Parturition reflex 10, 480, 646
Parvocellular neurons 457
Patch clamp technique 42
uses of 43
Patent ductus arteriosus 860
Paul-Bunne method 963
Pavlov pouch 355
Payer's patches 164
Peak expiratory flow rate 904, 967
Pelger-Huet anomaly 134
Pellagra 1290
Pelvis, renal 660
Pendred syndrome 485
Penicillamine 1228
Penile erection 631*fc*
Penis
blood supply of 631*f*
dorsal artery of 630
muscles of 631*f*
swelling and stiffening of 1073
transverse section of 631
Pentagastrin test 353, 357
Pepsinogen 323, 348
Peptic cells 349, 350
Peptic ulcer 358, 359*f*
Peptidases 423
Peptide 433, 444
fragments 171
hormone 441
synthesis 433, 434, 434*fc*
Pericardial fluid 737
Pericardium 736
layers of 737*f*
Pericytes 733, 818
Periglomerular cells 1221
Perineurium 222
Perinuclear cisterns 23
Peripheral nerves, basic structure of 222
Peristalsis 396, 407, 413
Peristaltic wave 399, 406, 415, 819
frequency of 406
Peritubular capillaries 663, 671, 672, 697
role of 687
Peroxisome 20
diseases of 20
Pertussis toxins 447
Petenkoffer's test 717
Petit mal epilepsy 1122
Peyer's patches 328, 331, 332
Phagocyte system, mononuclear 161*f*
Phagocytic cells 160, 332
Phagocytosis 38, 55, 143, 155, 160, 161, 173, 174, 190, 591, 1169, 1299
Phagolysosome 138
formation 138*f*
Phagosome 170
Phantom limb 1000
Pharynx 880
Phenolsulphthalein test 719
Phenomenon 1071, 1095

Phenyldiguanide 835
Pheromone 1221
Phillipson's reflex 1058
Phlebotomy 115
Phosphatases 445, 554
Phosphate 125, 559, 686, 713, 716
- absorption of 550, 564
- buffer 712
- buffer system 1267
- deficiency 549
- metabolism 547, 549
- reabsorption 564
- timer 445

Phosphatidylinositol 448
Phosphaturia 559
Phosphocreatine 1255
Phosphodiesterase 446f
Phospholipase 364
- activation of 448
- C 447, 557
  - pathway 464

Phosphoproteins, monomeric 449
Phosphorus 1291
- functions of 549
- metabolism 549f
- radio-isotopes of 65

Phosphorylase kinase 450
Phosphorylation 463, 477
- role of 445

Phototransduction, steps of 1180f
Phrenic nerve 936
Pigment epithelium 1169
Piloerection 1247
Piloerector muscles, activation of 300
Pineal gland 566
- functions of 568
- hormone of 566
- role of 1120

Pinealocytes 566
Pinna 1202
- role of 1215

Pinocytosis 55
Piriform cortex 1221
Pitch 1211
Pituitary
- disorders 620
- functions, posterior 1106
- gland 459
  - tumor of 492
- hormones, posterior 456
- hypothyroidism 494
- regulating hormones, anterior 454
- secretions 644
- target organ axis, hypothalamic 461fc
- tumor 466, 470

Placenta 599, 626, 638
- fetal part of 638
- formation 638, 638f
- syncytiotrophoblast of 642

Placental circulation 638
Planum temporale 1210
Plasma 63, 71, 73, 806, 928
- calcium 556, 557, 1250
- cell 145, 153, 168, 173
  - proliferation of 173
- cholesterol estimation 496
- composition of 73, 73t
- concentration 466, 685
- constituent of 73f
- estrogen 468
- flow, renal 718
- glucose 1109
- haptoglobin indicates hemolysis 101
- membrane 635
- osmolality 48, 476, 719, 1273
  - regulation of 660
- phosphate 466, 556, 557
  - concentration 549
  - level 562
- protein 71, 74, 75, 806
  - buffer system 1267
  - functions of 74
  - synthesis 868
  - types of 74
- recalcification time 208, 209
- skimming, phenomenon of 806f
- transfusion 870
- ultrafiltration of 676
- viscosity 89
- volume 65
  - determination of 73
  - measurement of 65

Plasmapheresis 73, 246
Plasmin 203
- activation of 203, 203f, 211
- functions of 203
- generation defects 204
- inhibitors 204

Plasminogen 204
- activator 203f, 204, 612
  - inhibitors 204
  - synthesis of 619
- deficiency 204

Plasticity, cortical 1147, 1153
Platelet 183, 185, 189
- activating factor 192, 437
- adhesion 191
- adhesiveness test 194, 208
- aggregation test 194, 208
- cellular constituents of 188f
- count 190t, 194
- deficiency 202
- formation of 185
- function of 202
- granules 188, 189t
- phospholipid 200f, 201, 205
- role of 205
- ultrastructure of 187f

Plexus of Auerbach 329
Plexus of Meissner 329
Pneumothorax
- causes of 890
- development of 890f

Poikilocytes 84
Poikilothermic animals 1237
Poiseuille-Hagen formula 805
Poliomyelitis 274, 1159
Polkissen cells 666
Polycythemia 109, 114, 115t
- types of 114, 115t
- vera 105, 114, 115

Polydipsia 478
Polymenorrhea 621
Polymerase chain reaction 34
Polypeptide 252, 335, 433, 460, 990
- hormone 626

Polyribosomes 92
- high concentration of 92

Polysynaptic spinal reflex 1057
Polythelia 652
Polyuria 478, 716, 719
Pontine reticulospinal tract 1066
Pontocerebellar tract 1091
Portal hypophyseal vessels 457
Post-conceptional pills 655
Postural hypotension
- acute 865
- chronic 865

Posture, regulation of 1056, 1062, 1066
Potassium 855
- absorption of 424
- channels, closure of 755
- ions 755
- salts 1227

Precursor cells 92, 559
Pregnancy 205, 282, 469, 486, 620, 634, 643, 650, 680, 788, 826
- diagnostic test 641
- ectopic 638
- induced hypertension 645, 862
- physiology of 634
- third week of 642
- toxemia of 645

Premature beats, atrial 771
Premenstrual syndrome 621
Premotor cortex 1062, 1079, 1080
Pre-ovulatory follicle 610
Presbyopia 1176
Pressure 238, 476, 1030
- aortic 780
- atrial 780
- gradient 46, 676
- overload 872
- sensation 997
- venous 814

Prickle cells 1234
Primordial follicular stage 608, 611

Procaine 231
Proerythroblast 81, 92
Progenitor cells 80, 80*f*, 91, 92, 94, 129, 1220
Progesterone 618, 625, 628, 642, 650
  influence of 619
  secretion 611
Prolactin 460, 468, 473, 644, 651
  action of 651
  episodic burst of 651
  inhibiting hormone 456
  secretion 466, 469, 571, 651
Promegakaryocytes 185
Promonocytes 131
Pronormoblast 92
Propranolol 493
Prosopagnosia 1152
Prostacyclin 193, 448, 572
Prostaglandin 162, 448, 572, 611, 617, 618, 646, 665, 681, 1119
  production of 617
  synthesis 572*fc*
Prostate 600
  benign hypertrophy of 600
  cancer 598, 1284
    theories of 627
  gland 594, 626
  hypertrophy 600
Protein 15, 96, 251, 252, 364, 408, 433, 434, 445, 716, 717, 899, 1241, 1285
  absorption of 423
  anabolic effect 465, 625
  binding 486
  buffers 75, 713
  C 199, 207
    activation of 199, 203, 203*f*
  channels, types of 40
  contractile 251
  creatinine ratio 717
  digestion 353, 364, 367, 409, 423
    and absorption of 422
    defects of 423
  energy malnutrition 1292
  functions of 1285
  glycation of 106
  integral 15, 16, 86
  intrinsic 15
  kinase 336, 445, 446, 477
    C activity 448
  metabolism 465, 491
  molecules, cross-linking of 39
  myeloma 717
  odorant-binding 1222
  peripheral 15, 16
  reabsorption 688
  rich food 1241
  structure of 1285
  synthesis 51, 465, 469, 565, 688, 795, 987
    steps of 33, 33*f*
  transmembrane 15, 15*f*
  transporter 423
Proteinuria 688, 717
Prothrombin 208
  activation 200
  consumption test 208
  time 208
Proton pump 711
  blocker 360, 402
  migrate 554
Pseudobipolar neurons 1024
Pseudohermaphrodite 583
Pseudohermaphroditism
  female 583
  male 583
Pseudohypoaldosteronism 693
Pseudohypoparathyroidism 444, 560
Pseudounipolar sensory neurons 1002
Psychic stimuli 1257
Pteroyl glutamic acid 1290
Pterygoids 398
Pterygopalatine ganglion 291*f*, 303
Ptosis 246, 309, 310
Pubarche 585
Puberty 462, 557, 577, 584, 620, 628, 650
  abnormalities of 586
  onset of 568, 584, 585
  precocious 568, 586, 627, 629, 1111
  stages of 585
Pubic hair 585, 625
  growth of 627
Pubic symphysis 626
Puborectalis muscle 418, 419
Pulmonary function tests 965
Pulp, white 154
Pulse
  deficit 799
  oximetry 928
  pressure 491, 643, 824, 832*f*, 1262
    method 790
  rate 799
Pulsus alternans 801
Pulsus bisferiens 800
Pulsus paradoxus 800
Punctate basophilia 86, 96
Pupil
  constriction of 1174
  dilatation of 409
  size of 1174
Purines 991, 993
Purkinje cell
  activity 1093
  layer 1090
  responses 1093*f*
Purkinje fibers 743
Pyelography, intravenous 720
Pyloric sphincter 405, 409, 410
  constriction of 405
Pyloric stenosis, hypertrophic 409
Pyogenic infections, acute 133
Pyramidal cells 222, 343, 980
Pyramidal tracts 1061
Pyrexia 1248
Pyridostigmine 246
Pyridoxine 1290
  deficiency 1290
Pyrimidines 993
Pyrogens 1249

Q

Quadriplegia 1069
Queckenstedt test 1159
Quinine 1227
Quinones 1287

R

Radford's formula 908
Radiation 786, 1241
Radioimmunoassay 439
Radioiodine 493
Radionuclide methods 849
Rahn-Otus method 970
Rapamycin 178
Raphe nucleus 1034
Raphespinal serotonergic pathway 1020
Raphespinal tract 1067
Ratchet theory 259
Rathke's pouch 457, 460
Raynaud disease 310
Receptor cell, olfactory 1221, 1221*f*
Rectum, physiology of 391
Red blood cell 83
  destruction of 99
  indices 107
Red cell 97
  abnormal 84, 85*f*
  biconcavity of 84
  breakdown 374
  composition 84
  count 84
  dimensions 83
  distribution width 107
  fall 88
  fragility 87
  functions of 87
  indices 88
  life span of 84
  macrocytic 84*f*
  macrocytosis of 110
  mass 72, 88, 643
  membrane 86
    structure of 16

metabolism of 86
production 110
structure of 83*f*
volume 63, 64, 73
Reflex 334, 1071, 1077, 1136, 1137
activities 397
arc 289, 479, 1055, 1056
Bainbridge 835
baroreceptor 829
bradycardia 833
chemoreceptor 833
circuit 1056, 1057
colonic 417
control 333, 798, 840
deglutition 398, 399
gastrointestinal 308
Hering-Breuer 943
hierarchy of 307
intestinal 342, 414
intestinointestinal 415
medullary 1075
movements 1073
pathway 399, 1076
peripheral 318
phenomenon 418
postural 1071, 1101
regulation 306
respiratory 943
responses 841, 1073, 1244
secretion 347
somatosympathetic 834, 834*f*
spinal 419, 632, 1054*f*, 1059, 1072
static postural 1075
vascular 842
Refractive index 1172
Refsum disease, infantile 20
Reissner's membrane 1212
Renal failure 715
acute 125, 720
causes of 720*t*
chronic 720
Renin 573, 667
angiotensin
aldosterone axis 668
mechanism 318
system 667, 668*fc*, 674, 868
secretion 674
regulation of 667
Renshaw cell 988, 989*f*, 1059
inhibition 988, 1059
Replacement therapy, renal 720
Reproductive organs 605*f*, 615, 616*f*, 626
Reproductive system 8, 492, 572
female 604, 624
male 588
Respiration 398, 399, 626, 797, 902, 942, 1257
artificial 961
hormonal control of 942

muscles of 887
regulation of 931
Respiratory
distress syndrome 900
dysfunction 971
failure 957, 958
system 8, 153, 491, 571, 572, 643, 709, 877, 879, 880*f*, 895*f*, 912*t*, 952
functions of 884
Rete testis 593
Reticular formation, functions of 1112
Reticulocyte 93, 96, 97
count 97
index 97
response 97
Reticulocytopenia 97
Reticulocytosis 97
Reticuloendothelial system 143
Reticulospinal tract 1043, 1045, 1062, 1066, 1067*f*, 1076
medullary 1066
Retina 1169
layers of 1170*f*
Retinohypothalamic fibers 1105
Retinoic acid 1286
Retinol 1286
Retrograde
degeneration 239
ejaculation 632
transport 219
Retrovirus 180
Rheumatic heart disease 179
Rhombencephalon 976
Rhythm method 655
Riboflavin 1289
function of 1289
Rickets 689
Rigor mortis 261, 271
Rinne's test 1218
Romberg sign 1012, 1038
Rothera's test 717
Rouget cells 818
Rouleaux formation 75, 88*f*
Rubrospinal tract 1062, 1065, 1065*f*, 1067*f*
Ruffini ending 998, 999*f*
Russell viper 211
Ryanodine receptors 255, 256

S

Saccades 1199
Safe period method 655
Saliva 159, 345
composition of 345
production 303
tonicity of 345
Salivary blood flow 345

Salivary gland 328, 343, 343*f*
innervation of 344
Salivary nucleus 293, 344, 346
superior 344
Salivary secretion 300, 341, 342, 345, 346*f*, 347, 398
control of 346
rate of 345
study of 342
Salt
appetite 1276
restriction of 863
sensitivity 862
wasting
cerebral 479
pulmonary 479
water drowning 918
Sarcolemma 243
Sarcomere 253, 269
structure of 253*f*
Sarcoplasmic reticulum 255, 255*f*, 277, 282, 741
role of 256*fc*
Sarcotubular system 254, 255*f*, 740, 740*f*
structure of 256*f*
Saturation
degree of 1283, 1284
kinetics 44, 46
Saw tooth appearance 771
Scala tympani 1206
Scala vestibule 1205
Scavenger cells 978
Schilling test 369
Schistocytes 85
Schizophrenia 1132
Schlesinger's test 717
Schwabach's test 1219
Schwann cell 217, 218*f*, 219*f*
role of 217
Sciatic nerve 335
Sclera 375*f*, 1166
Sclerosis, multiple 238
Sclerotomes 1004
Scrotum 600
cremaster muscle of 589*f*
Scuba 955
Scurvy 1288
Sebaceous glands 1234, 1235
Secrete testosterone 592
Secretin 354, 355, 367
inhibits gastric secretion 354
secretion, regulation of 337*fc*
stimulation test 368
Sella turcica 459
Semen analysis 597
Semicircular canal 1065, 1099
ampulla of 1100*f*
Semilunar valve 730, 738
aortic 738
pulmonary 738

Seminal vesicle 594, 632
Seminiferous tubule 590, 590*f*
  dysgenesis 582
Sensation 977, 995
  cortical 1011, 1034, 1039
  dimensions of 996
  subcortical perception of 1030
  types of 995, 996
Sense organ 996
Sensitization 989, 1060, 1135, 1137
Sensorineural deafness 1217
Sensory 1049
  abnormalities 1037
  aphasia 1145
  cortex 1033
  cortical areas 1033
  deficit 1038, 1151
  feedback 1070
  fibers 406, 1049
    numerical classification of 238*t*
  function tests 1039
  ganglia 1038
  homunculus 1034, 1035*f*
  laminae 1005
  loss 1037–1039
  modulation 996
  motor coordination 1006, 1031, 1043, 1067, 1068
  nerve conduction 1039
  neurons 222, 846, 977, 980
  organs 1236
  paroxysms 1123
  pathways 977, 1051
  system 1039
  unit 1001
    recruitment of 1001
Septal defect, atrial 860
Septic abortions 211
Serotonin 192, 396, 410, 570, 993, 1118
  receptors 570
  uptake inhibitor 621
Serous cells 343, 343*f*
Serpentine receptors 443
Sertoli cells 578, 581, 588, 590, 590*f*, 591*f*, 593*f*, 597, 602
  endocrine functions of 592
  functions of 591
  structure of 590
Serum gastrin level 357
Sex chromatin, demonstration of 578
Sex determination 134, 577, 578
  abnormalities of 581
Sexually transmitted diseases 653
Sheehan's syndrome 620
Shock 673, 855, 866, 869, 1072
  anaphylactic 179, 869
  cardiogenic 866, 869
  endotoxic 869
  hemorrhagic 847, 867
  hypovolemic 681, 866–868
  neurogenic 869, 918
  obstructive 866, 869
  pathophysiology of 866
  refractory 868
  septic 869
  spinal 726, 1072
  stage of 1072
  traumatic 868
  treatment of 869
  types of 869
Sialic acid 470
Sialolithiasis 347
Sialoproteins 677
Sialorrhea 347
Sick sinus syndrome 771
Sickle cell anemia 112, 114*f*
  pathogenesis of 113*f*
Sickle red cells 85
Signal transduction, steps of 445, 449
Simmond's syndrome 620
Single breath nitrogen technique 908, 909*f*
Singlet oxygen 138
Sinus
  arrhythmia 317, 322, 771, 797
    respiratory 771
  bradycardia 771
  hair follicle 999
  medullary 153
  tachycardia 771
Sinusitis 880
Sinusoid 370, 371
Sinusoidal capillaries 460
  structure of 817*f*
Skeletal muscle 245, 249, 259, 260, 263, 266, 268*f*, 270, 271, 401, 465, 489, 492, 740*f*, 1014, 1045, 1239, 1246, 1252, 1266
  basal tone of 1240
  blood flow 1260
  circulation 857
  contraction 258, 262, 262*fc*
  fiber 263
  pump 791, 791*f*, 814, 867, 1260
  relaxation 263*fc*
  structure of 249, 249*f*
Skin 159, 1014, 1233
  acidic pH of 160
  appendages 1235
  blood supply 1235
  changes 601
  color 568, 1234
  functions of 1236
  hyperpigmentation of 472
  layers of 1233
  lesions 420
  structure of 1233
  test 179
Sleep
  apnea
    obstructive 1123
    syndrome 945, 959
  cycles 1117
  disorders 1122
  disturbances 1122
  paralysis 1123
  potentiates growth 1117
  spindles 1117
  stages of 1117*f*
  theories of 1120
  wake cycle 436, 1120
Slow pain 1002, 1003, 1015, 1017
Smell, physiology of 1220
Smooth muscles 156, 247*f*, 249, 260, 276, 277*f*, 278, 278*f*, 281, 281*t*, 304, 329, 393, 401, 413, 570, 732, 818, 1073
  cells, vascular 666
  function 1073
  hypertrophy 282
  tone, bronchial 902
  types of 276
  vascular 823, 837, 842, 864
Snake bite 211
Sneezing 944, 1223
Snellen's chart 1189
Sodium
  absorption of 424
  bicarbonate 963
  channels 41
    closure of 754
  citrate 206
  depletion 1246
  dihydrogen phosphate 1267
  enters enterocytes 424
  fluoride 205
  influx of 228, 235
  ions
    influx of 228
    massive influx of 229
  potassium pump 43
Soft tissue hematomas 209
Soluble fibrinogen, proteolysis of 201
Somatic cell therapy 37
Somatic mutation theory 1296
Somatic system 289, 290
Somatomedin-C 1279
Somatostatin 339, 353, 436, 456
  secretion 359
Somatotrophs, tumor of 466
Sound
  frequency of 1211
  waves 1211, 1212
Space of Disse 371
Space of Mall 371
Spastic neurogenic bladder 726, 1073
Spasticity 1064

Special sense organs 995
Speech 884, 1096
audiometry 1219
production, theories of 1144
Spermatic cord, smooth muscle of 478
Spermatids 594
growth of 591
Spermatocytes 594
Spermatocytogenesis 594
Spermatogenesis 492, 582, 588, 593, 594, 597, 601
duration of 596
stages of 595f
steps of 594, 595f
Spermatogonia 594
Spermatozoa 594, 633
structure of 596
Spermiogenesis 594, 595, 597, 601
Sperms
abnormal 598f
ejaculation of 585
head, membrane of 636
motility 626
penetration of 636
production 603
transport of 634, 635
Spherical aberration 1174
Spherocytosis, hereditary 84, 112
Sphincter 397, 401, 723
gastrointestinal 332
of Oddi 332, 337, 362, 363, 378
role of 397
urethrae 723, 723f
vesicae 723, 1073
Spinal artery syndrome, anterior 1038
Spinal cord 296f, 630, 724, 955, 976, 993, 1002, 1002f, 1004, 1005f, 1007, 1009, 1016f, 1018f, 1038, 1062f, 1071
cardiovascular axis, medullary 828
central canal of 978
degeneration of 1011
dorsal horn of 1009
function of 976
hemisection of 1038
laminae 1005, 1005f
lesions 1038
pattern 1078
sacral segment of 418
segment 1002
transection 725, 840
tumor 1159
Spines, dendritic 216
Spinocerebellum 1089, 1092
Spinohypothalamic fiber system 1017
Spinothalamic fibers 1038
Spinothalamic tract 479, 1008, 1009, 1010, 1019, 1023
anterior 1008, 1009, 1010
fibers of 1012
Spironolactone 864
Splanchnic nerves, pelvic 307f
Spleen 154, 186
functions of 155
Splenic blood flow, regulation of 857
Splenic circulation 154f, 856, 857
Squamous epithelium 1233
Squamous mesothelial cells 331
Stannius ligatures 747, 747f
Starch, splitting of 345
Starling's curve 791f, 792f
Starling's forces 676, 696, 819
Steatorrhea 368, 376, 382, 388, 423
Stein-Leventhal syndrome 620
Stellate
cells 222, 980
ganglion 296
Stem cell 80, 80f, 91, 92, 185
multilineage 80
hemopoietic 76
Stensen's duct 342
Stercobilinogen 374, 376
Stereocilia 1213
Stereognosis 1011, 1035
Sterilization
female 656
male 656
Sternocleidomastoids 888
Steroid 433, 1022
hormone 563, 611, 617, 1284
synthesis 434
transport of 437
receptor, structure of 449f
Steroidogenesis 588, 593, 640
cells of 592
Steroids, rapid actions of 451
Stimulation
duration of 1228
parasympathetic 344–346, 346fc, 396, 413
test 356
Stimuli
external 37
types of 227
Stimulus
quality of 1059
strength of 1001
Stokes-Adams syndrome 773f
Stomach 328, 414
acidic
pH of 160
secretion of 328
distension of 354
functional anatomy of 348
innervation of 405
interior of 349f
mucous membrane of 349
nerve supply of 350
oxyntic cells of 96
parts of 404
receptive relaxation of 407f
wall, structure of 405
Stomatocyte 86
Stratum
basale 1234
corneum 1233
germinativum 1233, 1234
granulosum 1233, 1234
lucidum 1233, 1234
spinosum 1233, 1234
Streptokinase 851
Streptomycin 1217
Stress 472, 862
acute 1252
chronic 359
dysfunctions 1286
induced analgesia 1022
proteins 449
relaxation 281, 835
ulcer 359
Stretch reflex 1054–1056, 1058t, 1071, 1094
atrial 771, 829, 834, 834fc
cardiopulmonary 834
pulmonary 835
types of 1055
Striatum, subdivisions of 1085
Stroke 191, 1284
ischemic 847
treatment of 848
types of 847
volume 490, 643, 787, 790, 801
Stroma 153, 154, 1166, 1167
Strychnine 1227
Stuart-Prower factor, activation of 200
Submandibular and sublingual glands, innervation of 344f
Substantia gelatinosa 1005
Substantia nigra 1032
Substantia propria 1166
Succinylcholine 245
Succus entericus 384
Sucrase-isomaltase deficiency 422
Sudden cardiac death 324
Sulphosalicylic acid test 717
Superficial reflexes, loss of 1065
Superoxide anion 138, 1297
Suppressor T cells 166
Supraventricular tachycardia, paroxysmal 771
Supravital stain 93, 96
Surgery, abdominal 415
Swan-Ganz catheter 970
Sweat glands 300, 1234, 1235, 1248
Sweating 1242, 1246, 1247
Swelling 162
Sylvester-Brosche method 963

Sylvian fissure
 superior wall of 1035
 wall of 1033
Sympathetic system, stimulation of 436
Synapses 981
Synaptic transmission 981
Syncytiotrophoblast cells 641
Syncytium, atrial 740
Synthesis and secretion, regulation of 899
Syringomyelic syndrome 1038
Systemic allergy, acute 570

T

T cell 165, 170, 171
 activation of 172
 development of 165, 573
 receptor 165, 167, 170*f*
 types of 165
Tabetic syndrome 1038
Tachycardia 309, 409, 491, 768, 778, 799, 833, 834, 867, 1250
 anticipatory 1260
 atrial 771
 causes of 799
Tachykinins 444
Tactile agnosia 1011
Tamm-Horsfall protein 688
Tank and valve system 955
Tanner's method 585
Target cells 82*t*, 85
Taste
 buds 1224
  number of 1228
  structure of 1225*f*
 hallucination of 1229
 pathway 1225, 1226*f*
 physiology of 1224
 pore 1225
 salivary reflex 1229
 sensation 1229
 type of 1225
Taurocholic acid 379
Tear 159
 drop 85
Tectocerebellar tract 1091
Tectospinal pathways 1076
Tectospinal tract 1062, 1067
Tegmental system 1128
Telencephalon 975
Temporal lobe 1151
 epilepsy 1229
Temporary hemostasis 183, 189, 190
Temporary hemostatic plug 184, 190, 208
 formation 184
Tendon reflexes 1055
Tenia coli 416
Tension 273
 isometric 264
Testes 582, 588, 589
 descent of 601
 functions of 593
 Leydig cells of 599
 Sertoli cells of 602
 undescended 603
Testicular feminization syndrome 582
Testosterone 599, 600*f*
 synthesis, steps of 599*f*
Tetanus toxin 984
Tetrahydrofolate 1290
Tetralogy of Fallot 860
Tetrapyrrole rings 103
Tetrodotoxin 231
Thalamic nuclei 1018, 1026, 1027, 1029
 posterior 1022
Thalamic syndrome 1022, 1031, 1039
Thalamocortical loop 1031
 role of 1121
Thalamostriate projection 1083
Thalamus 454, 1026, 1026*f*, 1028*f*, 1043, 1222
 dorsal nucleus of 1029*f*
 functions of 1030
 intralaminar nuclei of 1029*f*
 midline nuclei of 1029*f*
 nuclei of 1027
 pulvinar of 1029*f*
 ventral nuclei of 1030*f*
Thalassemia 110, 113
Theca
 cells 579, 627
 externa cell 609
 interna cells 609, 623
 lutein cells 611
Thelarche 585
Thermal sensors 1243
Thermodilution method 790
Thermogenesis, nonshivering 1241, 1246
Thermogenic cutaneous vasodilation 490
Thermogenin, production of 491
Thermoreceptors 997, 1243
Thermoregulatory sweat test 315
Thermostat, sensitivity of 1239
Theta rhythm 1116
Thiamine 1288
 deficiency 1289
 functions of 1289
Thiazide diuretics 691, 708, 864
Thiol protease inhibitor 199
Thionamides 493
Thoracic
 cavity 889
 duct 152*f*
 ganglia 296
 pump 791
 wall compliance, measurement of 897
Thoracoabdominal breathing 892
Thoracolumbar outflow 288*f*, 293, 295
Thrombasthenia 194
Thrombin 189, 191, 202
 functions of 201
 inhibitor of 207
 time 208, 209
Thrombocytes 71
Thrombocytopenia 147, 190, 195
 gestational 195
Thrombocytosis 190
Thromboembolism 212
 pulmonary 970
Thrombohydroperoxides 1299
Thrombolysis 189, 190, 193
Thrombomodulin 193, 199
Thrombophlebitis 126
Thrombopoiesis
 regulation of 186
 stages of 185*fc*, 186*f*
Thrombopoietin 186
Thrombosis 211, 1299
Thromboxane 448
Thrombus, consolidation of 193, 202
Thymectomy 151, 246
Thymine 30*f*
Thymocytes 151
Thymopoietin 152
Thymosin 152, 573
Thymus 150, 152
 functions of 151
 lymphocytes of 151
 removal of 152
Thyroglobulin
 molecule, proteolysis of 485
 proteolysis of 483
Thyroid
 antibodies, detection of 496
 dwarf 1279, 1281
 dysfunctions 496*f*
 ectopic 481
 follicles 482
  appearance of 483*f*
 follicular cells, structure of 483*f*
 function tests 495, 496*f*
 gland 470, 481, 482*f*, 644
  growth of 471
 hormone 471, 482, 484*f*, 486, 490*fc*, 492*t*, 565, 667, 795
  decreases, free level of 486
  gene deficiency 462
  measurement of 495
  metabolism of 485
  replacement 495
  resistance 494

secretion of 483, 485, 486
synthesis 471, 483
peroxidase 484, 485
secretion 644
stimulating hormone 455, 460, 470
storm 494
Thyroiditis, autoimmune 495
Thyrotoxic myopathy 492
Thyrotoxicosis 493
Thyrotropin releasing hormone 455
Thyroxine 94, 334, 380, 409, 485, 793, 900, 1246, 1279
binding globulin 486
binding prealbumin 486
metabolism of 487*fc*
secretion 1246
Tic douloureux 1022
Tidal volume 643, 892, 966
Tissue 177, 490
fluid 156
hypoxia 107
insulation 1248
kallikrein 836
macrophages 133, 144
plasminogen activator 204
pressure theory 842
repair 163
thromboplastin 200*f*, 201, 210
Tongue 1228
floor of 481
Tonic
contraction 281, 404
discharge 827, 828
labyrinthine reflexes 1072, 1075, 1076, 1101
neck reflexes 1072, 1075, 1076
stretch reflex 1055, 1072
Tonsils 164
Toothache 1022
Total leucocyte count 148
Total lung capacity 893, 966
Toxic adenoma 493
Toxins, transport of 219
Trabeculae 153, 154
Trabecular bone 551, 559
Transairway pressure 891
Transcellular
fluid 64
osmotic gradient 686, 706
pathway 684, 684
Transcytosis 56, 818, 819
Trauma 211, 1218
Traumatic peripheral nerve injury 1022
Trephine biopsy 78
Tricuspid valve 730, 738
ring, bulging of 783
Triiodothyronine 485
Trilineage stem cells 128
Trisodium citrate 205
Tritium oxide 65
Trophoblast 637
cells 637
rapid proliferation of 637
Tropical sprue 424
Tropomyosin 252
Troponin 252, 252*t*, 451
protein complex 278
Trousseau's sign 560
Truncal vagotomy 360
Trypsin
activation of 367
inhibitor 364
Tryptophan 570
T-snare protein 984
Tubal ligation 656
Tubercle, olfactory 1222
Tuberculosis 179
Tuberoinfundibular system 1127
Tuberoinfundibular tract 1105
Tubular cells 688
proximal 712
Tubular epithelial cells 678, 717
Tubular fluid 666, 667
formation of 591
hypotonic 694
osmolality of 707
osmotic pressure 677
Tubular function 682, 683, 685, 694
proximal 685
tests 715, 718
Tubular glands 1234
Tubular hydrostatic pressure 678
Tubular reabsorption, proximal 689
Tubule
parts of 686
proximal 661, 686, 687*f*, 694, 706, 711
renal 712*f*
Tubulovesicular system 350
Tubulus rectus 589
Tumor
hypothalamic 466, 470
necrosis factor 131, 180
somatotroph 444
Tunica albuginea 589
Tunica externa 731
Tunica intima 731
Tunica media 731
Tuning fork tests 1218
Turbulent flow 805, 805*t*, 901
Turner's syndrome 31, 31*f*, 582, 582*f*
Twins, development of 636
Tympanic membrane 1203, 1217
Tyrosine kinase
cytoplasmic 468
system 450*f*

U

Ulcerative colitis 420
Ulcers
perforation of 359
trophic 1037
Umbilical cord 646
blood 78
Upper motor neuron 1045
paralysis 1057
Upper respiratory tract 879
Urease test 358
Ureter, peristaltic movements of 722
Urethral sphincters 723
Uric acid 718
Urinary
bladder 277, 722
functions of 723
buffers 710
system 8, 660*f*
tract 1074
infection 709
urobilinogen 376
Urine 160
acidification of 692, 694, 709, 1268
rate 710
alkalization of 709
concentration 661, 694, 702*f*
production 716
storage of 723
volume 715
determination of 719
Urobilinogen 101, 374, 717
Urochrome 716, 717
Urogenital sinus 601
Uterine
blood flow 624
cervix 615
dilation of 626
contraction 626, 646
endometrium, proliferation of 624
fluid 572
secretion 624
muscle 624
myometrial contractions 626
pathology 620
relaxation 642
size 624
smooth muscles 626
stretch of 282
Uterus 277, 605, 624, 626, 635
body of 605

V

Vagal
activity, inspiratory inhibition of 318
cholinergic fibers 352
control 322

fibers 363, 401, 405
inhibits, stimulation of 840
cholinergic 437
noncholinergic 437
stimulation 322, 357, 386, 756
facilitates 350
noncholinergic 339
promotes 409
tone 316, 318, 744, 840
function of 743, 744
Vagina 605
acidic pH of 160
Vaginal
contraction 633
discharge 619
epithelium proliferates 617
needle aspiration 640
sponge 653
wall, rhythmic contraction of 633
Vagosympathetic trunk 304
Vagotomy 318, 354, 357, 360, 409, 835
types of 360*f*
Vagovagal reflex 355, 367, 407
Vagus nerve 331, 335, 341, 353*f*, 354, 366, 399, 401, 407, 415, 417, 798, 830, 831, 1018
inhibits 798
role of 934, 1108
Vagus, dorsal motor nucleus of 293, 304
Valsalva maneuver 313, 314
Valsalva muscle 314
Valve
closure, aortic 785
pulmonary 730, 785
venous 734, 814
Valvular flap 722
Van Den Bergh test 376
Van Slyke gasometric method 970
Vas deferens 593
smooth muscle of 632
wall of 593
Vasa recta 663, 672, 700, 701
functions of 672
role of 703
Vascular endothelium, role of 205
Vascular resistance
peripheral 322
pulmonary 859, 860, 915, 916
Vascular system, divisions of 733
Vasectomy 599
Vasoconstrictor
fibers 852, 856, 857
system 827, 827*f*, 857
Vasodilation 793, 834, 836, 846
metabolic 1261
renal 644, 680
Vasodilator system 827, 827*f*, 857, 1261
Vasopressin 282, 475, 479
antagonists 708
secretion of 867
Veins 734, 813
functions of 813
varicose 814, 858
wall of 813
Vena cava 813
Venous pressure, peripheral 814
Ventilation 907, 910, 942*fc*, 966, 967, 1241
artificial 961
perfusion ratio 914, 918, 1258, 1259
pulmonary 1259
rate of 713
stage 879
Ventilatory functions, measurement of 967
Ventral
corticospinal tract 1062, 1063
posteromedial
nucleus 1225
thalamic nucleus 1226, 1226*f*
spinocerebellar tract 1091
Ventricles, distention of 792
Ventricular
depolarization 762, 764
diastole 778, 781
ejection 779
fibrillation 772
function curve 792*f*
hypertrophy 775, 807
muscle
fiber 754*f*
mass 792
myocytes 740
repolarization 762, 766
rhythm 747
septal defect 800
stretch reflex 834
syncytium 740
tachycardia, paroxysmal 772
Ventrobasal complex 1028
Venules 734, 813
Vertebral puncture 78
Vertebrobasilar system 845
Vertigo 1102, 1250
Vesicles 983
fusion of 170
transport of 477
Vesicular transport proteins, role of 53
Vessel
diameter 793, 803
prevents distension of 732
pulmonary 971
wall 863
Vestibular
apparatus 1097
function 1095
tests 1102
glands 633
movements 1199
nuclei 409
pathways 1101, 1101*f*
receptors 1078
reflexes 1101
Vestibulocerebellar tract 1091
Vestibulocerebellum 1089, 1092
Vestibulocollic reflex 1102
Vestibulo-ocular reflex 1093, 1102
Vestibulospinal tract 1043, 1061, 1062, 1065, 1066*f*, 1076, 1078
Viagra 632
Vibration, sense of 1010
Villi 331, 384
Vipoma 338
Viruses, transport of 219
Viscera, distension of 1019
Visceral reflex mechanisms, principle of 1238
Visceral smooth muscle, contraction of 571
Viscosity 749, 825, 902
Vision 1286
Visual
acuity 1188
cortex 1181, 1184
reflex 1102, 1188, 1191
Vitamin 489, 1285
A 423, 1169, 1286
deficiency 1287
dysfunctions 1287
functions of 1286
sources of 1286
toxicity 1287
absorption of 425
antiscorbutic 1288
B complexes 387
B1 1288
B12 94, 95, 369, 380, 388, 425, 852, 1291
absorption 351, 352, 425*f*
deficiency 425
storage of 425*f*
B2 1289
B6 1290
functions of 1290
C 96, 1288
deficiency of 1288
D 380, 423, 466, 553, 556, 557, 562, 563*fc*, 1284, 1287
deficiency 564
dysfunctions 1287
supplement 565
deficiency of 1287
functions of 1287
synthesis of 562
deficiency 489
E 423, 1287
functions of 1287
sources of 1287

K 387, 423, 1287
antagonists 206
synthesis 390, 1236
types of 1286*t*
Vitreous humor 1168, 1169
Voltage-gated calcium channels 753, 984
Vomiting 359, 409, 410, 1223, 1259
reflex 410*f*
von Willebrand disease 189, 210
von Willebrand factor 189, 191
deficiency of 210

W

Wallerian degeneration 238, 1003
Waste
materials, excretion of 328
products, elimination of 288
Water
absorption of 349, 387, 391, 424
and electrolytes, absorption of 424
diuresis 707, 716, 1276
hammer pulse 800
homeostasis 72
metabolism 465
reabsorption 381*f*, 478, 686, 693*f*, 706
types of 705
soluble
antioxidants 1298
substances 15
vitamins, absorption of 425
vapor-pressure gradient 1242
Weber's test 1218, 1219
Weber-Fechner law 1000
Wedge pressures 970
Wenckebach phenomenon 773
Wenckebach tract 742
Wernicke's aphasia 1145
Wernicke's area 1144
Wernicke's encephalopathy 1289
Westergren method 89
Western blotting 34, 35
Wet beriberi 1289
Wharton's duct 342
Whipple's disease 387
Wilson's terminal 761
Windkessel vessels 732
Wolff-Chaikoff effect 493
Wolffian duct, development of 601
Wolff-Parkinson-White syndrome 773
Wound healing 193, 201
Wrinkles, facial 985

X

X chromosome 123, 198, 577
Xanthines 708,793
Xanthurenic acid 1290
Xerophthalmia 1287
Xerostomia 347, 1228
X-linked
agammaglobulinemia 180
disorders 31

Y

Yellow marrow 76, 77
Yolk sac, mesoderm of 90

Z

Zellweger syndrome 20
Zollinger-Ellison syndrome 336, 359
Zona pellucida 609, 635, 636
part of 636
rupture of 637
Zonula adherens 25, 26*f*
Zonula occludens 24
Zygote 636
formation 636